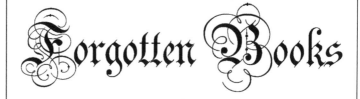

ISBN 978-1-5285-2095-9
PIBN 10903104

A
SYSTEM OF MEDICINE

BY MANY WRITERS

EDITED BY

THOMAS CLIFFORD ALLBUTT

M.A., M.D., LL.D., F.R.C.P., F.R.S., F.L.S., F.S.A.

REGIUS PROFESSOR OF PHYSIC IN THE UNIVERSITY OF CAMBRIDGE, FELLOW OF GONVILLE
AND CAIUS COLLEGE, HON. FELLOW ROYAL COLLEGE OF PHYSICIANS OF IRELAND

NEW AND CHEAPER EDITION

VOLUME VI

New York
THE MACMILLAN COMPANY
LONDON: MACMILLAN & CO., LTD.
1905

Norwood Press
J. S. Cushing & Co. — Berwick & Smith
Norwood Mass. U.S.A.

CONTENTS

DISEASES OF THE CIRCULATORY SYSTEM—*Continued*

ILLUSTRATIONS

PLATES

TABLES

LIST OF AUTHORS

Allbutt, Thomas Clifford, M.D., LL.D., F.R.C.P., F.R.S., Regius Professor of Physic in the University of Cambridge, Fellow of Gonville and Caius College, Consulting Physician to the Leeds General Infirmary.

Barlow, Thomas, M.D., F.R.C.P., Physician Extraordinary to the Queen ; Physician to H.M. Household ; Physician and Professor of Clinical Medicine, University College Hospital ; Physician to the Hospital for Sick Children.

Batten, Fred. E., M.D., Casualty Physician to St. Bartholomew's Hospital ; Assistant Physician to the Hospital for Sick Children ; Pathologist to the National Hospital for Paralysis and Epilepsy.

Beevor, Charles E., M.D., F.R.C.P., Physician to the National Hospital for the Paralysed and Epileptic, and to the Great Northern Central Hospital.

Bury, Judson S., M.D., F.R.C.P., Senior Assistant Physician, Manchester Royal Infirmary.

Carter, R. Brudenell, F.R.C.S., Kt. of Grace of Ord. St. John of Jerusalem ; Consulting Ophthalmic Surgeon to St. George's Hospital, and Ophthalmic Surgeon to the National Hospital for the Paralysed and Epileptic.

Clutton, H. H., M.C. Cantab., F.R.C.S., Surgeon and Lecturer on Surgery to St. Thomas's Hospital.

Fleming, R. A., M.D., Pathologist to the Royal Infirmary ; Lecturer on Medicine in the Medical School of the Royal Colleges, Edinburgh.

Gairdner, Sir W. T., K.C.B., M.D., LL.D., F.R.S., Physician in Ordinary to Her Majesty the Queen in Scotland ; Professor of Medicine in the University of Glasgow ; Physician to the Western Infirmary, Glasgow.

Gibson, G. A., M.D., D.Sc., Senior Assistant Physician, Royal Infirmary ; Consulting Physician to the Deaconess Hospital, Lecturer on Medicine in the Medical School of the Royal Colleges, Edinburgh.

Head, Henry, M.D., Assistant Physician to the London Hospital.

Hopkins, John, F.R.C.S., Medical Superintendent of the Central London Sick Asylum.

Horsley, Victor A. H., F.R.C.S., F.R.S., Surgeon to University College Hospital and to the National Hospital for the Paralysed and Epileptic.

Lewis, W. Bevan, Medical Superintendent and Director of the West Riding Asylum at Wakefield ; Lecturer on Mental Diseases at the Yorkshire College.

Mott, Frederick Walker, M.D., F.R.S., F.R.C.P., Physician in charge of Out-Patients to Charing Cross Hospital, and Pathologist to the Asylums Board of the London County Council.

Pitt, George Newton, M.D., F.R.C.P., late Fellow of Clare College, Cambridge; Physician and Lecturer on Pathology at Guy's Hospital.

Powell, Sir R. Douglas, Bart., M.D., F.R.C.P., Physician Extraordinary to H.M. the Queen; Physician, Middlesex Hospital; Consulting Physician, Brompton Hospital for Consumption.

Roberts, Frederick T., M.D., F.R.C.P., Professor of Medicine and of Clinical Medicine, University College, London, and Physician to the University College Hospital; Consulting Physician to the Brompton Hospital for Consumption.

Rolleston, Humphry Davy, M.D., F.R.C.P., late Fellow of St. John's College, Cambridge; Physician and Lecturer on Pathology to St. George's Hospital; Physician to Out-patients, Victoria Hospital for Children.

Russell, J. S. Risien, M.D., F.R.C.P., Assistant Physician to University College Hospital, and to the National Hospital for the Paralysed and Epileptic, Queen Square, London.

Sharkey, Seymour John, M.D., F.R.C.P., Physician and Lecturer on Medicine to St. Thomas's Hospital.

Sherrington, C. S., M.D., F.R.S., Holt Professor of Physiology, University College, Liverpool.

Turner, W. Aldren, M.D., F.R.C.P., Physician to the Hospital for Epilepsy and Paralysis; Demonstrator of Neuro-pathology at King's College; Assistant Physician, the West London Hospital.

Turney, Horace G., M.D., F.R.C.P., F.R.C.S., Assistant Physician to and Physician in charge of the Electrical Department at St. Thomas's Hospital.

Welch, Wm. H., M.D., Professor of Pathology, Johns Hopkins University, Baltimore.

White, W. Hale, M.D., F.R.C.P., Physician and Lecturer on Pharmacology and Therapeutics to Guy's Hospital.

ERRATA

In vol. iv. p. 118, line 1, *for* "A. J. M. Soc. 1884-88" *read* "A. J. M. Sci. 1884-85."

,, ,, 123, ,, 17, ,, "four" *read* "five."

,, ,, ,, ,, 28, ,, "257" *read* "250."

,, ,, 158, ,, 17, ,, "finally" *read* "finely."

,, ,, 383, footnote, ,, "1897" *read* "1877."

In vol. v. p. 37, line 23, ,, "wool-fir" *read* "fir-wool."

,, ,, 81, ,, 44, ,, "wood fir" *read* "fir-wool."

,, ,, 151, ,, 6, ,, "phthisical" *read* "physical."

,, ,, 230, ,, 5, ,, "infiltration" *read* "filtration."

,, ,, 318, ,, 4, add inverted commas at end of quotation.

,, ,, 269, ,, 7, *for* "studied" *read* "studded."

,, ,, 417, ,, 38, ,, "lymphocytes" *read* "leucocytes."

,, ,, 456, ,, 20, ,, "Co" *read* "CO."

,, ,, 1010, ,, 10, ,, "article" *read* "auricle."

In order to avoid frequent interruption of the text, the Editor has only inserted the numbers indicative of items in the lists of "References" in cases of emphasis, where two or more references to one author are in the list, where an author is quoted from a work published under another name, or where an authoritative statement is made without mention of the author's name. In ordinary cases an author's name is a sufficient indication of the corresponding item in the list.

DISEASES OF THE CIRCULATORY SYSTEM

(CONTINUED)

RIGHT-SIDED VALVULAR DISEASES

DISEASES OF THE PULMONARY VALVES

PULMONARY INCOMPETENCE.—This is the rarest of the valvular lesions of the heart, only 17 cases having been noted in the post-mortem room at Guy's Hospital out of 11,000 examinations during a period of twenty-three years.

One of the earliest papers on the subject was by Whitley (1857), who reported three cases. Blattmann (1887) collected 14, Barie (1891) 35, and Gerhardt (1892) 6 new cases; all of which were confirmed by necropsy. To this we have been able to add 41, of which 29 are unpublished cases from the records at Guy's Hospital.[1] The total number is therefore 99, besides some 30 published clinical cases which were not verified after death.

Etiology.—These cases may be divided into five important groups: A, Ulcerative endocarditis, 57 cases; B, Dilated pulmonary artery, 12 cases; C, Aortic aneurysm pressing on the pulmonary valves, 14 cases; D, Abnormality in the number of valves, 13 cases; E, Pulmonary stenosis, 14 cases; F, Unclassified, 5 cases.

A. **Infective endocarditis.**—This is by far the most frequent cause of the incompetence, being present in 57 cases.

The age distribution is as follows :—

0-10 years . . . 2 cases		41-50 years . . . 4 cases
11-20 ,, . . . 12 ,,		51-60 ,, . . . 4 ,,
21-30 ,, . . . 15 ,,		61-70 ,, . . . 1 ,,
31-40 ,, . . . 11 ,,		

Etiology.—There are several associated conditions which are of especial importance in connection with infective endocarditis of the pulmonary valve.

No obvious cause . . . 19 cases		Gonorrhœa . . . . 8 cases
Patent ventricular septum . 10 ,,		Puerperal fever . . . 4 ,,
Congenital pulmonary stenosis 8 ,,		Pyæmia . . . . . 4 ,,
Patent ductus arteriosus . . 3 ,,		Pneumonia . . . . 5 ,,

---

[1] I am indebted to my friend, Dr. Alfred Salter, for the great trouble he has taken in examining for me the records at Guy's Hospital, and for his collation of the notes on the cases of pulmonary and tricuspid lesions.

The stream, regurgitant through an aperture in the ventricular septum, or through a patent ductus arteriosus, tends to damage the endothelium of the wall on which it impinges, and thus gives rise to vegeta-

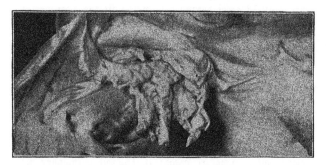

Fig. 1.—A pulmonary artery with a mass of pendulous vegetations attached to the right anterior cusps, while the greater portion of the posterior valve has completely ulcerated away, and what remained of the right anterior valve has been perforated by the pressure of the infective vegetations.

From a man aged 19, who had gonorrhœa four months before death, and was admitted with pyrexia, dyspnœa, and a double basic bruit. At the inspection there were also found advanced tubal nephritis, with apoplexies in the lung, and a small patch of pneumonia.

tions. This formation of vegetations opposite the aperture, and on the pulmonary valves, is well shown in several museum specimens.

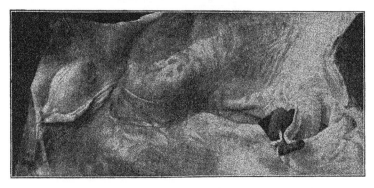

Fig. 2.—A pulmonary artery stretched over an aortic aneurysm; two cusps have adhered to the wall of the vessel and the aperture, which is apparent immediately below the juncture of two valves, leads into a saccular aneurysm of the aorta, an inch across, immediately above the aortic valves which had remained competent. The margin of the aperture is smooth, not much thickened, and is free from lymph.

From a man aged 39, who gave no history either of rheumatism or of syphilis. He had been short of breath for some years, but was only ill for three weeks.

It is remarkable how very rarely a diastolic bruit has been noticed in cases of congenital pulmonary stenosis, even when the cusps are fused into a rigid cone, which, it would appear, must have allowed some regurgitation. Probably the blood does not regurgitate vigorously enough to produce a bruit, owing to the low blood-pressure which results from the defective supply to the lungs. It is only when an ulcerative destructive process has been superadded that the incompetence has been noticed.

In cases of infective endocarditis due to gonorrhœa or puerperal infection the pulmonary valve is the one which is especially liable to be implicated. Of three cases, reported recently, gonococci were found in the vegetations in two and streptococci in the third.

In 16 out of 19 cases recorded at Guy's it is definitely stated that there was no history of any rheumatism, and in only one patient had its occurrence been noted. This differs from left-sided lesions, in which old rheumatic heart disease has often preceded the infective process.

Sometimes masses of vegetations block the orifice and prevent the closure of the valves; in a few cases, however, the process has consisted merely in a destruction of the cusps, clearing one or more away as if cut off with scissors. This is well shown in Fig. 1, where one cusp is retroverted and carries a pendulous mass of vegetations. The greater portion of the other cusps has ulcerated away, leaving only small pieces at the attached margin.

TABLE of Associated Lesions in 19 Cases.

Thickened mitral valve	3 cases
Mitral valve, Vegetations on	3 ,,
Aortic ,, ,, ,, ...	4 ,,
Tricuspid ,, ,, ,, ...	1 ,,
All four valves affected	4 ,,
Aneurysm on a branch of the pulmonary artery . .	2 ,,
Infarcts in the lung	5 ,,

. It is specially mentioned in some of the post-mortem reports of these cases that the spleen was small.

In three cases the pulmonary valves were also thickened; and in nine cases the pulmonary valves alone showed vegetations, although in one of them the mitral valve was thickened.

Symptoms (19 cases).—Hæmoptysis and dyspnœa were the symptoms chiefly noticed. In 8 cases the implication of the pulmonary valves was definitely diagnosed. This is a very large proportion when it is borne in mind that some of the cases were in surgical wards where the condition of the heart would not be systematically examined, and others were admitted shortly before death. In 5 carefully reported cases, only a systolic bruit appears to have been observed. In 3 cases it is definitely stated that no bruits could be heard. In others a diastolic, as well as a systolic, bruit was noted.

(**Acute endocarditis limited to the pulmonary valves.**—In only one case, out of 11,000 necropsies, were minute vegetations found on the pulmonary cusps, while the other valves were free. This was a case of a patient who died in 1894 of pernicious anæmia; but both aortic and mitral valves were incompetent from old sclerotic changes.)

B. **Dilatation of the pulmonary artery.**—We have collected 12 cases of pulmonary incompetence in which also the artery was found to be dilated. It has long been recognised that aortic incompetence may take place, although the valves remain healthy, when the first part of the aorta becomes dilated from any cause. It is an interesting question to consider whether dilatation of the pulmonary artery may, in the same way, be an efficient cause of pulmonary incompetence.

Pathological evidence.—*Conditions under which dilatation of the pulmonary artery takes place.*—An examination of museum specimens, which are collected from the more extreme cases, would show that the associated conditions are fibroid lungs, or bronchitis with emphysema; besides these groups, dilatation also occurs in some cases of pulmonary stenosis. But this conclusion is fallacious, as an examination of 5000 consecutive necropsies shows that mitral stenosis was present in 19 out of 21 cases in which dilatation of the pulmonary artery was noted, and is consequently the chief lesion to be considered. In the two remaining cases phthisis, and bronchitis with emphysema were present.

Clinical evidence.—Not infrequently, in advanced cases of mitral stenosis, pulsation may be observed in the second and third left spaces close to the sternum, which is now generally considered to be due to dilatation of the infundibulum and of the pulmonary artery. Gouraud, Crocker, Bamberger, Goodhart, and other observers, have insisted that the occurrence of diastolic bruits down the left side of the sternum in cases of advanced mitral stenosis, and also in cases of dilated pulmonary artery with emphysema or fibroid lung, is not very infrequent. Their presence they consider to indicate a certain amount of leakage through the pulmonary orifice. Notes of several cases are to be found among the Guy's clinical records, but in all, save two, there was no conclusive evidence of regurgitation at the necropsy. It may readily be granted, however, that incompetence would probably have to continue for a long time before it need produce structural changes.

Stokes' observation, made many years ago, remains true in the main, that even when the pulmonary artery is found dilated there are generally no changes in the cusps, nor any notable symptoms during life. I would qualify this last sentence by pointing out that a variable diastolic bruit may be detected occasionally. The orifice also may have been sufficiently stretched during life to allow leakage, and yet appear normal after death.

Sometimes these basic diastolic murmurs in cases of mitral stenosis lead to a diagnosis of slight aortic incompetence ; yet there can be little doubt that in such cases, when the aortic valves are found healthy, the murmurs are of pulmonary origin.

The difficulty of diagnosis is well illustrated by the following case of a dilated pulmonary artery, published by Mr. Holmes, in which the carotid artery was ligatured under the impression that the case was one of aortic aneurysm.

A woman, æt. 21, who had always been delicate, gave a history of phthisis in her family, and of an attack of acute rheumatism a year previously. She was admitted with a long, loud systolic bruit over the upper part of the left chest and a thrill in the second left space. Her chief symptoms were bronchitis, dyspnœa, and hæmoptysis. After being kept in bed for six months the left common carotid was ligatured, under the supposition that she had an aneurysm of the transverse arch of the aorta. She married and died twelve years later from acute phthisis.

P.-M.—There was found a greatly dilated pulmonary artery, with considerable stenosis of the orifice, due to the two cusps which were present being welded to form a funnel. The foramen ovale was patent, the other valves and the aorta healthy. The evidence pointed to the rheumatism having damaged valves previously defective.

1. There is therefore evidence, both clinical and pathological, that in advanced mitral stenosis the pulmonary artery may become distended.

2. In such cases a variable diastolic bruit down the left side of the sternum may be evidence of a functional incompetence of the pulmonary orifice. This is certainly of far more frequent occurrence towards the end of life than is generally recognised.

3. Almost invariably post-mortem evidence of any structural change at the orifice will be wanting.

We have only been able to find the three following cases in which there was both clinical and post-mortem evidence of pulmonary incompetence without any thickening of the valves :—

1. A man, æt. 34, who for six months had had a cough with dyspnœa. The cardiac impulse was feeble, but there was intense and extended fremitus ; and a loud musical diastolic bruit not transmitted to the arteries. Pulse small and feeble, not aortic in character. Distended jugular veins.

P.-M.—Pulmonary orifice 4 inches, aortic $3\frac{1}{4}$, tricuspid $6\frac{1}{4}$, mitral 5 inches (Stokes).

2. Man, æt. 34, with dyspnœa, cyanosis, and œdema.

P.-M.—General pleuritic adhesions. Right ventricle greatly dilated and hypertrophied. The pulmonary artery was greatly dilated, and its valves were incompetent (Rokitansky).

3. Man, æt. 28, with a history of acute rheumatism five years previously. At the apex a systolic and a fainter diastolic bruit was heard ; over the tricuspid a loud systolic bruit, and a dull diastolic sound ; and in the first, second, and third left spaces there was a short systolic with a variable diastolic bruit.

P.-M. — Aneurysmal dilatation of pulmonary artery ; valves thin, but elongated. Mitral stenosis and pulmonary incompetence (Galewski).

In nine other cases of pulmonary incompetence the artery was dilated, and this was in some of the cases the cause of the incompetence.

In two cases the cusps were reduced to two, and twice there were four cusps. One of these cases is of especial interest, as it was under Dr. Addison's care in 1857 ; the remarkable character of the to-and-fro basic bruit led Dr. Hermann Weber to diagnose the pulmonary origin of the disease. In the Guy's Museum there are two specimens in which the margins only of the incompetent valves are thickened, and in one of these the valves are retroverted; the associated lesions were mitral stenosis and fibroid lungs. In both cases a lesion of the pulmonary artery was diagnosed.

A similar case of thick incompetent pulmonary valves with an orifice 6⅛ inches in circumference, associated with advanced emphysema, has been recorded by Dr. Coupland.

In two remaining cases there was ulcerative endocarditis of the cusps.

C. **Aortic aneurysm pressing on the pulmonary artery** (14 cases).— An aneurysmal pouch of the aorta immediately above the valves, especially above the left posterior cusp, may press upon the pulmonary artery, or open into it close to the valves. The inflammation which is set up, as the wall yields, causes the free margin of one or even two pulmonary cusps to become blended and firmly adherent to the walls of the artery, and thus to become incompetent. The adhesion of the free margin of valves to the wall of the vessel where they are stretched over an aneurysmal pouch is shown in Fig. 2; on the right of the figure is seen the aperture through which the aorta had opened into the pulmonary artery. One pulmonary cusp has completely blended with the wall, and only the extreme end of the second has not been obliterated. As may be readily imagined, the incompetence in such a case is considerable.

This cause of pulmonary incompetence, which has been overlooked by most authors (Grawitz reports two cases), cannot really be very uncommon, as there are eight specimens at Guy's and two at St. George's Hospital, in which pulmonary cusps adhere to the wall, and had thus become useless.

The evidence of the incompetence is masked during life by the lesion of the aortic valves which is usually present.

D. **Abnormality in the number of pulmonary valves** (13 cases).— Eight cases with two cusps; four with four cusps; and one with five.

In most cases these abnormalities have been of congenital origin; the consequent imperfect closure of the orifice probably initiated sclerotic changes in the cusps which tended to progress as the incompetence became established.

In one or two cases the regurgitant stream through a patent ventricular septum has impinged on normal segments and caused two to adhere together.

Dilg has collected the scattered information on the subject of abnormality in the number of cusps, and finds recorded of

Two pulmonary cusps, 64 cases	Two aortic cusps, 23 cases
Four „ „ 24 „	Four „ . „ 2 „
Five „ „ 2 „	Five „ „ 1 case

He attributes the abnormalities to (i.) fœtal endocarditis; (ii.) defective site; (iii.) one of these, with endocarditis in later life.

Meckel noted that when the foramen ovale was patent there were often only two pulmonary segments.

When there are only two cusps one is usually abnormally large, and has arisen from the fusion of two. Normally in molluscs, osteoid fish, and reptiles, only two cusps form.

In fœtal chicks the anterior and inner cusps form the first, and the third cusp at a later period. Virchow, however, is of opinion that in many cases the union of two cusps is probably a change belonging to a later period of life.

E. **Pulmonary stenosis** (14 cases).—In eight of these cases there was ulcerative endocarditis; in two, a dilated pulmonary artery; and in one, only two cusps. There remain three cases, not included in the previous lists, in which a basic diastolic bruit had been noted indicating regurgitation through an orifice which was ultimately found to be congenitally stenosed.

F. The five following cases, which cannot be included in the previous groups, remain to be considered :—

(*a*) (Wunderlich.) Foramen in ventricular septum opening directly on a pulmonary valve.

(*b*) (Schwalbe.) A gummatous infiltration of the pulmonary artery, with adhesion of a valve to an aortic aneurysm.

(*c*) and (*d*) Two specimens in Guy's Museum, from patients aged 38 and 70, in whom there were only symptoms of bronchitis during life. In one, there are only two cusps, which are retroverted, one of them only being adherent to the vessel; in the other specimens one cusp is adherent along its margin, and the other two are elongated and thickened. The causation of these changes is obscure.

(*e*) A case of a man, æt. 27, who had had four attacks of rheumatism, after death the mitral orifice was found stenosed, the pulmonary and aortic incompetent, and the pericardium adherent (Gerhardt). One pulmonary flap was markedly retroverted.

In the preceding groups are included four other cases of mitral stenosis and cardiac failure, and four of mitral and tricuspid incompetence, which had induced pulmonary incompetence with thickening of the valves.

While discussing the etiology, I would draw attention to the remarkable fact that in cases of the most extreme mitral stenosis, in which a similar defect is ultimately set up in the tricuspid valve, the pulmonary cusps almost invariably escape, and do not show even a trace of thickening.

The proportion of cases with a history of acute rheumatism is small —not much over 10 per cent; and the influence of rheumatism is far less on this than on any other valve. We can find no specimen of acute rheumatic endocarditis of the pulmonary valves, although there is definite evidence that the poison may set up vegetations on the tricuspid valves.

The free margins of cusps were more or less adherent in eighteen cases, and retroverted in four.

The statement usually made that pulmonary incompetence is a congenital defect is not accurate; practically, a diastolic bruit is not audible in cases of pulmonary stenosis, unless infective endocarditis is present. Yet, on the post-mortem table, the matted valves may remain rigidly fixed. About one-fifth of the cases collected showed evidence of old pulmonary stenosis; or of abnormality in the number of the valves. There is practically no evidence that traumatism is a cause of incompetence.

In three cases calcareous nodules were present in the valve, independently of congenital lesions.

There is not the liability to the development of tuberculosis, as is the case with pulmonary stenosis.

Clinical aspects of pulmonary incompetence.—The cases may be divided into three groups :—

1. Those which present themselves with pyæmic symptoms, of which in recent years a correct diagnosis has been made in more than half.

2. Those with cardiac symptoms. The difficulty in such cases is to determine that the pulmonary is the valve involved. This is much increased, in many of the cases, by the presence of lesions elsewhere; for instance, aortic aneurysm or fungating endocarditis of several valves.

3. In a few cases there has been no evidence during life to indicate that the heart was affected, and no bruits were audible. Such cases must remain for post-mortem diagnosis.

Symptoms.—(i.) One of the first changes is a displacement of the cardiac impulse downwards and considerably to the left, in consequence of the right-sided enlargement which results from the pulmonary incompetence. The right ventricle dilates, and the dulness extends beyond the right side of the sternum. When the muscular accommodation is good the force of the impulse is increased, and the epigastric pulsation marked; sometimes a systolic thrill is palpable (Bamberger). When there is great cardiac failure they are absent. In some cases a distinct pulsation may also be felt in the second left space.

(ii.) On auscultation a diastolic bruit may be heard in the second left space and traced down the left of the sternum; but it is not transmitted to the vessels of the neck.

(iii.) The absence of a quick water-hammer pulse, and of marked pulsation in the main systemic vessels.

(iv.) As was first noticed by Bernhardt, the diastolic bruit is intensified by expiration.

(v.) Emboli occur in the lungs, and as a result hæmoptysis. This is present in one-third of the cases, chiefly in those due to infective endocarditis (Weckerle).

(vi.) Not infrequently both the aortic and pulmonary valves are incompetent. Can the murmurs due to the two lesions be distinguished ?

Gerhardt thinks that the latter is deeper in tone and rougher than the aortic, owing to the feeble pressure in the pulmonary artery.

(vii.) The murmur is intensified by the erect position.

(viii.) A capillary pulse can be detected in the pulmonary circulation. When a long, deep breath is taken, the vesicular murmur is jerky, and can be heard to wax and wane with the cardiac contractions over portions of the chest, such as the angle of the right scapula, where normally such tides never occur. This Gerhardt has also shown graphically by registering the variations of pressure in the tracheal column of air.

Although the number of diagnostic symptoms is not small, practically the difficulties of diagnosis may be enormous, because the lesion is excessively rare ; and it is generally complicated by other serious mischief.

The development of a diastolic bruit towards the end of life, especially in cases of mitral stenosis, probably is due to a relative pulmonary incompetence, but structural change is most exceptional. It should, moreover, be borne in mind that murmurs, which apparently have a distribution similar to that which we have described above as characteristic of pulmonary incompetence, may ultimately be found to have been produced at the aortic orifice.

Dyspnœa, cyanosis, and œdema are symptoms which generally appear as the heart fails. Of a specially suggestive import with these is hæmoptysis, which results partly from the sudden changes in the pulmonary pressure, and partly from emboli which have broken off from vegetations.

Prognosis.—Pulmonary incompetence is always a serious lesion. It is usually the result of an acute infective process, or is a final stage in other serious heart trouble. Apart from such complications, it would appear that patients with pulmonary incompetence may live for a considerable time ; it is the associated lesions which are the cause of death.

Treatment.—No special line of treatment is indicated unless there be reason to suspect a fungating endocarditis. In one or two cases brilliant results have already followed the repeated injection, subcutaneously, of antistreptococcic serum. When it is found possible to produce a much more trustworthy serum, we may look forward to controlling the infective process with good results.

PULMONARY STENOSIS.—This lesion, when the valves are united and form a perforated dome, is almost invariably congenital in origin, and has already been treated (*vide* vol. v. p. 703). Occasionally, however, we meet with cases—there are over ten on record—in which there is evidence that the stenosis has taken place after birth, and in others has considerably increased after birth as the result of an attack of rheumatism.

Paul reports the case of a man, æt. 36, admitted with advanced phthisis and hæmoptysis, who had enjoyed good health until the age of ten, when he was laid up for three months with endocarditis and acute rheumatism ; since then he had been troubled with palpitation and slight dyspnœa. The onset of phthisis was two years before his death. The right ventricle was hypertrophied, and there was a basic systolic bruit on the left side not propagated up into the vessels of the neck. After death it was found that the ductus arteriosus was closed; the pulmonary artery was not wasted, but the orifice was stenosed owing to adhesions between the valves. Paul considers that cyanosis is generally absent in the cases which are not of congenital origin. Besides these cases, the orifice or the lumen of the artery may be stenosed by the bulging of an aortic aneurysm, or by masses of fungating vegetations blocking the aperture to which reference has already been made.

DISEASES OF THE TRICUSPID VALVES

In order to define the causation of the lesions of the tricuspid valve as clearly as possible, and to determine the relative frequency of the symptoms of the various associated lesions, we have examined the clinical and post-mortem records of Guy's Hospital for the last twenty or thirty years, and have tabulated the tricuspid cases in which (i.) acute vegetations were found upon the valve, (ii.) the valvular cusps were thickened, (iii.) the cusps were affected with fungating endocarditis, (iv.) the cusps were incompetent, and (v.) the tricuspid orifice was stenosed.

1.. ACUTE VEGETATIONS ON THE TRICUSPID VALVES. — Fifty-four cases. The proportion of male to female cases was 4 to 3. The youngest patient was only three months old. There was only one other patient under ten years of age, and the number of cases for the succeeding decennia were 2, 15, 18, 4, 3, 3, 1.

On examining the records, we were struck at once by the frequency with which vegetations were also met with upon the mitral and aortic valves; and also by the still greater frequency with which old lesions of these valves were present. In 41 cases there was evidence of old mitral disease, and in 35 of recent vegetations on the mitral; in the majority of cases on damaged valves. In the same way the aortic valves showed evidence of old damage in 21 cases; and in 33 cases recent vegetations, but occurring more frequently on previously healthy valves than on those which had been diseased. In 17 cases there was recent pericarditis, and in 13 the pericardium was adherent. In only one case out of the whole series were the mitral valves stated to have been normal. In this case, however, acute pericarditis was present, and also vegetations on damaged aortic valves. On three occasions the vegetations were limited to the tricuspid valve; in two of these cases the mitral valves were thickened, and in the third there was thickening of the mitral, aortic, and pulmonary valves. Recent lymph over the surface of the pleura was found in 20 cases. With regard to the history of rheumatism, it was noted as present during the final illness in 21 cases; in 20 other cases there was a history of previous attacks, and in only 10 cases was it stated that there had never been any acute rheumatism. The evidence was therefore conclusive that the dominant cause of vegetations on the tricuspid is a severe rheumatic process; not invariably shown by acute joint troubles, but practically without exception by evidences of either acute or old mischief, involving the mitral, and very frequently the aortic valves; by inflammation of the pericardium in more than half the cases, and by acute pleurisy in nearly half the cases. An examination of the records for the past twenty years presents no evidence of any importance in favour of any other causation.

2. THICKENING OF THE TRICUSPID VALVES.—From the 148 cases in which thickening of the tricuspid flaps was noted, an examination of the records at once shows that these cases fall into three great groups :—

A. Those which are secondary to *rheumatism, or left-sided valvular disease.*

B. Those which are the result of *degenerative changes involving several organs.*

C. Those associated with *pulmonary stenosis of congenital origin.*

That these distinctions are fundamental ones, is at once proved by the relative age distribution; as we find that the majority of cases in the first group occur between the ages of 20 and 30, and five-sixths of the cases between the ages of 10 and 40.

In the second group, one patient, aged 27, with emphysema, was the only case in which the age was under 30 : the decennium in which the greatest number of cases occurred was between 50 and 60, and six-sevenths of the cases occurred between the ages of 40 and 70.

A. In the first group *mitral stenosis* was present in a very large number of the cases. In 48 there was a definite history of rheumatism; and in 20 left-sided heart lesions were present, although there was no history of rheumatism; they were, nevertheless, most probably due to it. As a sub-group of this class we would put the cases of mitral stenosis in which the kidneys were found to be granular, of which there were 11. This aptness of granular kidneys to induce mitral stenosis in a heart previously damaged by rheumatism was recorded by me many years ago; and it is interesting to find that interstitial changes in the kidneys tend to induce thickening of the tricuspid valve also. I shall show later that, in the more severe cases, this proceeds to stenosis. There were five cases in which the kidneys were granular, without the mitral orifice being stenosed.

B. The second group, that is, the *degenerative one*, may be divided into —(*a*) Cases with widespread degenerative fibroid change affecting several organs; such as the valves (aortic, mitral, and sometimes the pulmonary); the arteries; the kidneys; the liver; and the elastic tissues of the lung. Of such widespread degenerative change there were 15 cases; but, most probably, the succeeding groups should be considered merely as subdivisions, although the fibroid change is limited to one organ. (*b*) Cases of emphysema, obstructive lung disease, dilated bronchial tubes, or fibroid lung: of emphysema there were 25 cases; of fibroid phthisis, 7 ; of fibroid lung, 4 ; and of emphysema, with granular kidneys, 17. (*c*) Cirrhotic liver and perihepatitis, 3 cases. (*d*) Granular

kidneys, 16 cases, to which I have already referred. I would insist
that, pathologically, emphysema should not be considered solely as a
disease of the lung; but in many cases rather as part of a widespread degenerative change affecting more particularly the elastic tissues
of the body, and, through the change in the arteries, damaging the various
viscera. Amongst our groups of cases we note the association of emphysema
with bronchiectasis, fibroid lung, granular kidneys, and cirrhosis of the
liver; and, in eight cases, with thickening of the aortic and sometimes of
the mitral valves, in one case with marked aortic stenosis. Malignant
disease, which was present in four cases, had probably accelerated the
degenerative changes; twice there was also lardaceous disease.

C. The third group; associated with *pulmonary stenosis.* Six cases.

3. INFECTIVE ENDOCARDITIS OF THE TRICUSPID VALVES.—From the
records at Guy's Hospital, between 1860 and 1894, out of 15,000 post-
mortems we have collected 29 cases; 10 are also recorded in the Pathological Society of London's *Transactions,* making a total of 39.

The age distribution during the various decennia are 3, 11, 6, 6, 5, 3,
3, and 2; the youngest child being only three months old. The majority
of cases as usual were between the ages of 10 and 40. There were 20
male and 19 female cases.

Etiology.—Cause not determined, 10; pyæmia and inflammatory conditions, 15; pneumonia, 7; puerperal, 3; patent ventricular septum, 2;
pulmonary stenosis, 1; chorea for ten years, 1. In 2 cases in which
pneumonia was present pneumococci were found in the vegetations, but
otherwise there are no notes as to micro-organisms.

No definite history of rheumatism was found in 19, a definite
history in 7.

Associated valve lesions.—Other valves all healthy, 10; vegetations on
all valves, 3; only on pulmonary, 1; on aortic, 14; on mitral, 17 (valves
also thickened, 6); vegetations on sclerotic tricuspid valves, 8; sclerotic
aortic valves, 4; sclerotic mitral, 4 (and with vegetations, 6); acute pericarditis, 6; adherent pericardium, 5.

Murmurs.—No note, 14; no cardiac bruit, 4; no tricuspid bruit, 10;
loud systolic bruit, 5; diastolic bruit, 1.

In the majority of cases the valves were incompetent, yet in only
five cases was a systolic tricuspid murmur noted, and this corroborates the
fact, mentioned under tricuspid incompetence, that there is not necessarily
a systolic murmur when the right side is dilated; as although the
blood may flow back the muscle may often be too feeble to produce
a murmur.

4. TRICUSPID INCOMPETENCE.—This is by far the most frequent
right-sided valvular lesion.

Pathology.—When primary, it may result from fungating endocarditis,
due to puerperal fever, gonorrhœa, or pneumonia; and, occasionally,
from the regurgitant stream driven through an imperfect ventricular
septum. Eight per cent of cases of fungating endocarditis involve the
tricuspid orifice.

In a second group of cases the valves are thickened and shrunken, owing to chronic changes the result, sometimes, of rheumatism, but more frequently of chronic atheroma following increased ventricular pressure, and forming but one item in widespread fibroid degeneration. This increased ventricular pressure may result from (*a*) mitral incompetence, and, still more frequently, from mitral stenosis; (*b*) from chronic bronchitis and emphysema, cirrhosis of the lung, or bronchiectasis; and (*c*) in the final stages of granular kidneys or of chronic cardiac enlargement, whether the result of alcoholic poisoning or of arterial degeneration.

Third group.—The valves may be healthy, but the orifice dilated. This occurs in connection with some of the conditions above noted, but it is also frequently observed as the temporary result of cardiac dilatation, whether due to disease or over-exertion (Clifford Allbutt). The size of the auriculo-ventricular orifice varies with the efficiency of the muscular contraction, and a very slight increase in the size is sufficient to allow leakage through the tricuspid orifice. This is looked upon as a safety-valve action, and is considered of great importance in relieving the strain upon the heart on occasions of sudden exertion. This temporary incompetence is probably of frequent occurrence.

The size of the tricuspid orifice may become permanently enlarged as the secondary result of other lesions. According to Hamilton's measurements, tricuspid dilatation occurs with aortic incompetence with dilated orifice, and also with dilatation of the mitral, but does not occur if there is any stenosis; although the right side of the heart would, nevertheless, be dilated and hypertrophied. Hamilton's measurements also tend to show that bronchitis, emphysema, fibroid lung, chronic Bright's disease, and the like, do not tend to dilate the tricuspid orifice. The tricuspid orifice may be dilated up to as much as $6\frac{1}{4}$ inches. Some authors lay stress on the occurrence of tricuspid incompetence in connection with digestive disturbance, whether in the stomach or in other parts of the alimentary canal.

That tricuspid incompetence may occur during fœtal life is proved by the following case, in which Professor Peter heard a rough murmur followed by a sharp sound, instead of the normal fœtal sounds, when auscultating the abdomen of a pregnant girl, æt. 17, at full term. It was thought probable that the tricuspid was the valve affected; and at the necropsy the tricuspid valve was found covered with abundant vegetations and with shrunken flaps.

During a period of twenty-five years, out of over 11,000 necropsies at Guy's Hospital there were 405 cases of tricuspid incompetence, excluding cases of stenosis. In 12 cases the reports were imperfect.

They may be classified as follows:—

A. 200 cases. *Left-sided failure with valvular disease.*—Mitral regurgitation with mitral endocarditis or adherent pericardium, 64; mitral stenosis, 66; mitral and aortic disease, 61; valvular lesion not named, 9. The tricuspid incompetence occurs late and is unusual with aortic disease: it is more common and occurs sooner with mitral disease.

B. 71 cases.   *Left-sided failure without valvular disease.* — Bright's disease, 46; malignant disease, 8; cirrhosis of liver, 11; various, 6.

C. 56 cases.   *General muscular failure of the whole heart.* — Fibroid or fatty heart, 19; in the course of acute rheumatism, 17; in the course of acute fevers, 20 (pneumonia, 8; diphtheria, 6; typhoid, 2; typhus, 1; scarlatina, 1).

D. 7 cases.   *Right-sided failure with pulmonary valvular disease.* — Pulmonary stenosis, 5; pulmonary incompetence, 2.

E. 55 cases.   *Right-sided failure without disease of other valves.* — Bronchitis and emphysema, 21; cirrhosis of lung with and without tubercle, 18; bronchiectasis, 4; fatty or fibroid right heart, 12.

F. 4 cases.   No cause found.

An examination of the clinical reports for six years—235 cases, that is, 40 cases per year—gives the following results:—

In only 2 cases was dyspnœa not mentioned, and in these there is no note of its absence.

In 84 a systolic bruit was noted; in most reports there is no definite note about a tricuspid bruit.

In very few reports was the condition of the pulmonary second sound noted; in 10, of which 3 were cases of mitral stenosis, a diminution in intensity was remarked. Œdema was present in 200; ascites in 140; œdema alone in 76, and together with ascites in 124; ascites alone in 14, neither in 21; cyanosis in 107; venous pulsation in neck in 41; hepatic pulsation in 15.

Physical signs.—(i.) A *systolic bruit,* best heard in the fourth and fifth spaces to the left side of the sternum, traceable sometimes to the right and for a short distance upwards, but very rarely as high as the third rib on the left; not traceable beyond the apex; occasionally, however, best heard in the fifth space to the right of the sternum. Usually the bruit is very faint, but often of a character quite distinct from the systolic bruit at the apex. Occasionally it has been noted as loud, and it may be audible over a wide area.   The bruit is increased with expiration, and may cease during forced inspiration.   It is not audible in the back, a character distinguishing it from a mitral bruit.   In cases of relative incompetence the feeble contraction of the right heart may be insufficient to produce a bruit; hence in many cases its presence is variable, and very frequently no bruit has been heard during life, although at the necropsy the evidence of incompetence was indubitable.

(ii.) Regurgitation through the right auriculo-ventricular orifice tends to produce *dilatation of the right ventricle,* as does a corresponding lesion of the left side; but hypertrophy results much less readily, as there is much less muscle; and a hardening of the wall, which results from its venous engorgement, is the more notable change.   The cardiac dulness is increased to the right side of the sternum, and may even extend as far as the parasternal line; but in many cases this increase is masked by an emphysematous condition of the lung.

(iii.) Except in cases of extreme cardiac failure with advanced emphysema, *pulsation will be both visible and palpable at the epigastrium* and also to the right of the sternum.

(iv.) *Pulsation of the veins in the neck.*—This may be due to various causes, some of which are of no pathological import. For instance, the veins normally become distended during expiration, and in cases of dyspnœa this may be very marked.

Not infrequently a systolic impulse is transmitted to the veins by the underlying arteries. This impulse may be eliminated by compressing the proximal part of the artery only, and noting the cessation of the pulsation. A venous pulsation, presystolic in time, may be produced by the contraction of a vigorous right auricle driving the blood back past the valves at the root of the neck; and it is difficult to draw a sharp line between what is normal and abnormal in such pulsations. The true venous pulsation which alone is of importance as indicative of incompetence of the tricuspid valves, is, as was shown by Riegel and Gerhardt many years ago, always systolic in rhythm. It may be observed in the veins of the neck, particularly in the internal jugular, and more especially on the right side; the same phenomenon also occurs in the veins of the liver, and very exceptionally in the veins of the extremities. That the systolic distension of the internal jugular vein is due to regurgitation from the right side of the heart, may be readily shown on emptying the vessel by carrying the finger from below upwards over its surface and noting that it refills at once from below.

In arterial pulsation the distension is greater than the collapse, while the converse is true of venous pulsation.

The systolic jugular pulsation is due to the yielding of the valves at the root of the vein, due to the over-distension of the bulb of the jugular, the height of which above the clavicle varies in different individuals; but sometimes the pulsation is limited to the bulb. The pulsation is increased by pressure on the liver (Pasteur).

The pulsation is only marked so long as there is a vigorously acting ventricle, and becomes less obvious when this fails; hence the pulsation is often wanting in spite of tricuspid regurgitation.

(v.) *Pulsation of the liver.*—This is a true expansile pulsation of the liver, as may be shown by taking the liver between the two hands; it is not a mere transmitted pulsation through the diaphragm. Friedreich, Matot, and, in this country, Taylor and James Mackenzie have fully established the importance of this symptom; the left lobe, it may be noted, pulsates more than the right, as the blood more readily regurgitates into that part. The systolic bruit appears first, the hepatic pulsation next, and last, the venous pulsation.

(vi.) *Feebleness of the second pulmonary sound.*—This sound is intensified in cases of mitral stenosis or of any chronic lung mischief which impedes the pulmonary circulation—the very conditions which, as stated above, induce tricuspid incompetence. Hence the diminished accentuation of this sound is not infrequently of great value, as indicative of the fall in pressure brought about by the leakage through the tricuspid valve. It is especially valuable in those cases in which the patient has been under observation for some time, so that both the accentuation and, later, the diminution of the sound have been observed.

Symptoms.—*Cardiac dyspnœa.*—This, as pointed out already, is almost invariably present, and in the majority of cases in the form of orthopnœa; exceptionally, however, cases are met with, which are difficult to explain, in which the patient is most comfortable when lying down flat, and is distressed when the head is at all raised. In some of these cases at any rate this has occurred when the left ventricle was unaffected, while the right was dilated. The orthopnœa varies in degree, and comes on at night when the patient tries to sleep, or at any time on the least exertion; it is also much increased by flatulence. In advanced cases the patient is more or less cyanosed, with lividity of the lips, ears, face, and not infrequently of the extremities. The surface temperature falls, the pulse is small, irregular, and often impalpable, and the extremities are bathed in a cold sweat.

When there is much œdema of the lungs there is a troublesome cough with bloody foamy serous expectoration.

The œdema varies in amount, but is generally extreme towards the end, and is most marked in the dependent parts. Ascites is present in more than one-third of the fatal cases.

Diagnosis.—When the three cardinal symptoms—systolic epigastric bruit, systolic venous pulsation, and a feeble second pulmonary sound— are present, there can be no doubt as to the diagnosis; but in the earlier stages there may be great uncertainty. Duroziez has especially insisted upon the non-transmission of the tricuspid systolic bruit to the back as an important distinction from a mitral bruit. The various conditions under which leakages occur should be borne in mind in forming a diagnosis.

Prognosis.—This depends not only on the cause, but also upon the associated lesions which are almost invariably present. In but too many cases it is the final scene in cardiac failure. Hence the evil prognosis when the heart has long been struggling against the extra work thrown upon it; as the orifice does not yield until the muscle is exhausted and degenerate. The muscle no longer responds to digitalis, and diffusible stimulants do but postpone death.

On the other hand, where the leakage is due to over-exertion with acute dilatation of the right ventricle, the prognosis may be favourable.

Treatment.—In cases in which the incompetence has arisen from dilatation of the ventricle, and not from organic disease of the valves, there is no drug equal to digitalis. Under its use in such cases it is not infrequent for a tricuspid systolic bruit to disappear within twenty-four or forty-eight hours; the venous pulsation soon ceases to be systolic in rhythm, the pulse is slowed and diuresis increases; but the dyspnœa and œdema, if present, disappear more slowly. On the other hand, if the bruit and venous pulsation persist in spite of improvement in the other symptoms, the lesion is organic. The interesting observation has been made by Potain that occasionally in such cases for a few days hæmoptysis will follow the administration of digitalis. He offers the following explanation; namely, that the returning competence of the tricuspid valve throws a greater strain upon the pulmonary vessels, and thus causes a rupture of the smaller branches; but that later, as the right heart regains its power, the normal condition of the circulation becomes re-established, and the excessive arterial pressure in the lungs returns to the normal.

The patient must be kept in bed; digitalis may be given as Nativelle's digitalin in 1 milligram dose, and repeated in five days; or 0·25 mg. daily, and gradually increased : or it may be given in the form of a fresh infusion (Ʒj.) or ♏x. of the tincture every four or six hours, if preferred. Strophanthus and convallaria are of much less value. In cases of acute dilatation, where there is a rapid, irregular, feeble pulse, venesection, wet cupping, or leeches often render the greatest service, provided there is still vigorous epigastric pulsation. Cardiac dyspnœa may be greatly relieved by morphia and diffusible stimulants, by hot poultices to the heart, and sometimes by belladonna.

Paracentesis of the abdomen and the drainage of œdematous legs, either by acupuncture, Southey's tubes, or incisions, are not infrequently necessary before the end; and often give the patient a fresh lease of life for a time. Calomel in doses of 1 to 3 grains, three times a day for three days, is often capable of re-establishing the secretion of urine; but in cases of diseased kidneys even smaller doses should be given. Constipation is especially injurious and must be prevented, many patients, especially when the liver is large and tender, benefit by free purgation from time to time.

5. TRICUSPID STENOSIS.—Although this lesion is decidedly rare it is much more common than any lesion of the pulmonary valves. Both Niemeyer and Skoda state that they had never met with an example, and were only familiar with it through the specimens in the museum at Vienna. Flint also speaks of it as a rare curiosity, yet we have been able from the records of a single hospital to collect 87 fatal cases during a period of twenty-six years, out of 12,000 necropsies.

Etiology and pathology of tricuspid stenosis, 84 cases.

(1) *Age distribution.*—Only one patient was less than ten years old, and only two more than sixty.

Between 11 and 20 years, 16 cases
,,   21   30   ,,   31   ,,
,,   31   40   ,,   22   ,,
,,   41   50   ,,   10   ,,
,,   51   60   ,,   3   ,,
,,   61   70   ,,   2   ,,

From this it is clear that more than a third of the cases proved fatal between the ages of twenty and thirty, and more cases ended in death between the ages of thirty and forty than between ten and twenty ; this corroborates the conclusion that the lesion in the majority of cases is the result of severe rheumatism, but requires many years for its production.

(2) It is stated that this disease is generally due to a congenital lesion ;· yet it would appear that this inference has not a sufficient basis of facts to justify it. Undoubtedly hearts with congenital lesions, taken from still-born children or from children that only lived a few days, show tricuspid stenosis in a considerable proportion. Both Peacock and Rosenstein say that the lesion is almost invariably a congenital defect, yet an examination of the specimens in the London museums quite fails to bear out this statement. In many specimens of pulmonary stenosis. even of the most extreme degree, the tricuspid valve is normal or but slightly thickened—the explanation being that the associated abnormal patency of one of the septa relieves the right side of the heart from what would otherwise be an excessive pressure ; and whether we judge from the continuous records at Guy's Hospital for over twenty-five years, or from an examination of all the specimens which have been saved in the London museums, we should conclude that only a small minority of the cases are due to congenital defect.

This is still more marked if we exclude cases of still-born children, or those who have died within a few days of birth. Out of 87 cases dying in the hospital only one patient was under ten years of age, a fact which is quite opposed to the lesion being generally of congenital origin. In cases due to congenital lesions the tricuspid valve is more likely to be normal when the foramen ovale is patent, than when there is a perforation in the ventricular septum ; in the latter case there will be some thickening.

(3) *Sex.*—54 women ; 30 men.

(4) *The associated valvular lesions* were as follows :—(a) In every case except two there was *mitral stenosis*. An examination of the records shows that the stenosis of the mitral is far more severe than that of the tricuspid. Of the two cases in which mitral stenosis was absent, in one the valves were said to be thickened ; and in only one case of the whole series were they said to be healthy.

(b) *Aortic valves*—thickened, 25 ; stenosed orifice, 24 ; incompetent, 23 ; recent vegetations, 8.

(c) *Pulmonary valves* were thickened in 9 cases ; in 1 there were recent vegetations ; in 24 the pulmonary artery was atheromatous, in 3 it was thickened, and in 2 dilated.

The general conclusions to be drawn are—

(a) That, almost without exception, this stenosis is the sequel of preceding stenosis of the mitral orifice (omitting cases that did not last a week).

(β) In almost half the cases there is evidence of some change in the aortic valves also.

(γ) In a large number the aortic valves are thickened, not infrequently they are incompetent, and in a very fair number of cases there is a very marked stenosis.

(δ) In all such cases the evidence is in favour of the changes being the effects of rheumatism, extreme either in its severity or in the frequency of the attacks. In fact, rheumatism dominates the lesion to the exclusion of almost every other cause.

(5) *The relation of tricuspid stenosis to mitral stenosis.*—In 63 cases the mitral orifice admitted one finger only, or its circumference did not exceed 2 inches; showing that in two-thirds of the cases a severe form

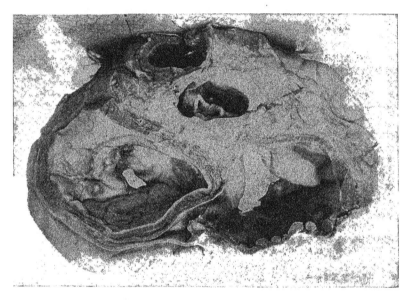

FIG. 3.—A transverse section of a heart viewed from above, showing underneath the extremely stenosed mitral orifice on the left; the moderately stenosed tricuspid on the right; with the aortic valves fused into a dome above.

From a man aged 19, who died in 1878 under Dr. Habershon. He gave no history of rheumatism. The chief symptom was hæmoptysis. There was an apical, diastolic bruit with a thrill, and a loud, basic systolic bruit. The heart weighed 16 ounces. The tricuspid orifice admits two fingers, and the cusps are much thickened. The mitral orifice is still more stenosed, with a calcareous deposit in its wall. The aortic valves are blended together into a dome-shaped septum, with a small central aperture, but were still capable of supporting a column of water.

of mitral stenosis predominated. The amount of the tricuspid stenosis in 44 cases was such that the orifice admitted two fingers only, that is, its circumference was not more than 3 inches. In 8 cases it was extremely small, admitting not more than one finger.

(6) *On the relation to rheumatism.*—In 24 cases there had been only one or two attacks of acute rheumatism. In 18 cases there had been more than two; in many cases the attacks had been numerous; in 6 there was a history of vague rheumatic pains. In 16 it is definitely

stated that there had been no rheumatism; but in 12 there had been one or two attacks of chorea.

(7) *Duration.*—In 3 cases there was a history of heart trouble for over twenty years. In 6 cases there was a history of symptoms for five to ten years; in 28 cases of symptoms for one to five years; in 3 cases for rather less than a year; and in 8 cases the symptoms had been observed for less than three months. Twice the patients were quite well within six weeks of death; twice within three weeks of death; once within ten days; and one patient was supposed to have been in good health until his death took place.

Duroziez considers that the length of life varies with the degree of stenosis; the average age at death, when the orifice would not admit more than one finger, being 32 years; and 42 when the orifice admitted two fingers.

(8) *On the size of the heart.*—In 6 cases the heart weighed less than 10 ounces; in 29 cases from 10 to 15; in 10 cases between 20 and 25; in one case it exceeded 30 ounces, and in three the weight was between 25 and 30 ounces.

(9) *Associated lesions.*—In 38 cases there was brown induration of the lungs, and in 37 marked pleuritic adhesions; in 33, effusion into one or both pleural cavities. The lung was œdematous in 13; in 12 there was recent inflammation over the surface of the pleura. In 27 there were pulmonary apoplexies, but in only 4 were thrombi found in the pulmonary artery. Twice there was bronchiectasis, twice emphysema, and only twice phthisis. Two cases were especially remarkable: in one it is stated that there was a complete absence of any induration of the lung, such as is usually met with in cardiac failure, yet there had been symptoms of mitral failure for two years, and the mitral orifice would only admit one finger. In another patient, who died from septic broncho-pneumonia with secondary peritonitis, there were no previous symptoms of any cardiac disease.

In the case in which the mitral valve was stated to be only thickened, but otherwise healthy and competent, there was emphysema with dilatation of the bronchial tubes. The tricuspid valve was thin and atheromatous, and its orifice contracted. The aortic valve was thickened and somewhat calcified, but competent; and there was a history of two attacks of hæmoptysis.

The pericardium was adherent in 38 cases; there was recent pericarditis in 10. The comparatively frequent occurrence of perihepatitis in these cases has not been previously noticed. It was noticed that in 23 of the cases the kidneys were granular, and in two there was acute nephritis. Especial attention was directed to the exclusion of cases of scarred kidneys, of which there were many; as some may have been the secondary results of the mitral stenosis. This entirely unanticipated result corroborates the views put forward in 1887 on the important influence which granular kidneys have in the production of mitral stenosis in adults; it would appear that they have also a potent influence in the production of stenosis of the tricuspid orifice. In three cases the suprarenals were caseous; twice there was acute peritonitis, once due to renal disease and once to thrombosis. In one case infective endocarditis was present.

(10) **Symptoms.**—The symptoms most frequently met with are dyspnœa, œdema, albuminuria, enlarged liver, and cyanosis ; the order being that of their relative frequency. Dyspnœa was met with in 73 cases; in 19 of these it amounted to orthopnœa. In 65 cases there was œdema, in 63 albuminuria ; in 47 the liver was enlarged ; and in 45 there was cyanosis. Ascites was only present 30 times. In 32 cases it is expressly stated that there was no cyanosis ; in 24 the liver was not enlarged ; and in 23 there was no albuminuria. In 15 cases there was no œdema.

An examination of the records brings out the remarkable fact that, of the symptoms œdema, cyanosis, and albuminuria, it was not at all infrequent for one to be absent, while the other two were present; and it has not been possible for us to determine the corresponding differences in the pathological lesions. Why one patient with mitral stenosis, or marked stenosis of his mitral and tricuspid valves, suffering with dyspnœa and œdema, should have no cyanosis, while another cyanosed and dyspnœic should have no œdema, it is difficult to say.

There are some other points of interest ; for example, in 12 cases the liver was cirrhosed, and in 11 cases there was perihepatitis with marked thickening of the capsule of the liver. The fact that 15 of the patients were free from œdema is of interest, as we also know that with pure mitral stenosis œdema is most exceptional. It is worth bearing in mind that in more than a quarter of the cases the liver was not found to be enlarged, and in 23 there was no albuminuria. It is difficult to understand why seven of the patients were free from dyspnœa, while more than one of them was not ill till within three weeks of death. Glycosuria was noticed only once. While certain deductions may with confidence be drawn from statistics based upon observations made by medical students, still undoubtedly the frequency of common symptoms must inevitably be underestimated. Among these series of cases, true expansile pulsation of the liver, due to associated tricuspid incompetence, was only recorded eight times ; there can be little doubt, however, that it was present more frequently, but had not been specially sought for.

Concerning the *bruits* which were heard : the difficulty of diagnosing cases may be realised when it is pointed out that in 20 cases—that is, in nearly a quarter of the whole—no bruits were specially noted in reference to the tricuspid area in the region of the ensiform cartilage. In 10 cases a systolic bruit, widely distributed over the cardiac area, was noted. In 5 cases no cardiac bruits were noted while the patients were under observation ; and in one case there was some doubt as to the presence of a cardiac bruit. In 28 there were bruits audible near the ensiform cartilage on the left, and sometimes on the right side of the sternum, which were distinct in character from those heard elsewhere. The bruits were described as high-pitched, as distinct in character, and sometimes as rougher than those heard in the mitral area; several times as very distinct, occasionally as loud, and sometimes as harsh. In scarcely any case is it stated that the bruit was of a lower pitch than the mitral, as has been suggested by certain German observers. In several of the cases the bruit has been limited to a very narrow area; and not infrequently a thrill has been palpable. In only 10 cases out of the whole series was a presystolic or mid-diastolic bruit heard in the tricuspid region. In some of these it was doubtful, and in 2 cases it was heard on one occasion only. It was, however, very definitely stated in some reports that the presystolic bruit was distinct in character, and its area of maximum audibility definite. In one case the registrar described the systolic bruits as distinct from the mitral, more harsh, and followed by a faint bruit which ran up to the second sound. When we bear in mind that a vigorously acting auricle is required for the production of the mitral presystolic bruit, we need not wonder that it is infrequent in cases of right-sided stenosis; the right side works at a very much lower pressure, because the auricle is thinner, and contains less muscular fibre which can hypertrophy. Most authors state that a presystolic bruit should be heard; but clinical experience shows that such a bruit does not occur in 10 per cent of the cases of tricuspid stenosis. A localised, definite systolic bruit is much more frequent; and in half the cases no characteristic bruit is detected. As a natural sequence of this it follows that the lesion usually remains undiagnosed, and, not infrequently, unsuspected. This must always be so.

Hæmoptysis was noticed in 20 cases; in 8 of these pulmonary apoplexies were found at the inspection. A jaundiced condition of the skin was noticed 14 times; petechiæ 4 times; extreme pulsation in veins of neck 4 times; and once extreme distension of the veins generally.

Our knowledge of the lesion is largely due to Dr. Bedford Fenwick, and later to Leudet, who in 1888 collected 114 fatal cases not due to congenital lesion; to these Ashton and Stewart, in 1895, added 17 more. Their conclusions practically agree with ours.

Of Leudet's cases, in 57 there was no preceding illness; and in 41 a history of rheumatism. The lesion was four times as frequent in women as in men. Two-thirds of the cases occurred between the ages of twenty and forty. A presystolic bruit was heard in 13 cases.

Leudet points out that mitral stenosis was almost always present, but gives 11 as the number of cases in which it was absent; this number should be considerably reduced. Of these cases there was infective endocarditis in five, and three were very imperfectly reported. One was a remarkable case, published by Professor Sir William Gairdner (in 1862), of a tumour which had invaded the orifice and given rise to a presystolic bruit; the stenosis was diagnosed ten years before death. In one case the aortic valves were involved, and, excluding the cases of ulcerative endocarditis, in only one case, that of Hayem's, were the other valves healthy.

Philip has recorded a case in which the tricuspid valve was involved alone; and Delépine one in which a mass of calcified clot blocked the tricuspid orifice, and another of infective endocarditis with calcification of the valve. Apparently calcification of vegetations has taken place in several cases of right-sided lesions, and probably is more rapidly produced there than on the left side.

General conclusions.—1. Tricuspid stenosis is rare, but not excessively so; and in adults is not of congenital origin.

2. It is almost invariably preceded by mitral stenosis, and in one-fourth of the cases there is also aortic stenosis. A very well-marked example is shown in Fig. 3, where there is marked stenosis of the mitral and aortic orifices and moderate stenosis of the tricuspid.

3. The degree of stenosis of the mitral is generally more severe than that of the tricuspid.

4. The principal cause is a severe form of rheumatic endocarditis, but a history of rheumatism is only obtainable in about half the cases.

5. The stenosis generally advances insidiously, and in exceptional cases has been present in patients feeling fairly well.

6. Dyspnœa is almost universal; œdema and albuminuria are present in two-thirds; enlarged liver and extreme cyanosis in one-half of the cases.

7. A presystolic bruit is only heard in a small fraction (one-eighth) of the cases; an epigastric systolic bruit is much more common, while in one-quarter no bruit is audible.

If we bear in mind that this lesion is almost invariably found in connection with mitral stenosis, this may not infrequently suffice to enable us to make an accurate diagnosis. Such stenosis arises most insidiously; and to determine the diagnosis we must sometimes be satisfied with the collateral symptoms of great cardiac failure—dyspnœa, œdema, and notable cyanosis.

Treatment.—The treatment is practically that already indicated for mitral stenosis and tricuspid incompetence, but the beneficial results are much less apparent.

G. Newton Pitt.

REFERENCES

1. Allbutt. *On Overwork and Strain of the Heart.*—2. Ashton and Stewart. "Report of a case of Tricuspid Stenosis, associated with Mitral Stenosis and Aortic Stenosis," *American Journal of Med. Sciences,* 1895, vol. cix. p. 177.—3. Barie. "Sur l'insuffisance des valvules de l'artère pulmonaire," *Arch. gén. de méd.* 1891, vol. clxviii. p. 183.—4. Blattmann. *Zwei Fälle von Insufficienz der Pulmonalarterienklappen-Glarus.* 1887; Dissertation, Zurich.—5. Bramwell. *American Journal of the Medical Sciences,* April 1886, p. 419.—6. Charcot-Bouchard. *Traité de médecine,* tome v. 1893.—7. Coupland. *Trans. Path. Soc. London,* 1875, vol. xxvi. p. 22.—8. Dilg. "Ein Beitrag zur Kenntniss seltenen Herzanomalien im Ausschluss an einen Fall von angeborner linkseitiger Conusstenose," *Virchow's Archiv,* B. xci. p. 193.—9. Duroziez. *Bull. soc. de méd. de Paris,* 1868 : *L'Union méd.* Paris, Dec. 1883.—10. Fenwick. *Trans. Path. Soc. London,* 1881, vol. xxxii. p. 42, and vol. xxxiii. p. 64.—11. Gairdner. *Clinical Medicine,* p. 602.—12. Geigel. "Ueber den Venenpuls," *Würzburg med. Zeitschr.* 1863.—13. Gerhardt. *Klinische Untersuchungen über Venenpulsation,* Leipzig, 1894; "Ueber Schlussunfähigkeit der Lungenarterienklappen," *Charité-Annalen,* 1892, p. 255.—14. Gouraud. *De l'influence pathogénique*

des maladies pulmonaires sur le cœur droit. Paris, 1865.—15. GRAWITZ. *Virchow's Archiv*, B. cx. p. 436.—16. HERRICK, J. "Tricuspid Stenosis," *Bost. Med. and Surg. Journal*, 18th March 1897.—17. HOLMES. *Clin. Soc. Trans.* vol. ix. p. 114, vol. x., and vol. xxi. p. 146.—18. KERSCHENSTEINER. *Münchener med. Woch.* 1897, p. 808, etc. (which contains several additional cases of ulcerative endocarditis of the pulmonary valves).—19. LEUDET. *Essai sur le rétrécissement tricuspidien.* Paris, 1888.—20. MORISON. *Dextral Valvular Disease of the Heart*, 1878.—21. PAPAS. *Thèse de Paris*, 1894.—22. PASTEUR. "A New Method of Estimating the Condition of the Right Side of the Heart," *Lancet*, 1886, i. 914.—23. PAUL. *Gazette heb. de méd.* 1871, No. 27, p. 431.—24. PAWINSKI. "Ueber relative Insufficienz der Lungenarterienklappen bei Mitral Stenose," *Archiv für klin. Med.* 1894.—25. PETER. *Maladies du cœur*, 1883, p. 612.—26. PITT. "Association of Mitral Stenosis, with Gout and Granular Kidneys," *Brit. Med. Journal*, 1887, vol. ii. p. 118.—27. POTAIN. "Insufficiance et rétrécissement tricuspidiens," *Semaine médicale.*, 1891, p. 346 ; "Des mouvements et des bruits qui se passent dans les veins jugulaires," *Soc. méd. des hôp.* March 1867.—28. RIEGEL. *Deutsches Archiv für klin. Med.* B. xxxi.—29. SANSOM. *The Diagnosis of Diseases of the Heart and Thoracic Aorta*, 1892.—30. SCHIPPMANN. "Ueber angeborene Stenose oder Atresia des Ostium dext.,' Virchow und Hirsch's *Jahresb.* 1899.—31. WHITLEY. "Disease of the Pulmonary Artery and its Valves," *Guy's Hospital Reports*, S. III. vol. iii. 1857, p. 252.

G. N. P.

ANGINA PECTORIS

Definition.—A sudden paroxysmal disturbance of the heart's function accompanied by severe pain, distressed breathing, and a vague or instant apprehension of death.

Angina, in its graver forms, is an appalling and a picturesque disease, about which a certain glamour has been cast by the many noble and distinguished lives it has stricken down. It is, however, a common malady, and its victims are not limited to the wise and great ; a malady which, with advancing civilisation, extended mean duration of life, and increased stress of mental occupation, must probably become yet more common.

History.—Although the symptoms of angina pectoris did not altogether escape the notice of authors before the last century, the disease was first definitely recognised and described by Heberden[1] in 1768. His description is a model of accuracy and lucid expression, and has remained up to the present time unsurpassed in exactness and graphic force. Fothergill and John Hunter in the previous year had described two cases of anginous cardiac failure, in which calcification of the coronary arteries was recognised as accountable for death ; but Dr. Edward Jenner, in 1799, was the first to regard coronary disease as the lesion of angina ; this view, further advocated by Parry and others, still holds good for the graver forms of the malady to which the name angina was then restricted.

---

[1] Professor Gairdner, in a note appended to his article in Reynolds' *System of Medicine*, and still more authoritatively in a letter contributed to the discussion on Sir R. Douglas Powell's paper on angina pectoris at the Medical Society of London in 1891 (*Transactions*, vol. XIV.), has controverted the statements that M. Rougnon, in a letter to M. Lorry, dated 1768, had anticipated Heberden in the description of angina pectoris. See, however. Osler (3A) on claims of Rougnon, Morgagni, and Seneca in this regard.

Some distinguished authors, even at the present day, still regard Heberden's angina as the only true form of the disease; but this view has
become less tenable as our knowledge of the physiology of the anginal
seizure and the pathological states which are concerned in its manifestations has advanced; and it is impossible at the present time, with due
regard to clinical consistency, thus to restrict our conception of the disease.

Reeder, in 1821, seems to have been the first to draw a distinction
between so-called true and false angina, but it could not be until physiological knowledge, especially of cardio-vascular innervation, was much
further advanced that Nothnagel and Eulenburg, and particularly the
former, were in a position to establish vasomotor angina as a definite
group of symptoms.

The observations of Landois (1865) and Ross (1885) and particularly
the researches of Gaskell on cardiac and vascular innervation have
rendered it possible of late years to give a better explanation of the
phenomena of angina, and have been of great service in suggesting
some successful methods of treatment.

Many other able writers, besides those first concerned in its recognition, have contributed to the advance of our knowledge of the symptomatology and pathology of angina pectoris in modern times, and to a still
more considerable advance in the rational therapeutics of the disease.

Angina pectoris manifests itself in three forms :—

(i.) In the first group are to be found those cases in which the
disease is a pure neurosis of the cardio-vascular system, a disturbance of
the innervation of the systemic or pulmonary vessels including sometimes
the vessels of the heart itself, causing their spasmodic contraction and
thus increasing the peripheral resistance to circulation. The sudden
excessive demand upon the propelling power of the heart thus occasioned
produces a more or less painful embarrassment of its action ; and in some
cases this embarrassment is increased by anæmia of the cardiac muscle
due to the coincident contraction of the coronary vessels. We speak of
this variety as *angina pectoris vasomotoria*, and we have to inquire into the
conditions which lead up to such disturbed innervation and its consequences.

(ii.) In another and graver class of cases we have precisely the
same mechanism of disturbed cardio-vascular innervation, but associated
with it a diseased heart, either a texturally damaged heart muscle or a
valvular defect, or both combined. This variety may be designated
angina pectoris gravior, or *secondary cardiac angina*.

(iii.) In a third group of cases we have a few tolerably well-
defined forms of disease of the heart, in which the organ itself is the
primary seat of the painful and often fatal symptoms. In these cases
also the cardiac lesion may be valvular or textural. We may distinguish
this third group by the designation *primary cardiac angina*. It includes
certain cases of obstructive cardiac disease, especially cases of aortic or
mitral narrowing, cases of textural degeneration and ischæmia of heart
generally dependent on coronary narrowing; and, lastly, although some-

what loosely, many cases of fatal syncope dependent upon degenerated heart, which are unattended with other anginal phenomena.

We have thus two fairly definite kinds of angina pectoris :—I. Vaso-motory angina. II. Angina pectoris gravior; which latter is divisible into (A) Secondary cardiac angina ; (B) Primary cardiac angina.

There are other cases of acute cardiac failure from causes which perhaps would not be included within the above headings, but they, for the most part, will find their place amongst other kinds of cardiac failure. The end may be with anginal suffering, but the disease may not be angina pectoris.

I. Angina Pectoris Vasomotoria

Syn.—*Pseudangina.*

Etiology.—*Age.*—Vasomotory angina may occur at any age, but it prevails most between puberty and middle life with a distinct accession of prevalence about the climacteric period. It may be met with in early life, and I have observed a considerable number of instances of the purest vasomotory angina in advanced life.

Sex.—The lighter forms of angina, which are more prevalent towards the earlier periods of life, are also much more equally divided between the sexes. For whilst the more idiopathically neurotic forms are more prevalent amongst women, those attacks attributable to an exhausted nervous system, from alcoholic and other excesses, are more commonly met with in men. Tobacco angina is more prevalent amongst men, and tends to balance the larger prevalence of the affection in women at the climacteric period and in association with anæmia. Again, with regard to this form of angina, the male sex is affected on the whole at an earlier age than the female ; I have never met with a case of pure vasomotory angina in an elderly man.

Hereditary tendency.—A very distinct hereditary tendency may be observed with regard both to the lighter, or more purely neurotic, and the graver forms of the disease. Eulenburg speaks of vasomotory angina as alternating in persons and in families with a history of insanity or epilepsy ; and certainly an instability of the nervous system and the occurrence of such diseases as asthma and the neuralgias may be fre-quently observed thus associated with it.

Climate ; Temperature.—Although it has not been shown that climate has any important influence upon the prevalence of angina pectoris, it is quite certain that cold, in the sense of getting chilled, is a most important cause, whether immediate or remote, of attacks of angina in all varieties ; but especially in the vasomotory forms. Riding or walking against a cold wind, sleeping in cold rooms, getting the extremities chilled, are causes frequently assigned. Sudden immersion in cold water, or remain-ing too long in water, will cause an attack in the predisposed ; and there can be little doubt that attacks of "cramp" in the water are sometimes anginal in nature. The effect of a chill is to contract the arterioles by over-stimulation of the vasomotor centres ; and its operation in inducing angina is thus equally favourable to the occurrence of either variety of the disease.

Occupation.—Probably all practising physicians will accept Huchard's statement that those occupations and professions — such as finance, politics, medicine—in which through nervous strain arterial tension ranges high, are favourable to arterial disorders. Prior to any organic alteration they favour the occurrence of vasomotory disturbance tending to angina. It is more doubtful whether laborious occupations, involving physical strain, dispose so much to angina as to more definite lesions of the cardiac valves and the main trunks of the arterial system.

Gout is a frequent causative element in vasomotory angina, but is commonly then associated with some permanent cardiac changes.

Influenza. — Amongst the pure neuroses of the recent influenza epidemics angina pectoris has been frequently met with. In my experience it has been generally vasomotory, and associated with a remarkable excess of urea in the urine.

Uræmia.—The anginal or " heart asthma " attacks of kidney disease do not come on until permanent and considerable hypertrophy and dilatation of the heart have ensued upon chronic high arterial pressure, and thus the cases come fittingly in the next category.

Tabes.—Cases of angina have been described as occurring amongst the "crises" of tabes. Huchard quotes several from Vulpian, Leyden, Groebel, and some that he has himself observed. He attributes such cases as are genuine to the aortic and cardiac lesions which are commonly associated with ataxy, and not to the affection of the nervous system itself. Huchard maintains that in the absence of such cardiac lesions, the more purely neurotic cases are not due to affections of the cardiac plexuses, but to thoracic or brachial neuralgia, girdle pains or gastric crises simulating anginal seizures.

Dyspepsia. Constipation.—Dyspepsia is a frequent exciting cause of anginal attacks, and particularly those forms of it which are attended with flatulent distension of the stomach or colon. It must be remembered, however, that flatulent distension is also a frequent concomitant of anginal paroxysms, no doubt as a reflected or associated nervous phenomenon.

Constipation is a very frequent cause of high arterial blood-pressure and favours attacks in this way.

Emotion. — Emotional disturbance, fright, pain, sudden shocks of sorrow will produce attacks, and are thus efficient causes. Exertion, especially when attended with excitement, will also bring on the lighter forms of angina in younger persons who are disposed to them.

Pathology.—In discussing the pathology of angina pectoris, we have to explain the mechanism of attack, to account for the most characteristic symptoms, and to provide the data for a differential diagnosis,—with especial regard to prognosis and treatment.

Angina pectoris vasomotoria cannot be said to have any pathology. It is a disordered innervation of the vessels, peripheral or visceral, resulting in their contraction, causing an increased pressure of blood in the cavities of the heart, and a consequently embarrassed action with pain and dyspnœa. The texture and valves of the heart are sound, although in cases which have extended over years there may be some secondary changes in the heart and vessels attributable to long-continued high pressure ; just as in asthma we find, after a time, secondary textural changes in the lung consequent upon the bronchial spasm which was originally a pure neurosis.

The nerves concerned are the sympathetic, the vagus, the depressor nerve, the vaso-constrictor and vaso-dilator nerves of the blood-vessels, and any nerve which conducts afferent impulses to the central nervous system.

The vasomotor nerves have their centre in the medulla, and consist of vaso-constrictor and vaso-dilator fibres. The vaso-constrictor fibres pass to the vessels by way of the sympathetic chain, which is reached through certain anterior spinal nerve roots and their rami communicantes ; while there is reason to suppose that the vaso-dilator fibres pursue a direct course from the spinal cord through the anterior spinal nerve roots without connection with the sympathetic system. The currents through both sets of nerves are efferent currents. The sympathetic is the motor nerve of the heart, its stimulation being attended with waste and oxidation (acidulation of muscle). The pneumogastric is the restraining nerve of the heart, its stimulation being attended with regulation and restraint of action, favouring nutrition and repair. The depressor nerve of the heart is an afferent nerve conducting impulses from the heart by way of the vagus nerve. Its impulses, arriving at the vasomotor centre in the medulla, influence the general blood-pressure through the vaso-dilator nerves, causing a gradual but marked fall which is especially brought about by dilatation of the abdominal vessels. The depressor nerve in some of the lower animals (rabbit) is a separate nerve for the greater part of its course, although it is ultimately connected with the pneumogastric and its superior laryngeal branch.

The writings of George Johnson, Broadbent, Nothnagel, Eulenburg, and Gaskell have made us familiar with vasomotor mechanism ; a due understanding of which, thanks especially to the labours of Gaskell, is now a matter of current physiological knowledge,—a knowledge, however, which had undoubtedly been in great measure anticipated by the clinical studies of George Johnson.

Stimulation of the vasomotor centres by the direct application of cold to the surface, or by a certain degree of irritation or stretching of the visceral terminations of corresponding afferent nerves, will cause constriction of the vessels. Central stimuli—emotion, pain, anger, fright—may supply the same motor impulses. Certain blood conditions, especially uric acid and its allies in excess, the absorption of ptomaines from the bowel, and the action of certain drugs of the digitalis class will have a similar effect. These latter conditions, however, operate rather by increasing the general arterial pressure, and thus rendering it easy, by a slight additional excitement, to produce that higher degree of contraction of peripheral vessels which shall cause acute cardiac embarrassment. Many neurotic states keep the vessel innervation in the same sensitive condition. The intra-cardiac pressure in the right or left ventricle, or both, is thus liable to sudden increase, the first effect being stimulation of the sympathetic nerve, and rapid and often disorderly efforts of the heart to overcome the resistance; which it can do, however, with but imperfect success. As the intra-cardiac pressure rises the depressor nerve becomes in turn excited, and inhibits sympathetic activity; the vessels are relaxed, the pressure is relieved, and the heart's action is restored to regularity.

It will be obvious, then, that fatigue and exhaustion must attend the excited and laboured action of the heart; and it has been shown by Gaskell that fatigue of cardiac muscle, as of other muscles, causes a tendency to cramp; and that accumulation of products of waste in the cardiac muscle tends to render its tissues unduly acid, an undue acidity which causes paralysis. Whilst these considerations are of no great practical importance in reference to attacks of pure vasomotory angina, unaccompanied by any organic disablement of the heart, beyond explaining the sense of fatigue and often of prostration that follows such seizures, they are of the utmost importance in the graver cases of the next category, and explain the fatal termination of many of them.

The pathology, so far as we may call it so, of angina pectoris vasomotoria has distinct relations then with ordinary high arterial blood-pressure, and with those local extreme degrees of vessel constriction which constitute Raynaud's disease. In the opposite direction we come, on the other hand, to cases of chronic high arterial pressure with secondary cardio-vascular changes. This is most completely observed in cases of chronic interstitial nephritis, in which vascular tension, at first a truly physiological and conservative condition involving increased cardiac effort, becomes chronic, and entails cardio-vascular hypertrophy; in cases in which the malady is fairly worked out on cardio-vascular lines (not cut short by more acute uræmic phenomena) the final symptoms are those of chronic cardiac distress with anginal paroxysms, such as may be frequently witnessed in the last months of chronic interstitial nephritis.

The effect of nicotine upon the small vessels and heart seems to be a matter of considerable uncertainty; Claude Bernard finding contraction of the vessels, whilst other experimental observers find dilatation to follow its use. This discrepancy seems to be very much a matter of dose: the physiological action of nicotine is, however, currently regarded as contracting the blood-vessels (Brunton). Clinically, one finds varied arhythmic disturbances of the cardiac function in those who are indulging too freely in tobacco (and much the same in coffee), which suggest that the pneumogastric nerve is most affected, and thus control of cardiac and vasomotor innervation is practically lost. And when Huchard himself speaks of the cardiac phenomena arising from the abuse of tobacco as "accélération ou ralentissement du pouls, intermittences et arythmie du cœur, lipothymies et syncopes, sentiment d'angoisse et d'anxiété précordiale, palpitations, battements tumultueux, arrêts subits et angoissants du cœur, instabilité extrême des functions circulatoires et état particulier que je propose d'appeler 'cœur irritable' des fumeurs" (p. 699), we cannot doubt that loss of pneumogastric control is the chief neurosis present. Under this loss of pneumogastric control it is easy for slight causes to bring about vasomotory anginal seizures. Huchard speaks of three forms of tobacco angina. One is purely functional, in which the heart is sound, but the coronary arteries are spasmodically narrowed, producing temporary anæmia of the heart muscle (l'angine spasmo-tabacique); secondly, there is organic narrowing of the vessels from arterial sclerosis due to chronic tobacco poisoning, which he calls "l'angine sclero-tabacique"—a more grave condition to be considered in our next category; thirdly, the arterial spasm is attendant upon dyspeptic causes of tobacco origin, "l'angine gastrique tabacique." These would also come under the head of functional or vasomotory angina. Huchard (page 712) quotes one fatal case in which no other reason for death could be found than a functional failure of the heart from excess of tobacco; and two other cases in which both patients, aged respectively 38 and 50, died of tobacco angina, but in which no autopsy was made; the absence of coronary sclerosis could not therefore be verified.

Symptoms.—Angina pectoris vasomotoria, false or spurious angina as it has been called, is a group of symptoms from which persons of either sex, of neurotic temperament or inheritance, may suffer in the first half of adult life; but which prevails more amongst women at or about the climacteric period, and in later life affects women rarely yet almost exclusively. In its marked degrees it is not a very common affection, merging on the one side into the attacks of mere perturbed heart's action so common in young people, and on the other gravitating into those cases of the second and much more serious category of angina in which vasomotory phenomena still play a most important part. The subjects of this form of angina are liable to disordered peripheral circulation; their extremities are habitually chilly; they get "dead" hands or fingers, local sweatings, and they suffer much from cold feet at night. The attack is apt to occur under the influence of some emotion; or it may be induced by walking or riding against cold winds; or, again, it may occur at night, and is then often attributable to coldness of the extremities. There are, however, generally some premonitory symptoms of defective surface circulation,—"creeps," "pins and needles," "deadness of hands,"—and these premonitory symptoms often affect particular sides or parts of the body in different people. Headache, chiefly frontal or supra-orbital, is frequently complained of about these times; and constipation is often present. The patients are commonly but not necessarily anæmic. Sometimes, in cases approaching the menopause, they are unduly plethoric. If they be under medical observation, it will be found that the pulse is habitually quick, and that, although the arterial pressure is very variable, the range of it is decidedly high. Marey's law that the high pressure pulse is slow does not always apply in clinical medicine, the reason no doubt being that with instability of vessels more or less irritability of heart is associated.

The heart presents nothing abnormal to percussion or auscultation, except that usually the second sound is unduly accentuated. The cardiac impulse is normal in position, and, at least in the earlier years of the malady, normal in character, except for a certain excitement of action usually noticeable in persons of this class. Amongst such persons, who are mostly of spare build, one finds a relatively large number of instances of mobility of the right kidney ; and undue pulsation of the abdominal aorta is also another occasionally associated symptom. The attack begins quite suddenly, with acute pain and a sense of distension or oppression in the region of the heart. Severe palpitation ensues, accompanied by more or less apnœa and sense of air hunger. Sometimes the heart appears to stop altogether, and the patient may fall down in a semi-faint with a cry of pain ; this is rare, but it was a marked symptom in a young married lady seen by myself in consultation with Dr. Sansom and Dr. F. Smith. If the pulse be observed at this stage it will be found small, perhaps very irregular or intermitting, and generally quick, though some of the cardiac impulses may fail at the wrist. The attack may last a few seconds or a few minutes only, during which time the surface is pale and cold, and the countenance pinched ; there may be clammy sweats, and the patient has a sense of extreme illness. A peculiar desire for air is generally a marked feature in these cases. After a few seconds the pulse becomes relaxed, if not rendered so by treatment ; the patient pants more or less convulsively, and tends to toss about or move to the window for air. This restlessness and tendency to seek fresh air by personal effort is very different from the still attitude of the subject of the graver angina. It is particularly noticeable in cases in which the severity of attack is not sufficient actually to stop the patient, who in such cases will often continue in exercise throughout an attack ; a thing never observed in grave angina, and therefore of some value in diagnosis in cases otherwise doubtful. A copious flow of pale urine is a usual sequel of all cases of angina presenting the vaso-constrictive element. The attack passes by and leaves the patient fatigued and alarmed, and there is a decided tendency to a serial recurrence of the attacks during the ensuing few hours or days, when they will cease for perhaps a considerable interval. The degrees of severity of symptoms are, as already said, very variable, and the diagnosis is, as a rule, not difficult.

I will now relate three cases to give a more clinical character to the above statement of symptoms :—

CASE 1.—A lady of forty-five, of active habits and neurotic temperament, complained that for the past four or five years she had been conscious of her heart's action ; that it had been occasionally disturbed, palpitating, and irregular, sometimes intermitting. She had had rheumatic fever fifteen years before, and was subject to occasional rheumatic pains. Her mother, without previous illness, had died almost suddenly of heart failure. As long as ten years ago she would occasionally, when in the midst of a sharp run out hunting, experience a severe pain at the heart, lasting for two or three minutes, and interfering with breathing. She would not stop for this pain, although it was severe, and it would pass away whilst still riding fast. She now complained of having similar attacks of pain ; sometimes as sharp as before, at other times more dull and of longer duration. Occasionally she has felt very giddy and ill, but never actually fainted. She suffered at times from numbness of the arms and a great sense of chilliness, requiring extra clothing even during sharp exercise. Sometimes quick walking would bring on an attack of the heart pain, but not always. This lady presented no symptoms of approaching menopause, such as flushings or perspirations, or irregularity of the catamenia. Her digestion and nutrition were good ; her pulse was quick, small, and of high tension, that is, when stopped by the strong pressure of one finger, the vessel beyond was still filled and pulsated from the peripheral side. The heart's apex was only just within the nipple line, the impulse was rather increased in force, the first sound muffled, but unattended with murmur ; its action intermitted about twice in each minute. Urine 1020, no albumin, phosphates, or sugar present.

It will be observed in this case that some noticeable cardiac signs were present, indicative of slight dilatation and hypertrophy. These conditions, however, were not due to the anginal seizures, or in any way responsible for them, but were attributable rather to the chronic high arterial pressure of which the seizures were incidental accessions.

The following case is a fair example of several cases of vasomotory anginal attacks which I have observed in persons, in my experience always women, beyond middle life :—

CASE 2.—A widow lady, aged seventy-two ; seen with Dr. Dickinson, of Sloane Street ; has had four children. Father died suddenly of bursting of an abdominal aneurysm ; mother of diabetes ; one brother of dropsy, probably renal ; one sister of consumption ; one sister of asthma, and a sister living has diabetes. The patient has passed uric acid calculi, and has had two attacks of broncho-pneumonia. She is a thin, bright-eyed woman, of vivacious manners and nervous temperament. For twelve years she has suffered from attacks of pain at the heart, which are brought on by physical exertion, by passing into a colder atmosphere, or by the excitement of seeing visitors, and frequently on beginning a meal. This pain is situated behind the sternum, and spreads upward to the throat and jaw, under the tongue and ears, thence to the shoulders and down the arms ; it is also felt to some extent in the back, but leaves the cranial vertex free, and never goes below the waist. The bowels habitually tend to be confined, but are kept regulated by cascara. The urine shows absence of albumin and sugar ; the pulse is hard, tense, and has been observed to become more so during the attacks ; rate 76. The heart sounds are normal, the action somewhat forcible. Since the beginning of 1894, these attacks, under trinitrine treatment, have to some extent become less frequent; but lately they have been replaced by attacks of palpitation, during which the pulse is soft and the heart's action very irregular ; these attacks are remedied by ether and strophanthus, and have taken place since the trinitrine was left off, and are, therefore, not immediately caused by that drug. I may add that this lady has no sign of disease of the heart, but on several occasions on which I have seen her, usually soon after an attack, the pulse has always been thready and incompressible ;

on one occasion, when a mild attack came on during my visit, it perceptibly hardened.

The following case is one which, whilst presenting decided symptoms of the form of angina now under consideration, is a better illustration of the so-called spurious angina, which cannot be separated from this variety :—

CASE 3.—Mrs. X., aged thirty-five, a lady of nervous temperament and inheritance, and married to an extremely nervous man, was seen in consultation with Dr. Sansom and Dr. Fred. J. Smith in March 1895. In the course of seven years she had had eight children, and during her eighth pregnancy suffered from dyspepsia, vomiting, and tachycardia, the heart's action reaching 135. In September 1895, after some extra fatigue on a blackberrying excursion, she was suddenly seized with great breathlessness and severe palpitation, attended with swelling of the veins of the neck, causing her to feel as though her head would burst, and pain over the cardiac region, with a feeling of great precordial (epigastric ?) distension. These symptoms were attended with such utter prostration of strength that she was obliged to lie down or she would have fallen, although there was no loss of consciousness. The symptoms subsided in two or three minutes, but pain and tenderness remained in the cardiac region. A few days later Dr. Smith found the heart normal in position, the first sound peculiarly sharp and short, and the rate very variable from minute to minute, being especially more rapid during forced expiration, and slowed by forced inspiration. More or less similar attacks were of frequent occurrence, caused chiefly by fatigue or excitement. The patient described an attack which occurred in the Christmas week of 1895, after some extra exertion in entertaining her children, as beginning in the limbs "with the circulation going the wrong way"; then a sense of the heart "turning over," and a feeling as though she were dying. To ordinary observers this seemed no exaggeration, and it was only by close examination that the absence of any cause of death was ascertained. During one exacerbation of the attack, witnessed by Dr. Smith, there was decided gaseous distension of the stomach. In the intervals of attack, sleeplessness, constipation, and coldness of the extremities were her most frequent complaints. Shortly before our consultation she had had a very severe attack, seizing her quite suddenly and causing her to fall down. On very careful examination no cardiac abnormality of any kind could be found. The pulse was rather quick, the pressure somewhat raised, varying in this respect even under examination. She was a tall, slender woman, with the neurotic characteristics already mentioned, and a somewhat patchy flush upon the cheeks. She has greatly improved in health, and in July 1896 went to Switzerland and walked the hills as well as her companions, provided she did not hurry. The attacks of heart pain continue from time to time, but they are never severe; movement of the left arm is apt to bring them on.

Diagnosis.—The diagnosis of these cases presents no great difficulty, and it is scarcely necessary to say that this is of very great importance in view both of prognosis and treatment.

(i.) We have to deal with a patient of a neurotic temperament and physiognomy; often, not always, at a period of life too young for the more serious kinds of angina. Although very ill for the time, the aspect to an experienced observer is not that of a fatal seizure.

(ii.) On sufficient recovery, or in an interval between the attacks, no cardiac lesion is to be found. There may be some modification of the rhythm or some accentuation of the second sound, but the position, dimensions, and sounds of the heart are within the limits of health, modified only by functional disturbance. This somewhat difficult decision must be established by most careful palpation, percussion, and auscultation in the intervals between the attacks.

(iii.) The ambulatory tendency in the attack is a decided point in favour of its vaso-constrictive origin.

(iv.) It will usually be found, in persons subject to these attacks, that the arterial blood-pressure, as detected by the character of the pulse, ranges high. It is, moreover, variable, and may vary during the time of examination. Other phenomena, indicative of instability of the vaso-motor nervous system, may be observed.

Prognosis.—The prognosis of angina vasomotoria is, as a rule, very favourable. Under varied moral, hygienic, and medicinal treatment, and with lapse of time, the younger patients get well. Climacteric cases, and a certain proportion of gouty cases also, end in recovery. A certain number of patients, however, lapse into the second category; or if they lose their heart attacks, they still advance to the gradual establishment of cardiac hypertrophy and, usually, mitral incompetence; these phenomena being attendant upon that chronic high arterial tension in the earlier stages of which the anginal paroxysms have intervened as incidental neuroses (*vide* Case 1). Lastly, in a very few cases death occurs in an attack. Some such cases have been recorded by Dr. Huchard, and amongst them must be included some of the cases of death in the water from cramp. In these latter, however, it is probable that the attack only proves fatal indirectly, the patient, rendered helpless by his cardiac seizure, being drowned.

Treatment.—The treatment of angina pectoris vasomotoria is prophylactic and medicinal. The mode of life of the patient must be considered, and there will usually be some defect to be remedied. Over-excitement, moral errors, dissipation, excesses in tobacco-smoking and alcohol are to be inquired for and corrected. Irregularity in meals, quick eating, and sitting down to meals when exhausted, are, through the dyspeptic troubles entailed, indirect exciting causes of the attack. Many persons towards middle life become overwhelmed with engagements and worries, which make their lives quite unnecessarily hurried, and anxious beyond their nervous powers of endurance; with a firm hand these extra causes of nerve strain must be pruned down, and, after a sufficient rest and holiday to recover from them, the patient may with advantage return to regular work. It is certainly our experience that it is not the routine labour of the day, but the multifarious occupations and engagements of our so-called leisure which, especially with the class of patients under consideration, exhaust the nervous energies and bring about neurotic disturbances; and it is often the worst treatment possible for such patients to cut them off from their business or professioual work. Their labours may be, however, curtailed somewhat in two directions: first, to secure a moderate amount of quiet open-air exercise daily, and, secondly, to ensure the return home in time to get an hour's quiet before dinner. When the heart's action is habitually quick, this hour should be spent lying down. On the other hand, the after-dinner hour should never be spent in sleeping, but rather in some quiet occupation, such as billiards. The dietary of the patient must be carefully inquired into, especially in those about the climacteric period, or who present gouty phenomena, or venous plethora. In the latter class of cases a course of waters at Buxton, Harrogate, Carlsbad, Homburg, or Nauheim will often be desirable to start a cure, which subsequent care in exercise and diet will maintain. Cases of venous plethora with disposition to superfluous adipose tissue about the cardiac vessels, and defective cardiac tone, are those to which Nauheim exercises are especially if not solely applicable.

Finally, after a careful diagnosis, the definite assurance to these people that their distressing and painful symptoms are not dependent upon cardiac disease, and are not of a dangerous nature, will do much to relieve the attacks by withholding that element of panic which tends to intensify them.

The medicinal treatment of vasomotory angina is of considerable importance. It consists in lowering any excess of arterial blood-pressure, which is not corrected by the hygienic and dietetic measures spoken of; a careful regulation of the bowels is of the first importance, and should include a small dose of mercury once or twice a week, followed by a saline. In highly neurotic persons, especially those about the menopause, a little hydrobromic acid and bromide of sodium may be prescribed for a time. Iron may sometimes be given in anæmic cases, but it is rarely well borne, and must be given in small doses. Arsenic is a valuable remedy, and may be usefully combined with valerian; for instance, as a tenth of a grain of arseniate of iron with two grains of extract of valerian after food three times daily. Neither quinine nor strychnine is, as a rule, well borne by these patients—hop, calumba, or chiretta are better tonics; but in the neuralgic bouts, to which they are subject, quinine and phenacetin may be usefully combined.

During the attacks we have to guard against the tendency to fly to stimulants and sedatives. Brandy or subcutaneous injection of morphia will give relief, but they leave the patient on a lower plane and less resistant to fresh attacks than before. Perhaps very hot water, slowly sipped, is the best domestic remedy; but such patients should have at hand a draught of soda, ammonia, or ammoniated valerian, cardamoms and chloric ether, to be slowly sipped on the oncoming of an attack. A minim or two of one per cent trinitrine solution may often be added to the draught with advantage, or a trinitrine lozenge taken at the same time. A rest in bed of twenty-four hours is usually necessary; and sometimes in anæmic or neurasthenic cases a more prolonged complete rest is desirable ; but it is important as soon as may be to get the patient back to the ordinary routine of life with the restrictions above laid down.

II. Angina Pectoris Gravior

A. Secondary cardiac angina.—**Etiology.**—The etiology of this group of cases of angina pectoris gravior is, in most respects, precisely the same as that of the preceding form of angina, in so far that it includes all the causes of vasomotor disturbance which, by constricting the arterioles, brings about cardiac embarrassment. Furthermore, however, we must take into account the causes of those diseases and degenerations of the heart which constitute the pathology of secondary cardiac angina, and place it, in contrast with the preceding group, amongst that most grave of cardiac disturbances—the true angina of Heberden.

Sex.—Whereas the vasomotor anginas were found to be more common amongst women, the graver forms of the present category are vastly more prevalent amongst men, according to Forbes and Walsh as ten to one. The reason for this increased prevalence amongst men is clear when we observe that all the causes tending to earlier degeneration of the vascular system, namely, physical toil, gout, syphilis, alcoholism, and so forth, are more prevalent amongst them ; and that the causes of increased arterial tension, for instance, mental strain and gout, are more frequent and abiding in them as they approach middle and late middle life.

Age.—The more serious cases of angina occur within the years of commencing and advancing degeneration, more particularly between forty and sixty ; in the earlier decade it has generally been hurried forward by some antecedent morbid diathesis, such as syphilis, alcoholism, or gout, predisposing to earlier degenerations. Dr. Dreschfeld states that the coronary arteries are often atheromatous when other arteries show as yet no sign of disease ; and this he attributes to the high pressure of the circulation in them. He relates one case in a boy of twelve, who died suddenly with this affection. Beyond sixty-five the field of liability to the disease has become somewhat exhausted, and the conditions of life become less favourable to its manifestation.

Heredity.—The tendency in families to the occurrence of the graver forms of angina is very decided, and this is explained by the fact that the disposition to cardiac and vessel degeneration and to those diseases, such as rheumatism and gout, which lead up to them, are all very hereditary.

Morbid factors.—Gout, syphilis, plumbism, alcoholism, and tobacco are concerned in the causation of angina in so far as they conduce to cardio-vascular degenerations ; and in this connection they are referred to elsewhere. They may all be said to be important factors in the pathological history of the lesions associated with angina. The uric acid diathesis, alcohol, and tobacco also favour a chronic or intermittent high arterial tension ; besides favouring arterial degeneration they cause disturbances of innervation which, in earlier life, tend to bring about the first variety of angina, and later to excite attacks in connection with degenerated conditions of heart.

Syphilis is not only a cause of local or general arteritis, but may lead to the formation of gummata or gummatous infiltration of the heart.

Dr. Dreschfeld has found that congenital syphilis attacks the aorta and coronary arteries more often than is supposed; causing endarteritis, which may lead to contraction of lumen.

Glycosuria.—Diabetes has not been shown to have any etiological effect in angina. Cases are met with in association with glycosuria, but are dependent rather on the degenerative changes consequent upon the gouty condition with which this state of urine is connected.

Uræmia.—In chronic uræmia, especially when due to contracted kidneys, anginal phenomena are very frequently manifested,—a fact which is not surprising when we recollect the persistent high blood-pressure which is a feature of this disease.

The most common proximate cause of the graver forms of angina is physical exertion. The ordinary history of the first attack is that it began during some effort, a quick walk up an incline, hurrying to catch a train, mounting a ladder, running a race, or after a fatiguing walk. The patient may often have exerted himself to the same or a greater extent before, but the time had come when the reserve power of the heart, weakened by insidious disease, had been overstepped.

Pathology.—The forms of heart disease which constitute the serious factor of this second group of angina are several. First, there is fatty infiltration of the heart, independent of coronary degeneration. Secondly, there are those forms which depend upon permanent constriction of the coronary arteries. I have elsewhere described coronary atheroma and the forms of heart disease secondary to it; namely, fatty degeneration, false or fibroid hypertrophy, fibro-fatty change, fatty infiltration of the heart, infarction of the heart, syphilitic arteritis extending to the cardiac substance. Thirdly, there are certain valvular diseases of the heart, especially aortic regurgitation, aortic stenosis, and mitral stenosis. Fourthly, diseases of the aorta, atheroma, and aneurysm.

Of these the three most commonly met with are simple fatty infiltration of heart, fibroid or fibro-fatty hypertrophy and aortic regurgitant valvular disease, often associated with dilatation of the vessel. Perhaps aneurysm ought also to be included. The patients are mostly men and at or a little beyond middle age.

(i.) The least grave form is simple fatty infiltration of the heart in which the fibres of the heart are not primarily diseased, but are merely more or less toneless and atrophied, being hampered in action by the intercalation of adipose tissue deposit, the result of imperfect metabolism. The patients are usually of sedentary habits and disposed to good living; they are generally gouty, and uric acid or its allies are the most common proximate causes of the vasomotor spasm that starts the cardiac attack. The mechanism is precisely the same as that considered under the preceding heading. The coronary vessels of the heart may or may not partake in the more general arterial spasm, but they are not diseased. In short, these cases have the same etiology as the preceding, with a weak heart in the background; the organ is more or less enlarged and its cavities dilated.

(ii.) The much more grave cases, in which the heart is enlarged and its walls thickened by fibroid or fibro-fatty changes, are almost all secondary to narrowing of the coronary vessels. The texture of the organ is impaired, its circulation is impeded, and cramp and paralysis of the muscle are apt to ensue upon any sudden accession of blood-pressure from vasomotor spasm causing dangerous or fatal angina. Thickening of the valves or aorta from chronic endarteritis is often associated with the textural changes in the heart muscle. With the establishment of mitral regurgitation the intra-ventricular pressure becomes lowered from reflux through the valve, and the anginal seizures are mitigated and sometimes cease altogether. The heart in these cases is always much thickened and dilated.

(iii.) Anginal seizures of the present category in association with aortic regurgitant disease are rather common. The incompetence of the aortic valves arises in one of the usual ways—from rheumatic endocarditis, traumatic lesions, or endarteritis from syphilis or strain. The excessive strain to which the small vessels are subjected with each beat of the heart following upon very complete relaxation may be a cause of vasomotor spasm in aortic regurgitation, as it is a frequent cause of capillary hæmorrhage. The valvular disease may not be associated with coronary narrowing or degenerative disease of the heart muscle; but the more marked the dilated hypertrophy of the ventricle, and the less, therefore, the reserve power of the heart, the more readily induced and the more dangerous in character do the attacks become.

Owing to the great reserve capacity of the left auricle and pulmonary veins, mitral regurgitation is incompatible with the mechanism of the vasomotory variety of angina pectoris now under consideration; and the establishment of mitral incompetence by progressive endarteritic changes and mechanical dilatation of the left ventricle, which may be observed to occur in the course of some cases of coronary angina, is accompanied by cessation of the anginal attack.

Excessive intra-cardiac pressure as a cause of angina is not, however, necessarily due to contraction of the vessels of the periphery. In cases of aortic and mitral stenosis, and in some other heart diseases, the ventricle is subjected to habitual strain in maintaining the circulation; and any extra exertion may overstep the limits of reserve power and bring about anginal symptoms.

An eminent example of the angina now under consideration was related by the late Dr. Anstie in the case of a boy who, whilst sharply running, suddenly cried out with severe pain in his chest, and died. On examination post-mortem he was found to have great narrowing of the aortic orifice.

In atheromatous disease of the aorta with dilatation, and especially with aneurysm, anginal seizures are not uncommon. In most cases aortic regurgitation is well marked and will account for the attacks; in some we have to seek for the explanation in disturbances of cardiac innervation through pressure upon or stretching of the cardiac plexuses.

B. PRIMARY CARDIAC ANGINA.—*Syncope anginosa.*—In a third group of cases the symptoms are solely dependent upon causes within the heart itself. These may be spoken of as cases of primary cardiac angina; or, if the apt term of Parry may be restricted to them, "syncope anginosa." Their essential pathology is cardiac cramp and paralysis, due to narrowing or occlusion of one or both coronary vessels.

Taking 45 cases of fatal angina enumerated by Forbes and adding to them 46 more recent cases, otherwise collected, in which autopsies were made, we find, of the total 91 cases, only 7 in which there was no organic disease of the heart and great vessels. Of the 84 remaining cases there were in 64 disease of the coronary vessels or heart structure (namely, of coronary vessels 51 cases, of heart alone 13 cases). Huchard, in an additional chapter to his most recent work, has given a careful précis of 145 autopsies of cases of angina pectoris in which disease of the coronary arteries has been found, and these cases he thus classifies :—

In 64 cases the lesion affected both coronaries.

In 37 cases the lesion affected the left coronary.

In 15 cases the lesion affected the right coronary.

In 12 cases seat of lesion not specified.

In 17 cases coronary disease present, but no statement as to the narrowing of the vessel.

In 128 out of 145 cases there was obliteration or stenosis of the vessels; in 5 by embolism, in 2 by compression, in the rest either by atheromatous narrowing or thrombosis.

It is thus evident in how large a proportion of cases of fatal angina coronary arterial disease is present in a marked degree; and that there is much to justify the opinion of some pathologists, from the time of Jenner to our own day, who maintain that coronary disease is the essential pathology of angina pectoris.

I have endeavoured to controvert this opinion by showing that the more important symptoms of angina pectoris are frequently met with without any coronary or other cardiac lesion (vasomotory angina pectoris); secondly, that in many cases of grave cardiac disablement, even including a considerable but indeterminate proportion of the cases of coronary disease above enumerated, the characteristic features of the anginal attack are dependent on the same vasomotor causes remote from the heart; that is, upon paroxysmal constriction of the peripheral vessels telling back upon the enfeebled heart, which latter, however, is concerned in the often fatal issue. Lastly, these cases having been eliminated, there remains a residuum of cases belonging to the present category in which the heart and the heart alone is the primary and final factor in the anginal seizures.

It will be obvious that cases thus separable for more precise pathological consideration must overlap and merge into one another; and that clinically it may sometimes be difficult to classify a given case precisely. This matters nothing if our pathological insight into the disease for prognosis and treatment be assisted by the recognition of the three types.

The heart is the large heart usual in such cases; its texture more or less fibroid or fattily degenerated. The coronary vessels, one or both, are narrowed or occluded by disease; they may be obstructed at their aortic origins by the degenerative endarteritis about them; or they may be converted into thickened calcified tubes; or, again, at some portion of them thick calcareous plates may almost close their calibre. Superadded to this condition thrombosis of the vessel may take place at any point. One of the vessels may be closed by an embolism, or a syphilitic growth may thicken its walls to complete occlusion. Patches of extreme anæmia, hæmorrhagic infarction, or softening affect the territory of muscle corresponding to the completely, or almost completely, occluded vessels. The mechanism of the angina in these cases is tolerably simple and precisely analogous to anginal seizures in muscles of less vital importance with which we have now for some time been familiar.

Cramp or spastic contraction of muscle may be caused by restricted arterial blood-supply; it is common under conditions of faulty metabolism, and it affects, by choice, those muscles which are most in use. Elderly or old people, whose arteries are degenerating and whose muscular blood-supply is wanting in elasticity of accommodation, not infrequently complain that after walking a certain distance they are pulled up by more or less severe cramps in the legs or thigh muscles. In other cases instead of cramp their muscles fail in power, and they can walk no farther. Sometimes after a tiring day they will wake up at night with cramp pains in the limbs.

Similarly, in the history of anginal seizures, we are occasionally met by the statement that the patient's earlier seizures occurred whilst walking perhaps faster or more laboriously than usual; that the attack caused him to stop short, and that only after a time could he with great care and caution get home. Subsequently a less effort will bring on a similar attack, and sometimes the attack will come on at night after a fatiguing day. In such cases the factors are probably the same as in those of cramp in the leg muscles, namely, restricted irrigation of muscle through narrowing of its arterial supply, impaired removal of waste products, cramp or paralysis; but the muscle involved is in the centre of life, and its temporary disorder is apt to have a fatal issue.

Under the name of "intermittent claudication," Bouley described loss of power in the limbs of the horse attended by painful cramps, which is attributable to the partial or complete occlusion of vessels supplying the parts; the blood-supply being only sufficient for the muscles during rest or slight exertion, but insufficient to secure the nutritive changes adapted to increased muscular exertion. Charcot, in 1858, described this condition of vessels as a cause of pain in the limbs in the human subject, and as a premonitory sign indicative of a tendency to senile gangrene. Sir Benjamin Brodie, however, twelve years before, namely, in 1846, had distinctly described this incapacity of rigid or thickened arteries to secure that fluctuating blood-supply to muscles which is necessary to repair the varying waste during rest and severe or slight exercise, as met with not only in the muscles of the limbs, but in other muscles also ; and he, in this connection, alludes to the observations of Jenner and Parry, which were supposed to prove that angina pectoris is due to ossification of the coronary arteries. We are indebted to Professor Osler for drawing attention to the fact that Allan Burns had nearly forty years before Brodie, namely in 1809, distinctly described the effect of constriction of vessels from disease in causing failure of power, with or without pain, in muscles during action. Burns compares a heart with narrowed coronary vessels to a limb round which a ligature has been applied with a moderate degree of tightness. Moderate and equable muscular action can in both cases be carried on without distress, but under any pressure of labour fatigue and exhaustion soon set in.

"In examining the bodies of persons who died from the disease (angina pectoris) in question," Brodie says, "I have sometimes found ossification of the coronary arteries to so great an extent, that they were converted into complete bony tubes while there was no disease of consequence elsewhere. When the coronary arteries are in this condition, they may be capable of admitting a moderate supply of blood to the muscular structure of the heart, and as long as the patient makes no unusual exertion the circulation goes on well enough. When, however, the heart is excited to increased action, whether it be during a fit of passion, or in running or walking upstairs, or lifting weights, then, the ossified arteries being incapable of expanding so as to let in the additional quantity of blood, which under these circumstances is required, its action stops and syncope ensues, and I say that this exactly corresponds to the sense of weakness and want of muscular power which exist in persons who have the arteries of the legs obstructed or ossified."

Whilst Brodie mentions intermittent pains as amongst the symptoms of this partially obstructed circulation, he does not speak of it as an essential or constant symptom ; and there can be no doubt that, as pointed out by Dr. Parkes Weber, the cramp pains and loss of power are both attributable to accumulation of waste products in the muscles ; that they can both be induced in healthy persons by over-muscular fatigue ; that they are more easily induced in muscles whose vascular supply is inadequate, and whose tissue renewal is therefore sluggish ; and, finally, that in angina pectoris from diseased coronary arteries the heart failure may or may not be attended with painful cramp. The key to the whole mechanism is supplied by Dr. Gaskell, who points out (a) that the lymph fluid of all tissues in a condition of inactivity is alkaline; (b) that the

natural activity of a muscular organ is invariably accompanied by dilatation of its blood-vessels ; and (c) he argues that, nervous influences apart,
this dilatation of blood-vessels is brought about by the diminished
alkalinity of the lymph fluid of the tissue during its activity which relaxes
their muscular coats.

Under conditions of diseased, rigid and narrowed vessels this arrangement for flushing tissues with blood while in action is obviously interfered
with. In the cases of syncopal attacks to which the name of "angina sine
dolore" has been given by Gairdner, the phenomena are those of paralysis
without cramp; some of these cases are, however, no doubt cases of extreme
fatty degeneration ; on the other hand, the syncope anginosa of Parry is
heart failure with cramp ; whilst there may be many intermediate attacks
of more or less severe cardiac cramp without actual syncope.

It is then certain that the same morbid condition of the coronary
vessels of the heart which constitutes the pathology of primary cardiac
angina may extinguish life, not with a paroxysm of acute anginal suffering
but with a prolonged intermission terminating in fatal syncope. These
syncopal attacks may be attended with some anginal phenomena, and
especially with that sense of failure and impending dissolution alluded to
in the letter from Heberden's "unknown" patient as occasionally replacing
his more ordinary anginal symptoms, and described by Gairdner as
characteristic of a group which he would separate under the term "Angina
sine dolore." It is to be remarked, however, that these attacks of painless
angina are not infrequently the final phenomena in the fatal issue of
angina pectoris, and, again, that they are not to be distinguished from the
attacks of prolonged and often fatal intermissions of heart's action observed
in cases of fatty degeneration. I would rather regard them, therefore, as
detached symptoms of the heart failure with which angina, in common
with some other heart affections, may terminate, than as constituting a
separate group.

We have now well-nigh traversed the field of anginal pathology, and
yet it may be complained that little has been said of neuralgia or neuritis
as a cause of the symptoms. Without venturing to deny the possible
occurrence of neuralgia, whether central or originating in the gray matter
of the cord or cardiac ganglia, or the possibility of a neuritis of the
cardiac plexus or nerves as causes of angina, I am convinced that they
are of the rarest occurrence in connection with this group of symptoms.
I have seen instances of neuritis, and perhaps of neuralgia of the cardiac
nerves in diphtheria, influenza, pericarditis, and so on, but in such cases
the symptoms are not those of angina. That angina pectoris, however,
is a neuralgic affection or an actual neuritis of the nerves of the heart
has been contended by many and distinguished authors ; that morbid
changes can and do arise in the nerves and plexuses connected with the
heart is perfectly well known, and that perversion of the cardiac rhythm
and pain connected with the heart's action may and do arise therefrom
are facts too obvious to need comment ; but the question is, how far it
can be shown that any appreciable number of cases of angina pectoris

have in this cause an exclusive mechanism. With regard to Nothnagel's views of the vasomotory origin of angina I am in full accord; but here the neurosis is a general or central one, in which the heart is only involved by a reflected mechanism, so to speak—although in some cases of tobacco angina the coronary vessels may themselves partake in the spasm and so embarrass cardiac circulation. But Anstie, Eulenburg, and others maintain that angina is a neuralgia or a neuritis affecting the cardiac nerves, exclusively or essentially. Eulenburg, excluding all organic changes as conditions sometimes associated but not essential, describes four varieties of cardiac neurosis as causes of angina, namely :—

(i.) Disease, injury, or irritation of the automatic nerve apparatus of the heart.

(ii.) Some such affection of the regulating apparatus of the heart.

(iii.) Similar influences affecting the sympathetic apparatus.

(iv.) Disturbances of the vasomotor nervous system.

The late Dr. Anstie, by ingenious reasoning and by comparison with other neuroses, maintained that angina is a pure neurosis, interchangeable in families and individuals with asthma and gastralgia, and due to an irritation of the vagus nerve, or to a primary affection of the spinal centres in the upper dorsal region rapidly involving the vagus through the cardiac plexus. If, however, we descend to the consideration of facts, there are few observations in favour of angina being a cardiac neurosis; whilst in all fatal cases, or in almost all, some definite lesion of the heart's texture or cardiac valves is present.

On the other hand, in almost all the cases of fatal angina pectoris in which nerve lesions have been found, other conditions have been present, which may be regarded as having played at least a more important part in the fatal issue. Thus, in Rokitansky's case, in 1841, in which the right phrenic and left vagus were found to present pigmented nodular changes, the patient died of syncope rather than of angina. Lancereaux, in 1864, found those cardiac ganglia which were adjacent to thickening of the coronaries to be granular. Putjakin found changes of the cardiac ganglia in angina; but he found similar changes in other cases of heart disease also, and quotes others who had found them in such cases. Haddon, in 1870, found the left phrenic nerve in a case of angina entangled in an enlarged gland and its elements changed; but the aorta was atheromatous and dilated. Peter, in 1883, found the cardiac plexuses undergoing inflammatory changes and disorganised; but old pericarditis and dilated and thickened aorta were also present. Raymond and Barth, in 1891, found similar changes in subjects who had never suffered from angina.

In the face of such facts, positive as regards the heart, negative or subordinate as regards the nerves, it seems to us futile to contend with Eulenburg, Austie, and others, that angina is a neuralgia of the heart in any other sense than that it is a painful affection of that organ. It is true that in the course of pericarditis anginoid attacks are sometimes, though rarely, met with, their gravity depending upon that of the cardiac lesion.

In influenza, towards the close of the illness, cardiac seizures of a decided anginal kind are not very uncommon ; but these seizures, in my experience, have been of the nature of vasomotory angina and associated with an enormous discharge of (previously retained) urea—enough to produce a dense precipitate of crystals on the addition of nitric acid. Fatal attacks of multiple neuritis in influenza, and attacks of general paralysis resembling diphtheritic paralysis, have also been met with, but not associated with angina pectoris (in my experience), as in multiple neuritis might well have been expected. Huchard thus summarises his conclusions with regard to the position of cardiac neuralgia and neuritis in the pathology of angina : " Angine de poitrine coronarienne et névrite cardiaque sont deux maladies distinctes. L'une est une affection artérielle, l'autre une affection nerveuse. Il n'y a pas deux angines, l'une due à la sténose coronarienne, l'autre due à la névrite cardiaque : il n'y a qu'une angine de poitrine, relevant de la lésion du coronaire " (p. 617).

The precise nature of the pains in angina has given rise to considerable discussion and is not yet perhaps fully understood. Setting aside pure neuralgia of the cardiac plexuses or of central origin as a possible cause of occasional attacks of anginal suffering, the origin of the pain is, as we have seen, most commonly either a stretching or compression of the peripheral nerves of the cardiac muscle or endocardium, or a cramp affecting a limited area of the cardiac muscle.

The intensity of the irritation may be only sufficient to affect the gray matter of the cardiac ganglia or (to use Dr. Sturge's expression) to cause a commotion in it ; in which case the pain remains localised in the heart, and consists of a more or less dull and distensile suffering or oppression.

In other cases the intensity of irritation may be so great, or the nervous susceptibility of the patient so great, that the painful impression passes beyond these narrow bounds and extends to the cord itself.

It has been shown by Dr. Head, partly from clinical observation and partly from a consideration of the work of Allen Sturge, Gaskell, Ross, Dean and Bradford, and Edgeworth on the cardiac innervation, that the sensory nerves of the heart are in relation with the spinal cord from the first to the eighth dorsal roots : namely, auricle, with fifth to eighth dorsal ; ventricle, second to fifth dorsal ; ascending aorta, first to third dorsal, and third and fourth cervical. In the early tubal form of the heart the auricles are placed below (posterior to) the ventricle, and their nerve supply is therefore lower in the cord.

It would appear, however, that the nerve roots most central to the paths of pain from the heart, which as a rule receive the first and most intense impressions, are the second dorsal roots—although the painful commotion may extend or overflow to higher or lower centres. The painful impressions upon the root centres are referred to the corresponding surface areas of nerve distribution, and taking the left ventricle as the most common primary seat of pain, and the second dorsal as the chief recipient of the disturbance when intense enough to pass beyond the cervical cardiac ganglia, we can account for the most common reflected surface pains. These are well illustrated in a record given to Ross, by an intelligent patient, of the reflected pains suffered during an anginal attack :—"The pain is described as starting at a point a little below mid-sternum, then shooting between the shoulders at the level of the second dorsal vertebra, and darting down the inside of the left arm to the elbow ; at the same time a feeling of great tightness was experienced over the second ribs below the clavicles on each side, and a degree of pain was similarly felt down the right arm." This distribution corresponds closely with the sensory distribution of the second dorsal nerve and its intercosto-humeral branch. In other cases the reflected pains extended to more or less of the whole area of sensory supply from the brachial plexus. It is observed by Head that during an attack of angina a notable degree of tenderness is felt over certain areas—the precordial, dorsal, and supra-orbital. This tenderness is neatly explained by Allen Sturge, who remarks that ordinary tactile sensations transmitted to irritated sensory roots become painful impressions ; and that in angina the sensory roots of the dorsal nerves corresponding with the left ventricle are undoubtedly irritated. The supra-orbital pains referred to by Head as constant in angina and in some other heart pains are most difficult to interpret precisely, as are similar pains well known in association with other visceral disturbances. My attention has not been attracted by these head pains in angina ; and, although of much pathological interest, they are naturally obscured by more urgent symptoms.

Symptoms.—(*a*) *Secondary cardiac angina ;* (*b*) *Primary cardiac angina.* —The symptoms of the two varieties of angina pectoris gravior have so much in common that it will save repetition if we include them in one description, and afterwards endeavour to discriminate between them in diagnosis and prognosis, and for the purposes of treatment, with the help of a few illustrative cases.

The patient, most commonly a man, and usually between 40 and 65 years of age, is quite suddenly seized whilst under excitement, or engaged in some exertion not unusual or excessive for him, or even whilst in bed after a somewhat fatiguing day, with severe pain in the precordial region. The character of the pain varies. It may be most acute and agonising, of a rending character ; or accompanied by a sense of constriction as though the heart were gripped or the thorax were severely pressed. Its onset is always sudden, but the pain is sometimes rapidly ingravescent rather than reaching its height at once. Having its principal seat within the precordial region, usually at the lower mid-sternum, the pain radiates in most cases upwards to the left shoulder and down the arm to the elbow or wrist ; sometimes similarly to the right shoulder or to the chin and throat, but rarely in a downward direction. This radiation is not essential, and varies with the intensity and seat of the pain. The countenance becomes pale and assumes an anxious, panic-stricken expression, sometimes betraying acute suffering, and that apprehension of death which is more or less a feature of the attack. A cold sweat bedews the brow and the coloration of the lips is livid. Whatever he may be doing, the subject of true angina stops short and rests—sitting, stooping, or leaning forward against any support that may be at hand. The breathing is disturbed, oppressed, and restrained by the pain, then panting or sighing; there is a sense of air hunger, and the patient will motion attendants aside, although himself he dare not stir; fanning is grateful to him. The pulse may be but little changed, yet it is sometimes tightened. It may be small, hard, thready and irregular. As a rule, it is not markedly quickened, sometimes decidedly infrequent; but in these latter cases on listening to the heart it will often be found beating twice to each radial pulsation. During the attack the heart sounds are, as a rule, distant, feeble, and of purely valvular character, the first sound resembling the second; adventitious sounds, such as murmurs, may or may not be present, but they have no necessary relation to the anginal paroxysm. The intensity of the attack may last only a few minutes and rapidly subside; but it sometimes returns in a series of wave-like recurrences through a period of an hour or more. There is often flatulent distension of the stomach, eructation of flatus giving some relief; but such distension is an attendant phenomenon arising during the attack, and has no necessary causative relationship to it. Much exhaustion ensues upon an attack, and a sense of having received a severe shock, from which, however, recovery takes place with varying rapidity; some patients resume their usual business the next day, some even continue the business in which they were at the time engaged. It is rare for a patient to faint with true angina, except in cases of fatal syncope.

It often happens that a patient having experienced a severe attack feels afterwards, on taking exercise, that at a certain point the premonitory symptoms of cardiac oppression and pain are felt; these become more severe as he proceeds on his walk, and oblige him to stop before all the completed phenomena of radiating pains and the rest are manifested.

Such being a description of the clinical features that may accompany an ordinary attack of angina, let us glance at the brief records of a few well-marked cases as they come before us for diagnosis and treatment.

CASE 1.—J. P., aged twenty-seven, a draper, had suffered from rheumatic fever at the ages of nine and fourteen, and several times since. He had been several times laid up with heart trouble, pain, and dyspnœa. He had never had dropsical symptoms. He was admitted into Middlesex Hospital on 5th October 1896 on account of paroxysmal pain chiefly referred to the lower precordial and upper epigastric regions. He presented no marked dyspnœa and no œdema. He was a fair-haired man of spare build, with visible pulsating carotids and a regular full collapsing pulse of 100 beats per minute. The heart's apex beat was in the 6th space, one inch outside the nipple line, was heaving in character and diffused over an extended area, the dulness extended upwards to the third rib, and laterally to an inch and a half beyond the right border of the sternum. A to-and-fro murmur was audible over the base of the heart, the diastolic being the more prolonged and conducted down the sternum in the usual manner.

The patient had frequent attacks of pain, sometimes three or four a day, of which paroxysms the following description is characteristic :—Whilst under examination in his usual condition on November 5th, an attack of pain came on, attended with quickened action· of heart and diminution in size and increase in tightness of the pulse—the diminution in size proceeding almost to extinction, a mere tightened thread being felt under the finger. Whilst the patient leaned forwards on the bed, forcibly pressing his chest against a chair placed in front of him, the action of the heart remained so powerful as to give a visible impulse to the chair, and the neck vessels were observed to throb strongly. Two amyl capsules were inhaled, with the result of immediate relief to the pain and restoration of the pulse to its full volume. The attacks were all similar in character, and were relieved by one or two minim doses of nitro-glycerine solution. He somewhat improved generally, was able to get about the ward, and finally left hospital at the end of November.

' This was an excellent example of aortic regurgitant heart disease with vasomotory angina; and it is most instructive to note the powerfully labouring heart, the strongly throbbing large vessels in contrast with the contracted and almost pulseless smaller vessels; and again the rapidly restored equilibrium of circulation under a remedy which relaxed the arterial spasm. The imminent peril of such a case could not be doubted, nor could the propriety of the term "angina" be questioned by any one who witnessed the paroxysm.

Case 2.—A gentleman, aged about fifty-four, engaged in anxious and pressing business, had been for some years the subject of gouty glycosuria; he had complained for the past five years that occasionally while walking over London Bridge he would be seized with sudden pain at the heart, causing him to stop instantly, and either stand still or lean against some support. After a few minutes he would get on slowly and carefully, being stopped once or twice on his way. He had had several of these attacks, and an ether and ammonia draught containing 1 minim of nitro-glycerine gave him relief. His heart was distinctly and considerably enlarged, but there was no murmur present, until two years later, when a mitral murmur appeared; since that time he has had no similar attack. I may say that this gentleman's mother died suddenly in a railway carriage, and his sister dropped dead of heart disease. My belief is that his mitral incompetence has served as a safety-valve against excessive intra-cardiac pressure, and so has kept him free from attack. This gentleman has quite recently died from a syncopal attack.

Case 3.—A man, fifty-eight years of age, a bootmaker, was admitted into hospital with signs of heart failure and a history of attacks of cardiac pain. ·There was a history of rheumatic fever in early life and of two attacks of rheumatic gout; also a doubtful history of syphilis. He had been in fair health up to three years before admission, when he began to suffer from sudden attacks of pain in the region of the heart, extending to the shoulder and down the left arm. The pain recurred at intervals of a few weeks, was generally attended with profuse sweating, and left the patient in a state of great prostration. Except at these times he did not feel ill, and he kept at his work until a very severe attack occurred three months before his admission; from this time he had suffered from cough, shortness of breath, and dyspnœa on lying down, and had been incapacitated for work. During the last month he had observed his legs becoming dropsical.

He was a gray-haired, largely built, spare man with livid coloration, œdematous trunk and extremities, and orthopnœa. The pulse was 120 per minute, weak, irregular, soft, and compressible, and physical examination revealed an increased area of cardiac dulness, especially to the right and downwards, and a weak and diffused impulse with muffled sounds, the first sound at the apex being prolonged without distinct murmur. The lungs were moderately emphysematous, with œdema at the bases, and there were signs of slight effusion into the right pleura. The liver was increased in size, the urine scanty, 1030, acid, and contained a trace of albumin. The case as it now presented itself was then one of enlarged, dilated, failing heart, with secondary congestive œdema of the tissues and organs in a man with a history of illness beginning with anginal seizures. On the eighth day after admission, at 4 A.M., the house physician was called to him, and found him pale, distressed-looking, and streaming with perspiration, suffering from a sudden seizure of great pain in the precordial region, and spreading as before to the shoulders and down the left arm, with short, laboured breathing ; the pulse was very small, scarcely perceptible, but very hard and thready. It became full and soft under nitrite of amyl, but the symptoms did not immediately abate, and he recovered but slowly in the course of a few hours. On the two following days he had similar attacks. the first slight, the second severe, and on the third day he woke at 4 A.M. as if in pain, groaned, and was dead in a few minutes.

On examination the heart was found greatly enlarged, the enlargement being principally on the left side ; the auriculo-ventricular orifices were dilated, the ventricles thickened, their texture firm. The valves were practically sound ; there were some atheromatous points in the aorta. The right coronary artery was notably contracted, slightly atheromatous, and at a little distance from its orifice occluded by fibrinous clot. The left artery, fully patent at its commencement, was considerably thickened, and at a point rather less than an inch inwards was closed by organised clot. This latter was the thrombosis of older date, although the clot in the right coronary did not appear to be of quite recent formation. The texture of the heart showed fibro-fatty degeneration.

CASE 4.—A military man, aged fifty-five, quite recently home from India, who had never previously complained of any heart symptoms, and had dined with familiar friends in apparent health and good spirits the evening before, was walking quietly with his wife when he was taken with pains in his chest, and was brought in a cab a short distance to my house. Observing him to be very ill, my servant showed him at once into a side room, where I found him sitting on a chair with his hand pressed to the cardiac region with pale pinched features beaded with perspiration, cold extremities, and small, thready, and irregular pulse ; a half-suppressed groan and the expression of his countenance indicated the severity of his sufferings. After a restorative and a tabloid or two of nitroglycerine, he was gently moved to a sofa in another room and was able to lie down. The pulse became more regular and less thready—it never had the complete characters of vasomotor spasm. I gave a little morphia subcutaneously, and left him, returning, however, every few minutes. Thirty-five minutes from the time of his entering my house I found that he had just vomited slightly. His pulse had become regular and of better force, and he expressed himself as for the first time feeling decidedly easier. He had hardly finished speaking, however, when with an exclamation of pain he partially raised himself with his hands clasped to his breast, and fell over on his left side livid, insensible, pulseless, and with breathing arrested in expiration. By slapping with cold water, and other means; some deep convulsive respiratory movements with loud groaning expirations were excited, but the pulse never returned. The jugular vein became slowly distended and could not be emptied by pressure towards the heart.

Under all the painful circumstances I could not but assist the friends in avoiding a post-mortem examination, and the exact lesion remains obscure ; but I cannot doubt that some sudden thrombosis of diseased coronaries started the cardiac spasm, and the notable manner in which the jugular became filled, resisting pressure onwards, suggested cardiac paralysis, beginning at the right heart, and spasmodic closure of the left cavities.

CASE 5.—Mr. G., aged fifty-one, a clerk, had suffered for three or four months from pain beginning in the left interscapular region, and passing to the precordial region on first walking in the morning. The pain is very severe and obliges him to stop. He does not get the pain if he walks very slowly and cautiously. He can also walk better about a room or even upstairs than in the air ; even a moderate pace or a slight incline causing dyspnœa out of doors. On first going out into the cold air the pain most readily comes on. The pain starts sometimes between the shoulders. If he continues to walk with it, it increases to a point of severity which obliges him to stop.· One night recently, while at Bournemouth, he was awakened in the middle of the night with severe pain in the centre of the chest, which obliged him to get out of bed and stand, he could not walk. The pain this time radiated to the right shoulder, not affecting the left. It yielded in half an hour to hot applications to the chest and a hot foot-bath. He is an intelligent business man of medium build. Father died suddenly of heart disease at sixty-eight ; mother of paralysis at sixty-seven. The pulse presented nothing notable in character or volume except that the left pulse was thought to be slightly smaller. The heart's apex beat was outside the normal line, its impulse unduly heaving, and the superficial dulness extended upwards to the lower margin of the third rib.

We have in this case clinical evidence of an enlarged and somewhat labouring heart, and of distinct anginal seizures. The mechanism of the seizures would seem to be twofold, namely, rise of the arterial pressure by such causes as chill to the surface, inhalation of cold air or flatulent distension of stomach stimulating the vaso-motor contraction of vessels including, perhaps, the coronaries ; and, secondly, a heart muscle badly supplied with arterial blood through defective coronary circulation becoming rapidly fatigued and deranged by any extra call upon it, whether this call were from constriction of the general circulation or from physical exertion. The family history on both sides points to degeneration of the vascular system.

CASE 6.—A merchant, aged sixty-seven, had some months previously suffered from a peculiar attack of giddiness, the ground appearing to move up to his eyes, when he sank powerless into a chair, and remained there a quarter of an hour, with no loss of consciousness. A few weeks later he was suddenly seized with intense darting pain in the region of the heart which made him call out, and was accompanied by a sensation of "tumble over" of the organ. He had frequently suffered from attacks of giddiness accompanied by slight pain in the left fronto-parietal region, which lasted for a little time beyond the giddiness. He had only once or twice, however, suffered from the more severe vertigo since that first described, and on three occasions only had he experienced the acute pain at the heart.

On examination a systolic mitral *bruit* was heard, and a slight systolic aortic murmur also. The action of the heart was quiet. Some degenerative changes were noted in the vessels.

Two years later this patient died suddenly within a few hours of a severe attack.

Diagnosis.—The diagnosis of angina pectoris gravior, with a sufficiently careful consideration of the symptoms and signs, can be made out with accuracy in almost every case.

The age, sex, and hereditary history of the patient ; the preceding health record with respect to such diseases as syphilis, alcoholism, gout, rheumatism ; the effects of strain as calculated to induce premature arterial degeneration ; the evidence of such degeneration in the radial or other vessels,—bearing in mind the fact that in the coronary vessels such changes sometimes arise earlier than in other vessels ; an exact estimate of the dimensions, functions, and valve sounds of the heart, which determine its muscular and valve integrity or otherwise; these are the points upon which diagnosis depends. Any evidence that the heart has yielded before the blood-pressure, or that it has become hypertrophied yet with signs of failing circulatory power as registered at the pulse, or that the mitral or aortic valves have become thickened or incompetent, furnishes us, in the presence of attacks of painful heart failure, with proofs that such attacks are of the graver form of angina.

In discriminating cardiac pain from that of hepatic or renal colic, of flatulent colic in the stomach, and of rheumatic neuralgia of the chest walls, it may be briefly observed—

(*a*) That renal colic is a pain often of sudden appearance, of considerable duration, situated in the flank on one side, reflected downwards towards the groin or testicle, and accompanied or followed by characteristic changes in the urine. There are no heart phenomena.

(*b*) Hepatic colic is also often of very sudden and agonising onset, the pain being situated at the epigastrium or right hypochondrium, reflected across the abdomen and through to the right scapula, sometimes to the right shoulder-tip. The associated phenomena are nausea and vomiting, sometimes jaundice. The cardiac phenomena are nil, or only such as are attributable to acuteness of suffering. I have met with one case in which hepatic colic was complicated with an attack of fatal angina, which it apparently excited.

(*c*) Flatulent colic of the stomach may be associated with angina and in some cases may excite it. Otherwise the phenomena observed are localised in the stomach, and consist of flatulent distension with eructations of wind ; the pains are epigastric, hypochondriac (left), and inter-scapular.

(*d*) Neuralgic rheumatism of the chest walls presents features rather suggestive of pleurisy; the pain is unilateral, increased on breathing, and the dyspnœa arises directly from the restraint of pain unqualified by restlessness and gasping symptoms of air hunger.

(e) The passage of a clot through the heart into a branch of the pulmonary artery is attended with symptoms at the moment indistinguishable from angina. The paroxysm is, however, almost immediately followed by cough and the expectoration of dark, more or less clotted blood, significant of pulmonary embolism.

In our endeavour to distinguish between vasomotory and primary cardiac forms of angina pectoris gravior—a diagnosis of some importance, both in regard to prognosis and treatment, and often presenting very considerable difficulty—we have to keep in view the following points :—

1. The presence of a high and especially of a variable degree of blood-pressure in the intervals between the attacks, and of a tightened radial vessel during the attack, would be decided evidence in favour of vasomotor spasm as an important symptomatic factor in the case.

2. The presence of an aortic regurgitant valve lesion or of aneurysm, or the recognition of a weak and large heart from fatty infiltration, as distinguished from fatty degeneration of the cardiac muscle, would be strongly presumptive evidence of the angina being of the secondary cardiac form (Case 1).

3. The recognition of dyspepsia, of constipation, of present gouty phenomena, or of mental emotion as factors in the causation of the attacks in any given case, would also favour the diagnosis of its vasomotory incidence.

On the other hand—

4. The absence of the vasomotory phenomena referred to ˙under headings 1, 2, 3 would suggest primary cardiac angina; but it must be remembered that under the circumstances of an attack in a person of nervous temperament, some increase of arterial tension may well be present and intensify the symptoms.

5. That the earlier attacks came on during exercise not of a violent kind, and that the symptoms steadily increased during exercise, obliging the patient to stop, would suggest primary cardiac angina (Cases 2, 3).

6. The presence of a large fibroid hypertrophied heart failing before a normal blood-pressure without any murmurs being as yet present, would signify primary cardiac angina (Case 3).

7. The presence of an apex murmur, showing incompetence of the mitral valve in cases of the kind under consideration, indicates degenerative thickening of the mitral and probably also yielding of the ventricle before the blood-pressure : regurgitant escape of blood from the ventricle militates against the mechanism of vasomotory angina. Hence mitral murmur in association with angina is in favour of the attack being of primary cardiac origin (Case 2). ˙ An aortic systolic murmur would point in the same direction.

8. Sudden syncopal attacks with or without pain, and generally fatal, are usually of primary (coronary) cardiac source (Case 4). It is to be remarked that such attacks are frequently preceded by more recognisable anginal seizures coming on during exercise (Case 10).

Prognosis. — The prognosis of angina pectoris gravior is always serious, but varies according to the nature of the heart condition which lies behind the symptoms.

(*a*) In cases in which the heart condition is one of muscular atony with a variable degree of adipose infiltration and mechanical dilatation of the weakened ventricle, the prognosis is decidedly encouraging. Doubtless some of the cases pass in later life into group *c*.

(*b*) In cases of valvular disease of the heart with vasomotor spasm, the attacks, although much more hazardous, are not commonly fatal; and are susceptible of great relief from treatment.

(*c*) When, still in cases of secondary cardiac angina, a recognisable element of arterial spasm is present, but with a large fibroid or fibro-fatty heart in the background, in which the coronary vessels are presumably diseased, a sudden fatal termination may be feared; although even in such cases the end may be averted by judicious care and treatment.

(*d*) In cases in which the symptoms are of primary cardiac origin a fatal termination within a short period is inevitable.

Treatment.—In popular and even in professional estimation heart disease is too often used in a sense of very exaggerated prognostic significance, and when the name Angina is used a fatal issue is a foregone conclusion. Yet, as a matter of experience, with the more enlightened and rational treatment of modern times, and the use of some new remedies and the better handling of old ones, there is no class of serious diseases which are so amenable to remedial measures as those of the heart.

It may truly be said that we have enlarged the field of angina, including therein a large class of cases which were not contemplated in the description of Heberden and Parry, and which would be excluded by some modern writers of great authority, such as Sir William Gairdner. This matter has been duly considered; all merely functional diseases of the cardiac vascular system are excluded from the present category of angina pectoris gravior, and yet we shall find that treatment is not merely to be regarded as palliative or expectant.

Treatment is of undoubted value in angina. Much may be done, not only to relieve symptoms but to remedy the conditions which underlie them. Taking first the anginal paroxysm, there are certain prominent symptoms that call urgently for relief, if relief be possible, namely :—

(i.) Pain. (ii.) Arterial spasm if present. (iii.) Stenocardiac and cardiac muscle failure. (iv.) Shock and air hunger.

Pain is almost always due to one or both of two conditions, namely, distension or muscular cramp of the ventricle. When first called to a patient in the midst of a paroxysm there is no time for careful examination even did the condition of the patient permit of it. A tightened, thready pulse, with obviously labouring or it may be paralysed heart, urges upon us the immediate use of the vascular antispasmodics, nitrite of amyl or nitro-glycerine. Five to twenty minims of nitrite of amyl may be inhaled, or one to five minims of a one per cent solution of trinitrine given. If there be violent or forcible heart action, stimulants are better avoided; but if there be flatulent distension, a draught of aromatic ammonia, soda, cardamoms, and chloric ether may be given with the amyl inhalation or the nitro-glycerine drops; if such means be not to hand, some very hot water with a little peppermint essence or brandy may be sipped slowly.

In cases where there is marked heart failure, ether by preference, or brandy, in doses of 20 drops to ʒj., in which one to two minims of trinitrine (one per cent solution) may be dissolved, should be injected hypodermically. When the pain is not relieved by this treatment, arterial spasm having thus been eliminated as its cause, the use of subcutaneous morphia is indicated; due care being exercised with regard to the dose in view of the possible presence of kidney disease; if this factor be excluded, the degree of pain would regulate the dose, and the combination of atropine would be useful as a heart stimulant.

The free use of oxygen inhalation is of very great value in all cases in which cardiac failure is a marked feature. The remedy has a double value in satisfying and relieving the air hunger (due to impaired circulation through the lungs), which is often so marked a feature; and in securing the circulation through the usually constricted coronary vessels of over-oxygenated blood, which stimulates nutritive changes in the muscle and secures the removal of effete and half-changed material which embarrass its function. In administering the oxygen, however, all personal co-operation on the part of the patient must be avoided; the naso-oral muzzle must never be used, but the gas must be directed over the mouth and nostrils by means of a glass funnel attached to the tubing held a few inches away so as to leave the patient to breathe a highly oxygenated air at his ease. Oxygen inhalation is particularly indicated in those cases in which morphia is found necessary; and, when the paroxysm is over and sleep induced, the gas should be allowed from time to time to fortify the air immediately about the patient's mouth and nose. It is best to let the patient choose his position for himself, and to adopt that which is most comfortable and helpful to him.

After the acute seizure is over, the whole case must be carefully investigated with a view to an accurate diagnosis; and the treatment to be adopted must depend upon the conclusion arrived at.

It is needless to say that in all cases the causes of angina must be reviewed, and all pernicious factors in the case in hand, such as excess in diet, tobacco, alcohol, and other habits, forbidden.

The treatment of the different forms of heart disease will be found under the proper headings; that suited to the vasomotory factor in any given case has been already touched upon. It only remains, therefore, to make one or two further observations with regard to treatment.

In the first group of cases of angina pectoris gravior, in which the heart is large, wanting in power, and embarrassed in action by fatty depositions about its surface and fibres, and is labouring against a high arterial resistance which is prone to acute increase, the line of treatment is a restricted but fairly nitrogenous dietary in three regular moderate meals ; root vegetables, sweets and starchy foods, and all sweet wines and beers being avoided. Fluid should be taken very sparingly at meal times, and supplemented by a draught, preferably of hot water, taken between meals or shortly after food, and again either at bedtime or in the early morning, with a view to the excretion of effete materials.

Regulated open-air exercise is of the utmost importance—beginning with regulated level walks, proceeding to gentle inclines, and so on, but never overstepping the limits of cardiac power. Unquestionably Oertel's treatment for cardiac weakness and the Nauheim baths and exercises are valuable in this form of malady. It is only to be regretted that the latter treatment has been so "boomed" into popularity for every conceivable form of heart disease and imaginary heart ailment as to discredit its use in appropriate cases.

The most important drug treatment of these cases consists in the judicious administration of mild mercurial laxative and saline aperients to reduce arterial blood-pressure ; iodide of potassium is also sometimes valuable to this end. It is in this stage of the disease that Prof. Bradbury advises the use of erythrol tetranitrate, which he finds to exercise a more persistent influence upon the blood-pressure than other preparations of the kind. In addition, strychnia and acid tonics, taken once or twice a day only, are sometimes of value.

In cases of valvular disease of the heart appropriate remedies must be employed. When digitalis is employed it is often advantageous to combine with it small doses of nitro-glycerine ($\frac{1}{200}$ to $\frac{1}{100}$ gr.), or of erythrol tetranitrate, to slacken the arterial resistance.

In cases of coronary disease and consequent secondary nutritional changes in the heart there is still much to be done : (a) by regulating the daily life of the patient, physically and mentally, on the capacity of his circulatory powers, and by insisting upon a leisured and level life, free from excitement, hurry, and physical exertion or fatigue, and yet occupied up to within the limits of his capacity.

(b) Small nutritious meals always to be preceded by a period of quietude or complete recumbent rest, and followed by an interval of quietude, but not of sleep. A digestive and carminative medicine may be given before the chief meals.

Arsenic is the most appropriate drug for these cases, and oxygen inhalations from time to time, and especially in the night, are very valuable in those where respiration becomes shallow and inclined to the Cheyne-Stokes type during sleep. In the latter cases strychnia is the most valuable cardiac tonic. Small doses of digitalis or strophanthus are indicated when the cardiac power is much reduced and its rhythm irregular ; caffein is also of great value, especially when the urinary secretion is scanty. The liver function must be stimulated from time to time by a mercurial laxative. Let it be said in fine, that he who would treat angina pectoris in its multiform degrees with all the success that can be looked for, must take the cases in hand on broad lines in accordance with the well-defined principles of medicine, pursuing such lines into such detail as may be appropriate to each case.

R. Douglas Powell.

REFERENCES

Historical and general : 1. Eulenburg. *Ziemssen's Cyclopaedia*, vol. xiv. p. 31 ; 1878.—2. Forbes. *Cyclopædia of Practical Medicine*, vol. i. p. 81 ; 1833.—3. Gairdner. Reynolds' *System of Medicine*, vol. iv. p. 535 ; 1877.—4. Huchard. *Maladies du cœur*, 1893, p. 589.—4a. Osler. *Lectures on Angina Pectoris*, 1897, p. 5.—5. Stokes. *Diseases of Heart and Aorta*, 1854, p. 481. References to earlier and some current literature will be found in the above.
Experimental observations with reference to angina : 6. Charcot. *Progrès médical*, série 2, tome vi. p. 115 ; 1887.—7. Cohnheim. *Lectures on General Pathology*, New Sydenham Society, vol. i. p. 35 ; 1889.—8. Porter. *Journal of Physiology*, vol. xv. p. 121 ; 1894.—9. *Idem. Journal of Experimental Medicine*, vol. i. p. 46 ; 1896. 9a. Brunton. *Pharmacology*, 1887, and *Lectures on the Actions of Medicine*, 1897, p. 321. References to earlier experimental writings will be found in the above.
Organic nerve lesions as causative of angina : 10. Eulenburg and Guttman. *Physiology and Pathology of Sympathetic System of Nerves*, 1879, p. 97.—11. Haddon. *Edin. Med. Journ.* vol. xvi. p. 45 ; 1870.—12. Lancereaux. *Gazette médical*, série 3, vol. xix. p. 432 ; 1864.—13. Peter. *Traité clinique et pratique des maladies du cœur*, Paris, 1883, p. 671.—14. Putjakin. *Virchow's Archiv*, vol. lxxiv. p. 461 ; 1878.— 15. Raymond and Barth, quoted by Fraenkel. *Verhand. d. Congress für innere Medicin*, Wiesbaden, Bd. x. S. 228 ; 1891.
Neuralgia a cause of angina : 16. Anstie. *Neuralgia and its Counterfeits*, p. 70 ; 1871.—17. Eulenburg. *Ziemssen's Cyclopaedia*, vol. xiv. p. 41 ; 1878.—18. Gaskell. *Journal of Physiology*, vol. iv. p. 43 ; 1882.—19. Head. *Brain*, vol. xix. p. 218 ; 1896.—20. Huchard. *Maladies du cœur*, 1893, p. 598.—21. Ross. *Brain*, vol. x. p. 355 ; 1888.—22. Sturge. *Brain*, vol. v. p. 492 ; 1883. Eulenburg contains references to earlier writers, Laennec, Trousseau, Romberg, Friedreich, etc.
Vasomotor angina — the disease a vasomotor neurosis (?) : 23. Eulenburg. *Ziemssen's Cyclopaedia*, vol. xiv. pp. 34 and 48 ; 1878.—24. Gairdner. Reynolds' *System of Medicine*, vol. iv. p. 575 ; 1877.—25. Nothnagel. *Deutsches Archiv für klinische Medicin*, 1867, p. 309.—26. Douglas Powell. *Medical Society's Transactions*, vol. xiv. p. 267 ; *Lumleian Lectures*, Lect. i. 1898.—Eulenburg and Gairdner give the views of Cohen, Traube, Romberg, and Landois.
Intermittent claudication a factor in pathology of angina : 27. Bouley. *Archiv. gen. de méd.* vol. xxvii. p. 425 ; 1831.—28. Brodie. *Lectures on Pathology and Surgery*, p. 360 ; 1846.—29. Burns. *Diseases of the Heart*, p. 138 ; 1809.—30. Charcot. *Mém. de la soc. de biolog.* and *Gaz. méd. de Paris*, 1859.—31. *Idem. Progrès médical*, p. 99 ; 1887.—32. Fraenkel. *Verhand. d. Congress für innere Med.* Wiesbaden, 1891.—33. Huchard. *Maladies du cœur*, 1893, pp. 608 and 644.—34. Osler. *Loc. cit.* Lects. iv. and vi.—35. Potain. *L'Union médical*, vol. lvii. p. 181 ; 1894. —36. Weber, Parkes. *American Journal of Medical Science*, p. 531 ; 1894.
Toxic and epidemic angina : 37. Beau. *Gaz. des hôpitaux*, p. 330 ; 1862.—38. Gelineau. *Gaz. des hôpitaux*, p. 454 ; 1862.—39. Griffiths. *Compt. rendu acad. des sciences*, vol. cxx. p. 1128 ; 1895.—40. Huchard. *Maladies du cœur*, p. 683 ; 1893.— 41. Whittaker. *Twentieth Century Pract. of Med.* vol. iv. p. 442 ; 1896.

R. D. P.

DISEASES OF THE MEDIASTINUM AND THYMUS GLAND

INTRA-THORACIC GROWTHS AND TUMOURS

DISEASES OF BLOOD-VESSELS AND LYMPHATICS

DISEASES OF THE MEDIASTINUM AND THYMUS GLAND

Introduction—Clinical Investigation.—It is desirable at the beginning of this article to refer briefly to the normal anatomical relations of the part known as the mediastinum. Under this name is included the median space within the thoracic cavity which lies between the lungs, and is bounded on each side by the reflexions of the pleuræ passing from the front to the back of this cavity. It has been arbitrarily subdivided; usually into three portions, namely, *anterior*, in front of the pericardium; *middle*, which is occupied mainly by the heart enclosed in the pericardial sac; and *posterior*, limited by the posterior aspect of this sac and roots of the lungs anteriorly, and the spinal column behind. Some anatomists recognise further a *superior* division, extending from the upper opening of the chest to about the level of the upper end of the pericardium and the roots of the lungs. It is hardly necessary to indicate precisely the several structures contained in each division of the mediastinum; it will suffice to state that, setting aside the heart and pericardium, the important contents of the space to be borne in mind from a pathological point of view are the thymus gland or its remains in the anterior division; the arch of the aorta and its descending portion, with the innominate and commencement of the left carotid and subclavian arteries; the superior vena cava, innominate, and azygos veins, and the termination of the inferior vena cava within the pericardium before it enters the right auricle; the pulmonary vessels; the trachea and its bifurcation, with the main bronchi; the pneumogastric nerves, with the left recurrent laryngeal and cardiac branches, phrenic, and splanchnic nerves, and the cardiac plexuses; the roots of the lungs, including the pulmonary vessels and bronchi with their primary divisions, and the anterior and posterior pulmonary plexuses; the œsophagus; the thoracic duct; and the lymphatic glands and vessels. The loose cellular tissue which is also present in the mediastinum must not be forgotten. With regard to nerves; although the sympathetic trunk is not exactly within the mediastinum, it certainly may be implicated in diseases of this region; and the same remark applies to the right recurrent laryngeal, which originates higher up than the left, about the level of the root of the neck. The lymphatic glands within the thorax have been differently grouped, but the following arrangement answers well for practical purposes; namely, (i.) *Anterior mediastinal* or *sternal*, in the loose cellular tissue between the sternum and pericardium; (ii.) *Superior mediastinal* or *cardiac*, in front of the upper part of the pericardium, the arch of the aorta, and the left innominate vein; (iii.) *Posterior mediastinal*, along the course of the aorta and œsophagus; (iv.) *Bronchial*, which are situated in front of and behind the bifurcation of the trachea, along the main bronchi, and in the angles of their chief branches at the roots of the lungs.

It requires but little consideration to realise the difficulty of determining what should be included under diseases of the mediastinum, and any arrangement adopted must be a somewhat arbitrary one, modified by the views of the individual writer. The affections of the principal contents of this region just enumerated are dealt with, in their appropriate connections, in other parts of this work; and it is entirely beyond the province of the present article to discuss them at any length. It has been deemed expedient, however, to incorporate what is of practical importance in relation to morbid conditions of the thymus gland, instead of dealing with this organ separately; and the lymphatic glands will also call for a special notice. Moreover, it has been thought desirable, in the discussion of mediastinal tumours, to give a general account of intra-thoracic growths, and thus to bring in here those originating in the lung or pleura, as well as those which are more strictly mediastinal.

While avoiding, then, as far as possible any trespass on the domain of other articles in this work, it must be clearly recognised that in a considerable proportion of the cases which come within the category of mediastinal diseases, the morbid conditions either originate in, or sooner or later (and often at an early period) implicate in some way one or more of the important structures already referred to. Further, such diseases as aneurysm necessarily encroach in various degrees upon the mediastinum, and in a sense might fairly be included amongst its diseases, especially as they often lead to secondary morbid changes in this region; but custom has established that they shall not be so included, and they will therefore only be incidentally alluded to as causes of certain mediastinal disorders.

Seeing that the clinical phenomena, upon which our recognition of the presence and nature of morbid conditions of the mediastinum is founded, are to a large extent due to the effects of these upon the contents of this region, upon adjacent intra-thoracic structures, and upon the walls of the chest, it will materially help in the general study of these conditions, as well as in their clinical investigation in individual cases, to start with a definite and comprehensive knowledge of what these effects might be under various circumstances. They are of different kinds, and may be summed up in the following way : (i.) Mere general encroachment on the thoracic space, interfering with the breathing capacity more especially, but not obviously affecting any one particular structure more than another. (ii.) Mechanical effects on individual structures; namely, diffused compression, especially affecting the lung or heart; local direct pressure, causing obstruction of hollow tubes and vessels, or irritation followed by paralysis of nerves; stretching or traction; and displacement, as the result of pressure or dragging. (iii.) Inflammatory changes, due to irritation or pressure. (iv.) Implication or invasion of structures in particular morbid processes, such as acute inflammation, fibrotic changes, or growths. (v.) Atrophy, degeneration, or actual destruction of tissues, leading to perforation of tubes or vessels, ulceration or gangrene, erosion of bones and cartilages, removal of soft tissues, division of nerves, and other more or less serious lesions.

Summary of clinical phenomena and methods of investigation. —It may be assumed that any one who is acquainted with the anatomy and physiology of the thoracic contents, and who has duly studied the clinical investigation of this region, will have acquired a comprehensive knowledge of the symptoms which may result from interference with the more important individual structures, and will fairly understand the nature of the phenomena which are likely to be produced by the disturbances just indicated. For this and other reasons it is not intended to discuss this part of the subject in detail; but it may afford a clearer perception of its general clinical aspects, and at the same time save unnecessary repetition, to present a preliminary summary of the phenomena which have to be borne in mind, and to point out the course of investigation which it may be requisite to follow in dealing with particular cases of mediastinal disease. In the normal state we are unconscious of the existence of any of the structures which occupy this region; nor, with the exception of the heart, do they give any external indication of their presence. Their morbid conditions may be revealed by one or more of the following groups of clinical signs, to which attention will now be briefly directed. They may be arranged under the heads of — I. Symptoms of local origin; II. General symptoms; III. Physical and special signs; IV. External manifestations.

I. *Symptoms of local origin.*—Under this head come all phenomena usually classed as symptoms, as distinguished from physical signs, which are directly due to the effects of the mediastinal disease upon the thoracic structures; and they always need careful study, for they are of the greatest importance in diagnosis. These symptoms are usually both subjective and objective; and they include not only the local disturbances commonly associated with chest affections, but also certain phenomena which may be observed in more or less remote parts of the body.

(a) Painful and other morbid sensations.—Different kinds of pain are often complained of in connection with mediastinal affections, and pain is not uncommonly a very pronounced symptom. There may, however, be rather a sense of uneasiness, discomfort, irritation, tightness or oppression, weight, and the like, or of subjective heat, than actual pain. The symptom may be part of the disease itself, but generally results more from its effects upon adjoining structures. Hence it varies much as regards its site, extent, intensity, characters, and other particulars;

again it may be constant, or occasionally intermittent, or prone to exacerbations. The most important forms of pain to be borne in mind are those due to direct interference with nerves, causing neuralgia or neuritis, when it is of shooting or lancinating type; to inflammatory changes, especially pleurisy; or to erosion of bones, the pain being then heavy, grinding, gnawing, or boring in character. Probably it is occasionally due to muscular cramp. It may be distinctly localised in the chest walls, and shoot along the course of one or more of the intercostal nerves, or run up the neck; or more or less of the brachial plexus may be involved, so that painful or other sensations, such as tingling and numbness, are referred to the upper extremity, even to the fingers. In exceptional instances pain is felt in the abdomen or back in connection with mediastinal disease. Local tenderness over more or less of the chest is often noticed, and occasionally there is remarkable superficial hyperæsthesia.

(*b*) Disorders of respiration.—As might be expected, breathing is extremely apt to be affected by morbid conditions of the mediastinum; and the disturbances thus produced always demand special study and consideration in individual instances. To sum up all such disturbances indiscriminately under the term "dyspnœa" is specially wrong and misleading in this class of cases, for they present great variety; and as there are often different kinds of respiratory disorder even in the same case, it is of essential importance to understand their significance. The factors which may lead to such disorders are many, and not uncommonly several of them act together. Without entering into details, it must suffice to state that these factors are chiefly direct interference with, or implication of one or both lungs, diminishing their breathing surface or power; obstruction of the trachea or a main bronchus; bronchitis; pleural or occasionally pericardial effusion; obstruction of the pulmonary vessels, either preventing a due supply of blood to the lungs, or causing pulmonary congestion and œdema; compression, displacement, or other kind of embarrassment of the heart; and implication of the vagus or recurrent laryngeal nerves, the pulmonary plexuses, or the phrenic nerves. In exceptional cases the movements of breathing are directly prevented or diminished by physical changes involving the chest walls or diaphragm, or by muscular paralysis. It would not serve any useful purpose to describe at length the several respiratory disorders which may be associated with mediastinal diseases, for, as a matter of fact, all varieties and degrees of such disorders are met with, from mere shortness of breath, or somewhat hurried breathing, to the most urgent and terrible orthopnœa, or even fatal apnœa; and it will be more practical to discuss this part of the subject in relation to the particular affections of this region. It may be pointed out, however, that the dyspnœa is often definitely obstructive, due to pressure on the trachea or a main bronchus; or is associated with muscular laryngeal disorder affecting the glottis, and resulting from nerve disturbance within the thorax. The breathing is not uncommonly noisy and stridulous, or accompanied with audible wheezing, and the sounds thus heard during the act may be highly significant. In many instances also the respiratory disorder is more or less paroxysmal; and under certain circumstances it may assume the characters of "spasmodic asthma." The sensations accompanying the disturbances of breathing are not uncommonly pronounced, and may be very distressing; while the aspect of the patient reveals the effects of the interference with the respiratory function—a point which will be dealt with later. Hiccup, due to irritation of the phrenic nerves, may be a prominent symptom.

(c) Cough; Expectoration; Hæmoptysis.—Cough is another very common symptom in mediastinal diseases, but varies much in its severity. It is only, however, when it assumes certain peculiar characters that it becomes significant. It may be irritable and teazing, almost constant or paroxysmal, and either quite dry or attended with slight and difficult mucous expectoration. Pressure upon the trachea renders the cough peculiarly stridulous; or it may have the spasmodic and clanging, hoarse, husky, or aphonic character associated with different degrees of interference with the laryngeal nerves. Bronchitis is a very frequent factor in the causation of cough in mediastinal diseases.

Expectoration, when present, as a rule gives no positive information in relation to affections of the mediastinum. In most cases it is simply bronchitic. Should an abscess in this region open into the air-passage, a quantity of pus would probably be expectorated; or exceptionally the sputum may be fœtid or gangrenous. Under certain circumstances very careful examination of materials thus discharged occasionally reveals the presence of portions of morbid growths, which might be of great diagnostic significance. Special kinds of expectoration have been described; but these will be more conveniently noted in connection with the particular diseases to which they belong. Hæmoptysis, in various degrees and of different kinds, is not uncommon in connection with mediastinal complaints; and the. intimate admixture of blood with the sputa may give rise to peculiar appearances. Hæmorrhage may be the first symptom, or it may be repeated; it is occasionally so grave as to prove directly fatal.

(d) Alterations in voice.—These are also important phenomena to be watched for and studied, as indicating direct interference with the trachea, or revealing implication of the vagus or laryngeal nerves in different degrees. Thus, there may be a peculiar reedy quality of voice, a change in pitch, more or less huskiness or hoarseness, or weakness to absolute aphonia. These symptoms present considerable variety in different cases, and may also change in the same case from time to time; intermitting aphonia is sometimes observed. It may be noted that pressure on the inferior laryngeal nerves may not only lead to muscular disturbance affecting the glottis, but may also set up chronic changes in the larynx, such as laryngitis or ulceration, which naturally tend to aggravate the symptoms.

(e) Cardiac and arterial symptoms.—As a consequence of embarrassment of the heart in various ways, or of disturbance set up through the vagi nerves or cardiac plexuses, the action of this organ is liable to be affected. Thus the patient may be conscious of cardiac disorder, and complain of palpitation ; and such disorder may be evident at once to the clinical observer. It may be paroxysmal. Occasionally the heart may be markedly slowed or quickened. Should either of the main arterial branches be obstructed—innominate, left carotid, or left subclavian—there will be corresponding changes in the carotid or radial pulse, or both, on the affected side ; as evidenced by retardation of the beat, diminution of its strength and fulness, or, it may be, even complete obliteration of the pulse.

(f) Symptoms of deficient blood aeration and venous obstruction.— These are amongst the most common and striking evidences of morbid conditions occupying the mediastinum, and the phenomena resulting from venous obstruction often afford much information as to its situation, and as to the vein which happens to be interfered with. The difficulty is usually associated either with the superior vena cava, one or other innominate, or the azygos vein ; and it may not only be due to pressure, but also to blocking by thrombosis or a growth. Only under very exceptional circumstances is the inferior vena cava obstructed. The symptoms are both objective and subjective, and those due to imperfect aeration of blood may be added to those consequent upon local venous stasis.

The objective symptoms are merely those which ordinarily result from venous obstruction, and consequent mechanical congestion ; namely, more or less change of colour in the direction of lividity or cyanosis ; swelling, chiefly from œdema, which may be soft, or of a firm and brawny character ; increased visibility, dilatation, tortuosity, and varicosity of the superficial veins, venules, and capillaries ; and possibly hæmorrhage from rupture of vessels. Their significance lies in the localisation and distribution of the phenomena, and often in their intensity ; though their absolute and relative degree is subject to much variety. They are also likely to be increased by any exertion, and in the stooping posture. When the superior vena cava is affected, the whole head, face, ears, neck, both arms, and the chest present these appearances, contrasting remarkably with the lower half of the body. The aspect of the patient is very striking, and the condition can hardly be mistaken for anything else. Not only are the features discoloured, bloated and swollen, but the eyes may be prominent and staring, as if starting from their sockets, and the conjunctivæ injected, suffused, or œdematous ; exceptionally distinct exophthalmos may be noticed. On examination it may be found that the tongue and throat are similarly affected. In well-marked cases there is a distressing appearance of semi-strangulation, with a very anxious expression. The neck is obviously enlarged and tumid-looking, and has in some instances a peculiar spongy or .elastic feel. In certain cases the swelling may be partly due to dilatation of the subcutaneous veins above the clavicle. The vascular phenomena are chiefly seen over the thorax, involving especially the mammary and superior epigastric veins. The intercostal veins and the subcutaneous veins near the spine may also be dilated, which is suggestive of occlusion of the vena azygos. Those of the arms may be much enlarged. It is stated that enlargement of the superficial veins is sometimes obviated by the formation of deeper-seated anastomoses returning the blood by the iliac veins. When either innominate or one of the subclavian veins is implicated alone, the resulting phenomena are correspondingly limited and unilateral. Cases have been noted in which pressure on these veins by mediastinal conditions has been followed by venous distension on the opposite side. In some instances the obstruction is at first unilateral, and afterwards becomes bilateral. The chief form of hæmorrhage likely to occur is epistaxis; but it may also take place under the conjunctiva, or into the cerebral meninges. In the very exceptional cases in which obstruction of the inferior vena cava is caused by mediastinal disease, the chief consequences are œdema of the legs and abdominal walls, ascites, albuminuria, and enlargement of the superficial veins, especially over the abdomen.

The subjective symptoms to be noted in this connection are chiefly associated with the brain, being indicative of cerebral congestion; namely, headache, vertigo, tinnitus or deafness, visual disturbances, and somnolence, which sometimes passes into temporary attacks of stupor or unconsciousness; these may be brought on by exertion or stooping. Epileptiform seizures have been noted occasionally. It is believed that spinal symptoms may result from obstruction of the vena azygos, in the form of sensory and motor disturbances affecting the limbs and lower part of the body.

(g) Disorders of deglutition.—More or less dysphagia is not uncommon in certain forms of mediastinal disease. It may be of different kinds, and attended with pain or other unpleasant sensations associated with the attempts at swallowing. It is sometimes influenced by posture. The difficulty is naturally likely to be prominent when the disease starts in or implicates the œsophagus; but it may also result from pressure upon this tube, diffused or localised, or from nervous disturbance, being then of reflex origin, when the dysphagia is sometimes intermittent.

(h) Special nerve symptoms.—Pressure upon the brachial plexus not only causes sensory disturbances in the arm, but may lead ultimately to paralysis and muscular atrophy. As the result of different degrees of interference with the sympathetic trunk, contraction of the pupil or, more rarely, dilatation is observed on the affected side; and the temperature and nutrition of the same side of the face and head are exceptionally affected, as results of vaso-motor influence.

(i) Spinal symptoms.—In extremely rare instances a morbid condition starting in the posterior mediastinum makes its way through the vertebral column, and affects the spinal meninges, or ultimately even the cord itself. The symptoms are first those of irritation of this structure, and of the spinal nerves corresponding to the seat of mischief, followed by evidences of inflammatory or destructive changes, which may end in complete paraplegia.

(*k*) Subcutaneous emphysema.—As a symptom, accumulation of air in the subcutaneous tissue of the neck and chest, or even spreading more widely, may be an indication of a similar condition in the mediastinal cellular tissue, as the result of some perforative lesion in this locality injury, or other causes.

II. *General symptoms.*—But little need be said under this head at present, as the general symptoms in mediastinal cases must necessarily depend very much on the nature of the individual disease, and they can be more conveniently discussed in that relationship. They are referred to here mainly to emphasise the necessity of duly considering them in the investigation of these complaints. There is one symptom, however, belonging to this category which needs particular notice and attention, as it may be the direct result of certain mediastinal affections, and sometimes reaches an extreme degree, namely, wasting. This condition is especially likely to follow any œsophageal obstruction interfering with the taking of food. It is also believed to be produced by closure of the thoracic duct, preventing the passage of the chyle and lymph into the circulation; the supposition is a reasonable one, but a doubt has been expressed whether the connection has ever been actually demonstrated. It may be noted as a remarkable fact that in some cases of grave mediastinal disease the general system suffers in but a very slight degree, and this fact may be of diagnostic significance.

III. *Physical and special signs.*—The systematic study of mediastinal disease by the ordinary methods of physical examination, and in other ways, is obviously of the highest importance in its clinical investigation, and, indeed, is indispensable in every case. In many instances the phenomena thus revealed are quite pathognomonic, and indicate at once the nature of the morbid condition. The fact must be recognised, however, that there is no class of chest cases which present greater difficulties in their physical diagnosis, and the examination should therefore always be conducted with the utmost care and thoroughness. Indeed, it not uncommonly happens that the knowledge and skill of the most experienced clinical observers are severely taxed, and the aid of expert specialists is often essential for the complete clinical investigation of these cases.

The details of this part of the subject can only be satisfactorily discussed in relation to the several mediastinal diseases, and at present it will be sufficient to point out the general course of procedure which may be called for under different circumstances.

(*a*) Physical examination of the chest according to the usual methods naturally comes first, and often reveals all that it is necessary to know. The signs to be looked for in relation to mediastinal diseases are— (α) Those of the morbid condition itself, such as a solid growth. (β) Those of its effects upon neighbouring structures, the most important being displacement of organs, especially the heart; and various degrees of collapse, distension, congestion and œdema, consolidation, or actual destruction of one or both lungs. (γ) Those of serous effusion; pleuritic in the large majority of cases, rarely pericardial. These conditions are not uncommonly mixed up in various ways and degrees, and consequently the physical signs are sometimes exceedingly complicated and difficult to describe or explain.

(*b*) The sputum has already been referred to, as a mere symptom; but in the present connection it is important to point out that a more thorough and systematic examination of any materials expectorated, especially by the aid of the microscope, sometimes affords valuable help in the diagnosis of mediastinal diseases, and may give very definite information as to their nature.

(*c*) It is also worth while in certain cases to pay special attention to the arteries and veins which may be affected by morbid conditions in the mediastinum, and to study them by particular methods. Thus, the sphygmograph may be of service in the examination of the arteries ; while the effects of cough and respiratory movements upon the veins may also be of much significance. The *pulsus paradoxus* is frequently associated with certain forms of mediastinal disease.

(*d*) The methodical examination of the main air-tube, especially by the aid of the laryngoscope, should always be carried out in cases of suspected mediastinal affections ; and the signs thus recognised are in not a few cases most instructive. It may be necessary not only to investigate the larynx and vocal cords, but also the trachea, even down to its bifurcation. Such investigation requires in difficult cases the help of a thorough expert in the use of the laryngoscope, and this fact must be duly recognised. Under certain circumstances it is desirable to examine the œsophagus by instrumental methods ; but this procedure always demands great caution, and it is generally safer to call in the aid of an experienced surgical manipulator.

(*e*) For particular purposes, and especially in obscure and difficult cases, the use of the exploratory trochar or aspirator may be of conspicuous service in the diagnosis of mediastinal affections. At the same time, this method of investigation must not be adopted rashly or needlessly, but should always be carried out on rational and intelligent principles.

(*f*) Skiagraphy may possibly help in the diagnosis of some cases of mediastinal disease.

IV. *External manifestations.*—Under this head it will suffice to state that certain morbid conditions starting in the mediastinum may make their way outwards through the chest walls, sometimes involving or even perforating the skin ; thus their nature may be clearly revealed to sight and touch. It may further be added that the appearance of enlarged glands in the neck or axilla may be of special significance in the diagnosis of certain of these conditions.

Special Mediastinal Diseases

The preceding general discussion of the mediastinum and its clinical investigation will, it is hoped, have prepared the way for the consideration of the individual morbid conditions affecting this region; these will now be dealt with in the following order :—I. Abnormal mediastinal contents. II. Acute simple mediastinitis and œdema. III. Suppurative and gangrenous mediastinitis—Mediastinal abscess. IV. Chronic indurative mediastinitis. V. Tuberculous disease of the intra-thoracic lymphatic glands and thoracic duct. VI. Mediastinal emphysema. VII. Special conditions of the thymus gland. VIII. Intra-thoracic new growths, malignant and non-malignant—Mediastinal tumour.

I. ABNORMAL MEDIASTINAL CONTENTS.—There is a definite class of cases, of extremely exceptional occurrence, and as a rule most difficult to recognise clinically, but which nevertheless demand brief notice in order to render the consideration of morbid conditions of the mediastinum complete ; they might possibly be made out more frequently during life were they not so entirely forgotten. They are the cases in which certain structures, which ought not to be there, have gained access into this space, and are found in it. Such an event happens practically only in cases of diaphragmatic hernia, either congenital or acquired from injury or other causes, when one or more of the abdominal contents find their way into the chest. The stomach is the organ most frequently thus displaced ; then come in order the colon (almost as frequently), the spleen, the small intestines, liver, duodenum, pancreas, cæcum, and extremely rarely the kidneys. In the large majority of cases two or three organs form the hernia, to which may be added more or less omentum. It usually occupies the left side of the chest. A case came under my observation many years ago in which the stomach was thus displaced in an aged woman. The left half of the chest has been found filled with coils of intestine as high as the second rib. The most marked effects of diaphragmatic hernia are displacement of the heart and compression of the lung, but the œsophagus has also been seriously interfered with.

Clinical signs and diagnosis.—Congenital diaphragmatic hernia has usually been found on dissection of a fœtus or still-born child ; or death occurs very soon after birth. Exceptionally life may be prolonged for some years ; and it is affirmed that individuals born with this condition have lived even to old age. Cases have also been recorded in which a hernia into the thorax had not caused any symptoms to attract attention ; but as a rule some disturbances are produced. Under any circumstances the diagnosis must be extremely difficult and uncertain ; and it is only practicable to point out the data upon which such a diagnosis might possibly be made. A knowledge or history of certain injuries, or a strain likely to affect the diaphragm, might be of some value. The actual occurrence of the hernia has sometimes caused almost immediate or very rapid death, from shock and compression of the lung; or has been attended with the phenomena of an acute internal strangulation. Usually there are more or less urgent or grave chest symptoms, especially dyspnœa; and among other symptoms noted are a feeling as if something had given way, sudden pain, a sense of oppression, cough, cardiac disturbance, faintness or signs of shock, and inability to lie on the sound side. Therefore, when such symptoms occur suddenly, and cannot be explained, the possibility of diaphragmatic hernia should be borne in mind. The next group of phenomena deserving attention are those associated with the displaced organs, of which nausea and vomiting are often very pronounced. In the majority of chronic and established cases, in addition to more or less thoracic symptoms, those associated with the alimentary canal have been prominent; and they have been attributed to dyspepsia, including chiefly various pains, aversion to food, thirst, flatulence, heartburn, colic, and constipation alternating with diarrhœa. The troubles are generally worse after meals and exertion; but in some instances a heavy meal has given relief. Exceptionally the patient has felt conscious that the food has not gone to the right place. Death has occurred from compression of the œsophagus, and consequent complete dysphagia.

Physical examination may afford some aid in the diagnosis of the presence of abnormal contents in the mediastinum. The signs to be chiefly looked for are depression or hollowness of the abdomen, indicating displacement of some of its contents; fulness and impaired movement of the affected side of the chest, with abnormal percussion and auscultatory signs in connection with the lung; the presence of gurgling sounds over the same region, due to movements of the stomach or intestines; and marked displacement of the heart towards the right. Such displacement has been mistaken for " ectopia cordis."

A remarkable case of diaphragmatic hernia has been recorded by Drs. Hale and Goodhart,[1] in which, in a gentleman aged 49, the symptoms simulated those of cancer with dilatation of the stomach. When first seen he complained of heat and pain at the ensiform cartilage; he was continually bringing up mouthfuls of dark-coloured mucus, and at intervals vomited enormous quantities of the same; he suffered also from obstinate constipation. He improved somewhat under treatment, but the symptoms returned, with copious vomiting of yeasty, fœtid fluid. Emaciation became rapid and extreme. Two days before death tympanitic resonance was noted behind up to the angle of the scapula, with retraction of the abdomen. Post-mortem a diaphragmatic hernia was found, with a distinct hernial sac in the posterior mediastinum; the hernia consisted of the greater part of the stomach enormously dilated, pylorus, duodenum, greater part of the pancreas, a large loop of the transverse colon, and the lesser omentum.

Treatment.—In the large majority of cases of mediastinal hernia

---

[1] The case mentioned in vol. iii. p. 577 was diagnosed by a member of the patient's family—a layman—who put his ear to the chest when the symptoms occurred.—ED.

treatment must be entirely symptomatic, and no definite. rules can be laid down. How far operative interference may be justified, and what particular procedure should be adopted, are questions which can only be decided in relation to individual cases, and they belong to the province of modern surgery.

II. ACUTE SIMPLE MEDIASTINITIS AND ŒDEMA.—It cannot be doubted that under certain circumstances an acute inflammatory process affecting the mediastinal cellular tissue occurs, which does not go on to suppuration, but either subsides and undergoes resolution without leaving any ill effects, or lays the foundation for permanent changes, such as will be described under chronic mediastinitis, by which the fact of its having occurred is revealed later. Several supposed cases of this kind have been recorded from time to time, and attributed to injury. the sudden suppression of long-continued discharges or of the menstrual flow and other causes , but, apart from traumatism, such a connection is very questionable. From a practical point of view it is far more important to note that this condition is not infrequently associated with other acute intra-thoracic inflammatory diseases, especially pericarditis and pleurisy. resulting either from the same cause or from extension ; and the possible combination should be duly borne in mind and looked for. Local mediastinitis might also be produced by some neighbouring irritation ; for example, in connection with periostitis or bone disease, or a tumour.

Mediastinitis of the kind now under consideration would be characterised by increased vascularity, and by the presence of more or less serous fluid or fibrinous exudation in the cellular tissue. Probably the lymphatic glands are sometimes involved. Local mediastinal œdema may possibly occur apart from actual inflammation, and of course it may be a part of general dropsy. Should the lymph become organised more or less thickening would remain, with adhesion of the pericardium or pleura to the chest wall and to each other. *Clinically* this complaint can only be recognised when it affects the anterior mediastinum, and even then a positive diagnosis can hardly be made with certainty. It might be suspected from the intensity and superficialness of post-sternal pain, with tenderness ; but the only positive sign is the presence of a "mediastinal crepitation," or a quasi-friction sound, elicited by deep respiration, or possibly of cardiac rhythm. I am convinced that such phenomena are sometimes the result of an acute mediastinitis. If the case is not fatal they subside after a time, and subsequently those indicative of chronic mediastinitis may supervene. No special *treatment* is required for this affection, which must be dealt with on general principles.

III. SUPPURATIVE AND GANGRENOUS MEDIASTINITIS—MEDIASTINAL ABSCESS.—Suppuration and gangrene involving the mediastinal structures must be considered together, as in individual cases there is no definite line of demarcation between them. Mediastinal suppuration, usually terminating in an abscess, and occurring either as an acute or chronic condition, should not be forgotten in relation to chest affections, although it is very rare. Gangrene is extremely rare, and is only met with under special circumstances, being the result of an acute septic or putrid inflammation of some of the lymphatic glands, ending in sloughing, and involving the mediastinal cellular tissue in the destructive process. Suppuration also frequently starts in the glands; but it may begin in the cellular tissue, and abscesses beginning in the thymus body may likewise be included in the group now under discussion. The suppurative and gangrenous changes are of course directly set up by the micro-organisms which usually originate these processes. In the gangrenous conditions not only are streptococci and staphylococci found, but also spirilla and amœbæ.

Etiology.—Mediastinal suppuration is on the whole most commonly associated with tuberculous disease of the lymphatic glands, which will be separately considered (p. 84). Apart from this group of cases it may occur under the following circumstances:—(i.) From injury. Abscess in the mediastinum has been attributed to a blow on the chest; and suppuration may certainly result from wounds, though it appears to be exceptional as the result of gun-shot wounds. In this category may be included cases originating from injury by a foreign body introduced through the œsophagus, though such injury generally leads to gangrene. (ii.) Secondarily to disease of bone or periosteum; as caries of the sternum or spine, or post-sternal syphilitic nodes. (iii.) As the result of burrowing of pus from above. In this connection mediastinal suppuration may be associated with a similar condition in the cellular tissue of the neck or "angina Ludovici" [vide vol. iv. p. 737], suppurating tuberculous glands, retro-pharyngeal abscess, and suppuration starting in the thyroid gland. As already stated, a mediastinal abscess may originate in the thymus gland. Under this head it may also be mentioned that purulent mediastinitis has occasionally followed the operation of tracheotomy for certain conditions. (iv.) From general septic causes. Thus mediastinal abscess may occur in cases of erysipelas, pyæmia, or even of typhoid fever, measles, and other exanthems. (v.) By extension from pneumonia or pleurisy of low type. (vi.) Extremely rarely from suppuration of a hydatid cyst in the mediastinum, or of a dermoid cyst. (vii.) As a consequence of "taking cold" or a chill, it is alleged; but although in exceptional cases no other cause can be suggested, this mode of origin is very doubtful.

Gangrenous mediastinitis may result from some of the causes just mentioned as producing the suppurative variety, especially extension from above. In the very large majority of cases, however,—indeed with rare exceptions,—it is directly due to ulceration and perforation of the œsophagus. In this way it has followed injury by a foreign body; sword-swallowing, or the unskilful passage of an œsophageal bougie; the effects of corrosive fluids; perforation in connection with diseases of the œsophagus, —namely, various forms of inflammation, ulceration, stricture, malignant disease, dilatation, and diverticula; perforation from without, as a consequence of surrounding inflammation, or of degeneration and breaking-down of the mediastinal glands themselves. Exceptional cases of mediastinal gangrene have been reported, associated with pulmonary gangrene, due to extension ; gangrene of the larynx ; malignant endo-carditis. It is also stated that the glands have been found primarily affected. It is important to note that diseased lymphatic glands in the chest, which have been lying dormant for years, do, very rarely, become the seat of some fresh infection, which may lead to acute suppuration or gangrene.

With regard to remoter causes, mediastinal abscess appears to be far more frequent in men than women ; and in comparatively early life— from twenty to thirty. Occupations involving pressure on the chest or liability to injury may possibly have some predisposing influence.

Anatomical characters.—When mediastinitis goes on to suppuration, the pus may be infiltrated or lodged in the meshes of newly-formed fibrous tissue, or be collected in one or more definite abscesses. Either the anterior or posterior mediastinum may be affected, or both ; the pus passing from one division to the other. According to Hare's statistics, including all cases abscess is far more common in the anterior mediastinum, even when of a scrofulous nature. The amount of pus varies considerably, and it is sometimes very large. As a result of extension, pleurisy, usually purulent, or acute interlobular suppurative pneumonia may be set up. An abscess may make its way to the surface or up towards the neck, or may burst into the œsophagus, pericardium, pleura, lung, trachea, or a bronchus ; and has even been known to ulcerate into the arch of the aorta, causing fatal hæmorrhage. Very exceptionally pus has burrowed from the posterior mediastinum between the pillars of the diaphragm, and pointed in the iliac or femoral region.

The cavity caused by the sloughing of infected mediastinal glands is described as usually situated at the bifurcation of the trachea, behind and below the right bronchus. "It is rarely more than an inch or so in diameter, in one case only it measured $2\frac{1}{2}$ inches. Its walls are soft, dark, smooth, and regular, not sinuous like the walls of a gangrenous cavity in the lung ; its contents are grayish, fœtid, and may contain the remnants of a gland, or what remains of the gland may be found still adherent to the walls of the cavity" (Stephen Paget). Gangrenous media-stinitis may lead secondarily to gangrenous pleurisy or pyo-pneumothorax ; to putrid bronchitis or broncho-pneumonia, from perforation of one or both bronchi ; or to pulmonary gangrene, usually diffuse, sometimes superficial. Very rarely the great vessels give way ; or the œsophagus may be per-. forated in a different place from that which caused the disease originally. Very large ichorous collections may result from perforation of traction-diverticula associated with this tube.

Symptoms and signs.—Mediastinal suppuration may be almost latent from first to last ; but, on the other hand, the clinical phenomena and course may be sufficiently definite for diagnostic purposes, or even quite characteristic. As regards local symptoms, in acute cases one of the most frequent and prominent is pain, though this varies a good deal in individual instances, according to the position of the abscess and other circumstances. In most cases it has been described as post-sternal, and accompanied with marked superficial tenderness; but it may be deep-seated between the shoulders, or pass from one point to the other. The pain is generally seated in the region affected, but not uncommonly it seems to radiate through the entire chest, and may be centred in some part quite away from the actual seat of mischief. When the abscess is in the posterior mediastinum it is said that sometimes, owing to pressure on the nerves at their exit from the spine, the painful sensations are referred to their peripheral endings on the front of the chest, thus giving a wrong impression as to the seat of the disease. The pain as a rule increases steadily until suppuration takes place, and the pus finds an outlet in some direction. Occasionally it remits, or even assumes a paroxysmal character. Exceptionally it is accompanied with a feeling of pulsation.

A mediastinal abscess, when of considerable size, or so situated as to interfere with the structures in this space, gives rise to more or less of the symptoms of irritation or pressure. As a rule these are slight or moderate; but occasionally they are very pronounced, and may even mask the pain. The most common are some form of dyspnœa, wheezing respiration, and cough, either short and dry, or distinctly paroxysmal, and presenting laryngeal or tracheal characters, with mucous expectoration. The voice may be husky. Occasionally hæmoptysis occurs. There is also not uncommonly a certain degree of venous obstruction, and now and then the signs of this difficulty are very obvious; there may even be arterial pressure also, with obliteration of the pulse on the affected side. Dysphagia is not common, but there may be some degree of pain and difficulty in swallowing. Owing to implication of the vagus nerves, disordered cardiac action and gastric symptoms, with vomiting, may supervene. Pain and numbness in one arm have also been noticed, due to nerve irritation or pressure. The patient may be unable to lie down on account of a feeling of suffocation, or for other reasons. In individual cases it has been noted that dyspnœa was induced by pressure on an external prominence formed by a mediastinal abscess; or that interruption of discharge through a fistulous opening was followed by palpitation, faintness, and cough.

Acute suppurative inflammation in the mediastinum will be accompanied by more or less of the usual general symptoms: namely, chills or rigors, sometimes repeated; pyrexia, which tends to assume a hectic type; and sweating. Such symptoms, with local pain, may be present for some days before any definite indications of mediastinal abscess appear. Soon various degrees of wasting and weakness ensue, and in prolonged or chronic cases these symptoms, with anæmia, become prominent.

A definite mediastinal abscess is likely to give rise to *physical signs* more or less distinct and characteristic. The signs to be more particularly looked for at first are fulness or prominence over the upper sternal region, sometimes with superficial redness and slight œdema, and corresponding dulness. When the abscess is in the posterior mediastinum it is affirmed that one or two of the dorsal spines may project. Occasionally the tracheal sound is unduly conducted to the surface over the affected area. Should an abscess make its way to the surface and point, the fluctuation of pus will be felt ; and it is said to be frequently noted at the borders of the sternum or at the suprasternal notch (Hare). An important point to be borne in mind is that a mediastinal abscess sometimes presents an obscure or even distinct pulsation, conducted from the aorta, and may thus simulate an aneurysm, for which indeed it has been actually mistaken. In a few instances the pus has partially detached the pleura from the costal cartilages, and presented externally as a round, soft and fluctuating tumour.

Course and terminations. — The progress and end of a case of mediastinal suppuration depend very much on the course of certain events. An abscess may burst externally or be evacuated by operation ; or it may lead to inflammation of the internal periosteum of the sternum, and subsequent caries of the bone itself. Sometimes it gives way into the cellular tissue of the mediastinum, when death ensues. It is probable that a small collection of pus may be partially absorbed, the remains becoming caseous or calcified. As already mentioned, an abscess may make its way downwards, and come to the surface in the abdominal wall or thigh. Should it open into the trachea, either bronchus, or a lung, a quantity of matter may be coughed up ; or death may speedily follow from suffocation. When rupture takes place into the œsophagus, the pus may be discharged by vomiting, and subcutaneous emphysema may then supervene. Death from hæmorrhage has resulted from a mediastinal abscess opening into the aorta. When it communicates with either of the serous cavities, or sets up inflammation in connection with these structures, the effects will be evident, and they add seriously to the danger. Acute mediastinal abscess may run its course in a few days, or last two or three months or more. It may also end in the chronic variety, which, in whatsoever way it begins, may persist for years. Death sometimes occurs during a paroxysm of dyspnœa ; or it may result from exhaustion due to the disease itself, or to intercurrent complications.

The occurrence of gangrene in the mediastinum can only be revealed when a communication is established with the air-passages or lung. Then the breath or the gas driven out by the act of coughing emits a foul odour, and sloughing materials may possibly be expectorated. There is nothing, however, to distinguish such symptoms from those indicating pulmonary gangrene, and the two conditions may be associated. It is said that the breath sometimes becomes fœtid very early in the course of gangrenous mediastinitis. As the result of extension or perforation grave accidents are likely to ensue ; while the general symptoms will probably be of a well-marked septic type.

Diagnosis.—The recognition of the morbid conditions of the mediastinum now under discussion is in some cases impossible, and is often surrounded with great difficulties. An important factor in diagnosis is the discovery of some disease with which such conditions are likely to be associated, and in this connection periosteal or bone disease, affecting the sternum or vertebræ, is worthy of special attention. So long as a mediastinal abscess does not come to the surface it might be confounded with a tumour in this region, but the general history and course of the case ought, as a rule, to clear up any obscurity or difficulty in this direction. Should the abscess approach the surface it may be recognised by the usual objective signs. The possibility of confounding such a condition with an aneurysm, when pulsation is present, must be particularly borne in mind; but there is rarely any great difficulty from this point of view. The fluctuation of an abscess may, it is affirmed, be simulated by that of a dermoid cyst. As already intimated, the diagnosis between mediastinal and pulmonary gangrene is practically impossible. The complications and untoward events which may supervene in cases of this class must be watched for from a diagnostic point of view, and they can generally be made out by their usual symptoms and physical signs.

Prognosis.—Mediastinal suppuration is obviously a very dangerous condition, and ends fatally, sooner or later, in a considerable proportion of cases. No definite rules for prognosis can be laid down, but each case must be dealt with on its own characters, and according to general principles. In individual instances there may be hopeful elements, and the modern advances in surgical treatment no doubt make the prognosis less grave at the present day than formerly. It is better when an abscess occupies the anterior mediastinum than when the posterior division is affected: in the latter case there is much less chance of the pus coming to the surface, definite treatment is often impossible, and serious complications are more likely to arise, owing to the matter burrowing into vital structures. Some of the untoward events which have already been mentioned are necessarily fatal, and the supervention of complications adds greatly to the danger. Mediastinal gangrene may be regarded as practically hopeless. On the other hand, the advance of an abscess to the surface is a favourable indication. It has occasionally happened also that communication with a bronchus has ended in recovery, the pus being in course of time completely evacuated. Some remarkable instances have been recorded of very large collections of pus in the mediastinum, which were cured or greatly benefited by treatment, and in which the patients either lived for many years afterwards, or ultimately succumbed to other and independent diseases.

Treatment.—In the early stages of acute mediastinitis, ending in suppuration, the treatment can only be conducted on the general principles applicable to inflammatory conditions. Of course the patient should be kept absolutely at rest in bed, and suitably dieted; nourishing articles of food being soon required, as well as alcoholic stimulants judiciously administered. Poultices or other applications may be useful to relieve pain; and other symptoms must be attended to as they arise. Leeching and counter-irritation have been recommended, but it is doubtful whether they can be of any real service, and lowering measures may certainly be ultimately to the disadvantage of the patient, whose strength generally has to be sustained in every possible way. With regard to medicinal treatment there are no definite indications at first; but a saline mixture may be given, or perhaps antipyretic or cardiac drugs may be useful in some instances. Subsequently quinine and acids, or other tonics, are chiefly needed, or perhaps stimulant remedies ; but no particular rules can be laid down. Of course the general functions must be attended to. In dealing with chronic mediastinal abscess a general tonic and nutrient plan of treatment is invariably indicated.

When suppuration in the mediastinum is definitely recognised, or even reasonably suspected, and especially if a localised abscess can be made out, surgical treatment is obviously called for, if it can be carried out ; but the difficulties are often great, and may be insurmountable. It is quite beyond the province of this article to discuss in detail the surgical measures which may be required ; a few general remarks must suffice. Should an abscess come to the surface, and especially if symptoms are urgent, it must be evacuated as speedily as possible, by free opening and drainage, with the employment of antiseptic precautions and applications. Possibly the aspirator may be of service, especially when there is a large quantity of pus in the mediastinum, which it may not be desirable to draw off all at once, lest the sudden removal of pressure within the chest lead to syncope. Before the abscess can be properly emptied, it might be necessary to remove one or more rib cartilages. Another operation which is practised under certain circumstances, and which in several cases has proved most successful, is trephining the sternum. This may be called for, even on suspicion of abscess in the anterior mediastinum, if there are alarming symptoms in the direction of cardiac failure or suffocation. When the suppuration is associated with caries or necrosis of the sternum or spine, operative interference may aim at the removal of the diseased bone, as well as at the treatment of any abscesses or sinuses associated therewith. When the posterior mediastinum is the seat of a purulent collection, surgical measures are practically inadmissible ; and the same remark applies to gangrenous mediastinitis. It may happen that the secondary results of either abscess or gangrene in connection with the pleura may call for operative treatment, in the way of removing fluid or gas. Should an abscess open into the air-passage, the discharge of the pus should be encouraged by the act of coughing, and antiseptic inhalations employed.

IV. CHRONIC MEDIASTINITIS—INDURATIVE OR CALLOUS MEDIASTINO-PERICARDITIS.—Before considering the important group of cases in which chronic inflammation of the mediastinal tissues is a prominent feature, brief allusion may be made to its occurrence under other circumstances. There may be a localised change of this nature, associated with degeneration and pigmentation of glands as life advances, especially in those who have lived in large and smoky cities or towns, or have worked at dusty trades. The glands become shrunken and tough, fibrous, or calcified, and may set up a chronic inflammatory process around, leading to thickening and adhesion. It is only in exceptional cases that any ill effects ensue, from pressure on the trachea or a bronchus, the œsophagus, or one of the great vessels. In rare instances a fibrous growth of considerable thickness is thus produced. These changes may give rise to traction-diverticula of the œsophagus, by dragging on its walls. More or less extensive chronic mediastinitis is often associated with prolonged suppuration, tuberculous disease of the glands, or tumours of various kinds; but its effects are, as a rule, then of quite secondary importance, and are obscured by the primary affection. It may also possibly occur in connection with actinomycosis.

The more pronounced forms of chronic mediastinitis are usually intimately connected with pericardial adhesions, and are dealt with from this point of view in the article on "Diseases of the Pericardium" [vol. v. p. 779]. Dr. Thomas Harris, of Manchester, in his excellent monograph on *Indurative Mediastino-Pericarditis*, published in 1895, has given a tabular abstract of cases reported up to that time, as well as the details of others observed by himself, and has discussed the subject in an able and comprehensive manner. The complaint was thus named by Kussmaul, who first brought it into prominent notice in 1873. It was, however, known before that period, as I can testify from personal experience and observation at the Liverpool Northern Hospital; and Sir Samuel (then Dr.) Wilks had drawn attention to the subject in relation to pericardial adhesions in *Guy's Hospital Reports* for 1871, and described several cases As a matter of fact chronic mediastinitis in its various degrees is much more common than is usually supposed, or than is recognised in ordinary practice. The records of the subject, however, are almost entirely founded upon fatal cases in which a necropsy was made.

The particular conditions to be referred to in the present connection are (a) the rare variety which has been especially termed *chronic mediastinitis*, in which the morbid changes are entirely external to the pericardium, and confined to the mediastinum; (b) *pericarditis externa et interna*, where, although the pericardium is more or less adherent to the sternum, costal cartilages, and lungs, as well as internally, there is little or no general mediastinitis; and (c) that form to which the term *indurative mediastino-pericarditis* more properly belongs, where, along with an adherent pericardium, there is extensive and marked increase of fibrous tissue in the mediastinum. Clinically it is impossible to draw any definite line of demarcation between the several groups.

Etiology and Pathology.—The origin of the mediastinal changes associated with pericardial adhesion has been already discussed in relation to that condition, to which reference may be made. In the present article it must suffice to offer a few remarks on the general bearings of the subject. A certain proportion of cases can be definitely traced to an acute chest affection, of which acute pericarditis formed a prominent feature; but it is highly probable that, in some instances at any rate, there has been at the same time an acute mediastinitis, or an adjacent pleurisy, which formed the starting-point of the subsequent mediastinal lesions. I have met with a few cases during their acute stage strongly supporting this view, and it is only by particularly careful examination of the chest that the signs can be verified. Should these grave cases, in which the pleuræ as well as the pericardium are extensively involved, end in recovery, mediastinal mischief is very likely to remain. Occasionally a history of an acute illness can be obtained, especially scarlet fever or measles, but without any record of disease in the chest; though no doubt in such instances pericarditis had occurred as a complication of such an illness. In many cases no definite history of an acute origin can be obtained, but at the same time such an origin is revealed by the results of the necropsy. Indeed it must be familiar to all how often pericardial adhesions thus discovered cannot be traced to any definite acute attack. Another important fact to be remembered is that the attacks of pericarditis may be repeated, when the probability of mediastinal implication is much increased; of this course of events I have met with some striking instances, and have watched their progress for some time.

Occasionally chronic mediastinitis follows injury of various kinds, and has even been attributed to prolonged pressure on the sternum in connection with some handicraft; but I have never personally met with a case in which such a mode of origin could be positively ascertained.

In some instances mediastinitis is chronic from the outset, being then almost always associated with tuberculous disease, either affecting the glands or connected with pulmonary phthisis. Possibly it may arise in old cases of bronchitis and emphysema, especially when these conditions are engendered by the inhalation of irritating particles. It has also been attributed to syphilis and bone-disease. Once a chronic inflammation of the mediastinal tissues has started, I believe that it tends to advance; and thus what was originally a very limited and slight change may ultimately become pronounced and extensive.

Age and Sex.—Speaking of indurative mediastino-pericarditis, Dr. Harris (21) writes —:"I think many physicians have an impression that the affection occurs more commonly in children than in adults. Such an impression may be correct; but if so, a large number of cases in children must have escaped having been placed on record, or have not been followed by a post-mortem examination." Of the 22 cases included in his tables, verified after death, he observes that 9 occurred in persons under 18 years of age, and 13 in persons over that age; only 2 patients were over 30. Dr. Harris, therefore, concludes that "the affection would appear to be rather more common in adults than in children." On further analysing these tables, however, I note that the eldest of the patients under 18 was really only 16; that four ranged from 14 to 12, and that the remainder were aged respectively 10, 8, 6¼, and 2.` Moreover, of the cases under 30, no less than eight ranged from 19 to 22; two others being 24 and 26. These facts seem to bear out the view, which certainly accords with my own experience, that at any rate the foundation of indurative mediastino-pericarditis, as well as of *pericarditis externa et interna*, is generally laid in childhood or in early life, although their effects may not become evident until a later date. Simple chronic mediastinitis has quite a different history, for it occurs later in life, and this fact is easily explained. Of the three cases mentioned in Harris' tables the youngest was 37. As regards *sex*, all the varieties of chronic mediastinitis are decidedly more common in males than females. In Harris' tables 20 out of the 25 cases were males.

Anatomical characters.—The essential and characteristic change in chronic mediastinitis of any kind is an increase, more or less pronounced, of fibrous tissue in the mediastinal space, which tends to promote adhesion of the different intra-thoracic structures to each other or to the chest wall, and to compress or contract certain of them, thus leading to secondary consequences, usually of a grave nature. This change is, as already stated, generally associated with pericardial adhesions, and we have, as a rule, to deal in individual cases with their combined pathological effects, which it may be impossible to discriminate. In some instances also one or both lungs are adherent to the chest walls, it may be extensively or universally. In the present connection we have only to consider the mediastinal conditions. These changes vary a good deal in situation, extent, and exact characters. In a fair proportion of cases they are limited to the anterior mediastinum, rarely to the posterior or middle, or to the lateral boundaries; but the entire space is not uncommonly involved. They may merely amount to adhesion of the pericardium to the sternum and rib-cartilages, or to one or both lungs at the same time, with little or no thickening. In other instances there is marked increase of the fibrous tissue, which sometimes attains a great thickness, or even forms definite masses. The material is firm and tough, and often very dense, indurated, or callous—hence the terms "indurative" or "callous" mediastino-pericarditis. There may be considerable fibrous mediastinitis, however, without any internal pericardial adhesions. In this condition the external adhesions of the pericardium are very dense and strong; and it may be impossible to separate this sac from the chest wall or adjoining structures without forcibly tearing them asunder. In the midst of the fibrous material the remains of lymphatic glands are often found, usually caseous.

One of the most important pathological effects of chronic mediastinitis is that it often leads to compression of certain mediastinal structures, or to other physical interference with them. It is most likely to involve the large vessels, especially the veins. In several instances the superior vena cava has been implicated, and sometimes occluded. Many years ago a remarkable case came under my observation, with all the symptoms of complete closure of this vessel, in which the necropsy revealed no more than a limited mediastinal fibrous thickening surrounding the vein. Other intra-thoracic veins may be implicated singly. The aorta has been found narrowed and twisted in some instances. The pulmonary vessels may also be compressed, and in all Kussmaul's cases hæmorrhagic infarcts were found in the lungs, which probably were associated with this condition. In one of this observer's cases the ascending part of the arch of the aorta, the trunk of the pulmonary artery, and the superior vena cava were all compressed to a marked degree. Thrombosis may add to the difficulty in the vessels, and help to obstruct them. Pressure upon the inferior vena cava may possibly aid in causing enlargement of the liver, and also dropsy. The main air-passages often escape altogether, and are seldom much narrowed, but may be somewhat compressed. The œsophagus, again, is rarely inter-fered with to any material degree, and as a rule escapes. In exceptional instances the left vagus or recurrent laryngeal nerve has been involved in mediastinal fibrous thickening.

Extreme cases are occasionally met with in which all the intra-thoracic structures are matted together, as well as to the chest wall, by thick and dense adhesions,—pericardial, pleuritic, and mediastinal ; so that at the necropsy the contents of the thorax have to be torn away and removed in a mass. Even after their removal it is very difficult, and may be impossible, to separate them or to dissect them out properly. On opening the chest these cases sometimes give the impression at first sight of the presence of an intra-thoracic tumour. In connection with mediastino-pericarditis, should the pleuræ be partially or entirely free from adhesion, effusion is often found on one or both sides. The lungs are congested or affected in other ways.

The remote effects of the morbid conditions now under consideration must be duly recognised. They are mainly those resulting from marked obstruction of the venous system which, in the case of mediastino-pericarditis, are of general distribution, being then due chiefly to cardiac difficulty , but there may also be the local consequences of the mediastinal changes as affecting particular veins. From the general venous obstruc-tion the usual effects ensue, especially in connection with the liver, spleen, and kidneys ; in inveterate cases they become very pronounced. In exceptional instances of mediastino-pericarditis a slight form of chronic peritonitis is produced, and this occurred in one of Harris' cases ; the explanation of this is not always evident, but he suggests that it might be set up as a result of chronic venous congestion. There may also be an associated hepatic and splenic capsulitis.

Clinical history.—It will be readily understood that no definite or independent description can be given of the symptoms and physical signs of chronic mediastinitis. As a matter of fact, the condition frequently cannot be recognised during life ; or its clinical phenomena are so inti-mately blended with those of pericardial agglutination and its con-sequences that they cannot be separated. Indeed, in cases of well-marked indurative mediastino-pericarditis the symptoms are practically of cardiac origin in the main ; leading not only to certain forms of dyspnœa, dis-turbance of the heart's action, and other chest symptoms, but also to those of general venous obstruction, as evidenced by dropsy and other phenomena elsewhere described in relation to adherent pericardium. When all the structures are matted together, it becomes still more difficult to make out what share each particular factor has in the causation of the symptoms. The explanation of the occurrence of ascites in some instances of mediastino-pericarditis, before the anasarca, or out of all proportion to it, is not always evident ; but it may be due to a chronic peritonitis resulting from venous congestion. In one of the cases collected by Harris, it was found to be due to acute tuberculosis of the peritoneum. Personally, I have usually attributed it to cirrhotic changes in the liver, resulting from the prolonged congestion; but he does not seem to favour this view. There may, of course, be an independent alcoholic cirrhosis. Occasionally mere cardiac dilatation originates ascites without œdema of the legs. The urine is generally deficient in quantity and dark-coloured; it may be albuminous.

The symptoms more directly due to the chronic mediastinal changes, if any, result mainly from their effects upon the structures in the space. There may be pain behind the sternum, or a sense of oppression or dragging, and an inability to expand the chest in deep breathing. Signs of local venous obstruction are those most likely to occur, with enlargement of the superficial veins; and there may be the characteristic evidences of occlusion of the superior vena cava. Definite symptoms referable to the aorta, trachea, or œsophagus are rare. In one of Harris' cases there was limited œdema of the left arm, and paralysis of the left vocal cord due to implication of the recurrent laryngeal nerve. As the left vagus nerve was also involved, it was a question whether the dyspnœa in this case was partly due to this cause.

Jaccoud lays much stress on posture in relation to indurative mediastino-pericarditis. In a case observed by him the patient had to sit up in bed with the trunk markedly bent forward, because in the erect posture, and still more in the recumbent, the dyspnœa and intra-thoracic pain became much worse. I quite agree with Harris, however, that this symptom is by no means diagnostic, and that many exceptions are observed in both directions.

Physical signs.—Here again it is impossible to give any description apart from the pericardial and cardiac conditions, already discussed under adherent pericardium. In fact the signs are mainly associated with the heart; but others are often present also due to pleuritic and pulmonary complications. Possibly the anterior part of the chest may be somewhat depressed as the direct result of chronic mediastinitis; and it certainly interferes with respiratory movements. Further, a considerable mass of fibrous tissue, with enlarged glands, may undoubtedly add to the dulness over the upper part of the sternum, which is then likely to be very pronounced, and accompanied with much sense of resistance. The sign to which attention has been specially called by Dr. George Perez, of Orotava,—namely, a creaking or other sound audible on auscultation when the patient moves the arm,—is well worthy of attention, and may give definite evidence of the presence of chronic mediastinitis. The value of the *pulsus paradoxus*, and of inspiratory swelling of the veins in the neck, in relation to the diagnosis of indurative mediastino-pericarditis, has been fully discussed in the article on adherent pericardium. Examination of the abdomen will reveal ascites or enlarged liver when present; but the spleen is usually small and contracted.

Chronic mediastinitis can sometimes be followed up from its acute origin; but as a rule it comes under observation for the first time as a

chronic case.   Its duration varies considerably, even after the disease has
been discovered.   It may last from a few months to several years.
Indurative mediastino-pericarditis generally tends to go from bad to
worse, causing much suffering.   Death usually results from progressive
cardiac dilatation and failure.   The fatal termination may be hastened
by pulmonary or pleuritic disease, or other complications.

Treatment.—Unfortunately nothing can be done directly to influence
the morbid conditions associated with chronic mediastinitis of any form.   It
is of no use whatever to go on applying iodine or such remedies to the
chest indefinitely, or to carry out any other plan of treatment for the
supposed purpose of promoting absorption of the fibrous tissue in the
mediastinum.   Various measures are often called for to relieve symptoms;
the chief indication being to study the cardiac action, and to endeavour to
assist it in such ways as may be requisite or practicable.   Each case must
be dealt with judiciously, rationally, and individually; and the treatment
will frequently require much attention in various directions.   The
dropsical conditions often require operative interference, and the fluid
may have to be removed again and again, both from the subcutaneous
tissue and serous cavities.

V. Tuberculous disease of mediastinal lymphatic glands and
thoracic duct.—The lymphatic glands occupying the mediastinum are
liable to different morbid changes, most of which are sufficiently noticed in
other parts of this general article.   At present attention will be briefly
directed to *tuberculous* or so-called scrofulous disease of these structures.   In
the large majority of cases it is the bronchial glands which are mainly or
entirely affected, especially those situated at the bifurcation of the trachea,
the condition being known as "bronchial phthisis"; but occasionally those
more particularly termed mediastinal, it may be the anterior mediastinal,
are chiefly or alone implicated; and they sometimes attain a very large
size.   In rare instances the thoracic duct has been found to be the seat
of tuberculous disease.

Etiology.—The intra-thoracic glands are usually involved by secondary
infection from neighbouring structures, especially the lung or pleura;
occasionally from bone.   The disease may also extend directly from the
neck, or from the abdomen, along the lymphatics through the diaphragm;
or may result from remote infection.   Although this statement has been
disputed, there can be no doubt that the glands are attacked primarily
in a certain proportion of cases.   Such a mode of origin is far more
frequent in children than in adults; in the latter it is very exceptional.
It also occurs more commonly in the acute than in the chronic form
of tuberculosis.   Sometimes at the autopsy of a case of pulmonary and
bronchial phthisis it is impossible to determine where the mischief began.
Implication of the thoracic duct is always a secondary event.   With
regard to primary tuberculous disease of the bronchial glands, it is by
no means improbable that they may be directly infected by the tubercle
bacillus when in a healthy state.   They are far more likely to be

attacked, however, when previously irritated or inflamed from any cause; especially if such disturbance should continue for some time, or if the inflammatory process should end in suppuration or caseation. Possibly a cold or some traumatic cause may be the starting-point of mediastinal tuberculosis.

Intra-thoracic tuberculous disease of glands is, in my opinion, more likely to arise in those who present a marked hereditary tendency thereto; but in many of the patients no' such tendency can be traced. The complaint is far more common in children and young subjects than in adults, but the relative proportion of cases at particular ages has been variously stated by different observers. No doubt conditions which impair the general health, such as want of proper food, unfavourable hygienic surroundings, and the like, may act as remote causes in children, as well as lowering illnesses. Tuberculosis of the bronchial glands sometimes follows an acute illness, or it may be a sequel of whooping-cough. The thoracic duct is but rarely definitely affected; but this may happen from extension, or in acute cases.

Anatomical characters and pathological changes.—In the early stage, or when involved in acute tuberculosis, the glands in rare instances merely present discrete gray granulations. As a rule, however, the growth is infiltrated, there being a general inflammatory process which is of a tuberculous nature—*lymphadenitis tuberculosa*—as proved by the presence of abundant tubercle-bacilli. The two conditions may be associated. The affected glands are swollen and enlarged, sometimes considerably, and by their aggregation they may form masses or tumours of great size. They are of soft consistence, and may present a medullary appearance. In different parts they may be pale and opaque, or highly vascular. The usual tendency is for the tuberculous glands to undergo caseous degeneration, either in spots or extensively; and this change may take place very rapidly. The late Dr. Wilson Fox believed, however, that a fibroid transformation sometimes takes place, even of the tuberculous granulations themselves, "with thickening of the reticulum and septa, until large tracts of the glands may be converted into a glistening semi-cartilaginous substance with only scattered nuclei here and there distributed through it. These glands are commonly at the same time intensely pigmented; they are hard and resistant, and may even, by shrinking, become smaller than natural." This eminent physician and pathologist found such changes, and especially pigmentation, particularly in the bronchial glands. Cheesy spots may be evident in parts. Schüppel has given a different explanation to account for these appearances; namely, that the tubercle granulations always become caseous, and that the induration is due to a secondary growth of connective tissue, the caseous matter disappearing by absorption.

A further change which is prone to take place in glands which have become caseous is that they break down, and pus is formed; this being the common origin of chronic or so-called "cold" abscess in the mediastinum. Such a collection of pus may open externally, or into the various structures already mentioned in relation to mediastinal abscess generally, especially the trachea or a main bronchus, or the œsophagus. It is important to bear in mind also that a tuberculous abscess may perforate the aorta or pulmonary artery, causing fatal hæmorrhage. In one case the trachea, œsophagus, and pericardium were simultaneously perforated. Suppurating glands are occasionally embedded in the lung, and it may then be very difficult or impossible to distinguish them from pulmonary cavities. Ulceration associated with caseous glands may take place without actual suppuration, and this may also lead to perforation. Cases have been recorded in which a gland has ulcerated into the trachea, and then, becoming detached, has caused sudden death from suffocation by impaction in the rima glottidis. In the majority of cases the material resulting from caseation of the glands becomes inspissated, and being encapsuled by fibrous tissue, may remain inert for long periods. Such a condition, however, is always a source of danger, lest it should act as a centre of infection; or acute suppuration may be set up at any time. The final change which tuberculous glands in the mediastinum may undergo is calcification; encapsuled cretaceous material or calcareous masses remaining as the sole evidence of the previous existence of the disease.

With regard to the thoracic duct, it has been found in some cases, by Ponfick and others, to be the seat of extensive tuberculous infiltration, with ulceration; this condition being an obvious source of general infection. Perforation of the duct by a mediastinal gland has also been observed in rare instances.

Clinical history and Diagnosis.—The phenomena associated with tuberculous disease of the mediastinal glands present considerable variety in individual cases; and as the more characteristic of them are described in relation to other subjects in this article, of which such disease forms a part, it will only be necessary to deal here with the clinical history in general terms. It can be easily understood that the glands may not be sufficiently affected to give rise to any obvious or trustworthy symptoms, and in a fair proportion of cases no doubt this happens. Moreover, when they become involved secondarily, in connection with pulmonary phthisis, there are often no special indications of the event, or they are obscured by those of the lung trouble. Again, there may only be the usual chest symptoms; namely, pain, disturbance of breathing, cough, and expectoration of no definite significance. When the bronchial glands are affected, and attain a sufficient size, the characters of the breathing and cough will reveal more or less obstruction of the main air-passages, or nerve irritation; and it is to the phenomena thus originated that special attention must be paid in early diagnosis, particularly in children. Any tendency to obstructive, noisy, or stridulous respiration; to attacks resembling spasmodic asthma; or to spasmodic cough of a "croupy" quality, or resembling that of whooping-cough, should always suggest mediastinal glandular disease as a possible cause. The voice may also be affected; and other pressure symptoms may be present. At the same time there may be signs on physical examination of deficient entrance of air into one or both lungs; changes in the normal percussion sounds; tactile and auscultatory phenomena indicating unusual conduction of breath sounds, and of vocal or tussive vibrations and sounds from the main air-tubes, especially in one or both interscapular regions, and the sounds often have peculiar characters. In short, there are the signs of the presence of some unusual solid collection in the mediastinum, which culminate in those of a distinct mediastinal tumour, in relation to which they will be more fully discussed. Extensive tuberculosis of the anterior mediastinal glands will give rise to marked dulness over the sternum. Dr. Eustace Smith has described in children a venous hum, audible at the root of the neck when the head is thrown back, which he attributes to pressure by enlarged glands on the venous trunks.

Another class of phenomena which may occur in connection with tuberculous mediastinal glands are those due to the formation of an abscess, and its communication with the trachea or a bronchus. This event may be immediately followed by urgent symptoms; and if not fatal there will be expectoration of purulent or caseous material, accompanied with the development of signs of a cavity. On examination of the sputum tubercle bacilli will probably be detected in abundance. Hæmoptysis may also occur. In old chronic cases calcareous particles may be expectorated. Should the abscess come to the surface there will be the usual objective evidences of this condition. It must be remembered that it may possibly open in other directions, and that fatal hæmorrhage may happen from perforation of a great vessel.

Mediastinal tuberculous disease will be attended with the ordinary general symptoms of this complaint, and they are likely to be pronounced; namely, fever, wasting, anæmia, night-sweats, general debility, and loss of appetite. Occlusion of the thoracic duct may cause extreme emaciation, but it is impossible in these cases to recognise this condition definitely during life. The presence of pulmonary phthisis, or of tuberculous lesions in other parts of the body, will materially help in a doubtful case in the diagnosis of the nature of a morbid condition giving rise to mediastinal symptoms or physical signs. The complaint sometimes runs an acute course, but is generally chronic. It is important to observe that the symptoms, after having been prominent, may gradually subside, and practical recovery ultimately ensue.

Treatment.—Mediastinal tuberculosis is in many cases so intimately associated with the same condition in the lungs or other parts, that any independent treatment is quite out of the question. Even when it exists alone, the indications to be carried out are merely those applicable to tuberculous disease in general. It is very doubtful whether any of the vaunted "specific" methods of treatment now in vogue can have any positive beneficial effect upon this complaint when it involves the mediastinal glands. Should an abscess form, and come to the surface, or open internally, it must be treated on ordinary principles. How far operative interference is practicable or permissible, and what measures should be carried out, must be determined by the circumstances of each individual case; and for guidance in this part of the subject reference must be made to surgical works.

VI. MEDIASTINAL EMPHYSEMA.—Accumulation of air in the mediastinal cellular tissue is of extremely rare occurrence, but it is nevertheless a definite morbid condition in connection with this region, and cannot be ignored in this article. In the large majority of cases it is of traumatic origin, or occurs during or after the performance of tracheotomy for different purposes. In this way it may be associated with diphtheria. The air then gains access into the anterior mediastinum beneath the deep cervical fascia. Very exceptionally mediastinal emphysema results from rupture or perforation of the trachea or a bronchus, or of the lung and pleura, in connection with ulceration, abscess, gangrene, tuberculous disease, or extreme pulmonary emphysema, either vesicular or interstitial. The condition is said to have been produced by a violent paroxysm of whooping-cough. Gas may also find its way into the mediastinum as a consequence of perforation of the œsophagus. Moreover, it may be present from decomposition, occurring either during life or after death. [Cf. et B. aerogenes capsulatus (Welch).]

The amount, distribution, and characters of a gaseous accumulation in the mediastinum vary much under different circumstances. In certain conditions it has an offensive smell. When a persistent leakage of air takes place through an opening in an air-tube or in the pleura, it enters with each inspiration; but a valve-like action prevents its escape during expiration, so that the chest becomes rapidly more and more filled and distended, the lungs are compressed, and death speedily ensues. When an escape of gas occurs into any part of the mediastinal space, it is likely to find its way to the other divisions. A limited emphysema has been described, named *extra-pericardial*, in which the air accumulates around the pericardium, interfering with the cardiac movements.

Clinically mediastinal emphysema may be recognised under certain circumstances, especially if it originate from injury or tracheotomy. Symptoms of interference with the intra-thoracic structures would rapidly supervene; while the chest would become distended, and yield signs indicating that this distension was due to accumulation of gas. It might be difficult to determine the situation of the gas, especially as the mediastinal condition may be associated with pneumothorax; but the extensive distribution of hyper-resonance or tympanitic percussion-sound, or its presence over the front of the chest, would help the diagnosis. The air in the cellular tissue may give rise to a very peculiar and characteristic dry crackling sound, produced by deep respiration, or by moving the arms, and audible on auscultation. It might farther make its way to the cellular tissue of the neck or front of the chest, or even more extensively, thus causing subcutaneous emphysema, which would be an additional help in diagnosis.

Treatment can only be conducted on general principles, especially to combat symptoms; nothing definite can be done for the mediastinal emphysema itself. Possibly some kind of operative interference might be indicated under special circumstances. It is important to take due precautions to prevent the occurrence of this complication during or after the performance of tracheotomy.

VII. SPECIAL CONDITIONS OF THE THYMUS GLAND.—The thymus gland has been already referred to as the possible seat of origin of a mediastinal abscess; and it will call for notice again in relation to tumours in this region. At present I only intend to offer a few remarks upon certain other pathological relations and morbid conditions of this curious organ.

1. Persistent thymus.—The thymus body or gland is a structure which normally is only present during early life. It is quite obvious at birth, when it weighs on an average about half an ounce, but varies with the weight of the infant; it increases in size and weight up to the age of two years, when it reaches its maturity; remains more or less perfect until eight to twelve years of age; and then undergoes rapid wasting, accompanied with fatty degeneration, shrivelling up so that at the age of twenty no trace of it can be discovered, or but an insignificant vestige. Occasionally, however, this body is persistent, and it has been found of some size as late as forty years of age. In an ordinary way the condition now under notice does not give rise to any symptoms; but it may nevertheless be of pathological significance, as, for instance, when a persistent thymus is associated with exophthalmic goitre. Moreover, it may be the starting point of malignant disease encroaching upon the mediastinum, or of other growths.

2. Enlarged or hypertrophied thymus.—This is a far more important morbid condition of the thymus body, and may occasion marked or even grave symptoms. It occurs in childhood, and also later in life. An enlarged thymus may exist alone, or be associated with exophthalmic goitre, leucocythæmia, lymphadenoma, or other maladies. The increase in size is not due to any new growth, but is entirely or in the main a mere hypertrophy or hyperplasia of the gland-structures. The body has been found in individual cases to weigh as much as 620 grains in a boy aged fourteen; 380 grains at twenty-five; and 356 at twenty years of age. Several instances of enlarged thymus have been reported of late years, and the subject is now receiving more attention than formerly. An interesting case was recently brought before the Pathological Society by Dr. H. D. Rolleston (39), in which a boy aged six years, three weeks before death, became subject to cough and stridor, the physical signs being limited to dulness behind the sternum. There was swelling of the neck and fulness of the veins with enlargement of the glands, but no urgent dyspnœa. A mediastinal growth was diagnosed, which was supposed to be lymphadenoma or lympho-sarcoma. After death a large tumour was found in the position of the thymus compressing the vagi, but not invading the parts around; there were no secondary growths. Histologically it presented the structure of normal thymus in parts; elsewhere there was an

abnormal amount of leucocytes without reticulum. Death was sudden, and was attributed to dilatation of the heart arising from compression of the vagi.

In a very interesting case of exophthalmic goitre, in a woman aged twenty-two, who was admitted into my ward at University Hospital in October 1895, which ended fatally, the thymus gland was found to be considerably enlarged, and weighed 1¼ oz. It reached down to the middle third of the pericardium. The following is the description of the organ given by my house-physician, Mr. T. W. Starkey :—" Lobulations were distinctly marked on the surface of the thymus body, which was divided into two halves by a fibrous septum. Smaller septa spread out from this one, dividing it into smaller lobes. On section it was dark red in colour. Microscopically the gland presented all the typical characters of a normal thymus in a young child, and showed no trace of fatty degeneration. The concentric corpuscles were rather more numerous than is ordinarily seen in a specimen of thymus gland, but did not differ otherwise."

Clinically an enlarged thymus gland is sometimes revealed by respiratory disorder. It may compress the trachea, and thus cause more or less obstructive dyspnœa ; or it is affirmed that it may cause spasm of the glottis—the so-called " thymic asthma "—also known as Copp's or Millar's asthma. Death from suffocation in young children has been attributed to this condition. Should the organ implicate the vagi nerves, cardiac disturbance or dilatation may be produced, as in Dr. Rolleston's case. An enlarged thymus may cause impaired resonance or definite dulness over the upper part of the sternum. In my case there were no definite symptoms or signs pointing specially to any enlargement of this body. How far general or remote symptoms might arise from the physiological effects associated with a persistent or hypertrophied thymus cannot at present be determined, so far as I am aware.

3. Among **miscellaneous morbid conditions** to which the thymus gland is liable may be mentioned syphilitic disease, which is said to set up an inflammatory change ; tuberculous deposit ; fatty degeneration ; and formation of calculi or concretious in its substance. These are merely of pathological interest, and cannot be recognised clinically.

Treatment.—Little or nothing of a definite character can be said under this head. Whether any actual benefit can be derived from the administration of the thymus gland or its extract, when this organ is supposed to be the seat of disease, I do not know. It has been given, with favourable results, it is said, in defective development, rickets, exophthalmic goitre associated with anæmia and debility, leucocythæmia, chlorosis, and pernicious anæmia. Its administration appears to cause increased formation and excretion of uric acid. When urgent dyspnœic symptoms arise from an enlarged thymus, the performance of tracheotomy gives little or no relief, and under such circumstances the operation has been performed of exposing and partially removing the body. When it is the seat of suppuration or a tumour, the principles of treatment are similar to those dealt with in other parts of this article which are concerned with such conditions.

VIII. Intra-thoracic new growths, malignant and non-malignant — mediastinal tumour.—As already indicated in the introductory remarks to this article, it is intended to discuss under this head not only growths which are actually mediastinal in origin, but also certain morbid formations which start in the lung or pleura, and tend to form tumours within the chest. By such an arrangement a comprehensive view of a somewhat complicated subject can be presented, in its pathological and clinical aspects, with much practical advantage, for the following reasons:—In the first place, it is impossible in a considerable proportion of cases to draw any definite clinical line of demarcation between growths associated with the mediastinum, lung, or pleura respectively. Secondly, the different structures are often affected together; it may be almost simultaneously, but usually as the result of direct extension or secondary implication, so that no actual distinction can be made between them; and it may even be impossible on post-mortem examination positively to determine the starting-point of an intra-thoracic tumour. Thirdly, in their morbid anatomy the growths affecting the various parts usually present many features in common; though there are exceptions in this respect. Of course I do not propose to deal with those pulmonary and pleuritic new formations which are discussed, in their appropriate connections, in other parts of this work; such as tubercle, syphilitic products, or hydatids. It may be stated generally that mediastinal growths are much more common than those originating in the lung or pleura; and it is in very exceptional cases only that the structure last mentioned is attacked primarily.

Pathology.—It must be taken for granted that the reader is already sufficiently acquainted with the general pathology of the various morbid growths which give rise to intra-thoracic tumours, and with the different meanings of their nomenclature. There are, however, certain points demanding notice which may be conveniently considered under the above comprehensive heading, and to these attention will now be directed.

Summary of growths.—In the study of intra-thoracic tumours obviously the first step is to obtain a comprehensive knowledge of the nature of the morbid growths of which they may consist. According to the usual classification these formations are primarily divided into *malignant*, and *non-malignant* or *benign;* but this arrangement cannot be strictly carried out on an anatomical or histological basis, as certain of them, which are structurally alike, may under different circumstances belong to either category. Without further comment they may, for practical purposes, be enumerated as follows:—(i.) *Carcinoma*, in its several varieties; these being all essentially malignant. (ii.) *Sarcoma*, in the form of round-celled, spindle-celled, and small-celled or *lympho-sarcoma*. Some of these growths are benign, while others manifest very distinctly the characters of malignancy   (iii.) *Lymphoma* and *lymphadenoma*, which some pathologists regard as identical, others as distinct.   (iv.) *Fibroma, fibro - cellular* and *fibro - plastic* growths. (v.) *Teratoma* or "dermoid cyst." (vi.) *Hydatids*. These are discussed elsewhere in relation to the lungs [vol. ii. p. 1137], and they are extremely rare in the mediastinum. (vii.) *Syphilitic gumma.* This subject is also dealt with in connection with lung-affections [vol. v. p. 316], and it will suffice to say that exceptionally they are met with in the mediastinum, embedded in dense fibrous material.   (viii.) *Tuberculous glands,* which occasionally attain such a size as to form a mediastinal tumour of considerable dimensions   (ix.) *A miscellaneous group,* including *lipoma,* or *steatoma , chondroma* of soft parts, *osteo-chondroma,* or *enchondroma ; myeloid* tumour *, hæmatoma.*   Intra-thoracic tumours occasionally present a mixed structure, but reference will be made later to these combinations.

Most of the growths in the foregoing list are quite rare , and the large majority of intra-thoracic tumours which are of practical importance, and which can be recognised during life, are either carcinomatous or sarcomatous.   It is to these formations, therefore, that attention must be more especially directed.

Seat of origin —In the next place, it is desirable to get a general notion of the structures from which intra-thoracic growths may originate ; though later this question will have to be considered more particularly in relation to special morbid formations.   Taking them as a whole, these growths may start from : (a) Either lung, which is not very common (b) The pleural or subpleural tissue, in comparatively few cases   (c) The thoracic wall,—a tumour growing inwards from the periosteum covering the sternum ; or from the cartilaginous or bony framework.   This seat of origin applies more particularly to osteo-chondroma or enchondroma, but sarcoma may arise from the sternal periosteum.   (d) The lymphatic structures, especially the glands.   A large proportion of intra thoracic growths have their starting-point in these structures.   Not only may the glands within the chest be thus primarily affected, but it is important to note that those at the base of the neck may be implicated first, the mischief extending thence directly into the thorax.   The anterior mediastinal glands, and those associated with the trachea and main bronchi, are frequently involved; or the growth may begin in the lymphatic structures in the root of the lung   Cases have been reported in which cancerous growths were supposed to have started in the thoracic duct.   (e) The important tubes occupying the mediastinum.   Thus tumours, which subsequently become mediastinal, may have their seat of origin in the œsophagus, the trachea, or a main bronchus.   (f) The cellular tissue or fat of the mediastinum.   A steatoma of sarcomatous type or "lipoma sarcomatodes" has been described as originating in the fatty tissues.   (g) The pericardium or subpericardial tissue ; or, very rarely, the adventitia of the large blood-vessels   (h) The thymus gland. Numerous cases have been reported in which a tumour in the mediastinum, especially its anterior division, began in a persistent thymus.   Virchow has particularly insisted on this mode of origin of such tumours. (*i*) A growth starting in the thyroid gland may possibly extend into the chest, and become a mediastinal tumour.

General grouping of cases.—It is customary to divide cases of intra-thoracic tumour, as they come under observation in practice, into *primary* and *secondary*, these terms having the signification usually recognised in relation to new growths. For practical purposes, however, it may be useful to make a further subdivision, and I venture to suggest the following as indicating the circumstances under which such growths may occur in the chest.—

(i) They may be strictly *primary*, starting from some definite intra-thoracic structure Mediastinal tumours far more frequently belong to this category than do those of pulmonary origin; and, according to Kaulich, nearly half of all mediastinal tumours are primary. Growths thus originating may (*a*) remain throughout confined to the structure first attacked. which applies to many benign growths; (*b*) spread so as to implicate other structures within the chest, this being the usual course of events in the case of malignant growths, (*c*) extend directly to the surface or into the abdominal cavity; or (*d*) give rise to secondary formations in more or less remote parts.

(ii) As already stated. tumours beginning on the inner surface of the chest wall may grow inwards and encroach upon the thoracic space, or even implicate some of its contents. But, further, a growth starting outside the chest. in the mammary gland for instance, occasionally penetrates the wall, so that ultimately it becomes intra-thoracic also. Whether originating from within or from without, we now and then meet with cases in which all the structures seem to be involved in a common mass.

(iii.) Of the *secondary* group, the following subdivisions may be recognised:—(*a*) Primary malignant disease within the chest, not giving rise to any obvious disturbance, may be the source of infection, and originate a secondary growth forming a distinct tumour with all its consequences. A very interesting example of such a case occurred recently at University Hospital in my ward, to which reference will be made hereafter, in which a mass of glands formed a tumour giving rise to very pronounced symptoms, the primary mischief having been a limited area of malignant disease near the lower end of the œsophagus, which during life had been entirely latent. (*b*) Direct extension from the abdomen into the chest takes place now and then, leading to secondary implication of some of the thoracic contents. Such extension is most likely to come from the peritoneum, very rarely from the stomach, liver, or kidney. (*c*) An independent secondary malignant tumour may grow within the chest, in cases where a primary disease of this nature exists in some other more or less distant part of the body. Such primary disease is generally quite obvious clinically, but not always, and it may not be discovered till after death; possibly not even then. Instances occasionally come under observation where, along with an intra-thoracic tumour, many structures are involved, so that it is impossible to determine the original seat of the mischief. (*d*) An important group of secondary formations within the thorax are those in which a recurrence of malignant disease is thus revealed ; as in cases where one or more growths of this nature have been removed by operation from other parts of the body. Of this group I have met with many striking examples.

(iv.) It appears to me desirable to recognise separately a class of cases in which a mediastinal tumour is merely part of a general disease affecting the absorbent glands, and involving these structures in various parts of the body, it may be even universally. There has been a good deal of discussion as to the exact nature of the changes which affect these glands within the chest, and with reference to their nomenclature ; but at any rate there is a very definite form of lymphadenoma known as Hodgkin's disease, to which the above description fairly applies. This disease may certainly begin in the intra-thoracic glands, or they may be involved by extension from the glands of the neck, or at a period more or less remote after the primary implication of distant glands. In either case, however, the enlargement of these structures is a manifestation of a general or constitutional disease, often of wide distribution ; and it may give rise to a distinct mediastinal tumour. Tuberculous glands in the chest might also in some instances be included in this category.

Special growths.—With regard to the majority of new growths within the chest already enumerated, nothing more need be said, but there are a few the pathology of which, in relation to the structures occupying this region, demand further consideration, especially carcinoma and sarcoma. It will be convenient to discuss these morbid formations separately, in connection with the lung, pleura, and mediastinum respectively.

1. **Carcinoma.**—(*a*) *Lung.*—Pulmonary cancer is rare under any form, and particularly so as a primary disease, being in the large majority of cases secondary. The common form of primary cancer in the lung has been generally classed by writers on the subject as medullary or encephaloid, being of soft consistence ; but the characteristic growth in this organ has also been described as a *cylindrical-celled carcinoma*, developing from the bronchial epithelium. Scirrhus is less frequent. The growth may become melanotic ; or, exceptionally, it is of an epithelio-matous nature, the primary variety being squamous, the secondary columnar. Colloid cancer is extremely rare in the lung, and always secondary. Extension of cancer from adjacent structures to this organ happens only very occasionally. When it is secondary, the chief seats of the primary growth are said to be the mammary gland, the bronchial glands, the œsophagus, the stomach, the liver, the peritoneum, the testes, and the bones ; it may, however, be part of a widely-diffused malignant disease. It occurs not uncommonly after removal of a tumour of the breast. The secondary pulmonary growths in such cases will probably be of the same kind as that of the original tumour. Thus epithelioma may follow a similar disease affecting the lip, tongue, œsophagus, trachea, uterus, or vulva.

(*b*) *Pleura.*—Primary cancer of the pleura is extremely rare ; but it does occur as a diffuse endothelial growth, either with very limited implication of the lung, if any, or with secondary development in this organ. It is generally supposed to originate from the endothelium of the lymphatic vessels ; but in a case recorded by Dr. Joseph Coats the author regarded it rather as arising from the surface epithelium or endothelium. Dr. Harris has recorded two cases which he believed to be primary malignant disease of the pleura (22), and has discussed the subject in a very interesting manner. He points out the difficulties which surround it, and truly says that "although the pleura may be affected with a malignant growth in such a way that it appears to have probably arisen there, it is quite possible that the appearances are misleading, and that although the pleura is the only seat where a malignant growth is found, or the chief seat of the growth, the primary seat may have been elsewhere, and may, for various reasons, have escaped detection even after a careful post-mortem examination." Of his two cases one presented the characters of a cylindrical-cell endothelioma, the other of a squamous epithelioma.

More frequently the pleura is implicated secondarily by extension from the lung, which is very likely to happen, or from the mediastinum. Such implication may, however, possibly be independent, and not traceable to direct extension. A tumour growing from the lung, mediastinum, or chest wall sometimes finds its chief expansion within the pleural cavity, filling the whole of its interior, and simply compressing the lung.

(*c*) *Mediastinum.*—There is a decided difference of opinion as to the real nature of the majority of mediastinal tumours, and especially as to the comparative frequency of primary carcinomatous and sarcomatous growths in this region. Most writers on this subject have regarded carcinoma as the least common of such tumours, and it has even been stated that as a primary growth it is almost unheard of. Sir R. Douglas Powell (35) affirms that even secondary cancer is rare, except when it travels inwards from the breast. Dr. Lindsay Steven, of Glasgow, in his very able and interesting treatise on "Mediastinal Tumours," expresses his strong opinion that cancer is not anything like so frequently met with as sarcoma, especially lympho-sarcoma. He writes : "Cancer is a disease which can only originate, except in very rare and exceptional circumstances indeed, in connection with epithelial tissues, and more particularly in those epithelial tissues which are especially prone to injury or irritation. For this reason the most likely place for a primary carcinoma to develop within the chest is the posterior mediastinum, where we have the epithelial structures of the trachea, bronchi, and œsophagus to afford a starting-point for the disease." In further dealing with this subject, however, Dr. Steven admits the possibility of cancer primarily originating in other than the epithelial tissues of the mediastinal space, though this must be an occurrence of the rarest kind. He further discusses the difficulty sometimes experienced in distinguishing between sarcomatous and carcinomatous growths (endothelioma and alveolar sarcoma), as regards their histological structure; and adds in relation to the mediastinum, that "while strongly of opinion that cancerous tumours in this region, in the great majority of cases, originate in epithelial tissues, I am still aware of the difficulties which apparently cancerous tumours not so originating raise. I think it not at all improbable that very often the appearance of a cancerous tumour in the mediastinum may be caused by a sarcoma forming a stroma for itself out of the loose connective tissue amongst which it has frequently to grow." Dr. Steven gives an account of an interesting case of primary cancer originating in the right bronchus, which was supposed during life to be one of pulmonary phthisis. He rightly states, however, that a much more frequent starting-point for primary cancer of the posterior mediastinum is the epithelium of the œsophagus; and such a growth by its increase and extension may ultimately give rise to definite symptoms and physical signs of mediastinal tumour, of which I have met with more than one striking example. As already stated, the thoracic duct is believed to be the original seat of cancer in exceptional instances.

In opposition to the views just considered, some writers place cancer first, especially in relation to tumours occurring in the anterior mediastinum. Dr. Hare, founding his conclusions on the cases collected by him, supports this opinion both as regards primary and secondary mediastinal growths. Out of 520 cases he classes 134 as of this nature, and writes: " The tissues in which cancer may arise in the mediastinum are exceedingly numerous; indeed, those which it does not attack can scarcely be mentioned. Undoubtedly the lymph-glands at the base of the neck, or those which accompany the trachea and bronchi, are frequent seats for its beginning, and in quite a large class of cases a persistent thymus seems to form a nidus, particularly for a growth in the anterior mediastinum. The lymph-tissues at the root of the lungs, the pericardium and sub-pericardial connective tissue, the periosteum of the sternum, the fat and connective tissue of the mediastinum, and the adventitia of the blood-vessels, may give rise to the growth. The lung tissues themselves may also, and do frequently exhibit cancerous tendencies, and the mediastinum is frequently filled by a tumour projecting from the lung, or by metastasis to the tissues of the area itself."

Individual experience of mediastinal tumours is necessarily limited, and no positive opinion can be founded upon such experience as to the relative frequency of cancer in this region; but I have met with a sufficient number of cases to give me the impression that it is at any rate a less rare form of growth than is generally recognised. At the same time the statement made by Hare as to the structures from which it may arise can hardly be maintained, if modern views as to the origin of carcinomatous growths are to be accepted. Moreover, there can be no doubt, as has been often pointed out, that many tumours formerly described as cancerous would now be removed from this category; a criticism which fairly applies to some of the cases collected by Hare.

With regard to secondary mediastinal cancer, there is but little to be said.

As an independent condition resulting from so-called "metastasis," and following carcinoma in some remote organ or structure, it is much less common than pulmonary cancer, and as a matter of fact it is extremely rare. Of course the mediastinum is liable to be encroached upon by a tumour starting from the lung or pleura, or from other structures in the immediate vicinity. In the case of the lung, the bulk of extension of a carcinomatous growth may be mediastinal. Other classes of cases of secondary cancer are those which either follow a similar disease in the breast, in its later stages offshoots passing directly through the chest wall and invading the pleura and mediastinum, or the complaint breaking out again after the removal of this organ by operation; or those which result from extension of the mischief, through the lymphatics of the diaphragm, from the peritoneum, stomach, liver, or kidneys. From a practical point of view, however, such modes of origin are mere pathological curiosities.

Different statements have been made as to the nature of carcinoma in the mediastinum. According to Douglas Powell (35), scirrhus is the most frequent form; such is also my experience. Encephaloid or epithelioma may occur as secondary growths. On the other hand, Hertz affirms that it is usually medullary, and rarely scirrhus or epithelioma. With regard to the 134 cases of supposed mediastinal cancer collected by Hare, in only 61 was the nature of the growth stated. Among these encephaloid is decidedly more frequent than scirrhus, in the proportion of more than 2 to 1; and as exceptional growths are mentioned colloid, endothelioma, melanotic cancer, and sarcoma carcinomatodes.

2. Sarcoma.—Whatever view be held as to their relative frequency, sarcomatous growths must be recognised as one of the most important groups of intra-thoracic tumours, whether primary or secondary. Moreover, not uncommonly they manifest very distinctly the characters of malignancy, especially in the later stages. The varieties that may be met with are round-celled, spindle-celled, and lympho-sarcoma; the last-mentioned being of special consequence as a primary growth. Steven affirms that of all malignant tumours sarcomata are more likely to be soon complicated by the development of secondary tumours within the chest, and my experience certainly agrees with this statement. Sarcoma of any kind very rarely occurs in the lung primarily; but this organ may be involved by extension, and secondary growths of this nature from remote sources of infection are decidedly more frequent in the lung than in other intra-thoracic structures. Hare, however, speaks of the lungs as being very rarely affected by primary or secondary sarcomatous formations. A secondary growth from the mediastinum generally extends through the glands at the root of the lung, and then along the bronchial tubes and blood-vessels to the lung-tissues. Wilson Fox affirmed that sarcoma in the lung is only secondary, and usually to sarcoma of bone, the lung being the place of selection. Separate pulmonary nodules may be found after mediastinal lympho-sarcoma. Next to the mediastinal tissues the pleura appears to be the chief point in the chest where sarcoma occurs as a primary growth; and Hare states that in nearly every case of secondary mediastinal sarcoma it has been primary in the pleura. Several cases have been reported in which this kind of tumour had arisen from the subpleural tissue, and afterwards encroached upon the mediastinum. Such mediastinal tumours seem to be not uncommon in very young children. Dr. R. S. Thomson showed a case of this kind at the Glasgow Pathological and Clinical Society, in which a tumour was believed to be of subpleural origin, and was composed of "small spindle-celled sarcomatous tissue combined with a large amount of very fibrous connective tissue."

The mediastinum is the seat of origin of the large majority of sarcomata within the chest; and, as already mentioned, many eminent authors regard lympho-sarcoma as the most frequent primary mediastinal growth. Powell (35) goes so far as to say that a primary sarcoma in this region is almost invariably lymphomatous. It is a matter of general agreement that the glands are the usual starting-point for the growth, especially the anterior mediastinal or bronchial; but this is by no means invariably the case. The fact is fully recognised that it is often difficult at the necropsy to say precisely where a mediastinal tumour has originated; but its situation and characters (even when there are large nodulated masses), as well as its histological structure, are very suggestive of glandular origin. Writing on this point Steven holds the name lympho-sarcoma to indicate "that variety of sarcoma which both by its naked-eye appearances and its histological characters is to be looked upon as originating in connection with the lymphatic glands—that is, a sarcoma of the lymphatic glands. In this sense a lympho-sarcoma is to be regarded as a variety of sarcoma, in the same way as a cylinder-celled epithelioma as a variety of epithelioma originating in connection with the cylinder-celled structures of the intestinal mucous membrane. Thus, a lympho-sarcoma may originate in one gland, or in a part of one gland, and in its growth may surround and involve neighbouring glands, which may be quite recognisable in the midst of the tumour tissue." Steven strongly argues against any relationship between mediastinal lympho-sarcoma and Hodgkin's disease, even though certain other glands should become affected; and with this view I fully agree. He writes: "With an enormous mass in the mediastinum pressing more or less upon the main lymphatic channels, at or near the points where they pass into the venous system, we need not wonder if a number of the lymphatic glands become enlarged. But this, indeed, is a very different thing from a general morbid process affecting all the lymphatic glands of the body altogether independently of any secondary pressure effects." A lympho-sarcoma in the mediastinum may be associated with a similar condition in the neck. In one case mentioned by Wilson Fox there was a very large sarcomatous mass in the lung and another in the mediastinum.

In addition to the pleural and subpleural tissue already mentioned, it seems certain that a sarcomatous growth may arise from the sternal periosteum, and from the remains of the thymus body. Dr. Rolleston has described a tumour originating from this gland (40), which presented the structure of a hæmorrhagic adeno-chondro-sarcoma.

Secondary mediastinal sarcoma is very unusual, and, according to Hare, even when this growth is extensively distributed the mediastinum seems to escape. He states that next to the pleura come the abdominal viscera as the primary seat; and that the secondary tumour may arise either from direct extension through the diaphragm along the œsophagus, or from metastasis. Steven thinks it not at all unlikely that if a secondary sarcomatous mass does fill the mediastinum it has spread from the lung. It may, however, follow a similar disease in the arm or leg, or in any part of the body; and may occur after amputation for sarcoma of bone, of which I have met with some interesting and striking examples. Hare observes that "where the disease is primary in an arm, the secondary growth not infrequently occurs in the mediastinum, comparatively speaking, while sarcoma in the leg, as a general rule, attacks secondarily the abdominal viscera rather than the tissues above the diaphragm." I am not aware whether this statement holds good, but certainly, according to my experience, there are remarkable exceptions to such a rule. Primary mediastinal sarcoma, especially lympho-sarcoma, is apt to be followed by secondary metastatic growths in distant organs, so that a case may ultimately become more or less complicated. Nodules of a similar structure may thus form in the liver, spleen, and kidneys. The tumour in the mediastinum secondary to sarcoma in remote parts, generally belongs to the round-celled or spindle-celled varieties of this growth; but it may be osteoid or enchondromatous, and the same remark applies to the lung.

3. **Miscellaneous growths.**—It is necessary to offer a few general remarks, from a pathological point of view, about some of the other kinds of tumour mentioned in the list previously given, but which are of exceptional occurrence. With regard to *lymphoma* and *lymphadenoma*, Hare gives a table of twenty-one cases of mediastinal growths which he includes under these names; but Steven is decidedly of opinion that a number of these cases might with perfect accuracy have been relegated to the table of lympho-sarcoma. Most pathologists do not make any distinction between these names, but Hare regards them as of different significance, and states "that as a general rule lymphoma is more frequently benign than is lymphadenoma, and is in a very large proportion of cases solitary rather than multiple." It is quite possible, I think, that from local causes a group of lymphatic glands in the chest may become so enlarged as to constitute a tumour; and, of course, as already stated, these glands may be involved either primarily or secondarily in cases of Hodgkin's disease; it seems hardly possible, however, to indicate any definite histological differences between the two kinds of growth.

Fibroma is a definite variety of tumour to be borne in mind in relation to the mediastinum, though it is very rare. Hare collected seven cases. It may start from the sternum or the cellular tissue. It does not occur in the lung, but *fibro-plastic* growths have been described in this organ, both primary and secondary. Mediastinal fibroma is solitary, and seldom reaches any large size, but it may do so. It is of very slow growth.

The structure may be fibro-cellular or fibro-fatty, but is generally dense and fibrous. *Fibro-sarcoma* has also been described. Steven gives an account of a case which he regarded as a fibrous tissue tumour of the mediastinum, and which he names "malignant fibrosis," associated with pronounced rheumatic manifestations; and he believed the growth to be of rheumatic origin.

Teratoma or *dermoid cyst* is another variety of mediastinal tumour which, though of very infrequent occurrence, must not be forgotten. Hare collected ten cases, and states that the mediastinum occupies the fourth position as the site of this condition. Examples have been since reported from time to time, and out of forty-two cases of mediastinal growth, collected by Rumpf in 1894, five were dermoid cysts. The cyst originates as an embryonal development during fœtal life, either from dipping in of the skin of the neck, or out of remnants of germinal folds. It does not, however, give any clinical indications of its presence until long after birth; every patient reported in Hare's list was over twenty years of age. He explains this by the fact that while the cyst is a product of a fœtal life, the walls keep on developing and secreting after the child is born; and as a consequence the cyst must increase and with it the signs of its presence. It is affirmed that a teratoma never originates in the lung, and if found in this organ must have extended from the mediastinum. Such a tumour has, however, been operated upon in the lung by Mr. Godlee and others; and a specimen was recently brought before the Pathological Society, by Dr. Cyril Ogle, in which a dermoid growth was embedded in the lung, and apparently grew from the wall of a dilated large bronchus, but it probably originated in the mediastinum. In structure the tumour consists of a unilocular or multilocular cyst, containing sebaceous glands and matter, sweat-glands, hair, teeth, and sometimes fragments of bone or cartilage; the former in some instances closely resembling the superior maxilla. In a specimen exhibited before the Pathological Society, by Dr. Hale White, in 1890, the cyst, which was about the size of a Tangerine orange, and attached to the pericardium, was filled with a dirty yellowish fluid containing cholesterin and oil-globules, with a large quantity of solid sebaceous material, and some hairs loosely attached to its interior.

It is hardly necessary to make any special observations with regard to such growths as *hydatids, syphilitic gumma*, and *tuberculous glands* in the mediastinum. They have to be remembered as possible varieties of tumours in this region, but their nature and origin are well understood, and they do not call for any description here. Syphilitic growths may certainly originate in the bony structures and extend inwards. While tuberculous glands are very common in the chest, it is only in exceptional cases that they attain such a size as to be regarded as tumours. Most of the others mentioned in the preliminary list are mere pathological curiosities. *Myeloid, osteoid, enchondroma*, and *ossifying enchondroma* are now and then met with as primary growths in the lung, but when they do occur they are chiefly secondary. Chondroma of the soft parts is almost unknown, except when associated with sarcoma or other growth. *Osteo-chondroma* or *enchondroma* may grow inwards from the cartilaginous or bony structures forming the thoracic walls. A case of enchondroma of the right lung and lymphatic glands has been reported by Dr. Dalton.

ETIOLOGY.—Several of the more important questions relating to the causation of intra-thoracic growths and tumours have been discussed in the preceding section, and it will only be necessary to draw attention here to a few additional points. It must be acknowledged that the precise etiology of primary growths in this region is very obscure ; and in a large proportion of cases no definite or even probable cause can be traced. Hereditary proclivity may account partly for some malignant tumours ; or they may fairly be looked upon in many instances as manifestations of a special diathesis, favoured by local circumstances ; this particularly applies to cancerous growths. By some pathologists lympho-sarcoma is included among specific new formations or infective tumours, but others are opposed to such a view. Syphilitic and tuberculous forma-tions are of course mere local developments of these conditions ; and, as already stated, fibroma is regarded by Steven as a rheumatic manifestation. The growth last mentioned may, however, be associated with caries of the sternum or vertebræ ; and in some instances it can only be regarded as an exaggerated local result of chronic mediastinitis. Individual cases of tumour in the chest have been attributed to prolonged pressure in connection with occupation, a blow or other injury, or taking cold ; but the real influence of such antecedents is very difficult to estimate. It is quite possible that in some instances local irritation or injury of different kinds, which is not evident, may have an effect in starting a growth under favouring circumstances, and this especially applies to those originating in the œsophagus. Hare thinks that "sarcoma is much more frequently produced by pressure on the chest by foreign bodies, or like causes, than is cancer, probably owing to the fact that the tissues par-ticularly favourable to sarcoma are the ones most generally affected by such causes." The idea of infection by the breath has been advanced to account for some malignant growths in the lung, but is hardly tenable.

The influence of *age* and *sex* in relation to intra-thoracic growths, especially those of a cancerous or sarcomatous nature, demands brief notice, but there are marked discrepancies between the conclusions of different observers. With regard to *age*, it may be affirmed that no age is exempt, even from early childhood—though very exceptionally—to advanced life,—70 years or more. Among Hare's cases one is men-tioned of encephaloid in the mediastinum where the patient was only 4 years old ; and a case has been reported by Dr. Angel Money in an infant 18 months old. Cancer of the lung, according to Walshe's tables (quoted by Wilson Fox), is most common in middle and advancing life ; and Walshe expressed the opinion that if the mortality from this disease could be compared with that of the population living at each decade, it would be found regularly to increase up to the eightieth year.

In these tables the largest proportion of cases are between 20 and 30, and 40 and 50 years of age; and 46 per cent are below 40: in one instance the patient was under 10, and twelve more were under 20. Taking all mediastinal tumours together, of fifty-five cases collected by Eger, 67 per cent were under 40. Douglas Powell (35) states that true cancer in this region rarely occurs before middle life. Hare concludes that most mediastinal growths occur in adults. Hertz says that they are chiefly met with in the young and middle-aged, from 20 to 40; most cases from 20 to 30. It is generally agreed that lympho-sarcoma and other sarcomatous growths occur at an earlier period of life than cancer; and undoubtedly the largest number of cases of this kind are met with in the decade from 20 to 30. Powell says that, in contrast to true cancer, they are more prevalent before than after middle life.

In relation to *sex* Walshe maintained that there is no difference. Cancer of the lung appears on the whole to be more frequent in males. Taking all mediastinal growths together, the general conclusion is that there is a large preponderance in males; and this conclusion is supported by the cases collected by Hare, in which this point was noted, both as regards cancer and sarcoma, the proportion being more than two to one; it applies also to the other tumours in this region. Douglas Powell, however, states that sarcoma is more frequent in females, cancer rather more prevalent in males (35).

ANATOMICAL CHARACTERS.—It is a difficult matter to determine how far it is desirable to enter here into the consideration of the morbid anatomy of intra-thoracic growths; obviously the limits of this article forbid much detailed description of the several varieties, or of their histological structure; and it will only be necessary under this heading to deal specially with cancer and sarcoma, sufficient account having already been given of the characters of such of the exceptional kinds of tumour as seemed to require more than mere enumeration.

Some cases of morbid growth within the chest can hardly be spoken of as tumours, seeing that they take the form of infiltrations; but even these may produce considerable masses, and their effects may be very pronounced and definite. They vary much in their situation, extent and size, rapidity of development, and as regards the structures which they involve during their progress, as well as in the way in which they affect them; and these differences depend to a great degree on the nature of the particular growth, as exemplified by hard and soft cancers, lympho-sarcoma, and such limited and slowly-increasing tumours as fibroma or teratoma. With these preliminary observations I now proceed to call attention to the more important facts relating to the morbid anatomy of growths in the lung, pleura, and mediastinum respectively.

1. Lungs.—New growths in these organs may take the form either of infiltrations or distinct tumours, or these modes of arrangement may be associated in the same case. Most of the non-malignant varieties belong to the group of tumours, being either encapsuled, or surrounded by more or less condensed pulmonary tissue. In a case reported by

Clifford Allbutt, however, a primary myeloid growth appeared as an infiltration.

Cancer affecting the lungs may be met with under either of the varieties already mentioned, or rarely two kinds are present in the same case. The general distinction between separate tumours or nodules and infiltration must be recognised in growths of this nature, though they present considerable differences in detail in different cases. Primary cancer is not infrequently confined to a single lung, and it is usually stated the right lung especially, though statistics differ on this point; secondary cancer as a rule affects both organs. The latter, moreover, generally assumes a tuberous or nodulated form, and is most abundant near the periphery; while the infiltrated variety is in the majority of cases primary, being limited to one lung. It will be convenient to deal further with the more important points relating to this class of morbid conditions under the following heads. It may be remarked that such names as "cancerous pneumonia" or "cancerous phthisis" ought not to be employed at the present day.

(*a*) *Mode of distribution and extension.*—When malignant disease in the lung occurs in the form of separate tumour, there may be but one such growth, of large size, which generally extends from the root into the central portion; but it may be quite distinct. In other cases the growth is multiple and disseminated, varying in size from a hazel nut or walnut to a Maltese orange; such cases might be described as the "nodular" and "tuberous" group. These growths are at first isolated; but in their progress and development, which in the softer varieties is sometimes very rapid, they often become so incorporated together, that a large portion or even a whole lung may ultimately be involved. In a third group malignant disease presents a miliary appearance and mode of dissemination in the pulmonary tissues—"miliary carcinomatosis"—resembling tubercle, but differing from this morbid growth in that the apices and upper parts of the lungs are not specially implicated, and may be quite free. The cancerous material is then more or less thickly scattered through the lung, in small nodules, ranging in size from a lentil or millet seed to that of a pea. A class of cases occasionally met with consists of those in which the growths are chiefly subpleural, occurring either as flattened masses, from a quarter of an inch to an inch in diameter, semi-transparent or dull white, and compared to drops of wax; or extending more deeply into the lung, and acquiring a cupped, umbilicated, cupulated, or mushroom-like appearance. From these growths bands may also proceed into the interior of the organ for a variable distance.

The infiltrating form of cancer was described by Wilson Fox under two chief types. One is a general infiltration of the pulmonary tissues, which may fill large tracts of the lung with an almost uniform mass, in which, however, traces of the lobular tissue of the lung are still preserved; the other is more uniform, and in appearance and firmness may closely resemble the gray pneumonia attending tuberculisation. These conditions may involve the whole or nearly the whole of a lung. In the other variety the infiltration proceeds in the course of the interlobular septa, from which the growth may extend directly into the pulmonary tissue, or along the bronchi and blood-vessels, contracting their calibre, and greatly thickening their walls. These modes of extension may coexist.

While recognising the general distinction between tumours and infiltrations, it must be understood that they may occur together in various combinations. "The mode of extension of true cancer into the alveolar tissue of the lung is probably in all cases practically identical . . . namely, by the growth from the alveolar and interlobular tissue of hetero-logous cells and stroma, which replace and destroy the natural elements; and the same holds true for the growths which occur in the peribronchial and perivascular sheaths, and which thence extend into the walls of the air vesicles " (Wilson Fox).

(b) *Effects on the lung.*—Cancer of the lung is likely to cause either an increase or a diminution in the bulk of the organ, but it may remain of normal size. Enlargement is usually associated with more or less thickly disseminated growths, or when these are incorporated together; but is occasionally observed in connection with infiltration. The latter more commonly tends to produce contraction and puckering, with altera-tion in shape. The lung may be so contracted and puckered as to give it an appearance resembling that of a hobnailed liver. These changes are especially pronounced when there is a great thickening of the pleura, and when hard cancer extends inwards along the septa and bronchi, or in bands from subpleural tumours. There is always increase in weight, which may be very considerable, and the lung feels remarkably heavy. The effect of malignant disease upon the pulmonary tissues not actually involved is usually to cause congestion and compression, but they may be quite normal. Possibly inflammation may be set up occasionally, or even suppuration around cancerous masses. In one of Steven's cases, a primary cancer at the root of the lung had set up a widespread gray hepatisation. The condensation of lung is sometimes very marked, and the investment of a tumour by a "condensed zone" may give it the appearance of being "encysted," a condition which certainly does not occur in connection with malignant growths here; though it may with sarcoma in other parts of the body. In individual cases the compressed lung has been described as forming a kind of cap to a tumour growing from below, or as a thin layer covering a tumour occupying nearly the whole substance of the organ. Hæmorrhages or infarctions occasion-ally supervene; and diffuse pulmonary apoplexy has been found around tumours growing in the lung. It may happen that a tumour projecting from a lung presses on the main bronchus, and produces the changes in different degrees which result from such pressure from any cause. With the extension of cancer into the pulmonary tissue all distinctions of its structures tend to disappear; but the vessels and bronchi resist the longest. The lymphatic vessels around isolated tumours may be dis-tended with cancerous matter; and it is affirmed that the disease may be limited to these vessels, and may nowhere extend into the tissue of the lung.

(c) *Secondary changes.*—Malignant growths in the lung sometimes undergo destructive changes, which must be duly recognised. They may thus become the seat of fatty degeneration and softening; or abscesses may form, followed by cavities. Suppuration around cancerous masses may give rise to an appearance like metastatic abscesses, and the lung may be found riddled with cavities. Such abscesses in rare instances have dissected the pleura from the lung over a considerable area, or have even perforated the pulmonary pleura. A cancerous cavity in the lung has been found as the sole disease. A destructive process with suppuration may take place at the base of a lung, and simulate empyema. Extravasation of blood into malignant pulmonary growths occurs not uncommonly.

(d) *Morbid appearances and characters.*—Taking into account the differences in the nature, extent, and arrangement of malignant growths in the lung, the changes they may undergo, and their effects upon the pulmonary tissues, it will be readily understood that the appearances presented on section must necessarily vary a good deal, and no general description can be given. It would not serve any useful purpose to enlarge on this point, and it will suffice to mention some of the special appearances noted in individual cases,—in addition to those already described. It may be observed that the growths themselves differ much in physical characters as regards colour, vascularity, and consistence, according to their nature. Some are soft and easily broken-down or even pulpy; others are very hard and resistant. Soft infiltrations along the interlobular septa may look like purulent infiltration; when hard and dense they may give to large tracts a reticulate appearance, the condensed pulmonary tissue being mapped out in more or less regular spaces between the thickened septa. In extensive cancer the lung has been described as "transformed into a white, solid, lardaceous mass, totally destitute of nerves, blood-vessels, and bronchial tubes," and I have met with two specimens closely answering to this description. Another variety is that in which the organ is converted into a dense substance resembling a section of fresh pork, in which the lobular structure is still very conspicuous, but the blood-vessels and bronchi are either compressed or obliterated. "The latter appearance is not uncommon in some forms of sarcomata; whereas in cancerous growths the infiltration is often more gray in colour, mingled with pigment, or interspersed with areas of greater vascularity—a characteristic which predominates in some of the forms of so-called 'fungus hæmatodes'" (Wilson Fox). In exceptional instances a malignant growth in the lung is distinctly melanotic, or exhibits the characters of colloid cancer. The occurrence of hæmorrhage or degenerative softening will probably materially alter the original appearance of tumours in the lung. Cavities resulting from their destruction present irregular, anfractuous, ragged, and ulcerous walls which show no tendency to limitation or reparative changes.

Sarcomata in the lung may appear as independent growths, or as an evident extension from a mediastinal tumour of similar nature. Steven, writing of mediastinal sarcoma, draws attention as a very striking feature to the readiness with which it spreads in upon and works up the pulmonary tissue in an irregular and crab-like manner, simulating cancer. Very frequently the encroachment takes place along the bronchial tubes, which may be entirely destroyed; but sometimes the tumour moulds itself directly to the edge of the lung and begins to work it up. He has also observed in a museum specimen appearances suggestive of the tumour growing into pulmonary cavities. Hare describes growths secondary to mediastinal sarcoma as being "found scattered through the lung tissue, varying in size from a walnut to an orange, and having, as a general rule, a soft and spongy character, although this may, in some cases, be replaced by the variety known as multiple osteoid sarcoma, in which the tumour is so hard as to be cut only with great difficulty with a knife." Sarcomata in the lung may form very large tumours. They are, as a rule, soft and friable, white or yellowish white, and in general appearance resemble encephaloid cancer more or less. They may, however, present different degrees of firmness, due to intermixture of the fibrous element. In a case described by Dr. Arthur Davies the whole left side of the chest was filled by a hard mass of new growth, scarcely any lung substance being visible. The left lung cut with difficulty, and presented a mottled appearance and yellow colour; the growth was most distinct along the pleural cavity. Microscopic sections showed it to be round-celled lympho-sarcoma, which completely filled up the alveoli.

2. **Pleura.** —Malignant growths involving this structure, whether primary or secondary, assume different forms. There may be a general uniform infiltration, greatly increasing the thickness of the membrane, and affecting in some cases almost exclusively the parietal pleura, sparing the bones and muscles, but invading and thickening the mediastinal tissues with a growth of scirrhous character. Another variety is the tuberiform, in which enormous fungoid masses project from the surface into the pleural sac, and may become so pedunculated as to lose all apparent connection with the lung, hanging like grapes from the pleura, to which they may be attached by a narrow pedicle. In other instances scattered nodules are found on both the visceral and parietal membrane; or both nodules and infiltration may be present together. Prolongations from the pleura into the interior of the lung may or may not take place. The growth is likely to extend into the interlobar pleura, binding the lobes of the lung together. Pleural effusion is said to be common, and not infrequently hæmorrhagic; but, on the other hand, the sac may be entirely obliterated by the dense adhesions between the surfaces. In one of Dr. Harris' cases very great difficulty was experienced in removing the lung from the body, the growth having to be cut away from the chest wall, and the diaphragm removed with the lung and the growth. The organ was completely encapsuled by a mass of very firm, hard, white, new growth, with

trabeculæ like bands of fibrous tissue, which varied in thickness from half an inch to two inches, being thickest over the diaphragm. The interlobar pleura was also invaded by the new growth and everywhere thickened. The pleural cavity was practically obliterated. The lung was compressed, but still contained air; it was not infiltrated by the growth, nor was there any extension from the hilum along the course of the bronchi. The naked-eye and microscopical appearances were those of a primary cylindrical-celled endothelioma of the pleura. In Dr. Harris' second case the left pleural cavity was entirely obliterated, and the lung firmly adherent. The pleura was found everywhere thickened by a fine white new growth, which not only encased the lung but also extended into that organ from the hilum along the bronchi, and by delicate bands from various parts over its surface. The lymphatic glands in the hilum and mediastinum were likewise involved. The thickening was not nearly so great as in the first case, but generally ranged from one-eighth to a quarter of an inch. The growth presented on microscopical examination all the features of a squamous epithelioma (.22).

3. **Mediastinum.**—The first point to be noticed in relation to the morbid anatomy of mediastinal growths is their situation, in respect of the divisions of the space in which they are found. According to some writers, primary cancer is most frequent in the posterior mediastinum; and Steven properly points out that, considering the origin of cancer in epithelial tissues, this is the most likely place for a primary carcinoma to develop within the chest, where we have the epithelial structures of the trachea, bronchi, and œsophagus to afford a starting-point for the disease. Hare's statistics, however, give three to one in favour of the anterior mediastinum alone, while this lead is considerably increased if the cases starting from the anterior mediastinum and penetrating the other mediastinal divisions be taken into consideration. He maintains that all primary growths are far more frequent in the anterior division than in other parts of the mediastinum. Wilson Fox stated that primary tumours are nearly twice as often in the anterior as the posterior mediastinum. The latter division comes next in order; or there may be independent growths in both parts. The middle mediastinum is very rarely affected alone. Extension from one division to another is not uncommon, and occasionally the entire space is ultimately involved by carcinoma or sarcoma. In exceptional cases the growth may be fairly described as occupying the superior mediastinum. When sarcoma is secondary, it appears to affect most frequently the posterior or middle division. As already pointed out, the mediastinum may be invaded by a growth originating in the lung, pleura, or subpleural tissue, or in the chest wall.

The size, extent, shape, and rapidity of growth, as well as the characters of mediastinal growths, vary considerably according to their nature, already sufficiently discussed. Hence no comprehensive description can be given. In general terms they may be classified as solitary tumours of different sizes; multiple small or large tumours united into one mass, usually irregular or lobulated; and diffuse infiltrations. Hæmorrhage into their substance, or degenerative changes, with softening, may alter materially their original characters. The softer growths are likely to make rapid progress; and those which begin in the glands, once they break through their capsules, tend speedily to infiltrate the mediastinal space generally. A tumour starting in the mediastinum may grow upwards into the neck, or downwards into the abdomen.

While it is not practicable to give any general description of mediastinal tumours, it appears desirable to point out the chief characters of lympho-sarcomatous growths in this region. They usually give rise to an irregularly lobulated tumour, evidently composed of agglomerated glands, often of considerable size, superficially firm to the touch, and sometimes surrounded entirely or partially by a dense fibrous tissue or capsule. The growth may, however, be remarkably adherent to surrounding structures. On section it is generally white or yellowish-white, but may be very vascular, or even exhibit minute hæmorrhages scattered through its substance. Its consistence is usually soft and friable, and a white creamy juice sometimes escapes on section. A lympho-sarcoma may, however, be hard and cartilaginous, as in a case of Dr. Mott's. Microscopical examination shows small round or oval-shaped cells, with a delicate connective tissue stroma.

Effects of intra-thoracic tumours upon adjacent structures.—In the introductory remarks to this article a summary is given of the different ways in which the neighbouring structures may be affected by diseases of the mediastinum. The effects thus produced assume a peculiar importance in relation to intra-thoracic tumours, whatever their origin may be, but more especially when they encroach upon the mediastinal space, and therefore call for somewhat detailed consideration in the present connection. It will be readily understood that these effects differ widely according to the situation, anatomical relations, and dimensions of a growth; while there may be more than one tumour. Moreover, they vary materially with the nature of the growth, and before dealing with individual structures it is desirable to offer a few general remarks on this point. Localised non-malignant tumours merely lead to such physical consequences as their situation happens to involve, as the result of pressure or irritation; and they do not tend in any way to implicate adjacent structures. "Malignant growths, be their variety what it may, have certain peculiarities as to their development when in the mediastinum which they do not possess elsewhere, at least to so marked a degree. For example, mediastinal cancer does not confine itself as a general rule to any one or two tissues, but makes its onward march, involving whatever may come in its path" (Hare). When of a hard scirrhous nature, however, it tends to remain circumscribed; encephaloid, on the other hand, spreads rapidly and over a considerable area, usually soon attacking different healthy structures in its progress. Steven affirms that cancer, as a rule, does not become so bulky as a sarcoma; while in its growth it steadily infiltrates, and causes ulceration of everything coming into contact with it. This may occur, moreover, with a minimum of growth of the tumour as regards its bulk. Hence it happens that cancer not only invades, but causes ulceration and perforation of tubes or vessels, severs nerves, erodes bones, and produces like destructive effects. In his very instructive and interesting discussion of the local relation-ships of mediastinal sarcoma, this writer brings into prominence certain important peculiarities. He first mentions that the effects of a sarco-matous tumour may vary a good deal according to the form which is present. A subpleural sarcoma may simply cause pressure effects, crush-ing the organs aside without involving them to any great extent. This is explained by the fact that it is prone to present itself as a single rounded mass, with a very considerable fibrous basis. Mediastinal lympho-sarcoma exhibits well-marked local malignancy, which plays an important part in determining the relationship of the tumour. One of the features of these growths, which Steven regards as perhaps the most characteristic, is the manner in which they mould themselves round the great tubular (trachea and œsophagus) and vascular structures of the upper portion of the thoracic cavity, without actually implicating them. He describes the aorta, and large arteries springing from it, as often com-pletely buried in the midst of the tumour; but, as a general rule, by careful dissection the morbid tissue can be pretty completely separated from the arterial wall. The veins suffer much more severely than the arteries, and may present well-marked intravenous growths of the morbid tissue. Dr. Maguire has expressed the opinion that "lympho-sarcomata have little, if any, tendency to destroy the endothelium lining the vessels which they invade, whereas ordinary sarcomata ulcerate into the vessels and cause hæmorrhages." With this opinion Steven does not agree. He describes changes in the bronchi which will be more conveniently referred to later on. The relationship of a lympho-sarcomatous growth to the nerve trunks of the thorax which it happens to implicate is of a similar nature. They are often found to pass into and to become buried in the midst of the tumour, but they are merely surrounded, and may be flattened but not destroyed. In a case of lympho-sarcoma of the neck Steven was able to find and to dissect out the pneumogastric nerve.

Another peculiarity of lympho-sarcomatous tumours of the media-stinum, upon which Steven lays stress, is their tendency to grow in the direction of least resistance. He calls attention to the manner in which sarcomata of this region insinuate themselves in and out between the different structures in their neighbourhood, and adds, "Bulky and lobulated as most lympho-sarcomata of the interior of the thorax are, they do not simply crush the organs aside, as many other varieties of tumour would do. You find processes of the growth peeping out beneath the arch of the aorta, pushing their way upwards beneath the clavicles into the triangles of the neck, insinuating themselves between, and applying themselves around the great vessels of the root of the neck and the bronchial stems; and all this without there necessarily being any actual incorporation of the surrounded structures and tissues into the substance of the tumour itself, at least in the first instance. In this way the growth of a thoracic sarcoma differs in the most marked manner from that of a primary cancer within the chest." My experience agrees with his, that sarcoma occupying this region never causes erosion of bone.

It will now be convenient to indicate the possible effects of intra-thoracic growths upon the more important structures connected with this region, so far as these have a practical bearing upon the clinical history and progress of individual cases.

Apart from tumours originating in the respiratory apparatus itself, and setting aside functional disorders which arise from interference with nerves, this system is very liable to be directly affected in some part or other by mediastinal growths. The trachea is often compressed, and may be so narrowed as to leave only a small fissure; or it is surrounded by lympho-sarcomatous tissue which can be separated from the tube. It may, however, become itself involved by a cancerous growth, but is very rarely perforated. In a case already referred to, however, which came under my care, such perforation had taken place, and this event proved of great importance in relation to diagnosis. Obstruction may occur at the bifurcation of the trachea. A main bronchus is often interfered with by pressure, being flattened, and its channel becoming much narrowed or even obliterated; or it is directly implicated in a growth at the root of the lung, which may penetrate it, or, as already described, may extend along its divisions into the substance of the organ. Moreover, independent small tumours may develop in these structures, projecting into their interior, of which cases have been reported by the late Dr. Bristowe, Dr. Theodore Williams, and other observers. With regard to lympho-sarcoma Steven writes: " The bronchi very frequently suffer severely from the local malignancy of lympho-sarcomatous mediastinal tumours. The whole normal histological structure of the bronchial wall may entirely disappear, nothing being left but a channel, more or less narrowed, through the tumour tissue. . . . It is not at all unlikely that in many cases the bronchial tubes may be very considerably dilated, the bronchiectasis being partly due to the local action of the tumour on the bronchial wall, and partly to paralytic conditions induced by pressure on nerves and plexuses."

The conditions which may be produced in the lung itself by mediastinal tumours, besides its secondary implication, demand special attention. They vary a good deal under different circumstances. Either organ may be merely compressed, sometimes so completely as to become practically airless. More or less collapse also usually results from obstruction of the main bronchus. On the other hand, distension of the air-vesicles occurs from the slighter degrees of pressure; or there may be a combination of collapse and distension in different parts of the same lung; while if one organ is compressed or collapsed the opposite one will probably undergo compensatory enlargement. Bronchiectasis may follow compression of bronchi. In rare instances interlobular and subpleural emphysema has been observed. Another group of pulmonary conditions which may be associated with a mediastinal tumour are congestion, œdema, and sometimes hæmorrhage. Congestion may arise merely from grave interference with the respiratory function ; or it may be hypostatic in patients confined to bed. Œdema and hæmorrhage have been attributed in most cases to pressure on and obstruction of the pulmonary veins. The hæmorrhage may be in the form of partially discoloured infarcts, or it may consolidate the greater part of a lung. Thrombosis of the branches of the pulmonary artery occasionally occurs, or this vessel may be invaded by a growth.

Lesions of an inflammatory nature not uncommonly involve one or both lungs in cases of mediastinal tumour ; and destructive changes may take place, occasionally ending in gangrene. As the result of obstruction of the air-tubes, bronchitis with excessive secretion is very common, and the secretion may be extremely dense and adhesive. Purulent material may collect in bronchi or dilated bronchi, giving rise to the appearance of scattered puriform spots, general purulent infiltration, abscesses, or cavities. Pneumonia, with red or gray hepatisation, is sometimes produced, and catarrhal pneumonia may follow collapse. Destructive and gangrenous lesions have been attributed to various causes, including chiefly obstruction of the bronchial arteries ; compression or invasion of the pneumogastric nerve, or of the pulmonary plexus at the root of the lung ; direct pressure on the pulmonary tissue ; implication of the pulmonary arteries ; and accumulation of retained secretions in the bronchi. The last-mentioned was believed by Wilson Fox to be the most probable cause in the majority of cases, and he thought it " may account for some of the occasional cases where gangrene or abscess has been found in the lung on the side opposite to that affected by the cancer, and of which the most probable explanation would appear to be in the hypothesis of the gravitation of these secretions at the bifurcation of the bronchi from one side to the other." With regard to the mode in which interference with nerves is supposed to produce its effects on the lungs, they have been referred to direct nutritive disturbances (Budd) ; paralysis of the bronchial tubes (Gull) ; or the passage of food or saliva into the larynx, as the result of paralysis, these materials thus gaining access into the bronchial tubes. The last seems to be the most probable explanation, and this cause has actually been found after death, while inflammatory changes in the lung following experimental section of the pneumogastric nerve have been shown to be induced in this way. The various organisms which are known to produce the changes in the lung now under consideration, will of course have ample scope for their action in many cases of intra-thoracic tumour, and it is to these organisms that the lesions just mentioned must be directly attributed.

The pleura must always be borne in mind in mediastinal tumour, altogether apart from its primary or secondary implication by a morbid growth, or the projection of such a growth into the pleural space.

Effusion into this cavity is common, and in a certain proportion of cases it is sero-sanguinolent or hæmorrhagic; but too much reliance must not be placed on this latter point from a clinical aspect, for the fluid is in most cases perfectly clear. In very rare instances it is bilateral. Pleural effusion may result either from pressure on the pulmonary veins or vena azygos, or from irritation and consequent inflammation. All malignant tumours in the mediastinum have a great tendency to excite inflammation of the serous membranes with which they come immediately into contact; and it appears to be usually of a very acute and inten e character, the effusion hence being sanguinolent, and the fibrinous exudation being often very abundant. Empyema is extremely rare, but may occur. Possibly pulmonary hæmorrhage resulting from a tumour may cause rupture of the pleura and consequent hæmothorax.

The structures next to be considered in relation to the effects of intra-thoracic growths are the pericardium, heart, and great vessels. The pericardium is very liable to be involved in the progress of a tumour, and it may become completely surrounded and incorporated, or nodules form in its interior. Pericardial effusion is not uncommon; and acute pericarditis of a severe type may supervene, sometimes hæmorrhagic, very rarely purulent. The cardiac walls may be invaded from the pericardium, or direct extension of a growth has been known to take place from the superior vena cava into the right auricle, or from the pulmonary vein into the left auricle. The heart is often displaced in various directions by a tumour within the chest, sometimes considerably; and the organ may be thus much embarrassed. Occasionally it appears to be compressed by a surrounding growth.

The aorta and its branches are much less frequently and severely interfered with than the veins, but one or more of the large arteries may be compressed or even obliterated. The aorta has even been perforated by a cancerous growth, leading to fatal hæmorrhage. Allusion has already been made to Steven's description of this vessel and its branches being buried in lympho-sarcomatous tissue, which can be completely separated by careful dissection.

The large intra-thoracic veins are very liable to suffer from the effects of tumours, being often compressed or obliterated, or sometimes directly invaded. Steven observed in some of his specimens that lympho-sarcoma exhibited well-marked intravenous growths, and to this he attaches considerable importance. The superior vena cava or either of its larger branches may be implicated, and very rarely the inferior vena cava. The vena azygos is occasionally affected; but this vessel may also be greatly dilated as the result of an impediment in the superior vena cava.

With regard to the nerves, the pneumogastric or recurrent laryngeal are much the most commonly affected. Within a comparatively recent period I have met with two cases, in one of which the right, and in the other the left recurrent nerve was involved in a tumour. The phrenic is very rarely implicated. In most cases the nerves are merely flattened out by pressure; but when they pass through a growth all traces of them may be lost. The pneumogastric has been found, however, to traverse a tumour unchanged, as in Steven's case. Infiltration of cancer cells between the nerve fibres and other structural changes have been described. The pulmonary plexus may be interfered with, as already mentioned. No doubt the sympathetic trunk may be implicated; and also some of the nerves forming the brachial plexus.

The œsophagus is not only the starting-point for not a few cases of mediastinal tumour, but is also liable to be compressed, and its calibre thus seriously narrowed. The tube is seldom penetrated, but this event may happen. In lympho-sarcomatous cases, although surrounded by the tumour, it may not be materially interfered with. Compression or implication of the thoracic duct occasionally occurs, and it is said that when this duct is obliterated chylous ascites may follow.

The invasion of the chest wall by intra-thoracic tumours has been previously referred to. The sternum and ribs seem to be usually only pushed forward; erosion and destruction of bone or cartilage may indeed result from pressure, but are chiefly met with in cases of cancer. Very exceptionally a tumour encroaches upon the vertebral canal, and affects the spinal cord or its membranes. The diaphragm is not uncommonly implicated during the progress of an intra-thoracic growth, and may be extensively infiltrated.

CLINICAL HISTORY.—The preceding discussion of the morbid anatomy of intra-thoracic growths, and of the diverse effects which they may produce in connection with the various structures, will make it at once evident that it is by no means an easy matter to give any comprehensive description of their clinical history, or of the phenomena by which their presence is revealed in individual cases. These phenomena are met with in the most varied combinations, and it is hardly possible to find any two cases exactly alike. They naturally come under the usual broad divisions of symptoms, and physical or other signs revealed by the different methods of skilled examination. In the following discussion it will be convenient to recognise this distinction; while the plan of clinical investigation outlined in the introductory remarks to this article will form a practical basis for their systematic consideration. In this way it will be possible at any rate to present a fairly comprehensive account of the phenomena which may be met with under different circumstances; and at the same time an opportunity will be afforded of emphasising those which are of most frequent occurrence, and most important from a diagnostic point of view; and of explaining when necessary their immediate causation and significance.

Taking a comprehensive survey of cases of intra-thoracic growth or tumour as they come before us in practice, they may be primarily arranged under certain groups, to which attention will be directed before considering the symptoms and physical signs in detail.

(i.) In the first place, it is important to note that growths sometimes develop in the lungs, or even in the mediastinum, which are either entirely latent, or occasion such slight disturbance that they do not attract sufficient attention to lead to examination of the chest. Moreover, presuming that such examination be made, it reveals nothing at all, or possibly signs so indefinite as to appear to be of little or no consequence. Under the circumstances the nature of the case can only be cleared up when a necropsy is made. Small, isolated, secondary pulmonary growths obviously need not be accompanied with any symptoms whatever; and in the majority of cases limited enchondromatous, osteoid, or fibro-plastic growths in the lung are similarly latent. A mediastinal tumour, when of small dimensions, or so situated as not to interfere with the functions of any important structure, may likewise be altogether unrecognised during life. Even a growth of some size in this region, especially in the anterior mediastinum, has thus remained undetected under circumstances where other conditions giving rise to prominent or grave symptoms have obscured its presence.

(ii.) In a second group of cases, although symptoms are either entirely absent, or are so slight and indefinite as scarcely to attract notice, yet physical examination of the chest at once reveals the existence of a tumour, it may be of large dimensions and of rapid growth. Such a condition of things is practically met with only where secondary malignant disease is limited to the lung; and some remarkable instances of this nature have come under my notice, in which very extensive pulmonary growths, easily detected by physical signs, gave rise to no symptoms whatever, except some degree of shortness of breath on exertion, and occasional cough of no special character.

(iii.) Occasionally it happens that a mediastinal growth of small dimensions, it may be a mere nodule, from its situation originates pronounced symptoms, thus simulating one of considerable size; while physical examination yields no results, or none of a definite or trustworthy character. Cases beginning in this way are likely, however, after a time to. present more or less characteristic physical signs, either associated with the tumour itself, or due to its effects on some of the thoracic contents.

(iv.) There is an important class of cases of intra-thoracic growth which come under clinical observation under the aspect of a chronic pleurisy with more or less effusion. This may happen not only where the pleura is itself the seat of mischief, but also in connection with pulmonary and mediastinal growths; so that the real nature of the disease is altogether overlooked or misunderstood, unless the concomitant circumstances of the case or the general symptoms excite suspicions which may ultimately lead to the correct diagnosis.

(v.) When malignant growths develop on an extensive scale in one or both lungs, but do not encroach on the mediastinum, they will probably give rise to more or less pronounced pulmonary symptoms and physical signs; and such cases come under observation as those of lung disease. The phenomena are, however, not uncommonly anything but characteristic; and various other pulmonary affections may be simulated. Thus the symptoms are in some instances merely of a bronchitic, emphysematous, or asthmatic character, with very indefinite physical signs. " Acute general infiltrating cancer may run a course almost indistinguishable from that of acute pneumonia, commencing with rigors, herpetic eruption, high fever, with rapid consolidation of the lung and albuminuria. Disseminated cancer, limited to the lung, may be equally marked by simple dyspnœa of an intense kind, cough, indeterminate expectoration, emaciation, with only the physical signs of bronchitis ; or, in some cases, with imperfect consolidation of the lungs ; or, in others, with pleural effusion ; and these symptoms may equally occur whether the growth exist in large masses or in the miliary form. In other cases of this class the disease, with almost identical symptoms, runs an acute course, marked by fever, sweating, and rapid emaciation, occasionally combined with delirium or coma, and having a deceptive resemblance to tubercular meningitis " (Wilson Fox). Other pulmonary complaints which may be simulated by malignant growths in the lungs are chronic pneumonia, acute tuberculosis, and tuberculous phthisis with the formation of vomicæ. While fully recognising the difficulties which may thus arise in the diagnosis of growths limited to these organs, it must be noted that in some instances the clinical phenomena, if duly studied and understood, are at least suggestive ; while in others they are sufficiently distinctive or even quite characteristic.

(vi.) The last group to be mentioned consists of those which present themselves as obvious cases of mediastinal tumour, both as regards symptoms and physical signs ; though, as already pointed out, these phenomena present great variety as to their exact nature, mode of onset and progress, degree, and combinations. Whether the growth has started in the mediastinum or has encroached upon this region from the lung or other parts, the clinical signs are more or less of a similar kind ; and, as a rule, in the class of cases now under consideration, are at any rate sufficiently characteristic to point to the fact that the space is occupied by some abnormal mass or infiltration. Of course a mediastinal tumour may have existed for some time before its presence is revealed clinically ; or it may have been preceded by phenomena merely indicating pulmonary or pleuritic disease, the case sooner or later assuming a mediastinal character.

Symptoms.—Having thus attempted to give a comprehensive summary of the chief aspects under which intra-thoracic growths present themselves clinically, my next object is to endeavour to discuss from a practical standpoint the symptoms which have to be studied in connection with these morbid conditions. It is customary to make a clinical distinction between cases in which growths are strictly pulmonary, and those where they are mediastinal ; but, as already intimated, there is really no definite line of demarcation between them, and in a very large proportion of instances they are more or less combined. It cannot, therefore, serve any useful purpose to try to separate them, which would only involve unnecessary repetition and confusion ; but in going through the symptoms systematically I shall point out any particular differences to which it may be desirable to call attention.

A. *Symptoms of local origin.*—The phenomena coming in this category will now be discussed according to the arrangement adopted in the introductory summary.

(*a*) Painful and other morbid sensations.—Cases of secondary growths in the lung are usually characterised by the absence of any pain in the chest; this symptom may not be complained of from first to last even in primary cases; but is likely to be present when a tumour comes to the surface and irritates the pleura, or extends into the mediastinum. Pain is usually regarded as a frequent symptom in connection with mediastinal tumour, and may be the earliest or even the only one; some writers, however, have collected a number of cases in which well-marked pain was quite exceptional, or came on late in the course of a case; so that it is by no means an essential symptom. It may be due to any of the causes already indicated, and different kinds of pain may be met with in the same case. It varies in its site according to circumstances. When a growth occupies the anterior mediastinum, and presses upon the sternum, the pain will be post-sternal; in other cases it is referred to a greater or less area on one side, or to the back of the chest. It is frequently of a darting or lancinating character, shooting in different directions, as up the neck, towards the abdomen or loin, or to the opposite side of the thorax. In some instances it has been described as of a pressing or grinding character. Pain in the head is not uncommon. When the brachial plexus is involved, painful sensations are experienced in the shoulder or arm, on one or both sides, even down to the hands or fingers. Pain is not necessarily constant, being sometimes intermittent or paroxysmal. It varies greatly in degree, and is occasionally very severe, or even agonizing. As the result of implication of the intercostal nerves intense pain over one side of the chest has been observed, with corresponding sweating and herpetic eruption. More or less local tenderness on pressure or forcible percussion may be present; and occasionally there is very marked superficial hyperæsthesia or hyperalgesia. Pain associated with mediastinal tumour is sometimes increased at first by bodily exertion.

In some instances the subjective sensations hardly amount to pain, but are described rather as a feeling of uneasiness or discomfort in the chest, oppression, pressure, fulness, constriction, and the like. Numbness, tingling, or other paræsthesiæ are sometimes felt in the upper extremity, as the result of pressure upon the brachial plexus. Abnormal sensations may also be referred to the throat, as of a foreign body; or there may be pain on swallowing.

(*b*) Disorders of respiration.—The phenomena coming under this head are amongst the most common and prominent symptoms in cases of intra-thoracic growth; whether limited to the lung, or encroaching upon the mediastinal space. Not infrequently some form of dyspnœa first attracts attention; while its undue proportion to other symptoms and physical signs may be of considerable diagnostic importance, or it may even be practically the only symptom for long periods. Sometimes, indeed, death takes place before any other phenomena appear. The disturbances of breathing differ much in their nature and degree, especially in cases of mediastinal tumour, when they may result from any of the factors already discussed, which often act in various combinations. Hence they demand in every instance particularly careful and systematic investigation. When properly studied and understood the phenomena observed are often highly significant, or even quite characteristic.

In the case of pulmonary malignant disease, so long as the mischief is confined to the lungs, the evidence of interference with respiration will depend chiefly on the extent to which these organs are implicated and their functions interfered with, and on the arrangement of the growth. In secondary cases, however, there may be very extensive growths, with but little obvious disturbance of breathing. Dyspnœa is also absent in some cases of infiltration, but it may form a prominent feature when any considerable area has been affected, and also in most of those where cancer, though diffused, has been found limited to the interlobular septa, or has extended around the bronchi; and it has been present, though in a less marked degree, where the growth has assumed the form of diffused tumours or of the miliary type (Wilson Fox). According to the late Sir Risdon Bennett (2), the dyspnœa in disseminated malignant disease seems chiefly due to feeble circulation and general debility.

Taking a comprehensive survey of intra-thoracic growths, it may be stated that the disturbance of respiration generally comes on in an insidious and progressive manner, until it ultimately becomes very severe, and assumes grave characters. Not uncommonly it is at first paroxysmal, occurring only at intervals, which may be prolonged; and, even when constant dyspnœa is established, it may present paroxysmal exacerbations from different causes, and amount to partial suffocation. Occasionally the presence of a tumour in the chest is revealed by an acute or sudden onset of dyspnœa. Here again the disturbance of breathing differs in its characters, as well as in its severity, and it usually changes in these respects during the progress of a case. It may only amount to more or less shortness of breath, or breathlessness on exertion; and under any circumstances this is usually one of its prominent features. In advanced cases the least movement or effort causes great distress. The frequency of respiration, when the patient is quiet, differs a good deal in individual cases, and is not uncommonly quite normal; thus no particular importance can be attached to this point. The breathing may, however, be persistently quickened. In some instances it is obviously laboured; while in others distinct asthmatic attacks occur, one of which may end fatally. These paroxysms of "spasmodic asthma" may be associated with enlarged mediastinal glands in children, as pointed out by Goodhart; they are attributed by him to a spasm of the whole lung due to interference with the mediastinal nerves. Similar attacks may certainly be met with in cases of other kinds of mediastinal tumour, and it has been said that they are specially indicative of malignant growths.

The most significant respiratory disorders associated with intra-

thoracic growths, which are to be specially watched for, are those indicating definite tracheal or bronchial obstruction, or implication of the vagus
or inferior laryngeal nerves.   In the former case there will be an obvious
and constant obstructive difficulty, attended probably with noisy or stridulous breathing, or with wheezing or whistling sounds of various kinds; the
phenomena being often highly characteristic.   Interference with nerves, no
doubt, affects the respiration in different ways, but it must be particularly
noted that dyspnœa may thus arise due to muscular disturbance, whether
spasmodic or paralytic, affecting the glottis ; and this is likely to assume
a paroxysmal character, though under certain circumstances it may be
always present more or less.   When the phrenic nerve is involved the
diaphragm will be affected, but the difficulty in breathing induced in this
way could only be made out by investigating its movements.   Possibly
under these circumstances hiccough might be a prominent symptom.

The subjective sensations associated with the respiratory difficulties
in cases of intra-thoracic tumour are often very pronounced, giving rise
to much evident suffering and distress.   The patient also frequently presents a more or less cyanotic aspect, which may be entirely due to such
difficulties, along with cardiac embarrassment ; but this condition is generally associated with and aggravated by the effects of venous obstruction,
as we shall see hereafter.   In a considerable proportion of cases orthopnœa
is established sooner or later, any attempt at the recumbent posture causing urgent and intense fits of dyspnœa.   Some patients are obliged
ultimately to sit up in a chair constantly, never daring to go to bed, and
at the best only having fitful snatches of slumber.   They may instinctively and habitually, even during sleep, lean forwards or sidewards,
in order to take off pressure from the air-tubes.

(c) Cough ; Expectoration ; Hæmoptysis.—Cough is another symptom
which is almost always present during some part of the course of a case
of intra-thoracic growth, and it comes on not uncommonly at a very
early period.   It is, however, not absolutely essential, and may hardly
amount to more than a voluntary attempt on the part of the patient to
get rid of some persistent feeling of obstruction or accumulation of mucus.
As regards the lungs, small isolated tumours in these organs do not give
rise to any cough ; and in other cases of intra-pulmonary growths cough
may present no special characters.   In connection with mediastinal tumour
cough differs much in severity, but tends to increase, and to become more
and more troublesome as the case progresses.   It is often of a teasing
and irritable character, giving the impression of being due to irritation of
the main air-passage or bronchi.   The more significant kinds of cough
are the stridulous or wheezy variety, indicative of pressure on the trachea
or a main bronchus ; or the paroxysmal and spasmodic type, associated
with laryngeal muscular disorder or organic changes, and of croupy or
clanging quality, or accompanied with various degrees of huskiness or
hoarseness, in some instances being almost entirely aphonic.   The different sounds produced during the act of coughing in connection with
mediastinal tumour are highly suggestive to the accustomed ear.   The

paroxysms are in some instances very distressing, and are attended with grave disturbance of breathing.

Not uncommonly cough associated with intra-thoracic growth is practically dry; and this may be a suggestive point in diagnosis, when the cough is irritable or paroxysmal. Even when expectoration is present, in the very large majority of cases ordinary examination of the sputum does not afford any reliable information. Often only a small quantity of viscid, tenacious mucus is discharged; or the expectoration is simply bronchitic, muco-purulent, or bronchorrhœal, the last being probably the result of a congestive condition. When destructive changes occur in connection with growths in the lung, leading to the formation of cavities, the sputum may be of a purulent character; and occasionally it is distinctly fœtid, as the result of gangrene, or possibly of the decomposition of retained secretions or morbid products. In the general inspection of sputum in relation to intra-thoracic growths, especially pulmonary, the chief matter is to look for fragments of such growths or of caseous substance, which are occasionally found; but no positive opinion as to their nature could be arrived at without microscopical examination, a point which will be dealt with later. The late Dr. Hyde Salter described characteristic sputa resembling washed-out pieces of meat, but I have never met with anything of this description. The stridulous breathing and peculiar cough now described, like many others of the symptoms, are found also in aortic aneurysm, and are described in the article on this subject.

Hæmoptysis requires separate consideration. The expectoration is frequently streaked with blood, but this is of no special significance when associated with violent cough. In the case of intra-pulmonary growths hæmoptysis is an important, and may be the earliest symptom; and it is in some instances repeated. It has been affirmed that large hæmorrhages are even more common in pulmonary cancer than in phthisis, and may prove immediately fatal. According to the late Risdon Bennett, however, copious hæmoptysis, except in connection with extensive destruction of lung tissue, is not common in cancer of the lung. In former times much importance was attached herein to expectoration resembling red-currant jelly or prune-juice, due to the intimate admixture of blood. When present, it seems to be highly characteristic, but according to modern observations it is of extremely rare occurrence. With regard to mediastinal tumour, my experience agrees with that of Sir Douglas Powell (35), that hæmoptysis is not an important sign of this condition; but sanguineous expectoration may be observed when the growth has invaded the lung, and sometimes profuse hæmoptysis then occurs, which may be followed by considerable though temporary amelioration of symptoms. In only a few of the cases collected by Vincent Harris were the sputa tinged with blood. It is important to note, however, that when a mediastinal growth perforates the trachea it may bleed into its interior, and thus give rise to definite hæmoptysis; as happened in a case under my observation to which I have already referred.

(*d*) Alterations in voice.—So long as a growth is confined to the lung or pleura, it does not affect the voice. A mediastinal tumour is likely to originate symptoms coming under this category, but their frequency varies a good deal according to different statistics. An intermittent aphonia has been observed amongst the earliest phenomena, sometimes along with paroxysmal dyspnœa. A change in the quality and pitch of the voice, as well as more or less hoarseness, may certainly result from direct pressure on the trachea, or invasion of its channel. By far the most frequent and important symptoms of this kind, however, are those due to implication, in various ways and degrees, of one of the vagus nerves or its inferior laryngeal branch. A certain degree of hoarseness may be present without any obvious paralysis of the vocal cords, being then probably due to irritation or spasm. Pronounced hoarseness and weakness of the voice, culminating in aphonia, are chiefly associated with paralysis of the cords, but this may be only unilateral. These symptoms were very prominent in two cases under my observation, in one of which the right inferior laryngeal nerve was involved in a growth, in the other the left or recurrent branch. In some instances actual morbid changes in the larynx give rise to alterations in the voice. Thus the laryngeal muscles occasionally become atrophied; or laryngitis, œdema of the glottis and vocal cords, or ulceration may be set up; or there may be independent malignant disease of the larynx, causing thickening of its structures.

 (*e*) Cardiac and arterial symptoms.—So long as a growth is confined to the lung, disturbance of the heart's action is seldom complained of, except such as may be due to weakness of its muscular walls. Palpitation and obvious cardiac disorder are, however, not uncommon in cases of mediastinal tumour, owing to displacement or embarrassment of the organ, implication of its substance along with the pericardium, pericardial effusion, interference with the pulmonary circulation, or nerve disturbance due to the vagus trunk or cardiac plexus being involved. The condition last mentioned may also cause either greatly increased frequency, or, on the other hand, marked slowness of the pulse; and these disorders may occur at intervals. Different kinds of irregular action are observed in some cases. Anginal attacks, or a tendency to syncope, have also been noted. The pulse is in most cases increased in frequency. Should a mediastinal growth interfere with either of the main branches of the arch of the aorta, the corresponding pulses will be affected—carotid, radial, or both—in the way of retardation, or of more or less feebleness to complete extinction. Inequality of the radial pulses may disappear, owing to the pressure becoming equalised during the growth of the tumour. It must not be forgotten that in exceptional cases a growth makes its way into the aorta, and fatal hæmorrhage occurs. It is a question whether arterial obstruction may help in causing œdema of one arm, but when this condition is present the veins are generally implicated also. Gangrene of the legs has been noted in a case in which the descending aorta and inferior vena cava were both pressed upon. The *pulsus paradoxus* has been observed in some cases of mediastinal tumour.

(*f*) Symptoms of deficient blood-aeration and venous obstruction.—As already stated, more or less cyanosis may result from interference with the respiratory functions, and this may happen in cases of intra-pulmonary growths, as well as in those which are mediastinal. The latter, however, may give rise to definite signs of local venous obstruction without any evidence of deficient blood-aeration. Most commonly the objective and subjective phenomena coming under this category are the outcome of the combination of both these causes. These phenomena have been previously described in detail in this article, in the introductory remarks on the clinical investigation of mediastinal diseases; and it will suffice here to offer a few remarks bearing upon their relation to tumours in this region. They are of much importance in this class of cases, and often afford valuable information as to the presence and situation of a mediastinal growth. The evidences of venous obstruction may appear a considerable time before any other symptoms; especially swelling of the neck and face, which sometimes comes on suddenly, and is usually bilateral, but occasionally unilateral. Not uncommonly the patient has first noticed that he cannot button his shirt on account of enlargement of the neck; or puffiness of the eyelids has attracted attention at the outset. Sometimes the swelling began in one arm. In other instances lividity of the face is the earliest indication of venous engorgement. Sooner or later, in a considerable proportion of cases of mediastinal tumour, all the signs of this condition become prominent, as indicated by the cyanotic colour, oedematous swelling, distension and tortuosity of superficial veins, and so on. They are usually bilateral, and give rise to a highly characteristic appearance. Powell (35) describes a slightly staring, suffused, and anxious expression of countenance as most common; but in marked cases there is an aspect of semi-strangulation most painful to witness. The changes may be unilateral or localised, and the jugular vein on the compressed side may remain distended during inspiration, while that on the opposite side becomes emptied. Any of the consequences of cerebral congestion are apt to arise, and epistaxis or other hæmorrhages may occur. Exophthalmos is an exceptional phenomenon which has been noticed in association with enlarged thyroid, or with cancerous growths around this organ. It is affirmed that local oedema and venous varicosity may entirely disappear before death, and not be discoverable after death. Signs of obstruction of the inferior vena cava are extremely rare in cases of mediastinal tumour. It may interfere with the vena azygos, and originate corresponding symptoms.

(*g*) Disorders of deglutition.—Dysphagia is an important symptom of mediastinal tumour, not only when it starts in the œsophagus, but also when this tube is compressed by or involved in a growth. Douglas Powell (35) states that it is a much more common and abiding symptom in this condition than in aneurysm, and such appears to be the general experience. Dysphagia may be amongst the earliest, and is sometimes the only prominent symptom for a considerable time, as I can testify from my own experience. The difficulty is occasionally influenced by posture, and may be intermittent when of reflex nervous origin. Deglutition may be painful, or attended with other unpleasant or even distressing subjective sensations. Ultimately the œsophagus may become the seat of complete obstruction or stricture, and a pouch-like dilatation may form above the tumour. In the very exceptional cases in which the tube is perforated by a growth from the lung or mediastinum, vomiting of blood may possibly occur.

(*h*) Special nerve symptoms.—As a result of pressure by a tumour upon the brachial plexus, not only may sensation in the arm be affected, but in exceptional cases muscular paralysis and wasting are produced. Vomiting has occasionally been attributed to interference with the vagus nerve. Owing to pressure on the sympathetic trunk, contraction of the pupil, generally on one side, has been observed, which may be associated with ptosis; occasionally, on the contrary, there is dilatation. Possibly unilateral vaso-motor disorders may be noticed in the face and head. All these phenomena, however, are extremely rare in connection with mediastinal tumour.

(*i*) Spinal symptoms.—It is believed that numbness and paræsthesiæ in the legs may result from congestion of the spinal cord, due to interference with the vena azygos by a mediastinal tumour. What is more important, however, is that in rare instances the cord and its membranes become themselves involved during its progress, giving rise to spinal pain, and eventually to paraplegia or other phenomena. Growths in connection with the cord may, however, be primary, being followed by secondary development in the lung or mediastinum, and then the spinal symptoms occur at an early period.

Having thus given an account of the local symptoms which may be associated with pulmonary and mediastinal growths, the fact must again be emphasised that in individual instances they present great differences as regards their time and mode of onset and succession, degree, exact characters, combinations, and progress. Signs of pressure or irritation may develop early, and at first in an irregular or intermitting manner; or they may not come on until a late period. Sometimes they occur in distinct groups; but often they seem to be capriciously associated. Douglas Powell (35) describes pressure-symptoms as insidious in cases of mediastinal growth, but more persistent and less variable than those of aneurysm. They may, however, come on very rapidly or almost suddenly. The practical point to be insisted upon is, that the clinical observer must regard and study every case separately and individually, and, taking a comprehensive grasp of the phenomena presented for his consideration, endeavour to understand them, and to interpret their significance — by no means always an easy task. It may be stated generally that the more pronounced symptoms when the tumour occupies the anterior mediastinum are those of venous obstruction and interference with the arterial circulation, which accounts for their great frequency; while in the case of posterior mediastinal growth the air-passages, œsophagus, and nerves are more affected.

B. *General and remote symptoms.*—Under this head it will be convenient to mention not only the symptoms which are more strictly general, but certain others, not immediately associated with the chest, affecting particular organs or systems. Here again remarkable differences are observed in different cases. The general system may not be materially affected even when there is obvious and extensive malignant disease of the lungs, or a large mediastinal tumour ; while, on the other hand, when the local evidences of intra-thoracic disease are indefinite or absent, constitutional symptoms may be very pronounced. In some forms of growth there is no reason why such symptoms should be produced, but as a rule they are likely to be more or less prominent, either on account of the nature of the tumour itself, the changes it undergoes, or its effects upon vital structures. They are both subjective and objective, but of no specially defined character ; and it will be most convenient to refer briefly to each of the general symptoms which may require attention in relation to intra-thoracic growths. The subjective feelings of the patient must not be overlooked, and sometimes a sense of fatigue and weariness, aching in the limbs, or indisposition for exertion have been among the first symptoms complained of. More or less weakness, culminating in exhaustion or prostration, is likely to be associated with the objective constitutional conditions now to be described. Amongst them wasting, with proportionate loss of weight, demands the first consideration, as it is very common, and should be particularly watched for. In some cases wasting is not sufficiently marked to attract attention, but probably there is always more or less loss of weight in connection with malignant disease of the lung, or a definite mediastinal growth. Sometimes emaciation is remarkably rapid ; in other instances it is more slowly progressive, but ultimately reaching a marked or extreme degree. It is when the œsophagus is obstructed that wasting is most pronounced ; and emaciation in cases of mediastinal tumour has also been specially attributed to pressure on the thoracic duct. A gradual and increasing deterioration of the blood, leading to marked anæmia, is one of the most prominent phenomena in many instances, and this symptom may appear at an early period. Exceptionally a leukæmic condition is met with. In the great majority of cases there are no indications of the so-called " cancerous cachexia," even though the disease be malignant. Sometimes the finger-ends are clubbed. With regard to pyrexia, it is as a rule practically absent ; and, indeed, in connection with cancerous and sarcomatous growths the temperature is often below the normal. During the progress of rapid malignant disease, however, fever is likely to occur, and in the last stages it may be of a hectic type. When lymphadenomatous growths develop within the chest in connection with Hodgkin's disease, there may also be considèrable pyrexia, with a peculiar range of temperature. Fever may, moreover, be associated with tuberculous formations, or even with a dermoid cyst. When the temperature is raised, it seldom follows any particular type ; and, apart from complications, the elevation is only slight or moderate as a rule. Night-sweats are sometimes troublesome.

The general symptoms in exceptional cases closely simulate those of pneumonia or phthisis. Impairment or loss of appetite, dyspeptic symptoms, insomnia, or other disturbances not uncommonly add to the patient's troubles in cases of intra-thoracic growth, and contribute to the general wasting and weakness. Diarrhœa is present occasionally. Free diuresis has been observed in the early stages of intra-thoracic tumour; and albuminuria may result from obstruction of the inferior vena cava.

C. *Physical and special signs.*—The phenomena coming under this category are obviously of essential importance in the recognition of pulmonary and mediastinal growths; but their study in this class of cases often taxes to the utmost the practical knowledge and skill of the clinical investigator, both in carrying out the several methods of examination, and in duly estimating the value and teaching of the signs which they reveal. Hence it is particularly necessary to understand clearly at the outset the course of procedure to be followed, and to adopt it systematically in each individual case, so far as may be required. In the following remarks I propose to consider the subject on the lines previously indicated in the introductory portion of this article, and thus to endeavour to present some comprehensive outline of its practical bearings. Of course cases do occur in which, even when symptoms are prominent, or, it may be, characteristic, physical or other special modes of examination give little or no help; while, on the other hand, the signs thus elicited may at once reveal the presence and situation of an intra-thoracic growth or tumour, which does not give rise to any appreciable symptoms, or, at any rate, to none of diagnostic significance. In most instances they afford valuable corroborative evidence in relation to diagnosis, or they clear up various points which cannot be otherwise demonstrated.

I. **Physical examination of the chest.**—The examination of the thorax by the usual methods will, as a matter of course, first receive attention in any case of suspected intra-thoracic tumour; yet it may not reveal anything when a growth is of small size, lies deep in the lung, or is otherwise so situated as not to affect the normal physical signs of this region. Any one who has had much experience in these cases, and who is aware of the almost endless diversity in the combinations of physical conditions within the chest which they present under different circumstances, cannot fail to realise the difficulty of attempting anything like a systematic and comprehensive description of the abnormal signs which may be met with. Personally I feel deeply conscious of this difficulty, and it will be impossible within the limits of this article to do more than to give a general summary of the phenomena to be looked for in connection with intra-thoracic growths, and to explain, so far as is practicable, their relation to these growths, or to their associated conditions affecting the serous membranes, lungs, heart, vessels, and so forth. It is most important at the outset to understand clearly what these associated conditions may be, and to be prepared to recognise them in individual cases. These have, however, been fully discussed already, and cannot be further referred to here. Although it is customary to describe separately the signs indicative of pulmonary and mediastinal growths, it appears to me to be more convenient and practical to consider them together, and I propose to do so according to the plan which I am accustomed to adopt in recording thoracic physical signs.

1. *Superficial structures.*—(a) The chief phenomena to be noted under this heading are those indicating venous obstruction within the thorax. They have already been referred to under symptoms, but it must be remembered that as physical signs they not uncommonly require more or less careful investigation in cases of mediastinal tumour, and this applies particularly to dilated superficial veins, which by their situation and distribution often reveal clearly, not only that one or more of the intra-thoracic veins are obstructed, but also which of them it happens to be. In this investigation attention must of course be paid to the parts above the limits of the thorax and to the arms, as well as to any enlarged veins over the abdominal surface. In order to determine the degree of venous difficulty, and how far the signs depend on interference with the respiratory functions, it may be desirable to observe how the distended veins are affected by deep breathing and vigorous cough. The phenomena now under consideration are obviously not to be expected when growths are strictly limited to the lung or pleura; but they may supervene in cases where the disease originates in either of these structures, if afterwards it encroaches upon the mediastinum.

(b) It will be convenient here to draw attention to the great importance of carefully looking and feeling for implication of the superficial lymphatic glands in relation to intra-thoracic growths, and of noting their characters should they be found enlarged. Those to be more particularly studied are the supra-clavicular, the infra-clavicular, and the axillary glands. The cervical glands are said to be specially liable to be affected in cases of lympho-sarcomatous growths, but they may also be involved in those of a cancerous or tuberculous nature.

(c) The third point to be noticed in relation to the superficial thoracic structures is whether they are themselves involved in any morbid growth? An intra-thoracic tumour may follow primary malignant disease of the breast, and the two conditions may thus be met with together. On the other hand, a tumour in the mammary gland has been observed secondary to one in the lung. It is extremely rare for centrifugal perforation of the chest wall to take place, even when it is much pushed out; but this event does occur exceptionally, its structures becoming implicated, though practically only in cancerous cases. A growth of this nature may involve the sterno-clavicular joint, or the intercostal spaces, or may penetrate the sternum. I have met with two or three remarkable cases in which the thoracic walls have been extensively infiltrated, along with intra-thoracic growths; or in which disseminated sarcomatous collections have appeared in the superficial tissues in similar cases. The external manifestations spoken of in the preceding remarks are recognised by inspection and palpation; and it must be remembered that not only are they important in diagnosis, but they may also materially modify the signs elicited by other methods of examination.

In addition to the special points referred to in the investigation of the superficial structures, it must be noted that these structures are in many instances much wasted, as a part of the general emaciation.

2. *Shape and size of chest.*—Intra-thoracic growths are very apt to affect the shape and size of the chest in different ways, though there may be no obvious change in these respects, even when other signs of tumour are well marked. As the outcome of the study of cases which have come under my personal observation, I submit· the following summary of the deviations from the normal which may be met with ; though they present numerous diversities in detail in individual instances. In order to obtain more definite and correct records of dimensions and conformation, it may be desirable to take measurements of the chest, or to make cyrtometric tracings.

(*a*) The thorax is sometimes generally enlarged, though the two sides are seldom quite symmetrical. This may happen when a growth interferes with the trachea only to such a degree as to cause accumulation of air and consequent distension of both lungs, constituting one of the forms of so-called emphysema. I have also known it occur when one lung was practically converted into a large solid tumour distending the side, while the opposite organ had undergone compensatory enlargement. Possibly a similar condition of things might result from a large pleural effusion associated with a morbid growth. Pericardial effusion or displacement of the heart might also help in making enlargement of the thorax more general in cases of tumour on the left side.

(*b*) Unilateral enlargement of the thorax, affecting practically the whole side, though not necessarily to the same degree in all parts, is in some instances a very striking sign of intra-thoracic tumour. This happens usually when one lung is extensively involved, or if there is a large pleuritic effusion, while the opposite lung remains of its normal size. I have, however, known the side to be practically distended throughout in connection with a very large mediastinal tumour, or with one interfering in a minor degree with the main bronchus, thus causing accumulation of air in the lung. When the enlargement is due to a solid growth, the intercostal spaces are not prominent, though the normal depressions may be more or less obliterated, so that the surface feels unusually smooth.

(*c*) The opposite condition of unilateral retraction of the thorax is most common in cases of infiltrated cancer of one lung, or when a main bronchus is so obstructed by a growth as to lead to collapse of the organ. Pleuritic adhesions may help to cause retraction ; but it must be borne in mind that there may even be some fluid in the pleura, and yet the side be smaller than normal. It is an interesting fact that retraction has been noticed on the side opposite to that on which a lung was the seat of morbid growths, in consequence of the bronchus of the healthy lung having been compressed, and collapse thus produced.

(*d*) A local prominence or definite bulging of some part of the thorax is one of the changes to be specially looked for in connection with a circumscribed tumour coming to the surface, whether originating in the lung or mediastinum. Its situation and extent will necessarily vary ; but it is most often noticed in front, at the upper part, and involving the sternum more or less. Bulging may, however, be observed laterally or posteriorly. The intercostal spaces will be affected in the same way as when a solid growth produces a more general enlargement. It may also be mentioned here that a tumour sometimes extends upwards towards the neck, giving rise to a prominence in this direction.

3. *Movements of respiration.*—It may be stated generally that the effect of a growth within the chest, whether inside or outside the lung, is to interfere more or less, and often to a marked degree, with the respiratory movements, which always demand careful investigation in a particular case, in order to determine the actual nature and significance of the disorder, and the conditions upon which it depends. Obviously if one or both lungs are extensively involved, their movements will be proportionately limited ; while a large mediastinal tumour will probably directly prevent pulmonary expansion. Other factors to be specially borne in mind are spasmodic laryngeal disorders ; various degrees of obstruction of the trachea or a main bronchus ; the different secondary effects on the lungs ; pleuritic conditions ; and interference with the movements of the chest wall or diaphragm. As a rule, the most striking disorder of breathing, as determined by physical examination, is deficiency or abolition of inspiratory expansion of the chest, elevation being often excessive. This is occasionally general, but usually unilateral or local. When one lung is embarrassed, the opposite one may act excessively, so that the contrast between the movements on the two sides becomes very pronounced. Sometimes retraction of the lower part of the chest is observed during deep inspiration, this being as a rule unilateral ; but it may be bilateral when considerable areas of both lungs are occupied by growths, or when the main air-tube is affected. In connection with laryngeal or tracheal obstruction I have seen the lower part of the sternum and the contiguous rib cartilages on both sides fall in markedly with each inspiration, even in adults. Depression of the supra-sternal, supra- and infra-clavicular, and epigastric regions is occasionally observed. In some instances the breathing is entirely abdominal. In connection with an emphysematous condition of the lungs expiratory retraction may be affected more than inspiratory expansion. When retraction of one side is associated with a growth in the lung, some degree of movement of the intercostal spaces may in most cases still be observed ; but in cases attended with bulging they are practically motionless. The frequency and rhythm of respiration are often affected in connection with intra-thoracic tumour, but these deviations present no common or regular type.

4. *Tactile sensations.*—The feeling on digital palpation over a tumour within the chest which reaches the surface is often that of abnormal firmness and resistance, and this may be very pronounced. Exceptionally

a sensation of indistinct fluctuation is noticed. Vocal fremitus frequently
persists in the case of pulmonary growths, and may even be intensified
in different parts, when the growths are diffused or there is moderate
infiltration ; or when the pulmonary tissue is more or less condensed or
consolidated. Should, however, a lung be the seat of dense infiltration,
or be converted into one large solid tumour, the vocal fremitus will
be diminished over a corresponding area on one side, or even entirely
abolished. On careful palpation in the class of cases last mentioned
it may sometimes be noted that there are islets here and there over
which the fremitus can still be felt. Another combination that may
be met 'with is the total abolition of vocal fremitus over the seat of
a tumour, with exaggeration over condensed lung. This applies more
particularly to cases of mediastinal tumour, and it may be stated
generally that such a growth always tends to impair or suppress this
tactile sensation over the area which it occupies, but it may be increased
at its confines. Pleuritic conditions and emphysema must always be
remembered as modifying the vocal fremitus. Cough fremitus is
affected in the same manner as that associated with the voice. Rhonchal
fremitus, due to conditions of the bronchi, and often resulting indirectly
from obstruction of the trachea or a main bronchus, is not uncommonly
met with in cases of intra-thoracic tumour ; and when unilateral or
localised it may be of considerable diagnostic significance. It will be
convenient to mention here that in exceptional instances a more or
less distinct pulsation is felt over an intra-thoracic tumour, possibly
simulating that of an aneurysm. The movement is transmitted from
the heart or aorta. The cardiac impulse is sometimes felt over a considerable area of a lung infiltrated with cancer. In connection with
mediastinal tumour a double impulse has been noticed, which may be
felt by observer and patient as a sort of inward succussion (Walshe).
The pulsation conducted from the aorta has been described as of a
"knocking" character, and is, as a rule, essentially different from that
of an aneurysm.

5. *Percussion signs.*—It is highly important in relation to intra-thoracic
tumours to bear in mind when carrying out the method of percussion,
and to endeavour to realise, not only the sounds which are thus elicited,
but also the sensations which are felt by the fingers during the act. Not
uncommonly the latter afford most useful information.

The *percussion-sounds* demand the first consideration, but they vary
a good deal under different circumstances, so that it is by no means an
easy matter to give any definite description of the abnormal signs coming
under this category. They may not present any obvious deviation from
the healthy standard, especially in the case of small single or scattered
growths confined to the lung, which are likely to be entirely obscured by
healthy or emphysematous pulmonary tissue. Mediastinal tumours also,
when of small size or occupying certain situations, may not affect the
percussion-sound in the least, either in themselves, or by their effects
upon the air-tubes or lungs.

In further considering this part of the subject an endeavour will be made to classify the changes in the percussion-sounds which may be met with in different cases.

(*a*) A remarkable and general rise of pitch in the percussion note over both lungs has been described by Fraentzel in a case where a growth chiefly extended along the lymphatics of these organs. A similar change, of unilateral distribution, may certainly be associated with a diffuse growth in one lung, when not too abundant. In connection with tumours lying deep in the lung the sound may be hyper-resonant or actually tympanitic.

(*b*) In a second class of cases the striking change in the percussion sound is an increase in the extent of the pulmonary resonance, with hyper-resonance or possibly a tympanitic note ; this may be either generally distributed over the chest, or unilateral. This indicates distension, either of both lungs, from a certain degree of obstruction of the trachea by a mediastinal tumour, or of one lung from similar obstruction of a bronchus, which may occur both in pulmonary and mediastinal cases. Under these circumstances a tumour, even of some considerable size, may be entirely obscured as regards its own percussion signs.

(*c*) The percussion-sound to be more particularly looked for as evidence of the existence of an intra-thoracic growth is more or less pronounced dulness ; and when such a growth comes to the surface the dulness is of the most marked and absolute kind. Obviously its situation and extent will vary in different cases. In some instances the whole of one side of the chest is completely dull and toneless, and this change may be conspicuous at the first examination ; of this I have met with some striking examples. In other cases it increases progressively while under observation. This extensive dulness may be due to the conversion of the entire lung practically into a solid mass, or to the coexistence of a pulmonary with a mediastinal growth, completely filling one side of the chest. Implication of the pleura, whether primary or secondary, is likely also to be attended with widespread dulness ; and the possible effect of pleural effusion upon the percussion-sound must always be borne in mind, even in cases of limited tumour, which it may completely mask. As subsidiary causes of extensive unilateral dulness in some instances, associated with a growth, must be mentioned pulmonary collapse, or secondary consolidation of the lung due to inflammatory changes. The sound elicited over the corresponding regions of the thorax would, however, probably not be so absolutely dull as over the tumour itself, though it might be very difficult to distinguish between them. Pericardial effusion, if present, would also add to the dulness. When the superficial structures of the chest are involved in a growth, this condition will certainly contribute to the impairment of resonance, sometimes to a considerable degree. Unilateral dulness may be associated either with retraction or enlargement of the side. In the latter case, when the combination is due entirely to a pulmonary growth, careful percussion may bring out isolated spots or islets which are more or less resonant, and correspond to unaffected portions of lung tissue. The opposite lung is often hyper-resonant, but it may itself be the seat of less extensive growths, and the percussion-sound would probably be modified accordingly. It must further be noted that dulness may extend from the affected side across the sternum to its opposite margin, or even for some distance beyond. When the heart is displaced, this organ will also add to the dulness in the situation in which it happens to be located.

In the large majority of cases of intra-thoracic growth the dulness is limited in its area, though varying in its locality according to the situation of the disease. When the mischief is confined to the lung and pleura, this sign may be observed either over the upper part of the chest in front, in the mid-region posteriorly, or at the base. It is of most importance in relation to mediastinal tumour, and the following points are worthy of special attention in cases of this nature. As a rule the dulness, which is absolute, is observed in the upper and anterior region. It is then often mainly post-sternal, and in all cases crosses the middle line, though it encroaches more towards one side than the other, so that it is unsymmetrical. The dulness varies much in size, but may extend over a considerable superficial area. Its shape is irregular, and it may present a distinctly sinuous border. On careful percussion towards the lung the circumference of the area of dulness is found to be bounded by the pulmonary note, which is considered very characteristic of mediastinal tumour as distinguished from primary lung disease. In some instances the dulness is not observed in front, but posteriorly; and occasionally it is limited to the interscapular region. I have met with cases of lympho-sarcoma in which the upper part of the chest, both front and back, was extensively dull.

Extension of dulness across the middle line of the sternum has also been looked upon, when present, as an important sign of cancer of the lung; but it is by no means invariable. Similar extension posteriorly may be very difficult to recognise. With regard to the heart and liver, it may be impossible to draw any line of demarcation between the dulness due to a tumour and that associated with these organs; but such distinction can sometimes be made out by careful percussion, or possibly by "auscultatory percussion." It may be stated generally that dulness due to an intra-thoracic growth is in no way affected by change of posture.

(d) In exceptional cases the percussion-sound elicited over a localised intra-thoracic tumour, whether pulmonary or mediastinal, is peculiar. Thus it may be of high-pitched, tubular, or amphoric quality, either owing to conduction of the sound from the trachea or a main bronchus, or in connection with cavities resulting from the breaking down of cancerous growths in the lung, especially in the infra-clavicular region.

(e) Lastly, it is always necessary, in studying the percussion-sounds associated with tumours within the chest, to be prepared to recognise different modifications over different regions. Thus there may be marked dulness in one part, while in other parts, or even over the rest of the side, the note is hyper-resonant, tympanitic, or amphoric. In rare instances a cracked-pot sound may be elicited over some portion of the thorax.

The *sensation* felt on percussion over a tumour or growth within the chest which reaches the surface is usually one of remarkable hardness and resistance. This will vary in its extent according to the area occupied by the growth; and when the whole side is dull the feeling is often of great service in revealing that we have to deal with a dense solid mass, and in distinguishing it from the dulness due to fluid effusion.

6. *Auscultatory signs.*—Under this heading it is only intended to discuss the auscultatory signs connected with the respiratory apparatus. These also present much variety in different cases; not only individually and in their combinations, but also over different parts of the chest. In many instances, however, they afford most valuable information, especially when studied in their association with other physical signs.

(*a*) Respiratory sounds.—These are not necessarily affected in cases of intra-thoracic growth, whether inside or outside the lung; even when the existence of such a growth is revealed by other definite signs. The following are the chief alterations which may be met with. When both lungs are distended the breath-sounds will probably be weak all over the chest, but may be accompanied with stridor. A similar condition affecting one lung may cause high-pitched, harsh, or stridulous respiration on the corresponding side; but, as the obstruction of the bronchus increases, the tendency is towards weakening and finally abolition of the sounds, until they become entirely inaudible over the area of lung corresponding to the distribution of the obstructed tube. These changes may be noted successively during the progress of a case under observation, and when associated with normal, increased, or high-pitched resonance are very significant. With regard to growths in the lung, cancer infiltrating the septa may only give rise to harsh breathing, or harsh breathing above and indeterminate breathing below, which in the later stages may pass into simple weak breathing. Diffused miliary nodules may also only cause harsh breathing, with prolonged expiration. When a lung becomes converted into a solid mass, with the bronchi and alveoli filled up, the respiration will be practically inaudible over the whole side, or it may be feebly heard here and there, or possibly some circumscribed hollow breathing may still continue in the infra-clavicular region, or the sound may be bronchial or tubular in the interscapular region. I have had the opportunity of watching a few cases in which the breathing on one side, at first harsh, then weaker but of tubular quality, became by degrees more and more obscured, until finally it was completely suppressed. Implication of the pleura, or pleuritic effusion, will also help to weaken or abolish the respiratory sounds, often very extensively. Should the opposite lung be healthy and free to act, puerile breathing will probably be observed on that side.

When a portion of lung is consolidated, or a definite tumour exists in its substance, the breath-sounds are generally bronchial or tubular, and may be excessively loud, being conducted from the larger air-tubes ; in exceptional instances they may even approach a cavernous quality. Different changes in the respiratory sounds may be observed over different parts of the same lung. Thus, with a tumour in its upper part and collapse below, it may be bronchial above and weak or inaudible towards the base.

As regards mediastinal tumour, when of not too large a size, and situated in the upper sternal region or in the posterior division, the respiratory sounds over such a tumour are likely to be bronchial or tubular, and may be intensely so. I have known the breathing in a case of tumour even of considerable size assume a distinctly amphoric quality, audible practically over the upper half of the posterior aspect of the chest on one side. When it attains large dimensions and involves the lung, the respiratory sounds are generally suppressed over a corresponding area, and should the lower lobe be at the same time collapsed they will be inaudible over the whole side.

Should cavities form, either in the lung or mediastinum, the respiratory sounds will probably exhibit a corresponding hollow quality, but this is by no means always the case. Cavernous respiration in different parts of the chest was noted in a case of Stokes's with dissection of the pleura from the lung by abscesses originating in cancer.

(b) Adventitious sounds.—Intra-thoracic growths seldom give rise directly to any signs coming under this category, unless they should happen to break down and form abscesses or cavities, especially in the lungs, with which bronchi communicate. Under these circumstances various râles might be heard, more or less moist, and perhaps having a hollow character. As the result of pressure on the main air-passages, different kinds of rhonchi, sonorous and sibilant, are often audible, and when accompanied with stridulous breathing are very suggestive, especially if of unilateral distribution. These sounds, as well as mucous râles, may indicate definite bronchitis. In cases of infiltrating cancer of the lung, and also where there are diffused miliary nodules, dry or moist râles may be present. Coarse crepitation has been described over lung nearly solid from cancer and coexistent pneumonia, due to abscesses forming in the pneumonic parts, or to dilated bronchi. Pleuritic friction-sound may be audible from time to time in some cases. Possibly a mediastinal adventitious sound might be elicited by movement of the arms in connection with certain tumours occupying this region.

(c) Vocal resonance.—It is desirable to study the voice, as well as the cough and whisper, in relation to growths in the chest ; but the signs coming under this category present many varieties, and their indications must be determined on general principles. If the lung is the seat of consolidation up to a certain point, the vocal resonance will be increased ; and it may be very loud, bronchophonic, or even pectoriloquous. In connection with a definite tumour, whether within or outside the lung, conducting the vibrations from the main air-passages, it may be very intense, and sometimes of ægophonic or amphoric quality. It is a striking fact that the vocal resonance may be thus exaggerated when the fremitus is greatly impaired, or even altogether absent. Occasionally distinct whispering pectoriloquy can be heard over a tumour. In the upper part of the chest and interscapular region collapse of the lung may help to intensify the vocal resonance; but in the lower region this condition would tend to diminish or annul it. Over a cavity pectoriloquy and whispering pectoriloquy would probably be heard, and the voice might have peculiar characters.

When consolidation of the lung by new growth becomes excessive, the vocal resonance becomes impaired, and it may ultimately be suppressed, practically over a whole side; though perhaps still audible in spots here and there. Sometimes, in connection with an infiltrating pulmonary growth, it is intensified or pectoriloquous above, but absent below. A similar combination may be met with associated with a tumour in the upper part of the chest and condensed lung below. When, however, a tumour attains a very large size, the vocal vibrations may in time become entirely suppressed throughout. Pleuritic thickening or effusion will necessarily produce their usual effects in the way of impairing or abolishing the vocal resonance. The study of this sign is of little or no use when there is pulmonary distension, though this condition tends to weaken it. The cough may not only present similar changes to those of the voice, but sometimes it is useful in bringing out or modifying adventitious sounds in the air-tubes or lungs.

7. *Cardio-vascular signs.*—Examination of the heart sometimes affords useful signs in intra-thoracic tumour, and always demands attention. As already stated, the pulsation of this organ can sometimes be felt extensively over lung infiltrated with cancer. On the other hand, it is often indistinct and the apex-beat indefinite, because the heart is covered by distended lung, or by a growth which pushes it towards the back of the chest. Displacement is one of the most important evidences of tumour to be looked for in relation to this organ. As might be expected, such displacement is usually less marked in cases where growths are limited to the lung, but it is sometimes observed in such cases to one or other side, even to a considerable degree. A mediastinal tumour not uncommonly causes more or less lateral displacement. More important, however, from a diagnostic point of view, is the fact that the heart is often pushed downwards or towards the ensiform cartilage. Pleuritic effusion will tend to cause the usual displacement, but this may be prevented by cancerous growths at the base of the heart. Collapse of the lung may lead to elevation of the apex-beat, but not necessarily, even in extreme cases. The organ is occasionally dragged over towards the side of the disease in cases of retraction, but usually it is pushed in the opposite direction by a tumour. Murmurs, generally systolic, have been described in several instances over an intra-thoracic tumour, or along the course of the aorta or pulmonary artery. A systolic murmur, audible in the back, was noted by Kaulich, associated with a dilatation of the aorta on the cardiac side; the vessel being compressed

and narrowed beyond this.   Pressure on this artery does not, however, necessarily give rise to a murmur.   Double murmurs are of very uncommon occurrence (Walshe).   In exceptional instances a pericardial friction-sound is heard.   Of course it is always necessary to be on the look-out for signs indicating pericardial effusion, or implication of the pericardium and heart-substance in a growth; though the latter condition would be very difficult to demonstrate positively.

With regard to the arteries, any disorders of the circulation associated with these vessels can usually be easily recognised by inspection and digital examination.   Possibly the sphygmograph might be of service in some cases.   The veins must receive due attention, but this point has already been considered in relation with the superficial structures.

II. Special Examination.—Having thus far considered the signs to be studied by the ordinary methods of physical examination in relation to intra-thoracic growths, it will now be convenient under this general heading to indicate the phenomena which may be revealed by special modes of investigation, which are only called for under particular circumstances.

1. *Examination of the sputum.*—In addition to the general examination of the sputum already referred to, it is important in certain cases to subject any materials expectorated to careful investigation with the microscope, and the help of an expert pathologist may be required.   This may reveal not only the presence of the distinctive elements of malignant growths, associated it may be with definite fragments, but also of blood-corpuscles when blood is not otherwise evident.

2. An *exploratory puncture* of the chest, by means of a fine trochar or the aspirator, is called for under particular circumstances, and may yield valuable information.   In the first place it may reveal at once that we have to deal with a solid mass, and not with a collection of fluid.   The needle may be felt to penetrate and to be fixed in solid tissue.   If no fluid is obtained, the needle-point should be carefully examined, in case a small fragment of growth may be found sticking to it.   If only a few drops of blood come away, and the needle does not seem to move freely in a cavity, the fear of malignant disease is heightened (Stephen Paget).   One of Harris' cases of malignant disease of the pleura (22) illustrates a possible fallacy deserving of notice.   In using an exploring syringe he happened to hit upon a very small cavity in the pleura, and withdrew a syringeful of perfectly clear pale yellow fluid.   He took the case to be one of chronic pleurisy with much effusion, but only about an ounce could subsequently be obtained, and the necropsy revealed that the pleural space was entirely obliterated except at the point where the needle was introduced.   Of course fluid may be obtained in quantity from the pleural cavity in not a few cases of intra-thoracic growth, especially when of a malignant nature; and in some instances the tumour may afterwards be more readily recognised.   If the fluid thus withdrawn be hæmorrhagic, this is regarded as an important diagnostic point in favour of malignant tumour, but it must be remembered that in a considerable proportion of

such cases it is quite clear, and resembles an ordinary effusion. In rare instances it presents a chylous appearance, and possibly this may result from obliteration of the thoracic duct. Whether any characteristic structures indicating malignant disease can be detected on microscopical examination in fluid removed from the pleural cavity is a matter of doubt, but cancer cells may possibly be found.

3. *Laryngoscopic examination* is in some cases of the greatest value in the clinical investigation of intra-thoracic tumour. It may disclose—(*a*) Motor disorders affecting the vocal cords, due to nerve-implication, which may be present without any prominent symptoms. (*b*) Organic changes in the larynx, resulting indirectly from the tumour, not forgetting wasting of the muscles, or local malignant disease associated with a similar growth in the chest. (*c*) Morbid conditions of the trachea. In exceptional instances tracheal stenosis has been seen with the laryngoscope. In a case under my care at University Hospital, already referred to in other relations, my friend Dr. Herbert Tilley was able to observe during life, by the aid of this instrument, that a growth had penetrated the trachea ; the autopsy proved that his observation was perfectly correct. Special *œsophageal examination* may also be demanded under suitable circumstances.

4. How far *skiagraphic* investigation is likely to be of service in the diagnosis of intra-thoracic growths is at present a question upon which no definite opinion can be given. In one doubtful and difficult case under my care in which the Röntgen rays were employed, no help in diagnosis was obtained. It seems highly probable, however, that in course of time skiagraphy will prove of much assistance in this class of cases.

5. *Abdominal examination.*—It is desirable to draw special attention to the necessity for examining the abdomen in relation to intra-thoracic growths. A mediastinal tumour occasionally extends towards the epigastrium in such a way as to give rise to a prominence in this region. More frequently there may be evidence of displacement of organs downwards, especially the liver, stomach, or spleen. The liver may be also enlarged from congestion. Ascites may be associated with obstruction of the inferior vena cava ; and any fluid removed from the peritoneum may possibly be chylous in appearance, in consequence of obstruction of the thoracic duct. An important object of abdominal examination, especially in doubtful cases, is to look for malignant disease in this region, either primary or secondary ; and in such examination the more obscure organs must not be forgotten, such as the pancreas and suprarenal capsules, as well as the absorbent glands. In females it may be desirable to make a special investigation directed to the generative organs.

Course, duration, and terminations.—The preceding discussion of the clinical history of intra-thoracic growths will have made it clear that individual cases present great variety in their course and mode of progress, and it is impossible to make any absolute statements on this subject. As a rule the onset of symptoms is more or less gradual, but which first attract attention, and in what combinations they appear, depends on the nature and situation of the tumour, its associated morbid changes, and other circumstances. It may happen that extensive malignant disease within the chest is first discovered on physical examination, the mischief having progressed for a considerable time in a latent manner. The course is generally chronic but progressive, though marked differences in the symptoms are often observed in individual cases as they advance: fresh incidents may arise, and pronounced exacerbations may appear from time to time; or, on the other hand, striking intermissions, especially as regards the respiratory disorders, may last for weeks. The physical signs also frequently undergo remarkable changes. The *duration* of chronic cases varies a good deal within certain limits. Carcinoma of the lung is said to last as a rule from 6 months to 2 years, and seldom goes beyond 4 years. Walshe, in a small number of cases, found the mean duration to be 13·2 months; the maximum being 27 months and the minimum 3·5 months. No trustworthy general conclusions can be formed as to the duration of mediastinal tumour, and each case must be studied individually in relation to this point. Of 42 cases collected by Eger, the duration in 32 was from under 2 months to 12 months, and the extreme limit was 7 years. There is no reason why non-malignant growths, whether pulmonary or mediastinal, may not continue for many years, provided they do not seriously interfere with the functions of vital structures. In malignant cases of any kind the duration would be much influenced by the existence of growths elsewhere.

While the large majority of cases of intra-thoracic growth run a more or less chronic course, it is important to bear in mind that occasionally the progress of events is acute from first to last, and that the existence of a tumour, which may perhaps have been present for a considerable time previously, is now and then revealed by some sudden grave symptom or symptoms, the subsequent progress being very rapid. Again, cases known to be chronic may end by some acute or sudden change. Several cases are on record in which pulmonary cancer ran an acute course of from two to six weeks from the first appearance of symptoms; sometimes with phenomena closely simulating tuberculous phthisis, severe acute bronchitis, or pneumonia. Jaccoud has recorded a remarkable case of mediastinal tumour in which death occurred on the ninth day from the first onset of dyspnœa, but the tumour had probably existed for some time. I believe I have seen a case of a similar kind, but a necropsy could not be obtained.

The *termination* in cases of intra-thoracic growth, with rare exceptions, must inevitably be fatal, sooner or later; and this applies with special force to all forms of malignant disease, though in some instances, especially when tumours are of an osteoid or fibro-plastic nature, and of secondary origin, they do not appear materially to hasten the fatal result, death being due to the primary disease. "The ordinary course of growths limited to the lung is that of a gradual death by means of

mingled conditions of asphyxia, hectic, and exhaustion in relatively varying degrees, in which, however, asphyxial symptoms usually predominate,
being sometimes rapidly intensified by the supervention of acute œdema
of the lung" (Wilson Fox). Mediastinal tumour may end gradually
from apnœa and venous stasis, progressive weakness and exhaustion,
inanition from œsophageal obstruction, cardiac failure, or other causes;
and these symptoms may be variously combined. The chief events
which lead to sudden or very speedy death are hæmorrhage, either
taking place internally or revealed by hæmoptysis, which is very rare;
an asthmatic paroxysm; asphyxia, due to an abscess opening into the
bronchi, and choking the tubes in the opposite lung; cardiac paralysis
with consequent syncope, attributable in different instances to direct
implication of the heart and pericardium, thrombosis of the pulmonary
artery, or compression of the pneumogastric or recurrent laryngeal
nerves; and cerebral vascular lesions. It may happen that no definite
cause can be found. Death may be hastened by different complications,
or by operations performed for the relief of urgent symptoms or other
purposes. Of course in some cases the fatal result is not due directly to
the morbid conditions in the chest, but to disease elsewhere.

Diagnosis.—It is generally understood and insisted upon by most
writers on the subject that the diagnosis of intra-thoracic growths presents many and multifarious difficulties, and that in some instances they
are practically insuperable. If there be no definite symptoms or
physical signs to draw attention to the presence of such a growth, it
would probably never be suspected; while in cases where the clinical
phenomena and course resemble those of some of the more common pulmonary diseases, mistakes might easily be made; under such
circumstances the most experienced and accomplished physicians and
clinical observers have fallen into error. At the same time, I believe
the tendency is to exaggerate these difficulties; and my experience has
led me to the conclusion that in a considerable proportion of cases, of
mediastinal growth at any rate, a definite diagnosis can be made, sufficient
for all practical purposes, granted adequate knowledge and skill in the
investigation, and that such investigation be carried out intelligently and
methodically. Douglas Powell (35) affirms that when attention is seriously
drawn to the case by the symptoms, the diagnosis, as a rule, is not difficult, and I am inclined to agree with him. Moreover, not uncommonly
cases which at first excite no suspicion, or are more or less obscure,
become quite characteristic during their subsequent progress. There are
certain distinct points to be briefly discussed in relation to the diagnosis
of intra-thoracic growths and tumours, and it will be convenient to deal
with them separately. It may be affirmed generally that an important
factor in the recognition of these morbid conditions is that the practitioner should never forget the possibility of their occurrence in any
case, and should particularly bear them in mind when thoracic symptoms
or physical signs are observed which are of an unusual character.

1. The first question for consideration is, what are the data upon

which a positive diagnosis of intra-thoracic growth can be made? In not a few cases the fact that the patient has malignant disease elsewhere, or has previously been operated upon for such disease, is of much importance; and when any chest symptoms supervene under such circumstances, the development of secondary mischief in this region should be particularly watched for. Even the occurrence of pain, especially if localised or lancinating and of a severe character, should always be regarded with suspicion, and frequent examination made. The danger of regarding such pain as simply neuralgic or neurotic, because no physical changes can be detected, must be carefully guarded against. In doubtful cases very minute search should be made for unsuspected primary growth. When symptoms or physical signs, or both, are suggestive, or, it may be, more or less characteristic of tumour within the chest, the point now under consideration is of great value in corroboration of the diagnosis. The same remark applies to the development of lymphadenomatous growths in the thorax in connection with obvious Hodgkin's disease. Again, the extension of a tumour towards the neck, implication of glands in this region or of the superficial structures, or the occurrence of secondary malignant disease in other parts of the body are important factors in arriving at a positive diagnosis. Secondary nodules of cancer or sarcoma may appear in different parts of the body, over bones, or in the subcutaneous tissue, as well as in organs; and these appearances are highly significant; though in my experience they have not appeared until a late period, when the diagnosis was but too evident. It should be noted that the points just considered are always important in diagnosis, when cancer or sarcoma within the chest has to be distinguished from other diseases.

The more immediate clinical phenomena upon which a positive diagnosis of intra-thoracic growth is founded are the different symptoms of local origin, and the physical or special signs to which they give rise, aided in some cases by the general symptoms. The phenomena presented by individual cases, although they occur in such diverse combinations, and cannot be definitely classified in groups, are often highly characteristic or even pathognomonic; and in a considerable proportion of instances their intelligent study, on the lines already discussed, can leave little or no room for doubt. When growths are confined to the lung or pleura, the difficulty of diagnosis is obviously much greater than when they occupy the mediastinum, either entirely or partially; and under such circumstances it may be almost impossible to come to a positive conclusion, especially when the disease is primary; though due consideration of the case in all its aspects may at any rate lead to a suspicion of its nature. In not a few instances, however, pulmonary malignant disease can be fairly recognised by the signs of extensive and marked consolidation of the lung, attended either with enlargement or retraction of the side, and, it may be, showing little or no disposition to break down. Among the symptoms which may be significant, associated with such conditions, are severe pain in the side, disproportionate or paroxysmal dyspnœa, and repeated hæmoptysis, especially if the blood resembles currant jelly. Evidence of obstruction of one bronchus, or any indication of pressure signs, would materially assist the diagnosis. When the disease is secondary the local phenomena are not uncommonly highly characteristic.

When a tumour occupies or encroaches upon the mediastinum its positive diagnosis is founded, as a rule, upon the abnormal physical signs which either directly or indirectly it originates ; accompanied with different phenomena resulting from its mechanical or pathological effects, and indicative of irritation, pressure, or other kind of interference with adjoining structures. It would involve needless repetition to refer to these again in any detail, even if space permitted. It must suffice to state that the chief symptoms to be looked for are the more characteristic disorders of breathing ; the peculiar kinds of cough ; the changes in the voice ; the phenomena indicating venous or arterial obstruction ; dysphagia ; and special nerve-symptoms. It is in the investigation of the diverse combinations of symptoms and physical signs met with in this class of cases that individual experience and skill in clinical observation are of such great advantage. Occasionally it happens that a fairly confident diagnosis may be founded on the symptoms alone, if aneurysm can be excluded. It must be borne in mind that the positive diagnosis should aim not only at the recognition of a tumour in the chest, but also as far as possible of the other morbid conditions in this region to which it may have given rise.

In some instances the general symptoms may be of more or less value in the diagnosis of intra-thoracic growth, but often they are of little or no positive significance. Occasionally one or other of the special modes of investigation previously described afford most useful information, and clear up any previous difficulty in arriving at a definite opinion. We have seen that cases which are obscure at first may, when properly watched during their progress, reveal phenomena which become more and more characteristic, until at last the diagnosis is quite easy. This fact is well exemplified by cases of growth beginning in the lung, and afterwards extending into the mediastinum. The appearance of a tumour through the chest wall is of course pathognomonic ; but this is an event which very rarely happens, and as a rule only in cases previously obvious enough.

2. Assuming a positive diagnosis of intra-thoracic growth to have been made, it is desirable to endeavour to determine within due limits the situation which it occupies, and the structures which it involves. If a tumour is limited either to the anterior or posterior mediastinum, the localisation of the physical signs, and the differences in the mechanical effects produced, will probably make this fact clear. A growth confined to the lung is not likely to cause pressure-symptoms, but may do so. When it has attained a large size, and has implicated various structures, it is often very difficult to ascertain the exact state of things with any approach to certainty ; under such circumstances, however, it is not a

matter of much practical moment. It must be remembered that there
may be more than one tumour in the same case ; the phenomena may
then be very complicated, and, unless this possibility is borne in mind,
are more difficult to understand clearly.

3. One of the most important points to be discussed in the present
connection is the differential diagnosis between intra-thoracic growth and
other morbid conditions affecting this region. This matter not uncommonly presents considerable difficulties, when symptoms and physical
signs of different kinds are associated with the thoracic structures ; and
unless particular care is exercised mistakes may readily be made. In
dealing with this aspect of the subject it will be convenient to consider
separately the more important diseases and conditions in relation to
which the differential diagnosis is likely to give trouble.

(a) *Lung affections.*—The ordinary diseases of the lungs do not, unless
under certain exceptional circumstances, give rise to pressure-symptoms ;
and the presence of any such symptoms constitutes, as a rule, a broad
distinction between these affections and an intra-thoracic tumour. It
must always be borne in mind, however, that the various pulmonary
morbid conditions already described may be secondary to a growth in
this region ; and their true interpretation may, without due care, be
then easily overlooked. The chief danger of error arises when definite
pressure-signs are absent or not prominent, even though a tumour exists ;
and it is most important that the clinical observer should be constantly
on the look-out for phenomena of this nature, which, even when slight,
may be of the greatest value in diagnosis. The following are the
principal pulmonary conditions in which difficulties are likely to arise,
though it must not be supposed that in actual practice they are of
frequent occurrence ; as a matter of fact cases coming under the present
category which give trouble in diagnosis are quite exceptional ; still it is
well to be prepared for them :—

(a) Acute pulmonary diseases.—It has already been pointed out that
acute disseminated or infiltrating cancer in the lungs may closely simulate
other acute pulmonary affections ; namely, bronchitis, pneumonia, tuberculous phthisis, or acute tuberculosis. It should also be mentioned that
the course of events may much resemble that of tuberculous meningitis,
cerebral symptoms being prominent, which may or may not be associated
with cerebral cancer. It is impossible to lay down any definite rules for
establishing a diagnosis in cases of this kind, and it must suffice to warn
the practitioner of their possible occurrence. The probability is that
even the most experienced would under the circumstances fall into error,
and fail to recognise the nature of the disease. Wilson Fox refers particularly to acute caseous pneumonia, affecting chiefly the base, and con-
solidating the whole or the greater part of one lung, as in some cases
presenting a striking resemblance to infiltrating cancer when the latter
does not retract the side. "The most distinctive features are the high
fever, the more abundant expectoration, and the rapid emaciation.
Diarrhœa, if present, would be still more in favour of the diagnosis of

caseous pneumonia. Cancerous infiltration is more likely to be mistaken for caseous pneumonia than that the converse error should occur." I have not in my personal experience met with any acute case exemplifying this difficulty.[1]

(β) Emphysema and chronic bronchitis. — These conditions, both individually and in combination, demand special attention in relation to the diagnosis of intra-thoracic growths. Cases in which they exist are usually dealt with in such an off-hand and casual manner that, when they are associated with other more serious diseases, their significance is very apt to be misunderstood; and I have known very grave errors in diagnosis to result therefrom. True vesicular emphysema may exist before and along with a tumour, whether within or outside the lung; but it must be always borne in mind that a condition of so-called "emphysema," which is really due to distension of one or both lungs with air, owing to pressure on the main air-tube, may be the result of such a tumour, and one of the evidences of its presence. Bronchitis may be similarly produced, or be associated with disseminated or infiltrating cancerous growths in the lungs. Without due attention and consideration the underlying causative conditions may easily be overlooked; especially as their more characteristic physical signs may be completely obscured by the emphysema and bronchitis. Should these affections be unilateral or localised, one of the causes to be particularly looked for is interference with the corresponding main bronchus or some of its divisions; and amongst them a tumour must not be forgotten. It may happen that, on careful examination, signs of a growth may be detected even when the lungs are much distended. It is, moreover, very important to be on the alert to note even slight audible peculiarities in the breathing, cough, or voice, suggestive of pressure on either of the large air-passages. In very obscure cases of this kind the presence of excessive dyspnœa or cyanosis should lead to the suspicion of growth; as well as repeated hæmoptysis and absence of fever with marked bronchitis. The diagnosis is rendered more probable if no other cause of this complaint can be discovered; and if there is no cardiac disease.

(γ) Pulmonary collapse. — When this condition affects one lung extensively, it may be difficult to determine whether it be due to a tumour obstructing a main bronchus, or to some other cause. The diagnosis must then be founded on due consideration of the case in all its aspects, including the past history, as well as the present state; and it seldom happens that a fairly definite opinion cannot then be arrived at, especially after watching the progress of events for a while.

(δ) Chronic phthisis.—There is a real danger of mistaking cancer affecting the lung for chronic tuberculous disease, although, of course, only in the very exceptional cases when the growth happens to involve

---

[1] A patient died of primary cancer of the left lung in Addenbrooke's Hospital a few months ago (1897). As she was in hospital during an examination week she was seen by some six physicians of large experience. Four of them took the case to be caseous pneumonia, two of them made the correct diagnosis. A remittent febrile temperature had been present since admission.—ED.

the upper part of the organ, and especially if it should break down and form a cavity or cavities. The local and general symptoms may be very similar in both classes of cases; and even diarrhœa may be a prominent symptom in those of cancer. Steven records a case where a primary cancer of the mediastinum, originating in the tissue of the right bronchus, simulated pulmonary phthisis, and was thus diagnosed. On the other hand, old chronic tuberculous disease occasionally presents certain phenomena which may be very suggestive of cancerous growth; such as laryngeal symptoms due to implication of one of the inferior laryngeal nerves. The first point in diagnosis is always to remember that there is a possibility of confounding the two kinds of morbid conditions, especially in elderly patients. Implication of both apices, with absence of pressure-symptoms and presence of fever, would be practically positive evidence of tuberculous mischief. Extensive consolidation of one lung, without signs of softening or cavities, but with gradual suppression of the respiratory sounds and extension of dulness across the middle line, are strongly in favour of malignant disease. Prolonged absence of pyrexia is also very suspicious; as well as "unusual" symptoms; such as extreme debility, marked anorexia, and a slow, feeble pulse, coupled with a limited amount of disease at one apex (Wilson Fox). With regard to hæmoptysis, it is nearly as frequent in cancer as in phthisis, some say more frequent; and the evidence it may afford is not very trustworthy. Frequently recurring hæmoptysis in a man past middle age, and without signs of emaciation, was noted by Stokes as characteristic of malignant disease. In unilateral phthisis hæmoptysis is said to be rarely profuse, or often repeated, but I have met with not a few exceptions to this statement. The curability of this symptom in any given case is in favour of tuberculous disease rather than cancer. It has been stated that enlargement of the supra-clavicular glands is probably associated with malignant disease, while enlargement of the submaxillary glands is in favour of tubercle; but this distinction cannot be positively relied upon in diagnosis. Systematic examination of the sputum would be likely to afford valuable information in doubtful cases, if any could be obtained. Its absence, or presence in very small quantity with no special characters, might under certain circumstances point rather to cancer. The detection of tubercle-bacilli would indicate tuberculous disease.

(ε) Chronic pneumonia.—I have met with two cases of what I believed to be extensive unilateral chronic pneumonia, in which the lung was not retracted, but appeared even to be enlarged, where the phenomena were very like those of a pulmonary growth. The prolonged duration of the cases was one of the points in favour of this diagnosis, but in neither instance could a necropsy be obtained. By far the more important condition, however, to be mentioned under this head is the fibroid or cirrhotic lung, which may be confounded with infiltrating pulmonary cancer causing retraction of the side, or with certain cases of mediastinal tumour associated with collapsed lung. In most instances the history would materially help in the diagnosis; and probably any obscurity would be cleared up sooner or later by the course of events. The differences in the physical signs are, as a rule, sufficiently distinctive, though by no means wholly to be trusted. Those in favour of malignant disease are absolute dulness with much resistance, especially if it extends across the middle line; suppression or marked weakness of breath-sounds; absence of adventitious sounds; abolition of vocal fremitus and resonance; and depression of the liver—if the retraction is on the right side. As the cirrhotic lung is often accompanied with cavities or dilated bronchi, bronchial or tubular breathing is likely to be audible, with moist râles, which may be of more or less cavernous quality. Severe pain in the side is in favour of cancer; as well as pyrexia in a case of considerable chronicity, and where the disease is manifestly advancing.

(b) *Pleuritic conditions.*—Difficulties in diagnosis between intra-thoracic growths and morbid conditions of the pleura present themselves from different aspects, and it must always be borne in mind that they are not uncommonly associated in the same case; while the pleura may also itself be involved in a growth, either primarily or secondarily. Speaking generally, it may be stated that pleuritic changes rarely give rise to any evidence of centripetal pressure, and this is often an important point in diagnosis in doubtful cases. A difficulty might possibly arise in making a diagnosis between an adherent and much-thickened pleura, with condensation of the lung and retracted side, and the effects of a tumour or a pulmonary growth; but due consideration of the history of the case, and of the existing symptoms and physical signs, ought to leave little room for doubt. Cancer beginning in the pleura may be attended with phenomena very like those of a chronic pleurisy with little or no effusion, and unless one were always on the look-out for such a possible condition a mistake might be easily made. Progressive and rapid wasting and weakness, without fever, should lead at any rate to a suspicion of the nature of the disease.

One of the most important matters to be referred to in the present connection is the danger of mistaking a malignant tumour, whether originating in the pleura or lung, so extensive as to occupy the whole of one side of the chest, where pressure-symptoms are practically absent, for a chronic pleuritic effusion or an empyema, especially with thickened pleura. Many cases have been recorded where such a mistake has been made, but it is rare to fall into the opposite error. I have met with a few well-marked instances of this kind, in one of which pleural effusion had been diagnosed, and can fully appreciate the difficulties they may present; but it has so happened in my experience that the diagnosis was fairly clear, as the growth was obviously secondary, and from other circumstances. In doubtful cases certain symptoms are worthy of consideration. Thus marked pyrexia would be in favour of pleurisy or empyema, and its absence would suggest cancer. Repeated hæmoptysis, especially of the red-currant jelly type, would be strongly in favour of the latter; as well as profuse offensive expectoration, and fœtor of the breath, if a perforating empyema could be excluded. A careful search for enlarged glands in the neck might materially help in clearing up the diagnosis in doubtful cases.

In distinguishing between the conditions at present under consideration, physical signs demand special attention and study, and to these reference will now be made. (a) Œdema of the subcutaneous tissue of the chest is suggestive of intra-thoracic tumour, though it does rarely occur in connection with empyema. In the latter case, however, it is almost always unilateral, and the superficial veins are not enlarged. When the œdema is more extensive over the thorax, and involves the neck, face, or arm, and is accompanied with any appearance of cyanosis, or with dilated veins, the diagnosis is strongly in favour of growth. (β) The affected side is more or less enlarged as a whole in both kinds of cases, but extreme enlargement would be rather indicative of pleural effusion. In this condition the dilatation is likely to be uniform, and any want of regularity, or a local bulging, would suggest a tumour. Empyema may, however, cause a limited prominence. Another point of distinction is that fluid tends to make the intercostal spaces prominent, while a growth will only lead to stretching without protrusion, or may affect them but little. (γ) A feeling of fluctuation over any of the intercostal spaces is in favour of fluid, but this sign is liable to fallacy. On the other hand, I have distinctly noted in some cases of intra-thoracic growth a remarkable degree of resistance on palpation, which differed from the feeling yielded by effusion. (δ) Careful investigation of the vocal fremitus may afford indications in diagnosis, on the lines previously discussed ; especially as revealing, in connection with tumour, islets where it can be felt, while it is generally abolished or markedly deficient. (ε) The percussion signs demand particular study. In both conditions dulness is very pronounced and extensive, but there are certain points relating to the percussion-sound which may be of diagnostic significance in difficult cases. Those in favour of tumour are extension of dulness from above downwards, if the case happens to have been under observation, or it may be less marked below than above ; . absolute and general dulness, without such a degree of enlargement of the side or other signs as would point to an effusion sufficiently large to produce this effect; irregularity and inequality in the degree of dulness in different parts of the chest, possibly with resonant spots, not varying with change of posture ; and its irregular extension across the middle line at the upper part of the thorax. It has been stated that the absence of Skodaic resonance under the clavicle, in a case of extensive unilateral dulness, is characteristic of malignant disease as distinguished from pleuritic effusion ; but I can affirm from my own observations that such a distinction cannot be relied upon in either direction. The marked sense of resistance elicited on percussion is often highly significant of a solid intra-thoracic growth, as compared with the feeling associated with fluid. (ζ) Auscultation signs are also worthy of attention. Breath-sounds and vocal resonance may be practically abolished over the whole side both in pleural effusion and intrathoracic tumour, but in the latter condition they will probably be audible in some parts, at any rate; and there may be bronchial breathing and bronchophony over considerable areas where dulness is pronounced. Absence of respiratory sounds and vocal resonance below, with auscultatory phenomena indicative of condensed lung above, would probably point to effusion. Undue conduction of the heart sounds is much in favour of a solid growth. (η) Displacement of organs, and especially of the heart, is likely to be decidedly more marked in cases of pleural effusion than of tumour. Moreover the latter tends to push the heart more downwards than laterally, and this is especially characteristic when the left side is affected. (θ) The exploring needle or trochar must of course always be used in doubtful cases, and it may clear up any obscurity at once. The possible fallacy exemplified by Harris' case, already referred to, must, however, not be forgotten, though its repetition would be extremely improbable. (ι) It is always well to examine the opposite lung should the diagnosis not be clear. This organ might yield signs indicating the presence of growths in its substance, which would be highly suggestive. I have known such signs of material help in arriving at a decided opinion in a doubtful case.

I have thus discussed in some detail the probable differences between a growth filling one side of the chest and a large pleural effusion, because the subject is an important one. It must be understood, however, that singly the peculiarities in the signs mentioned are not absolutely conclusive; but it seldom happens that a careful consideration of the whole of the phenomena observed, coupled with the history of the case, will not indicate a definite diagnosis. The presence of pleuritic adhesions may modify the signs in various ways, and thus add considerably to the difficulty in arriving at a satisfactory conclusion.

It must be remembered that an intra-thoracic tumour may be associated with a pleuritic effusion, and then, if there are no obvious pressure-signs, the diagnosis is likely to be extremely difficult, and may be impossible. The question as to the hæmorrhagic nature of the effusion in connection with malignant disease has already been discussed; and it must suffice to state that should such an effusion be obtained by paracentesis in a middle-aged or elderly patient, cardiac disease being excluded, it should excite grave suspicion. The fluid must be carefully examined for cancer elements. Its rapid reaccumulation is in favour of cancer, but this may also be a prominent feature in tuberculous cases. Want of relief of dyspnœa after the removal of the effusion may point to malignant disease. Physical examination after evacuation of the fluid sometimes affords positive evidence of the presence of a tumour. An important sign is the persistence of dulness over the upper part of the chest, especially if it extends beyond the middle line in front; phthisis and pneumonia being excluded. The results of paracentesis are not uncommonly, however, far from conclusive. The general dulness may continue, or pulmonary resonance return, with or without restoration of the breath-sounds.

It may be noted that the dulness of a mediastinal tumour has been simulated by an encysted empyema situated between the anterior edge of the lung and the pericardium, or passing round the root of the lung. A difficulty in diagnosis might possibly thus arise.

(c) *Pericardial conditions.*—Under ordinary circumstances it seems hardly possible that a pericardial effusion resulting from pericarditis could be confounded with a mediastinal tumour. Exceptional cases have occurred in which a cancerous tumour has been mistaken for such effusion, and unsuccessful attempts at paracentesis have been made. In the article on "Diseases of the Pericardium" allusion is also made to a case in which repeated tapping of a supposed cyst in the chest was performed, which proved to be a chronic pericardial effusion. One of the difficulties which may be met with arises from the fact that this condition sometimes causes symptoms of pressure. Moreover, it may be associated with a tumour, and the combination might be very puzzling. As regards physical signs, the diagnosis between pericardial effusion and a mediastinal growth is chiefly founded on the situation, shape, and outline of the dulness; the position of the apex-beat of the heart; and the effects of change of posture upon these signs. When the two conditions exist together it is said that the diagnosis may be aided by the observation that the cardiac sounds are better heard at a distance from, than immediately over the heart. A hæmorrhagic character of any fluid removed by paracentesis would be very suggestive of cancer.

Another condition in which the pericardium is involved, where a difficulty might certainly arise in the diagnosis from tumour, is "indurative mediastino-pericarditis." It is impossible to lay down any definite distinctions, and the diagnosis can only be made from a comprehensive and intelligent consideration of all the circumstances relating to the particular case. I have recently had under my observation a case in which there was marked retraction of the right side, with bulging on the left over the precordial region, and pronounced dulness. The signs and symptoms were very suggestive of tumour, but the conclusion I arrived at was that the conditions were the remains of pleurisy and pericarditis, and consisted in dense adhesions and thickening, accompanied with mediastinal changes. The patient is, however, still alive, and the diagnosis is unverified. Skiagraphy did not afford any help in this case. The possible implication of the pericardium and heart in a mediastinal growth must be borne in mind, but its diagnosis would be extremely difficult.

(d) *Mediastinal conditions.*—In addition to the mediastinal changes just described, associated with those affecting the pericardium, others must be borne in mind as possibly simulating tumour, especially abscess giving rise to pressure-symptoms. The history of the case, perhaps of injury; the characters of the pain, with tenderness; evidences of local inflammation or suppuration; general symptoms indicative of pyrexia, it may be of a hectic type; and the progress of events would probably enable a satisfactory diagnosis to be arrived at. A growth, however, might set up inflammation and abscess. In this connection may also be noticed certain conditions of some of the mediastinal contents, and of the thoracic walls. An enlarged and persistent thymus may give rise to marked phenomena of a tumour in the anterior mediastinum. Syphilitic disease may also simulate this condition. Thus a post-sternal node sometimes originates pronounced pressure-symptoms, at the same time causing dulness. Syphilitic ulceration and stricture of the lower end of the trachea or a main bronchus is another aspect of this disease which may present difficulty in diagnosis, especially when accompanied with enlarged glands, of which I have recently met with a very striking instance. The distinction between such a condition of things and a small mediastinal tumour merely interfering with one or both of these tubes, and not giving rise to any physical signs, may be almost impossible. A history of syphilitic infection, and the effects of treatment, often help the diagnosis materially, but not always. When dysphagia is a prominent symptom, where there is an evident growth, it may be a question whether it is œsophageal in origin, or an independent mediastinal growth causing pressure on the tube. The former is the more probable; but cases which have come under my notice have proved to me that it may be impossible to come to any positive and certain conclusion on the point, especially when œsophageal cancer gives rise to pressure-symptoms, which, however, is not a question of great moment. Examination with a bougie might perhaps afford some help. It will suffice to mention caries and cancer of the spinal column as possible conditions which may resemble intra-thoracic tumour in some respects, so as to put the practitioner on his guard against overlooking the real nature of the disease in such cases, and to prepare him for further developments which may clear up any initial obscurity in the diagnosis.

(e) *Aortic aneurysm.*—I have left to the last one of the most important diseases which embarrass the diagnosis of mediastinal growth. A difficulty in distinguishing between these two conditions arises chiefly under the following circumstances :—There may be definite indications of direct pressure on the trachea, but no signs to explain whether the cause of the pressure be an aneurysm or a solid tumour; but the probability is, as a rule, in favour of the former, so far as my experience goes. In another class of cases the question arises as to the nature of a pulsating tumour. I have known pulsation associated with a large aneurysm to be so diffused and indistinct, and accompanied with such extensive dulness, that it was supposed to be a transmitted movement from the aorta through a growth. On the other hand, such a growth may actually conduct an aortic pulsation to the surface, and there may even be a murmur; an aneurysm being thus simulated. Very rarely, also, a communication forms between the aorta and a cystic tumour within the chest; or a pulsating cancer is met with. In my experience the difficulties encountered in this direction have been as a matter of fact extremely exceptional, due attention being paid to the points of distinction usually recognised, as regards the characters of the pulsation and other signs; but they do occur, and must not be ignored. Another condition which I have known to cause error in diagnosis is where an aneurysm has undergone a curative process, and become practically a solid mass. Such a condition might easily be mistaken for a growth if the practitioner were unacquainted with the history of the case.

The discussion of this aspect of the subject would not be complete without a general summary of the points to be more particularly attended to in making a diagnosis between a mediastinal growth and an aneurysm within the chest, especially in doubtful cases.

(a) Among general matters age and sex are worthy of note. The fact that the patient is a female and under twenty-five years of age is in favour of a growth; while in a male adult aneurysm would rather be thought of. In old persons cancer would be the more probable. This point, however, must not be pushed too far. Hereditary tendency to malignant disease, a history of a previous tumour in the patient, or still more its actual presence in some other part of the body, or evidence of implication of glands, would of course afford strong indications in this direction. Occupations or violent forms of exertion favouring aneurysm, either past or present, would point to this complaint; and a history of syphilis might also be suggestive, as well as the condition of the arteries generally. (β) Symptoms always demand due consideration, particularly pressure phenomena. Severe pain, especially in the back, is most common in aneurysm, but can hardly be relied upon. Frequent hæmoptysis, with red-currant jelly expectoration, points rather to tumour. Douglas Powell (35) affirms that pressure-symptoms are insidious in cases of tumour, but more persistent and less variable than those of aneurysm. Thus dyspnœa tends to increase more gradually, while paroxysmal dyspnœa is less common, except, perhaps, in the later stages of the disease. In discussing this question in diagnosis, Steven emphasises the importance of distinguishing between pressure effects pure and simple, and pressure effects accompanied by structural alterations in the neighbouring tissues set up by the vital action of the tumour. Aneurysm and benign growths give rise to the former group, while the latter are associated with malignant intra-thoracic tumours, in connection with which the signs of pressure are therefore relatively more numerous and more frequent than with aneurysm. He writes: "In aneurysm we can often demonstrate only one pressure effect —for example, recurrent nerve pressure—whereas in solid growths we often have a large number—for example, localised œdema, varicosity, dyspnœa, obstructed bronchi, hoarseness, etc., in one and the same case." Most writers are agreed that the effects of pressure upon the larger intra-thoracic veins are more common and more pronounced in connection with solid tumour than aneurysm. Steven says: "Varicosity of veins and localised œdema are relatively rare in cases of aneurysm, because the veins, though pressed upon and dislocated, are not very likely to be crushed against resistant points, and so the blood still circulates through them." Conversely, it has been affirmed that the phenomena resulting from pressure on the air-passages, nerves, and œsophagus are most frequently observed in tumours. Steven insists upon the fact of spasmodic asthma—that is, spasm of the whole bronchi rather than of the vocal cords—being a symptom very specially indicative of the presence of a malignant growth within the chest. He also concludes that, in our ordinary clinical experience, irritative and paralytic nervous symptoms are perhaps not so frequently associated with solid as with aneurysmal tumours. My personal experience has convinced me that we must be careful not to rely too implicitly on the supposed distinctions between the pressure-symptoms of aneurysm and a solid tumour respectively; though in some instances they certainly do afford useful indications. (γ) Physical and other special signs obviously require intelligent and careful study in doubtful cases. As a rule the differences are obvious enough. It is when a pulsatile movement is associated with a mediastinal growth that the chief difficulty arises. This pulsation, however, is not expansile or heaving; and the site of its maximum intensity does not correspond so closely as in aneurysm with that of the most marked dulness. The gradual approach of a pulsation towards the surface is very suggestive of the latter disease. Great superficial area of dulness, altogether out of proportion to the amount of impulse, is in favour of tumour; but I have known this sign to mislead. Other data pointing to aneurysm are limitation of the signs to the region of the arch of the aorta; the presence of thrill; a marked diastolic shock; accentuation of the second sound over the prominence of the tumour, or a diastolic murmur; cardiac hypertrophy; and marked retardation in the pulsation of the distant arteries. In exceptional cases examination of the sputum, or of the main air-tube by means of the laryngoscope, might help the diagnosis. The development of pleuritic and pericardial effusion would be in favour of malignant growth. Skiagraphy may be expected in course of time to assist materially in the diagnosis between aneurysm and a solid tumour within the chest, and, indeed, is said to have done so already.

4. Supposing the diagnosis of the presence of an intra-thoracic tumour to have been made, and aneurysm excluded, the next procedure is to attempt to determine its nature, and this may be fairly easy. When a growth is secondary, it may be concluded that this is similar to the primary disease, if its nature is known. The association of a tumour within the chest with obvious tuberculous or syphilitic disease, or with diffused lymphadenoma, would suggest like conditions. In primary cases the main point is to determine whether a tumour is benign or malignant, and this is, as a rule, not a difficult matter if due consideration be given to all the data. Benign growths usually only give rise to pressure effects pure and simple. From their greater frequency one would always be inclined towards the diagnosis either of carcinoma or some kind of lympho-sarcoma. In elderly subjects, and if a growth could be traced originally to the lung or pleura, the former would be more especially indicated. As regards primary tumours in the mediastinum, the diagnosis of their nature may be quite easy or very difficult in different cases, and much will depend upon individual experience and acumen. The comparative frequency of cancer and lympho-sarcoma

cannot be relied upon, especially as observers differ on this point. Lympho-sarcoma must always be borne in mind, particularly in young subjects. The appearance of fulness and nodular or glandular projections beneath the clavicle and in the neck is, according to Steven, especially character-istic of this variety of growth. Speaking of the differential diagnosis between sarcomatous and cancerous tumours of the mediastinum, this writer remarks : " As a general rule lympho-sarcomatous growths are bulky tumours, often giving rise to very definite physical signs, and causing multiple pressure effects, which there is usually very little difficulty in recognising. Such tumours also very readily grow towards the front of the chest. Primary cancers of the mediastinum, on the other hand, are usually smaller and more limited tumours, and in respect of their general size or bulk are often incapable of giving rise to physical signs capable of detection." Should such a growth break down and communicate with the air-passages, its nature might be revealed by examination of the sputum. The secondary development of growths in other parts of the body might clear up any obscurity in the diagnosis in doubtful cases ; as well as the progress of the general symptoms.

The special diagnosis of exceptional tumours within the chest, not already referred to in this connection, can only be made by exclusion of the more common varieties, and by detailed consideration of the clinical and pathological features of each individual case, but it is often impossible. The presence of a pronounced rheumatic diathesis, and the discovery of subcutaneous nodules, might suggest fibroma. This variety grows very slowly, and even when it originates marked pressure-symptoms, years often elapse before it causes death, the surrounding tissues accommodating themselves to existing conditions. Teratoma must be remembered as a possible condition, but it presents no pathognomonic symptoms or signs, unless a fistulous communication should form with the cyst, and its characteristic contents be discharged. Hydatid tumour of the mediastinum must not be forgotten, but is extremely rare.

5. The last point to be noted in relation to the diagnosis of intra-thoracic tumours, and which can only be mentioned, without any discussion, is that the practitioner must be prepared for the possibility of cases coming before him, of which he knows nothing, under an acute or sudden aspect, owing to the effects of such a tumour upon the contents of the thorax, rapidly and unexpectedly produced. Under such circumstances it would probably be impossible to come to any definite or positive conclusion as to the actual state of things.

Prognosis.—Unfortunately but little can be said under this head, and that of a very unfavourable nature. The prognosis is always very grave in relation to intra-thoracic growths, and as a rule practically hope-less, especially if the disease is malignant. The probability also is that the patient will pass through much suffering during the progress of the growth. The question of duration must depend upon the nature of the tumour, its situation, effects, and symptoms, rapidity and mode of development, and other circumstances ; and it is generally quite impossible to give any definite opinion on this point. Benign growths may last a very long time. The prognosis is obviously more hopeful in such tumours as may be amenable to treatment under favourable conditions, such as those of a syphilitic or tuberculous nature, or a dermoid cyst. Possibly complete recovery may be brought about in some of these cases, but at the best the outlook is always serious, and under any circumstances a very cautious opinion should be given as to the ultimate cure.

Treatment.—It will only be practicable to indicate the general principles upon which the treatment of intra-thoracic growths, whatever their seat of origin, must be founded, and to mention some of the more important measures which may be called for. Obviously our remedies can only be palliative in the large majority of instances, and each case must be dealt with individually. The desire to afford relief will often tax the therapeutic knowledge and resources of the practitioner to the utmost, and his efforts will but too frequently end in disappointment. The first principle to be enforced is that, considering the conditions with which we have to deal, it will be for the welfare of the patient that we should not be too active in treatment, or employ irritating applications and such things energetically or for a long time without any definite purpose; and that we should not resort to the more powerful and effectual palliative measures at our command at too early a period, but reserve them until the urgency of the symptoms calls for their rational employment.

Any hope of curative treatment by medicinal methods can only be entertained in the case of tuberculous or syphilitic morbid conditions; or possibly of fibroma associated with the rheumatic diathesis. A tumour due to tuberculous glands must be dealt with according to the usual principles applicable to that complaint, which have already been described in this article. Syphilitic conditions would be the most hopeful from a curative point of view; and the free administration of iodide of potassium, or perhaps the judicious employment of mercurials, might prove highly beneficial. I have no experience as to the effects of anti-rheumatic remedies in the treatment of fibroma. The notion of absorbing lympho-sarcomatous or cancerous tumours by medicines or injections is out of the question, at any rate so far as our present knowledge goes.

Nor can a much more hopeful view be taken of any operative measures for the removal or cure of intra-thoracic tumours. Those ordinarily met with are practically beyond the reach of any operation, especially considering their relation to the vital structures with which they are more or less intimately associated. How far the more heroic surgeons of the present day would be inclined to interfere in particular instances must be left to their individual judgment and skill. The only conditions which, as a rule, might rationally call for operative treatment are tuberculous disease forming an abscess approaching the surface, teratoma, and possibly hydatids occupying the anterior mediastinum, or osteo-chondroma or enchondroma growing from the sternum. In the treatment of teratoma the sternum has been trephined, and the cyst punctured and injected with iodine.

In the large majority of cases of growths within the chest, the only definite treatment that can be adopted is of a palliative kind, intended for the relief of symptoms, and for dealing with secondary morbid conditions or complications to which they may give rise. The chief symptoms which may demand attention are pain, dyspnœa of various kinds, cough, hæmoptysis, cardiac disorder, restlessness, and insomnia. These must be treated on general principles, but, sooner or later, they often baffle us completely. Rest and posture are frequently important factors in treatment, and should always be intelligently considered in individual cases. Among the agents and methods which may be particularly helpful in affording relief may be mentioned opium or morphine internally, or subcutaneous injection of morphine, with or without atropine; hydrate of chloral; ether internally or by inhalation; possibly nitrite of amyl; application of leeches to the chest, or even venesection if there be much venous obstruction and cyanosis; and inhalation of oxygen. Certain medicines may be helpful for bronchitic conditions. Poultices or irritant applications to the chest may be of service, but they must be employed judiciously. It is often not desirable to attempt to check hæmoptysis, even if it were possible. Should dysphagia be a prominent symptom it is practically beyond the reach of treatment. Œdema of the arms may be relieved in some cases by the very careful and accurate application of a soft flannel bandage from the fingers to the shoulders, as advised by Steven. Puncturing the skin, or the introduction of Southey's tubes, must only be resorted to as a last resource, and when absolutely needed.

There are two points in treatment which must be referred to separately, as they may demand special consideration in particular cases. The first is the performance of tracheotomy for the relief of urgent or paroxysmal dyspnœa. This operation can only be of service when the paroxysms depend chiefly on laryngeal spasm from nerve irritation. Unfortunately, however, there is usually at the same time direct pressure on the trachea or main bronchi, so that tracheotomy gives no relief. At the best the operation will probably be very difficult to perform, on account of the conditions present. The other point is the mode of dealing with pleural effusion, and possibly with pericardial effusion also. In my opinion it is not desirable to remove pleuritic effusion as a matter of course in cases of this nature; and Sir Douglas Powell expresses the opinion that it should not be interfered with unless it is definitely increasing the dyspnœa; its tendency being to retard the progress of the growth. On the other hand, there should be no hesitation about taking more or less of the fluid away if it is obviously adding to the difficulty of breathing or other ills; and this procedure may afford the greatest relief, as in a case of Sir W. Broadbent's, where two quarts of blood-stained fluid were removed. The fluid should be taken away slowly, and it is not necessary to withdraw the whole of it; but as much as six or seven pints have been removed. There may be danger of hæmorrhage from the growth or its adhesions. As a rule the effusion returns speedily, and frequent repetitions of paracentesis may become necessary, sometimes at very short intervals. In exceptional cases profuse serous expectoration has followed the operation. Should the fluid become purulent or semi-purulent, incision and drainage may be called for. Paracentesis of the pericardium may possibly be demanded for urgent symptoms, but this can only afford temporary relief. It has happened in some instances of mediastinal malignant disease that the fibrinous element has so predominated in pleuritic and pericardial effusion that tapping was of little or no service. Secondary cancerous nodules have sometimes been observed at the site of paracentesis.

The general condition and the remoter symptoms or complications occurring in the course of cases of intra-thoracic malignant growth must be dealt with on ordinary principles. The patient must take as nourishing a diet as possible, the appetite should be maintained, and the functions of the alimentary canal attended to. Stimulants may be given as required. The general surroundings should be as comfortable and cheerful as circumstances permit, and everything done that can alleviate the sufferings of the patient, which often become very distressing before death closes the scene.

FREDERICK T. ROBERTS.

REFERENCES

1. ALLBUTT T. CLIFFORD. *Trans. Royal Medical and Chirurgical Society*, vol. xlix. p. 165.—2. BENNETT, Sir RISDON. Quain's *Dictionary of Medicine*, 2nd ed. vol. i. p. 1202, "Malignant Disease of Lungs."—3. *Idem. Loc. cit.* vol. ii. p. 22, "Diseases of Mediastinum."—4. *Idem.* Lumleian Lectures at R. Coll. Physicians, 1871, *On Cancerous and other Intra-thoracic Growths.*—5. BRISTOWE, J. S. *Path. Soc. Trans.* vol. xi. p. 32.—6. BROADBENT, Sir W. H. *Clinical Soc. Trans.* vol. xi. p. 136.—7. BRUCE, J. MITCHELL. Quain's *Dictionary of Medicine*, 2nd ed. vol. i. p. 835, "Morbid Growths in the Heart." —8. BUDD *Trans. Royal Medical and Chirurgical Society*, vol. xliii. p. 228.—9. COATS, J. *Glasgow Medical Journal*, July 1889, p. 15.—10. COCKLE. *Intra-thoracic Cancer*, 1865. —11. DALTON, N. *Path. Soc. Trans.* vol. xxxv. p. 82.—12. DAVIES, A. T. *Path. Soc. Trans.* vol. xl. p. 46.—13. EGER. *Zur Pathologie der mediastinal Tumoren*, Diss. Inaug. Breslau, 1872.—14. FOX, WILSON. "Diseases of Mediastinum," in *Treatise on Diseases of the Lungs and Pleura*, edited by S. Coupland, 1891, p. 1021 *et seq.*, with very full bibliography. The present article contains many quotations and references obtained from Dr. Wilson Fox's valuable work.—15. FRAENTZEL. *Charité-Annalen*, 1876, vol. iii.—16. GODLEE, R. J. *Trans. Royal Medical and Chirurgical Society*, vol. lxii.— 17. GOODHART, J. F. *Brit. Med. Journal*, 1879, vol. i. pp. 542, 580.—18. GULL, Sir W. W. *Guy's Hospital Reports*, new series, vol. v.—19. HALE and GOODHART. *Clin. Soc. Trans.* vol. xxvi. p. 105.—20. HARE, H. A. *The Pathology, Clinical History, and Diagnosis of Affections of the Mediastinum*, Fothergillian Prize Essay, 1889.—21. HARRIS, T. *Indurative Mediastino-pericarditis*, 1895.—22. *Idem. Journal of Pathology and Bacteriology*, vol. ii. p. 179, "Malignant Disease of Pleura."—23. HARRIS, V. D. *St. Bartholomew's Hospital Reports*, vol. xxviii. p. 73.—24. HERTZ. Ziemssen's *Cyclopaedia*, vol. v.—25. JACCOUD. *Leçons de clinique médicale.*—26. KAULICH. "Ueber maligne Neoplasmen im vorderen Mediastinal-Raum," *Prager Vierteljahr.* 1868, vol. c.—27. KUSSMAUL. *Berlin. klin. Wochen.* Jahrgang x. 1873.—28. MAGUIRE, R. *Brit. Med. Journal*, 1888, vol. ii. p. 1047.—29. MAIN, E. *Twentieth Century Practice of Medicine*, vol. vii. "Disease of Mediastinum."—30. MONEY, ANGEL. *Brit. Med. Journal*, 1888, vol. ii. p. 1046.—31. MOTT, F. W. *Path. Soc. Trans.* vol. xl. p. 47, "Malignant Growth involving Pericardium."—32. OGLE, C. *Path. Soc. Trans.* vol. xlviii. p. 37.—33. PAGET, S. *Surgery of the Chest*, 1896, "Some Diseases of Bronchial Glands and Posterior Mediastinum," p. 336; "Intra-thoracic New Growths," p. 398.—34. PEREZ,

GEORGE. "Mediastinal Friction. On a New Auscultatory Sign in connection with Mediastinal Affections," *Brit. Med. Journ.* 1896, vol. i. p. 82.—35. POWELL, Sir R. DOUGLAS. *Diseases of Lungs and Pleura,* 4th ed.—36. *Idem.* Reynolds' *System of Medicine,* vol. v. "Mediastinal Tumours."—37. RENDU. "Des tumeurs malignes du médiastine," *Archives générales de méd.* 1875.—38. RIEGEL. *Virchow's Archiv,* Bd. xlix. —39. ROLLESTON, H. D. *Path. Soc. Trans.* vol. xlviii. p. 200.—40. *Idem. Journal of Pathology and Bacteriology,* vol. iv. p. 228.—41. RUMPF. *Ueber Neubildungen im Mediastinum,* Inaug. Diss. Freiburg, 1894.—42. SALTER, HYDE. *Lancet,* 1869.—43. SCHÜPPEL. Quoted by Wilson Fox in his treatise, footnote on p. 615.—44. SEITZ. "Der klinische Diagnose der bronchial Drüsen-erkrankungen," *Wien. klin. Woch.* 1894.—45. SMITH, EUSTACE. *Diseases of Children,* 2nd ed. p. 191.—46. STEVEN, J. LINDSAY. *Mediastinal Tumours,* 1892.—47. STOKES, W. *Diseases of the Chest.*—48. THOMAS, R. S. *Glasgow Med. Journal,* vol. xxx. p. 483.—49. THORNTON, PUGIN. Quain's *Dictionary of Medicine,* 2nd ed. vol. ii. p. 1030, "Diseases of Thymus Gland." —50. VOELCKER, A. F. "On some Effects produced by Caseous Bronchial Glands in Children," *Practitioner,* June 1895.—51. WALSHE, W. H. *On Cancer,* 1846.—52. *Idem. Diseases of Lungs,* quoted by Wilson Fox.—53. WHITE, W. HALE. *Path. Soc. Trans.* vol. xli. 283.—54. WILKS, Sir S. *Guy's Hospital Reports,* 1871.—55. WILLIAMS, C. T. *Path. Soc. Trans.* vol. xxiv. p. 23.

F. T. R.

DISEASES OF BLOOD-VESSELS

THROMBOSIS

Definition.—A thrombus is usually defined as a blood-coagulum, formed in the heart or vessels during life. This definition applies to most cases; but, in order to meet the objections of those who do not concede that all thrombi are genuine coagula, and to give due prominence to the participation of blood-platelets and corpuscles, a thrombus may be more broadly defined as a solid mass or plug formed in the living heart or vessels from constituents of the blood. Thrombosis is the act or process of formation of a thrombus, or the condition characterised by its presence.

Structure of thrombi.—The formed elements which may enter into the composition of fresh thrombi are blood-platelets, fibrin, leucocytes, and red corpuscles. These elements may be present in varying number, proportion, and arrangement, whence there results great diversity in the appearance and structure of different thrombi.

The two main anatomical groups of thrombi are the red and the white thrombi. Many of the mixed thrombi may be regarded as a variety of the white thrombus. In addition there are thrombi of relatively minor importance composed wholly or chiefly of leucocytes, of fibrillated fibrin or of hyaline material.

Red thrombi.—These are formed from stagnating blood, and in the recent state do not differ in appearance and structure from clots formed in shed blood. They are made up of fibrillated fibrin and of red and white corpuscles in the same proportions as in the circulating blood, or the white corpuscles may be somewhat in excess. If any part of such a red thrombus be exposed to circulating blood, white material, consisting of platelets with fibrin and leucocytes, is deposited upon it. This deposit may aid in distinguishing the thrombus from a post-mortem clot.

White and mixed thrombi.—Most thrombi are formed from the circulating blood, and are white, or of a mixed red and white colour. The white or gray colour is due to the presence of platelets, fibrin, and leucocytes, occurring singly, or, more frequently, in combination. The admixture with red corpuscles is not an essential character of the thrombus, although it may be sufficient to give it a predominantly red colour.

Fresh white human thrombi, when examined microscopically, are seen to be composed of a granular material, usually in islands or strands of varying shape and size, around and between which are fibrin and leucocytes with a larger or smaller number of entangled red corpuscles. The granular matter, to which the older observers attached comparatively little importance, and which they interpreted as granular or molecular fibrin or the detritus of white corpuscles, is now known to be an essential constituent of the white thrombus, and is composed chiefly of altered blood-platelets. Intact polynuclear leucocytes are usually numerous in the margins of and between the masses of platelets, and may be scattered among the individual platelets. Not less important is the fibrillated fibrin, which is generally present in large amount. It is particularly dense in the borders of the platelet-masses, and stretches between them in anastomosing strands, or as a finer network containing red and white corpuscles. Within the accumulations of platelets in fresh thrombi fibrin is often absent, or is in small amount. These various constituents of the thrombus often present a definite architectural arrangement, and soon undergo metamorphoses which will be described subsequently.

Thrombi of the kind just described, and as we find them at autopsies on human beings, are completed products, and it is difficult, indeed generally impossible, from their examination to come to any conclusion as to the exact manner of their formation; particularly as regards the sequence and relative importance of their different constituents. So long as the knowledge of the structure of thrombi was limited to that derived from the study of these completed plugs, the coagulation of fibrin was generally believed to be the primary and essential step in their formation; although Virchow pointed out the greater richness in white corpuscles as a feature distinguishing them from post-mortem clots.

Zahn, in 1872, was the first to make a systematic experimental study, mainly in frogs, of the mode of formation of thrombi. He came to the conclusion that the process is initiated by the accumulation of white corpuscles which, by their disintegration, give rise to granular detritus. This is quickly followed by the appearance of fibrin, which was readily accounted for by Weigert on the basis of Alexander Schmidt's well-known suggestion of the origin of fibrin ferment from disintegrated leucocytes. Zahn's views, anticipated in part by Mantegazza in 1869, and confirmed by Pitres in 1876, gained prompt and wide acceptance.

Continued experimental study of the subject, however, especially upon mammals, led to opposition to Zahn's conclusions, and favoured the opinion, now generally accepted, that the ordinary white thrombus starts as an accumulation not of leucocytes but of blood-platelets. The investigators chiefly concerned in the establishment of this doctrine are Osler (1881-82), Hayem (1882), Bizzozero (1882), Lubnitzky (1885), and Eberth and Schimmelbusch (1885-86).

There is no difficulty in producing thrombi experimentally by injury, either mechanical or chemical, to the vessel-wall; or by the introduction of foreign bodies into the circulation. If the early formation of such a thrombus be observed under the microscope in the living mesenteric vessels of a dog, as was done by Eberth and Schimmelbusch, it is seen that the first step consists in the accumulation of blood-platelets at the seat of injury. These plates, in consequence of their viscous metamorphosis, at once become adherent to each other and to the wall of the vessel, and thus form plugs which may be subsequently washed away into the circulation, but which sometimes so increase in size as to obstruct the lumen of the vessel completely. Red and white corpuscles may be included in the mass of platelets; but their presence at this stage is purely accidental; they are not to be regarded as essential constituents of the thrombus in its inception.

The microscopical examination of young experimental thrombi confirms the results of these direct observations, and affords information as to their further development. To obtain a clear idea of this development, thrombi should be examined at intervals of minutes from their beginning to those half an hour old or older. I reported the results of such an experimental study in 1887. The material composing the youngest thrombi formed from the circulating blood appears macroscopically as a soft, homogeneous, gray, translucent substance of viscid consistence. Microscopically it is made up chiefly of platelets, which are seen as pale, round, or somewhat irregular bodies, varying in size but averaging about one-quarter the diameter of a red corpuscle.

Leucocytes, which may be present in small number at the beginning, rapidly increase in number, and within the first fifteen minutes to half an hour they are usually in such abundance that at this stage of its formation they must be considered an essential constituent of the thrombus. They tend to collect at the margins of the platelet-masses and between them. These leucocytes are nearly all polynuclear, and usually present no evidence of necrosis or disintegration.

With the accumulation of leucocytes, fibrillated fibrin, which at first was absent, makes its appearance; being, as pointed out by Hanau, especially well marked and dense in the margins of the masses of platelets. Within these masses it is usually absent. The rapidity with which leucocytes and fibrin are added to the masses of platelets varies much in different cases. At the end of half an hour the thrombus may be composed of platelets, leucocytes, and fibrin with entangled red corpuscles, in essentially the same proportions and with the same arrangement as in the human thrombi already described; or even after several hours it may still consist almost wholly of platelets.

The prevailing view is that platelets exist in normal blood, where they circulate with the red corpuscles in the axial current. In accordance with this view, many observers, following Eberth and Schimmelbusch, explain the beginning of a white thrombus by the accumulation of pre-existing platelets upon a foreign body, or, in consequence of slowing or other irregularities of the blood-flow, on the damaged inner wall of the heart or vessels. Contact with the abnormal surface sets up an immediate viscous metamorphosis of the platelets, whereby they adhere to each other and to the foreign body or vascular wall. Eberth and Schimmelbusch designate this process as conglutination, and distinguish it sharply from coagulation, which they regard as a later event in the development of the thrombus.

Those who hold with Löwit, that platelets do not exist in normal blood, believe that they are produced at the moment of formation of the thrombus, as the result of injury to the blood; and many who believe that they are in normal blood not as independent elements, but as derivatives from leucocytes or red corpuscles, consider it probable that those in the thrombus are formed, at least in part, in consequence of such injury. Although there are observations which suggest that platelets may be derived from leucocytes, there is no evidence that the masses of platelets found in incipient thrombi come from leucocytes previously attracted to the spot.

Strong evidence has been recently presented, by Arnold, F. Müller, and Determann, in favour of the origin of platelets from red corpuscles. Wlassow, working in Ziegler's laboratory, finds that the white thrombus is formed primarily by the destruction of red corpuscles, and is composed at the very beginning of shadows of red corpuscles, corpuscular fragments both with and without hæmoglobin, granular material and platelets of nucleo-proteid substance; all derived from disintegrating red corpuscles. A similar view is entertained by Mosso, Klebs, Arnold, Ziegler, and F. Müller.

The accumulation of leucocytes in the young thrombus may be explained partly by mechanical causes,—the most evident being the projecting, irregular, sticky substance of the platelet masses associated with slowing and eddies of the blood-stream,—and partly by chemiotactic influences.

Whatever difficulties there may be, in accounting for the fibrin, relate to the general subject of coagulation of the blood (see Professor Foster's article in vol. vi. p. 403) rather than to the special conditions of the thrombus. As to the participation of platelets in the production of fibrin, opinion is divided; and upon this point the study of thrombi has not afforded conclusive evidence one way or the other. The usual absence of fibrin within the platelet masses for a considerable time after their formation may be thought to speak against the generation of fibrin-ferment by the platelets. But if, as is probable, the platelets contain nucleo-proteid, it would be reasonable to suppose, in accordance with current physiological ideas, that they can yield one of the fibrin factors; and it may be that in these compact masses there is not enough fibrinogen furnished by the plasma to generate an appreciable amount of fibrin. The characteristic dense ring of fibrin immediately around the platelet masses, where there is abundant fibrinogen, could be interpreted in favour of the liberation of fibrin-ferment by the collected platelets. By the time, however, that the fibrin appears, leucocytes have also accumulated in the same situation; and they, either alone or together with the platelets, may be the source of the ferment; although, as already stated, the leucocytes in young thrombi generally show apparently intact nuclei and cytoplasm.

Does the recognition of the described mode of development of a white thrombus necessitate a radical break, such as that made by Eberth and Schimmelbusch, with the old and still common conception that a thrombus is essentially a blood coagulum? This question applies only to the first stage of formation of a white thrombus, for the completed thrombus is undoubtedly a coagulum. It is, however, of both scientific and practical interest to inquire whether coagulative phenomena usher in the process of thrombosis or are merely secondary. A decisive answer to this question cannot be given until we are better informed than at present concerning the chemistry and morphology of coagulative processes, and the source and properties of the granular material constituting the youngest thrombi. The possibility that this material is already coagulated, and falls into the category of the coagulative necroses, has been suggested by Weigert; but without any proof of this view. There' is greater probability that the accumulation and metamorphoses of the so-called platelets in beginning thrombi represent a preparation for coagulation or a first step in the process. As Hammersten has pointed out, two chemical phases are to be distinguished in the process of coagulation; namely, the formation of fibrin ferment from its zymogen, and the transformation of fibrinogen into fibrin under the influence of this ferment. Morphological phases may also be distinguished, and the platelet stage of thrombus formation may be interpreted as the first morphological phase of coagulation in circulating blood. According to Wlassow a similar morphological phase may be recognised in the clotting produced by whipping shed blood. It would lead too far afield to enter here into a discussion of the arguments in favour of this view; but much in its support is found in recent chemical and morphological studies of extravascular and intravascular coagulation, and of the anatomical and chemical characters of blood platelets.[1] It does not appear, therefore, that we are called upon at present to make any such radical revision of the traditional conception of white thrombi as coagula, as has been advocated of late years by some writers.

Leucocytic thrombi.—As has already been explained, leucocytes, although they do not usher in the process of ordinary thrombosis, make their appearance at an early stage, and often accumulate in such numbers as to constitute a large part of the thrombus. My studies of experi-

---

[1] This recent work has been critically reviewed by Lòwit in Lubarsch-Ostertag's *Ergebnisse*, 1897.

mental and human thrombi have led me to assign to them a more important part in the construction of white thrombi than that indicated by Eberth and Schimmelbusch. Whether the regular mural white thrombi ever arise as a collection of leucocytes, in the manner described by Zahn, is uncertain. Such a mode of development, if it occurs, is, I think, exceptional. Intravascular plugs, however, occur, which are made up wholly or predominantly of polynuclear leucocytes. These are found mainly in small vessels in acutely inflamed regions, where they are to be regarded as inflammatory and probably chemiotactic in origin. Leucocytic masses may also be found after death in small vessels in leucocythæmia, and in diseases with marked leucocytosis; but it is probable that these are not genuine obstructing plugs.

Purely fibrinous thrombi.—As will be described subsequently, fibrin usually increases in amount with the age of the thrombus. The masses of platelets may be replaced by fibrin, and leucocytes may degenerate; so that many old, unorganised thrombi consist of practically nothing but dense fibrin, in places hyaline. I do not, however, desire now to call especial attention to these old, metamorphosed thrombi.

One sometimes finds in inflamed areas, less frequently under other circumstances, the vessels, particularly those of small size, partly or completely filled with fibrillated fibrin, presenting such an arrangement and configuration as to indicate coagulation during life. Neither leucocytes nor platelets need take part in the formation of these plugs of pure fibrin, although sometimes they are present. K. Zenker has well described the microscopical appearances in these cases. Whorls or brush-like clumps of fibrin may spring at intervals from the wall of the vessel, where they are attached especially to necrotic endothelium or to points devoid of endothelium. The fibrin may be disposed regularly, often in stellate figures, around definite centres in which, perhaps, a necrotic cell or fragment, endothelial or leucocytic, or a clump of platelets can be demonstrated. The fibrin is often notably coarse. The affected vessels are not usually filled completely with fibrin, and they can be artificially injected. In croupous pneumonia such fibrinous masses are regularly present, both in capillaries and larger vessels of the hepatised area. These purely fibrinous coagula are of anatomical rather than clinical interest.

Hyaline thrombi.—These are of more interest and importance than the purely fibrinous and leucocytic thrombi just described. The presence of hyaline material in old white thrombi will be spoken of subsequently. To von Recklinghausen we especially owe the recognition of hyaline thrombi as a distinct class. They are found especially in the capillaries, but may occur also in the smaller arteries and veins. The capillaries are filled with a refractive, homogeneous, translucent, colourless or faintly yellow material, which stains well with Weigert's fibrin dye. The same material may partly or completely fill the smaller arteries and veins. Balls, as well as cylindrical masses, of this hyaline substance may be found, especially in the cerebral vessels.

This hyaline thrombosis has been observed in a variety of conditions, partly general, partly local. It occurs especially in infective and toxic diseases. Kriege found extensive hyaline thrombosis in the small vessels after freezing the rabbit's ear. Von Recklinghausen had previously attributed to this cause spontaneous gangrene of both feet occurring in an old woman who had suffered repeatedly from slight frost-bites; and he likewise found the same hyaline vascular plugs in cases of mortification following experimental ergotism. Capillary hyaline thromboses are common in the lungs in pneumonia, and in hæmorrhagic infarcts. In general infective and toxic states they may be present in the liver, the lungs, and, above all, in the kidneys.

The most striking examples of this form of thrombosis, with which I am acquainted, are encountered in the renal capillaries, chiefly of the glomeruli, of swine dead of hog-cholera; or of animals infected with the hog-cholera bacillus. In extreme cases there is complete anuria; and it may be impossible to force more than a minimal amount of injecting fluid into the renal vessels. Sections stained with Weigert's fibrin-stain look as if the capillaries had been injected with Berlin blue. Ribbert found similar hyaline thrombi in the kidneys of rabbits inoculated with the S. pyogenes aureus. I have repeatedly found them in various experimental infections, and in human infections. They occur in eclampsia. Bacteria are not necessarily present, so that toxins are probably the underlying causative factor, and for this there is experimental evidence.

Klebs and others have thought that the hyaline material is derived from coalesced and altered red corpuscles. Red corpuscles may in fact be so crowded together, and apparently coalesced, as to appear as nearly homogeneous yellowish cylinders (globular stasis). The genuine hyaline thrombi have the staining reactions of fibrin, and are often continuous with ordinary fibrillated fibrin in larger vessels. Transitions between fibrillated fibrin and the hyaline material can sometimes be seen; but it is often impossible by any staining to resolve the latter into a fibrinous network. If the recent views previously mentioned concerning the origin of platelets from red corpuscles and the participation of these corpuscles in the process of coagulation be accepted, there would be no difficulty in adopting Klebs's hypothesis as to the origin of hyaline thrombi from red corpuscles. Von Recklinghausen and Kriege find evidence that the hyaline substance is derived from leucocytes.

Growth, Metamorphoses, and Organisation of Thrombi.—Thrombi in their growth assume various characters to which special epithets are applied. A thrombus formed from the circulating blood is at first parietal or mural, but by continued growth it may fill the vessel and become an occluding or obstructing thrombus. A primitive or autochthonous thrombus, caused by local conditions, may be the starting-point of a continued or propagated thrombus, extending in the course of the thrombosed vessel and perhaps into communicating vessels. A secondary or encapsulating thrombus is one which starts from an embolus of thrombotic material. A continued thrombus is also often spoken of as secondary. Thrombi are, with rare exceptions, adherent, at least in places, to the wall of the vessel or the heart. Mural thrombi appear more or less flattened against the vessel wall, or they may project in a globular or polypoid form into the lumen. Their free surface is generally rough. Loose thrombi in the heart are called ball-thrombi.

The thrombus grows in length chiefly in the direction of the current of blood; but it may grow in the opposite direction. The intact and growing end of the thrombus is a flattened blunt cone, usually not adherent to the wall of the vessel; it is sometimes compared in shape to a serpent's head. A venous thrombus extends in the direction of the circulating blood, not only as far as the next branch, but frequently a greater or less distance beyond it, in the form of a mural thrombus. A thrombus is at first soft in consistence and moist; but by contraction and extrusion of fluid it becomes more compact, firmer, drier, and more granular in texture.

Mural thrombi, especially small ones, such as fresh vegetations on the cardiac valves, may occur without any definite arrangement of the constituent elements. Such thrombi may consist almost wholly of platelets; but it is most exceptional not to find at least some admixture with leucocytes and fibrin coagulated *intra vitam*.

The larger white and mixed thrombi often present a typical architecture. The stratified structure has long been known and emphasised. More recently Zahn has directed especial attention to the rib-like markings on the free surfaces,[1] and Aschoff to the internal architecture of white and mixed thrombi. Microscopical sections of these thrombi often show an exquisitely trabecular structure due to irregularly contoured, anastomosing columns and lamellæ, of varying size and shape, which spring at intervals from the wall of the vessel and extend, usually in an oblique or twisting direction, toward the free surface of the thrombus, upon which their extremities form the network of whitish lines or the transverse ribs noted by Zahn. If the thrombus be detached from the inner wall of the vessel, similar projecting lines and dots can be seen on its attached surface and often on the inner lining of the vessel. This trabecular framework of the thrombus is composed of masses of platelets with cortical layers of fibrin and leucocytes, as already described. The whole arrangement is aptly compared by Aschoff to branching coral stems. The spaces between the trabeculæ contain blood which during ·life may be fluid or may have coagulated; or they may contain only fibrin and leucocytes, or an indefinite mixture of platelets, fibrin and red and white corpuscles. Between the lamellæ and columns bands of fibrin with or without platelets, often stretch loosely and in a curved manner, the concavity of the curve looking toward the axis of the vessel. Aschoff explains the coral-like architecture and the ribbed surface of the thrombus partly by the oscillatory or

---

[1] A number of writers before Zahn observed the markings on the surfaces of thrombi. Bristowe in 1855 spoke of the "peculiar ribbed appearance" of the surface of cardiac thrombi (*Trans. Path. Soc. London*, vol. vii. p. 141).

wave-like motion of the flowing blood, which, as previously suggested by Zahn, may account for the ribs, and partly by slight irregularities of surface level normally present in the inner lining of vessels. Zahn finds an analogy between the ribs of a ,thrombus and the ripple-marks in sand at the edge of the sea, or at the bottom of flowing streams. Before Zahn, Wickham Legg, in 1878, described the surface of a cardiac thrombus as "marked by lines resembling the impressions made by the waves on a sandy shore."

The usual explanation of the red and white stratification of mixed thrombi is that the thrombus is deposited in successive layers, of which the red are formed rapidly and the white more slowly. There are manifest difficulties in such an explanation. It is more probable that the red layers are cruor clots formed from blood brought to a standstill. Blood entering crevices, spaces, and clefts resulting from the irregular mode of growth of the thrombus, or from its contraction, or from the blood-stream, often with increase of pressure in consequence of the thrombotic barrier, undermining and splitting the white substance, at first soft and later brittle, of the thrombus, may readily stagnate and clot. Indications of such a splitting of the thrombus by the circulating blood are often seen in horizontal white lamellæ covering red layers and present within them : these lamellæ are apparently split off from the general framework and bent in the direction of the blood-current. The typical architecture of the thrombus may not appear, or may be obscured or destroyed by displacement of its parts through the blood-stream, especially when this is forcible : hence it is often missed in arterial thrombi. White thrombi are, as a rule, microscopically mixed thrombi; and in colour there is every transition from these to thrombi so red that careful examination is required for the detection of the white substance.

In long propagated venous thrombi smaller white thrombus-masses often alternate in a longitudinal direction with longer red ones. The explanation of this is that a primary white thrombus is formed, often starting from a valvular pocket. This becomes an occluding thrombus, and the column of blood reaching to the nearest branch, or to the confluence of two important veins, is brought to a standstill, and forms a red, obstructing thrombus. At the extremity of this, where the blood enters from the branch, another white occluding thrombus may be formed, to be followed again by a red thrombus, and so on. Thrombi are sometimes described as red in consequence of failure to detect the small white autochthonous part of the thrombus. In fact the term mixed thrombus is applied to three different appearances of thrombi : (a) an intimate mixture of gray and red substances ; (b) stratification in successive gray and red layers, and (c) red propagated clots consecutive to autochthonous white or mixed thrombi.

In old thrombi various metamorphoses have occurred which obscure or obliterate the typical structure and architecture of the younger ones. The masses of platelets, although they may persist a long time, become finely granular, sometimes almost or quite homogeneous in texture. They are invaded by fibrin, especially along the edges of spaces and clefts which appear. Notwithstanding these profound changes a certain configuration and a differentiation in staining properties often enable us to recognise the sites of the original columns and lamellæ of plate- lets. The leucocytes, often at an early date, undergo fatty degenera- tion and necrosis, their nuclei disappearing both by karyolysis and karyorrhexis. The leucocytic detritus adds to the granular material of the thrombus. The red corpuscles are decolourised and fragmented. The hæmoglobin is in part dissolved and, after organisation begins, is partly transformed into amorphous and crystalline hæmatoidin. These pigmentary transformations impart a brownish red colour to red and mixed thrombi. Fibrin increases in amount and becomes coarse and dense. The part of the thrombus adjacent to the vessel-wall is often converted into compact concentric layers of fibrin at a period when masses of platelets are well preserved nearer the lumen. The hyaline material, which is very frequently found in layers and clumps in old thrombi, may be derived both from fibrin and from platelets; perhaps also from red corpuscles and leucocytes. It may stain well by Weigert's fibrin-stain, or only faintly, or not at all. Small spaces and canals, often containing nucleated cells, may be present in the homogeneous fibrin or hyaline substance (canalised fibrin of Langhans).

Of special importance are the liquefactive softenings which may occur in old thrombi. These are distinguished as simple or bland, septic or purulent, and putrid softenings.

The simple softenings occur in bland thrombi, being especially common in globular cardiac thrombi which, when old, regularly contain in their interior an opaque whitish or reddish thick fluid. This in old days was mistaken for pus, and hence the name puriform softening (purulent cysts). The liquid or pulpy material is the result of granular disintegration and liquefaction of the solid constituents of the thrombus, and consists of necrotic fatty leucocytes, albuminous and fatty granules, blood pigment and altered red corpuscles; the varying red tint of the fluid depending upon the number of red corpuscles originally present in the thrombus. Occasionally acicular crystals of fatty acid are present. This form of softening is probably due to the action of some ferment; it occurs in ordinary bland thrombi, and is distinguished from the infec- tive forms. It is not generally supposed that micro-organisms are in any way concerned in the process: bacteria, however, have been found of late years repeatedly in these thrombi; and it may be that they are not so absolutely unconcerned in simple thrombotic softening as is generally thought to be the case.

There is no question as to the participation of bacteria in the other forms of softening. Septic or purulent softening, met with most fre- quently in infective thrombo-phlebitis, is a true suppuration; being the result of the accumulation of polynuclear leucocytes with fermentative liquefaction of the thrombus. The leucocytes are attracted in part from the blood of the thrombosed vessel and in part from the vasa vasorum and surrounding capillaries and veins. Pyogenetic bacteria, most frequently streptococci, are present in the thrombus and the walls of the vessel. Putrid softening is due to the invasion of putrefactive bacteria. Here the thrombus is of a dirty brown or green colour, and of foul odour.

These various softenings often lead to the separation of thrombotic fragments to be transported by the circulation as emboli,—bland, septic, or putrid according to the nature of the process.

White thrombi in veins, far less frequently in arteries, may undergo calcification, forming phleboliths or arterioliths. They are generally approximately spherical, and lie loosely or slightly adherent in the lumen. They are found most frequently in the veins around the prostate and bladder of men, in the plexus pampiniformes of women, and in the spleen.

One of the most interesting adaptive pathological processes is the so-called organisation of thrombi, which is the substitution for the thrombus of vascularised connective tissue. The thrombus itself takes no active part in the process, but behaves as a foreign body. It is gradually disintegrated and absorbed, largely through the activities of phagocytes. The new tissue springs from the wall of the vessel or the heart; the tissue-forming cells being derived both from the endothelium and from other fixed cells in the wall. New vessels spring from the vasa vasorum. Lacunar spaces in the thrombus, or between the thrombus and the vascular wall, may become lined with endothelium, and also serve as channels for the circulating blood. These new vessels may establish communication with the lumen of the thrombosed vessel above or below the thrombus, or on both sides. The new tissue, which at first is rich in cells, becomes fibrous, and contracts. The result may be a solid fibrous plug, or a cavernous structure with large blood-spaces; or, by disappearance of the septa, a restoration of the lumen, with perhaps a few fibrous threads or bands stretching across it, as in the normal cerebral venous sinuses.

There are great diversities in individual cases as to the rapidity of onset and the course of the organising process; these differences depending upon various circumstances, the most important of which are the location of the thrombus, the condition of the wall of the vessel or heart, the general state of the patient, and the presence or absence of infection. In favourable cases the process may be well under way within a week. The wall of the vessel, or of the heart, may be so diseased as to be incapable of furnishing any new tissue; as is usually the case in aneurysmal sacs, and often in varices and in cardiac disease. The presence of pyogenetic bacteria prevents or delays the process of organisation. This process is a proliferative angeiitis. It is this angeiitis which leads to the closure of a vessel after ligation. If the ligature be applied aseptically, and without injury to the internal coats, usually no thrombus is formed, or only a very small one. The formation of a thrombus is of no assistance in securing obliteration of a ligated vessel, in fact it impedes the development of the obliterating endarteritis.

The causes of organisation of thrombi are probably to be sought partly in the influence exerted by the thrombus as a foreign body, and partly in slowing or cessation of the blood-current and lowering of the tension of the vessel-wall (Thoma, Beneke). Whether, in addition, growth of cells may be determined by chemical substances derived from the thrombus is uncertain.

Etiology.—The recognition of the three classes of causes assigned for thrombosis, namely, alterations in the blood, mechanical disturbances of the circulation and lesions of the vascular or cardiac wall, is not of recent date. The dyscrasic theory is the oldest. John Hunter introduced and Cruveilhier elaborated the conception of primary phlebitis with consecutive plugging of the vein; and Baillie, Laennec, Davy and others emphasised stasis as a cause of intravascular clotting. Virchow's name, however, is the one especially associated with mechanical explanations of thrombosis. The experiments of Brücke, showing the importance of integrity of the vascular wall in keeping the blood fluid, led to general recognition of the part taken by alterations of this wall in the etiology of thrombosis.

While it is generally agreed that slowing and other irregularities of the circulation, contact of the blood with abnormal surfaces, and changes in the composition of the blood are concerned, singly or in combination, in the causation of thrombosis, there is much difference of opinion as to the relative importance of each of these factors, and as to the part of each as a proximate, as a remote, or as an accessory cause.

Slowing and other irregularities of the circulation.—Diminished velocity of the blood-current is not by itself an efficient cause of thrombosis. The circulation may be at a low ebb for a long time without the occurrence of thrombi. A stationary column of blood included in an artery or vein between two carefully applied aseptic ligatures within the living body may remain fluid for weeks (Glénard, Baumgarten). Slow circulation, however, in combination with lesions of the cardiac or vascular wall, or with the presence of micro-organisms or other changes in the blood, is an important predisposing cause of thrombosis, and frequently determines the localisation of the thrombus. This is evident from the relative infrequency of thrombi upon diseased patches of the inner coat of large arteries in contrast with their frequency upon similar patches in the small arteries and in the veins; and in general from the predilection of thrombi for those parts of the circulatory channels in which the blood-flow is normally, or as the result of disease, slow. Extensive injury to the walls of arteries may be experimentally produced without resulting thrombosis.

Eberth and Schimmelbusch find that under normal conditions the platelets circulate with the red corpuscles in the axial blood-current, but make their appearance in the outer still zone when the rapidity of the circulation is sufficiently diminished. Moderate slowing is attended by the accumulation of white corpuscles in this zone, while a further slackening of the stream is characterised by fewer leucocytes and more platelets in the peripheral layer. Mere slowing of the circulation, however, does not suffice to form thrombi; there must be some abnormality of the inner lining of the vessel-wall, with which the platelets are brought into contact, in order to induce the viscous metamorphosis of these bodies essential in the formation of plugs. Hence Eberth and Schimmelbusch conclude that it is only by the combination of slowing of the circulation with changes in the inner lining that the formation of white thrombi can be explained.

Von Recklinghausen attaches more importance to a whirling or eddying motion (Wirbelbewegung) than to mere slowness of the circulation. He has pointed out that eddies are produced when the blood enters normally or pathologically dilated channels from smaller ones, or passes into a cul-de-sac, or over obstructions; and he has considered in an interesting way the special conditions causing this motion and its influence upon the production of thrombi. This irregularity of the blood-current will be referred to again in considering the localisation of venous thrombi (p. 181). Von Recklinghausen's observations make a valuable contribution to our knowledge of the mechanical disturbances of the circulation which favour the development of thrombi.

Thrombi attributed to slowing of the blood-current, often combined with eddying motion of the blood, are called stagnation-thrombi. Of these two groups are distinguished: (a) those due to local circulatory disturbances, as from interruption or narrowing of the lumen of vessels by ligation or compression, or from circumscribed dilatations, as aneurysms or varices; and (b) marantic thrombi resulting from weakened heart's action, with consequent feebleness of the general circulation. Virchow gave the name "marantic thrombi" to all or nearly all thrombi complicating or following anæmic and cachectic states, general infective diseases— as enteric fever, typhus fever, and the like, and certain constitutional diseases. He considered a condition of marasmus, or great prostration, to be the common underlying factor. As we shall see subsequently, there are serious objections to this explanation of these thromboses, which indeed constitute the class of chief medical interest. The designation "marantic thromboses" for this group is still, however, in common use. Although it is proper in these groups of thrombi to emphasise the mechanical disturbances of the circulation as an important accessory factor, it is evident, from what has been said, that the class of stagnation-thrombi cannot be maintained in the strict sense originally advocated by Virchow. Other factors, especially lesions of the walls of the heart or vessels, enter decisively into their causation.

Contact of the blood with abnormal surfaces. Lesions of the cardiac and vascular walls.—It is universally recognised that the influence of the endothelial lining of the vascular channels in maintaining the fluid state of the blood is of the first importance. This influence appears to be partly physical and partly chemical. The smooth, non-adhesive character of the inner surface of the heart and vessels is the physical property which comes primarily into consideration. Whereas the introduction of such foreign bodies as threads, or bristles with rough surfaces, into the circulation is an efficient cause of thrombosis, perfectly smooth, indifferent bodies, as small glass balls, may be introduced without causing any coagulation (Zahn). Freund has shown that blood collected with proper precautions in vessels lined with oil or vaseline remains fluid for a long time. Mere contact with a foreign surface, therefore, does not suffice to induce clotting; the result depends upon the character of this surface. Freund concludes that the essential thing is that the surface shall be such as to permit adhesion to occur between it and the corpuscles, particularly the red corpuscles; the normal lining of the blood-vessels being characterised by the absence of this adhesive property. Without adopting Freund's theory of coagulation, which does not here concern us, we can apply, with much satisfaction in the explanation of many thrombi, his observations concerning the importance of adhesive surfaces in causing coagulation. There should also be taken into consideration the damage known to be inflicted by adhesive contact with abnormal surfaces upon platelets or red corpuscles; if these be regarded as the source of the granular material and platelets in thrombi.

Changes, therefore, which impair or destroy the smooth, non-adhesive surface of the normal inner lining of the vessels play an important part in the etiology of thrombosis; and thrombi thus caused may be called adhesion-thrombi. The efficiency of these lesions in causing thrombi is increased if, by projection into the lumen, they obstruct the blood-flow; or by their rough, irregular surface set up an eddying motion of the blood.

Although we have very little definite information about any chemical activities of the normal vascular endothelium concerned in the preservation of the fluidity of the circulating blood, there is evidence that lesions of the intima, through chemical as well as physical influences, may incite thrombosis. That necrotic endothelial and intimal cells may liberate fibrin-ferment is in accordance with both physiological and pathological observations relating to the origin of this ferment from dead or disintegrated protoplasm in general. Reference has already been made to observations of Zenker indicating the coagulative influence of necrotic endothelium, and of the intima deprived of endothelium.

Strong support for a belief in the participation of chemical substances in the causation of certain thrombi due to intimal lesions is to be found in contrasting the effects of mere traumatism with those of traumatism combined with infection of the intima. This has been especially brought out in the experimental studies of valvular lesions of the heart. Aseptic laceration of the cardiac valves generally leads to but slight production of thrombi upon the injured surfaces; whereas the same traumatic lesions, combined with the lodgment and growth of pyogenetic bacteria, are usually attended by the formation of considerable thrombotic vegetations. The differences in the result can hardly be explained by differences in the physical characters of the lesions in the two cases; but we have no definite knowledge concerning the nature and mode of action of the chemical bacterial products concerned in causing the thrombi. We may draw the conclusion that lesions of the intima, apart from their more manifest characters, may possess certain specific properties especially favourable to the production of thrombi.

The most important of the structural changes of the vascular and cardiac walls which cause thrombosis are those due to inflammation, atheroma, calcification, necrosis, other degenerations, tumours, compression, and injury. Here again may be emphasised the importance of retardation and other irregularities of the circulation in rendering these various lesions effective causes of thrombosis. The aorta, for example, may be the seat of most extensive deforming endarteritis, with irregular projecting calcific plates and ragged atheromatous ulcers, without a trace of thrombotic deposit. The forcible pulsating current prevents the adhesion and accumulation of the formed elements constituting the beginning thrombus, or quickly washes them away. The presence in some instances of white mural thrombi in the aorta upon an intima apparently but slightly damaged indicates the importance of certain specific, although little understood, characters of intimal lesions in association with changes in the blood.

Foreign bodies, which have penetrated the blood-channels and set up thrombosis, have been observed repeatedly in human beings, especially in the heart and abdominal veins. Such accidents have followed swallowing fish-bones, needles, nails, bits of wire and the like. A blood-clot or thrombus in a vessel, or projecting into the lumen from a wound of the vessel, may itself be looked upon as a foreign body, and lead to further extension of the thrombus. There seems to be a certain self-propagating power in a thrombus. Similar effects are produced by the entrance of large parasites, such as distomata, by the invasion of tumour-masses, and by the penetration of parenchymatous cells into the circulatory channels (p. 260).

Infective thrombi. Thrombo-phlebitis.—Phlebitis, as a cause of thrombosis, has reacquired within the last few years so much importance that it is here singled out from other lesions of the vascular wall for special consideration.

In the first half of the present century, mainly through the influence of John Hunter and of Cruveilhier, thrombosis was by many regarded only as an expression of inflammation of the inner lining of the vessels. The material composing the thrombus was considered to be, at least in part, an exudate of coagulable lymph from the inflamed vascular wall. Virchow, by his monumental work on thrombosis and embolism, dating from 1846, reversed this order of things, and made, for the great majority of cases, the thrombus the primary and essential phenomenon, and the inflammation of the wall, if present, a merely secondary effect. Phlebitis disappeared, as a chapter, from works on internal medicine, and thrombosis took its place. Within recent years, and again chiefly through the work of French investigators, the pendulum has swung

back, and phlebitis has once more come to the front as a common
and important cause of thrombosis, and resumed an important place in
many systematic treatises on medicine.   This rehabilitation of phlebitis is due mainly to bacteriological investigations of thrombosed
vessels, especially of the so-called marantic thrombi of infective and
cachectic diseases.

The distinction between bland thrombi and infective thrombi is an
old and important one.   The thrombi in septic and suppurative phlebitis,
concerned especially in pyæmic processes and surgical affections, were for
a long time the chief, indeed almost the only recognised representatives
of the class of infective thrombi.   There has been a gradual extension of
the domain of infective thrombosis, until now many thrombi, previously
classified as bland, are considered to be of infective origin.   This is
notably true of a large number of thrombi, formerly and still often
called marantic, complicating many infective diseases, wasting and
cachectic conditions, and anæmia.   In 1887 Weigert stated that by
means of his fibrin-stain he had found unsuspected micro-organisms in
marantic thrombi with surprising frequency ; and since then there have
been numerous similar observations, as well as not a few negative ones.
In France the studies of Cornil and his pupils, especially Widal, and
of Vaquez have had the greatest influence in developing the doctrine of
the mycotic origin of this class of thrombi, and particularly that of
primary phlebitis as the cause of these thromboses.   It should not be
forgotten that Paget, in 1866, contended for the primarily phlebitic
nature of thrombosis in gout.

Phlegmasia alba dolens of the puerperium is the prototype of this
class of thromboses.   In the articles on various infective diseases, particularly enteric fever (see vol. i. p. 817) and influenza (vol. i. p. 683),
attention has been called to the occurrence of thrombosis as a complication or sequel.   Similar thromboses occur in pneumonia, typhus,
acute rheumatism, erysipelas, cholera, scarlatina, variola, tuberculosis,
syphilis,—in fact with greater or less frequency in nearly all acute and
chronic infections.   Likewise in chlorosis, gout, leukæmia, senile
debility, and chronic wasting and cachectic diseases, particularly cancer,
thrombosis is a recognised complication.   The more important associations of thrombosis with these various diseases will be considered more
in detail subsequently (p. 191).

These various thromboses, occurring very rarely as primary affections, usually secondary to infective or constitutional diseases, compose
the great majority of those of medical, as distinguished from surgical
interest.   Clinically and anatomically they undoubtedly have much in
common.   Is there any common etiological point of view from which
they may be regarded ?   Virchow thought so in calling them marantic
thrombi, and attributing their causation to enfeebled circulation.
The same causative factor still remains the underlying one with those
who, like Cohnheim, interpolate nutritive changes in the endothelium
between the slow circulation and the beginning of the thrombus.

Impaired circulation cannot serve as a common etiological shelter for this whole class of thromboses. There is no definite and constant relationship between the condition of the circulation and the occurrence of these thrombi. While many appear during great debility, others of the same nature, and often in the same disease, occur when the heart's action is not notably weak. Thrombosis may ensue early in influenza. It is oftener a sequel than an accompaniment of enteric fever. On the other hand, the circulation may be extremely feeble for days without the appearance of thrombosis.

Many of these so-called marantic thrombi are unquestionably of infective origin. Vaquez, in his monograph on phlebitis of the extremities, published in 1894, has brought together the results of the observations of others, and especially those of his own and Widal's investigations, which demonstrate that bacteria are often present in these thrombi and in the adjacent vascular wall. Since the appearance of Vaquez' monograph there have been a number of confirmatory observations. Widal emphasises the importance of searching for bacteria in fresh thrombi, and in the autochthonous part of the thrombus and the adjacent wall of the vessel. The largest contingent of positive results has been furnished by the examination of puerperal thrombi,—many of which indeed are examples of septic thrombo-phlebitis, and of the marantic thrombi of chronic pulmonary tuberculosis; but bacteria have also been found in thrombi complicating or following typhoid fever, influenza, pneumonia, cancer, and other infective and cachectic conditions.

In relatively few instances has the specific micro-organism of the primary disease, as the typhoid or the tubercle bacillus, for example, been present in the thrombus; more frequently secondary invaders, especially streptococci and other pyogenetic bacteria, have been detected: so that the thrombosis is considered to be oftener the result of some secondary infection than of the primary one. Colon bacilli have been found in typhoidal and other thrombi; but as these bacteria are found so commonly in the blood and organs after death from all sorts of causes, no great importance can be attached to their mere demonstration without some further evidence of their pathogenetic activity. As might be expected, streptococci are the bacteria found most frequently in puerperal thromboses. Singer believes that gonorrhœal infection is also a possible factor.

Not only in thrombi of infective diseases but also in cachectic thromboses have bacteria, and here again most frequently pyogenetic forms, been demonstrated. Nor is this surprising when we consider the frequency of secondary infections in chronic diseases, especially as a terminal event; as has been clearly brought out in the analyses, by Flexner, of the autopsies at the Johns Hopkins Hospital, where bacteriological examination is a routine procedure at the post-mortem table. Many of these infections are unsuspected during life.

The supposition that in all of these cases the bacteria are accidentally or secondarily present, and in no way concerned in the causation of the thrombi, is extremely improbable. They are often in such number, in such arrangement and associated with such lesions, that they must have multiplied in the thrombus and in the vessel wall.

The problem whether the bacteria have led to thrombosis by first invading the vascular wall and setting up inflammation is not solved by the mere demonstration of their presence. Certainly, in some instances, this sequence of events is plainly indicated by the microscopical appearances; but in many it is impossible to decide to what extent inflammatory changes in the wall antedated the thrombus, for the latter, especially when infected by bacteria, induces a secondary angeiitis. Opportunities to study very recent infective marantic thrombi with reference to this point are not common.

In a case, which I examined, of multiple venous thrombosis complicating leucocythæmia, there was a primary mycotic endophlebitis with secondary thrombosis. There was a secondary streptococcus infection. In the intima of the thrombosed vessels were numerous scattered foci in which large numbers of streptococci were present. In these areas there was necrosis of endothelial and other intimal cells, with proliferation of surrounding cells and many polynuclear leucocytes. These foci formed little whitish elevations capped with platelets, fibrin, and leucocytes; the whole presenting an appearance similar to that of endocardial vegetations. There was marked nuclear fragmentation both in the infected intima and in the thrombus. Fresh mixed thrombi, containing fewer streptococci, were connected with these phlebitic vegetations. Although the vasa vasorum were hyperæmic, and were the seat of a moderate migration of leucocytes, streptococci were absent from the adventitia; and the appearances spoke decidedly for the direct penetration of the streptococci from the circulating blood into the intima. I have examined three other similar cases. A similar form of mycotic endophlebitis has been described by Vaquez (endophlébite végétante). In other cases the intima is more diffusely inflamed. After a short time there is no distinct line of demarcation between the thrombus and the intima, and all of the coats of the vessel are more or less inflamed.

Although the bacteria found in the intima may gain access from without through the vasa vasorum, or the lymphatics, it is probable that in the class of cases here under consideration they more frequently enter directly from the blood circulating in the main channel. There may be very extensive bacterial inflammation of the venous wall, even with bulging of the intima into the lumen, without any thrombosis.

We do not possess sufficiently numerous and careful bacteriological examinations of the thrombi of infective and wasting diseases to enable us to say in what proportion of cases they contain micro-organisms. It is certain that in many instances such examinations have yielded negative results. It is quite possible that in some of these negative cases bacteria, originally present, have died out; but although by some authors much use is made of this explanation, it is not in general a satisfactory one. Many of the examinations were of thrombi sufficiently recent to exclude this possibility.

To explain these non-bacterial cases, the French writers assume the existence of a primary toxic endophlebitis, the toxins being either of bacterial origin or derived from other sources. Ponfick, many years ago, called attention to the occurrence of degenerations of the vascular endothelium in infective diseases; and there can be no doubt of the frequency of both degenerative and inflammatory changes of the intima in toxic and infective conditions.

A lesion which I have seen in the intima of veins (less frequently of arteries) in typhoid fever, diphtheria, variola, and other infective diseases, is a nodular, sometimes a more diffuse, accumulation of lymphoid and endothelioid cells beneath the endothelium. These cells, as well as the covering endothelium, may undergo necrosis; indeed the appearances sometimes suggest primary necrosis with secondary accumulation of wandering cells and proliferation of fixed cells. These foci are not unlike the so-called lymphomatous nodules found in the liver in typhoid and other infections. They may unquestionably be the starting-point of thrombi, as has been shown by Mallory in his study of the vascular lesions in typhoid fever. Although this form of endophlebitis or endarteritis resembles that demonstrably caused by the actual presence of bacteria in the intima, bacteria are often absent, even in the fresh lesions; so that it is reasonable to suppose that the affection may be caused by toxins. I think that this toxic endangeiitis is of importance in the causation of thrombosis complicating infective and cachectic states.

There are, however, instances of so-called marantic thrombosis where no visible alteration of the intima can be made out at the site of the thrombus, or only the slight fatty degeneration of the endothelium which is such an extremely common condition that it does not afford a satisfactory explanation.

It is obvious that bacteria are likely to find especially favourable opportunities to gain lodgment, and toxic substances to do injury, in situations where the blood-current is slow and thrown into eddies; but the localisation in these situations of thromboses complicating infective and chronic diseases has perhaps been unduly emphasised. These thromboses may occur elsewhere, even in the aorta and larger arteries. Pre-existing diseases of the veins, especially chronic endophlebitis and varicosities, are conditions predisposing to infective and cachectic thromboses.

While we are justified in assigning a far more prominent place to the agency of micro-organisms and to primary phlebitis in the etiology of thrombosis than, until recent years, has been customary since Virchow's fundamental investigations, recent attempts to refer all thromboses, formerly called marantic, to the direct invasion of micro-organisms and to phlebitis go beyond demonstrated facts. We have not at present any satisfactory bacteriological and anatomical substratum for so wide a generalisation. The whole field, although difficult, is an inviting and fruitful one for further investigation. The clinical arguments in favour of the phlebitic origin of thrombosis will be considered below (p. 212).

What has been said regarding the relation of phlebitis to thrombosis complicating infective and constitutional diseases applies also to that of arteritis to the similar arterial thromboses which, although less common than the venous, are more frequent than was formerly supposed; this will appear when we take up the association of thrombosis with particular diseases (p. 191).

It is of course understood that the preceding remarks on the relation of phlebitis and arteritis to thrombosis relate only to the medical thromboses, and not to the septic and suppurative thrombophlebitides of the surgeon, of the bacterial origin of which there is no question; although these latter may be concerned in diseases, such as suppurative pylephlebitis, which are in the province of the physician.

Chemical changes in the blood. Ferment-thrombi.—The old ideas of chemical changes in the blood as causes of intravascular clotting, embodied in such terms as acre coagulatorium, hyperinosis, inopexia, are now of historical interest only. There appears to be no definite and constant relation between the amount of fibrin obtainable from the blood, or the rapidity of its coagulation in the test tube, and the occurrence of thrombosis in human beings. Peripheral thrombosis is a less common complication of pneumonia and acute articular rheumatism, which are characterised by high fibrin-content of the blood, than of enteric fever and certain cachectic states in which the fibrin-content is approximately normal or reduced.

In dogs whose blood was rendered incoagulable by injection of "peptone" (albumose) Schimmelbusch produced platelet-thrombi experimentally. On the other hand, Sahli with Eguet observed no collection of platelets or formation of thrombi around hog's bristles or silk threads inserted into the jugular veins of rabbits having incoagulable blood from injection of leech extract; although control experiments regularly gave positive results. These latter experiments show that chemical changes in the blood may influence the process of thrombosis.

The main support of the belief entertained by some that the liberation of fibrin-ferment in the general blood-stream is an important cause of human thrombosis, is based on the results of experiments which demonstrate that the injection of various substances into the circulation may cause intravascular clotting. The most important of the substances which have been observed to produce this effect are laky blood (Naunyn), biliary salts (Ranke), ether (Naunyn, Hanau), fresh defibrinated blood (Köhler), emulsions or extracts from cells, especially lymphoid cells (Groth, Wooldridge), transfusion of blood (Landois, Ponfick), and snake-venom (C. J. Martin, art. "Snake-poison and Snake-bite," vol. iii. p. 819). The coagulating effect of laky blood is attributable to the stromata of red corpuscles rather than to dissolved hæmoglobin (Wooldridge). The coagulating principle here, as well as of the various tissue-extracts, is believed to be a nucleo-proteid which, by combination with calcium, forms the fibrin-ferment. It is to the presence of this ferment or the subsequent liberation of the ferment that the dangerous intravascular clots following the injection of defibrinated blood or the transfusion of foreign blood are due. The coagulative effect of snake-venom under certain conditions is referred by Halliburton to proteoses free from phosphorus, and therefore not nucleo-proteids. The action of snake-venom upon coagulation is probably analogous to that of various toxic albumoses, bacterial and vegetable. They are in general to be ranked among anti-coagulating substances ; but the result varies with the dose, the manner of injection, and other circumstances. Wooldridge has shown that thromboses are particularly prone to occur in the territory of the portal system after the injection of various substances favouring coagulation. Fibrin-ferment may be used up in the process of intravascular clotting, so that after this has taken place the remaining blood may be incoagulable.

Interesting as these experimental results are to the physiologist, and with reference to the theories of the coagulation of blood, it is difficult to utilise them in any satisfactory way in the explanation of ordinary human thrombosis. Most of the experimenters make no statement as to the microscopical structure of the intravascular clots, which are described generally as soft, dark red masses ; and they seem to identify them with ordinary human thrombi, being apparently not familiar with the researches on the peculiar constitution of the latter. Some of the substances used for the experiments cause precipitates in the blood, and many are very destructive to the red corpuscles. Hanau, however, has shown that masses of platelets may be present in these clots.

Conditions analogous to those set up in these experiments may occur in human beings ; but they are, so far as we know, most exceptional. Especially do we lack satisfactory observations, in cases of thrombosis in human beings, of increase of fibrin-ferment in the blood. Considerable quantities of fibrin-ferment, more than are likely to be liberated under any probable circumstances in man, can be injected into the circulation without causing coagulation. Still it is possible that the mechanism by which this excess of fibrin-ferment is neutralised and coagulation prevented may be paralysed under certain conditions. There are certain instances of rapidly-formed red thrombi in vessels with apparently normal walls which, in the absence of other explanation, it would be very convenient to refer to ferment-intoxication. Köhler and Hanau consider that many thrombi, especially those complicating infective and cachectic states, are best explained by supposing a liberation of fibrin-ferment in the blood, and they call them, therefore, ferment-thrombi.

Hayem designates as thrombi from precipitation (thromboses par précipitation) many which others call ferment-thrombi ; especially those following injection of various destructive substances into the circulation, and those caused by burns and freezing.

Silbermann and others assert that thrombosis, particularly multiple capillary thrombosis, plays an important part in extensive superficial burns, and in poisoning with various substances destructive to the blood corpuscles, such as anilin, potassium chlorate, arsenic, phosphorus, sublimate, carbonous oxide, illuminating gas. These views need further confirmation before they can be accepted, as several observers have obtained only negative results in searching for thrombi in the same class of cases.

Notwithstanding the lack of a substantial basis of demonstrated facts for the opinion that human thrombosis is often caused by liberation of fibrin-ferment in the general blood-stream, it would be quite unreasonable to suppose that chemical changes of the blood are without influence upon the occurrence of thrombosis in man. Indeed, in infective and toxic conditions such changes are doubtless the underlying factors. Both the circulatory disturbances and the alterations in the vascular wall to which we attribute the production of thrombi are the result of damage done to the heart and vessels by bacterial and other toxins. More than this, there is good reason to believe that alterations in the formed elements of the blood, caused directly or indirectly by toxic substances, are of great significance in the etiology of thrombosis. The platelets are in all probability cell-derivatives; and we may well suppose that damage inflicted upon leucocytes and red corpuscles may favour their production, and that, in consequence of abnormal composition of the plasma, the platelets themselves may more readily undergo viscous metamorphosis, and form plugs. In view of recent observations in favour of the origin of platelets from red corpuscles, the studies of Ehrlich, Maragliano, von Limbeck, and others, concerning degenerations and increased vulnerability of these corpuscles in various diseases, are of interest with reference to thrombosis; but it must be confessed that we cannot at present make more than a hypothetical application of these results to the explanation of certain forms of thrombosis. To discuss here further the hypotheses upon this subject would be barren of any useful result.

Increase of blood-platelets.—In view of the essential part taken by blood-platelets in the formation of thrombi, it is important to inquire whether thrombosis can be brought into any relation with a pathological increase of these elements. Some observations of the existence of such a relationship are highly suggestive.

Especial difficulties are encountered in the efforts to enumerate the platelets on account of their small size and their viscid consistence, which causes them to clump together. Brodie and Russell give, as the norm, one platelet to 8·5 red corpuscles; or about 635,000 per cubic millimetre. This estimate is considerably higher than that obtained by others, probably, however, by less accurate methods. Van Emden gives as the average for human beings in health 245,000; which corresponds fairly well with the figures of Hayem, Cadet, Afanassiew, Muir, Fusari, and Determann, but is lower than those of Laker and Prus.

There is considerable divergence of statement as to the number of platelets in different diseases. This number is markedly increased in chlorosis (Muir), of which thrombosis is a well-recognised complication. The platelets are increased in post-hæmorrhagic anæmia (Hayem), which is one of the remoter causes of thrombosis. There is evidence that hæmorrhage after childbirth, and in the course of various diseases, favours the occurrence of thrombosis. Several observers have found the platelets reduced in number in pernicious anæmia, which, unlike chlorosis, is rarely, if ever, complicated by thrombosis (Hayem, Birch-Hirschfeld, Beugnier - Corbeau). In purpura hæmorrhagica there is extreme diminution of platelets, sometimes amounting to total absence (Denys, Hayem, Ehrlich, van Emden), which constitutes the only demonstrated morphological change of the blood in this disease. In febrile infections there is often a correspondence between leucocytosis and the number of platelets. Thus in influenza, pneumonia, erysipelas, meningitis, and septic infections the number of platelets is often increased, in severe cases sometimes diminished; whereas in enteric fever and malaria it is diminished (Hayem, Reyne, Türk, Muir, van Emden). The disappearance of leucocytosis is sometimes followed by increase of platelets. In view of the greater frequency of thrombosis as a sequel than in the course of many acute diseases, the recognition by Hayem of a platelet crisis (crise hématoblastique) is interesting. After the crisis or subsidence of certain infective diseases Hayem observed a rapid and marked increase in the platelets. This was noted after pneumonia and enteric fever. Platelets are said to be often increased toward the end of pregnancy and after delivery (Hayem, Cadet). In various cachectic conditions, in tuberculosis, and, in general, in states of bad nutrition, increase is the rule. Dr. Muir finds that in spleno-medullary leucocythæmia the platelets are notably increased, but not in the lymphatic form (art. "Leucocythæmia," vol. v. p. 640). In chronic passive congestion, due to heart disease, the platelets are said to be diminished (van Emden). An increase of platelets in various conditions in which they are usually diminished can often be attributed to complications. Upon the whole there is much in support of the view that increase of platelets is an index of lowered resistance of the red corpuscles.

It is fair to say that some of the foregoing statements regarding the condition of the platelets in various diseases need further confirmation, and that in general the subject is difficult and has been insufficiently investigated. Nevertheless we cannot fail to have our attention arrested by a parallelism, in many instances, between disposition to thrombosis and increased number of platelets; although in others no such relationship is apparent. It must suffice to call attention to this parallelism, for we are ignorant of the underlying factors.

It hardly need be said that the mere increase of platelets is insufficient to explain the occurrence of thrombosis. We are brought back here, as elsewhere, to disturbance of the circulation and changes in the vascular walls as the determinants of the localisation of thrombi; while we must recognise changes in the chemistry and morphology of the blood as important predisposing causes.

Localisation.—Thrombosis may occur in any part of the circulatory system. We distinguish therefore arterial, venous, capillary, and cardiac thrombi. Lymphatic vessels may likewise become plugged with fibrin, leucocytes, or foreign material; such as tubercle, cancer, or red corpuscles.

Arterial thrombi.—The majority of arterial thromboses are caused by some local injury or disease of the arterial wall, or by the lodgment of an embolus. Especially important are the arterio-sclerotic thromboses of the brain, heart, and extremities.

Here may be mentioned the varying relations of arterial thrombosis to *gangrene* of the extremities. Thrombosis of arteries, as well as of veins, may be secondary to varieties of gangrene which are not caused by primary plugging of the arteries. Senile gangrene is caused either by embolism, which may lead to thrombosis, or by arterio-sclerosis, usually associated with thrombosis. In various infective and chronic wasting diseases gangrene may result from primary arterial thrombosis of the class often called marantic. Many of these thromboses are infective in origin; but we have not sufficient information to warrant the assertion that all are caused by micro-organisms.

Of especial interest is the relation of thrombosis to certain forms of so-called "spontaneous" gangrene which may occur in middle life, or even in the young, and are often preceded by definite symptoms indicative of gradual occlusion of the arteries. Von Winiwarter concluded from his examinations of several cases that the primary disease is an obliterating endarteritis resulting in complete closure of the affected vessels. Zoege von Manteuffel, however, finds that thrombosis participates, in an interesting way, in the gradual occlusion of the arteries. According to him, by the deposition and organisation of successive layers of parietal thrombi, the arteries, which are usually the seat of a primary sclerosis, gradually become filled with vascularised connective tissue. Haga considers this endarteritis thrombotica to be syphilitic. Hoegerstedt and Nemser believe that, in general, the deposition and organisation of parietal thrombi are common and important processes in angio-sclerosis. Von Recklinghausen has described hyaline thrombosis of small arteries in spontaneous and arterio-spastic gangrene.

The *action of infective agents* in the causation of focal and diffuse diseases of the arteries is receiving constantly increasing attention. The occurrence of acute and chronic arteritis as a result of various infective diseases—as enteric fever, typhus fever, acute articular rheumatism, variola, scarlatina, pneumonia, endocarditis, septicæmia, syphilis, tuberculosis, leprosy—is now so well established that it is reasonable to believe that the arterial thromboses complicating or following these diseases are often referable to an infective arteritis.

It cannot be doubted that not a few cases reported in literature as primary arterial thrombosis are to be attributed to embolism which was overlooked. The possible sources of emboli for the aortic system can be usually controlled much more readily than those for the pulmonary arteries; for the latter sources embrace all the systemic veins. These veins may contain mural thrombi, or in places occluding thrombi, which give no signs of their presence. The possibility that an entire thrombus may be detached and transported by the blood-current, so that its original location cannot be determined, is also to be considered. But, after all has been said, it is carrying scepticism to an unjustifiable extreme to refuse to admit the occurrence of primary arterial thrombosis in infective, cachectic, and anæmic states, under circumstances where the localisation cannot be attributed to arterio-sclerosis or other pre-existing arterial disease. Mr. Jonathan Hutchinson has recently reported observations of rapid thrombosis of arteries without obvious disease of the walls.

The most frequent site of arterial thrombosis is in the extremities, and far more frequently in the lower than the upper. Arterial thrombosis, unlike venous, occurs on the right side as often as on the left. Other situations, more or less common, are the cerebral, pulmonary, coronary of the heart, mesenteric arteries, and the aorta and its primary branches.

Venous thrombi.—These may result from local causes, such as traumatism, compression, phlebitis, phlebo-sclerosis, varix (266), inflammation or other lesion of surrounding parts, and connection of venous terminals with septic or gangrenous foci.

Vascular thromboses due to general causes are, in the great majority of cases, situated in veins; and to this group the chief medical interest attaches. In special characters of the venous circulation we must seek the explanation of the greater effectiveness of these general causes in veins than in arteries. The physiological peculiarities, partly general and partly local, which come especially into consideration, are—the slower mean speed of the blood in veins than in arteries ; the low blood-pressure ; the flow from smaller into larger channels ; the absence of pulsation ; the presence of valves ; fixation of the venous wall in certain situations to fasciæ and bone ; the existence in some places of wide sinuses and ampullar dilatations ; the agency of certain subsidiary forces, such as muscular contraction and movements of the limbs, in assisting the flow in the veins ; the composition of venous blood, particularly the higher content of CO_2, and perhaps the functions of the capillaries and small veins in the production and absorption of lymph. It is obvious, without detailed explanation, that some at least of these special characters must render the venous system much more favourable than the arterial to the occurrence, under the general conditions known to dispose to thrombosis, of retardation of the blood-current; eddying motion of the blood, and damage to the vascular wall from impoverished and insufficient blood-supply, or prolonged contact with micro-organisms and toxic substances, the agency of which in the etiology of thrombosis has already been considered.

The best evidence that these mechanical conditions determine the localisation of the majority of thrombi of infective, anæmic, and cachectic diseases is afforded by the marked preference of such thrombi for situations where these conditions are in the highest degree operative. The tendency of venous thrombi to start from valvular pockets has already been mentioned. It is important to note that thrombi due to general causes, unlike those starting from local septic foci, do not begin in the rootlets, but originate usually in the main venous trunks of a member. The very large veins are unusual primary seats of marantic thrombi. Beginning as a rule in a sinus or medium-sized vein, the thrombus may grow centrally into large veins; as from the femoral into the iliacs and vena cava, and peripherally into small veins, not, however, generally reaching the smallest veins. The favourite starting-point of so-called marantic thromboses of the cerebral sinuses is in the middle of the superior longitudinal sinus at the top of the cranial cavity, whence the thrombus may extend forward, but tends especially to grow toward the torcular Herophili, and into other sinuses and into the cerebral veins. There is, however, no rigid rule in this matter. The plug may begin in other sinuses, or even in the cerebral veins.

In extensive thromboses, such as occur especially in veins of the thigh and leg, it is sometimes difficult to determine the point of origin of the thrombus, and the exact manner of its propagation. Often, however, decisive information can be gained by careful attention to features indicative of the age of thrombi, as already described (p. 163). Thus the autochthonous part of the thrombus is gray, or reddish gray, and firmly adherent; the continued part often red and more loosely attached, and the older parts frequently softened or liquefied in the centre. By observation of such points as these, the common assumption that a thrombus, occupying continuously both large and small veins, began in the most distal veins and grew thence into the larger channels, can often be shown to be erroneous. An occluding thrombus may lead to such disturbances of the circulation as to cause the formation of discontinuous multiple thrombi on both the central and the peripheral sides, and these may become connected by red or mixed thrombi. In short, the modes of extension of thrombi are sometimes complicated, and not readily unravelled.

The so-called law of Lancereaux was enunciated by him in 1862 as an explanation of the common site of thrombi in the cerebral sinuses, and at the summits rather than at the peripheries of the extremities; his rule is as follows :—"Marantic thromboses are always formed at the level of the points where the blood has the greatest tendency to stasis, that is, at the limit of the action of the forces of cardiac propulsion and of thoracic aspiration." There are serious physiological objections to the physical conceptions of the circulation underlying this so-called law, which in any event cannot be accepted in the exclusive form given to it by Lancereaux. Wertheimer has shown that the effect of thoracic aspiration upon the venous circulation extends to remote parts of the saphenous vein by the side of the tendo Achillis. As the collective sectional area of the veins steadily diminishes from the capillaries to the heart, the average speed of the blood must be greater in the large veins than in the small ones, if the circulation is to continue for any length of time; and this remains true even when the energy of the blood-current is feeble.

Much more satisfactory, it seems to me, is the explanation offered by von Recklinghausen, of which mention has already been made (p. 167). This explanation places the chief emphasis upon the eddying movement (Wirbelbewegung) of the outer lines of flow of the blood-stream when there are counter-currents, or when the blood with retarded flow passes from smaller into larger channels or over obstructions, or especially into spaces relatively too wide for the received volume of fluid. Especially favourable for the appearance of this irregularity of the circulation are the ampullar dilatations just above the insertion of the venous valves, the intracranial sinuses, and the femoral vein near Poupart's ligament, which, in consequence of fixation to bone or fasciæ, cannot readily adjust themselves to a lessened volume of blood, and in which counter-currents are set up by the obtuse or right angles at which blood is received from some of the tributary veins. The trabeculæ which cross the cerebral sinuses may be a contributory factor. Similar irregularities of the blood-flow must occur with feeble circulation in other situations, as in the pelvic venous plexuses, where wide channels are intercalated between smaller ones, in the recesses of the heart, and in aneurysms and varicose veins. Von Recklinghausen has pointed out that the plexus-like arrangement, the entrance of small veins into large ones, and the close apposition of artery and vein render branches of the renal veins in the kidney susceptible to irregular blood-currents.

The greater frequency of venous thrombosis in the left leg than in the right is attributable to the more difficult return-flow from the former, in consequence of the greater length and obliquity of the left common iliac vein and its passage beneath the right common iliac artery. It has been suggested that pressure upon this vein by a distended sigmoid flexure or rectum may likewise contribute to slowing of the blood-current upon this side. The preponderance of thromboses of the left axillary and brachial veins over those of the right is attributed in a similar way by Parmentier; that is, to the greater length and obliquity of the left innominate vein.

As has already been urged, these mechanical disturbances of the circulation are not, by themselves alone, efficient causes of thrombosis. They simply make certain parts of the vascular system seats of election for thrombi. It is quite possible to exaggerate their function in the etiology of thrombosis. The presence of micro-organisms or other changes in the blood may induce lesions of the vascular wall in any part of the circulatory system; and primary thrombi may be formed in situations apparently the most unpromising, so far as the circulatory conditions are concerned ; as for instance in the pulmonary veins and in the venæ cavæ near the heart.

Capillary thrombi.—The blood in the capillaries remains fluid, even with extensive venous and arterial thrombosis, unless necrosis or gangrene of the tissue ensue, in which case, as in infarctions, the capillaries are always plugged. The interesting fibrinous and hyaline thromboses of the capillaries have already been considered (p. 160).

Cardiac thrombi.—There is no stranger chapter in the history of pathology than the story of cardiac polypi, from the first observation of fibrinous clots in the heart by Benivieni, in the fifteenth century, until the end of the last century. It is full of warnings against the uncritical use of post-mortem findings. The cardiac polyps of the old writers were, for the most part, nothing more than ordinary colourless post-mortem clots. Nor has the error of confounding these with genuine thrombi wholly disappeared from medical literature even at the present day. These moist, pale, yellowish, smooth, elastic, uniform, more or less translucent, fibrinous clots, softer or firmer according to their content of serum, non-adherent though entangled with muscular columns and trabeculæ, often showing moulds of the valves or other projecting surfaces with, at least, some red cruor clot at their most dependent parts—such clots, membranous, polypoid, band-like, or filling the right cavities of the heart and sending worm-like offshoots into the vessels, should never be mistaken for the drier, opaque, gray or reddish gray, granular, more friable, usually much smaller, adherent, often centrally softened or stratified thrombi.

Although there is a common impression that these fibrinous clots are formed during the death agony, I know of no good reason for such a view. It is much more probable that they are analogous to the buffy coat of clots in shed blood, and are formed after death, when coagulation does not set in until the red corpuscles have settled from the plasma. Liberation of fibrin-ferment, fibrin-content of the blood, sedimentation-time of red corpuscles and coagulation-time,[1] all variable elements, are the leading factors which determine the production of these colourless clots. Most striking examples of colourless clots are found after death from pneumonia and acute articular rheumatism, where the fibrin-content is high, the sedimentation-time rapid, and the coagulation-time slow. The whole doctrine of death from "heart-clot" in these and other acute diseases is based, in my opinion, upon mistaken interpretation of fibrinous post-mortem clots.

The *fresh vegetations* of endocarditis are not generally included in the consideration of cardiac thrombi. Still they are genuine thrombi, and

---

[1] By "fibrin-content" is meant the amount of fibrin yielded by the blood, and is not of course to be understood as implying the pre-existence of fibrin in the blood. The rapidity of coagulation is an element which is more or less independent of the total yield of fibrin. Red corpuscles settle from plasma or from serum with varying degrees of rapidity in different specimens of blood. Clots also vary much as to their contraction and the separation of serum. Although in using such an expression as "coagulability of the blood" these factors are often confounded, it is important that they should be distinguished.

there is no more favourable situation for the study of the formation of mycotic thrombi than the acutely inflamed heart-valve. The first step is the invasion of bacteria, as a rule directly from the blood in the cardiac cavities, into the endothelial and subendothelial layers. The surrounding cells undergo rapid necrosis with karyorrhexis; and simultaneously are deposited upon the damaged spot masses of conglutinated platelets followed by leucocytes and fibrin, these masses forming the vegetations. Proliferation of the subendothelial and adjacent cells quickly follows, polynuclear leucocytes migrate into the area, and before long new vessels with organisation of the thrombus make their appearance. A process essentially the same may occur not only in the mural endocardium but also in arteries and veins (vegetative arteritis, vegetative phlebitis, p. 172).

Putting aside these endocardial vegetations, it has been customary to consider the conditions leading to cardiac thrombosis as essentially identical with those of peripheral venous thrombosis, but there are differences. Cardiac thrombi are found especially in association with chronic diseases of the heart, lungs, arteries, and kidneys; in all of which, with the exception of pulmonary tuberculosis, peripheral venous thrombosis is uncommon. On the other hand, most of the acute infective diseases, as enteric fever, influenza, pneumonia, which are so important in the etiology of venous thrombosis, are in general of less relative importance in the causation of cardiac thrombosis, although it may occur in these diseases. In cachectic states, especially phthisis and cancer, the conditions as regards the incidence of cardiac and of venous thrombi are more nearly identical, for here thrombi are often enough found in the heart; particularly when there is well-marked fatty degeneration. Cardiac thrombosis stands in no such peculiar relation to chlorosis and gout as does venous thrombosis, although its occurrence in these diseases is not unknown. The great field for cardiac thrombi is afforded by diseases of the valves and walls of the heart, and especially by dilatation of one or more of its cavities with cardiac insufficiency (asystole of the French school); conditions which, in spite of the great retardation of the venous flow, are not often attended by peripheral venous thrombosis, unless in association with diseases known to dispose to the latter.

The seats of election for cardiac thrombi are the auricular appendices and the ventricular apices between the columnæ carneæ; the particular situation varying as the cause may affect the whole heart, or only one side, or one cavity. In cardiac insufficiency from general or local causes these recesses and pockets must offer the best possible conditions for slowing of the blood-current, and especially for the formation of eddies. That there is no actual stasis of the blood is shown by the gray or reddish gray colour of the thrombi.

The familiar *globular thrombi* (végétations globuleuses of Laennec) are by far the commonest form of cardiac thrombus. Varying in size usually from a pea to a hazel-nut they may attain the size of a hen's egg. They are usually multiple, and neighbouring ones are connected by an adherent subtrabecular thrombotic meshwork or membrane, of which they constitute sessile or pedunculated spheroidal or ovoid projections. Their surface may be smooth, or marked by delicate lines or ribs; and their interior is usually converted into an opaque, gray, or brownish red grumous fluid, so that the whole resembles a cyst with puriform contents. The liquefaction is of the bland variety already described (p. 164). Although the projecting covering of these cysts is often only a thin shell it rarely bursts. These thrombi may, however, be the source of emboli. Hearts containing these thrombi are often the seat of fatty degeneration. Usually no localised mural disease is to be detected with the naked eye beneath these thrombi, although the microscope generally shows degeneration or defect of the endothelium. It is most exceptional for any trace of organisation to be present in these globular thrombi.

Calcification of cardiac thrombi is a rare event. Delépine has described very fully a cardiolith, and has collected reports of similar cases. Some of these are probably pheboliths in or derived from varicose veins which Wagner, Zahn, and Bostroem have described in the wall of the heart, particularly in the septum auriculorum.

Somewhat different as a rule are the *mural thrombi* found on areas of circumscribed disease of the heart wall; as on infarctions, fibroid patches,[1] and gummata, and in partial aneurysm. These may be identical in appearance with the ordinary globular cysts; but often they are flat or polypoid, stratified, and more intimately incorporated with the cardiac wall.

Cardiac thrombi may be in the shape of massive or of elongated polypoid formations, occupying a large part of one of the cavities, and extending even through valvular orifices into adjacent cavities or vessels. One of the cavities, usually a dilated auricle, may be nearly filled with a massive laminated thrombus, as in a case reported by Osler which I examined. There is much resemblance between the clot in these cases and that found in aneurysms.

Apart from endocardial vegetations not much is known of *infective thrombi* in the heart, although it is probable that they occur more frequently than is suspected. In a child dead of scarlatina I found, in association with streptococcal mitral endocarditis, softened thrombi containing streptococci in the right auricular appendix. There are a few scattered reports of the discovery of bacteria in cardiac thrombi. Particularly interesting are the observations of Weichselbaum, of Birch-Hirschfeld, and of Kotlar, of tubercle bacilli in white cardiac thrombi. Birch-Hirschfeld found in a case of extensive genito-urinary and chronic pulmonary tuberculosis a white organised thrombus in the appendix of the right auricle which contained many tubercle bacilli and numerous tubercles. In these and similar cases there is difficulty in determining

---

[1] It is interesting to note that in 1809, Allan Burns in his classical work on *Diseases of the Heart*, in recording his observations on angina pectoris with calcification of the coronary arteries and polypi in the left ventricle, called attention to the relations between disease of the coronary arteries and cardiac thrombosis. He thus anticipated Weber and Deguy, and other recent writers, who have emphasised the occurrence of cardiac thrombi in angio-sclerotic hearts.

whether the bacteria are the direct cause of the thrombosis, or are secondary invaders. Kotlar interprets his case as the development of miliary tubercles in an organised thrombus.

As there are unquestionable instances of finding emboli derived from venous thrombi in the right heart, the possibility of a thrombus arising secondarily from such an embolus in this situation may be admitted; but I know of no convincing example.

Ball-thrombi, loose in the left auricle, are rare forms of cardiac thrombi. The first observation which I have found of such a thrombus was published by William Wood in 1814, in Edinburgh. As in other typical cases, the loose thrombus was in the left auricle and there was extreme mitral stenosis. The patient, a girl 15 years old, had the regular symptoms of chronic valvular disease. Death was not sudden. Wood thus describes the appearances : "The substance occupying the sinus venosus of the left auricle, when particularly examined, was found to be of a darkish red colour, in form completely spherical, measuring rather more than an inch and a half in diameter. It felt firm, but elastic ; the surface was everywhere smooth and polished, but having a singularly clotted appearance. Rolling loosely in the auricle, it had no connection with surrounding parts. When cut open, after having been kept for some days in diluted alcohol, it was found to consist of a sac, one-eighth of an inch in thickness, formed of an immense number of firm, smooth laminæ, which could be easily separated from each other. Within the cavity formed by this sac was contained a quantity of coagulated blood." Adherent to the wall of the auricle near the mitral valve was a firm, oval thrombus on the free surface of which was a superficial concavity which formed a "kind of socket for the loose ball to roll in." This last feature is a unique observation.

In 1863, Dr. J. W. Ogle reported a typical instance of ball-thrombus in the left auricle with extreme mitral stenosis, and accompanied the report with an admirable drawing. In 1877 Dr. Wickham Legg reported likewise, to the London Pathological Society, two cases of ball-thrombi in the left auricle with mitral stenosis. He refers to Ogle's specimen which he re-examined, and to a fourth specimen in the museum of St. Thomas's Hospital. One of his cases is unique in the presence of two ball-thrombi in the left auricle. This patient was brought dead to the hospital, and presumably died suddenly in the streets. Von Recklinghausen's brief description, in 1883, of two cases of ball-thrombi is quoted in the subsequent German records on the subject as the first observation of this interesting form of cardiac thrombus ; although there were much fuller previous accounts of at least four cases, with mention of a fifth, in Scotch and English records extending back as far as 1814 ; those of Ogle and Legg being certainly very accessible in the *Transactions of the London Pathological Society*. Macleod's case of loose thrombus in the right auricle is properly excluded by von Recklinghausen from the class of ball-thrombi. If the conception of a ball-thrombus be simply that of a loose thrombus too large to pass through

the valvular orifice, then van der Byl's case, reported in 1858, should be
included in this class.   He found in a case of sudden death "an irregular, shaggy-looking mass sticking" in the extremely contracted mitral
orifice.   When floated out in water this assumed a sac-like appearance,
was about the size of a pigeon's egg, and completed a broken thrombotic
sac in the auricular appendix.   This embolus must have been freshly
detached, and had not assumed the typical spherical or ovoid shape of the
ball-thrombus.   There have been later reports of ball-thrombi, by Hertz
(two cases), Osler (two cases), Arnold, von Ziemssen, Redtenbacher, Krumbholz, Rosenbach, Stange, and Eichhorst (three cases mentioned without
any details), making twenty, without including Macleod's and van der
Byl's cases.[1]   Of these, fifteen are reported with sufficient details for
analysis.   This form of thrombus, therefore, although rare, is not so
much of a curiosity as has been generally supposed.

The three characters, in my opinion, should enter into the definition of
a ball-thrombus : (i.) entire absence of attachment and consequent free
mobility ; (ii.) imprisonment in consequence of excess in the diameter of
the thrombus over that of the first narrowing in the circulatory passage
ahead of it ; and (iii.) such consistence and shape that the thrombus must
not of necessity lodge as an embolus in this passage.   The third point
does not prejudice the question of the possibility of a ball-thrombus
lodging as an embolus ; but it excludes from the group such detached,
shaggy, irregular masses (as in van der Byl's case) as must necessarily be
caught at once as emboli in the narrowed passage in front.   According
to this definition a ball-thrombus might, theoretically at least, occur in
any circumscribed or sac-like dilatation of the circulatory system ;
indeed von Recklinghausen considers loose phleboliths and cardiac ball-
thrombi as analogous.

All of the cardiac ball-thrombi—as thus defined—hitherto reported,
were in the dilated left auricle ; and, with one exception, were associated
with mitral stenosis.   In Stange's case there was aortic stenosis, with
slight insufficiency of the mitral valve without stenosis.   The agency of
mitral stenosis in the production of ball-thrombi is not only that it
prevents the escape of detached thrombi which might pass the normal
orifice, but also that it favours the formation of thrombi in the left
auricle, particularly in the appendix ; and doubtless also, through the
particular disturbance of the circulation, aids in their detachment,
increases the tendency to their rotary motion, and prevents the complete
emptying of the left auricle during systole, thus rendering more difficult
the lodgment and fixation in the valvular orifice of thrombotic masses
which at first may be irregular in shape.

The thrombi have varied in size from that of a small walnut to that

[1] I have also not included Schmorl's case, mentioned by Stange, as it is evidently identical
with that of Krumbholz, nor Fürbringer's case of numerous globular thrombi, the largest
the size of a cherry, in the right auricle, although he reports it as belonging to the group of
ball-thrombi.   He is evidently under a misconception of the nature of ball-thrombi.   There
was not the slightest reason why these small bodies, many of them indeed minute, if they
were really loose during life, should not have travelled on with the blood-stream.

of a hen's egg; in Wood's case the thrombus was over an inch and a half in diameter, and in Ogle's the weight was more than four drachms. In ten the shape was spherical; in four ovoid; in one (probably of recent separation) a somewhat irregular flattened hemisphere. In six the surface was smooth and polished; in six marked by granules, lines, ribs, or little depressions; in two smooth and knobbed; and in one (Redtenbacher's) beset with very fine, gray, fibrinous villi. Nine were centrally softened; four solid throughout; and for two there is no statement on this point. The colour was gray or reddish gray; in Wood's "darkish red." In the majority of cases it is said there were adherent thrombi in the left auricle, usually the appendix; and where this is not expressly stated they may have been present. In five cases only was there a rough or projecting spot on the surface of the ball indicative of the previous attachment; and in two this spot was not at all smoothed off: so that the detachment was evidently very recent, possibly indeed during the autopsy, as in one of the two loose balls in Legg's first case. Krumbholz says that the surface of his thrombus was covered with endothelium. In none, however, was any distinct evidence of organisation detected, for von Ziemssen's statement on this point is too indefinite to be considered.

Ogle, in 1863, clearly recognised the mode of production of a ball-thrombus " by the constant and free agitation of a fragment of fibrinous coagulum separated from some part of the endocardium, and uniformly increased by fresh material at its circumference precipitated from the surrounding blood-stream." Von Recklinghausen has given the fullest and most satisfactory explanation of the spherical shape and smooth surface, in noting that at least some ball-thrombi have a globular shape when first detached; and that irregular bodies, of the consistence of thrombi, rotating in a cavity and growing by successive accretions, assume a spherical shape by a process of moulding, and not by the grinding or breaking off of corners and projections, as was suggested by Hertz to account for the smooth roundness of ball-thrombi. In two or three instances where the ball-thrombus has consisted of a central irregular nucleus enveloped in a concentrically laminated capsule, it has been assumed that the former represents the original detached part, and the latter successive accretions during free rotation in the auricle. While suggestive of such an interpretation, this structure may, however, exist in still adherent globular thrombi. It seems to me probable that most ball-thrombi are smooth and at least approximately spherical when first detached. It is difficult to say how much a thrombus may have grown after its separation.

In nearly all cases the loose thrombus apparently came from the left auricular appendix, where adherent thrombi were rarely missed when it is expressly stated that they were searched for. In Wood's case the dark red colour, central blood-clot, and polished surface suggest the possibility that the loose body was a separated polypus resulting from hæmorrhage in the wall of the auricle or from a varix; and this opinion is strengthened by the socket-like depression in the adherent thrombus, for it is not clear how such a socket could be formed by a thrombus loose in the auricle; but it might have been the impression left by a polypus attached at some other point.

As regards the clinical significance [1] of cardiac ball-thrombi, Wickham Legg expressed the notion which would probably at first occur to most persons. "A loose thrombus," he says, "in the left auricle would at any time be ready to act as a ball-valve, and stop the circulation in the mitral orifice"; and in this opinion he was strengthened by the presumably sudden death of his patient. Von Recklinghausen, however, who at the time knew only of his own two cases and the two of Hertz, in criticising a similar opinion expressed by the latter, brought forward several arguments opposed to this notion. The main points of his argument are that instances of sudden death are not infrequent in extreme mitral stenosis without ball-thrombi; that lodgment of the thrombus in the mitral orifice has not been observed, and, even if it were found lying loosely over the orifice at the autopsy, that this would not indicate its position at the moment of death; that the funnel of the stenosed mitral orifice is elliptical in cross-section and shallow, so that a rolling sphere of the consistence of a ball-thrombus could neither completely occlude it nor get wedged in it, nor, if the ball should enter the shallow funnel, is there anything to hold it there, so that the next moment it would roll out. To these points may be added Arnold's argument that the thrombus cannot be horizontally pressed by the auricular contractions against the orifice; for during its systole the dilated auricle does not completely empty itself of blood through the stenosed orifice.

The histories of the cases of cardiac ball-thrombus support in general the position of von Recklinghausen. No symptoms were observed which may not occur in mitral stenosis. Death was gradual in all except four. In only one of these four cases of sudden death was there any conclusive evidence that the thrombus was the cause. This was Dr. Osler's second patient upon whom the autopsy was made in my laboratory by Dr. Flexner. The patient, a woman aged 20, was seen in good condition a few hours before death. At 4.30 A.M. she was found by the nurse very cyanotic, she gave a gasp or two, and died in a few moments. At the autopsy were found marked hypertrophy and dilatation of the left auricle, right ventricle, and to a less extent right auricle; without dilatation or hypertrophy of the left ventricle. The segments of the mitral valve were thickened, adherent, and drawn down by great shortening of the chordæ tendineæ, so as to form the wall of a distinct funnel. There were no fresh vegetations and no œdema. The stenosis was not extreme, the mitral orifice readily admitting the index finger. The other valves and the coronary arteries were normal. An ovoid ball-thrombus, resembling a thick chestnut, measuring 4 × 3·5 × 3 ctm., was found, upon

---

[1] In order to complete without interruption the description of ball-thrombi I introduce here their clinical significance, although the consideration of the symptoms of thrombosis is taken up subsequently.

opening the heart, occupying with its smaller end and completely blocking the funnel-shaped mitral orifice, from which it was readily removed
by the fingers. At one pole of the thrombus was an irregular, roughened
spot indicating a former attachment, probably to a thrombus in the
appendix. There can be no reasonable doubt that the thrombus in this
case was the cause of the sudden death, which is certainly not a common
occurrence with such moderate uncomplicated mitral stenosis at the age
of this patient. Indeed sudden death is less common in uncomplicated
mitral stenosis than in aortic valvular disease ; as the former occurs often
in young women, and is usually unassociated with disease of the coronary
arteries. In the three other instances of sudden death with ball-thrombus
the ages were 21, 22, and 39 years respectively. Only in one of these
was the thrombus a perfect sphere ; so that it would appear that an oval
thrombus is more likely to plug the mitral orifice than a spherical one.
This view is strengthened by the fact that of the four observations of
ovoid thrombi in three death was sudden. In the light of our case it
seems clear that a ball-thrombus may "act as a ball-valve and stop the
circulation in the mitral orifice," as suggested by Legg; but it is certain
that this is an exceptional occurrence.

Under the name of cardiac *pedunculated polyps* various formations have
been described. Some of these are ordinary unorganised or partly
organised polypoid thrombi, about which nothing more need be said ;
but others are very remarkable structures which occupy an entirely
exceptional position, not only among cardiac thrombi but among thrombi
in general. In the older records some of the latter were described as
fibromatous or myxomatous polyps,—two as hæmatoma ; but in the later
reports most have been recognised as organised thrombi. They are often
called true polyps in distinction from the false polyps of the older
writers.

The literature of the subject begins with Allan Burns in 1809.
References to many of the cases will be found in the papers of Hertz,
zum Busch, and Pawlowski. Among the noteworthy observations since
Hertz are those of Czapek, Voelcker, Bostroem, and Ewart and Rolleston. I have found records of thirty-three cases, at least twenty of
which were well-characterised, organised, pedunculated polyps. Twenty-
five sprang from the wall of the left auricle, usually the septum ; four
from the right auricle ; four from the left ventricle.

The following are the more notable features of these curious formations :—In many instances no cause whatever could be found for their
occurrence. The hearts containing them were often otherwise entirely
normal, with the exception of changes manifestly secondary to the polyp,
such as nodular fibroid thickening of the mitral segments and dilatation
and hypertrophy of the left auricle and right ventricle. Unlike other
cardiac thrombi they are solitary formations, and often unassociated
with ordinary thrombotic deposits. The vast majority of these polyps
spring from the septum of the left auricle near the fossa ovalis with
short pedicle, sometimes narrow, sometimes broad. They are firm or

gelatinous, elastic, ovoid or pear-shaped formations, in several instances hanging down into the left ventricle with a constriction corresponding to the mitral orifice. The surface is usually glistening, smooth, and covered by a distinct membrane which often resembles the endocardium. It may present calcific, atheromatous, or pigmented patches; and upon it may be irregular knobs and depressions. The colour is described as yellowish, gray, dark red or brownish red; the colour often varying in different parts of the polyp. A prevailing dark red colour has been observed in a large number of the cases. In distinction from nearly all other cardiac thrombi, these polyps are more or less organised by connective tissue and vessels; the organisation in some being little marked, in others so far advanced that the structure resembles that of a fibroma or myxoma. The central part is often unorganised or less organised than the base and periphery. In the incompletely organised forms the substance of the polyp is composed of red corpuscles, fibrin, granular detritus, yellow blood-pigment, leucocytes, and other cells between the blood-vessels and fibrous septa. Laminated fibrin may be present in the peripheral layers. Unless ordinary thrombi are likewise present, emboli are usually missed. A further distinction from the ordinary cardiac thrombi is that many of these polyps, by encroaching upon the mitral orifice, are of as much clinical as anatomical interest; the diagnosis during life in these cases being mitral disease, usually stenosis.

We have no satisfactory explanation of these pedunculated polyps. The ordinary causes of thrombosis are generally absent. Their commonest site of origin, the septum of the left auricle near the oval fossa, is not a usual situation for ordinary thrombi. They stand in no demonstrable relation to patency of the foramen ovale or to circumscribed endocarditis in this situation.

Bostroem has suggested that an explanation may be found in the existence of varicose veins which have been observed repeatedly in the septum, usually near the posterior quadrant of the foramen ovale. A difficulty with this explanation is that nine out of ten of the varicosities observed by Wagner, Zahn, Rindfleisch, and Bostroem were on the right side of the septum. In one instance, however, Bostroem found in the left auricle a spherical, dark red polyp, 13 mm. in diameter, attached by a short narrow stem to the septum on the posterior lower margin of the completely closed foramen ovale. This proved to be a varix containing a phlebolith. In another case a similar thrombosed varix had broken from its pedicle on the septum of the right auricle, and was lodged as an embolus in a branch of the pulmonary artery. He suggests this as a possible source of ball-thrombi. Of still greater significance is Bostroem's demonstration in an old museum specimen, labelled "thrombosis of the right auricle (pedunculated cardiac polyp) peripherally organised," of an enormous completely thrombosed varix almost filling the right auricle. In still another case he proved conclusively that a broad-based, nearly spherical polyp, occupying a large part of the right auricle, was a hæmorrhage in the wall of the auricle. Choisy and

Nuhn long ago interpreted the polyps, which they observed, as the result of hæmorrhage in the septum of the left auricle.

In the light of Bostroem's interesting investigations, more attention than has been customary should be given to the possibility that pedunculated polyps are the result of hæmorrhage or are thrombosed varices. Most competent investigators, however, have unhesitatingly pronounced the polyps which they have examined to be organised thrombi. It would appear, therefore, that the nature of these formations is not always the same. At any rate the great majority of the typical pedunculated polyps, to which the preceding description applies, occupy a position quite apart from ordinary cardiac thrombi. As already remarked, by no means all of the cases described as true cardiac polyps belong to this peculiar group. Some, as in Krumm's case, are ordinary partly organised thrombi attached to diseased patches of the heart wall.

Association with Certain Diseases.—Thromboses may be divided, as regards their clinical relations, into the following groups: (i.) those resulting from direct injury of vessels, including the penetration of foreign bodies; (ii.) referable to diseases of the vascular wall, as to angio-sclerosis, syphilitic arteritis, aneurysm, varix; (iii.) caused by lesions of neighbouring parts; (iv.) thromboses of arteries and veins whose terminal branches end in septic and gangrenous areas; (v.) complications or sequels of (a) infective diseases, (b) cachectic and anæmic states, (c) cardiac disease, (d) certain constitutional diseases; (vi.) idiopathic and primary infective thromboses. Several of these groups, being mainly of surgical interest, will not be considered here. The thromboses embraced in the fifth and sixth groups are of such special medical interest that it is proper in this article to give them particular attention; although it is manifestly impossible within reasonable limits to take up all in detail. Some of them are noticed in other parts of this work.

Enteric fever.—*Cardiac thrombosis* is a rare complication of enteric fever. In 2000 fatal cases of enteric fever in Munich there were only eleven instances of acute endocarditis (Hölscher). Girode, Viti, Carbone, and Vincent have found the typhoid bacillus in endocardial vegetations; and vegetative endocarditis has been produced experimentally by intravascular injections of pure cultures of the typhoid organism combined with injury to the valves. More frequently the endocarditis has been due to secondary infection. In rare instances in the course of enteric fever globular thrombi are formed in the auricular appendages and ventricular apices; and these, as well as the endocardial vegetations, may be the source of emboli.

Arterial thrombosis is a still rarer event, but, in consequence of its gravity, an important one. Bettke, in 1420 cases, found four of gangrene of the extremities; but in 2000 Munich autopsies no instance is recorded, a result in contrast with fifty-nine of thrombosis of the femoral vein in the same series. Keen, in his admirable monograph, has collected and analysed 115 cases of gangrene associated with enteric fever, and due to plugging of the arteries. In twenty-one cases arterial thrombosis was observed without gangrene, the absence of which is much more common with thrombosis of arteries of the upper extremity than of the lower. The earliest appearance of the gangrene was on the fourteenth day ; the latest in the seventh week.   In the great majority of cases the thrombus was seated in the arteries of the extremities ; and in those of the lower far more frequently than of the upper.   In eight out of eleven cases of arterial thrombosis of the lower extremities, collected by Barié, the posterior tibial artery was concerned.   In contrast with venous thrombosis the right side is the seat as often as the left.

Other arteries, as the pulmonary, the superior mesenteric, and the cerebral, may become thrombosed.   Four fatal cases of typhoidal thrombosis of the middle cerebral artery, or its branches, have been reported (Huguenin, Barberet and Chouet, Vulpian and Osler) ; and other cases have been recorded in which the diagnosis of cerebral thrombosis was made from the symptoms.   In Osler's case, in which Dr. Flexner and I examined the brain, the middle cerebral artery was open ; but the ascending parietal and parieto-temporal arteries and their branches were occluded by adherent, firm, mixed thrombi.   The adjacent brain substance was studded with punctiform hæmorrhages, but not much softened.   Typhoid bacilli were widely distributed in the body.

The arterial thrombosis may be secondary to embolism ; but in the great majority of cases it has been reported as autochthonous.   In the older records the thrombosis has been usually regarded as marantic ; whereas the tendency now is to refer it to an infective arteritis ; a view which is probable, although we have few conclusive observations in its support.   Rattone and Haushalter claim to have demonstrated the typhoid bacillus in the walls of occluded arteries ; and Gilbert and Lion, Crocq, and Boinet and Ramary have produced an acute aortitis experimentally, by injuring the vessel wall and then injecting typhoid bacilli into the circulation.   The bacteriological studies are too meagre and unsatisfactory to warrant any definite statements as to the specific cause of arterial thrombosis in enteric fever.

The far commoner venous thrombosis of enteric fever has been adequately considered by Professor Dreschfeld in vol. i. p. 817 ; and the points bearing on its causation have been presented under Etiology. Richardson has called special attention to the "marantic" thromboses of intracranial veins complicating enteric fever.

Influenza.—Nearly all of our knowledge of thrombosis in influenza dates from the pandemic of 1889-90, which led to the recognition of countless complications, among which those of the circulatory system occupy a less prominent place than the respiratory and nervous. *Arterial thrombosis*, although far from common, is still not an extraordinarily rare complication or sequel of influenza.   It is more common in this disease than in any other acute infection.   In a few instances it appeared as early as the third to the fifth day, but in most during convalescence.   Over forty cases of arterial thrombosis or of gangrene accompanying or following influenza have been reported.   References to many of these will be found in the monographs of Leichtenstern and of Lasker; but their lists are far from complete. In a partial collection of the cases I find that the popliteal artery was occluded in six; the femoral in four; the iliacs, the axillary, the brachial, the pulmonary, and the renal each in two; and the central artery of the retina (embolism being probably excluded) in one. The cerebral arteries were repeatedly invaded. In several instances there were multiple thrombi. Symmetrical gangrene following bilateral plugging was observed in a number of cases. Gangrene was observed in all the cases of occlusion of the arteries of the lower extremities, but not regularly with that of the upper.

It is difficult to say in how many cases the occlusion was due to embolism. Endocarditis is a rare but recognised complication of influenza, and globular cardiac thrombi have also been observed. In the great majority of cases it seems clear that there was primary arterial thrombosis.

Venous thrombosis is a far commoner result of influenza; and has been the subject of a special memoir by Chaudet, and of numerous articles in the medical journals of all countries. Twenty-five cases are recorded in Guttmann and Leyden's collective investigation, and many additional ones are to be found in the vast literature on influenza. Dr. Goodhart, in his article on "Influenza" (vol. i. p. 683), notes the frequency and the occasional diagnostic value of this complication, which may appear during the course of the disease or weeks afterwards, and in mild as well as severe cases. In the great majority of instances the femoral vein was attacked; but the veins of the upper extremity were thrombosed more frequently than in other acute infective diseases. Leichtenstern notes the acute onset and course in some of the cases. There are records of thrombosis of the cerebral sinuses in influenza. Klebs and Kuskow describe capillary thrombi in the lungs.

Few observers are satisfied with the explanation of either the arterial or the venous thromboses of influenza as marantic. Leyden suggests as a cause increase of blood-platelets from disintegration of leucocytes. Evidences of such disintegration, or of masses of platelets in the blood, have been noted by Klebs, Chiari, and Bäumler. Maragliano observed the onset of necrobiotic changes of the red corpuscles in influenza almost immediately after withdrawal of the blood. French writers for the most part attribute the thrombosis to infective arteritis or phlebitis (artérite grippale, phlébite grippale). Rendu, however, in his case of arterial thrombosis rejects this explanation; as he found the walls of the thrombosed arteries entirely normal (nothing is said of a microscopical examination), and he attributes the thrombosis to feeble circulation. In his case there was also a thrombus with softened centre in the left ventricle, and the occlusion of the artery may have been due primarily to an embolus. Gerhardt attributes the gangrene in his case to spasm of the arteries, considering it therefore analogous to symmetrical or arterio-spastic gangrene. In support of the more probable view that the thrombosis is the result of some change in the vascular

wall, directly referable to infection or intoxication, Kuskow observed
with great frequency degeneration, proliferation, and desquamation of
the vascular endothelium in influenza.   In a fatal case of influenzal
phlegmasia alba dolens Laveran found streptococci in the blood.   These
organisms have often been found in the blood and organs of those
dead of influenza.

In a remarkable case of multiple thrombotic vegetations present in
large numbers in the pulmonary artery, especially in the left main
branch, and also on the pulmonary valves (other valves normal), Flexner
in my laboratory found in the thrombus, chiefly enclosed within polynuclear leucocytes, very numerous, extremely delicate bacilli, which
were identified as the influenzal bacilli of Pfeiffer.   This establishes the
occurrence of an acute arteritis and thrombosis due to the bacillus of
influenza.

Pneumonia.—The sixteenth century error of mistaking for ante-
mortem coagula the firm, yellowish white cardiac clots, intimately
intertwined with the columnæ carneæ, and found after death from
pneumonia more frequently than from any other disease, has not wholly
disappeared at the end of the nineteenth century ; for coagulation of
blood in the right heart is still occasionally spoken of as a special danger
in pneumonia.   Genuine ante-mortem thrombi in the cavities of the
heart occur in pneumonia, but they are rare ; being much less common
than in many diseases in which death from "heart-clot" is not mentioned
as a special danger.   Acute valvular endocarditis is a well-recognised
complication of pneumonia.   Mention has already been made of coagula
in pulmonary vessels directly connected with the inflamed lung (p. 160).

Benedikt, Brunon, Rendu, Leyden, and Blagden have observed
gangrene of the extremities consecutive to arterial thrombosis in
pneumonia.   Blagden's patient was a woman 92 years old.   In
Leyden's case there was thrombosis of the lower end of the abdominal
aorta.   Gangrene of the extremities in pneumonia may also be the result
of embolism ; of this event Osler has observed an instance.

Venous thrombosis, although more frequent than arterial, is scarcely
mentioned in text-books as a complication or sequel of pneumonia.
Few cases have been reported.   Da Costa, in a valuable article on the
subject, reports three personal observations, and has collected from the
literature six additional ones, and two which are doubtful.   In addition to
these, I have found reports of cases by Barbanceys (two cases), Lépine,
Fabriès, Valette, Mya (two cases), and Lee Dickinson (seven cases), making a
total of twenty-three cases of venous thrombosis in pneumonia.   The femoral
or internal saphenous veins were those invaded, the affection being oftener
on the left than on the right side.   There were at least three deaths
from pulmonary embolism consecutive to the thrombosis.   The affection,
if one may draw any conclusion from so small a number of cases, is
more common in women than in men.   Of 367 cases of pneumonia,
observed by Dickinson, peripheral venous thrombosis occurred in seven, of
which four were in young women, two of these being chlorotic.   In

several instances of influenzal thrombosis pneumonia had occurred. Laache ranks pneumonia next to influenza and enteric fever as regards the frequency of occurrence of peripheral thrombosis; but this event is far commoner in the last two diseases. The affection occurs during convalescence, rather than in the course of pneumonia; and presents the same general characters as the phlegmasia alba dolens of enteric fever. Da Costa very plausibly attributes it to a primary infective phlebitis. Mya, in one of his cases, found pneumococci in large numbers in the thrombus.

Acute articular rheumatism.—There was a time when rheumatic phlebitis ranked in importance next to the puerperal form; but it is now recognised that most of the cases of thrombosis attributed by the older writers to rheumatism had nothing to do with acute articular rheumatism. Schmitt and Vaquez have sifted the reported cases, and they find that, while phlebitis or venous thrombosis is to be recognised as a complication of genuine acute rheumatism, it is a rare one. The infrequency of this event is noteworthy in view of the fibrinous state of the blood and the frequency of acute endocarditis. Gatay has reported a doubtful case with negative result of the bacteriological examination of the thrombus. Legroux reports an instance of thrombosis of the brachial artery without gangrene in acute articular rheumatism.

Appendicitis.—Mention may be made of the occurrence of thrombosis with appendicitis, as this affection is of medical as well as surgical interest. Besides the septic thrombo-phlebitis of the mesenteric and portal veins, thrombosis of the iliac and femoral veins may occur on the left side as well as on the right. The published reports indicate that this is more common on the right side; but in the 131 cases of appendicitis in the service of my colleague Professor Halsted, with the notes of which Dr. Bloodgood has furnished me, there were four instances of peripheral venous thrombosis, all of the left leg; one being limited to the calf. Three of these were in chronic appendicitis, the operation being between the attacks. Mynter, who has also observed thrombosis of the left femoral vein, attributes it to great prostration and weak circulation. It is interesting to note the analogy of appendicitic thromboses to puerperal thromboses, where we also have septic and suppurative thrombi in veins immediately adjacent to the inflamed organ, and less manifestly infective thrombi in the veins of the lower extremities. It is probable, however, that the latter thrombi in appendicitis, as well as in the puerperal cases, are frequently caused by bacteria, and oftenest by streptococci, which are concerned in both affections with great frequency. In one of Mynter's cases sudden death was probably due to pulmonary embolism following thrombosis of the femoral vein.

Other acute infective diseases.—It would lead too far to continue a detailed inquiry into the association of thrombosis with other acute infective diseases. It must suffice to specify typhus fever, relapsing fever, dysentery, erysipelas, suppurative tonsillitis, diphtheria, variola, scarlatina, measles, Asiatic cholera. In many instances thrombosis, as associated with specific infective diseases, has been due to a secondary septicæmia, streptococci being the commonest secondary invaders. The disposition in or after typhus fever to arterial as well as to venous thrombosis should be especially emphasised. Thrombosis has been added to the growing list of complications of gonorrhœa (Martel, Perrin, and Monteux and Lop).

Tuberculosis.—The consideration of thrombosis directly referable to tuberculous processes adjacent to vessels need not detain us. The occurrence of intimal tubercles, where the evidence is conclusive that tubercle bacilli have penetrated the inner lining of vessels directly from the circulation in the main channel, may be mentioned not only as a cause of thrombosis, but also as an interesting illustration of this mode of infection of the vascular wall. Several instances of endocarditis caused by the tubercle bacillus have been described, and mention has already been made of tuberculous cardiac thrombi (p. 184). Michaelis and Blum have produced vegetative tuberculous endocarditis experimentally, by injuring the valves in rabbits and then injecting tubercle bacilli into the ear veins. Particularly demonstrative of infection taking place through the vascular endothelium are the rare instances of tuberculous foci in the aortic intima, without invasion of the outer coats, and without tuberculosis of neighbouring parts. Two instances of this form of aortic tuberculosis have been observed in my laboratory, and described by Flexner and Blumer. I have recently examined a section, in the possession of Dr. Gaylord, of a superficial tuberculous focus in the intima of the aorta with an exquisite platelet and fibrinous thrombus containing tubercle bacilli attached to the nodule. A similar case has been described by Stroebe. These rare instances are cited because they furnish conclusive proof that bacteria may penetrate the inner lining of vessels from the main channel, even where the blood-current is forcible; and may set up inflammation of the intima with secondary thrombosis. Hektoen's interesting observations of changes in the intima of vessels in tuberculous meningitis furnish additional evidence along the same lines.

Arterial thrombosis, outside of the forms to which reference has just been made, and which are of pathological rather than clinical interest, is a rare event in tuberculosis. Most common are the instances of thrombosis of the pulmonary artery or its main branches in phthisis. Dodwell mentions an instance of thrombosis of both popliteal artery and vein. Vaquez, in chronic pulmonary tuberculosis, describes an interesting case of thrombosis of the left subclavian, axillary and brachial arteries with gangrene of the arm: he found streptococci in the plug and in the wall of the vessel, including the vasa vasorum, but no tubercle bacilli.

On the other hand, peripheral venous thrombosis in advanced phthisis is a comparatively common and well-recognised ailment. In the great majority of cases veins of the lower extremities, the left oftener than the right, have been plugged; but the thrombus may be in the inferior vena cava, or other veins, or the cerebral sinuses. Dodwell, in his valuable paper on this subject, places the proportion of cases of phthisis with this complication at about 3 per cent. In about 1300 necropsies of phthisical patients at the Brompton Hospital there were twenty cases of thrombosis of veins of the lower extremities (1·5 per cent).

The peripheral venous thromboses of advanced phthisis are usually cited as typical examples of the marantic or cachectic form. Dodwell, however, while recognising enfeebled circulation as a factor, is inclined to refer the thrombosis to some unknown change in the vascular wall set up by a complicating septicæmia. He emphasises the infrequency of venous thrombosis with the acute and the very chronic forms of phthisis, and its relative frequency with an intermediate type with remittent or continued fever. He also noted association with intestinal and laryngeal ulceration in a larger percentage of the thrombotic cases than the average. As is well known, secondary septicæmias, usually streptococcal, are very common in phthisis.

There are several records of bacteriological examination of the peripheral thrombi in phthisis, which show that they may be of mycotic origin. Vaquez found tubercle bacilli, without other micro-organisms, in a thrombus of the left profunda and femoral veins. They were present also in the wall immediately beneath the endothelium, but were absent from the media and adventitia. Sabrazes and Mongour in two instances found tubercle bacilli both in the plug and in the wall of a thrombosed iliac vein: they were associated with micrococci. More frequently micrococci, presumably pyogenetic, have been found, without tubercle bacilli, in the thrombi and vascular walls: examples of this are recorded by Vaquez. Notwithstanding these suggestive bacteriological findings it would be quite premature to conclude that all the peripheral venous thromboses of phthisis are referable to direct infection of the venous wall by bacteria. In a rather old thrombus of the iliac and femoral veins in phthisis I failed to find any micro-organisms, either by culture or by microscopical examination.

Hirtz has called attention to the occurrence of phlebitis in the initial stage of phthisis. Some cases so reported have appeared to be chlorotic in origin.

Cachectic states.—Of other marasmic or cachectic states, in which thrombosis is somewhat frequent, may be especially mentioned those resulting from cancer, dysentery, chronic diarrhœa, gastric dilatation, prolonged suppurations especially of bone, anæmia from loss of blood, and syphilis. The association of thrombosis with syphilis has been recently discussed by Barbe. Phthisis has just been considered. It is especially in the young and the very old that these conditions are most likely to produce thrombosis. Thromboses of the cerebral sinuses, and of the renal and other veins, in marasmic infants, particularly after diarrhœa, are well recognised. Peripheral venous thrombosis is more often associated with the waxy kidney than with other forms of Bright's disease. The thrombi occasionally found in the renal veins in chronic diffuse nephritis are probably due to local causes, and not to cachexia.

There is a French thesis by Rigollet on thrombosis in malaria, and Pitres, Bitot, and Regnier have likewise called attention to the subject. It is doubtful whether there is any relation between malaria and thrombosis. In over 2000 cases of malaria observed in Professor Osler's service at the Johns Hopkins Hospital no instance of thrombosis was found. (Personal communication by Dr. Thayer.)

Trousseau attached some diagnostic significance to the occurrence of thrombosis in cancer. There have been instances of latent cancer of the stomach in which peripheral venous thrombosis was the first symptom to attract attention, as indeed it was in Trousseau himself who died of gastric cancer. Gouget has reported a case of widespread venous thrombosis, of eight months' duration, which was the only affection observed during life. At the autopsy a small cancer of the stomach was found. Dr. Osler has told me of a personal observation of very extensive multiple thrombosis associated with cancer of the stomach.

The principal seats of cachectic thromboses are the auricular append-ages, between the columnæ carneæ of the right heart, in the veins of the lower extremities, the cerebral sinuses, the pelvic veins, and the renal veins. Lancereaux has strongly urged that this form of thrombosis never occurs in the arteries. Doubtless in not a few reported cases embolism has not been satisfactorily excluded; but older observations of Charcot and von Recklinghausen, and several recent ones, leave no doubt of the occurrence of genuine so-called marantic or cachectic thrombi in arteries, even in the aorta.

While pre-existing vascular disease, particularly angio-sclerosis and varicose veins, are predisposing conditions, these plugs are often seated upon intimæ which show very slight alteration. Indeed competent observers have repeatedly described the vessel wall beneath marantic thrombi as normal. While secondary septic infections often participate in the causation of cachectic thromboses, the view that all have this origin is at present unsubstantiated. It is clear that enfeebled cir-culation is of importance in their causation; but, for reasons already stated, there must be some additional element, which, in many cases at least, cannot well be other than changes in the composition of the blood. The nature of these changes is not known. Possibly increase of platelets, or a special vulnerability of cells, perhaps of the red corpuscles from which platelets are de ived, may be concerned.

Cardiac incompetency.—I have already had occasion in this article to speak repeatedly of the importance of feebleness of the general circula-tion in the causation of thrombosis. Thrombi in the heart itself have been considered (p. 182). In this respect attention is called to the occurrence of peripheral venous thrombosis in chronic passive congestion due to cardiac incompetency, chiefly from valvular disease. Especially noteworthy, in view of the slow venous circulation and the frequency of cardiac thrombi in this condition, is the infrequency of peripheral thrombosis. Hanot and Kahn, in reporting an instance of thrombosis of the right subclavian vein, say that they were able to find in the French literature, which is exceptionally rich in clinical contributions to the subject of thrombosis and phlebitis, only five additional observations of peripheral venous thrombosis in cardiac disease. I do not think that this complication is quite so rare as would appear from this statement; for, without any systematic effort to collect cases, I have found records of eighteen additional ones—Ramirez (two cases), Baldwin, Nicolle, Hirschlaff (two cases), Robert, Ormerod, Mader, Huchard (two cases), Cohn (three cases), Cheadle and Lees (three cases reported by Poynton); and I have observed two instances of femoral and iliac thrombosis associated with mitral regurgitation.

The most notable fact concerning these twenty-six cases is that seventeen were thromboses of veins of the neck or upper extremity or both, far more frequently of the left than the right side; and one of the innominate veins. In one of Cheadle and Lees' cases the innominate, subclavian, axillary, and internal and external jugular veins upon both sides, the left inferior thyroid, and the upper two-thirds of the superior vena cava were thrombosed; and in another of their cases both internal jugulars and both innominates were completely plugged, and there was a mural thrombus in the upper part of the superior vena cava. It may be that femoral thrombosis is more common in heart disease than would appear from these figures; it is less likely to be reported than thrombosis of the neck and arms, and, on account of the œdema attributable to cardiac insufficiency, may more readily be overlooked both at the bedside and the autopsy table. When, however, we consider that Bouchut places the ratio of thromboses of the upper extremity to those of the lower at 1 to 50, the relatively large number of the former associated with cardiac disease is certainly most striking. The clinical histories seem to show that thrombosis is more likely to occur in the cases with tricuspid regurgitation than in others; but it is certainly even then a very rare event. In several cases there was some complication, especially pressure on the veins and tuberculosis. The explanation of the greater frequency of the thrombosis on the left than the right side has already been given (p. 181).

The relative freedom from peripheral venous thrombosis in cardiac disease, in spite of conditions of the circulation apparently favourable to such an occurrence, may perhaps be attributable partly to the reduction in platelets in this condition (which has been noted by van Emden), and partly to the absence of von Recklinghausen's "Wirbelbewegung" (p. 181), an irregularity of the circulation which occurs especially in vessels too wide in proportion to the amount of blood which they receive. Hanot and Kahn refer the thrombosis to a cachectic state developing in the last stages of cardiac disease. Huchard likewise attributes it to cardiac cachexia associated with secondary infection. Cheadle and Lees' three cases are referred by Poynton, who reports them, to rheumatic infection. The bacteriological examination was negative.

As will appear later (p. 275), there is evidence that arterial plugging associated with mitral stenosis is due oftener to primary thrombosis than is generally supposed.

Chlorosis.—The association of thrombosis with chlorosis is of peculiar interest. Professor Allbutt, in his article on "Chlorosis" (vol. v. p. 508), has sketched the more essential features, but has referred some points for consideration here. In the older literature there are reports of plugging of the veins in young women which undoubtedly pertain to chlorosis. Thus William Sankey, in 1814, says: "I have met with two cases in young women, not after parturition; both were severe and well marked; both had obstructed menses." But Trousseau, with his pupil Werner, in 1860 was the first to draw distinct attention to this association. References to the more important records, up to 1898, will be found in the recent article by Schweitzer, from Eichhorst's clinic.

Although thrombosis is not a common complication of chlorosis, it is sufficiently frequent to indicate a special tendency to its occurrence in this disease; a tendency calcu'ated to arrest attention on account of the age and the class of the patients, the obscure causation, and the unexpected and calamitous termination which it may bring to a disease ordinarily involving no danger to life. Some idea of the frequency of chlorotic thrombosis' is perhaps afforded by the statements that von Noorden observed 5 instances in 230 chlorotics, and Eichhorst 4 in 243. The list of reported cases was brought by Proby in 1889 to 21, by Bourdillon in 1892 to 32, and by Schweitzer in 1898 to 51. I have found reports of 30 additional cases not included in these lists, and am indebted to Dr. W. S. Thayer for an unpublished personal observation; making a total of 82. (References will be found at the end of this article.) I have also seen 12 other cases mentioned, but without sufficient detail for statistical analysis; and I have come across several references to articles on the subject not accessible to me. Slavic and Italian literature has not been searched, and the American to only a small extent. I have no doubt that mention or reports of over 100 cases of thrombosis chlorotica could be gathered by thorough overhauling of medical books and periodicals. Thirty-one of my cases are from French literature, twenty-five German, eighteen English, three Scandinavian, two American, and one Italian. It would, however, be quite unwarrantable from this literary inequality to infer any difference in the incidence of the affection according to race or country.

The statistical study of these eighty-two cases brings out a number of interesting points, of which some only are directly pertinent to this article. Thrombi in the heart are very rarely mentioned in the post-mortem reports. There were only four instances of primary arterial thrombosis, two being of the middle cerebral arteries (Vergely); one of the pulmonary (Rendu) without thrombosis elsewhere, and one of the right axillary (Tuckwell) with gangrene of the hand and recovery.

Dr. Tuckwell reports his case as one of embolism ; but it is usually included among the arterial thromboses, and probably with as much or as little right as the others.

All the remaining 78 cases were venous thromboses. There was thrombosis of the cerebral sinuses in 32 cases (39 per cent), 6 (19 per cent) of these being associated with thrombosis of the lower extremities. In four instances thrombi extended from the sinuses into the internal jugular veins. Unquestionably sinus-thrombosis is represented by too high percentage figures in my list, for the obvious reason that reports of an affection of such gravity and such interest, especially to neurologists, are much more likely to get into print than those of ordinary femoral thrombosis. Still the figures are impressive, and indicate that sinus-thrombosis is not of great rarity in chlorosis ; to which malady a leading place among the causes of spontaneous thrombosis of the cerebral veins and sinuses in women must be conceded.

In 51 of the 82 cases there was venous thrombosis of the extremities (62·2 per cent—too low a percentage as already explained) ; 50 being of the lower and three of the upper, of which only one was limited to the upper extremity. Of the 50 cases of thrombosis of the lower extremities (which are probably involved in at least 80 per cent of all chlorotic thromboses), the process was bilateral in 46 per cent, and unilateral in 54 per cent—34 per cent being left-sided and 20 per cent right-sided. The usual preference of femoral thrombosis for the left side is shown by the beginning of the affection in the left leg in 64 per cent of the thromboses of the lower extremities, in the right leg in 29 per cent, and on both sides simultaneously in 7 per cent. There is in the list one case (Kockel's) with meagre history, in which no mention is made of thrombi outside of the upper part of the inferior vena cava ; death ensued from pulmonary embolism. This I have not included among the thromboses of the extremities.

So large a proportion of thromboses involving both lower extremities merits emphasis as a characteristic of chlorotic thrombosis. So again the repeated observations of multiple and successive thromboses, relapses and recurrent attacks (it may be after weeks or after years), all point to the peculiar and widespread tendency to thrombosis in some cases of chlorosis. The most remarkable example of this is Huels' case, in which various large veins of the extremities, trunk and neck became thrombosed in quick succession, until finally only the jugular and right subclavian veins remained free. The patient recovered. In five cases examined after death the inferior vena cava was plugged ; and in a few of those who recovered the symptoms indicated extension of the thrombus from the iliacs into this vein.

While the prognosis of chlorotic sinus-thrombosis is extremely bad, Bristowe and Buzzard each report an instance of recovery. Such a possibility has been questioned, but I see no reason to doubt it. Not very infrequently after death in one or more of the intracranial sinuses thrombi are found which had occasioned no recognisable symptoms during life, and no lesions of the brain.

A fatal issue of uncomplicated thrombosis of the extremities is due almost always to pulmonary embolism, which occurs oftenest in the second to the fourth week after the onset, and usually after some movement of the body. In my collection of cases there are thirteen instances of pulmonary embolism (25 per cent of the fifty-two cases with venous thrombosis outside of the cerebral sinuses). All but two terminated fatally. In some other cases there were symptoms suggestive of embolism ; and doubtless emboli lodged in smaller pulmonary arteries without giving any indication of their presence. After making due allowance for the undoubtedly disproportionate representation of embolism of the large pulmonary arteries in published records, this catastrophe remains sufficiently frequent to impart a certain gravity to the prognosis even of simple femoral thrombosis in chlorosis.

There are almost as many hypotheses of chlorotic thrombosis as of chlorosis itself. None of these introduces any factors which have not been considered already under etiology. The principal causes which have been assigned, either singly or in combination, may be grouped as follows : (i.) feeble circulation due to weakness of the heart, sometimes intensified by congenital hypoplasia of the blood-vessels (Virchow) ; (ii.) alteration of the vascular endothelium, especially fatty degeneration (Eichhorst, Renaut) ; (iii.) primary phlebitis of unknown causation (Vaquez) ; (iv.) increase of platelets (Hanot and Mathieu, Buttersack) ; (v.) some fault in the composition of the blood, variously defined as lowered specific gravity, deficiency of salts (?) (Renaut), presence of extractives derived from muscular activity (Proby), increase of fibrin-ferment (Birch-Hirschfeld) ; (vi.) secondary infection (Villard, Rendu, Oettinger, von Noorden).

It is not necessary here to discuss all these views in detail. The data for estimating their value have for the most part already been presented in this article. Such primary lesions of the vascular wall as have been noted in the thrombosed veins have usually been trivial, and are common enough without thrombosis. There is at present no bacteriological basis for the infective supposition. Villard's much-quoted observation is unconvincing ; in his case a small piece of a peripheral thrombosed vein was excised and examined by Nepveu for micro-organisms with negative result. Villard adds that Bossano found micro-organisms in the blood, but gives no details ; and there is no evidence that these micro-organisms may not have come from the skin. Perhaps more weight should be attached to a few observations in which some source of infection, such as furuncle, was present. Proby, Löwenberg, von Noorden, and other observers have examined the thrombi and blood of chlorotics without finding any micro-organisms. Nevertheless von Noorden and others are favourably disposed to the infective hypothesis, on clinical grounds. Sometimes the onset of chlorotic thrombosis is ushered in by a chill or chilly sensations ; usually there is fever, which may be well marked; and in general the symptoms are thought by some to indicate infection. It does not seem to me imperative to interpret these symptoms as necessarily indicative of infection by micro-organisms.

There are difficulties with all of the hypotheses which have been suggested. I think that there may be some significance for the etiology of chlorotic thrombosis in the increase of platelets noted by Hanot and Mathieu, and by Hayem; and determined more accurately by Muir.[1] I shall also venture to suggest that there may be some nutritive disturbance of the red corpuscles, in consequence of which they disintegrate more readily from slight causes, and produce the granular material, chiefly platelets, which constitutes the beginning white thrombus; and in support of this opinion I will call attention to Maragliano and Castellino's observations of the lowered resistance of chlorotic red corpuscles. Another element which may enter into the causation is some little understood irregularity of the circulation, other than retarded flow, which is manifested in the venous thrills and hums; and which may in certain situations, where thrombi most frequently form (sinuses, femoral vein), lead to the eddies shown by von Recklinghausen to be of importance in the causation of thrombosis; although I confess that the fulness of the veins in chlorosis does not support this suggestion.

Gout.—Since the publication of the classical paper on gouty phlebitis by Paget in 1866, followed by those of Prescott Hewett and Tuckwell, this affection has been well recognised (see art. on "Gout," vol. iv. p. 161). Its causation is unknown. Paget with much reason regards the ailment as a primary phlebitis with secondary thrombosis; and in this he has been followed by most writers on the subject. Although deposition of urates has been found in the sheaths of veins, there is no evidence that gouty phlebitis is caused in this way. Sir W. Roberts, on p. 172 of the article just quoted, ingeniously suggests that the presence of scattered crystals of sodium biurate in the blood may constitute foci around which thrombi may be formed.

Idiopathic thrombosis.—Paget says that the occurrence of phlebitis in elderly persons without any evident external cause warrants the suspicion of gout; and that this is perhaps the most common form of idiopathic phlebitis. There remain, however, rare instances of apparently spontaneous thrombo-phlebitis, occurring in previously healthy individuals, which cannot be explained in this way. Daguillon has observed and collected a number of such cases.

Primary infective thrombosis.—There are rare instances of arterial and venous thrombosis, generally widespread, which present the characters of an acute infective disease without anatomical lesions other than the

---

[1] Buttersack has recently described the presence in the blood of chlorotics of cylindrical masses of platelets identical with the first form of Litten's blood-cylinders. These he considers to be capillary platelet-thrombi, which have been washed out by the circulating blood. While they may occur in other conditions, Buttersack associates them especially with chlorosis. It remains to be determined whether this cast-like arrangement of platelets is not the result of the mode of preparation of the specimen of blood.

thrombo-phlebitis, or thrombo-arteritis, and the changes consecutive to the vascular obstruction and to the vascular or general infection. The thrombosis may be referable to a primary infective angeiitis, or to a general infection with changes in the blood and circulatory disturbances. The former class of cases may be considered analogous to mycotic endocarditis, the localisation being in the vascular intima instead of in the endocardium. In the latter group, which probably is not strictly separable from the former, the veins or the arteries are plugged with thrombi, which are often extensive and multiple. The venous is more common than the arterial form. Vessels both of the extremities and of the viscera may be invaded. The affection appears as an acute infective fever with the special localisation of the process in the blood-vessels.

As belonging to the group of primary infective thrombo-phlebitides I should interpret a case reported by Dowse. A woman, 43 years old, previously in good health, was suddenly seized with chills, fever, and great prostration, accompanied by the rapid onset of severe pain and œdematous swelling of the right leg. Death occurred after two and a half weeks. At the autopsy the iliac, femoral, popliteal, and deeper veins were found to be filled with mixed, adherent, predominantly red thrombus. The tissues around the thrombosed vessels were suffused with blood.

Osler has reported an instance of the arterial form of primary infective thrombosis. A man, aged 20, who had recovered from typhoid fever two years previously, presented fever, rapid pulse, diarrhœa, and abdominal pain, followed by gangrene of both legs extending to the middle of the thighs. He died about two weeks from the beginning of the illness. At the autopsy was found thrombosis of the femoral and iliac arteries, of the lower two inches of the abdominal aorta, and of two large branches of the splenic artery. The spleen was enlarged, and contained large infarcts, one the size of an orange, which had given rise to peritonitis. There were infarcts also in the right kidney. Numerous micrococci were found in the splenic infarct, and in the exudate covering it. The heart, the intestine, the brain, and the lungs showed no lesions.

Effects and Symptoms.—The lesions and the symptoms produced by thrombi are referable to the obstruction of the circulation caused by the plug, and to the local and constitutional effects of irritative or toxic substances which may be present in the thrombus or vascular wall. It is obvious that these effects must vary with the functional importance of the part supplied by the obstructed vessel ; with the rapidity, extent, and completeness of the obstruction ; with the location of the plug in heart, artery, capillary, or vein ; with the size of the vessel ; with the readiness of establishment of a collateral circulation ; with the nature of the thrombus, and with associated local and general morbid conditions. Thus the obstruction of each important vessel produces its own anatomical and clinical picture. The thromboses of certain vessels, as the intracranial sinuses, the portal vein, the femoral vein, are well characterised, distinct affections, which receive separate consideration in medical books. But I know of no modern work which presents in a systematic and thorough way the anatomical and clinical characters of occlusion of each of the important vessels of the body; although scattered through medical literature is a large and to a considerable extent unutilised casuistic material for such monographic treatment. In this article, treating of the subject as a whole, the more general considerations concerning the effects of thrombosis, with special reference to certain common and clinically important localisations which do not receive separate treatment elsewhere in this work, will be presented. Widely different are the effects according as the thrombosis is cardiac, arterial, capillary, or venous.

Of cardiac thrombosis.—If the presence of globular cardiac thrombi could be determined during life, it would be generally recognised as an index of grave impairment of the heart's action. But, apart from furnishing emboli, ordinary globular thrombi are not known to occasion any symptoms. There may be instances when during life cardiac thrombi may be suspected as more probable sources of emboli, particularly of those causing pulmonary infarction, rather than either endocardial vegetations or venous or arterial thrombi; but beyond conjecture the diagnosis can hardly go. Gerhardt attributed to the pressure of thrombosed auricular appendages upon the pulmonary artery or aorta murmurs heard over the arterial orifices of the heart; but other causes of such murmurs are commoner and better recognised. The encroachment of massive thrombi and of pedunculated polyps upon the orifices of the heart may occasion murmurs, thrills, and symptoms indistinguishable from those of valvular disease. In three such cases, involving the mitral orifice, von Ziemssen observed gangrene of the feet, which he was inclined to refer to arterial thrombosis rather than to embolism; but this symptom has not the diagnostic value which he assigns to it, for in other cases it was present only exceptionally, and it may occur in ordinary mitral stenosis. Unless the orifices are encroached upon, the mere presence even of large thrombi usually occasions little or no disturbance of the heart, or none which can be distinguished from that of associated valvular or mural disease. The clinical features of ball-thrombi have already been considered (p. 188).

Of arterial thrombosis.—The effects of arterial thrombosis are so much like those of embolism that it will be convenient to defer the detailed consideration of their manifestations in common to the article on embolism (p. 235), and here to speak only of the more distinctive features and clinical types of arterial thrombosis.

Whether the occlusion of an artery be by a thrombus or an embolus, the result, apart from possibly infective properties of the plug, depends upon the possibility of establishment of an adequate collateral circulation. If the anastomoses are such as to permit the ready development of a collateral circulation, an arterial branch may be plugged without any mechanical effects. In the case of certain visceral arteries, as the terminal cerebral, branches of the splenic, and of the renal, a collateral circulation sufficient to nourish the part supplied by the occluded artery cannot be established, even with a slowly-forming thrombus. In some situations, however, arteries whose abrupt obstruction by an embolus may cause the gravest lesions and symptoms, may be closed gradually by thrombus without serious consequences. This has been observed in thrombosis of various arteries of the extremities, neck, and trunk; as the femoral, the iliac, the carotids, the mesenteric, the cœliac axis, a main division of the pulmonary artery, and even the aorta. But in order to secure whatsoever advantage may accrue from its slower formation, the thrombus must find other conditions favourable for the development of a collateral circulation ; and often enough these conditions, of which the most important are integrity of the arterial walls and vigour of the general circulation, are absent. Furthermore, thrombosis is often rapid in attack, and hence, whether the plug be a thrombus or an embolus, the result is frequently the same.

In the differential diagnosis between arterial thrombosis and embolism emphasis is properly laid in the former upon the more gradual appearance of the symptoms of vascular occlusion and pre-existing arterial disease, and upon sudden onset and the detection of some source for an embolus, particularly cardiac disease, in the latter (see Diagnosis of Embolism, p. 253). But mistakes in diagnosis are sometimes unavoidable; for all the clinical phenomena which attend the one may occasionally be associated with the other form of arterial obstruction. Nor can the distinction always be made, with the desired precision, at the autopsy, although generally this is decisive. Hence cases are reported as arterial thrombosis which are doubtless embolism, and conversely.

Within recent years primary arterial thrombosis, occurring independently of chronic diseases of the arteries, has been recognised as a more frequent and important affection than had been generally supposed since the acceptance of Virchow's doctrine of embolism. Of especial medical interest are the primary arterial thromboses, arising oftener as a sequel during convalescence than as an accompaniment of various infective diseases, particularly of enteric fever and influenza. The associations and localisation of these thromboses, as well as the prevailing view that they are infective and referable to an acute arteritis, have already been considered.

Arterial thrombosis of the extremities.—When, as is usual, arteries of the lower extremities are affected, the first symptom is pain in the limb. This is often severe and paroxysmal, and is increased by pressure at certain points in the course of the vessel. The obliterated artery may be felt as a hard, sensitive, pulseless cord ; and below it pulsation may be feeble or cease altogether. Before obliteration the pulsations may be of wider amplitude than normal, in consequence of lack of arterial tone (Gendrin, Barié). The leg, especially about the foot and ankle, becomes pale, cold, mottled with blush-red spots, numb and paretic. With loss of tactile sensation there is often increased sensitiveness to painful impressions. There may be diminution or loss of muscular reaction to both galvanic and faradic currents. There may be increased moisture of the skin, and some œdematous swelling of the affected leg. Unless adequate collateral circulation be speedily developed the termination is gangrene. While the extent of the gangrene is in relation to the seat of the obstruction, it varies also according to the collateral circulation; so that with occlusion of the femoral or iliacs it may affect only the foot or even a toe; or with closure of the popliteal or tibial arteries it may extend as high as the point of obstruction. The gangrene is usually dry; but if septic inflammation or closure of the veins occurs it is likely to be moist. Recovery may follow with loss of the gangrenous part; or death may result from exhaustion, from extension of the mortification, from septicæmia and toxæmia.

The rarer arterial thrombosis of the upper extremities may likewise lead to gangrene; but here the chances for restoration of the circulation through the collaterals are much better.

I have already referred to the relations of thrombosis to senile, spontaneous, and other forms of gangrene (p. 178). Heidenhain and Naunyn hold that arterio-sclerotic thrombosis is the usual cause of diabetic gangrene; but further investigations into the causes of this form of gangrene are needed. Thrombosis of the abdominal aorta presents a group of symptoms which will be described under Embolism (p. 273).

The complex of symptoms called by Charcot "intermittent claudication" may be observed with thrombosis of arteries of the lower extremities, or of the iliacs or abdominal aorta; but it is more common with arterio-sclerosis. The term "intermittent claudication" (boiterie) is used by French veterinarians to describe similar symptoms in horses affected with thrombosis of the iliac arteries, which is not a rare disease in these animals. In these cases the lower extremities receive enough blood for their needs during repose, but not during active exercise. The slighter manifestations consist only in some muscular weakness and numbness of the legs after exercise; but in more severe cases, after walking a quarter of an hour or perhaps less, occur great muscular weakness, numbness, and pains and cramps in the legs, which may become cold, exsanguinated, sometimes cyanosed in the periphery, and almost pulseless. All of these symptoms disappear after repose, perhaps of but a few minutes' duration. Charcot's syndrome has in a number of reported cases been a precursor of arterio-sclerotic gangrene, but it may exist for years without this event. The phenomena are unilateral or bilateral, according to the seat of the arterial obstruction. Spasm of the arteries is evidently an important element in the pathogeny of intermittent claudication.

Other evidences of inadequate collateral circulation with arterial thrombosis of the extremities may be muscular atrophy and so-called trophic disturbances, which are generally the result of traumatism or of some infection in the member whose natural resistance is lowered by the imperfect blood-supply.

Thrombosis of the visceral arteries may produce lesions and symptoms identical with those following embolism, such as sudden death from thrombosis of the pulmonary artery, of the coronaries of the heart, or of the basilar; ischæmic cerebral softening, and infarctions of the lungs, heart, spleen, kidneys, retina, and intestine, with their attendant symptoms.

Thrombosis of the pulmonary artery.—It is especially to be noted that thrombosis of the pulmonary artery, both in its principal divisions and in the smaller branches, is often entirely latent, both as regards resulting lesions in the lungs and the symptoms. Thrombosis of the main trunk or primary branches may, however, produce sudden or rapid death; or a sub-acute or chronic affection characterised by dyspnœa, cyanosis, hæmoptoic infarctions and incompetency of the heart, as in a case reported by Blachez.

Dr. Newton Pitt believes that thrombosis of the pulmonary arteries is far more frequent than is generally supposed, even going so far as to say "that thrombosis in the pulmonary artery, so far from being very rare, possibly occurs more frequently than in any other vein or artery in the body." This opinion is based partly upon failure to find a source for an embolus; in the right heart or systemic veins, and partly upon absence of folding, fracture, or other appearances of the plug suggestive of an embolus, as well as upon association with general conditions known to dispose to thrombosis. A similar remonstrance against the current interpretation of so many plugs in the pulmonary arteries as embolic in origin was made by Bristowe in 1869. In my experience sclerosis and fatty degeneration of the intima of the pulmonary vessels is not particularly uncommon; and I also believe that primary thrombosis of the pulmonary arteries, particularly of medium-sized and smaller branches, is more frequent than is usually represented in text-books. Still, for reasons to be considered under Embolism (p. 262), the evidence seems to me in favour of the usually accepted opinion that the majority of plugs found in the pulmonary artery and its main divisions in cases of sudden death are emboli.

Thrombosis of the coronary arteries of the heart.[1] *Cardiac infarction.*— Although the general subject of infarction from arterial occlusion is reserved for the article on embolism, infarction of the heart is caused so much more frequently by thrombosis than by embolism that it is more appropriately considered here.

Thrombosis of the coronary arteries is in the great majority of cases an incident of angio-sclerosis of the heart, an affection of great clinical importance. It may also result from acute or chronic endaortitis near the orifices of these arteries, and possibly from acute inflammation of the coronary arteries. Thrombotic vegetations, springing from the aortic valves, have been known to block the mouth of one of the coronary arteries.

---

[1] I regret not to have noticed that this subject had been presented by Sir R. Douglas Powell in vol. v. p. 899. The paging cannot now be altered.

There has been much discussion concerning the existence of anastomoses of the coronary arteries. It has been demonstrated that anastomoses exist between the main trunks of these arteries, the most important being those between the auriculo-ventricular branch of the left coronary and branches of the right coronary in the sulcus on the posterior surface of the heart, forming a horizontal or equatorial auriculo-ventricular circle (Haller), and those between the anterior and the posterior interventricular branches near the apex of the heart, forming a vertical or meridional circle. There are also anastomoses on the surface of the left auricle between branches of the left coronary and those of the left bronchial artery. There are, however, no anastomoses between the branches of the coronary arteries after they have penetrated the myocardium, these intramuscular branches being anatomically terminal arteries.

These anastomoses do not usually suffice for the nutrition of the heart after rapid occlusion either of the main trunks or of intramuscular branches. Thrombosis of one of the coronary arteries may be the cause of sudden death. Barth reports the case of a robust young man, aged thirty, who died suddenly when in apparently the best of health. At the autopsy it was found that the mouth of the right coronary artery was blocked by a thrombus, the size of a pea to a bean, attached to a small atheromatous patch of the aorta, close to the opening of the right coronary. By a singular fatality this first and only atheromatous patch to be found anywhere in the otherwise perfectly healthy body had formed at the particular point where the small thrombus springing from it stopped one of the streams feeding the very fountain of life.

Porter has shown experimentally that the frequency of arrest of the heart after closure of the coronary arteries is in proportion to the size of the artery occluded; and that when arrest occurs it is preceded by a fall of aortic pressure and an increase of the diastolic intraventricular pressure. This increased intracardiac pressure checks the flow of blood in the coronary veins, and thus interferes with the coronary circulation in the entire heart.

There are, however, many recorded cases which demonstrate that the main trunk of one of the two coronary arteries may be plugged by a thrombus without causing sudden death. In an instance reported by Dr. Percy Kidd the patient suffered from extremely irregular and weak action of the heart, shortness of breath, and paroxysms of dyspnœa; and gradually sank from cardiac failure. The right coronary artery, about three-quarters of an inch from its origin, was blocked throughout by a firm, partly decolourised, adherent thrombus. The left coronary, particularly its descending branch, was greatly narrowed by sclerosis. There were no infarctions or fibroid patches in the heart. Chiari has reported an instance of thrombotic occlusion of the main stem of the right coronary giving rise to an embolus which lodged in the main trunk of the left coronary artery. Sudden death was caused by the latter. In areas supplied by the right coronary were ischæmic infarctions showing reactive inflammation. These, as well as the symptoms and the appearance of the thrombus, indicated that the main trunk of the right coronary artery had been closed for at least several days before death.

If the patient lives long enough, the usual, but not absolutely imperative, anatomical result of thrombosis either of the main trunks or of intramuscular branches of the coronary arteries, is infarction in the area supplied by the occluded artery. As the descending or anterior interventricular branch of the left coronary is by far the most fre-. quent seat of sclerosis and consequent thrombosis, the infarct is most commonly situated in the lower part of the interventricular septum and of the anterior wall of the left ventricle. The size of the infarct corresponds in general to that of the occluded artery; but, as a rule, the infarct occupies only a part, sometimes but a small part, of the area previously supplied by the obstructed vessel. Unlike infarcts in most other situations, those of the heart are not, as a rule, typically wedge-shaped, but are often irregular in outline, and sometimes appear as if several smaller areas of infarction had coalesced; indeed there may be multiple, detached infarcts resulting from occlusion of a single artery. Both pale, anæmic infarcts and hæmorrhagic infarcts occur in the heart, but the former are the more common. Fresh, anæmic infarcts are swollen, firm, of an opaque yellowish-white colour, and often present in the margin a zone of hyperæmia and hæmorrhage. Microscopically, they are the seat of typical coagulative necrosis; the muscle fibres being devoid of nuclei, indistinctly striated or homogeneous, and of brittle consistence. The term myomalacia cordis, introduced by Ziegler, is not a good designation of most fresh infarcts of the heart. The infarct usually reaches the endocardium, which then presents a mural thrombus; and it may extend to the pericardium and cause a localised fibrinous pericarditis. A reactive inflammation leading to the ingrowth of granulation tissue appears in the margin of the infarct, which, in course of time, is absorbed and replaced by scar tissue, unless it become infected and suppurate.

Cardiac infarction may be the cause of rupture of the heart, or of a parietal aneurysm; or may result simply in a fibroid patch. It is more common than would appear from the meagre attention usually given to the subject in text-books, and is of much anatomical and clinical interest.

The symptoms associated with coronary thrombosis are those of the angiosclerotic heart, so that it is hardly possible to make a positive diagnosis of thrombotic occlusion of the coronary arteries. Irregular, often slow pulse, shortness of breath, precordial distress, angina pectoris, sudden death, all these may occur from sclerosis of the coronary arteries, either with or without thrombosis. Fibroid myocarditis is often present and directly referable to arterial obstruction; but the changes in the myocardium are probably of much less clinical importance than the underlying disease of the coronary arteries. R. Marie has recently published a valuable monograph on infarction of the myocardium and its consequences, with a full consideration of the previous literature and the addition of many new observations.

Thrombosis of the mesenteric arteries will be considered with embolism of these arteries (p. 268).

Thrombosis of the cerebral vessels will be described in the part of this work treating of diseases of the brain in the next volume.

Here may be mentioned the interesting observations of recent years concerning the dependence of certain diseases of the spinal cord upon affections of the blood-vessels of the cord, arterial thrombosis being an especially important factor in many of these cases.

Capillary thrombosis.—In consequence of the abundant anastomoses, it is only when all or nearly all of the capillaries of a part are thrombosed that any mechanical effects result. Such extensive capillary thrombosis is more frequently the result than the cause of necrosis of a part. According to von Recklinghausen, superficial, often extensive, necrosis of surfaces, as of the skin and mucous membranes, may be caused by widespread hyaline thrombosis of capillaries resulting from the energetic action of thermic, chemical, and even mechanical agents. In frostbites and burns there may be extensive local hyaline thrombosis of capillaries and small vessels. I have already referred to my observations of anuria in swine, caused by extensive hyaline thrombosis of the renal capillaries (p. 161). Although in many cases I have seen similar hyaline thromboses in human kidneys, they were never so extensive as to seem likely to cause recognisable symptoms. Several years ago I drew attention to the presence of hyaline in capillaries and arterioles in the walls of some fresh gastric ulcers, and since then I have been able to repeat the observation in three or four instances.

Effects of venous thrombosis.—Thrombosis is so pre-eminently an affection of veins that chapters in text-books treating of the general subject usually pay scant attention to its occurrence in other parts of the circulatory system. In the veins thrombosis occupies the field of intravascular plugging almost alone, for it is only in the portal system, and in the rare instances of retrograde transport, that embolism enters into consideration; such extraordinary occurrences as embolism of the azygos vein, resulting from thrombosis of the inferior vena cava, reported by Löschner, being mere pathological curiosities.

The direct effects of venous thrombosis, as of arterial, are referable to the mechanical obstacle to the circulation and to the properties of the thrombus. The mechanical effects result from inadequacy of the collateral circulation. The free venous anastomoses in many parts of the body prevent any disturbance of the circulation as a result of venous occlusion by simple or benign thrombi. Such innocuous thromboses are particularly common in the pelvic veins. In some situations veins, whose rapid occlusion may cause serious lesions and symptoms, may be slowly plugged by a thrombus without manifest harm. For example, it is not uncommon to find at autopsy the main trunks of the renal veins completely thrombosed, without consequent alteration of the kidney or corresponding symptoms during life ; although we know that ligation of these veins causes hæmorrhagic infarction of the kidney with albuminous, bloody urine.

Frequently, however, the contrast between the effects of ligation and those of thrombosis of veins is in the other direction ; the thrombosis being followed by venous congestion, and the ligation of the same veins being without evident disturbance of the circulation. The latter difference is not always easy to explain ; but the factors to which we can often appeal with more or less success, in attempting to account for the absence of sufficient collateral circulation with venous thrombosis, are the extent of the occlusion, general debility, feebleness of the circulation in consequence of coexistent anæmia, infection, cachexia or constitutional disorder, generally high venous pressure and low arterial pressure, lack of muscular movement and perhaps of other subsidiary forces aiding venous circulation, phlebosclerosis, inflammation or some less evident affection of blood-vessels called upon for extra work, and irritative or toxic properties of the thrombus. The importance of these, and perhaps other accessory conditions, in explaining the passive congestion of many venous thromboses in human beings is made evident, not only by the inability to produce similar effects experimentally by correspondingly slight or moderate degrees of venous obstruction, but also by the varying effects of thrombotic processes with the same localisation and extent in different persons and under different conditions. Thus femoral thrombosis may be attended by absolutely no œdema or passive congestion, or may occasion extreme degrees of œdema and venous congestion.

The consequence of the passive hyperæmia caused by venous thrombosis is local dropsy. This constitutes the characteristic symptom of uncompensated venous obstruction by a thrombus, as local necrosis does that of uncompensated arterial thrombosis. In addition to the œdema, there may be diapedesis of red corpuscles, but this occurs to a perceptible degree only when the obstruction to the venous flow is extreme, or the capillaries unusually permeable. Such hæmorrhages are very rare in peripheral venous thrombosis, but are common with thrombosis of the portal and mesenteric veins, the cerebral veins and sinuses, the splenic, the retinal, and some other visceral veins. Actual necrosis may likewise result from thrombosis of the mesenteric, cerebral, and splenic veins; but, if it occurs at all with thrombosis of veins of the extremities, it is extraordinarily rare, and probably due to complications.

In addition to these effects, due directly to the blocking of the venous circulation, even so-called benign or simple thromboses often set up an acute inflammation in the venous wall and surrounding part ; or, as already explained, this inflammation may antedate the thrombosis. These chemical, as distinguished from mechanical, effects consist chiefly in arterial hyperæmia, inflammatory œdema, pain, implication of nerves, and constitutional symptoms, such as chills, fever, and quickened pulse. The occurrence of these irritative or toxic effects, even with the so-called marantic thromboses, is an argument (in addition to those already considered) in favour of the infective nature of many of these plugs, and of their primarily phlebitic origin. But while undoubtedly significant of such an interpretation, it can hardly be considered conclusive; for it is possible that certain thrombi may possess irritative properties not attributable to the presence of micro-organisms or their products, and that the phlebitis, as well as the periphlebitis, may be secondary. However this may be, the old distinction between benign and infective thrombi no longer appears so sharply marked as was once supposed.

In rare instances the venous medical thromboses associated with anæmic, infective, cachectic, and constitutional diseases are plainly septic, and give rise to phlegmons, and perhaps pyæmia or septicæmia. The suppurative or septic thrombophlebitis, which with its attendant pyæmia was in præ-antiseptic days such a common and formidable wound complication, belongs to the surgeon's domain, or, in puerperal sepsis, to the obstetrician's. (See arts. " Pyæmia " and " Puerperal Septic Disease " in vol. i.) To the borderland of medicine and surgery belong certain septic thrombophlebitides of visceral veins, of which the most important medical group, those of the portal system, has been considered by Professor Cheyne (vol. i.), and by Dr. Davidson in his article on "Suppurative Hepatitis" (vol. v. p. 123). Thrombosis of the umbilical vessels, which may occur either before or after birth, may be either simple or septic. The latter is an important affection, the consideration of which belongs to treatises on diseases of infants.

There is perhaps no pathological phenomenon which, on the face of it, appears simpler of explanation than the local œdema consequent upon venous obstruction, but which, the more it is investigated, turns out to be, or at least is made to appear to be, more complicated. The explanation which naturally occurs to one, and which is often given, is that the œdema is due simply to increased filtration of serum from the blood, in consequence of the rise of intravenous and intracapillary pressure resulting from the obstruction to the venous circulation. It is certain that this simple explanation does not suffice, at any rate for most venous thromboses, and that factors other than the mere rise of blood-pressure in the veins and capillaries are concerned; but as to the nature of these other factors there is great difference of opinion. The whole problem is wrapped up with that of the hypotheses of lymph-formation and lymph-absorption, so lively at the present day, into the discussion of which it is impossible here to enter. Corresponding to the two classes of these hypotheses, we have mechanical hypotheses and vital or secretory hypotheses of the œdema of passive congestion. The mechanical explanations are at least easier of comprehension. Cohnheim attributed this form of œdema to increased venous and capillary pressure, combined with increased permeability of the capillary wall due to malnutrition.[1] Starling and

[1] Cohnheim is sometimes quoted as considering increased pressure a sufficient explanation of mechanical œdema, although in his *Allgemeine Pathologie*, Bd. i. p. 494, he expressly recognises as an additional factor "unknown influences on the part of the living vessel-wall." As I had opportunity, when working in his laboratory on a problem concerning œdema, to

Cohnstein, with full knowledge of the later work, to which they have made important contributions, are advocates of a similar explanation.

Doubtless several factors, although not all necessarily operative in the same case, are concerned in the causation of the œdema of venous thrombosis. Those which seem to me most apparent are the following: (i.) increased intra-venous and intra-capillary pressure, with consequent increased transudation of serum (not alone sufficient, for tying the femoral vein or inferior vena cava generally causes no œdema); (ii.) increased permeability of the capillary walls, which may be due to various causes, such as stretching from larger content of blood, starvation and asphyxia of capillary endothelium from lack of fresh supply of nutriment and oxygen, and injury from abnormal composition of blood in anæmic, infective, cachectic, and constitutional disease, or from inflammatory irritants; (iii.) diminished absorption of lymph in consequence of lack of muscular movement, of imbibition of the capillary walls with fluid, and especially of retarded capillary and venous flow; (iv.) arterial dilatation from irritative or inflammatory influences emanating from adjacent thrombosed veins, probably also from the asphyxiated tissues, and acting either directly upon the arterial wall, or directly upon vaso-motor nerves, or reflexly (here the conditions resemble those in Ranvier's well-known experiment of tying the inferior vena cava or femoral vein, and producing vaso-motor paralysis by section of the sciatic nerve); (v.) sometimes a watery condition of the blood rendering it easier of filtration. Experiments of Dr. Lazarus-Barlow indicate that changes in the chemical composition of the tissues and tissue-fluids are also a factor in the production of the œdema.[1] The influence of hydrostatic pressure is evident from the greater frequency of œdema with thrombosis of the lower than of the upper extremities, and from the effect of position upon the amount of the œdema. While these various factors can be conceived as essentially physical and chemical in their action, the living capillary wall upon which they act, either directly or indirectly, is to be thought of as something different from a dead animal or artificial membrane.

Opposed to these mechanical explanations are the secretory hypotheses of œdema, of which Hamburger and Lazarus-Barlow are leading exponents. Of especial importance is the work of Lazarus-Barlow upon the œdema of passive congestion. He finds all the physical explanations inadequate; and, upon the basis of interesting experiments, he concludes that a principal factor is increased secretion of lymph by the capillaries incited by starvation of the tissues and accumulation of waste metabolic products. His *Manual of General Pathology* may be consulted for a full presentation of his views and a criticism of the mechanical hypotheses of œdema.

become familiar with his views on this subject, I may be permitted to say that he often spoke of increased permeability of the capillary wall as an essential factor in the explanation of the œdema of passive congestion.

[1] To these changes, as the cause of alterations in osmotic pressure, Loeb (*Pflüger's Archiv,* 1893, lxxi. p. 457) assigns the chief importance in the production of œdema.

The œdema of phlegmasia alba dolens is by no means all due to venous congestion. Much, sometimes most of it, is an inflammatory œdema spreading from the thrombosed veins. This is evident partly from the hard, brawny, painful, at times warm character of the swelling (œdema calidum); and partly from its location in the part of the extremity nearest the affected veins. The œdematous swelling may begin above and extend downwards, instead of in the usual direction from below upwards. The hydrarthrosis often associated in moderate degree with phlegmasia is probably also referable to an inflammatory serous exudate rather than to passive transudation from venous obstruction. It occurs especially in the knee-joint.

Thrombosis of veins of the extremities.—Clinically the most familiar form of venous thrombosis is that of the extremities ; the lower much oftener than the upper. Its various sites and clinical associations have already been considered (pp. 179 and 191). The affection may be entirely latent ; or may be recognised by a slight or moderate unilateral œdema without general or other local symptoms ; or may be in the form of well-marked phlegmasia alba dolens ; or rarely may assume a severely infective character, with chills and high fever ; or, exceptionally, may lead to phlegmon and pyæmia or septicæmia. There is every transition between the extremes. The latent and milder types occur especially with tuberculosis, cancer, and other cachexiæ ; the more severe manifestations with phlebitis of the puerperium, infective diseases, and chlorosis ; but there are many exceptions to this rule.

In the more acute and well-characterised cases the general symptoms are chiefly manifest at the onset ; and consist in moderate elevation of temperature, rarely preceded by a distinct chill, oftener by chilly sensations and quickened pulse. Increased frequency of the pulse may antedate the rise in temperature, and the pulse may remain rapid after the temperature falls. This disproportion between pulse and temperature is of diagnostic value (Mahler, Wyder, Singer),[1] but it is not always present. These general symptoms of the initial stage, which may persist for days, are often overlooked ; or they are masked by an existing febrile disorder. They are probably present in some degree, even in mild cases, oftener than the clinical records show.

The characteristic symptoms are the local ones in the affected leg. Pain, often paroxysmal, is usually the first to attract attention ; but sometimes it is the œdema. The pain may be severe. It is more or less generalised, with especial tenderness in the groin, the inside of the thigh, the popliteal space, and the calf. Often it is first noted and may remain localised in the calf ; as is true of the œdema also. There may be sensations of numbness or of "pins and needles." The cardinal symptom, œdema, sometimes descending sometimes ascending, gives rise to the firm, painful swelling of the limb, covered with tense, shiny, smooth, white or mottled skin, marked often by dilated veins, whence

---

[1] Singer (*Arch. f. Gynäk.* 1898, lvi. p. 218) has made a careful study of the pulse-curve in puerperal thrombosis. A step-like acceleration of the pulse-curve often precedes other manifestations of thrombosis by several days.

comes the name milk-leg or white leg. The œdema in typical phleg-masia alba dolens is hard and elastic, pitting but little on pressure. Occasionally the skin has a more livid, cyanotic hue, or it may be of a brighter red. In the more acute cases the surface temperature is elevated; in others it is often lowered. Muscular movements are naturally restrained, and it is said there may be actual paresis. The thrombosed vein, if accessible to palpation, can often be felt as a hard, tender cord; but it is best not to attempt to gain this information, which in most cases is of little practical importance. The sensation obtained from palpating the vein may be misleading in consequence of the peri-phlebitis, or of the soft character of the thrombus. Certainly, in view of the manifest danger of detaching an embolus, only the gentlest manipu-lations are permissible. If the thrombosed vein be superficial, it may sometimes be seen as a line of livid redness beneath the skin. It is not always tender on palpation.

The great and usually the only danger from peripheral thrombosis is fatal pulmonary embolism. It occurs oftenest between the second and fourth weeks, but may occur earlier or later. The danger may be con-sidered to be past at the end of six weeks, if the local symptoms have subsided; although there are exceptional instances of pulmonary embolism at a later period. It is to be noted that pulmonary embolism may result from latent and mild forms of venous thrombosis as well as from those of the well-marked examples; it is, however, rare with the cachectic thromboses of tuberculosis and cancer. Small pulmonary emboli usually cause no lesions or symptoms, yet they may give rise to hæmorrhagic infarction, or embolic pneumonia.

Nervous phenomena are sometimes so prominent as to have led to the recognition of a neuralgic type of phlebitis (Graves, Trousseau, Quenu). There may be even a mild peripheral neuritis associated with the venous thrombosis. This is probably caused by the direct action of inflammatory irritants spreading from the inflamed veins; but it has also been attributed to thrombosis of small veins in the nerve-trunks, to the bathing of the nerves in the œdematous fluid, and to reflex irrita-tion. Occasional sequels of femoral thrombosis, for the most part very rare, are varicose veins, leg ulcers, persistent chronic œdema, elephant-iasis, muscular hypertrophy, muscular atrophy, and club-foot.

There has been much discussion on the possibility of gangrene being caused by thrombosis of the femoral or iliac veins. Cases have been reported in which no other cause of the gangrene was found than venous thrombosis; but with peripheral venous thrombosis this is such an exceptional occurrence that it seems clear that, when gangrene results, complicating factors—such as arterial disease, pressure upon arteries, arterial spasm, great feebleness of the circulation or septic inflammation—must be associated with venous thrombosis. It is true that surgeons are familiar with gangrene after ligation of the femoral vein, but here also the result is exceptional and attributable to some complication. Braune, upon anatomical grounds, attempted to demonstrate that gangrene is to be expected after closure of the femoral vein near Poupart's ligament, but the clinical evidence does not support this view. Galliard has reported a case and has collected from the records others in which gangrene had followed venous without arterial thrombosis.

The thromboses of the upper extremities are usually of shorter duration and milder type than those of the lower; unless referable to some persistent cause, such as the pressure of a tumour. They are often accompanied by some cervical œdema.

Thrombosis of the inferior vena cava.—Since the days of Richard Lower occlusion of the inferior vena cava has been the subject of much experimental and clinical study. There are reports of at least 140 cases of this affection in human beings. The principal records are cited in the monographs of Vimont and Thomas, although the bibliography is by no means complete. Thrombosis of this vein is rarely autochthonous. Usually it is continued from the femoral or pelvic veins through the iliacs, or is due to some abdominal disease, as the pressure of a tumour. It may occur without any symptoms or without symptoms suggestive of the diagnosis. The characteristic symptoms are œdema of both lower extremities and of the abdominal walls, and the development of a typical collateral circulation. When the renal veins are likewise occluded there may be albuminous, bloody urine; but with thrombosis of these veins this symptom is oftener lacking than present. The diagnosis rests especially upon the appearance of dilated anastomosing veins coursing upwards from the groins and flanks over the abdominal walls and lower part of the thorax. These tortuous, varicose veins, sometimes as big as the little finger, make a very striking and characteristic picture. The superficial veins concerned in carrying on the collateral circulation are the inferior and superior superficial epigastric, the long thoracic, the superficial circumflex iliac, the external pudic, the lumbo-vertebral anastomotic trunk of Braune and numerous unnamed anastomotic veins. The direction of the circulation is of course from below upward. In addition there is a deep collateral circulation through various visceral veins with dilatation of the azygos veins. Sometimes the circulation is almost wholly through the deep collaterals, and there may be little or no dilatation of the visible superficial veins. In fact, in not a few cases, by the absence of visible dilated collaterals, the diagnosis is rendered difficult or impossible. Schlesinger has observed and collected a number of cases where the œdema was in one leg only. This may be due to the previous establishment of a collateral circulation on one side from a former iliac thrombosis, or to unilateral iliac thrombosis with parietal thrombosis of the vena cava, or to congenital duplication of the vena cava.

Thrombosis of the renal veins.—This affection is fairly common. It may be an extension of a thrombotic process in the vena cava, or on the other hand the latter may be secondary to renal thrombosis. Marantic thrombosis of the renal veins is not unusual in infants with cerebral symptoms, or exhausted by diarrhœa. In adults thrombosis of the renal veins is observed not very infrequently in chronic

Bright's disease, particularly the waxy kidney; and in malignant tumour of the kidney. The renal veins rank among those predisposed to marantic thrombosis. I once made an autopsy on a case of primary genito-urinary tuberculosis in which a caseous mass had broken into a renal vein which contained an adherent grayish-red thrombus extending into the vena cava. Tubercle bacilli were present in the caseous mass and the thrombus. There was acute miliary tuberculosis. The lesions and symptoms which one would expect to find with thrombosis of the main trunk of the renal vein are oftener absent than present. The various collateral veins, communicating through the capsule and along the ureters with the lumbar, diaphragmatic, adrenal, spermatic, and other veins, suffice for adequate return flow. Still a number of cases have been observed with more or less hæmaturia and albuminuria which have been referred to thrombosis of one or both renal veins, and genuine hæmorrhagic infarction may occur.

Thrombosis of the mesenteric veins.—Thrombosis of veins in the intestinal wall is often associated with ulcers and other morbid conditions in the intestine. The thrombus may extend into the small mesenteric veins, or the latter may be attacked independently. These small thrombi are important chiefly as a source of infective emboli transported to the liver.

Thrombosis of the large mesenteric veins is less frequent than embolism or thrombosis of the mesenteric arteries. I have reported an instance of this affection, and have found reports of 31 additional cases with pronounced symptoms, and of a few cases without symptoms referable to the thrombus and without intestinal lesion. The references will be found at the end of this article. The superior mesenteric vein was thrombosed much oftener than the inferior. In many cases with symptoms, the thrombosis was ascending and secondary to inflammation, ulceration or some other disease of the intestine; in some instances it was descending from thrombosis of the portal or splenic vein; in a few it was secondary to enteric fever or some marasmic or cachectic state; in one it was attributed to a calcific plate adjacent to the vein, and in one it followed splenectomy. The symptoms are the same as with occlusion of the mesenteric arteries (see art. "Embolism," p. 268), but as a rule are even more violent in character and rapid in course. They are as follows: sudden onset of very intense, colicky, not definitely localised abdominal pain; distended, tender, tympanitic abdomen; vomiting, which may be bloody; obstipation or bloody diarrhœa; and rapid collapse with cold sweat and subnormal temperature. The diagnosis is likely to be acute ileus, and laparatomy to be performed. Death generally occurs within two or three days. The symptoms may, however, be less violent, and the course less rapid than those mentioned. At the autopsy are found hæmorrhagic infarction and gangrene of the intestine, hæmorrhages in the mesentery, bloody fluid in the peritoneal cavity, and sometimes, although not regularly, peritonitis. The cases without symptoms have been usually thromboses of slower formation, but this does not appear to have been always the case.

In a case reported by Dr. Rolleston, the superior mesenteric vein was filled with softened, canalised clot; and in addition the inferior mesenteric vein, the internal and external iliac veins on both sides, and the splenic vein were completely thrombosed, and a partly occluding thrombus extended into the portal vein. The thrombus in the superior mesenteric vein was regarded as the oldest. There was old and recent inflammation of the intestine, but no intestinal infarction.

Of interest is the relation of thrombosis of the mesenteric veins to portal thrombosis. In several instances of the latter thrombosis of the mesenteric veins occurred without hæmorrhagic infarction of the intestine. Doubtless the explanation is that a sufficient collateral circulation had been established after the portal thrombosis to prevent the usual effects of a subsequent mesenteric thrombosis. That this, however, is not always the case is shown by the sudden or more gradual termination of some instances of portal thrombosis with hæmorrhagic infarction of the intestine, in consequence of the extension of the thrombus into mesenteric veins. This has occurred especially in the more acute cases of portal thrombosis, but it may occur also in those of several months' duration. Acute portal thrombosis may cause hæmorrhagic infarction of the intestine without mesenteric thrombosis; or the infarction may be over a larger extent of intestine than corresponds to the thrombosed mesenteric veins. On the other hand, the infarcted area may be much smaller than that supplied by the thrombosed vein. The symptoms may be of slower development and of milder type when thrombosis of the mesenteric veins is secondary to portal thrombosis than when it is primary. The sequence of events in Fitz's case is interesting—globular thrombi in the left ventricle, embolism and infarction of the spleen, secondary thrombosis of the splenic vein, extension of the thrombus into the superior mesenteric vein, hæmorrhagic infarction of the intestine terminating fatally. There was no obstruction in the mesenteric arteries.

Pylethrombosis.—The septic variety of thrombosis of the portal vein (suppurative pylephlebitis) having been described (vol. i. p. 610, and vol. v. p. 127), it remains to speak here of simple portal thrombosis, often called without much propriety adhesive pylephlebitis. This is a well-characterised, although usually not readily-diagnosed affection. It is caused most frequently by compression either of the intrahepatic branches of the portal vein in cirrhosis, syphilis, or tumours of the liver; or of the main branches or trunk by fibrous perihepatitis, chronic peritonitis, swollen lymph-glands, impacted gall-stones or tumours. Other causes are diseases of the walls of the portal vein, either primary or propagated from some neighbouring focus; extension of a thrombus from the splenic or mesenteric veins; pancreatic disease; gastric cancer; ulcer, or other gastric or intestinal disease; infective and toxic diseases; puerperal eclampsia (Schmorl); marasmus, and traumatism. Sclerosis and calcification of the wall of the portal vein deserve more attention as causes of portal thrombosis than they have usually received.   To the 12 cases collected by Spiegelberg and Borrman in which this was the cause, is to be added A. A. Smith's case, in which I made the autopsy.   There was extensive calcification and thrombosis of both splenic and portal veins in a man about 60 years old, who died of gastric hæmorrhage.   He had previously vomited blood on several occasions.   There was rapidly increasing ascites. Calcification of the media of the portal vein may occur without marked affection of the intima.   Marantic portal thrombosis is very rare, and, according to Schüppel, occurs chiefly as a terminal event without characteristic symptoms.   Nonne, however, in reporting a case of marantic thrombosis from Erb's clinic, interprets several previously reported instances with marked symptoms as belonging to this variety. The thrombus may become organised and the vein converted into a fibrous cord, as in a case reported by Osler.

The symptoms are those of portal obstruction—ascites, hæmatemesis and enterorrhagia, splenic enlargement, dilatation of superficial abdominal veins, and progressive marasmus.   The caprices of venous thrombosis are evident here as elsewhere.   Characteristic symptoms may be entirely lacking, or one or more of the important symptoms may be absent. Ascites has been absent or slight, especially in cases with abundant hæmorrhages from the stomach and bowels.   In general, however, the rapid onset, the intensity of the evidences of portal obstruction, and especially the quick return of ascites after tapping are characteristic of obliterating portal thrombosis ; and by observation of these points a correct diagnosis has repeatedly been made.   These acute symptoms are of most diagnostic value when they appear in persons previously in apparent health, as has been observed with phlebosclerotic thrombosis ; or in the course of some disease not itself a cause of obstruction to the portal circulation.   When, as in cirrhosis of the liver, the symptoms unfold themselves gradually, the diagnosis is manifestly impossible, or at best no more than mere conjecture.

I have added traumatism as a possible cause of portal thrombosis on the basis of a diagnosis made by Dr. Delafield, while I was resident physician in his service at Bellevue Hospital.   A lad, who had received a severe blow on the abdomen, was admitted with extreme ascites which had come on within two weeks after the injury.   He was repeatedly tapped, the clear fluid reaccumulating at first with great rapidity after each tapping, afterward more slowly, until in the course of months there was complete recovery.   In the meantime enlarged veins made their appearance over the upper part of the abdomen.

Jaundice is not a symptom of portal thrombosis, although repeatedly observed as a complication.   The channels for establishment of a collateral circulation are the same as in cirrhosis of the liver, with the exclusion of those which communicate with the portal vein itself, at or beyond the site of occlusion.

Under certain exceptionally favourable conditions recovery may take place ; a satisfactory collateral circulation being established, with perhaps opening of channels through the organised thrombus. The usually fatal termination may be from hæmorrhage or exhaustion, sometimes within a few weeks or even days from the onset. I know of no instance, in man, of death within a few hours after occlusion of the portal vein, such as occurs regularly, with great fall of arterial blood-pressure, after ligating this vessel in rabbits and dogs. As already mentioned, hæmorrhagic intestinal infarction may be caused by portal thrombosis (p. 219).

There has been much discussion on the occurrence of changes in the liver which can be attributed directly to stoppage of the portal circulation. In the majority of cases of portal thrombosis the liver has been the seat of atrophic cirrhosis, but most modern authors have regarded the thrombosis as secondary to the cirrhosis. Dr. Samuel West, however, in 1878, took strong ground in favour of the reverse being sometimes the case; and he found support in the experimental results of Solowieff. The later experiments of Cohnheim and Litten have been widely accepted as indicating that obstruction of the portal vein is without effect upon the hepatic structure and functions. Bermant has recently gone over the entire experimental and anatomicoclinical evidence, and has reached the conclusion that stoppage of the portal vein may lead to atrophic cirrhosis. The case which he reports speaks strongly in favour of this view; for only the right branch of the portal vein was thrombosed, and the cirrhosis was limited to the corresponding lobe of the liver. Nevertheless, cases of portal thrombosis, some not of short duration, have been reported by Frerichs, Leyden, Alexander, and others without any alteration in the liver; and I have observed two such cases in which the symptoms of portal obstruction extended over several months.[1]

Thrombosis of the splenic vein.—Primary thrombosis of the splenic vein and its radicles is rare. I have seen an instance of autochthonous thrombosis secondary to calcification of the wall of the splenic vein. Thrombosis of veins within the spleen, extending sometimes into the main trunk, is common with infarction, abscess, and certain other morbid processes in this organ. Thrombosis of the main trunk may be caused by suppurative or hæmorrhagic pancreatitis, or by cancer of the pancreas. As has already been mentioned, thrombi may extend from the portal or mesenteric veins into the splenic, as well as from the latter into the former. There is the possibility of thrombosis secondary to retrograde embolism of the splenic vein.

Köster has reported the rare complication of enteric fever with thrombosis of the radicles and main trunk of the splenic vein; the evidence being conclusive that the oldest part of the thrombus was in the spleen. The evidences of occlusion of the main vein appeared at the beginning of convalescence. The spleen was enormously swollen and the pulp of a diffuse reddish-black colour. The capsule and surround-

---

[1] Chiari (*Centralb. f. allg. Path. u. path. Anat.* 1898, ix. p. 854) has recently described endophlebitis, with thrombosis, of the radicles of the hepatic vein. There were symptoms of portal obstruction.

ing tissues were suffused with blood.   As there were thrombi in the small mesenteric veins near the ulcerated ileum, there was a possibility of retrograde embolism; but Köster thinks it more probable that the process originated within the spleen.

Thrombosis limited to the extra-splenic part of the vein may be completely or nearly compensated by the collateral venous circulation, so that no changes or only a moderate passive congestion occur in the spleen.

Thrombi occupying intrasplenic veins may cause hæmorrhagic infarction.   Dr. Rolleston has observed two instances of anæmic infarcts of the spleen in association with thrombosis of the splenic vein.   Litten probably goes too far in attributing most genuine hæmorrhagic as distinguished from pale infarcts of the spleen, to venous thrombosis rather than to arterial embolism.

Extensive necrosis and hæmorrhagic infarction may be caused by torsion of the pedicle of a movable spleen.   A perhaps unique instance of this occurrence was observed in the Johns Hopkins Hospital, and has been described by Osler.

Obliteration of the superior vena cava.—Since the admirable studies by Duchek (1854) and by Oulmont (1856) of the causes and symptoms of obliteration of the superior vena cava a considerable number of instances of this condition have been reported.   By far the most frequent cause is the pressure of a mediastinal tumour, of swollen lymph-glands, or of an aneurysm.   Less common is the growth of a cancer or other malignant tumour into the lumen of the vein.   Banti reports a curious case of generalised tuberculosis in which nearly the whole length of the superior vena cava was completely filled by a neoplastic tuberculous mass projecting into the right auricle.   The outer walls of the vein were intact. The condition seems to have been analogous to the tuberculous cardiac thrombi already described (p. 184).   Primary thrombosis of the superior vena cava is so rare as to be a pathological curiosity.   Poynton has reported an instance of thrombotic occlusion of the upper two-thirds of the superior vena cava in association with chronic and acute valvular endocarditis, and in a second case of valvular disease he found a mural thrombus in this vein.   In both cases there was tricuspid insufficiency (p. 199).   The characteristic symptoms are œdema and cyanosis of the upper half of the body—face, neck, arms, and thorax—and dilatation of deep and superficial veins, especially marked over the anterior wall of the thorax and upper part of the abdomen.   In a case exhibited by Dr. Osler to the Johns Hopkins Hospital Medical Society, the anterior surface of the chest was covered with large, spongy bunches of enormous varicose veins, in one of which a phlebolith could be felt.   Other symptoms, which may be present, are œdema of conjunctival and buccal mucous membranes, exophthalmos, watery secretion from the conjunctivæ, nosebleeding, and such signs of venous congestion of the brain as headache, vertigo, and ringing in the ears, especially on bending over.   In the light of the whimsicalities of venous thrombosis it is hardly necessary to add that the symptoms may be less marked, and may deviate from what might naturally be expected.

Thrombosis of the innominate, subclavian, and jugular veins.—The more important literature of this subject is cited in the papers of Pohl, Hirschlaff, and Helen Baldwin. The occurrence of these thromboses in cardiac disease, and from compression, has already been mentioned (p. 199); other rare causes are infection, empyema, acute rheumatism, tuberculosis, marasmus, and traumatism. The symptoms are the usual ones of venous congestion, œdematous swelling, pain in the regions from which the veins convey blood, dilatation of collaterals, and, in the case of the cervical veins, recognition of the thrombosed vein by palpation, which, however, should be done with great care.

Thrombosis of the pulmonary veins may be mentioned as a rare source of embolism in the aortic system. It is usually secondary to some pulmonary disease, as gangrene, malignant tumours, abscess, infarction, tuberculosis, pneumonia. It has been observed with extensive emphysema of the lungs (Schmale).

Thrombosis of the cerebral sinuses will be considered in connection with diseases of the brain in the following volume.

O. Wyss has described a remarkable instance of extensive hæmorrhagic myelitis caused by widespread hyaline and platelet thrombi in veins within the spinal cord. The thrombosis was secondary to a glioma of the dorsal cord. Rosin has likewise observed thrombosis of veins extending the whole length of the spinal cord, consecutive to a tumour of the cervical cord.

Multiple thromboses.—Finally may be mentioned the cases in which many veins in different parts of the body become thrombosed, as in Huels's case of chlorotic thrombosis; and Osler's, of thrombosis secondary to cancer of the stomach, already cited (pp. 201 and 198). Erlenmeyer has described as "jumping thrombosis" (springende Thrombose), in distinction from the ordinary creeping form, cases in which the process attacks first one vein and then another, in a different region, until finally various veins in the extremities, trunk, and brain may become plugged.

Treatment.—The treatment of thrombosis of the extremities is about all that needs special consideration in this article. In view of the part played by enfeebled circulation and secondary infections in the causation of thrombosis, prophylactic measures should be directed toward maintaining good nutrition, strengthening the heart's action, and warding off secondary infection, so far as may be, or treating accessible foci of infection antiseptically.

In the absence of any available medicinal treatment known to have any direct control over the process of thrombosis, the general indications for treatment are to secure as speedily as possible an adequate collateral circulation, in order to ward off the danger of tissue-necrosis or gangrene from arterial thrombosis and the effects of passive congestion from venous thrombosis; and, above all, in the case of venous thrombosis, to guard against the detachment of emboli. These indications are best met by absolute rest, suitable position and immobilisation of the thrombosed extremity, and nourishing diet.

With venous thrombosis of a lower extremity the patient should lie on the back with the limb elevated on an inclined plane, or in a trough well lined with cotton wool. The limb should be kept warm by wrapping in cotton wadding, and hot fomentations of lead-water and laudanum, or some similar preparation, may be applied. If the condition of the heart indicate it, digitalis or other cardiac tonic may be given. At the height of the process the pain may be so intense as to require the use of opium or some of its derivatives.

It is all-important to know what not to do. The patient should be cautioned against moving the leg, especially against any sudden jerk. Palpation of the affected veins should be of the gentlest sort, and is better omitted altogether. All unnecessary movements and manipulations should be avoided. Nothing is gained, and harm may be done by resorting, before all danger of embolism is passed, to the old-fashioned treatment of rubbing in mercurial or belladonna ointment. The length of time that the patient should remain quiet in bed will vary according to the severity of the case. Although the thrombotic process does not usually progress after the tenth or twelfth day, it is a general rule that the patient should not be allowed to walk in less than forty days. A large number of the deaths from pulmonary embolism have occurred when the patient first walks, or goes to stool, or takes a bath.

Light bandaging of the lower part of the leg assists the circulation ; but, if applied at all, it should be with only minimal compression. After the danger of embolism is passed, massage and bandaging may be employed to advantage, or a long elastic stocking worn.

If gangrene result from arterial thrombosis, the time and site of operation should be determined upon surgical principles.

WM. H. WELCH.

REFERENCES[1]

Structure of Thrombi.—1. ARNOLD. *Virchow's Archiv*, 1897, l. p. 445.—2. BIZZOZERO. *Virchow's Arch.* 1882, xc. p. 261.—3. DETERMANN: *XVI. Congr. f. inn. Med.* 1898, p. 237.—4. EBERTH and SCHIMMELBUSCH. *Die Thrombose nach Versuchen u. Leichenbefunden.* Stuttgart, 1888.—5. HAMMERSTEN. *Ztschr. f. physiol. Chem.* 1896-97, xxii. p. 333.—6. HANAU. *Fortschr. d. Med.* 1886, iv. p. 385.—7. HAYEM. *Compt. rend. de l'Acad. des sc.*, July 18, 1882.—8. KLEBS. *Allg. Path.* Th. ii. Jena, 1889.—9. KRIEGE. *Virch. Arch.* 1889, cxvi. p. 64. —10. LÖWIT. *Arch. f. exp. Path. u. Pharm.* 1887, xxiii. p. 1, and xxiv. p. 188.—11. LUBNITZKY. *Arch. f. exp. Path. u. Pharm.* 1885, xix. p. 185.—12. MANTEGAZZA. *Gazz. med. lombard.* 1869.—13. MOSSO. *Virch. Arch.* 1887, cix. p. 205.—14. MÜLLER, FR. *Ziegler's Beitr.* 1898, xxii. p. 498.—15. OSLER. *Seguin's Arch. of Med.* Feb. 1881.—16. *Idem.* *Centralbl. f. med. Wiss.* July 29, 1882.—17. *Idem.* *Cartwright Lectures*, 1886.—18. PITRES. *Arch. d. phys. norm. et path.* 1876, p. 230.—19. VON RECKLINGHAUSEN. *Handb. d. allg. Path. d. Kreislaufs u. d. Ernährung.* Stuttgart, 1893.—20. RIBBERT. *Die path. Anat. u. d. Heil. d. durch Staph. pyog. aur. hervorgeruf. Erkrank.* Bonn, 1891.—21. VIRCHOW. *Gesammelte Abhandlungen.* Frankf. 1856.—22. WEIGERT. *Virchow's Archiv*, 1877, lxx. p. 483, and 1880, lxxix. p. 87.—23. *Idem.* "Thrombose," in *Eulenburg's Real-Encyclopädie.*—

---

[1] The references are only to authors cited in the text, and are not intended to be a complete bibliography of the subject. The references to authors cited under different headings in the text will usually be found only under the first heading in which the reference appears.

24. WELCH. "The Structure of White Thrombi," *Trans. Path. Soc. of Phila-delphia*, 1887, xiii.—25. WELCH and CLEMENT. "Remarks on Hog Cholera and Swine Plague," *Proc. 30th Annual Convention, U.S. Vet. Med. Assoc. etc.* Chicago, 1893.— 26. WLASSOW. *Ziegler's Beiträge*, 1894, xv. p. 543.—27. ZAHN. *Virchow's Arch.* 1875, lxii. p. 81.—28. ZENKER, K. *Ziegler's Beitr.* 1895, xvii. p. 448.—29. ZIEGLER. *Lehrb. d. allg. Path. u. spec. path. Anat.* 9te Aufl. Bd. i. p. 149.
Growth, Metamorphoses, and Organisation.—30. ASCHOFF. *Virch. Arch.* 1892, cxxx. p. 93.—31. BENEKE. *Ziegler's Beitr.* 1890, vii. p. 95.—32. LEGG, WICKHAM. *Tr. Path. Soc. Lond.* 1878, xxix. p. 50.—33. THOMA. *Lehrb. d. path. Anat.* i. Stutt-gart, 1894.—34. ZAHN. *Virchow-Festschrift. Internat. Beitr.* ii. p. 199.
Etiology.—35. BAILLIE, MATTHEW. *Trans. Soc. Improvement Med. and Chir. Knowledge*, 1793, i. p. 119.—36. BAUMGARTEN. *D. sogen. Organisation d. Thrombus.* Leipz. 1877.—37. BEUGNIER-CORBEAU. *Gaz. méd. de Liège*, 1890, p. 348.—38. BIRCH-HIRSCHFELD. *Congr. inn. Med.* 1892, p. 28.—39. BRODIE and RUSSELL. *Journal of Physiol.* 1897, Nos. 4-5.—40. BRÜCKE. *Brit. and For. Med.-Chir. Rev.* 1857, xix. p. 183.—41. COHNHEIM. *Vorles. üb. allg. Path.* Bd. i. Berl. 1882.—42. CRUVEILHIER. *Anat. path.* Paris, 1829-42.—43. DAVY, JOHN. *Researches, Physiological and Ana-tomical.* London, 1839.—44. DENYS. *Centralbl. f. allg. Path. u. path. Anat.* 1893, iv. p. 174.—45. EGUET. *Mitth. a. Klin. u. med. Inst. d. Schweiz*, 1894, ii. Hft. 4.— 46. VAN EMDEN. *Fortschr. d. Med.* 1898, xvi. pp. 241 and 281.—47. EHRLICH and LAZARUS. *Die Anämie*, 1. Abth. Wien, 1898.—48. FLEXNER. *Journ. Exp. Med.* 1896, i. p. 559.—49. FREUND. *Wien. med. Blätter*, 1886, p. 296.—50. *Idem. Wiener med. Jahrb.* 1888, p. 259.—51. GLÉNARD. *Contrib. à l'étude des causes de la coag. spontan. du sang.* Thèse. Paris, 1875.—52. GROTH. *Ueb. d. Schicksale farbloser Blutkörperchen*, etc. Inaug.-Diss. Dorpat, 1884.—53. HALLIBURTON. *Journal of Physiol.* 1893, xiii. p. 806 ; xv. p. 90, and (with PICKERING) xviii. p. 285.—54. HAYEM. *Du sang et de ses altérations anatomiques.* Paris, 1889.—55. HAYEM. *Wien. med. Zeit.* 1897, Nos. 17-19.—56. HUNTER, JOHN. "Obs. on the Inflam. of the Intern. Coat of Veins," *Trans. Soc. Improvement Med. and Chir. Knowledge*, 1793, i. p. 18.—57. KÖHLER. *Ueb. Throm-bose u. Transfusion.* Inaug.-Diss. Dorpat, 1877.—58. LAENNEC. *De l'auscult. médiate*, etc. Paris, 1819.—59. LANDOIS. *Die Transfusion d. Blutes.* Leipz. 1875.—60. VON LIMBECK. *Prag. med. Woch.* 1890, xv. pp. 351, 365.—61. MALLORY. *Journ. of Exp. Medicine*, 1898, iii. p. 611.—62. MARAGLIANO and CASTELLINO. *Ztschr. f. kl. Med.* 1892, xxi. p. 415.—63. MARTIN, C. J. *Journal of Physiology*, 1893, xv. p. 380.— 64. MUIR. *Journal of Anatomy and Physiology*, 1890-91, xxv.—65. NAUNYN. *Arch. f. exp. Path. u. Pharm.* 1873, i. p. 1.—66. PAGET. *St. Barth. Hosp. Rep.* 1866, ii. p. 82.— 67. PONFICK. *Deutsche Klinik*, 1867, Nos. 20-26.—68. *Idem. Virch. Arch.* 1874, lx. p. 153.—69. *Idem. Virch. Arch.* 1875, lxii. p. 273.—70. RANKE. *D. Blutvertheilung u. d. Thätigkeitswechsel d. Organe.* Leipz. 1891.—71. SAHLI. *Centralbl. f. inn. Med.* 1894, p. 497.—72. SCHIMMELBUSCH. *Ueb. Thrombose im gerinnungsunfähigen Blute.* Inaug.-Diss. Halle, 1886.—73. SILBERMANN. *Virch. Arch.* 1889, cxvii. p. 288.— 74. SINGER. *Arch. f. Gynäk.* lvi. p. 218.—75. TURK. *Klin. Untersuch. üb. d. Verhalten d. Blutes bei Infectionskrankh.* Wien, 1898.—76. VAQUEZ. *De la thrombose cachectique.* Thèse. Paris, 1890.—77. *Idem.* "De la phlébite," in *Clin. méd. de la Charité*, Paris, 1894, p. 751.—78. WEIGERT. *Fortschr. d. Med.* 1887, v. p. 231.—79. WIDAL. *Étude sur l'infection puerpérale.* Thèse. Paris, 1889.—80. WOOLDRIDGE. *On the Chemistry of the Blood and other Scientific Papers.* Arranged by Victor Horsley and Ernest Starling. Lond. 1893.
Localisation.—81. ARNOLD. *Ziegler's Beitr.* 1890, viii. p. 29.—82. BENIVIENI. *De abditis nonnullis ac mirandis morborum et sanationum causis.* Florent. 1507.—83. BIRCH-HIRSCHFELD. *Deutsch. med. Woch.* 1892, p. 267.—84. BOSTROEM. *Deutsch. Arch. f. kl. Med.* 1895, lv. p. 219.—85. BURNS, ALLAN. *Obs. on some of the most frequent and important Diseases of the Heart.* Edinb. 1809.—86. ZUM BUSCH. *Ueb. d. Zusammensetzung d. Herzthromben.* Inaug.-Diss. Freiburg, i. B. 1891.—87. VAN DER BYL. *Tr. Path. Soc. Lond.* 1858, ix. p. 98.—88. CHOISY and NUHN, cited from No. 93.—89. CZAPEK. *Prager med. Woch.* 1891, xvi. p. 458.—90. DELÉPINE. *Tr. Path. Soc. Lond.* 1890, xli. p. 43.—91. EWART and ROLLESTON. *Tr. Clin. Soc. Lond.* 1897, xxx. p. 190.—92. HAGA. *Virch. Arch.* 1898, clii. p. 26.—93. HERTZ. *Deutsch. Arch. f. kl. Med.* 1885, xxxvii. p. 74.—94. HOEGERSTEDT and NEMSER. *Ztschr. f. kl. Med.* 1896, xxxi. p. 130.—95. HUTCHINSON, JONATHAN. *Arch. of Surg.* Apr. 1898, p. 100.—96. KRUMBHOLZ. *Arb. a. d. med. Klinik zu Leipzig*, 1893, p. 328.—97. KRUMM. *Deutsch. Arch. f. kl. Med.* 1895, liv. p. 189.—98. LANCEREAUX. *Traité*

d'anat. path. t. i. p. 604. Paris, 1875-77.—99. KOTLAR. Prag. med. Woch. 1894, xix. pp. 78 and 97.—100. LEGG, WICKHAM. Tr. Path. Soc. Lond. 1878, xxix. p. 49. —101. MACLEOD. Edinb. Med. Journ. Feb. 1883, p. 696.—102. MANTEUFFEL, ZOEGE. VON. Deutsch. Ztschr. f. Chir. 1898, xlvii. p. 461.—103. OGLE. Tr. Path. Soc. Lond. 1863, xiv. p. 127.—104. OSLER. Johns Hopkins Hosp. Rep. 1890, ii. p. 56.—105. Idem. Montreal Med. Journ. 1897, xxv. p. 729.—106. PARMENTIER. Arch. gén. de méd. July 1889.—107. PAWLOWSKI. Ztschr. f. kl. Med. 1894, xxvi. p. 482.—108. VON RECKLING-HAUSEN, No. 19, and Deutsch. Arch. f. kl. Med. 1885, xxxvii. p. 495.—109. REDTEN-BACHER. Wien. kl. Woch. 1892, v. p. 688.—110. ROSENBACH. Die Krankh. d. Herzens, Hft. i. p. 180. Wien u. Leipz. 1893.—111. STANGE. Arb. a. d. path. Inst. z. Göttingen, 1893, p. 232.—112. VOELCKER. Tr. Path. Soc. Lond. 1893, xliv. p. 31.—113. WAGNER. Arch. d. Heilk. 1861, ii. p. 364.—114. WEICHSELBAUM, cited from No. 83.—115. WERTHEIMER. Arch. de physiol. 1895, 5. S. vii. p. 107.—116. VON WINIWARTER. Arch. f. kl. Chir. 1878, xxiii.—117. WOOD, WILLIAM. The Edinburgh Med. and Surg. Journ. 1814, x. p. 50.—118. ZAHN. Virch. Arch. 1889, cxv. p. 55.—119. V. ZIEMSSEN. Congr. f. inn. Med. 1890, p. 281.

Association with Certain Diseases.—Enteric Fever.—120. BOINET and ROMARY. Arch. d. méd. exp. 1897, ix. p. 902.—121. CARBONE. Gaz. med. di Torino, 1891, No. 23.—122. CROCQ. Arch. d. méd. exp. 1894, vi. p. 583.—123. GILBERT and LION. Bull. méd. 1889, p. 1266.—124. GIRODE. Bull. méd. 1889, p. 1392.—125. HAUS-HALTER. Mercredi méd. Sept. 20, 1893. — 126. HÖLSCHER. Münch. med. Woch. 1891, pp. 43, 62.—127. KEEN. Surgical Complications and Sequels of Typhoid Fever. Philadelpha, 1898 (consult for other references to Arterial Thrombosis in Enteric Fever).—128. RATTONE. Morgagni, 1887, xxix. p. 577.—129. VINCENT. Mercredi méd. Feb. 17, 1892.—130. VITI. Atti d. r. Accad. d. fisiocrit. di Siena, 1890, 4. S. ii. p. 109.

Influenza.—131. BÄUMLER. Congr. f. inn. Med. 1890, p. 305.—132. CHAUDET. La phlébite grippale. Paris, 1892.—133. CHIARI. Prager med. Woch. 1890, p. 124.— 134. GUTTMANN and LEYDEN. Die Influenza-Epidemie, 1889-90. Wiesbaden, 1892.— 135. KLEBS. Deutsch. med. Woch. 1890, p. 278.—136. KUSKOW. Virch. Arch. cxxxix. p. 406.—137. LASKER. Inaug.- Diss. Freiburg, 1897.—138. LEICHTENSTERN, in Nothnagel's Spec. Path. u. Therap. Bd. iv. Th. ii. Abth. i. Wien, 1896.—139. LEYDEN. Charité-Annalen, xvii. and xviii.—140. RENDU. Bull. méd. 1892, pp. 50, 296.

Pneumonia.—141. BARBANCEYS. Études sur la coag. d. sang dans les veines. Thèse. Paris, 1870.—142. BLAGDEN. St. Barth. Hosp. Journ. 1897-98, v. p. 122.—143. DA COSTA. Philadelphia Med. Journ. 1898, ii. p. 519.—144. DICKINSON, LEE. Brit. Med. Journ. 1896, i. p. 149. — 145. FABRIÈS. Sem. méd. 1888, p. 144.—146. LAACHE. Deutsch. med. Woch. 1893, p. 785.—147. LEYDEN. Centralbl. f. in. Med. 1837, p. 25.—148. OSLER. The Principles and Practice of Medicine, p. 124. New York, 1898.—149. Traité de médecine, t. v. pp. 374, 432 (for other references to arterial and venous thrombosis in pneumonia).

Acute Articular Rheumatism. — 150. GATAY. Contrib. à l'étude de la phlébite rhumatismale. Thèse. Paris, 1895.—151. LEGROUX. Gaz. hebd. de méd. 1884, p. 140.—152. SCHMITT. De la phlebite rhumatismale. Thèse. Paris, 1884.

Appendicitis.—153. MYNTER. Appendicitis and its Surgical Treatment, Philadelphia, 1897.

Tuberculosis.—154. BLUMER. Amer. Journ. Med. Sc. 1898, ii.—155. DODWELL. Amer. Journ. Med. Sc. 1893, i. p. 641.—156. FLEXNER. Johns Hopkins Hosp. Bull. 1891, p. 120.—157. HEKTOEN. Journ. Exp. Med. 1896, p. 112.—158. HIRTZ. Mer-credi méd. 1894, No. 40.—159. MICHAELIS and BLUM. Deutsche med. Woch. 1898, p. 550.—160. STROEBE. Centralbl. f. allg. Path. u. path. Anat. 1897, p. 998.—161. SABRAZES and MONGOUR. Rev. méd. de l'est, 1897, p. 306.

Cachectic States.—162. CHARCOT. Union méd. 1865, xxvi. p. 165.—163. GOUGET. Bull. de la soc. anat. 1894, No. 13.—164. PITRES, BITOT, and REGNIER, cited from No. 77.—165. VON RECKLINGHAUSEN, No. 19.—166. RIGOLLET. De la phlebite paludéene. Thèse. Bordeaux, 1891.

Cardiac Incompetency.—167. BALDWIN, HELEN. Journ. Am. Med. Assoc. 1897, August 21, p. 371.—168. COHN. Klinik d. embol. Gefässkrankh. Berlin, 1860.—169. CHEADLE and LEES. Lancet, 1898, ii. p. 206 (reported by Poynton).—170. HIRSCHLAFF. Inaug.-Diss. Berlin, 1893.—171. HUCHARD. Rev. gén. de clin. et de thérap. 1897, xi. p. 787.—172. KAHN (and HANOT). Arch. gén. de méd. 1896, ii. p. 469.—173. MADER. Jahrb. d. Wien. k.-k. Krankenanst, 1895, 1897, iv. p. 252.—174. NICOLLE.

Normandie méd. 1897, xii. p. 68.—175. ORMEROD. *Tr. Path. Soc. Lond.* 1889, xl. p. 75.—176. RAMIREZ. *Gaz. méd. de Paris*, 1867, No. 47, p. 716.—177. ROBERT. *Bull. de la soc. anat.* 1880, v. p. 314.
Chlorosis.—178. BALL. *Trans. Assoc. Amer. Physicians*, 1889, iv. p. 52.—179. VON NOORDEN, in Nothnagel's *Spec. Path. u. Therap.* Bd. viii. Th. ii. Wien, 1897.— 180. SCHWEITZER. *Virchow's Arch.* 1898, clii. p. 337. (The three preceding articles contain the principal references to chlorotic thrombosis. The following Nos. 181 to 192 are the references to cases not found in them.)—181. AUDRY. *Lyon méd.* 1892 and 1893.—182. DICKINSON, LEE. *Tr. Clin. Soc. Lond.* 1896, xxix. p. 63.—183. DUCKWORTH and BUZZARD. *Brit. Med. Journ.* 1896, i. p. 149.—184. GAGNONI. *Riforma med.* 1897, xiii. p. 472.—185. GUINON. *Bull. et mém. soc. méd. des hôp. de Paris*, 1896, xii. p. 297.—186. GUTHEIL. Inaug.-Diss. Freiburg, 1892.—187. HAYEM. *Bull. méd.* 1896, p. 261.—188. POWELL, DOUGLAS. *Lancet*, 1888, ii. p. 1124.—189. Dr. THAYER's case was of a chlorotic young woman with thrombosis of left femoral, iliac and uterine veins. Death from pulmonary embolism.—190. VAQUEZ. No. 77.—191. VERGELY. *Bull. méd.* 1889, p. 1175.—192. VILLARD. *Assoc. franç. pour l'avancement des sciences*, 1891, ii. p. 791. Paris, 1892.—193. BUTTERSACK. *Ztschr. f. kl. Med.* 1897, xxxiii. p. 456.—193a. SANKEY, W. *Ed. Med. and S. Journ.* 1814, p. 401.
Gouty, Idiopathic and Primary Infective Thrombosis.—194. BARBE. *La France méd.* 1898. (Syphilis.)—194a. DAGUILLON. *Contrib. à l'étude clin. de la phlébite primitive.* Thèse. Paris, 1894.—195. DOWSE. *Lancet*, 1879, ii. p. 268.—196. OSLER. *Trans. Assoc. Amer. Physicians*, 1887, ii. p. 135.—197. PAGET. No. 66.—198. TUCKWELL. *St. Barth. Hosp. Rep.* 1874, x. p. 23.

Effects and Symptoms.—*Cardiac, Arterial, and Capillary Thrombosis.*—199. BARTH. *Deutsch. med. Woch.* 1896, p. 269.—200. BLACHEZ. *Gaz. des hôp.* 1866, No. 13. —201. BRISTOWE. *Tr. Path. Soc. Lond.* 1870, xxi. p. 143.—202. CHARCOT. *Compt. rend. soc. de biol.* 1858, Paris, 1859, 2. S. v. pt. 2, p. 225.—203. CHIARI. *Prager med. Woch.* 1897, Nos. 6, 7.—204. GERHARDT. *Würzburg. med. Ztschr.* Bd. iv. and v. —205. HEIDENHAIN. *Deutsch. med. Woch.* 1891, p. 1087.—206. KIDD, PERCY. *Tr. Path. Soc. Lond.* 1886, xxxvii. p. 197.—207. MARIE, R. *L'infarctus du myocarde et ses conséquences.* Paris, 1897.—208. NAUNYN, in Nothnagel's *Spec. Path. u. Ther.* Bd. vii. Th. vi. p. 216. Wien, 1898.—209. PITT, NEWTON. *Tr. Path. Soc. Lond.* 1893, xliv. p. 52.—210. PORTER. *Journ. Exp. Medicine*, 1896, i. p. 46.—211. WELCH, in *Pepper's System of Medicine*, ii. p. 505.—212. VON ZIEMSSEN. No. 119.

Venous Thrombosis.—213. COHNHEIM. *Vorles. üb. allg. Path.* Bd. i. pp. 150, 492.— 214. COHNSTEIN, in *Lubarsch-Ostertag's Ergebnisse*, 1896, ii. p. 563. Wiesbaden, 1897 (consult for literature on theories of œdema).—215. GALLIARD. *Méd. moderne*, 1894, v. p. 861.—216. HAMBURGER. *Virch. Arch.* 1895, cxli. p. 398.—217. LAZARUS-BARLOW. *Phil. Trans. Roy. Soc.* vol. clxxxv. B. 1894, p. 779.—218. *Idem. A Manual of General Pathology.* London, 1898.—219. LÖSCHNER. *Prager med. Woch.* 1888, No. 22.—220. SCHLESINGER. *Deutsch. med. Woch.* 1896, p. 460.—221. STARLING. *Lancet*, 1896, i. p. 1407.—222. THOMAS. "Beitr. z. Differ.-Diagnostik zwischen Verschluss d. Pfortaders u. d. unteren Hohlvenen," *Bibliotheca medica*, Cassel, 1895.—223. VIMONT. *Contrib. à l'étude des oblitérations de la veine cave infér.* Thèse. Paris, 1890.—224. WELCH. *Journ. of Exp. Med.* 1896, i. p. 35.—225. KÖSTER. *Deutsch. med. Woch.* 1898, p. 325. (This and the papers cited by K. contain references to 16 cases of thrombosis of mesenteric veins.) The additional cases with symptoms are Nos. 226 to 239.—226. BARTH. *Bull. méd.* 1897, Oct. 27, p. 989.—227. BOUCLY. Thèse. Paris, 1894.—228. BURGESS. *Sheffield Med. Journ.* 1892-93, i. p. 317 (3 cases).—229. DELATOUR. *Annals of Surgery*, 1895, xxv. p. 24.—230. FITZ. *Trans. Ass. Amer. Phys.* 1887, ii. p. 140.—231. GARMSER. Inaug.-Diss. Kiel, 1895.—232. LEECH. *Quart. Med. Journ.* Sheffield, 1897-8, vi. p. 370.—233. LILIENTHAL. *Matthew's Quart. Journ. Rectal*, etc. Louisville, 1898, v. p. 158.—234. LUND. *Hospitalstidende*, Mar. 23, 1898.—235. M'WEENY. *Lancet*, Dec. 23, 1893.—236. NORDENFELDT. *Hygiea*, 1897, lix. pt. 2, p. 228.—237. SMITH. *Dublin Journ. of Med. Sc.* 1894, xcvii. p. 274.—238. WATSON. *Boston Med. and Surg. Journ.* 1894, cxxxi. p. 556.—239. WESTHOFF. Inaug.-Diss. Kiel, 1895. (Cases without symptoms are reported in Nos. 240-243.)—240. COHN. *Embolische Gefässkrankh.*—241. FRERICHS. *Klinik d. Leberkrankh.*—242. ROLLESTON. *Trans. Path. Soc. London*, 1892, xliii. p. 49.—243. SPIEGELBERG. *Virchow's Arch.* cxliii. p. 547.— 244. BALDWIN, HELEN. *J. Amer. Med. Assoc.* 1897, xxix. p. 371.—245. BANTI. *Sperimentale*, 1891, p. 408.—246. BERMANN. *Ueb. Pfortaderverschluss u. Leberschwund.* Inaug.-Diss. 1897.—247. BORRMANN. *Deutsch. Arch. f. kl. Med.* 1897, lix. p. 283.

—248. COHNHEIM and LITTEN. Virch. Arch. 1876, lxvii. p. 153.—249. DUCHEK. Viertl.-Jahrs. f. d. prakt. Heilk. 1854, xli. p. 109.—250. ERLENMEYER. Deutsch. med. Woch. 1890, p. 781.—251. HIRSCHLAFF. Inaug.-Diss. Berlin, 1893.—252. LITTEN, in Nothnagel's Spec. Path. u. Therap. Bd. viii. Th. iii. p. 41.—253. NONNE. Deutsch. Arch. f. kl. Med. 1885, xxxvii. p. 241.—254. OSLER. Johns Hopkins Hosp. Bull. 1891, ii. p. 40.—255. Idem. Journ. Anat. and Physiol. 1878, xxix. p. 107.—256. OULMONT. Soc. méd. d'observ. Paris, 1856, iii. pp. 361, 468.—257. POHL. Inaug.- Diss. Göttingen, 1887.—258. ROLLESTON. Trans. Path. Soc. London, 1892, xliii. p. 49.—259. ROSIN. Verhandl. d. XVI. Congr. f. innere Medicin, 1898, p. 415.—260. SCHÜPPEL, in Ziemssen's Handb. d. spec. Path. u. Therap. Bd. viii. I. 2, p. 279.—261. SCHMALE. Ueber Thrombose d. Pulmonalvenen bei Emphysem. Inaug.-Diss. Würz- burg, 1889.—262. SMITH, A. A. N. Y. Med. Journ. 1880, xxxi. p. 16.—263. SOLO- WIEFF. Virch. Arch. 1875, lxii. p. 195.—264. WEST. Tr. Path. Soc. London, 1878, xxix. p. 107.—265. WYSS, O. Verhandl. d. XVI. Congr. f. innere Medicin, 1898, p. 399.—266. The relations of thrombosis to varix are considered in an interesting paper by Mr. Wm. H. Bennett (Lancet, 1898, ii. p. 973).

W. H. W.

EMBOLISM

Definition.—Embolism is the impaction in some part of the vascular system of any undissolved material brought there by the blood-current The transported material is an embolus. Embolism may occur likewise in lymphatic vessels.

Historical note.—Rudolf Virchow is the creator of the doctrine of embolism. There is scarcely another pathological doctrine, of equal magnitude, the establishment of which is so largely the work of a single man. Not but that there were foreshadowings of this conception before Virchow, notably by Bonetus and van Swieten in the seventeenth and eighteenth centuries, and by Allibert and François in the early part of the present century. A few observers and experimenters, indeed, anti- cipated some of Virchow's results. The wonder is that until Virchow's time the idea of embolism remained so foreign to medical thought; so obvious and necessary a corollary does it seem to be of the discovery of the circulation of the blood. Between the years 1846 and 1856 Virchow constructed the whole doctrine of embolism upon the basis of anatomical, experimental and clinical investigations, which for completeness, accuracy, and just discernment of the truth must always remain a model of scientific research in medicine. These discoveries introduced new chapters and necessitated a recasting of many old ones in pathology. A number of important morbid conditions, among which pulmonary embolism and cerebral embolism may be especially mentioned, were now for the first time clearly recognised. Virchow's studies of thrombosis and his demon- stration that not all intravascular, ante-mortem clots are formed at the place where they are found, and that infarcts are not the result of inflam- mation and capillary phlebitis, put an end to the false and to us at present almost incomprehensible ideas then prevailing as to the overshadowing importance of phlebitis in pathological processes. Especially was the doctrine of metastasis, which in old days was one of the most mystical in medicine, greatly expanded and at the same time placed upon an intelligible and firm foundation.

The new fields opened by Virchow have been industriously cultivated by a multitude of workers. The additions to our knowledge have been many and valuable, but they have related mainly to details, and can scarcely be said to have led to new points of view. The works of Bernhard Cohn and of Cohnheim may be signalised as among the most important of the contributions since Virchow's early publications. Cohn's remarkable book, published in 1860, is extraordinarily rich in anatomical, experimental, and clinical facts, and it is well for any one who believes that he has a new observation or opinion concerning embolism to consult it before venturing on publication; a precaution which has evidently been often neglected by writers on the subject.

Varieties of emboli.—Substances of the most varied character, solid, liquid or gaseous, may enter the circulation and be conveyed as emboli. Unless some special epithet be used, an embolus is generally understood to be a detached thrombus, or part of it, including under this designation endocarditic vegetations. Other possible sorts of emboli are fragments of diseased heart-valves, calcific masses, bits of tissue, tumour-cells, parenchymatous cells, animal or vegetable parasites, fat, air, pigment-granules and foreign bodies. Emboli of air, of fat, and of parenchymatous cells will be considered separately. An important classification, as regards their effects, is into bland or aseptic emboli and toxic or septic emboli.

Sources of emboli —Emboli in the lungs come from the systemic veins, the right heart or the pulmonary artery; those in branches of the portal vein come from the radicles or trunk of this vein; those in systemic arteries from the pulmonary veins, the left heart, or some artery between the heart and the location of the embolus. Sources of aberrant emboli, resulting from unusual modes of transportation, will be considered subsequently (p. 231).

Various features in the structure and disposition of thrombi bearing upon the detachment of emboli have been described in the preceding article. Here may be especially recalled the continuation of an occluding venous thrombus in the form of a partly obstructing thrombus beyond the entrance of an important branch, and the occurrence of softening in the interior of older thrombi; phenomena evidently favourable to the detachment of fragments. Globular thrombi in the right heart, particularly in the auricular appendix, are a fruitful source of the emboli which cause pulmonary infarction in heart disease. Vegetations of the aortic and mitral valves, particularly of the latter, furnish the great majority of emboli in the aortic system. Thrombosis or embolism of an arterial trunk—as of the internal carotid, splenic, femoral—is often followed by the conveyance of fragments of the plug into branches of the artery. When the plug in the main trunk is an embolus, this secondary embolism is described by Cohnheim as "recurrent"—an epithet which · has also been applied to retrograde embolism, and, therefore, to avoid confusion, had better not be used in either sense.

The detection of the source of an embolus is often unattended by any difficulty ; but sometimes it requires prolonged and painstaking search, and occasionally even such a search is unrewarded. The greatest difficulties are encountered when the source is in some peripheral venous thrombus which has caused no symptoms and is unattended by lesions suggestive of its location. An entire thrombus may be dislocated and transported as an embolus.

Site of deposit.—Emboli are carried along by the blood-current until they are caught on some obstruction, or become lodged in a channel too narrow to permit their further passage. It is evident that embolism can scarcely occur except in the arterial system, pulmonary and systemic, and in branches of the portal vein. The rare instances of embolism of systemic veins will be considered under aberrant embolism (p. 231). An extremely rare occurrence, of which several instances are recorded, is the blocking of the tricuspid or mitral orifice by an embolus. The result is, of course, sudden death. Very often an embolus is caught at an arterial bifurcation, which it rides with a prolongation extending into each branch (riding embolus). This may happen where the diameter of each branch is greater than that of the embolus. It is not uncommon for several emboli to enter successively the same branch of the pulmonary artery.

Any artery open to the circulating blood may receive an embolus of appropriate size. The course followed by an embolus in its travels is determined by purely mechanical factors, of which the most important are the size, form, and weight of the plug; the direction, volume, and energy of the carrying blood-stream ; the size of branches and the angles at which they are given off; and the position of the body and its members. In accord with these principles we find emboli in the lower lobes of the lungs oftener than in the upper ; and in the right lung oftener than in the left, the right pulmonary artery being larger than the left. Emboli from the left heart are more frequently carried into the abdominal aorta and its branches than into the carotid or subclavian arteries. The left carotid, arising directly from the aortic arch at its highest point, is in more direct line with the aortic blood-stream than is the right carotid, and is therefore a commoner recipient of emboli. The left common iliac artery is also somewhat more directly in the line of the current in the abdominal aorta, and, therefore, receives emboli somewhat more frequently than the right.

The order of frequency in which emboli are found in the different arteries may be given about as follows :—pulmonary, renal, splenic, cerebral, iliac and the lower extremities, axillary and upper extremities, cœliac axis with its hepatic and gastric branches, central artery of the retina, superior mesenteric, inferior mesenteric, abdominal aorta, coronary of the heart. There is, however, considerable difference of statement on this point. As a matter of fact this list, like similar ones, does not inform us of the frequency with which the different arteries of the body receive emboli ; for it is evident that it is based almost entirely upon embolic manifestations, and not upon the mere presence of emboli. If estimates of frequency be based only on infective emboli, the order would be in several respects different, the hepatic artery, for example, standing higher in the list, and the cerebral lower—sufficient evidence that the customary data for determining the frequency of embolism in different arteries relate only to such emboli as leave behind some record of their presence. Infective emboli, however, do not inform us of the incidence of embolism in different arteries; for these produce abscesses or other lesions in certain special situations, and not in every place where they may lodge; a fact which is brought out clearly in the experimental injections of bacteria into the circulation of animals. It seems to me very probable that, of the systemic arteries, those going to the lower extremities must be more frequent receptacles of emboli than either the splenic or the renal; but the smaller plugs in the former usually leave no readily demonstrable record of their presence, whereas in the latter they always do.

Aberrant embolism.—Certain exceptions to the general rules already stated concerning the sources and direction of transportation of emboli may be grouped under the heading of aberrant or atypical embolism, the latter epithet being the one employed by Scheven to designate paradoxical embolism, and retrograde embolism.

Zahn gave the name "paradoxical embolism," and his assistant Rostan the name "crossed embolism," to the transportation of emboli derived from veins into the systemic arteries without passing through the pulmonary circulation. Cohnheim was the first to note the passage of venous emboli through an open foramen ovale into the aortic system; and since then there have been enough observations of this so-called paradoxical embolism to prove that, although not frequent, it is really of practical importance, and not merely a curiosity. Zahn and Rostan found an open foramen ovale in about one-fifth of their autopsies, which is a considerably smaller percentage than most pathologists, who have investigated the subject, have found. An opening in the form of an oblique slit is certainly very often present in the oval fossa (in 34 per cent of all cases according to Firket), and it has been demonstrated by actual observation that, under certain conditions, this form of opening suffices for the transit of emboli. In three cases an embolus was found by Zahn and Rostan actually engaged in the opening, and two or three similar observations have been made by others.

I have found records of twenty-eight cases of paradoxical embolism, and there is no reason to suppose that this list is complete. The evidence upon which the diagnosis is usually based is an open foramen ovale and the presence in the systemic arteries of coarse emboli, for which the only source to be found is on the venous side or in the right auricle. While in some of the cases there may be room for scepticism as to the venous origin of the arterial embolism, there can be none for Schmorl's observation, in a case of traumatic laceration of the liver, of plugs of hepatic tissue in the left auricle and the main trunk of the renal artery, with an open foramen ovale admitting a finger. Conditions favouring the occurrence of paradoxical embolism are, according to Zahn, increased pressure in the right auricle and lowered pressure in the left. Under these circumstances the opening in the oval foramen is widened, and its walls bulge toward the left auricle. Rostan and Hauser have seen thrombi extending from the right auricle through the oval foramen into the left.

The best explanation of certain tumour metastases without pulmonary implication is by paradoxical embolism. Here, however, there is sometimes another possibility; for, as Zahn has demonstrated, tumour cells not of large size may pass through the pulmonary capillaries. Although the lungs are an excellent filter, their capillaries are certainly so wide that they may permit the transit of emboli too large to pass through capillaries elsewhere in the body.

The first conclusive observation of retrograde transport of an embolus in a human being was made by Heller, in 1870, who found, in a case of primary cancer of the cæcum and ileum, a loose plug of cancerous tissue in a branch of an hepatic vein. The only metastatic growths were in the mesenteric, retroperitoneal, and mediastinal lymphatic glands. Long before Heller, however, the conception of retrograde transport of venous emboli was familiar to pathologists ; especially in the discussions of the explanation of metastatic hepatic abscesses in cases where the lungs are not involved and the atrium of infection does not communicate with the portal system. The experimental side of the subject was diligently cultivated. The general trend of opinion among pathologists, however, was opposed to the acceptance of the doctrine of retrograde transport, under conditions occurring in human beings, until the publication of von Recklinghausen's article on the subject in 1885. He reported a convincing observation of embolism of the renal veins with masses of sarcoma, derived from a primary growth of the tibia, and also of retrograde embolism from the left auricle into the pulmonary veins. Since this publication there have been a number of equally conclusive demonstrations of the retrograde transport of venous emboli, and the subject has been taken up again on the experimental side. Retrograde venous embolism is an interesting, but, so far as at present known, a rare occurrence.

The difficulty of making sure that a suspected thrombotic embolus in a systemic vein is not an autochthonous thrombus is doubtless the reason why most of the reports of retrograde transport relate to emboli of tumour-cells or parenchymatous cells. In addition to Heller's and von Recklinghausen's cases already mentioned, reference may be made to Arnold's observation of masses from a primary mammary carcinoma filling the superior longitudinal sinus, with invasion of the wall of the sinus from within by the new growth, but without any intracranial tumour outside of this wall ; or indeed any metastasis elsewhere in the body except in the axillary and cervical lymph-glands : and also to Ernst's case of primary angio-sarcoma of the left kidney, growing into the renal vein, with a loose plug of sarcomatous tissue distending a branch of a coronary vein of the heart without connection with a metastatic growth. Bonome's observation of cancer of the thyroid with metastatic nodules in the liver, developing from plugs in the hepatic veins, should probably also be included in the list, as well as two cases of Bonome, reported by Lui, in one of which a cancerous embolus secondary to cancer of the rectum was found in a branch of the superior mesenteric vein; and in the other a similar retrograde embolus, secondary to adeno-carcinoma of the liver, was met with in the right pampiniform plexus.

To Schmorl's and Lubarsch's cases of emboli of liver-cells in the cerebral and the renal veins may be added two observations from my laboratory, of which one has been reported by Flexner, of clumps of liver-cells in branches of the renal vein in cases with extensive hepatic necroses.

That retrograde transport of ordinary venous thrombi may occur, is demonstrated by Arnold's discovery in a large branch of an hepatic vein of a riding embolus identical in appearance with a thrombus which occupied the right ovarian vein and extended some distance into the inferior vena cava. Cohn accepted, for a limited class of cases, backward conveyance of venous emboli; and in this sense interprets an observation of thrombosis of the superior longitudinal sinus, with a plug in the right axillary vein identical in appearance with an undoubted embolus in the pulmonary artery. Von Recklinghausen has furnished evidence of the retrograde transport of infective emboli into the renal veins.

From these cases it is seen that retrograde embolism of particles of tumour, of tumour-cells, of parenchymatous cells, and of ordinary bland and infective thrombotic fragments has been observed. Experiments have demonstrated that, under certain conditions, light as well as heavy particles may be transported in the veins in a direction contrary to that of the normal blood-current. The veins in which retrograde embolism in human beings has been found are the hepatic, the renal, the mesenteric, the pampiniform plexus, the coronary of the heart, the cerebral veins and sinuses, the axillary and the pulmonary. Experimental retrograde embolism has been produced in many other veins, including those of the lower extremities. While venous valves, when intact, are undoubtedly a protection against this occurrence, they are often imperfectly developed or insufficient. Emboli have been repeatedly observed in the cerebral veins and sinuses which should be protected by valves in the jugular veins.

Retrograde embolism is usually explained by a temporary reflux of the venous current in consequence of some sudden obstacle to the return flow to the right heart, as may occur with forced expiration and coughing. Whatever increases the pressure in the veins near the heart, and impairs the assistance to the venous stream afforded by the respiratory movements and the suction of the right heart, favours this backward movement. Increased intrathoracic pressure, stenosis of the respiratory passages, spasm of respiratory muscles, distension of the right heart, tricuspid insufficiency, slowing of the heart's beats from vagus-irritation, are among the conditions believed to dispose to retrograde transport.

Ribbert does not accept the reflux theory of retrograde embolism; partly for lack of any positive observation of such backward flow beyond the immediate neighbourhood of the right heart, and partly on account of the difficulty in explaining what becomes of all the blood which would be momentarily pressed back toward the capillaries.

His explanation is that in conditions of high venous stasis, emboli, sticking loosely to the venous wall, are not moved forward by the feeble current, but are slowly pressed backward, step by step, by pulse-waves in the veins. For this view he finds support in experiments which he has made. Observations, partly experimental, of Arnold and of Ernst, cannot readily be reconciled with Ribbert's explanation; so that, notwithstanding difficulties needing further elucidation, the reflux theory seems at present the more probable for most cases.

Of a different nature from the preceding form of retrograde transport is the conveyance of emboli by a blood-current reversed from its normal direction in consequence of obstruction of veins by compression or other causes. This kind of retrograde transport from more or less permanent reversal of the normal current is far more frequent in lymphatic vessels than in veins, and plays an important part in the metastases of tumours by means of the lymphatics.

Anatomical characters.—The appearances observed in embolised vessels vary with the shape, size, consistence, and nature of the embolus, and the duration of its impaction. Approximately spherical emboli, as a rule, completely close the lumen of the artery in which they lodge. Cylindrical, elongated, or flat emboli are usually caught as riders at an arterial bifurcation; and often at first leave more or less of the channels by their side open. Thrombi several inches long may be washed out of the femoral or other peripheral vein. Such a transported thrombus may be found in the trunk or a primary division of the pulmonary artery, folded two, three, or even four times upon itself, and pressed at different points into several of the main arterial branches at the hilum of the lung, as in an interesting case described by Fagge. In this way an embolus may completely plug a vessel three or four times its diameter. Irregularly-shaped emboli, if of soft consistence, may be pressed into an artery so as to block the lumen completely; but if of firmer consistence they leave at first some space for the blood to flow. Emboli may be of such consistence as to be shattered by impact with the arterial wall, the fragments blocking many or all of the small branches, and producing the same effect as if the plug had been arrested in the main trunk.

An embolus is the starting-point of a secondary thrombus which usually, although not always, completes the closure of the vessel, if this was not effected by the embolus itself, and extends on each side to the nearest branch. The same metamorphoses and process of organisation, with consecutive changes in the vascular wall, occur with emboli and encapsulating thrombi, as described in the previous article for primary thrombi. Non-absorbable emboli or parts of emboli, like foreign bodies, are encapsulated by cells and tissue.

In cases of recent embolism, the plug can generally be recognised as an embolus without much difficulty; but, in those of long standing, the anatomical diagnosis between embolism and thrombosis may be difficult, or even impossible. The criteria for the recognition of a fresh embolus are for the most part sufficiently self-evident. Such a plug lies loosely or is but slightly adherent to the vessel-wall. It often presents a broken or fractured surface which, in fortunate cases, may be made to fit on the corresponding surface of the thrombus from which it was originally broken off. It may be bent or folded, or show the marks of venous valves, or present ramifications which do not correspond to those of the artery in which it lies. It is of course of the first importance to find, if possible, the source of the embolus; and, when this is done, to make a careful comparison between the thrombus and the embolic fragment as to resemblances in structure and appearance.

After the embolus has become adherent and surrounded by a secondary thrombus, some of these differential criteria may still remain for a while; but, as time passes, the anatomical diagnosis becomes increasingly difficult. The embolus may perhaps still be distinguished from the surrounding thrombus by marked differences in its age and general appearance and structure, possibly by the presence of lime salts. An adherent plug which rides an arterial bifurcation is much more likely to be an embolus than a primary thrombus. In reaching a conclusion, weight must be given to the condition of the arterial wall; whether there be any local cause for thrombosis,—such as compression, aneurysm, arterio-sclerosis; and whether the microscope shows such secondary changes in the arterial wall as generally correspond to the apparent age and character of the adherent plug. The detection of a source for an embolus will be an important consideration. The clinical history may aid in the anatomical diagnosis; and all attendant circumstances, especially the existence elsewhere of undoubted emboli, should be taken into consideration. In some situations, as in branches of the renal or splenic arteries, primary thrombosis is so uncommon that the chances are all in favour of embolism.

It is evident from what has been said that in the older cases the anatomical diagnosis must often be based upon a weighing of probabilities, and that sometimes a positive conclusion cannot be reached.

Effects.—Bland or aseptic emboli produce chiefly mechanical effects referable to the obstruction to the circulation; toxic or septic emboli cause also other changes which may be described as chemical or infective. We shall consider first the mechanical effects.

The direct injury which may be inflicted upon the vessel wall by sharp calcareous emboli is, according to Ponfick, a rare cause of aneurysm. Embolic aneurysms, however, stand in much more definite relation to chemical properties of the embolus, as will be shown subsequently (p. 251).

Necrosis; Infarction.—The fate of a part supplied by an artery closed by a bland embolus depends altogether upon whether it is fed within a certain time after the obstruction with enough arterial blood to preserve its function and integrity. An embolus which does not completely plug the vessel may cause no appreciable interference with the circulation; but the closure of the lumen is usually soon effected by a secondary thrombus. The occlusion by a bland embolus of an artery with abundant anastomoses, such as those possessed by the arteries supplying bone, the voluntary muscles, the skin, the thyroid, the uterus, usually causes no circulatory disturbance of any consequence. Even in these situations extensive multiple embolism, or embolism with extensive secondary thrombosis, may cause local anæmia with its consequences.

Sudden death may be the result of embolism of the trunk or a main division of the pulmonary artery, of one of the coronary arteries of the heart, or of the bulbar arteries.

If an adequate collateral circulation be not established within the proper time the inevitable fate of a part, supplied by an embolised artery, is degeneration or death. Local death is the regular result of embolism of branches of the splenic artery, the renal artery, the basal arteries of the brain, the central artery of the retina, and the main trunk of the superior mesenteric artery. It is the usual result of embolism of one of the coronary arteries of the heart, if the patient survive long enough ; and it is the inconstant result, depending generally upon accessory circumstances, of embolism of the medium-sized and smaller branches of the pulmonary arteries, of cerebral arteries other than the basal, of the abdominal aorta, iliacs, main arteries of the extremities, and some other arteries. A collateral circulation may be established sufficiently to preserve the life of a part, but not to maintain its full nutrition ; under these circumstances it undergoes fatty degeneration or simple atrophy.

When the dead part is so surrounded with living tissue that it can be permeated with lymph, as is usually the case in the viscera, the mode of death is that described by Weigert, and named by Cohnheim " coagulative necrosis." Here the dead protoplasm, and to some extent intercellular substances, undergo chemical changes, believed to be in part coagulative ; and actual fibrillated fibrin may appear. If there be enough coagulable material present, the necrotic part becomes hard, dry, opaque, and somewhat swollen. For a time its general architecture, both gross and microscopic, is preserved ; but the nuclei and specific granulations disappear early, the former largely by karyorrhexis.

An area of coagulative necrosis resulting from shutting off of the blood-supply is an infarct. Its shape corresponds to that of the arterial tree supplying it, and is, therefore, as a rule, approximately conical, or that of a wedge, the base being toward the periphery of the organ. The wedge-shape is most marked in smaller infarcts ; large ones may be roundish or irregular in shape. The size depends upon that of the occluded artery. The colour is opaque, white, or yellowish, unless hæmorrhage is added to the necrosis. We thus distinguish anæmic, pale or white infarcts, and red or hæmorrhagic infarcts ; but, in the latter no less than in the former, the essential thing is the coagulative necrosis, the hæmorrhage being merely something added to the necrosis. This was not always clearly recognised, it being supposed at one time that the hæmorrhage was the characteristic feature of infarcts, and that pale infarcts were simply decolourised hæmorrhagic infarcts. The name "infarct" (from *infarcire*, to stuff), like many other old medical terms, is therefore now used in a sense at variance with its etymological meaning. In some situations, as the kidney and the retina, the infarct is nearly always pale ; in others, as the lungs and the intestine, it is as constantly hæmorrhagic ; and in yet others, as the spleen and the heart, it may be either white or red.

Where there is not a sufficient quantity of coagulable substance the area of coagulative necrosis does not become hard ; and it may be of much softer consistence than normal, as is the case with the ischæmic necroses of the brain and spinal cord. Necrosis of peripheral parts, as the toes, foot, leg, hand, is not of the coagulative variety ; for the dead part is not surrounded by living tissue to furnish the lymph which brings one of the factors essential for coagulation. This peripheral necrosis is called gangrene or mortification, and may be either dry or moist.

Collateral circulation ; local anæmia.—As the state of the collateral circulation is the decisive factor in bland embolism, it becomes important to learn the conditions under which establishment or failure of this circulation occurs. This subject is one eminently open to experimental study ; but more attention has been given to the anatomical than to the physiological side. In fact many writers seem to assume that the physiological factors can be so readily deduced from the laws of hydro-dynamics that it is only necessary to investigate the size, arrangement, and distribution of the vascular tubes. Nevertheless experience has shown abundantly the danger of accepting anything in the physics of the circulation which has not been put to an experimental test on the living body. The experimental study of the physiological conditions which determine the development of a collateral circulation has demonstrated that this problem is by no means so simple as has been often represented ; while some old errors have been corrected and new facts have been added, we are still far from an entirely satisfactory solution or any definite agreement of opinion. It is impossible here to do more than touch upon certain points bearing directly upon the subject in hand.

If an artery with slender anastomoses to its area of distribution, such as the femoral or the lingual in a frog's tongue, be tied, the immediate effect is stoppage of the circulation and anæmia of the part supplied by the occluded vessel, accompanied by contraction of the artery below the obstruction. Almost immediately, or within a short time, the blood begins to flow with greatly increased velocity through arteries arising above the point of ligation, but more rapidly only through those which send blood by anastomosing channels to the anæmic part. At the same time these arteries with quickened flow dilate. Formerly this vascular dilatation and increased flow were attributed to rise of blood-pressure above the ligature, but experiments have shown that in most situations this is a factor of relatively little moment. The rise of pressure cannot of course remain localised, and after ligation of the femoral artery amounts at most to only a few millimetres of mercury. Evidence of the relatively slight importance of this increased pressure is that the ligated artery actually contracts from the point of ligation to the first branch arising above the ligature (Thoma, Goldenblum); and that the phenomena of dilatation and increased velocity occur only in arteries which send blood to the anæmic area, although others which carry blood elsewhere may arise nearer to the point of obstruction (Nothnagel). Moreover, it is hardly conceivable that increased pressure above the ligature can persist for the days and weeks which may be necessary for the full development of the collateral circulation.

As the increased flow cannot be due to any change in the viscosity of the blood, it must be due to increase of the pressure gradient. Therefore, if it is not the result in any marked degree of rise of pressure above the obstruction, it must be caused by lowered resistance to the stream in the anastomosing vessels. A moment's reflection will show that this is a far more purposeful and better mode of compensation than one brought about exclusively by a rise of pressure which must act upon arteries in no way concerned in the collateral circulation. The difficulty is an entirely satisfactory and complete explanation of the lowered resistance. It seems impossible that it can be due to anything but a widening of the bed of the stream. Von Recklinghausen has pointed out that the stream-bed for the anastomosing arteries is enlarged, inasmuch as after occlusion of the main artery the blood can flow from these collaterals not only in its original bed, but also, with diminished resistance, into the stream-bed belonging to the closed artery. The pressure gradient is thus increased, and consequently the velocity of the current is quickened in the anastomosing arteries. The cause of the dilatation of these arteries is not so clear. Thoma states as his first histo-mechanical principle that increased velocity of the blood-current leads to widening of the lumen, and eventually, if the increase continues, to growth of the vessel wall in superficies. Admitting this to be true, it can hardly be considered an explanation. As the collateral circulation develops perfectly, and with the same phenomena, after severance of all connection of the part with the central nervous system, it is evident that vaso-motor influences which are under central control are not essential to the process.

Satisfactory as von Recklinghausen's explanation is, as far as it goes, there is evidence that it does not cover all of the facts, and that there is also some mechanism by which the vessels of an ischæmic part are opened wide for the reception of the needed arterial blood. The existence of such a mechanism has been recognised by Lister, Cohnheim, Bier, and others. I must refer especially to the recent papers of Bier for a full presentation of the evidence on this point, and shall merely mention, as a familiar illustration, the extreme arterial hyperæmia which follows the removal of an Esmarch bandage. This flushing of a previously ischæmic part with arterial blood has been usually attributed to paralysis of vaso-constrictor or stimulation of vaso-dilator nerves, but Bier has shown that it occurs under conditions where this explanation can be probably excluded.

Without following Bier in his somewhat vitalistic conceptions, or speculating regarding the explanation of the phenomenon, we must, I think, admit that deprivation of arterial blood sets up some condition of a part whereby the vessels which feed it are in some way dilated to receive any fresh arterial blood which can reach them. The existence of such an admirably adaptive, self-regulatory capacity must be an important element in the development of a collateral circulation, and it may be remarked that it is a physiological rather than an anatomical factor. Bier believes that this capacity is very unequally developed in different parts of the body; being highest in external parts, and feeble or absent in most of the viscera. He is also of the opinion that the arterioles and capillaries of external parts have the power, by independent contractions, of driving blood into the veins; and that, by contraction of the small veins, the capillaries of these parts are in large measure protected from the reception of venous blood.

A possible, but I think not fully demonstrated, variation in the power to lower the resistance to the collateral stream of arterial blood is not, however, the only physiological property which influences the varying effects following obstruction to the arterial supply of different parts of the body. In some situations there are physiological arrangements which seem calculated to increase the difficulty of establishing an adequate collateral circulation. Mall has shown that contraction of the intestine exerts a marked influence upon the circulation through this organ. In the light of his results, it is interesting to note that, immediately after closure of the main trunk of the superior mesenteric artery of a dog, the intestine is thrown into violent tonic contractions and remains in an anæmic, contracted condition for two or three hours; after which the spasm relaxes and the bloodless condition at once gives place to venous hyperæmia and hæmorrhagic infarction, which appears in the third to sixth hour after the occlusion of the artery (Mall and Welch). This intestinal contraction, which under these circumstances is equivalent to arterial spasm, is probably one, although not the sole, reason why, in spite of free anastomoses, occlusion of the arteries supplying the intestine is followed by necrosis and hæmorrhage. That the explanation is not to be found simply in the great length of intestine supplied by a single artery, is evident from the fact that, if the extra-intestinal arteries supplying a loop much more than 5 centimetres in length be suddenly closed, the loop becomes hæmorrhagic and necrotic (Mall and Welch, Bier). That the conditions are essentially identical in man is proven by the experience of surgeons, who have repeatedly observed the same results after separation of the mesentery close to the intestine over about the same length. The blood can enter at each end of the short loop arteries, whose branches anastomose freely within the walls of the loop with those of the closed arteries; there being a particularly rich arterial plexus in the submucous coat (Heller). But these anastomoses are insufficient to preserve the part; although, with reference to the extent of territory to be supplied, they are large in comparison with some of the trivial anastomoses which in external parts can respond effectively to the call for a collateral circulation to far larger areas. It must be left to future investigations to determine how far the inability of the intestinal vessels to compensate circulatory obstructions of a degree readily compensated in many other situations may be due, as claimed by Bier, to an inherent incapacity to lessen the resistance to the collateral stream, or to contraction of the muscular coats of the intestine, or to other causes. As Panski and Thoma have shown that slowing and interruption of the circulation in the spleen is followed, for several hours, by contraction of the muscular trabeculæ, it is probable that the development of a collateral circulation in this organ meets an obstacle similar to that in the intestine.

The various organs and tissues differ so widely as regards their susceptibility to the injurious effects of lack of arterial blood that local anæmias of equal intensity and duration may in one part of the body produce no appreciable effect, and in another cause the immediate abolition of function and the inevitable death of the part. In general, the more highly differentiated, specific cells of an organ are those which suffer first and most intensely. At one end of the scale are the ganglion cells of the brain, which, after the withdrawal of arterial blood for half an hour, and probably for a much shorter time, cannot be restored to life; and at the other end may be placed the periosteum, the cells of which may be still capable of producing bone two or three days after all circulation has ceased. So susceptible to local anæmia are the ganglion cells of the central nervous system, that not only is embolism of the branches of the cerebral arteries with only capillary communications, even of the minute terminal twigs in the cortex, always followed by necrotic softening, but also embolism of the anastomosing arteries in the pia very often causes softening of at least a part of the area supplied by the plugged artery. In the well-known Stenson experiment, temporary closure of the rabbit's abdominal aorta, just below the origin of the renal arteries, for an hour, results in the inevitable death of the ganglion cells in the central gray matter of the lumbar cord; and this notwithstanding the free anastomoses of the anterior and posterior spinal arteries. Many of the lesions which pass under the names of myelitis and hæmorrhagic encephalitis present the histological characters of ischæmic necrosis, although often no arterial occlusion can be found.

Perhaps, next to elements of the nervous system, the epithelial cells of the cortical tubules of the kidney are most susceptible to ischæmia. Litten has demonstrated that the temporary ligation of the renal artery of the rabbit for one and a half to two hours is followed invariably by necrosis of many of these epithelial cells. The cells in the walls of the blood-vessels and of connective tissue are relatively insusceptible to temporary slowing or cessation of the circulation.

It is evident from the preceding statements that the nature of the organ or tissue has a very important influence in determining whether local necrosis follows arterial embolism.

I have dwelt in some detail, although within the limited space necessarily inadequately, upon certain physiological characters of the circulation and of different organs and tissues, which appear to me deserving of more consideration than is usually given to them in discussions of the causes of embolic necroses and infarctions. It is, of course, not to be inferred that the number and size of the anastomoses are not of prime importance in determining the mechanical effects of. arterial embolism, but, important as they are, they are not the exclusive determinants of the result. There is no single anatomical formula applicable to the circulatory conditions under which all embolic infarcts occur. The nearest approach to such a formula is that embodied in Cohnheim's doctrine of terminal arteries, a name which he gave to arteries whose branches do not communicate with each other or with those of other arteries, although capillaries are of course everywhere in communication with each other. Terminal vessels in this sense are the renal, the splenic, the pulmonary, the central artery of the retina, the basal arteries of the brain, and in general all branches of cerebral and spinal arteries after they have penetrated the brain or the spinal cord, the intramuscular branches of the coronary arteries of the heart, and the portal vein.[1] Cohnheim's teaching was that infarction occurs always after embolism of a terminal vessel, except of the pulmonary artery, whose capillaries, under ordinary conditions, are numerous and wide enough, after obliteration of an arterial branch, to maintain a sufficient circulation; and of the portal vein whose capillaries communicate freely with those of the hepatic artery. Thoma and Goldenblum have shown that, contrary to Cohnheim's results, no infarction follows embolism or ligature of the frog's lingual artery, which is or can readily be made a terminal artery, provided the tongue be replaced in the mouth after the operation so as to avoid stretching and drying from exposure to the air. It is, therefore, quite possible in some situations for an adequate circulation to be carried on through merely capillary communications, although the conditions are of course less favourable than when there are arterial anastomoses. On the other hand, as we have seen, embolism of anastomosing arteries, such as the mesenteric and the cerebral, may be followed by necrosis or infarction; and it cannot be said that the anastomoses in all of these cases are so unimportant that the arteries are virtually terminal.

We may conclude then that, under ordinary conditions, embolism of an artery having abundant and large anastomoses has no important

---

[1] There is some confusion as to the sense in which the words "terminal arteries" should be used, and it must be admitted that later investigations have detracted from the precision given to this term by Cohnheim. Thus some do not recognise the pulmonary artery as terminal, because the lung is supplied likewise by the bronchial and several other arteries whose capillaries communicate with those of the pulmonary artery. But unless we make the extent of a second arterial supply the decisive point in the definition, we should have, for the same reason, to exclude the renal and the splenic arteries from the class of "terminal arteries." Then the conception of arteries which are "functionally" but not anatomically terminal, creates still further confusion.

mechanical effect; that embolism of an artery with few and minute anastomoses, especially embolism of an artery with only capillary communications, is in many situations followed by necrosis, this result being favoured by certain physiological conditions which have been considered; and that embolism of arteries with fairly well-developed anastomoses may in certain situations also cause necrosis. Among the factors influencing the result, other than those relating to the number and size of the anastomoses, are the varying susceptibility of cells to ischæmia, interference with the circulation by contraction of muscular constituents of a part, and perhaps some inherent weakness in the physiological part of the mechanism by which a vigorous collateral circulation is established.

The compensation of sudden occlusion of an artery, by means of the collateral circulation, generally presupposes vessels with fairly normal walls and a certain vigour of the circulation. When the arteries have lost their elasticity, or the general circulation is feeble, or there is some pre-existing obstacle to the circulation such as chronic passive congestion, the development of an adequate collateral circulation is rendered correspondingly difficult, and may be impossible. Hence embolism of arteries of the extremities is often followed by gangrene in the aged, in arterio-sclerosis, in heart disease, and in infective, anæmic, and exhausting diseases. There are some observations which suggest that arterial spasm may co-operate with embolism in causing local anæmia.

The agencies by which a sufficient collateral circulation is established may be thrown out of order to such a degree that embolism of arteries having even the most ample anastomoses may be followed by necrosis. Foci of cerebral softening have been observed after occlusion of the internal carotid or of one of the vertebral arteries; although the circle of Willis, the largest and most perfect anastomosis in the body, was open, and no vascular obstruction could be found beyond it. Here, doubtless, an important factor in this exceptional occurrence is the rapidity with which nerve cells die when insufficiently fed with arterial blood. Cohn narrates the interesting case of a young woman rendered extremely anæmic by repeated hæmorrhages from cancer of the tongue. In order to control the bleeding the right carotid was tied. The patient immediately, to all appearances, lost consciousness; acquired ptosis of the right, then of the left eye, drawing of the angle of the mouth to the right, and relaxation and almost complete paralysis of the left extremities. The pulse almost disappeared and the face became very anæmic. Respiration was unaffected. The ligature was at once removed, and at the same moment the patient awoke "as from a dream," and the symptoms just mentioned quickly disappeared. She said that she had not completely lost consciousness but was unable to speak, and that her will had lost control over the organs. She had lost so much blood that she died three hours later without again losing consciousness before death. At the autopsy the carotids and all of the cerebral vessels were found open, and there was no change in the brain except anæmia. In this case, the general anæmia was evidently so great that after closure of one carotid, which probably lasted not more than a minute or two, a sufficient supply of blood could not reach the brain through the circle of Willis.

Hæmorrhagic infarction.—The explanation of the accumulation and extravasation of blood in hæmorrhagic infarcts has been the subject of much speculation and experimental study. It is only in certain situations that infarcts are hæmorrhagic throughout; and, as already mentioned, these are no less necrotic than are the white infarcts. The necrosis and the hæmorrhage are co-ordinate effects of the disturbance of the circulation, neither being caused by the other. Virchow, in his early writings, suggested as possibilities, without definitely adopting any of them, most of the explanations which have since been advanced to account for the apparently paradoxical phenomenon that the occlusion of an artery may be followed by hyperæmia and hæmorrhage in the area of its distribution. Cohnheim, on the basis of experimental investigations published in 1872, came to the conclusion that the hyperæmia which may follow arterial embolism is the result of regurgitant flow from the veins, that the hæmorrhage occurs by diapedesis, and that this diapedesis is the result of some molecular change in the vascular walls deprived of their normal supply of nutriment. Although Cohn, in 1860, had shown conclusively, by numerous experiments on various organs, that the hyperæmia and hæmorrhage are not the result of regurgitant flow from the veins, Cohnheim's views were widely accepted until Litten, in 1880, in apparent ignorance of Cohn's work, repeated the experiments of the latter upon this point with the same results. The experiments of Dr. Mall and myself upon hæmorrhagic infarction of the intestine in 1887 convinced us that the blood which causes the infarct is not regurgitated from the veins. Cohnheim's results upon the frog as to the source of the blood in infarcts have not been confirmed by subsequent experimenters (Zielonko, Kossuchin, Küttner, Goldenblum, Thoma).

In situations where closure of an artery is followed by hæmorrhagic infarction, tying the veins also, so as to shut off all opportunity for reflux of venous blood, increases the hyperæmia and the hæmorrhage; and it may render an infarct hæmorrhagic which would otherwise be anæmic. On the other hand, if all vascular communication of a part be cut off except that with the veins, the part undergoes simple necrosis without hæmorrhagic infarction; and the result is the same even if the artery be cut open, so as to afford apparently the most favourable opportunity for backward flow from the veins. Or, expressed differently, if after closure of an artery all possibility of access of blood to the obstructed area through anastomosing arteries and capillaries be prevented, the veins remaining open, the part dies without hæmorrhagic infarction. Cohnheim was in error in supposing that hæmorrhagic infarction cannot occur where the veins are provided with valves, for it has been shown by Bryant, Köppe, and Mall that the small intestinal veins of the dog have effective valves; yet nowhere can hæmorrhagic infarction be more readily produced experimentally by arterial obstruction than in the intestine of this animal. It is, then, quite certain that the blood which accumulates in the capillaries and small veins, and is extravasated in hæmorrhagic infarction, comes in through the capillary, and, if they exist, the arterial anastomoses, and is not regurgitated from the veins.

It cannot be doubted that the red corpuscles escape by diapedesis, not by rhexis; but our experiments are in entire accord with those of Litten in failing to furnish any support to the prevalent doctrine that the hæmorrhage is the result of changes in the walls of the vessels caused by insufficient supply of arterial blood; in fact they seem to us more conclusive upon this point. If a loop of intestine be completely shut off from the circulation for three or four hours (by which time, after ligation of the superior mesenteric artery, hæmorrhagic infarction begins to appear), and the obstruction be then removed, the blood at once shoots in from the arteries with great rapidity, and distends the vessels.[1] If, as usually happens, the blood has not coagulated in the vessels, no hæmorrhagic infarction subsequently appears. If, immediately after the circulation has been fully re-established in the loop, the superior mesenteric artery be ligated, the intestine from the lower part of the duodenum into the colon becomes the seat of hæmorrhagic infarction in the usual time; but the infarction does not appear earlier and is not more intense in the part which had been previously deprived of its circulation for three or four hours than in the rest of the small intestine. It is true, as Cohnheim has shown, that re-establishment of a local circulation, after its stoppage for many hours or days, may be followed by hæmorrhages in the previously ischæmic area; but hæmorrhagic infarction after arterial occlusion begins long before it is possible to demonstrate this change in the vascular wall caused by lack of blood-supply.

In a part undergoing hæmorrhagic infarction the circulation is greatly retarded in consequence of the small difference between the arterial and the venous pressures. This result may be brought about by rise of the venous or lowering of the arterial pressure. If the veins are obstructed sufficiently to render the outflow nil, or very small, and the arteries are open, the infarction is intense, and occurs with high intracapillary pressure. In consequence of the free anastomoses of veins this mode of production of an infarct is rare, but it may occur after thrombosis of the mesenteric, the splenic, and the central retinal veins. Its explanation offers no especial difficulties. If the veins are open the arterial pressure must be reduced in order to furnish the conditions necessary for the production of hæmorrhagic infarction. This latter case is the one present in arterial embolism with hæmorrhagic infarction, and is the one especially needing explanation. The intracapillary

[1] Bier's experimental results concerning the absence of hyperæmia after temporary ischæmia of the intestine do not, according to our experience, apply to prolonged ischæmia, which we found to be followed by intense hyperæmia.

pressure in this case may vary, but will generally be low. The arterial pressure is so low that the lateral pulse-waves nearly or entirely disappear, so that the force which drives the blood into the capillaries is no longer the normal intermittent one, which experiment has shown to be essential for the long-continued circulation of the blood through the capillaries and veins. This reduction, or absence of lateral pulsation, to which, so far as I know, other experimenters have not called attention, I believe to be the factor of first importance in the causation of hæmorrhagic infarction following arterial embolism.

We are not sufficiently informed concerning the physical and vital properties of the blood and of the blood-vessels to be able to predict positively what would happen under such abnormal circulatory conditions as those named, and actual observation only can furnish a solution. The difficulties in making such observations under the requisite conditions are considerable. Dr. Mall and I, in examining microscopically, in a specially constructed apparatus, the mesenteric circulation of the dog after ligation of the superior mesenteric artery, observed that immediately after the occlusion the circulation ceases in the arteries, capillaries, and veins. In a short time the circulation returns, but with altered characters. The arteries are contracted, but may subsequently dilate somewhat; and the blood from the collaterals flows through them with diminished rapidity, and without distinct lateral pulsation. The direction of the current is reversed in some of the arteries. The movement of the blood in the capillaries and veins is sluggish and irregular. The direction of the current in some of the veins may be temporarily reversed, but we were unable to trace a regurgitant venous flow into the capillaries. The distinction between axial and plasmatic current is obliterated. Gradually the smaller and then the larger veins become more and more distended with red corpuscles, and all of the phenomena of an intense venous hyperæmia appear, so that one instinctively searches for some obstruction to the venous outflow. The red corpuscles in the veins tend to accumulate in clumps, and may be moved forward, or forward and backward, in clumps or solid columns. Stasis appears in the veins. This is at first observed only here and there and is readily broken up by an advancing column of blood; but it gradually involves more and more of the veins, and in some becomes permanent, producing an evident obstacle to the forward movement of the blood. The same phenomena of distension with red corpuscles, clumping, to-and-fro movement, and stasis appear gradually in the capillaries. An interesting appearance, sometimes observed in capillaries and veins, is that of interrupted columns of compacted red corpuscles with intervening clear spaces which are sometimes clumps of white corpuscles, sometimes of platelets, sometimes only clear plasma. With the partial blocking of the veins and capillaries, red corpuscles begin to pass through the walls of these vessels by diapedesis; and after a time the hæmorrhage becomes so great that it is difficult to observe the condition within the vessels. The venous outflow is diminished immediately or shortly after the closure of the superior mesenteric artery; it then rises, but later it continuously falls to a minimum.

An experiment which we made shows that the blood for hæmorrhagic infarction need not necessarily enter from the collaterals, and it sheds some light upon the condition of the circulation during the production of the infarct. We ligated all of the vascular communications of the intestine, with the exception of the main artery and vein, and then tied the intestine above and below, so that the included intestine was supplied only by the main artery and the blood returned by the main vein. Under these circumstances no infarction results. We then by a special device gradually constricted the main artery. In repeated experiments we found that not until the artery is sufficiently compressed to stop the lateral pulsations in its branches—the pressure in these being then about one-fifth of the normal—does hæmorrhagic infarction appear. Precautions were taken to make sure that the flow through the constricted main artery and its branches continued, and that the vein remained open. We have often measured the blood-pressure in branches of the superior mesenteric artery after ligation of this artery and during the progress of an infarction, and have found it to be generally one-fourth to one-fifth of the normal pressure. If the pressure on the arterial side falls below a certain minimum no hæmorrhage occurs in the infarction.

It is evident from the preceding description that the phenomena observed under these peculiar circulatory conditions are in large part dependent upon the physical properties of the blood, especially upon its viscosity and the presence of suspended particles which readily stick together; and differ in important respects from those which would occur under similar conditions with a thin, homogeneous fluid. The pressure gradient from arteries to veins of the ischæmic area is so low that the red corpuscles cannot fully overcome the resistance in the veins and capillaries. They accumulate in these situations, and probably undergo some physical change by which they become adherent to each other and to the vascular wall. The absence of the normal pulse-waves prevents the breaking up of these masses of corpuscles, the longitudinal pulse-waves sometimes observed having little or no effect in disintegrating the masses. In this way numerous small veins and capillaries become blocked, with a resulting rise of intracapillary pressure and diminution of outflow of blood through the veins. Von Frey has shown by interesting experiments that an intermittent pulsating force is necessary to prevent the speedy blocking of veins and capillaries with red corpuscles in carrying on artificial circulation with defibrinated blood through living organs. Kronecker has also demonstrated the influence of a pulsating force in increasing the venous outflow.

The diapedesis is due to the slowing and stagnation of the blood, and to the blood-pressure. Without a certain height of pressure there is no diapedesis; and, with a given retardation and stasis of the blood-current, the higher the intracapillary and intravenous pressure the greater the amount of diapedesis. The matter which needs explanation is that the diapedesis may occur with lower than the normal pressure, and through vessel walls apparently unaltered. This I attribute to the fact that the red corpuscles, in consequence of the slow circulation, have opportunity to become engaged in the narrow paths followed by the lymph as it passes out between the endothelial cells. Diapedesis is a slow process, and the channels for it are much smaller than the thickness of a red corpuscle. Unless the red corpuscles can get started on the path between the endothelial cells, they cannot traverse it; and unless the circulation is very much slowed, and the outer plasmatic current obliterated, there is no opportunity for the corpuscles to become engaged between the endothelial cells, provided, that is, the vascular wall be normal. With greatly retarded circulation there is opportunity, and when the way in front is blocked by compact masses of red corpuscles, and sometimes by actual thrombi, the only path open to the corpuscles is that followed by the lymph between the endothelial cells. This then becomes the direction of least resistance for their movement.

The reason why infarctions are hæmorrhagic in some situations and not in others offers difficulties chiefly in consequence of our ignorance of the exact circulatory conditions which lead to the production of infarction in different parts of the body. It is generally assumed that these circulatory conditions are everywhere essentially the same; but this is by no means proven. As we have already seen, the physiological conditions which influence the result are various. It may be, therefore, that the requisite intracapillary and intravenous pressure, or some other condition of the circulation essential for the production of hæmorrhagic infarction, is lacking when the infarction is anæmic. In general a high venous pressure favours hæmorrhage in an infarction, and a low arterial pressure opposes it. The pressure in the superior mesenteric and portal veins is higher than in any other veins of the body. Hæmorrhagic infarction of the lung occurs especially with high degrees of chronic passive congestion in which the venous pressure is elevated. Thrombosis of veins seems to be the cause of at least some of the hæmorrhagic infarcts of the spleen. Hæmorrhagic infarction of the kidney may be produced experimentally by ligating the renal veins.

The studies of recent years upon the formation of lymph have demonstrated that the blood-vessels in different regions differ markedly in their permeability, those of the intestine being probably the most permeable. It may be that this difference in the constitution of the vessels is an important factor in determining the extent of diapedesis under similar circulatory conditions. As pointed out by Weigert, however, the greatest influence appears to be exercised by the resistance offered by the tissues to the escape of red corpuscles from the vessels. Hæmorrhagic infarction occurs especially where this tissue-resistance is low, as in the loose, spongy texture of the lungs, and in the soft mucosa and lax submucosa of the intestine. The hæmorrhage is far less in the dense muscular coats of the intestine. The considerable resistance offered by the naturally firm consistence of the kidney is increased by the swelling and hardness resulting from coagulative necrosis of the epithelial and other cells of this organ; so that infarcts in this situation are nearly always anæmic in the greater part of their extent, although often hæmorrhagic in the periphery. The spleen is of softer consistence than the kidney; and here both white and red infarcts may occur, the latter especially with increased venous pressure. Although infarcts of the brain are soft, they are much swollen in the fresh state from infiltration with serum, so as to displace surrounding parts (Marchand). Here also there must be considerable resistance to the passage of red corpuscles through the vascular walls; but it is not uncommon for these softened areas to present scattered foci of hæmorrhage, and sometimes they are markedly hæmorrhagic. The intraocular pressure is probably a factor in making embolic infarcts of the retina anæmic. Embolism of arteries of the extremities with insufficient collateral circulation is often associated with extravasations of blood in the ischæmic areas.

Metamorphoses of infarcts.—A bland infarct is a foreign body most of the constituents of which are capable of absorption and replacement by connective tissue. The red corpuscles lose their colouring matter, some of which is transformed into amorphous or crystalline hæmatoidin. Polynuclear leucocytes, through chemiotactic influences, wander in from the periphery, the advance guard being usually the seat of marked nuclear fragmentation. This nuclear detritus mingles with that derived from the dead cells of the part. Granulation tissue develops from the living tissue around the infarct. Young mesoblastic cells wander in and assist the leucocytes in their phagocytic work. In the course of time the debris, which becomes extensively fatty, is disintegrated and removed; new vessels and new connective tissue grow in; and finally a scar, more or less pigmented according to the previous content of blood, marks the site of the infarct. In chronic endocarditis, depressed, wedge-shaped scars are often found in the spleen and the kidneys. They are rare in the lungs, not because hæmorrhagic infarcts in this situation usually undergo resolution like pneumonia or simple hæmorrhages, but because pulmonary infarcts generally occur under conditions not compatible with the prolonged survival of the patient. Partly organised infarcts are not uncommon in the lungs. In the brain, ischæmic softening may remain for a long time with apparently little change; but the common ultimate result is a cyst-like structure, which may be more or less pigmented, and is characterised by a meshwork of delicate neuroglia and connective-tissue fibres, infiltrated with milky or clear serum. Into the finer histological details of the process of substitution of an infarct by scar-tissue it is not necessary here to enter.

Chemical effects. Metastases.—Embolism and metastasis are sometimes employed as practically synonymous terms; but, in ordinary usage, by metastasis is understood any local, morbid condition produced by the transportation of pathological material by the lymphatic or blood-current from one part of the body to another.

We have already considered the coarser bland emboli in respect of their mechanical effects. Similar emboli, so small as to become lodged only in arterioles or capillaries, produce no mechanical effects unless, as rarely happens, numerous arterioles or capillaries are obstructed. The subject of transportation of pigment granules, and that of metallic and carboniferous dust, producing the various konioses, does not fall within the scope of this article. On account of certain special features, emboli of air, of fat, and of parenchyma-cells are most conveniently considered separately (pp. 254-259). There remain, in contrast to the dead and inert emboli to which our attention has been especially directed, those containing tumour-cells and parasitic organisms, or their products.

Masses of tumour growing into a blood-vessel may be broken off and transported as coarse emboli, producing all of the mechanical effects which we have described. There have been instances of sudden death from blocking of the pulmonary artery by cancerous or sarcomatous emboli, as in a case reported by Feltz. It is, however, as a cause of metastatic growths that emboli of tumour-cells have their chief significance. In individual cases it is oftener a matter of faith than of demonstration that the metastasis is due to such emboli, for opportunities to bring absolutely conclusive proof of this mode of origin of secondary tumours are not common. There have, however, been enough instances in which the demonstration has been rigorous to establish firmly the doctrine of the embolic origin of metastatic tumours. The evidence is that tumour-metastases are far more frequently due to capillary emboli than to those of larger size. Cancers and sarcomas furnish the great majority of emboli of this class; but in rare instances even benign tumours may penetrate blood-vessels and give rise to emboli, which exceptionally are the starting-points of secondary growths of the same nature as the primary. Mention has already been made of paradoxical and retrograde transport of tumour-emboli, as well as of the possibility of emboli of tumour-cells being so small as to traverse the pulmonary capillaries.

Certain animal parasites, as the Filaria sanguinis, Bilharzia hæmatobia, and Plasmodium malariæ, are inhabitants of the blood, or, in certain stages of their existence within the human body, are frequently found there. According to observations of Cerfontaine and Askanazy, the usual mode of transportation from the intestine of the embryos of Trichina is by the lymphatic and blood-currents. Echinococci have been known to pass from the liver through the vena cava; or primarily from the right heart into the pulmonary artery; and emboli from echinococci present in the wall of the left heart may be transported to distant organs (Davaine). The Amœba coli has been found in the intestinal veins; and, as stated by Dr. Lafleur in his article on "Amœbic Abscess of the Liver" (vol. v. p. 156), it is probable that this parasite can reach the liver through the portal vein.

On account of their frequency and serious consequences, infective emboli containing pathogenetic bacteria are of especial significance. Such emboli constitute an important means of distribution of infective agents from primary foci of infection to distant parts of the body, where the pathogenetic micro-organisms, by their multiplication and their chemical products, can continue to manifest their specific activities.   These emboli are often derived from infective venous thrombi connected with some primary area of infection.   The portal of infection may be through the integument, the alimentary canal, the respiratory tract, the genito-urinary passages, the middle ear, or the eye, with corresponding infective thrombo-phlebitis in these various situations.   Or there may be no demonstrable atrium of infection,. as in many cases of infective endocarditis, which constitutes an important source of infective emboli.   Emboli may of course come from secondary and subsequent foci of infection.

Coarse emboli are by no means essential for the causation of infective metastases, nor is it necessary that there should be any thrombosis to afford opportunity for the distribution of micro-organisms from a primary focus.   Bacteria may gain access to the circulation, singly or in clumps ; and such bacteria, without being enclosed in plugs of even capillary size, may become attached to the walls of capillaries and small vessels and produce local metastases.   In this way infective material coming from the systemic veins may pass through the pulmonary capillaries without damage to the lungs, and become localised in various organs of the body.

We cannot explain the various localisations of infective processes in internal organs of the body exclusively by the mechanical distribution of pathogenetic micro-organisms by the circulation.   We must reckon with the vital resistance of the tissues, which varies in different parts of the body, in different species and individuals, and with reference to different organisms.   Even the pyogenetic micrococci, which are capable of causing abscesses anywhere in the body, do not generally produce their pathogenetic effects in every place where they may chance to lodge. They have their seats of preference, which vary in different species of animal and probably in different individuals.

The mere presence of pathogenetic bacteria in an embolus does not necessarily impart to it infective properties.   This is true even of emboli containing pyogenic cocci.   I have in several instances observed in the spleen and kidney only the mechanical, bland effects of emboli derived from the vegetations of acute infective endocarditis, and have been able to demonstrate streptococci or other pathogenetic organisms in the original vegetations and in the emboli.   As has already been remarked concerning thrombi, the line cannot be sharply drawn between bland emboli and septic emboli, simply on the basis of the presence of bacteria ; although of course the septic properties must be derived from micro-organisms.

Infective emboli ar capable of producing all of the mechanical effects of bland emboli; to these are added the specific effects of the micro-organisms or their products.   These latter effects are essentially chemical in nature, and may occur wherever the emboli lodge, being thus independent of the particular circulatory conditions essential for the production of mechanical effects. The most important of these chemical effects are hæmorrhages, usually of small size, and of an entirely different causation from those of hæmorrhagic infarction; necroses; inflammation, often suppurative, and, in case of putrefactive bacteria, gangrenous putrefaction. The most important function of infective embolism is in the causation of pyæmia. This subject has been most competently presented by Professor Cheyne in vol. i. p. 601, who has left nothing which requires further consideration here.

Embolic aneurysms.—Both the first recognition and the correct explanation of embolic aneurysms, at least of the great majority of cases, belong to British physicians and surgeons. Tufnell, in 1853, called attention to the influence of emboli in causing aneurysmal dilatation. There followed observations by Ogle, Wilks, Holmes, Church, and R. W. Smith, before the appearance, in 1873, of Ponfick's important paper on embolic aneurysms. Ponfick explained their formation by direct injury to the vessel-wall, inflicted usually by calcareous, spinous emboli; a view which has since been confirmed only by Thoma. In 1877, Goodhart, in reporting a case, gave the first satisfactory explanation of the mode of production of most of these aneurysms. He pointed out their association with acute infective endocarditis, and referred them to acute softening of the arterial wall, caused by toxic emboli. Other observations followed; and in 1885 Osler reported a case which, although not embolic, belongs etiologically to the same general category. This was a case of multiple mycotic aneurysms of the aorta due to infective endaortitis associated with infective endocarditis. In 1886 and 1887 appeared the contributions of Langton and Bowlby, the most valuable in English literature, who fully confirmed and expanded in detail the views first briefly announced by Goodhart. Eppinger, in his extensive monograph on aneurysms published in 1887, presented the results of a minute and careful study of this class of aneurysm, which he calls aneurysma mycotico-embolicum, and reported seven personal observations. Of later papers on the subject may be mentioned those of Pel and Spronck, Duckworth, Buday, and Clarke.

The evidence is conclusive that aneurysms may be caused by the destructive action of bacteria contained in emboli or directly implanted on the inner vascular wall. The usual source for such emboli in relation to aneurysm is furnished by acute infective endocarditis; but as there is every transition from ordinary warty endocarditis to the most malignant forms, and as the same species of micro-organisms may be found in the relatively benign as in the malignant cases, no single type of endocarditis is exclusively associated with these aneurysms. As is demonstrated by Osler's case, the same result may follow a mycotic endarteritis not secondary to embolism.

Eppinger has shown that at least the intima and the internal elastic lamella, and usually a part, sometimes the whole, of the media, are destroyed by the action of the bacteria, when an aneurysm is produced

The site of the aneurysm corresponds to this circumscribed area of destruction, and therefore to the seat of the embolus, and is not above it, as some have supposed. The aneurysm is usually formed acutely, sometimes slowly. It may remain small or attain a large size. Multiplicity and location at or just above an arterial branching are common characteristics of embolic aneurysms. Favourite situations are the cerebral and mesenteric arteries and arteries of the extremities; but these aneurysms may occur in almost any artery. Arteries without firm support from the surrounding tissues offer the most favourable conditions for the production of embolic aneurysms.

Eppinger totally rejects direct mechanical injury from an embolus as a cause of aneurysm in the manner alleged by Ponfick; and Langton and Bowlby are likewise sceptical as to the validity of Ponfick's explanation beyond its possible application to some of his own cases. Certainly the great majority of embolic aneurysms are caused by pathogenetic organisms, and belong, therefore, to the class of parasitic aneurysms rather than to that of traumatic aneurysms. The affection is not a common one.

In this connection mere mention may be made of the interesting and very common verminous aneurysms of the anterior mesenteric artery of horses, caused by the Strongylus armatus.

General symptoms.—The symptoms of bland embolism are dependent mainly upon the degree and extent of the local anæmia produced by the arterial obstruction, and upon the specific functions of the part involved. In infective embolism there are additional symptoms referable to local and general infection. Here the constitutional symptoms usually overshadow those referable to the embolic obstruction and the local lesions.

It is not known that any symptoms attend the act of transportation of an embolus, even through the heart. In some situations there is sudden pain at the moment of impaction of the embolus (embolic ictus). This is more marked in large arteries, especially those supplying the extremities, than in smaller and visceral arteries. This pain has been attributed to various causes; but the most probable explanation seems to me to be irritation, by the impact of the embolus and by the sudden distension of the artery, of sensory nerves and nerve-endings in the vascular wall, present especially in the outer coat. It may be that the Pacinian corpuscles, which are particularly abundant in and around the adventitia of the abdominal aorta, the mesenteric arteries, the iliac and the femoral arteries, are susceptible to painful impressions. Embolism of the arteries named is characterised especially by the intensity of the pain, described sometimes as the sensation of a painful blow, at the moment of impaction of the embolus. Surgeons are familiar with the pain which attends the act of ligation of larger blood-vessels.

Of the pain which follows arterial embolism there are other causes, such as irritation of sensory nerves by local anæmia, altered tension of the part, presence of waste and abnormal metabolic products, structural changes in nerves, inflammation of serous membranes covering infarcts, and so forth.

Some writers have spoken of the occasional occurrence of a nervous or reflex chill at the time of the embolic act; but, without denying the possibility of such an occurrence, I think that chills associated with embolism have been due usually to infection rather than to vascular plugging.

Although Stricker has constructed a hypothesis of fever based largely upon experiments interpreted by him as demonstrating that the commotion mechanically set up by emboli causes fever, I am not aware of any conclusive observations which show that fever may be produced in this way in human beings. Independently of the intervention of pathogenetic micro-organisms, arterial embolism may, however, be accompanied by elevation of temperature. Direct invasion of thermic nervous centres is, of course, only a special case in certain localisations of cerebral embolism. Gangolphe and Courmont attribute the fever sometimes observed after arterial occlusion to the absorption of pyretogenetic substances which they find produced in tissues undergoing necrobiosis. Other possible causes of fever may be the reactive and secondary inflammations consecutive to embolism.

Only in external parts, or parts open to inspection, can the phenomena of mortification, or "local cadaverisation," as Cruveilhier designated the results of shutting off arterial blood, be directly observed. Here are manifest the pallor accompanied by patches of lividity, the cessation of pulsation, the loss of turgidity, the coldness, the annihilation of function, the local death. The hæmorrhages which result from arterial obstruction may, however, be evident, not in external parts only, but also by the discharge of blood from the respiratory passages, the intestine, and the urinary tract; as the result of pulmonary, intestinal, and renal infarction respectively. The phenomena following retinal embolism are open to direct inspection by the ophthalmoscope. In parts not accessible to physical exploration the symptoms are referable mainly to the disturbance or abolition of function, and, therefore, vary with the special functions of the part. They will be considered in connection with embolism of special arteries (p. 261).

Diagnosis.—The main reliance in the differential diagnosis of embolism from thrombosis, or from other forms of arterial obstruction, is the discovery of a source for emboli, the sudden onset and the intensity of symptoms referable to local arterial anæmia, occasionally the disappearance or marked improvement of symptoms in consequence of complete or partial re-establishment of the circulation, and to some extent the absence of arterio-sclerosis or other causes of primary arterial thrombosis.

Valuable as these characters are for diagnosis, they are neither always present nor infallible. For pulmonary embolism the source is to be sought in peripheral venous thrombosis or cardiac disease with thrombi in the right heart; for embolism in the aortic system, the usual source is the left heart, the great majority of cases being associated with disease of the aortic or mitral valves.   It may, however, be impossible to detect the source, and its existence does not exclude the occurrence of thrombosis or other forms of arterial occlusion.

Nor are the symptoms consecutive to embolism always sudden in onset.   An embolus may at first only partly obstruct the lumen of the vessel, which is later closed by a secondary thrombus ; or it may be so situated that a thrombus springing from it is the real cause of the local anæmia.   For example, an embolus lodged in the internal carotid artery usually causes no definite symptoms, but a secondary thrombus may extend from the embolus into the middle cerebral artery, in which case cerebral softening is sure to follow.   On the other hand, the complete closure of an artery may be effected by a thrombus with such rapidity as to suggest embolism.

While the sudden occlusion of an artery by an embolus often causes temporary ischæmia of greater intensity and over a larger area than the more gradual closure of the same artery by a thrombus, so that when the collateral circulation is fully established the disappearance or reduction of the symptoms may be more marked in the former case than the latter, there may be even in thrombosis very decided improvement in the symptoms with the development of the collateral circulation.

The existence of arterio-sclerosis, of course, does not exclude embolism ; but in case of doubt the chances are strongly in favour of embolism in children and young adults with healthy arteries, especially if cardiac disease be present ; the most common association in the latter cases being with mitral affections.

Notwithstanding all of these uncertainties, the diagnosis of embolism, when it produces definite symptoms, can be correctly made in the majority of cases.

Air embolism.—The majority of cases in which death has been attributed to the entrance of air into the circulation have been surgical operations and wounds about the neck, shoulder, upper part of the thorax and skull, where air has been sucked into gaping veins and sinuses by thoracic aspiration ; and cases in which air has entered the uterine veins, chiefly from the puerperal uterus, either spontaneously, as after abortions or detachment of placenta prævia, or after injections into the uterine cavity.   Jürgensen has reported cases in which he believes death was caused by the entrance of gas into open veins connected with diseased areas in the stomach and intestine.   Gaseous embolism has been assigned as the cause of symptoms and of death in caisson-disease and in divers ; and it has been observed in connection with the development of gas-producing bacilli in the body.

A large number of experiments have been made to determine the effects of air introduced into the circulation.   These have demonstrated that when the air is introduced slowly and at intervals, enormous quantities can sometimes be injected in a comparatively short time without manifest injury. Thus Laborde and Muron injected into the external jugular vein of a dog 1120 cc. in the space of an hour and a half without causing death ; and Jürgensen injected into the left femoral artery of a dog, weighing 43·5 kilo, 3550 cc. in the space of two hours and a half with only slight disturbance of the respiration and of the action of the heart. Under these circumstances the air-bubbles circulate with the blood, pass through the capillaries, and are speedily eliminated. Small amounts of air introduced directly into the carotids, the left heart or thoracic aorta, are often quickly fatal from embolism of the cerebral or coronary arteries.

The sudden introduction of large amounts of air into the veins is quickly fatal. Rabbits are much more susceptible to air embolism than dogs or horses. 50 cc. of air, and even more, can often be injected at once into the external jugular vein of a medium-sized dog without causing death ; nor can a dog be killed by simple aspiration of air into the veins, even when an open glass tube is inserted into the axillary or jugular vein and shoved into the thorax (Feltz). Barthélemy says that as much as 4000 cc. of air must be introduced into the veins of horses in order to cause death.

After death from entrance of air into the veins, the right cavities of the heart are found distended with frothy blood, and blood containing air-bubbles is found in the veins—especially those near the heart, and in the pulmonary artery and its branches. It is exceptional under these circumstances for air to pass through the pulmonary capillaries into the left heart and aortic system.

There are two principal explanations of the cause of death in these cases. According to one, associated especially with Couty's name, the air is churned up with the blood into a frothy fluid in the right heart, and on account of its compressibility this mixture cannot be propelled by the right ventricle, which thus becomes over-distended and paralysed. According to another hypothesis, supported by experiments of Passet and of Hauer, blood mixed with air-bubbles is propelled into the pulmonary artery and its branches, but the frothy mixture cannot be driven through the pulmonary capillaries, so that death results from pulmonary embolism. The paralysing influence upon the heart of obstruction to the coronary circulation from accumulation of air in the right heart and in the coronary veins must also be an important factor, as well as the cerebral anæmia. Probably all of these factors—over-distension of the right heart, embolism of the pulmonary artery and its branches and of the coronary veins, and cerebral anæmia—may be concerned in causing death, although not necessarily all in equal degree in every case.

We have no information as to the amount of air required to cause death by intravenous aspiration or injection in human beings. It seems certain that man is relatively more susceptible in this respect than the dog or the horse ; but it is probable that the fatal quantity of air must be at least several cubic centimetres, and that the entrance of a few bubbles of air into the veins is of no consequence. Many authors have entertained very exaggerated ideas of the danger of entrance of a small quantity of air into the veins.

A large proportion of the cases reported in medical records as deaths due to air embolism will not stand rigid criticism. I have had occasion to look through the records of a large number of these cases, and have been amazed at the frequently unsatisfactory and meagre character of the evidence upon which was based the assumption that death was due to the entrance of air into the circulation.

So far as I am aware, the first attempt to make a bacteriological examination and to determine the nature of the gas-bubbles found in the blood under circumstances suggestive of death from entrance of air into the vessels, was made by me in 1891. A patient with an aortic aneurysm, which had perforated externally and given rise to repeated losses of blood, died suddenly without renewed hæmorrhage. At the autopsy, made in cool weather eight hours after death, there was abundant odourless gas in the heart and vessels without a trace of cadaveric decomposition anywhere in the body. It was proven that the gas was generated by an anaerobic bacillus, which was studied by Dr. Nuttall and myself, and named by us Bacillus aerogenes capsulatus. This bacillus is identical with one subsequently found by E. Fraenkel in gaseous phlegmons, and with that found by Ernst and others in livers which are the seat of post-mortem emphysema (Schaumleber). It is widely distributed in the outer world, being present especially in the soil, and often exists in the human intestinal canal. Dr. Flexner and I have reported twenty-three personal observations in which this gas-bacillus was found, and since our publication we have met with several additional ones. The only points concerning these cases which here concern us are, that this bacillus not only may produce gas in cadavers, but may invade the living body, and cause a variety of affections characterised by the presence of gas. There is evidence that the bacilli may be widely distributed by the circulation before death, and that gas generated by them may be present in the vessels during life. In most cases, however, in which this bacillus was present, the gas found in the heart and blood-vessels was generated after death. I do not consider that there is satisfactory evidence that similar effects may be produced by the colon bacillus, as has been asserted. There is, however, a facultative anaerobic bacillus, very closely allied to the B. aerogenes capsulatus, which may also cause gaseous phlegmons and produce gas in the vessels after death.

Our observations have demonstrated that the finding of gas-bubbles in the heart and vessels a few hours after death without any evidence of cadaveric decomposition is no proof that the gas is atmospheric air, or is not generated by a micro-organism. In all such cases a bacteriological examination is necessary to determine the origin of the gas. In many cases reported as death from entrance of air into the veins, the evidence for this conclusion has been nothing more than finding gas-bubbles in the heart and vessels after sudden or otherwise unexplained death. In the absence of a bacteriological examination, the only cases which can be accepted as conclusive are those in which death has occurred immediately or shortly after the actually observed entrance of a considerable amount of air into the veins. There have been a number of carefully observed and indisputable instances in which during a surgical operation in the "dangerous region" life was imperilled or extinguished by the demonstrated entrance of air into wounded veins. After the audible sound of the suction of air into the vein, death was sometimes instantaneous; or it occurred in a few minutes after great dyspnœa, syncope, dilatation of the pupils, pallor or cyanosis, occasionally convulsions, sometimes the detection by auscultation over the heart of a churning sound synchronous with the cardiac systole, and the exit from the wounded vein of blood containing air-bubbles. These very alarming symptoms may disappear and the patient recover.

The evidence for this mode of death would seem to be almost as conclusive for a certain number of the sudden deaths following injections into the uterus, especially for the purpose of committing criminal abortion, and after the separation of placenta prævia. But I am sceptical as to this explanation of many of the deaths which have been reported as due to the entrance of air into the uterine veins. In the reports of Dr. Flexner and myself will be found the description of several cases of invasion of the B. aerogenes capsulatus, which without bacteriological examination would have the same claim to be regarded as deaths from entrance of air into the uterine veins as many of those so recorded. I have had the opportunity to examine the museum specimen of a uterus of a much-quoted case so reported, and I found in its walls bacilli morphologically identical with our gas-bacillus. Certainly all cases of this kind should hereafter be reported only after a bacteriological examination. Jürgensen's cases of supposed entrance of gas into the general circulation through the gastric and the intestinal veins are undoubtedly instances of invasion, either before or after death, of gas-forming bacilli.

Since Paul Bert's researches, the symptoms and death which occasionally follow the rapid reduction of previously heightened atmospheric pressure upon exit from a caisson or diver's apparatus, have been plausibly attributed to the liberation of bubbles of nitrogen in the circulating blood. This explanation of the phenomena is not, however, free from doubt, and it is difficult to bring conclusive evidence in its support in the case of human beings. Little weight can be attached at present to the reports of finding bubbles of gas in the blood-vessels of those who have died from caisson-disease, for these reports have not hitherto been accompanied by any bacteriological examination to determine the source of the gas.

Ewald and Kobert have made the curious observation that the lungs, are not air-tight under an increase of intrapulmonary pressure which may temporarily occur in human beings. They found in experiments on animals that small air-bubbles may appear under these circumstances.

in the pulmonary veins and left heart without any demonstrable rupture of the pulmonary tissue; and they argue that this may occur under similar conditions in human beings. The entrance into the circulation of a few minute air-bubbles in this way would doubtless produce no effects. Ewald and Kobert cite two or three not at all convincing published cases in support of the possibility of death resulting from the entrance of air through unruptured pulmonary veins. Very plausible is Janeway's hypothesis that the transitory hemiplegia and other cerebral symptoms, which have occasionally been observed to follow washing-out the pleural cavity with peroxide of hydrogen, or some other procedure by which air or gas may accumulate in this cavity under high pressure, are due to air embolism or gaseous embolism of the cerebral vessels.

Not less remarkable are the experimental observations of Lewin and Goldschmidt concerning air-embolism following injections of air into the bladder and its passage into the ureters and renal pelves. It has not been demonstrated that the same phenomenon can occur under similar conditions in human beings.

Fat embolism.—Fat embolism, first observed in human beings by Zenker and by Wagner in 1862, is the most common form of embolism; but its practical importance does not correspond to its frequency. It is of greater surgical than medical interest, inasmuch as the severer forms are nearly always the result of traumatism. The usual conditions for its occurrence are (i.) rupture of the wall of a vessel, (ii.) proximity of liquid fat, and (iii.) some force sufficient to propel the fat into the vessel.

Fat-embolism probably occurs in every case of fracture of bone containing fat-marrow. When the bone is rarefied, and contains an unusual quantity of fat-marrow, embolism resulting from its injury may be very extensive; as is illustrated by several fatal cases of fat-embolism following the forcible rupture of adhesions in an anchylosed joint. Ribbert has shown that fat-embolism may result from simple concussion of bone, as from falls or a blow. Inflammations, hæmorrhages and degenerations of the osseous marrow may cause it. It may likewise result from traumatic lesions, necroses, hæmorrhages, inflammation of adipose tissue in any part of the body,—of the brain, of a fatty liver, in a word of any organ or part containing fat. Injury to the pelvic fat during childbirth leads to fat-embolism. Oil-globules in the blood may come from fatty metamorphoses of thrombi, of endothelial cells and of atheromatous plaques. The lipæmia of digestion and of diabetes mellitus has not been generally supposed to lead to fat-embolism, but Sanders and Hamilton have observed capillaries filled with oil-globules after death from diabetic coma, and they attribute in certain cases dyspnœa and coma in diabetes to this cause.

In the great majority of cases, fat-embolism is entirely innocuous, and, unless it is searched for, its existence is not revealed at autopsy, and then only by microscopical examination. Plugging of capillaries and small arteries with oil may, however, be so extensive and so situated as to cause grave symptoms and even death. More moderate plugging may aid in causing death in those greatly weakened by shock, hæmorrhage, or other causes. The detection of fat-embolism in the pulmonary vessels may be of medico-legal value in determining whether injuries have been inflicted before or after death.

The deposition of fat-emboli is most abundant in the small arteries and capillaries of the lung, where in extreme cases the appearances of microscopic sections may indicate that considerably over one-half of the pulmonary capillaries are filled with cylinders and drops of oil. In rare instances of extensive injury the amount of fat in the blood may be enormous, so that post-mortem clots in the heart and pulmonary artery may be enveloped in layers of solidified fat. Some of the oil passes through the pulmonary capillaries and blocks the capillaries and arterioles of various organs; those which suffer most being the brain, the kidneys, and the heart. The extent of the embolism in the aortic system varies much in different cases, being sometimes slight, at other times extensive. Probably the force of the circulation determines the amount of fat which passes through the pulmonary capillaries. Oil once deposited may be again mobilised and transferred to other capillaries.

As already stated, it is only in the comparatively rare instances of extensive fat-embolism that effects of any consequence are produced. The fat itself is perfectly bland and unirritating, although it may be accidentally associated with toxic or infective material. The lesions and symptoms, when present, are referable mainly to the lungs, the brain, the heart, and the kidneys. These lesions are multiple ecchymoses (which in the lungs and the brain may be very numerous and extensive), pulmonary œdema, and patchy fatty degeneration of the cardiac muscle and of the epithelium of the convoluted tubules of the kidney. Pulmonary œdema, referable probably to paralysis of the left heart, is common with extensive fat embolism of the lungs. Death may undoubtedly be caused by fat-embolism of the cerebral vessels, possibly also by that of the coronary vessels.

The *symptoms* in the extreme cases are quickened respiration, rapid prostration, reddish frothy expectoration, the crepitations of pulmonary œdema, small frequent pulse, cyanosis, and—with cerebral invasion—coma, vomiting, convulsions, and occasionally focal cerebral symptoms. The temperature may either fall or rise. Oil-globules are often found in the urine, but it is still an open question whether these are eliminated through the glomerular capillaries, many of which are often filled with oil.

From the recent investigations of Beneke it appears that the oil is readily disposed of, in small part by saponification, possibly oxidation, and emulsion by means of the blood plasma; but in larger part through the metabolic and phagocytic activities of wandering cells which form a layer around the fat. The saponifying ferment — lipase — which Hanriot has discovered in blood-serum is probably one of the agents concerned in disposing of the fat.

Embolism by parenchymatous cells.—This is in general of more pathologico-anatomical than clinical interest, and therefore need not be considered here in detail. As has been shown by Lubarsch, Aschoff, and Maximow, bone-marrow cells, with large budding nuclei, usually undergoing degeneration, may often be found lodged in the pulmonary capillaries after injury to bone, in toxic and infective diseases, in leucocythæmia, and in association with emboli of other parenchymatous cells. I have seen them in large number in capillaries of the liver in a case of spleno-medullary leucocythæmia.

Next in frequency are emboli of liver-cells, which are found chiefly in pulmonary capillaries, but may pass through an open foramen ovale so as to reach capillaries of the brain, kidneys, and other organs. F. C. Turner in 1884 first observed liver-cells within hepatic vessels ; and later Jürgens, Klebs, Schmorl, Lubarsch, Flexner, and others noted their transportation as emboli after injury, hæmorrhages, and necroses of the liver, and with especial frequency in puerperal eclampsia. Secondary platelet-thrombi are usually formed about the cells.

Especial significance was attached by Schmorl to the presence of emboli of placental giant-cells (syncytium) in the pulmonary capillaries in cases of puerperal eclampsia ; but these emboli, although frequent, are not constant in this affection, and they may occur in pregnant women without eclampsia (Lubarsch, Leusden, Kassjanow).

To the group of parenchymatous emboli may be added the transport of large cells from the spleen to the liver through the splenic and portal veins. I have seen large splenic cells containing pigment and parasites blocking the capillaries of the liver in cases of malaria ; and also the well-known large splenic cells containing red blood-corpuscles in cases of malaria and of typhoid fever. The crescentic endothelial cells of the spleen may enter the circulation.

After traumatism and parenchymatous embolism fragments of osseous and medullary tissue may be carried to the pulmonary vessels as emboli (Lubarsch, Maximow). Emboli of large masses of hepatic tissue have been found in branches of the pulmonary artery by Schmorl, Zenker, Hess, and Gaylord as a result of traumatic laceration of the liver. Chorion-villi may be detached and very rarely conveyed as emboli to the lungs (Schmorl), or by retrograde transport to veins in the vaginal wall (Neumann, Pick). This is much more likely to occur from chorionic carcinoma and moles than from a normal placenta.

So far as known, emboli of marrow-cells, of liver-cells, of normal syncytial cells, and of splenic cells undergo only regressive metamorphoses, which lead to their eventual disappearance. The possibility that without the presence of any syncytial tumour in the uterus or tubes, emboli of syncytial cells may give rise to malignant tumours with the typical structure of those developing from syncytium, seems to have been demonstrated by a case reported by Schmorl ; but it can hardly be supposed that the displaced syncytial cells were normal. Emboli of liver-cells manifest a distinct coagulative influence (Hanau, Lubarsch); and in two instances Lubarsch attributed infarcts in the kidney and the liver to thrombi formed around these cells. Marrow-cells and syncytial cells may likewise cause, in less degree, secondary platelet and hyaline thrombi; but it does not appear that these thrombi have the importance in the etiology of puerperal eclampsia which is attached to them by Schmorl. With a few exceptions, no important lesions of the tissues or definite symptoms have been conclusively referred to emboli of these parenchymatous cells.

Although widely different in results, the transportation of tumour cells by the blood-current is a process similar to that of parenchymatous embolism, for which indeed cellular embolism seems to me a preferable designation. Benno Schmidt has found small branches of the pulmonary artery plugged with cancer-cells derived from gastric cancer or its metastases, both with and without growth of the cells into the walls of the plugged arteries. Such cells may reach the lungs by conveyance through the thoracic duct and innominate vein.

Embolism of special arteries.—I shall present the salient characteristics of the more important special localisations of embolism, so far as these have not been sufficiently considered in the preceding pages, or do not pertain to other articles in this work. Embolism of the central nervous system will be discussed in the next volume under Diseases of the Brain and Spinal Cord. The pyæmic manifestations of infective embolism have been described in the articles on "Pyæmia" (vol. i. p. 601) and on "Infective Endocarditis" (vol. i. p. 626 and vol. v. p. 876).

Pulmonary embolism.—The effects of pulmonary embolism vary with the size of the plugged vessel, the rapidity and completeness of its closure, the nature of the embolus, and associated conditions. Embolism of large, of medium-sized and small arteries, and of capillaries may be distinguished.

The most frequent source of large emboli is peripheral venous thrombosis, although they may come from the right heart. Sudden or rapid death follows embolism of the trunk or of both main divisions of the pulmonary artery. It may occur also from embolism of only one of the main divisions or from plugging of a large number of branches at the hilum of the lung.

Death may be instantaneous from syncope. More frequently the patient cries out, is seized with extreme precordial distress and violent suffocation, and dies in a few seconds or minutes. Or, when there is still some passage for the blood, the symptoms may be prolonged for hours or even days before the fatal termination. The symptoms of large pulmonary embolism are the sudden appearance of a painful sense of oppression in the chest, rapid respiration, intense dyspnœa, pallor followed by cyanosis, turgidity of the cervical veins, exophthalmos, dilatation of the pupils, tumultuous or weak and irregular heart's action, small, empty radial pulse, great restlessness, cold sweat, chills, syncope, opisthotonos, and convulsions. The intelligence may be preserved, or there may be delirium, coma, and other cerebral symptoms. Particularly striking is the contrast between the violence of the dyspnœa and the freedom with which the air enters the lungs and the absence of pulmonary physical signs; unless in the more prolonged cases it be the signs of œdema of the lungs. Litten found in two cases systolic or systolic and diastolic stenotic murmurs in the first and second intercostal spaces on the right or left side of the sternum. In prolonged cases the symptoms may be paroxysmal with marked remissions. Recovery may follow after the appearance of grave symptoms. There has been much and rather profitless discussion as to the degrees in which the symptoms are referable to asphyxia, to cerebral anæmia, or to interference with the coronary circulation. Doubtless all three factors are concerned, but the exact apportionment to each of its due share in the result is not easy, nor very important.

The diagnosis is based upon the sudden appearance of the symptoms, with a recognised source for an embolus. It is surprising to find in the larger statistics, as those of Bang and of Bunger, how often the thrombosis leading to fatal pulmonary embolism has been latent. Here the diagnosis cannot always be made; but in many cases it may be suspected, or be reasonably certain: as when the above-mentioned symptoms appear in puerperal women; during convalescence from infective fevers, as enteric fever, influenza, pneumonia; in marasmic and anæmic conditions, as phthisis, cancer, chlorosis; after surgical operations, especially those involving the pelvic organs; and in persons with varicose veins.

Even at autopsies the source for the embolus has sometimes been missed, but this has been due generally to inability or failure to make the necessary dissection of the peripheral veins, or to dislocation of the entire thrombus. Serre has published a series of cases of pulmonary embolism with latent thrombosis, showing the difficulties which may attend the discovery of the source, and the frequency with which patient search reveals the primary thrombus. The majority of plugs in the trunk or main divisions of the pulmonary artery, found in cases of sudden death, present the anatomical characters of emboli, associated perhaps with secondary thrombi; but there remain a certain number of cases of sudden or gradual death from primary thrombosis of the pulmonary artery, or from thrombosis extending into a main division from an embolus in a smaller branch (see Thrombosis, p. 208).

Bland embolism of medium-sized and small branches of the pulmonary artery in normal lungs, and without serious impairment of the pulmonary circulation, usually causes no symptoms and no changes in the parenchyma of the lungs. Even in lungs structurally altered, and with serious disturbances of the circulation, such embolism may be without effects. The explanation of the harmlessness of the majority of medium-sized and small pulmonary emboli is that the collateral circulation through the numerous and wide pulmonary capillaries is, under ordinary conditions, quite capable of supplying sufficient blood to an area whose artery is obstructed, to preserve its function and integrity; and that the pulmonary tissue, in contrast to the brain and the kidney, is relatively insusceptible to partial local anæmia.

Often enough, however, medium-sized and smaller branches of the pulmonary artery are occluded by emboli or thrombi under conditions where the pulmonary circulation is incapable of compensating the obstruction, and then the result is hæmorrhagic infarction of the lung. The most common and important of the conditions thus favouring the production of hæmorrhagic infarction is chronic passive congestion of the lungs from valvular or other disease of the left heart. It is especially during broken compensation of cardiac disease that hæmorrhagic infarction of the lungs occurs, sometimes indeed almost as a terminal event. Other favouring conditions are weakness of the right heart, fatty degeneration of the heart, general feebleness of the circulation, pulmonary emphysema, infective diseases.

The source of the embolus causing pulmonary hæmorrhagic infarction is oftener the right heart than a peripheral thrombus. Globular thrombi are often formed in the right auricular appendix and ventricular apex in uncompensated disease of the left heart, particularly of the mitral valve (see Thrombosis, p. 183). The infarction may be caused also by thrombosis of branches of the pulmonary artery, which are not infrequently the seat of fatty degeneration of the intima and of sclerosis in cardiac disease and in emphysema. Thrombi in larger branches often give rise to emboli in smaller ones.

Pulmonary infarcts are usually multiple, more frequent in the lower than the upper lobes, and occur on the right side somewhat oftener than on the left; corresponding thus with the distribution of emboli. Their size varies generally from that of a hazel-nut to a pigeon's egg; but it may be smaller or much larger, up to half or even an entire lobe. They are conical or of a wedge-shape, the base being at the pleura. Infarcts are rarely buried in the substance of the lung so as to be invisible from the pleural surface. Typical fresh infarcts are strikingly hard, sharply circumscribed, swollen, upon section dark red, almost black, smooth or slightly granular, and much drier than ordinary hæmorrhages. Examined microscopically, the air-cells, bronchi, and any loose connective tissue which may be included in the infarct are stuffed full of red corpuscles. The capillaries are distended, and in all but the freshest infarcts usually contain, in larger or smaller amount, hyaline thrombi, to which von Recklinghausen attaches much importance in the production of the infarct. Fibrin may be scanty in very recent infarcts, but in older ones it is abundant. The walls of the alveoli in the central part of the infarct are the seat of typical coagulative necrosis with fragmentation and solution of the nuclear chromatin. It is probable that the red corpuscles also undergo some kind of coagulative change, for otherwise it is difficult to explain the extremely hard consistence of the fresh infarct. It is possible that small pulmonary infarcts and very recent ones may occur without necrosis; but the ordinary ones are necrotic, and cannot therefore be removed by resolution; but, if the patient lives long enough and suppuration or gangrene of the infarct does not ensue, are substituted by cicatricial tissue (Willgerodt).

Ever since the first admirable description of hæmorrhagic infarcts of the lung by Laennec there has been considerable difference of opinion as to their explanation. The doctrine that they are usually caused by emboli, however, gradually gained general acceptance. This explanation has always had opponents, chiefly on the grounds that emboli often occur in the pulmonary arteries without infarction ; that infarction is not always associated with obstruction of the corresponding artery ; that some have believed that simple hæmorrhages may produce the same appearances, and that until recently attempts to produce pulmonary infarction experimentally have been without positive or at least sufficiently satisfactory results. Hamilton is strongly opposed to the embolic explanation, and attributes hæmorrhagic infarction of the lung to a simple apoplexy, resulting usually from rupture of the alveolar capillaries in chronic passive congestion. Grawitz, likewise, considers that embolism has nothing to do with the causation of pulmonary infarction, which he explains by hæmorrhage from newly-formed, richly-vascularised, peribronchial, subpleural, and interlobular connective tissue consecutive to the chronic bronchitis of cardiac and other diseases. He emphasises structural changes in the lung as an essential pre-requisite for infarction. Grawitz's attack especially has stimulated investigation which, in my opinion, has strengthened the supports of the embolic doctrine of hæmorrhagic infarction.

The evidence seems to me conclusive that pulmonary infarcts are caused by embolism and thrombosis of branches of the pulmonary artery. In the great majority of cases the arteries supplying the areas of infarction are plugged. Upon this point my experience is in accord with that of von Recklinghausen, Orth, Hanau, Oestreich, and many others. That these arterial plugs are secondary to the infarction is improbable, as hæmorrhages elsewhere, as well as undoubted ones in the lungs, often as they cause secondary venous thrombosis, rarely cause arterial thrombosis. Moreover, there is sometimes an interval of open artery between the plug and the infarct, a relation not observed with the undoubtedly secondary thrombosis of veins connected with the infarct, and not explicable on the assumption that the arterial thrombosis is secondary. The plug often has the characters of a riding embolus. Not a few of the plugs, however, are primary thrombi. The occasional occurrence of pulmonary infarction without obstruction in the arteries has as much, but no more, weight against the embolic explanation as the similar, and I believe quite as frequent, occurrence of splenic infarcts without embolism or thrombosis of the splenic arteries. Both the hæmorrhage and the necrosis of infarcts are essentially capillary phenomena, each being independent of the other ; and undoubtedly can occur, in ways little understood, in various regions, without plugging of the arteries.

The anatomical characters of pulmonary infarcts are essentially the same as those of hæmorrhagic infarcts of the spleen and other parts. The conical shape, the hard consistence, the peripheral situation, the coagulative necrosis are distinctive characters of pulmonary as of splenic infarcts. The necrosis cannot well be attributed to compression of the alveolar walls by the extravasated blood, for the capillaries in these are usually distended widely with blood. It has the general characters of the ischæmic necrosis of infarcts, except that it apparently occurs some-what later in the formation of the infarct and does not usually reach the periphery; phenomena which may be explained by the relative tolerance of the pulmonary tissue of partial ischæmia, and by a better peripheral circulation than is present in infarcts elsewhere.

Inasmuch as emboli do not ordinarily cause infarction in normal human lungs with vigorous circulation, it is not surprising to find that similar emboli under similar conditions do not cause infarction in the lungs of animals. It is not easy to reproduce experimentally in animals the conditions under which pulmonary infarcts occur in man; yet there have been several valuable contributions in recent years to the experi-mental production of pulmonary infarction: these have furnished an experimental basis, which, if not all that is to be desired, still marks a distinct advance for the embolic doctrine of hæmorrhagic infarction of the lung. Pulmonary infarcts, in all essential respects identical with those in human lungs, have been produced by experimental embolism or arterial occlusion by Cohnheim and Litten, Perl, Küttner, Mögling, Grawitz, Klebs, Gsell, Sgambati, Orth, Zahn, and Fujinami. Most of these experimental infarcts have been produced under conditions not very analogous to those of human infarcts; but the essential fact that typical hæmorrhagic infarction of the lung may be caused by arterial plugging has been experimentally established. Into the details of these experiments it is impossible here to enter.

Whether genuine hæmorrhagic infarcts of the lung may ever be caused by simple hæmorrhage from rupture of blood-vessels is perhaps an open question. At present this mode of their production seems to me undemonstrated and improbable, so that I hold that simple pulmonary apoplexies and genuine infarcts should be clearly dis-tinguished from each other. Neither the results of experimental introduction of blood into the trachea (Perl and Lippmann, Sommer-brodt, Nothnagel, Gluziński), nor the appearances of the lungs after undoubted bronchorrhagias, pneumorrhagias, and suicidal cutting of the trachea support the opinion that aspiration of blood from the trachea and bronchi causes genuine hæmorrhagic infarction. In only one of Sommerbrodt's numerous experiments was such infarction observed, and this he regards as accidental. The explanation of this exceptional result is probably the same as in Perl's experiment with thrombosis after venesection and anæmia.

I have seen, in two or three instances, nearly white or pale-red fresh anæmic infarcts in densely consolidated lungs.[1] Even when caused by bland emboli pulmonary infarcts are exposed to the invasion of bacteria from the air-passages; and such bacterial invasion may lead to sup-

---

[1] In very rare instances pulmonary infarcts are anæmic in consequence of extreme weak-ness of the circulation (87).

puration or gangrene.   Completely cicatrised pulmonary infarcts occur, but they are not common—life being usually cut short by the associated cardiac disease before the infarct is healed.

Hæmorrhagic infarction of the lungs may be entirely latent; often, however, the diagnosis can be made during life.   The affection may be ushered in by a chill or chilly sensation, increase of a usually existing dyspnœa, and localised pain in the side.   These symptoms are far from constant.   The characteristic symptom, although by no means patho-gnomonic, is bloody expectoration.   Profuse hæmoptysis was noted by Laennec, but is very rare.   The sputum contains dots and streaks of blood, or small dark coagula; or, more frequently, the blood is intimately mixed with the expectoration, which is in small masses and usually less viscid and darker red than that of pneumonia, although it may resemble the latter.   Blood may be present in the sputum for one or two weeks or even longer after the onset of the infarction.   It acquires after a time a brownish-red tint, and generally contains the pigmented epi-thelial cells usually seen in the sputum of chronic passive congestion. Circumscribed sero-fibrinous pleurisy is usually associated with pulmon-ary infarction.   Even with infarcts not more than four or five centi-metres in diameter the physical signs of consolidation and subcrepitant râles can sometimes be detected; usually in the posterior, lower parts of the lungs.   These signs are referable not only to the infarct, but also to the surrounding localised œdema and perhaps reactive pneumonia.   There may be moderate elevation of temperature.   When the characteristic bloody expectoration, together with signs of circumscribed consolidation, appears in the later stages of cardiac disease, or with peripheral venous thrombosis, there is generally little doubt of the diagnosis.   Yet similar expectoration may occur from simple bronchial hæmorrhages in intense passive congestion of the lungs without infarction.   The expectoration in cancer of the lungs may resemble that of pulmonary infarction.

The sudden appearance of pain in the chest, cough, and elevation of temperature, immediately after the hypodermic injection of undissolved preparations of mercury, is attributed to pulmonary embolism.   The symptoms disappear in a few days without serious consequences.   This complication has been rare in the experience of most of those who have employed this treatment of syphilis, but has led some to abandon the method.

The embolic pneumonias and abscesses caused by infective emboli are pyæmic manifestations, and have been considered in the article on "Pyæmia" in the first volume.

Splenic infarction.—Anæmic infarcts of the spleen, which are com-moner than the hæmorrhagic variety, are not usually in the recent state so pale and bloodless as those of the kidney; for the spleen is much richer in blood than the kidney, and in chronic passive congestion, during which the larger number of infarcts occur, the red pulp contains much blood outside of the vessels.   Many of these infarcts can be appro-priately described as mixed red and white infarcts.   Splenic infarcts vary greatly in size, but in general they are much larger than those occurring under the same conditions in the kidney, as comparatively large arteries in the spleen break up into numerous small terminal twigs. Averaging perhaps two to six centimetres in diameter, a single infarct may occupy one-half or more of the spleen. The recent infarcts are hard, swollen, and more or less wedge-shaped, with the base at the capsule, which is often coated with fibrin; or in older cases is thickened and adherent by fibrous tissue. The great majority are caused by emboli from the left heart or the aorta; but both hæmorrhagic and pale splenic infarcts occur without arterial occlusion; especially in certain acute infective diseases; oftenest in relapsing fever, but also in typhus, enteric fever, cholera, and septicæmia. The causation of the latter is unknown. Ponfick attributes them to venous thrombosis, which may be the cause of the hæmorrhagic infarcts; but it is difficult to understand how it can produce the pale anæmic infarcts. Bland infarcts are mostly absorbed and substituted by pigmented, occasionally calcified, scars, which when numerous may cause a lobular deformity of the spleen.

Splenic infarction is often entirely latent. Of the symptoms attributed to it chills and elevation of temperature belong usually to the accompanying acute or chronic endocarditis. Swelling of the spleen, which pertains to chronic passive congestion, is produced also by infarcts. The most diagnostic value attaches to the sudden appearance of pain in the region of the spleen, perhaps increased by lying on the left side, by deep inspiration, and by pressure; and to a perisplenitic friction rub, which can sometimes be detected. These symptoms are not very certain diagnostic points; but when they occur with some manifest source for a splenic embolus, and perhaps with recognised embolism in other organs, they justify a strong suspicion of splenic infarction.

Renal infarction.—There have been a few instances, especially after traumatism, of nearly total necrosis of a kidney from thrombosis of the renal artery, combined usually with thrombosis of the vein. Usually plugging of the main artery leads to multiple infarction with intervening intact areas. The capsular arteries suffice for the preservation of at least a narrow outer rim of renal tissue.

Renal infarcts are nearly always anæmic, in the recent state somewhat swollen, and of an opaque pale yellowish colour, with the base of the wedge just beneath the capsule and the apex toward the hilum, most frequently near the boundary between the pyramid and cortex. Three zones can often be distinguished :—the main central yellowish white mass of necrotic tissue ; next to this a narrow yellow zone of fatty cells, nuclear fragments, and disintegrating leucocytes ; and an outer, irregular, variable rim of hyperæmia and hæmorrhage which belongs partly to the infarct and partly to the surrounding tissue. The hæmorrhage may extend a variable distance into the infarct, and in very rare instances genuine hæmorrhagic infarcts occur in the kidney. Numerous scars from old infarcts may produce a form of atrophic kidney to which the epithet embolic is applicable. Thorel finds that a limited regeneration of the epithelium and even of uriniferous tubules may occur in healing renal infarcts.

Very large infarcts may so stretch the renal capsule as to induce severe pain. In a case diagnosed by Traube an infarct two inches in diameter, projecting well above the surface, caused intense pain and tenderness in the region of the infarcted kidney, with extension of the pain into the corresponding thigh. With the ordinary small infarcts pain is not usually a prominent symptom. The chief sign of diagnostic value is the sudden appearance of blood in the urine in association with disease of the left heart, aortic aneurysm, or other recognised source for a renal embolus. The amount of blood is usually only moderate or evident by microscopical examination of the urine. It is to be remembered that chronic passive congestion of the kidney is itself one of the many causes of hæmaturia.

Infective emboli, which are often capillary in size, cause multiple, often miliary abscesses in the kidney. This is the hæmatogenous variety of acute suppurative nephritis which occurs often in acute infective endocarditis and other forms of pyæmia. Here the pyuria and other renal symptoms are usually of less consequence than those of general infection.

Embolism and Thrombosis of the mesenteric and intestinal arteries.—Thrombosis of the mesenteric veins, which causes lesions and symptoms identical with those following embolism of the mesenteric arteries, has been considered in the preceding article (p. 218). Since Virchow's first description of embolism of the superior mesenteric artery, in 1847, at least seventy cases have been reported of embolism or thrombosis of the mesenteric arteries. The affection, although not common, occurs often enough and is of such gravity as to be of considerable clinical interest. In Watson's collection of cases there are eight which occurred within a single year in Boston. The casuistic literature upon the subject is fairly extensive. The articles of Litten and of Faber contain reports of most of the cases published up to 1875. The principal clinical features were carefully studied by Gerhardt and by Kussmaul in 1863-64. The papers of Watson and of Elliot in 1894-95 refer to about fifty reported cases, of which they have analysed those with satisfactory clinical histories with special reference to surgical treatment. The effects of occlusion of the mesenteric arteries have been experimentally studied by Beckmann, Cohn, Litten, Faber, Welch and Mall, and Tangl and Harley.

The principal conclusions drawn by Mall and myself from our experiments have been stated already in the discussion of the collateral circulation, and of hæmorrhagic infarction following embolism (pp. 239 and 245). It may here be repeated that, according to our experiments, the blood which produces the hæmorrhagic infarction enters by the anastomosing arteries and not by reflux from the veins ; that the hæmorrhage cannot be explained by any demonstrable change in the vascular walls, but is the result of retardation and stasis of the circulation and clumping of red corpuscles in the veins and capillaries, attributable in large part in cases of arterial obstruction to reduction or loss of lateral pulsation of the blood-current; that the ischæmia is increased by the tonic contraction of the intestinal muscle which follows for two or three hours' closure of the superior mesenteric artery; and that the sudden and complete shutting off of the direct arterial supply to a loop of intestine 5 to 10 ctm. in length is followed by hæmorrhage and necrosis of the loop, even when the vessels at each end of the loop are open. These results we obtained by experimentation upon dogs, but there is no reason to suppose that they do not apply to human beings. With the exception of Cohn, the other experimenters explain the infarction by regurgitant flow from the veins and alterations in the vascular walls.

The majority of the cases of hæmorrhagic infarction of the intestine have been due to embolism of the mesenteric arteries, the source of the embolus being usually the left heart, sometimes an atheromatous aorta or aortic aneurysm, and in one instance a thrombus in the pulmonary veins caused by gangrene of the lungs (Virchow). Several cases have been caused by autochthonous thrombosis resulting from arterio-sclerosis, aneurysm, pressure, or the extension of a thrombus from the adjacent aorta. It is probable that a certain number of the cases reported as embolic were referable to primary thrombosis of the mesenteric arteries, as no source for an embolus could be discovered, and the plugs in some of these instances were fresh adherent thrombi. As has been shown in the preceding article, primary thrombi may form in arteries which are free from atheroma or other chronic disease.[1]

In the great majority of the cases the obstruction was in the superior mesenteric artery. The few scattered instances of embolism or thrombosis of the inferior mesenteric artery indicate that this also may, very rarely, cause incomplete hæmorrhagic infarction of the corresponding part of the intestine, but that the collateral circulation here is better, and the lesions likely to consist only in small hæmorrhages in the intestinal mucosa. The inferior mesenteric artery may be obliterated without any manifest disturbance in the structure or function of the part of the intestine supplied by it.

The obstruction may be situated in the main stem or in any of the branches of the superior mesenteric artery. Intestinal infarction has been associated with embolism of the larger branches oftener than with that of the main stem. As the anastomoses through the arterial arches are so free, obstruction of single small branches is without mechanical effects. There have, however, been several instances of intestinal infarction caused by multiple emboli or extensive thrombosis of small branches of the superior mesenteric artery.

[1] Litten has reported two cases of hæmorrhagic infarction of the intestine from thrombosis caused by what he calls "latticed endarteritis" (gitterformige Endarteriitis) of the mesenteric arteries. So far as I can learn he has not furnished the fuller description which he promised in his article of nine years ago. Without such description there is room for the suspicion that Litten has mistaken the latticework markings sometimes seen after detachment of an adherent thrombus for a special form of endarteritis. It does not appear from his article that he has observed this "latticed endarteritis" except after removing adherent thrombi.

Intestinal infarction is not the imperative result of occlusion of the superior mesenteric artery, as infarction is of occlusion of branches of the splenic and renal arteries, and of the basal cerebral. Both the trunk and the principal branches of this artery may be gradually closed without serious effects. Tiedemann and Virchow have found the superior mesenteric artery completely obliterated by old, firm thrombi or connective tissue without any lesions in the jejunum or ileum. The most remarkable case is that of Chiene, who found in a woman sixty-five years old, with aneurysm of the abdominal aorta, complete obliteration of the cœliac axis and both mesenteric arteries, with an adequate collateral circulation through the greatly distended extra-peritoneal anastomosing arteries. In a number of instances plugging of large branches of the superior mesenteric artery has caused no more than hyperæmia and superficial ecchymoses, without genuine infarction of the intestine.

The rapid and complete closure of the superior mesenteric artery, however, is followed with great regularity, probably constantly, by hæmorrhagic infarction of the intestine. There have been several instances in which embolism or thrombosis of the trunk of this artery has caused hæmorrhagic infarction extending from the lower part of the duodenum into the transverse colon (Oppolzer, Pieper, Faber, Kaufmann), as in the experimental cases. More frequently the infarction is in the lower part of the jejunum and the ileum, corresponding to the occlusion of a principal branch or of several branches supplying this region. The infarction corresponds in general to the area of distribution of the plugged arteries, but it may occupy only a part of this area. In several instances a single small loop or several loops with intervening normal intestine have been infarcted.

As already intimated, the infarction may be complete or only partial. When completely infarcted, the wall of the affected intestine is thickened, œdematous, of a dark red colour from infiltration with blood and covered with lustreless peritoneum. The margins of the infarct are often sharply marked but may pass gradually into the normal bowel. The mucous membrane is necrotic, often defective, and may be coated with a diphtheritic exudate. In a few instances the intestine has been gangrenous over considerable areas, without typical hæmorrhagic infarction, or with the hæmorrhagic appearance adjacent to the gangrene. The lumen of the intestine contains black tarry blood. There is bloody fluid in the peritoneal cavity, and usually a fibrinous, sometimes a fibrino-purulent exudate on the peritoneum covering the infarction ; and there may be general peritonitis. The mesentery is succulent and hæmorrhagic, usually in patches, exceptionally in the form of large flat masses of extravasated blood. Areas of fat-necrosis may be present in the mesentery. The mesenteric veins are distended and the mesenteric glands often swollen and hæmorrhagic. Various intestinal bacteria, most commonly the colon bacillus, may make their way into the peritoneal cavity through the necrotic wall. Flexner and I have reported an instance of hæmorrhagic infarction of the jejunum in which evidences of pneumo-peritonitis, supposed to be due to perforation, existed during life. At the autopsy, made six hours after death, a large amount of gas was found in the peritoneal cavity without perforation. The B. aerogenes capsulatus was present in large numbers in the peritoneal exudate. This case demonstrates the generation of gas in the closed peritoneal cavity. In the intestinal mucosa were gas-blebs which were observed also in one of Faber's cases and in Jürgens' case of intestinal infarction.

The hæmorrhagic infarction is by no means always so completely formed as that just described. There may be no hæmorrhages in the mesentery. The extravasation of blood may be limited to the mucosa, or even to the submucosa, as in one of Ponfick's cases. In an instance of nearly complete thrombosis of the trunk of the superior mesenteric artery, reported by Councilman, there were paralysis, great distension and ecchymoses of the small intestine, but no infarction. Between mere venous hyperæmia with scattered, superficial hæmorrhages, and complete necrosis and infarction, there are all gradations, the controlling factors being doubtless the rapidity and extent of the arterial occlusion and the vigour of the general circulation.

There have been two or three instances in which the anatomical picture of hæmorrhagic infarction of the intestine has been present without discovery of any obstruction in the corresponding arteries or veins. Lycett reports an observation of hæmorrhagic infarction of the small intestine in an infant one month old without discoverable cause.

Hæmorrhagic infarction of the bowel may be insidious in its onset and course; and, in patients profoundly prostrated or with cerebral symptoms, it may occur without the attention of the physician being drawn to any abdominal trouble. Usually, however, the onset is abrupt, and grave intestinal symptoms are present. In the majority of cases, severe colicky pain and abdominal tenderness, either without distinct localisation or most marked near the umbilicus, are prominent and usually the first symptoms. The pain at the beginning is perhaps attributable to the violent, tonic spasm of the intestine which follows sudden occlusion of the superior mesenteric artery. After a few hours this spasm gives place to complete paralysis of the affected part of the bowel, and then the pain may be referable to peritonitis. The local anæmia, hæmorrhage, and necrosis seem, however, quite sufficient to account for the pain. Vomiting, which often becomes bloody and occasionally fæcal, is also usually an early and persistent symptom. By far the most characteristic symptom, which is present in the majority of cases but not in all, is the passage of tarry blood in the stools, which are frequently diarrhœal, and sometimes have the odour of carrion. In nearly all cases there is hæmorrhage into the bowel, but the blood is not always voided. Symptoms of intestinal obstruction—tympanitic distension of the abdomen, fæcal vomiting and obstipation—are in some cases prominent, and are readily explained by the complete paralysis of the infarcted bowel. The subnormal temperature, pallor, cold sweats and collapse,

which appear in most cases, are explicable in part by the intestinal
hæmorrhage, and in part by the shock of the destructive lesion. The
sensation of a palpable tumour, referable to a collection of blood in the
mesentery or to the infarcted bowel, has been noted in only three or
four cases.

The chief emphasis for purposes of diagnosis is to be laid upon the
occurrence of intestinal hæmorrhage, not explicable by independent
disease of the intestine or by portal obstruction, in combination with
other symptoms mentioned, and with the recognition of some source
for an embolus, perhaps of embolic manifestations elsewhere. In the
majority of cases the diagnosis has been intestinal obstruction, or acute
peritonitis. The symptoms closely resemble those of intussusception, in
which hæmorrhage from the bowel, although generally less abundant
than with embolism of the superior mesenteric artery, is common.
Fortunately the distinction of hæmorrhagic infarction from intestinal
obstruction is not of much practical importance ; for if the symptoms and
condition of the patient warrant it, an exploratory laparotomy is indicated in both conditions. Elliot, by the successful resection of four feet
of infarcted intestine, has brought hæmorrhagic infarction of the intestine
into the surgeon's domain.

The prognosis is grave ; and with complete infarction and necrosis of
the intestine it is almost necessarily fatal, unless surgical relief be available. Watson estimates that in about one-sixth of the cases the location and extent of the infarction are suitable for resection of the bowel.
It is impossible to say at present to what extent the prognosis of
hæmorrhagic infarction of the intestine is favourably modified by the new
possibilities of surgical interference. Gordon has successfully resected
two feet of infarcted intestine. This and Elliot's case are the only two
in which this operation has been performed ; so far as I am aware.

, When the infarction is incomplete, and is limited chiefly to the
inner coats of the intestine, recovery may doubtless take place. Cohn,
Moos, Lereboullet, and Finlayson have reported instances of recovery
after symptoms indicative of hæmorrhagic infarction. Packard attributed cicatricial areas found in the mesentery of an old man dead of
rupture of the ascending aorta to healed infarction ; but no previous history was obtained, and Packard's interpretation does not seem to me
to be free from doubt. Death may occur within 20 to 48 hours after the
onset, or the duration may be protracted over several days. Karcher
has reported the survival of a patient with mitral stenosis for two
months after the complete occlusion of the superior mesenteric artery by
an embolus, the symptoms being sufficiently characteristic to have permitted a probable diagnosis during life.

Intestinal ulcers due to embolism or thrombosis constitute a distinct
class, which has been studied especially by Ponfick, Parenski, and Nothnagel. Parenski relates an instance of operation for intestinal stricture,
which at the autopsy was found to be caused by cicatrisation of an ulcer
due to embolism of a branch of the superior mesenteric artery. Much

more common are ulcers caused by infective emboli lodging in the small arteries and capillaries in the intestinal wall; they are observed especially in acute ulcerative endocarditis and pyæmia. These emboli cause hæmorrhages, necroses, and miliary abscesses with resulting ulceration. The ulcers are usually multiple, sometimes numerous, and situated in the small intestine and cæcum. The intestinal ulcers occasionally associated with degenerative multiple neuritis are referred by Minkowski and Lorenz to thrombosis caused by disease of the small arteries, which has been repeatedly observed in this form of neuritis.

Embolism and Thrombosis of the thoracic aorta.—Unless there be some abnormal narrowing or obstruction of the aorta, it is hardly possible for an embolus to lodge in this vessel, except at the ostium or the bifurcation. An exception to this rule may result from the detachment of a large aneurysmal clot, which, as in three cases of abdominal aneurysm reported by Bristowe, may block the aorta at or just below the mouth of the aneurysm.

I know of but three instances of embolism of the mouth of the aorta— two reported by Cohn with instantaneous death, and one by Reid in which the patient lived an hour and a half after the first symptoms of partial obstruction.

In a very few instances the lumen of an atheromatous thoracic aorta has been seriously encroached upon, or even obliterated, by thrombotic masses. Such cases have been reported by Trost, Tewat, Carville, Armet, Chvostek, Jaurand, and Pitt. The thrombus may occupy the ascending, the transverse, or the descending aorta, and may occlude the mouths of the left carotid and subclavian arteries. If there remain a sufficient channel for the blood, as in Pitt's case, there is no resulting circulatory disturbance; otherwise there may be paralysis, œdema, gangrene of the lower extremities, and, if the left subclavian is obliterated, of the corresponding upper extremity.

Bochdalek and Lüttich have each described an instance of occlusion of the aorta in infants by the extension of an obliterating thrombus from a dilated ductus Botalli. Far more frequent is stenosis or atresia of the aorta at or near the attachment of this duct, due usually to persistence of the isthmus aortæ, as was first shown by Rokitansky. Of this latter condition about 100 instances have been recorded.

Embolism and Thrombosis of the abdominal aorta.—Graham in 1814 referred to a museum specimen in Glasgow, which had belonged to Allan Burns, of occlusion of the abdominal aorta just above the bifurcation by old laminated coagulum extending into the iliacs. I have found fifty-nine subsequent reports of occlusion of the abdominal aorta by embolism or thrombosis, and have seen references (which I have not consulted) to six or seven other cases.[1] I have not included in this list the detachment of clots from abdominal aneurysms, although Bristowe's three cases

---

[1] I have not included von Weismayr's case (*Wiener med. Presse*, 1894, p. 1774), as it was reported while the patient was living, and in the discussion some doubt was expressed as to the diagnosis; nor the brief mention made by Teleky, at the same time, of a similar observation.

demonstrate that this may occasion the same symptoms. The monographs and articles of Meynard, Cammareri, Selter, Roussel, Charrier and Apert, and Heiligenthal contain references to or reports of forty-seven cases; to these I have added twelve published cases not mentioned by them. The references are at the end of this article.

Three of the patients were living at the time of the reports, and in two fatal cases there was no autopsy. In the remaining fifty-four the plug occupied the lower end of the aorta and extended a variable distance into the arteries below. In thirty-one the plug did not reach higher than the inferior mesenteric artery; in ten the upper extremity lay between the inferior mesenteric and the renals; in three between the renals and the superior mesenteric; in two between the latter and the cœliac axis; in one just below the pillars of the diaphragm, and in seven the length of the plug is not stated. The upper part was often conical; so that, when the plug extended higher than the inferior mesenteric, it was often not obliterating until at or below this artery. In the great majority of cases only the last, or the last two, lumbar arteries were blocked by the thrombus. In several instances a thrombus, either independent or continuous with that in the aorta, occupied the lumbar, the mesenteric, the renal, or other branches of the aorta. In all instances the thrombus extended into the common iliacs, and in many into arteries lower down, sometimes even as far as the posterior tibial, the end being usually lower on one side than on the other.

It is difficult, indeed impossible, from the published descriptions, which are only too often incomplete and unsatisfactory, to determine accurately how many of the cases were referable to embolism and how many to thrombosis. Essentially similar cases have been interpreted differently in this respect by different observers. The plug was usually adherent, and only in relatively few cases were its anatomical characters such (or at least so described) as to indicate positively its nature as embolus or primary thrombus. The majority of cases with sudden or rapid invasion of characteristic symptoms were associated with cardiac disease, or disease of the upper part of the aorta; and would, therefore, naturally be interpreted as embolic. Still in many of these no satisfactory source for a large embolus was demonstrated. Some cases not less abrupt in onset were without any affection of the heart or of the aorta above the plug. The sudden appearance of symptoms of obstruction of the aorta, although strongly indicative of embolism, are not decisive upon this point. Barth, in 1848, described a case of obstruction of the aorta by a cylindrical thrombus extending from the superior mesenteric artery to the bifurcation, and leaving only a narrow channel for the circulation of the blood. There were no circulatory disturbances. If this narrow channel had been suddenly closed at one point, as might readily happen, the symptoms would probably have been those of embolism. It is evident that aortic thromboses secondary to only partly obliterative emboli riding the bifurcation of the aorta, or to emboli or thrombi in the iliacs or lower arteries, may occasion symptoms like those of primary thrombosis of the aorta. There are several instances of such secondary thrombosis of the aorta in my collection of cases.

Without much confidence in the accuracy of the classification in several instances, I have divided the fifty-nine cases into forty-five referable to embolism of the aorta at the bifurcation, and fourteen due to thrombosis; of the latter, seven were primary, six secondary to embolism of the iliacs, or possibly the femoral, and one to thrombosis of the arteries of the extremities. The source of the aortic embolus is believed to have been the heart in thirty-five cases; aneurysm of the ascending aorta in one; pressure of a tumour on the aorta in two; atheroma of the thoracic aorta in one; in six it was undetermined. The heart was found to be normal at the autopsy in eleven of the fifty-three cases; and in seven both the heart and the aorta above the plug were normal.

Mitral stenosis existed in twenty cases (two of these being caused by thrombi extending from the left auricle into the ventricle), acute mitral endocarditis in three, mitral endocarditis, not further defined, in four, mitral insufficiency without stenosis in one, thrombus in the left auricle without valvular disease in one, thrombi in the left ventricle, mostly without valvular disease, in eight, and large aortic vegetations in one.

The most interesting point in the etiology of plugging of the abdominal aorta, so far as it is permissible to draw conclusions from so few instances, is that nearly thirty-four per cent of the cases were associated with mitral stenosis. In many of these the stenosis was extreme. The question at once arises of the source of the embolus in these cases, for it cannot be supposed that an embolus large enough to occlude the lower end of the aorta could pass through the contracted mitral orifice. Some of the cases may be explained by a smaller embolus caught at the aortic bifurcation, or in an artery lower down, with secondary thrombosis of the aorta; but the sudden onset of motor and sensory paraplegia and of cessation of pulsation in both femoral arteries in a large number of cases seems to demand abrupt stoppage of the circulation through both common iliacs. A few observers who have realised the difficulty here presented have assumed that a large thrombus had formed in the left ventricle and been detached without leaving any trace behind; for only in two or three of the cases with mitral stenosis was there any evidence of a thrombus in the left ventricle or the aorta above the plug. This explanation must be regarded as purely hypothetical. The coexistence in a number of the cases of infarctions of the spleen, kidney, or brain has seemed to some writers strong evidence in favour of the embolic nature of the aortic plug. It is possible that the explanation even of the cases with acute bilateral symptoms referable to aortic obstruction and associated with marked mitral stenosis may be the lodgment of a small embolus followed by thrombosis of the aorta. Although in the classification above given I have placed nearly all the cases with mitral stenosis under embolism, I am nevertheless not disinclined in spite of the rapid onset of the symptoms, and frequently

coexistent infarctions, to interpret many of them as primary thromboses
of the aorta. The circulatory conditions with extreme, uncompensated
mitral stenosis seem favourable to the occurrence of arterial thrombosis; and, if this view be accepted for the plugging of the abdominal
aorta, the question arises whether thrombi frequently present in smaller
arteries in association with this form of valvular disease may not oftener
be primary than is generally supposed.

In a few cases congenital narrowing of the aorta was noted. In
three instances plugging of the abdominal aorta was associated with
embolism or thrombosis of arteries of an upper extremity. Coincident
thrombosis of the vena cava, iliac, or femoral veins was observed in a few
cases. In Jürgens' patient there was hæmorrhagic infarction of the
intestine. In several instances hæmorrhages were found at autopsy in
the mucous membranes of the bladder and uterus. Herter, in his experiments in my laboratory with ligation of the abdominal aorta in rabbits,
found hæmorrhagic infarction of the uterus to be so common a result of
this operation that, when it was desired to keep the animals alive for any
length of time, we abandoned the use of female rabbits for Stenson's experiment. It does not appear, however, that in human beings hæmorrhage
of the uterus is a common sequel of occlusion of the abdominal aorta.[1]
It is probable that if search were made in suitable cases in human beings
who have died of aortic thrombosis or embolism, the interesting muscular
changes described by Herter in the experimental cases would be found;
as similar changes had been previously discovered by Litten in an
instance of occlusion of the right iliac and femoral arteries. The most
important of these muscular alterations are vacuolisation, proliferation
of the sarcolemma nuclei, atrophy, and fatty and pseudo-waxy
degenerations.

Plugging of the abdominal aorta has occurred most frequently in the
course of chronic cardiac or arterial disease; but in some instances it
took place during or after an acute infective disease, as acute articular
rheumatism, puerperal fever, erysipelas, during convalescence from
enteric fever (Forgues), and after pneumonia (Leyden).

Of the fifty-nine cases thirty were females, twenty-seven males, and
in two the sex is not stated. Seventeen were between twenty and
thirty years of age, twelve between thirty and forty, eight between forty
and fifty, thirteen between fifty and sixty, one was nineteen, one sixty-
one, and the ages of seven are not given.[2] Marked atheromatous
changes in the arteries were noted in fourteen cases. Occlusion of the

---

[1] It may here be mentioned that Herxheimer, Popoff, and Chiari have each described an
instance of hæmorrhagic infarction of the uterus after extensive bilateral plugging of the
vessels supplying this organ.

[2] In Luttich's case already mentioned (p. 273) of thrombosis of the aorta in an infant
fourteen days old, a thrombus beginning 4 cm. below the insertion of the ductus Botalli
extended into the iliac arteries. Charrier and Apert include in their collection of reports of
thrombosis of the abdominal aorta two cases from Allibert's thesis of 1828, one three, and
the other three and a half years old, with gangrene of one leg. I have not counted these
three cases in my list.

abdominal aorta by embolism or thrombosis, therefore, is not especially a senile affection.

When one considers the manifold conditions under which the abdominal aorta may become partly or completely plugged by embolism or by primary or secondary thrombosis, it is evident that there can be no general uniformity of symptoms. The plug may be so situated as to interfere with the circulation in one leg more than in the other. Diversities arise from variations in the collateral circulation in different cases. Still the majority of patients have presented a well-characterised group of symptoms. In the larger number of cases the onset has been acute, in the minority insidious and gradual. The symptoms have often appeared simultaneously in both legs, but there may be a short or a long interval between the invasion of one and that of the other leg. In the more acute cases the leading symptoms are pain in the legs,—sometimes in the loins and abdomen, sudden or rapidly manifested paraplegia, anæsthesia of the legs, absence of femoral pulsation, and phenomena of mortification extending from the feet upward. In several instances the patients, while walking, have been seized with excruciating pain in the legs, and have fallen paralysed to the ground. The pain is often atrocious and more or less paroxysmal. There may be tenderness on pressure over the occluded aorta. In a few cases pain has not been a prominent symptom.

Although the paraplegia has been repeatedly described as instantaneous in its appearance, it is to be inferred from the histories of carefully observed patients that at least a short interval of time and sometimes several hours and even days elapse before it is complete. In forty-four cases in which there are definite statements about the motor power, there was complete or nearly complete paraplegia in twenty-four; incomplete paralysis of both lower extremities, described in some instances merely as weakness, in ten; paralysis of only one leg in five, and no paralysis in five. The paralysis seems to be usually of the flaccid variety, but in some cases the paralysed muscles are stiff. In Barié's patient the paralysed legs were completely rigid, and it may be inferred that a condition analogous to rigor mortis had set in. With complete paralysis the reflexes and electrical excitability are abolished. Paralysis of the bladder and rectum, with retention of urine and involuntary evacuations, was observed in several cases, but not in the majority.

Of the cases with satisfactory histories in only two was there no disturbance of sensation. In some there was only numbness or some reduction of sensation, but in most there was definite anæsthesia, extending in some instances no higher than the knee,—more frequently to the middle or upper third of the thigh, and in two cases as high as Poupart's ligament. There was sometimes complete analgesia, which, however, did not exclude sensations of spontaneous pain in the legs. In many cases, however, there was hyperalgesia, either in the anæsthetic area or above it.

The symptom of greatest diagnostic value is absence of pulsation in the arteries of the lower extremities. In three or four instances it was determined that the abdominal aorta below the navel was pulseless. Wilbur observed excessive aortic pulsation above the obstruction. The legs become cold, and their surface temperature may even fall below that of the room (Browne, Manz). Absence of bleeding upon incision and of reactive hyperæmia after application of heat have been noted. The skin, at first pale, soon acquires a livid mottling, and the superficial veins may be dilated. Œdema of one or both legs and cutaneous hæmorrhages are recorded in some of the histories. If the patient lives long enough gangrene usually ensues, and it may be manifest within twenty-seven to forty-eight hours. Gangrene was bilateral in at least twenty-four cases, and unilateral in seventeen. The extent of the gangrene varied greatly in different cases, being sometimes limited to the foot, sometimes reaching the middle of the thigh, and, in Bell's patient, involving the scrotum. Tympanites, diarrhœa, and albuminuria are common. Exceptional symptoms are the appearance of blood in the urine or stools, hæmatemesis, and priapism. Bedsores appeared in many cases, and may appear within a few days from the onset.

Death may occur within twenty-four hours from the beginning of the attack. Fourteen patients died within the first four days, with collapse and rapid, weak, usually irregular pulse. There may be marked improvement in the initial symptoms either in one or in both legs. The larger number of patients die after a variable interval, which may extend over several weeks or even months, from gangrene, decubitus, and sepsis.

Of the deviations from the type may be especially mentioned incomplete manifestation of symptoms on one or both sides, transitory affection of one leg, limitation of the symptoms to one lower extremity only (four cases), and affection of one leg followed after days, weeks, or months by that of the other (six cases). The two cases reported by Barth and by Jean are considered particularly characteristic of slowly forming thrombosis. Here the first symptoms were chiefly numbness and intermittent claudication, which, after a long interval, deepened into paraplegia without gangrene.

All but three cases terminated fatally, more frequently from the remote effects than from the immediate shock of occlusion of the aorta. The three instances of survival with marked amelioration of all the symptoms are reported by Gull, Chvostek, and Nunez. These cases began acutely with severe pains, paraplegia, disturbances of sensation, coldness and lividity of the lower extremities. The femoral pulse disappeared completely in Gull's and in Nunez's cases, but in Chvostek's it could still be felt, although it was feeble. In Chvostek's patient patches of superficial gangrene appeared ; but in the other two cases there was no gangrene. Nunez reports that after a year and a half there was no return of the femoral pulse on either side.

Since the demonstration by Schiffer and Weil, confirmed by Ehrlich and Brieger, Spronck, Herter, and others, that the paraplegia which follows immediately or very shortly after ligation of the abdominal aorta just below the renal arteries in rabbits (Stenson's experiment) is due to ischæmia of the lumbar cord, many have assumed that the same explanation applies to the paraplegia in human beings after occlusion of the abdominal aorta. If the rabbit's aorta be tied for an hour, and the ligature be then removed, the paraplegia and paralysis of the bladder and rectum are permanent, the gray matter of the lumbar cord undergoes necrosis, and a genuine myelitis affecting chiefly the gray but also the white matter ensues. The same experiment gives negative results with the cat and usually with the dog. In view of the great interest of the subject, it is, to say the least, remarkable how few of the reports of autopsies on persons dead of embolism or thrombosis of the aorta have anything to say about the condition of the spinal cord. Roussel and Heiligenthal observed no macroscopic changes in the spinal cord. In Bell's and Barié and du Castel's cases the cord was microscopically normal, save congestion in the latter. Broca, Legroux, and Malbranc noted with the naked eye changes in colour, from which no definite conclusions can be drawn. The only detailed report of a microscopical examination of the cord is that of Helbing, who found, in the lumbar region of a man who lived thirty-nine days after embolism of the abdominal aorta, degeneration of the anterior and posterior nerve-roots, more marked on one side than the other; and degenerations in the cord for the most part explicable by the changes in the nerve-roots. The lesions of the cord were quite unlike those found in experimental cases, and are interpreted by Helbing as essentially analogous to those after amputation, and not referable to ischæmia of the cord.

As the matter now stands, there are no direct observations to support the opinion that the paraplegia following embolism or thrombosis of the abdominal aorta in human beings is caused by ischæmia of the cord, so that the old explanation which refers it to ischæmia of the peripheral nerves and muscles has the most in its favour. The question of the possibility of this mode of production of paraplegia, however, seems to me still open, and it is to be hoped that hereafter fatal cases of this rare condition will not be reported without satisfactory microscopical examination of the spinal cord. The anatomical investigations of Kadyi and of Williamson at least do not exclude the possibility that the lumbar cord in human beings is dependent to a considerable extent for its blood-supply upon the lumbar arteries.

The diagnosis of ischæmic paraplegia from spinal paraplegia can generally be made without difficulty by the absence of femoral pulsation, by the coldness and lividity of the extremities, and by the occurrence of gangrene in the former.

Embolism of arteries of the extremities.—Of the arteries of the extremities the popliteal and the femoral are the most frequent recipients of emboli. The results of embolism of arteries supplying the extremities are essentially similar to those of arterial thrombosis, which have already been considered (p. 206). The modifications resulting from the sudden advent of embolism are sufficiently self-evident. There may be severe pain at the moment of impaction and at the site of lodgment of the embolus. The general principles involved in the differentiation of embolism from thrombosis have been presented under Diagnosis (p. 253).

Hepatic infarction.—As the effects of infective emboli in branches of the portal vein and of the hepatic artery have been considered elsewhere in this work (vol. i. p. 601, and vol. v. p. 123), only the possible mechanical effects of hepatic emboli require consideration here. Although the intrahepatic branches of the hepatic artery and of the portal vein are terminal vessels, their capillary communications are so abundant that, as a rule, embolism or thrombosis of the hepatic vessels causes no interference with the circulation in the liver. Experiments of Cohnheim and Litten and of Doyon and Dufourt have demonstrated that complete interruption of the circulation through the hepatic arteries of the rabbit and the dog is followed by necrosis of the liver. Chiari has observed an instance of necrosis of the entire liver caused by closure of the trunk of the hepatic artery beyond the origin of the pyloric branch.

In rare instances, and under circumstances at present not thoroughly understood, a condition somewhat resembling hæmorrhagic infarction may follow plugging, either by an embolus or a thrombus, of branches of the portal vein. Instances of this occurrence in human beings have been reported by Osler, Rattone, Klebs, Lubarsch, Köhler, Pitt, Zahn, and Chiari; the last-named having seen 17 cases, of which 15 were embolic. A somewhat similar condition was observed by Arnold after retrograde embolism of the hepatic vein. Pale wedge-shaped areas have been observed, but in most of the cases there were circumscribed dark red or reddish-brown wedge-shaped, rectangular or irregular areas

Köhler and Chiari found that the red colour is due mainly to dilatation of the intralobular capillaries, with atrophy of the liver-cells. Genuine coagulative necrosis is not present. The affected areas are patches of circumscribed red atrophy rather than typical hæmorrhagic infarcts. Zahn observed the same condition in a human liver after plugging of portal branches, and reproduced it experimentally by emboli of sterilised mercury injected into mesenteric veins. In his experimental cases the change in the liver did not begin until the eighth day, and was distinct after thirty-five days. It is probable that the areas do not undergo cicatrisation.

Rattone's theory, based upon experiments, that occlusion of branches of both the hepatic artery and portal vein is essential for the production of infarction of the liver, is not supported by the observations in human beings. Klebs, whose two cases followed injury of the liver, as was true also of Lubarsch's observation, attributes the infarction to extensive capillary thrombosis. Köhler considers that the essential factor is combination of occlusion of branches of the portal vein with obstruction to the return flow from the hepatic veins. Chiari believes that the second factor, to be added to the plugging of portal branches, is feeble flow through the hepatic artery, from weakness of the general circulation. Wooldridge, by injecting coagulative tissüe-extracts into the jugular vein of the dog, caused extensive clotting of blood in the portal vein and its branches, followed by numerous hæmorrhages and necroses in the liver; but the interpretation of these results as actual infarctions does not seem to me certain, inasmuch as these extracts in toxic doses produce a hæmorrhagic diathesis, and may cause necroses in various situations independently of thrombosis. The focal necroses so often met with in the liver in various infective and toxic states do not usually stand in any definite relation to closure of the vessels (Welch and Flexner).

Embolism of the coronary arteries of the heart.—This is far less frequent than thrombosis, but Marie's position, that scarcely more than one or two of the reported cases of coronary embolism are free from all criticism, seems to me too extreme. Metastatic abscesses in the heart are not particularly rare manifestations of pyæmia. To what extent they are caused by coarse infective emboli, or by the lodgment of isolated bacteria, or small bacterial clumps, does not appear to be established. The heart ranks next to the kidney as the most frequent seat of abscesses following intravascular injection of the pyogenetic staphylococci in rabbits.

Virchow, Chiari, Rolleston, Hektoen, and others have published observations of bland embolism of the coronary arteries. I have observed an instance in which the embolic nature of the plug seemed to me conclusively established. A woman, 36 years old, who had presented symptoms of mitral insufficiency, died suddenly after a paroxysm of dyspnœa and precordial distress lasting two or three minutes. I found an entirely loose grayish plug, 4 mm. long, with a rough irregular extremity, completely occluding the descending branch of the left coronary artery near its origin. There was no atheroma at the site of lodgment of the embolus, although there were a few patches in other parts of the coronary arteries. The segments of the mitral valve were thickened, retracted, and beset with both old and fresh vegetations, and globular thrombi were present in the left auricular appendix. There were also fresh vegetations upon the aortic valve. There were infarcts in the spleen and kidneys. There were no fibroid patches or infarction in the myocardium.

The effects of embolism of the coronary arteries are like those of thrombosis, which have already been considered (p. 208).

Embolism and Thrombosis of the retinal vessels.—Plugging of the retinal vessels is of general pathological as well as special ophthalmological interest, for it is possible to observe with the ophthalmoscope the circulatory disturbances in the retina. Ischæmia and stasis follow immediately closure of the central artery of the retina by an embolus. Vision is lost with characteristic suddenness. Both the arteries and the veins are narrowed, the latter being often unequally contracted. Subsequently the veins may dilate to some extent, especially in the periphery of the retina, and present ampulliform swellings. An interesting phenomenon is the appearance in the veins of an intermittent, sluggish stream of broken cylinders of red corpuscles, separated by clear spaces ; and by pressure on the eye-ball a similarly interrupted current may often be made to flow through arteries and veins.   This appearance of interrupted columns of blood is evidently similar to that observed by Mall and myself after closure of the superior mesenteric artery and previously described (p. 245).   After a short time the optic papilla becomes pale and gray, and the retina, especially in the neighbourhood of the papilla and macula, assumes an opaque, grayish white, œdematous aspect.   Hæmorrhages are exceptional.   A characteristic ophthalmo-scopic appearance is the cherry-red spot in the centre of the macula, caused by the red colour of the choroid shining through.   There may be more or less return of the circulation with improvement and even complete restoration of vision ; but the prognosis as regards sight is in general unfavourable, as atrophy of the retina and of the optic nerve is likely to ensue.   The prognosis is more favourable with embolism of branches of the retinal artery.   Here multiple hæmorrhages usually occur.

Thrombosis of the central retinal vein is distinguished from plugging of the artery especially by the abundant hæmorrhages.   With occlusion of the central artery the condition is anæmic infarction, and with plug-ging of the vein hæmorrhagic infarction.

There is some difference of opinion as to the relative frequency of embo'ism and of thrombosis of the central retinal artery.   Of 129 cases collected by Fischer, ninety-one had heart disease ; whereas Kern reports that of twelve cases in Haab's clinic only two had demonstrable cardiac disease ; and of eighty-three cases, collected from the records, in 66 per cent there was no demonstrable source for an embolus.   The latter author, therefore, regards the majority of plugs in the central artery of the retina as primary thrombi.   The generally accepted opinion, however, is that embolism is more common than thrombosis of the retinal arteries.

Treatment.—In the preceding pages mention has been made of the surgical treatment of hæmorrhagic infarction of the intestine and of gangrene of the extremities ; and under " Thrombosis " the importance of preventing so far as may be the separation of emboli has been empha-sised.   The general indications in the treatment of embolism are essen-tially similar to those already considered for thrombosis (p. 223).

WM. H. WELCH.

REFERENCES[1]

Historical.—1. COHN, B. Klinik d. embol. Gefässkrankh. Berlin, 1860.—2. B. COHNHEIM. Untersuch. üb. d. embol. Processe. Berlin, 1872. 3. Idem. Vorles. üb. allg. Pathol. Berlin, 1892.—4. VIRCHOW. Gesammelte Abhandl. Frankf. 1856.
    Aberrant Embolism.—5. ARNOLD. Virchow's Archiv, 1891, cxxiv. p. 385.—6. BONOME. Arch. per le sc. med. 1889, xiii. p. 267.—7. ERNST. Virchow's Archiv, 1898, cli. p. 69.—8. FIRKET. Acad. roy. de méd. de Belge, 1890.—9. FLEXNER. Bull.

[1] See footnote to References to Thrombosis, p. 224.

Johns Hopkins Hosp. 1896, vii. p. 173.—10. HAUSER. *Münch. med. Woch.* 1888, xxxv. p. 583.—11. HELLER. *Deutsch. Arch. f. kl. Med.* 1870, vii. p. 127.—12. LUBARSCH. *Fortschr. d. Med.* 1893, xi. p. 805.—13. LUI. *Arch. per le sc. med.* 1894, xviii. p. 99.—14. RIBBERT. *Centralbl. f. allg. Path.* 1897, viii. p. 433.—15. v. RECKLING-HAUSEN. *Virchow's Arch.* 1885, c. p. 503.—16. ROSTAN. Thèse. Genève, 1884.—17. SCHEVEN. Inaug.-Diss. Rostock, 1894.—18. SCHMORL. *Deutsch. Arch. f. kl. Med.* 1888, xlii. p. 499.—19. SCHMORL. *Path.-anat. Untersuch. üb. Puerp.-Eklampsie,* Leipz. 1893.—20. ZAHN. *Virchow's Arch.* 1889, cxv. p. 71, and cxvii. p. 1.
Anatomical Characters.—21. FAGGE. *Trans. Path. Soc. Lond.* 1876, xxvii. p. 70.
Effects.—22. ASKANAZY. *Virchow's Arch.* 1895, cxli. p. 42.—23. BIER. *Virchow's Arch.* 1897, cxlvii. pp. 256 and 444; 1898, cliii. pp. 306 and 434.—24. BRYANT. *Boston Med. and Surg. Journ.* 1888, cxix. p. 400.—25. CERFONTAINE. *Arch de biol.* 1894, xiii. p. 125.—26. DAVAINE. *Traité des entozoaires,* p. 406. Paris, 1877.—27. FELTZ. *Schmidt's Jahrb.* 1870.—28. v. FREY. *Arch. f. Physiol.* 1885, p. 533.—29. GOLDENBLUM. *Versuche üb. Collateralcirculation, etc.* Inaug.-Diss. Dorpat, 1889. —30. KOPPE. *Arch. f. Physiol.* 1890, Suppl.-Bd. p. 168.—31. KOSSUCHIN. *Virchow's Archiv,* 1876, lxvii. p. 449.—32. KÜTTNER. *Ibid.* 1876, lxi. p. 21; 1878, lxxiii. p. 476.—33. LISTER. *Bull. acad. de méd.* 1878, 2nd s. vii. p. 640.—34. LITTEN. *Ztschr. f. kl. Med.* 1880, i. p. 131.—35. MALL. *Johns Hopkins Hosp. Reports,* vol. i. p. 37.— 36. MARCHAND. *Berl. kl. Woch.* 1894, p. 37.—37. NOTHNAGEL. *Ztschr. f. kl. Med.* 1889, xv. p. 42.—38. PANSKI and THOMA. *Arch. f. exp. Poth.* 1893, xxxi. p. 303.— 39. PONFICK. *Virchow's Arch.* 1873, lviii. p. 528.—40. v. RECKLINGHAUSEN. *Handb. d. allg. Path. d. Kreislaufs, etc.* Stuttg. 1883.—41. THOMA. *Lehrb. d. path. Anat.* Th. i. Stuttg. 1894.—42. WEIGERT. *Virchow's Archiv,* 1877, lxx. p. 486; 1878, lxxii. p. 250; 1880, lxxix. p. 104.—43. *Idem. Centralbl. f. allg. Path.* 1891, ii. p. 785.—44. WELCH. "Hæmorrhagic Infarction," *Trans. Assoc. Amer. Physicians,* 1887, ii. p. 121.—45. ZIELONKO. *Virchow's Arch.* 1873, lvii. p. 436.
Embolic Aneurysms.—46. BUDAY. *Ziegler's Beitr.* 1891, x. p. 187.—47. CLARKE. *Trans. Path. Soc. London,* 1896, xlvii. p. 24.—48. DUCKWORTH. *Brit. Med. Journ.* 1890, i. p. 1355.—49. EPPINGER. *Pathogenesis, Histogenesis u. Aetiologie d. Aneurysmen.* Berl. 1887.—50. LANGTON and BOWLBY. *Med.-Chir. Trans.* 1887, lxx. p. 1117. (Consult for references to Ogle, Wilks, Holmes, Church, Smith, Goodhart, and other previous literature.)—51. PEL and SPRONCK. *Ztschr. f. kl. Med.* xii. p. 327.—52. THOMA. *Deutsch. med. Woch.* 1889, p. 362.—53. TUFNELL. *Dubl. Quart. Journ. Med. Sc.* May 1853.
General Symptomatology.—54. GANGOLPHE and COURMONT. *Arch. méd. expér.* 1891, iii. p. 504.—55. STRICKER. *Vorles. üb. allg. u. exper. Pathologie,* p. 770. Wien, 1883.
Air Embolism.—56. BERT. *La pression barométrique, etc.* Paris, 1878.—57. COUTY. *Études expér. sur l'entrée de l'air dans les veines.* Thèse. Paris, 1875 (also for reference to Barthélemy).—58. FELTZ. *Compt. rend.* 1878, lxxxvi. No. 5.—59. EWALD and KOBERT. *Pflüger's Arch.* 1883, xxxi. p. 160.—60. HAUER. *Ztschr. f. Heilk.* 1890, xi. p. 159.— 61. JANEWAY. *Trans. Assoc. Amer. Physicians,* 1898, xiii. p. 87.—62. JÜRGENSEN. *Deutsch. Arch. f. kl. Med.* 1882, xxxi. p. 441.—63. LABORDE and MURON. *Compt. rend. soc. de biol.* 1873, v.—64. LEWIN. *Arch. f. exp. Path. u. Pharm.* 1897, xl. p. 308.— 65. PASSET. *Arb. a. d. path. Inst. zu München,* p. 293. Stuttg. 1886.—66. WELCH and FLEXNER. *Journ. Exp. Med.* 1896, i. p. 5.—67. WELCH and NUTTALL. *Johns Hopkins Hosp. Bulletin,* 1892, iii. p. 81.
Fat Embolism.—68. BENEKE. *Ziegler's Beitr.* 1897, xxii. p. 343.—69. HANRIOT. *Compt. rend. acad. des sc.* 1896, cxxii. p. 753; cxxiii. p. 833; 1897, cxxiv. pp. 235 and 778.—70. RIBBERT. *Correspondenz-Bl. f. schweiz. Aerzte,* 1894, xxiv. p. 457.—71. SANDERS and HAMILTON. *Edin. Med. Journ.* 1879-80, xxv. p. 47.—72. WAGNER. *Arch. d. Heilk.* 1862, iii. p. 241; 1865, vi.—73. ZENKER. *Beitr. zu norm. u. path. Anat. d. Lunge.* Dresden, 1862.
Embolism by Parenchymatous Cells.—74. ASCHOFF. *Virchow's Arch.* 1893, cxxxiv. p. 11.—75. GAYLORD. *Proc. Path. Soc.* Philadelphia, 1898, N.S. i. p. 184.—76. HANAU. *Fortschr. d. Med.* 1886, iv. p. 387.—77. LUBARSCH. *Fortschr. d. Med.* 1893, xi. pp. 805 and 845 (consult for references to Turner, Jürgens, Klebs, Schmorl, Zenker, and Hess).—78. *Idem. Virchow's Arch.* 1898, cli. p. 546.—79. MAXIMOW. *Virchow's Archiv,* 1898, cli. p. 297 (also for references to Leusden and Kassjanow).—80. NEU-MANN. *Monatsschr. f. Geburtsh. u. Gynakol.* 1897, vi. pp. 17, 157.—81. PICK. *Berl. kl. Woch.* 1897, p. 1069 (also for Schmorl).—82. SCHMIDT, B. *Centralbl. f. allg. Path.* 1897, viii. p. 860.—83. SCHMORL. *Centralbl. f. Geburtsh. u. Gynäkol.* 1897, p. 1216.

Pulmonary Embolism.—84. BANG. *Jattagelser og Studier over døhdelig Embolie og Thrombose i Lungearterne.* Copenhagen, 1880.—85. BUNGER. *Ueb. Embolie d. Lungenarterie.* Inaug.-Diss. Kiel, 1895.—86. COHNHEIM and LITTEN. *Virchow's Archiv,* 1875, lxv. p. 99.—87. FREYBERGER. *Trans. Path. Soc. London,* 1898, xlix. p. 27. —88. FUJINAMI. *Virchow's Archiv,* 1898, clii. pp. 61, 193 (also for Oestreich).— 89. GLUZINSKI. *Deutsch. Arch. f. kl. Med.* 1895, liv. p. 178 (for references to Perl and Lippmann, Sommerbrodt and Nothnagel).—90. GRAWITZ. *Virchow's Festschrift der Assistenten,* Berlin, 1891.—90a. GSELL. *Mittheil. a. Klinik u. med. Inst. d. Schweiz.* iii. R. Hft. 3 (also for Hanau).—91. HAMILTON. *A Text-Book of Pathology,* vol. i. p. 683. London, 1889.—92. KÜTTNER. *Virchow's Archiv,* 1878, lxxiii. p. 39.—93. KLEBS. *Allg. Path.* ii. p. 20. Jena, 1889.—94. LITTEN. *Charité-Annalen,* 1878, iii. 1876, p. 180.—95. MOGLING. *Ziegler's Beitr.* 1886, p. 133 (see also reference 90).—96. ORTH. *Centralbl. f allg. Path.* 1897, viii. p. 589.—97. PERL. *Virchow's Archiv,* 1874, lix. p. 39.—98. SERRE. *De l'origine embolique des thromboses de l'artère pulmon.* Thèse. Lyon, 1895.—99. SGAMBATI. *Arch. ed atti d. soc. ital. di chir.* Roma, 1897, xi. p. 37.—100. WILLGERODT. *Arb. a. d. path. Inst. in Göttingen,* p. 100. Berlin, 1893.— 101. ZAHN. *Centralbl. f. allg. Path.* 1897, viii. p. 860.

Splenic Infarction. Renal Infarction.—102. PONFICK. *Virchow's Arch.* 1874, lx. p. 153.—103. THOREL. *Virchow's Arch.* 1896, cxlvi. p. 297.—104. TRAUBE. *Gesammelte Beitr. zu Path. u. Physiol.* ii. p. 347. Berl. 1871.

Embolism and Thrombosis of the Mesenteric Arteries.—105. BECKMANN. *Virchow's Arch.* 1858, xiii. p. 501.—106. CHIENE. *Journ. Anat. and Physiol.* 1869, iii. p. 65.—107. COUNCILMAN. *Boston Med. and Surg. Journ.* 1894, cxxx. p. 410.—108. ELLIOT. *Annals of Surgery,* 1895, xxi. p. 9.—109. FABER. *Deutsches Arch. f. kl. Med.* 1875, xvi. p. 527.—110. FINLAYSON. *Glasgow Med. Journ.* 1888, xxix. p. 414.—111. GERHARDT. *Würzb. med. Ztschr.* 1863, iv. p. 141.—112. GORDON. *Brit. Med. Journ.* 1898, i. p. 1447.—113. KARCHER. *Correspondenz-Bl. f. schweiz. Aerzte,* 1897, xxvii. p. 548.— 114. KAUFMANN. *Virchow's Arch.* 1889, cxvi. p. 353.—115. KUSSMAUL. *Würzb. med. Ztschr.* 1864, v. p. 210.—116. LEREBOULLET. *Rec. de mém. de méd.* 1875, xxxi. p. 417.—117. LITTEN. *Virchow's Arch.* 1875, lxiii. p. 289.—118. *Idem. Deutsche med. Woch.* 1889, p. 145.—119. LORENZ. *Ztschr. f. kl. Med.* 1891, xviii. p. 493.—120. LYCETT. *Brit. Med. Journ.* 1898, ii. p. 84.—121. MINKOWSKI. *Mitth. a. d. med. Klin. zu Königsberg,* 1888, p. 59.—122. MOOS. *Virchow's Arch.* 1867, xli. p. 58.—123. NOTHNAGEL. *Spec. Path. u. Therap.* xvii. p. 156. Wien, 1898.—124. OPPOLZER. *Allg. Wien. med. Ztg.* 1862, vii.—125. PACKARD. *Proc. Path. Soc. Philadelphia,* 1898, N.S. i. p. 288.—126. PARENSKI. *Wiener med. Jahrb.* 1876, p. 275.—127. PIEPER. *Allg. med. Centr.-Ztg.* 1865, p. 493.—128. PONFICK. *Virchow's Arch.* 1870, l. p. 623. —129. TANGL and HARLEY. *Centralbl. f. d. med. Wiss.* 1895, p. 673.—130. TIEDEMANN. *Von d. Verengung u. Schliessung d. Pulsadern in Krankheiten.* Heidelb. u. Leipz. 1843.—131. WATSON. *Boston Med. and Surg. Journ.* 1894, cxxxi. p. 552.— 132. WELCH and FLEXNER. *Journ. Exp. Med.* 1896, i. p. 35.

Embolism and Thrombosis of the Thoracic Aorta.—133. ARMET. Thèse. Paris, 1881.—134. CHVOSTEK. *Wiener med. Blätter,* 1881, p. 1513 (also for references to Trost, Carville, Lüttich, and Tewat).—135. BUCHDALEK. *Vrtljschr. f. d. prakt. Heilk.* 1845, viii. p. 160.—136. BRISTOWE. *Lancet,* 1881, i. pp. 131 and 166.—137. JAURAND. *Progr. méd.* 1882, x. p. 147.—138. PITT. *Trans. Path. Soc. London,* 1889, xl. p. 74.

Embolism and Thrombosis of the Abdominal Aorta.—139. CAMMARERI. *Morgagni,* 1885, xxvii. pp. 1, 113.—140. CHARRIER and APERT. *Bull. soc. anat. de Paris,* 1896, 5th s. x. p. 766.—141. GRAHAM. *Med.-Chir. Trans.* 1814, v. p. 297.—142. HEILIGENTHAL. *Deutsche med. Woch.* 1898, p. 519.—143. MEYNARD. *Étude sur l'oblitération de l'aorte abdom. par embolie ou par thrombose.* Thèse. Paris, 1883 (Meynard's case is identical with Barié's and du Castel's).—144. ROUSSEL. *Études sur les embolies de l'aorte abdom.* Thèse. Lyon, 1893 (the cases of Barié and of Desnos reckoned as separate cases by Selter and by Roussel are identical).—145. SELTER. *Ueb. Embolie d. Aorta abdom.* Inaug.-Diss. Strassburg, 1891. The references to my additional twelve cases of embolism or thrombosis of the abdominal aorta are Nos. 146 to 157 inclusive.—146. BALLINGALL. *Trans. Med. and Phys. Soc. Bombay,* 1857, N.S. No. iii. App. p. xxv.—147. BRISTOWE. *Trans. Path. Soc. London,* 1872, xxiii. p. 21.—148. CARTER. *Trans. Med. and Phys. Soc. Bombay* (1859), 1860, N.S. No. v. App. p. xxii.—149. GOODWORTH. *Brit. Med. Journ.* 1896, i. p. 1501.—150. KIRKMAN. *Lancet,* 1863, ii. p. 510.—151. MANZ. *Berl. kl. Woch.* 1889, p. 812.—152. NUÑEZ. *Gaz. med. de la Habana,* 1879-80, ii. p. 160.—153. OSLER. *Trans. Assoc. Amer.*

Physicians, 1887, ii. p. 135.—154. PETTIT. *New Orleans Med. and Surg. Journ.* 1880-81, N.S. viii. p. 1151.—155. SCHILLING. *Münch. med. Woch.* 1895, p. 227.— 156. SCHOLZ. *Ein Fall von Obturation d. Aorta abdom.* Inaug.-Diss. Tübingen, 1850. —157. WILBUR. *Amer. Journ. Med. Sc.* 1857, N.S. xxxiv. p. 286.—158. BARTH. *Bull. Soc. anat. de Paris*, 1848, xxiii. p. 260.—159. HERTER. *Journ. Nerv. and Mental Dis.* 1889, xvi. p. 197 (for references to Schiffer, Weil, Ehrlich and Brieger, and Sprouck).—160. HERXHEIMER. *Virchow's Arch.* 1886, civ. p. 20.—161. KADYI. *Ueb. d. Blutgefässe d. menschl. Rückenmarkes.* Lemberg, 1889.—162. LITTEN. *Virchow's Arch.* 1880, lxxx. p. 281.—163. POPOFF. *Arch. f. Gynäk.* 1894, xlvii. p. 12.—164. WILLIAMSON. *On the Relation of Diseases of the Spinal Cord to the Distribution and Lesions of the Spinal Blood-Vessels.* London, 1895.

Hepatic Infarction.—165. ARNOLD. *Virchow's Arch.* 1891, cxxiv. p. 383.—166. CHIARI. *Centralbl. f. allg. Path.* 1898, ix. p. 839.—167. COHNHEIM and LITTEN. *Virchow's Arch.* 1876, lxvii. p. 153. — 168. DOYON and DUFOURT. *Arch. de physiol.* 1898, 5th s. x. p. 522.—169. FLEXNER. *Johns Hopkins Hosp. Reports*, 1897, vi. p. 259. —170. KLEBS. *Virchow's Festschrift der Assistenten*, 1891, p. 8.—171. KÖHLER. *Arb. a. d. path. Inst. in Gottingen*, 1893, p. 121.—172. LUBARSCH. *Fortschr. d. Med.* 1893, xi. p. 809.—173. OSLER. *Trans. Assoc. Amer. Phys.* 1887, ii p. 136.—174. PITT. *Brit. Med. Journ.* 1895, i. p. 420.—175. RATTONE. *Arch. per le sc. med.* 1888, xii. p. 223.—176. WELCH and FLEXNER. *Johns Hopkins Hosp. Bulletin*, 1892, iii. p. 17.— 177. WOOLDRIDGE. *Trans. Path. Soc. London*, 1888, xxxix. p. 421. — 178. ZAHN. *Centralbl. f. allg. Path.* 1897, viii. p. 860.

Embolism of the Coronary Arteries.—179. CHIARI. *Prag. med. Woch.* 1897, Nos. 6 and 7.—180. HEKTOEN, *Med. News*, 1892, lxi. p. 210.—181. MARIE. *L'infarctus du myocarde*, p. 30. Paris, 1897.—182. ROLLESTON. *Brit. Med. Journ.* 1896, ii. p. 1566.

Embolism and Thrombosis of the Retinal Vessels.—183. FISCHER. *Ueb. d. Embolie d. Art. centr. retinae.* Leipzig, 1891.—184. KERN. *Zur Embolie d. Art. centr. retinae.* Inaug.-Diss. Zürich, 1892.

W. H. W.

PHLEBITIS

OPINIONS as to the affinities between phlebitis and thrombosis have varied from the earliest time at which pathology could have for us any meaning up to the present day. Hunter and his followers, with Cruveilhier at their head, laid the greatest stress on the inflammation of the vein; the latter asserting that whatever the form of the inflammation it is always accompanied by the formation of a clot —thrombosis, but that this coagulation of the blood is a secondary phenomenon. Thus phlebitis at that time held the primary position. In 1856 Virchow completely turned the tables, and was able to convince the vast majority of pathologists that thrombosis was the primary and essential condition. Since then bacteriology has shown that microbes play a most important part in causing phlebitis, and that thrombosis in such cases is a secondary result (*vide* Professor Welch's article, p. 169 in this volume).

With our present knowledge we may confidently assert that in all suppurating wounds, where organisms abound, the progress of infection is from without inwards; that the inflammation around the infected spot involves the outer coat of the vein, and from this onwards till endophlebitis is fully established; and that this endophlebitis is the cause of the thrombosis in this particular variety of the disease. Arguing from this as an established and easily demonstrated fact, we have been gradually induced to think that many of the so-called cases of primary thrombosis really depend upon an endophlebitis which may either have extended from the outer coat inwards, as in the septic phlebitis above mentioned, or be itself primary and due to a specific cause, such as acute articular rheumatism, or gout. We cannot, however, assume that this is always the case ; and Virchow's work on the coagulation of the blood as the cause of phlebitis may explain some of those cases of thrombosis which cannot at present be attributed to phlebitis (*vide* p. 173).

Etiology and Pathology.—The circumstances under which phlebitis may arise, and the different forms it may assume, must now be considered.

Traumatic phlebitis, simple or infective, may arise in any wound, or after any operation, in which a vein has been exposed. The simple form will pass unnoticed and be unaccompanied by thrombosis, if a large vein be not exposed or wounded and ligatured. The inflammation is part of the reparative process which ordinarily takes place in the healing of a wound, and does not spread. If a vein has been ligatured endophlebitis ensues, but it is strictly local for the obliteration of the vein at that spot. On the proximal side of the ligature this obliteration takes place, as far as the next collateral branch, without the formation of a thrombus, as in an amputation stump ; but on the distal side, as the vein is full of blood, a clot is formed which, after it has undergone softening and fatty degeneration, is again absorbed. The thrombus on this side of the ligature may indeed extend farther than the nearest collateral vein, but it has no evil consequences in its extension towards the periphery.

The infective phlebitis from a wound, on the other hand, is one of the most serious diseases with which we have to deal ; and, according to our present knowledge, admits of many clinical varieties from the different degrees of virulence which the infective organisms present, and the different susceptibility of the individuals infected. As the pyogenetic organisms, to which this infection is due, vary in their mode of growth, and in their virulence, there is a considerable variety in the clinical manifestations of an infected wound. We do not as yet know to which particular pyogenetic organism, or even to what group of such organisms, we are to attribute a particular train of symptoms. When a wound does not heal by first intention, we believe that it has been infected by such organisms of one kind or another ; whether by means of instruments, fingers, or ligatures, or, in the case of an accident, by the original injury. It is very difficult to fix upon a particular predominating organism among the many which will be detected in the laboratory. We recognise sometimes a very rapid and acute form of suppuration in which, from the intensity of the inflammatory processes which the organisms have produced, the tissues rapidly break down, and even sloughs come away. In other cases there may be merely a little pus, or even none at all, and a good deal of swelling. The difference in the progress of these cases, the one towards almost certain death, and the other possibly towards ultimate recovery, may be due to the varying degrees of virulence in the same organism, and of suitability of the soil for their cultivation. In either case a vein may be involved; the external coat is invaded by the same organisms which are the cause of the inflammation in the connective tissue, and the extension of this to the internal coat, and the consequent endophlebitis, give rise to thrombosis. For a time the coagulation of the blood in the vein may arrest the general dissemination of the infective process; but, in the more virulent forms of the disease, the thrombus is itself invaded by the bacterial infection, and softens down under its influence. Septic embolism may now take place with its characteristic symptoms of pyæmia, or this may be again prevented by farther thrombosis.

In many instances the progress of farther infection of the vein is permanently arrested by the formation of a healthy clot; yet too often, if the larger veins be the seat of the trouble, the auto-infection goes on till the whole length of a large vein, or series of veins—like the femoral and iliac veins—are filled with purulent fluid, with or without the consequent phenomena of embolism and pyæmia. Death is produced either by pyæmia, septicæmia, or the extension of the mischief to the vena cava; when, even if some arrest of the disease do take place, it is too late to hope for recovery.

A small vein, if it be shedding septic emboli into the circulation, is as mischievous as a larger one; for each embolus carries with it the organism of suppuration, and starts again—most often in the lungs—the disease originated at the primary seat of infection. In this way all the characteristic and fatal symptoms of pyæmia (see vol. i. p. 606) may be produced from what was at first a most insignificant wound or operation. Again, a suppurating wound may be surrounded by a barrier of inflammatory tissue which has arrested the progress of the infecting organism. This barrier of granulation tissue may have in its midst a vein, the walls of which are thus inflamed, and the lumen consequently filled with clot. But if this barrier and vein be not themselves invaded with organisms, we have after all to deal with a simple phlebitis, not with an infective or septic one; although the original cause was perhaps as septic as it well could be.

Other instances of suppurative phlebitis and thrombosis, which are not dependent upon injury or operation but yet arise from a definite form of suppuration, should here also be mentioned.

The lateral sinus and jugular vein may be infected in this way from acute or chronic suppuration of the middle ear, as will appear in later articles. The intervening bone is not necessarily diseased, though this is far from rare. The emissary veins may become involved in the area of infection, exactly as we have described above, and, by the extension of endophlebitis, may eventually produce the same result—endophlebitis and suppurative thrombosis—in the lateral sinus. Before this sinus is blocked by thrombosis, septic emboli may be thrown into the circulation producing the ordinary signs of pyæmia (see article "Pyæmia," vol. i. p. 601).

Pylephlebitis is another instance of the same kind. In this disease the portal vein becomes the seat of suppurative phlebitis and thrombosis from some suppurative and infective disease in its tributary branches; such, for example, as those coming from a suppurating appendix vermiformis. For this and for other visceral lesions of a similar kind, the reader must be referred to the appropriate section in which such conditions are more fully described ("Pylephlebitis," vol. i. p. 610). They are quoted here as instances to show the various modes in which suppurative phlebitis and thrombosis may arise.

We have now to consider those cases of phlebitis and thrombosis which are unattended by any suppuration, and which are not due to any injury or operation.

Rheumatic phlebitis most frequently attacks the veins of the lower extremities, and occurs before, during, or after an attack of acute or subacute articular rheumatism. It is, however, much more common during the convalescence, or after the acute attack has passed off. Sometimes when the phlebitis comes on, the general symptoms of rheumatic fever reappear. As a rule, pain in the part precedes the general swelling and the cord which is finally to be felt in the situation of the vein involved. It seems reasonable, therefore, to suppose that many of these cases are due to endophlebitis, with which both the clinical symptoms and the pathology of the disease would appear to agree.

Gouty phlebitis.—To Sir James Paget we are indebted for the first clear account of this condition. "It affects the superficial rather than the deep veins, and often occurs in patches, affecting (for example) on one day a short piece of a saphenous vein, and on the next day another separate piece of the same, or a corresponding piece of the opposite vein or of a femoral vein. It shows herein an evident disposition towards being metastatic and symmetrical; characters which, I may remark by the way, are strongly in favour of the belief that the essential and primary disease is not a coagulation of blood, but an inflammation of portions of the venous walls."[1] It occurs chiefly in the lower limbs of those who have a marked gouty constitution, or with gouty inheritance; it may arise during acute gout, in an interval between attacks of gout, in persons of more latent gouty habits, and, indeed, in persons of gouty inheritance in whom no gouty symptoms had previously appeared. It is also to be added that the heredity is very often expressed not only in the general features of gout, but also in the form of phlebitis itself. Although more frequent in middle and later life, it is far from unknown in younger persons.

[1] *Clinical Lectures and Essays*, by Sir James Paget, Bart., edited by Howard Marsh, 1875, p. 293.

After enteric fever, during the convalescent stage, obstruction of the veins in one of the lower extremities is not uncommon. The patient is often extremely weak, and the strength of his circulation is reduced to the lowest ebb. But, besides slowing of the blood-stream, there seems some accumulating evidence to show that the typhoid bacillus may be the cause of endophlebitis, as it is for the periosteal affections which occur and continue so long after the attack of fever has passed, and the patient has apparently recovered.

The *pressure of a tumour* is one of the causes ordinarily assigned for thrombosis. And yet how rare it is for a vein to be thus occluded by clot, unless the tumour be one of those that infiltrates the surrounding tissue as it increases in size,—namely, a malignant growth! Œdema from the pressure of a simple tumour is of course another matter, for this does not prove thrombosis, but only obstruction to the flow of blood. Malignant infiltration of the walls of a vein gives rise to endophlebitis ; the thrombosis is, in that case, secondary, and is itself invaded by the growth in its further extension.

During the convalescence of any serious illness, or in the late stages of a malignant disease causing *cachexia,* the obstruction of a vein is not uncommon. Although not always evident before death, the necropsy in a malignant case may prove that a secondary growth was the cause, in the manner described above. In the other instances where no obvious cause can be discovered, slackening of the circulation, accumulation of platelets and of white corpuscles along the sides of the vessel, and an alteration of the chemical composition of the blood may be the cause of the thrombosis, which is here supposed to precede the phlebitis. (See art. "Thrombosis," p. 166 *et seq.*)

The phlebitis and thrombosis which follow upon a varicose condition of the veins fall within the sphere of surgery.

Symptoms.—1. *Of simple phlebitis.*—The local symptoms of a non-suppurative phlebitis are ushered in by pain, which gradually increases in severity for some hours or days, and then slowly subsides ; unless there be further extension of the inflammation or a fresh attack elsewhere. On examination of the part at first no swelling is discovered ; but in the course of the day, or of a few hours more, some diffused swelling is felt : if the vein affected be a deep one, like the femoral, some days elapse, as a rule, before a distinct cord-like swelling is found. If it be one of the superficial veins, like the saphenous, it is more clearly defined, or more quickly recognised. Œdema of the parts beyond the seat of obstruction is well marked, especially in the foot when the common femoral is the vein concerned ; but it is entirely absent if the superficial veins alone are inflamed and obstructed. The œdema is generally of the soft variety, easily pitting on pressure, and extends from the foot to the knee. In cases in which the thrombosis has extended to the highest point in the main vein of a limb, such as the external and common iliac, and has farther induced coagulation in its chief collateral branches, the œdema is of a peculiarly hard and brawny consistence, like that which is seen in the " phlegmasia alba dolens " after parturition (see p. 215).   The length of time that the œdema lasts is very variable. In the soft œdema, where the obstruction is not so extensive or complete, a few weeks or months will be a sufficient time to reckon for the complete restoration of the circulation.   But in many cases of "solid œdema " the circulation is never completely restored ; the limb remains larger for the rest of life, and requires support to keep the swelling in check.   Redness of the skin over the parts affected is a very noticeable feature when the superficial veins are inflamed and thrombosed ; but in the case of the veins beneath the deep fascia it does not appear.   When this redness is seen over a superficial vein it is not in a fine line leading to an inflamed gland, as in lymphangitis, but a wide and diffused band.

Suppuration does not occur, even in thrombosis of the superficial veins, unless there be an abrasion of the skin or an ulcer through which organisms can have entered ; occasionally, however, fluctuation may be present when fluid blood lies between two near patches of thrombosis in a vein beneath the skin.

The general symptoms of simple phlebitis are those of a mild fever. The temperature rises at the onset, and reaches its highest point, generally about 102° F., on the second day, remains stationary for a few days, and then sinks to normal.   It is not, however, uncommon, especially after typhoid fever, for the onset to be marked by a rigor, and a temperature of 103° F., or higher ; but the rigor is not repeated, and in a few days the temperature falls.   If the temperature persist, either a fresh extension of the phlebitis is taking place, or, especially if at the same time it rises higher, suppuration is to be suspected after all. .

Complications.—One of the common features of simple phlebitis is the possibility of a relapse, when all the symptoms begin again.   It may be an extension of inflammation from the part first attacked, or a fresh attack at another part of the body.   This is especially frequent in gouty phlebitis, as I have already explained.

Embolism is the most serious complication to which a patient suffering from simple phlebitis is exposed.   These only too well-known accidents should always be recollected by every practitioner ; they are fully described in the previous article.   Cases have occurred in which a most sudden and distressing dyspnœa has taken place, and death seemed imminent ; but the patient has rallied nevertheless, and a patch of crepitation has been discovered at the base of one lung.   Another complication or sequel should also be borne in mind—namely, the persistence of œdema for months, years, or indeed for the rest of life, in some cases where the deep femoral vein had been thrombosed.

2. *Of suppurative phlebitis.*—The local symptoms are those of suppuration.   In most cases pus is already escaping from some wound or abscess cavity, and the known proximity of some large venous trunk causes great anxiety, if more acute general symptoms suddenly appear, or the ordinary febrile attack persists beyond the time during which

such an abscess or wound would cause such symptoms. Sometimes, however, there are scarcely any local symptoms, or they are so trivial as to escape observation till the acute general symptoms lead to a more careful examination. The special symptoms are those of high fever, with sharp rises and falls. Shivering, or a distinct rigor, may accompany the sudden rise of temperature; and the fall may be associated with profuse sweating. There may have been a high temperature for a week or more before the fever assumes this particular character; or the hectic may be the first indication of what is taking place. If the ordinary symptoms of phlebitis have already been present for some days, there can be no doubt as to the cause of the symptoms being infection from the thrombus; but in other instances a large inflammatory swelling may have existed without any distinct evidence of thrombosis or phlebitis. A re-examination may show that, after all, pent-up pus may be the more likely cause of this fever; yet if, after the evacuation of the pus, the same symptoms recur, the suspicion that the vein is involved in the suppuration will be confirmed.

Superficial veins do not give rise to the difficulty described above; for at one or other extremity of the inflammatory swelling the hard cord-like outline of the thrombosed vein can usually be felt. A deep vein, on the other hand, when infected by pyogenetic organisms, is, as a rule, surrounded by so much inflammatory exudation that it may be impossible to find the characteristic local signs of a thrombosed vessel. It is in such places as the groin, the axilla, or the neck that this difficulty arises; but, as has been already stated, the diagnosis must be made by the combination of local signs of deep suppuration with systemic infection. In the case of the ear, with suppurative thrombosis of the lateral sinus, there is often a deep swelling in the neck beneath the mastoid process, which is due in part no doubt to inflamed glands from chronic discharge from the ear; but it is also in many cases caused in great measure by the inflammatory swelling round the thrombosed jugular vein, and is one of the most marked indications, if it be not already too late, for surgical interference. The further progress of infective phlebitis and thrombosis is shown by the persistent character of the fluctuating temperature; if this cease, and the temperature, although high, no longer oscillates in a rapid and irregular manner, we may hope that, although suppuration is still going on in the tissues around, the vein is occluded on the proximal side by a healthy thrombus. Unfortunately this is not often the case; the temperature rises as before in the same sudden and uncertain manner and as quickly falls; variations from 105° to 99° F. in the course of an hour or two being not uncommon. When these variations cover as much as six degrees, septic embolism has probably begun already. Although with nearly every sudden rise of temperature which reaches as high as 104° F. or 105° F. a rigor may be expected, it does not by any means always occur; the sweating with the fall, however, is never absent. The stage at which these violent oscillations of temperature begin is very variable; they

are probably coincident with the disintegration of the infected thrombus ;
it is probable, therefore, that till this occurs there will be no certain
sign of suppurating phlebitis, but only the symptoms ordinarily present
in an infected wound.

When the sudden changes of temperature have been repeated again
and again in the course of a few days, or even, as in some cases, in the
course of twenty-four hours, there is little or no prospect of recovery,
unless indeed some surgical means can be adopted to shut off the pathway
by which the septic emboli are entering the general circulation.

The farther history of the case is that of pyæmia, which has been
described in the first volume of this work.

Treatment.—1. *Simple phlebitis.*—Rest in bed, with the limb slightly
raised, is the really important treatment for simple phlebitis in its early
stage. This does all that is possible to prevent the detachment of
any part of the clot. Although embolism is a rare event, the mere
possibility of such accidents to which allusion has already been made
should make us insist upon absolute rest till all the tenderness on pressure, and other signs of inflammation, have disappeared. Extract of
belladonna and glycerine in equal parts may be applied locally for the
relief of pain ; but all friction, as in the use of ointments, should be
avoided. The constitutional condition should be treated on general
principles ; if the pain be distressing, small doses of morphia may be given
subcutaneously. When the patient is fit to get up and to move about,
he may require an elastic bandage or stocking to prevent the œdema of
foot or leg, if the obstruction has been in the femoral vein. If much
muscular wasting has ensued from the extension of the thrombosis into
the collateral branches, massage may be ordered ; but great care must be
taken to forbid this until· all dangers of embolism have long passed
away.

2. *Suppurative phlebitis.*—As infective phlebitis in wounds and after
surgical operations is directly due to suppuration from the introduction
of organisms from without, it is clear that no one should undertake the
treatment of wounds who is not thoroughly familiar with the various
ways in which the organisms of suppuration may be introduced. "Prevention is better than cure."

But when suppuration has taken place, or an abscess has formed
(apart perhaps from all surgical interference), everything must be done
to stop the further progress of infection. The abscess must be opened,
a sinus slit up, or a counter-opening made, according to the surgical
necessities of the case. By such means suppuration may be prevented
from extending to the neighbourhood of a vein. A deeply-seated and
acute abscess is much to be feared as the forerunner of infective phlebitis,
and must be treated early if preventive surgery is to take its proper
place in our clinical work.

The treatment of suppurative phlebitis has entered upon a new era
since it has been shown that "lateral sinus pyæmia" from ear disease
may be arrested by the ligature of the internal jugular vein. The vein

is completely divided between two ligatures, the proximal end being ligatured as low down in the neck as possible, and the distal end turned but on the surface of the wound. The sinus is then exposed by trephining the mastoid, and the pus and decomposing clot are scraped out with a sharp spoon. If the distal end of the divided jugular vein has been turned out upon the neck, it can be used as an outlet for washing through from the opening in the lateral sinus. I have recorded a case in which pyæmic infection of the ankle joint had occurred before this operation was undertaken, and yet after the above proceeding had been carried out the boy recovered. The further details of these most interesting cases will be described in a later article ; but it is necessary here to state what has been successfully accomplished for a disease that is otherwise certainly fatal, to illustrate the same principles in dealing with other parts of the body. It is not likely, however, that in the extremities there will be many opportunities of applying this principle of cutting off the connection of a distant suppurating vein from the central organ of circulation ; and, as surgical methods of treatment steadily improve through all ranks of the profession, suppurative phlebitis in the extremities must diminish. The middle ear, on the other hand, will continue to supply such cases so long as the public refuse to treat their ears on modern antiseptic lines. Still, it should be impressed on all teachers of medicine and surgery, that this method of cutting short an attack of pyæmia, due to suppurative phlebitis, is as applicable to the extremities as it has been found to be serviceable in lateral sinus pyæmia. We must remember that reamputation was done many years ago with success for infective osteomyelitis of a stump, when pyæmia had apparently already begun ; it is possible, therefore, that at no distant date the division and double ligature of large venous trunks will be a recognised treatment of pyæmia in other parts of the body.

H. H. CLUTTON.

ARTERIAL DEGENERATIONS AND DISEASES

Introduction.—The aphorism "A man is as old as his arteries" suggests more than its literal meaning; it implies that the majority of morbid processes known as degenerations are associated with diseases of the coats of these vessels, or are even directly due to them. In a large proportion of male adults past forty years death is due to cerebral hæmorrhage, cerebral softening, cardiac degenerations, or aneurysm; and it is safe to assume that disease of the arteries plays a very important part in these results. The morbid process may be universal; it may affect primarily the large or the small arteries; it may be local; it may affect all the coats or one of them only. Among the most important determining causes of arterial disease are strain, syphilis, lead, alcohol, gouty diathesis, and laborious occupations, to all of which males are more exposed; no wonder then that men are more frequently the subjects of arterial disease than women.

Certain arteries of the body are more prone to particular morbid processes than others. Gout and Bright's disease, for example, are associated with changes in the walls of the small arteries; and, since the morbid matter is eliminated by the kidney, this organ especially suffers. Although syphilis may attack any of the arteries, it has a predilection for the vessels at the base of the brain; while the effect of mechanical strain due to laborious occupations is felt more especially by the aorta and large vessels.

Before passing to a full description of the various diseases of arteries it will be well to recall a few of the more important facts relating to their distribution and structure.

Distribution of arteries.—The more active the function of an organ the greater the arterial supply; and in every part of the body there is some relation of a special and useful nature between the arterial distribution and the structures which it serves: as is seen, for example, in the circle of Willis, which is a provision against temporary or permanent suppression of the blood-supply to the important cerebral arteries which arise from it; in the renal arteries, which arise at right angles to the aorta and break up within the kidney in such a way as to favour high blood-pressure in the glomeruli and velocity in the arteriæ rectæ; and in the coronary arteries, which arise in the sinuses of Valsalva, but, instead of running into the substance of the heart, are contained in grooves surrounded by loose fat, so that, while their place of origin ensures the necessary high blood-pressure, their ready distension during systole is un-impeded.

Another important consideration relating to the site and effects of arterial disease is the *dichotomous mode of division*, which explains the frequency of disease at the points of bifurcation. *Tortuosity* is another important factor in localising disease from internal strain. In certain organs, such as the brain, lungs, kidney, and spleen, the arteries are terminal, or virtually so; so in the defect of anastomosis with other branches, occlusion cuts off the area supplied by that branch from its blood, and the tissue undergoes necrosis.

General structure of arteries.—The arteries of the body may be roughly divided into large, middle-sized, and small; they possess three coats—internal, middle, and external.

(i.) The *tunica intima*, or inner coat, consists, from within outwards, of three distinct layers :—

(*a*) An endothelial lining, in contact with the blood, made up of delicate nucleated cells joined together by a cement substance, and arranged like a mosaic pavement. This endothelium, slightly modified in different situations, lines the whole cardio-vascular apparatus, and its integrity is of the greatest importance in preventing the coagulation of the blood in the living vessels.

(*b*) A subendothelial layer of branched connective tissue corpuscles with intervening cement substance.

(*c*) A continuous layer made up of a felt work of fine elastic fibres with small openings therein, the fenestrated membrane of Henle. This elastic lamina in the empty contracted artery has the appearance of a crinkled, bright, yellow line.

(ii.) The *tunica media*, or middle coat, consists, in the large arteries, of alternate layers of elastic fibres and unstriped muscle fibres arranged circularly. The larger the artery the more does the elastic element predominate; whereas in the arterioles the muscular coat is, relatively to the size of the vessel, much better developed; and elastic tissue is not present. If we consider the dynamics of the circulation this difference of structure is at once explained; the large arteries by their elasticity help to convert the intermittent force of the heart into a continuous pressure; the muscles of the small arteries, by a general tonic contraction under the control of the vaso-constrictor nerves, maintain the peripheral resistance to the outflow of blood, keeping the arterial system always over-full, while the elastic-buffer action of the large arteries, continually tending to overcome this resistance, causes a steady flow through the capillaries. [For further particulars, see vol. v. p. 474.]

(iii.) The *tunica adventitia*, or external coat, consists of connective tissue possessing a large number of interspersed elastic fibres, together with blood-vessels, lymphatics and nerves. The blood-vessels—vasa vasorum—serve to nourish the walls of the vessels; probably they enter the middle coat of the larger vessels : at any rate, it is not disputed that the tunica media is nourished by the blood of the vasa vasorum, and it is highly probable that even the inner coat is nourished by the transudation of lymph from them. I have pointed out (10) that the openings of the fenestrated membrane probably serve the purpose of allowing nourishment to enter from this source. The lymphatics are numerous, and in certain situations, as in the central nervous system, they form distinct perivascular sheaths. Vaso-motor nerves run by the side of the vasa vasorum (Fig. 4), and over many of the large vessels important plexuses of nerves exist; for example, the carotid plexus of the sympathetic and the cardiac plexus round the aorta.

Local variations in the structure of arteries.—A full account may be found in the admirable work of Ballance and Edmunds, who explain the variable thicknesses of the outer coat in different situations as an adaptation to resist the pressure of joints, and visceral and muscular movements : as examples they cite the common femoral, superior mesenteric and facial ; all of which have relatively thick outer coats.

Charcot says the arterioles of the encephalon present the same characters as those of the large arteries at the base ; namely, abundance

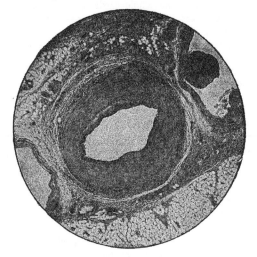

Fig. 4.—Photomicrograph. Section of small artery of great toe of healthy human subject showing the thick media. The adventitia with vasa vasorum injected. Magnified 30 diameters.

of muscular elements, a relative paucity of elastic fibres, and remarkable tenuity of the adventitia. He also points out the importance of the perivascular lymphatic sheath enveloping the small blood - vessels, especially the arterioles, and containing a transparent fluid.

Developmental defects of arteries.—A few examples will be cited under this heading : such as (a) defect of certain arteries with non-development of the corresponding organ ; (b) doubling of aorta ; (c) obliteration of aorta, which may recur at the junction of the ductus arteriosus, or at the isthmus of the aorta (junction of pulmonary artery with aorta) ; (d) congenital smallness of the arterial system described by Virchow in 1870 as the aortic hypoplasia of chlorotic girls. In these last three coats of the aorta are greatly thinned, and the calibre of the vessel is that of a child ; the internal coat presents a reticulated appearance, and scattered yellowish lines and patches indicating fatty degeneration are often seen. Such a vascular system is sufficient until puberty; but the additional requirements of the blood entailed by the development of the reproductive and other parts render it relatively insufficient. Virchow attributes the frequency of palpitation and cardiac hypertrophy in chlorotic women to these congenital arterial defects (vol. v. p. 487). Beneke, in 1867, began a series of researches on cadavers of different ages; he measured the volume of the organs and the circumferential measurement of the arteries; his average results show that the size of the arteries, contrary to what one observes in the case of the heart, increase in a regular ratio to the age. The heart is twelve times less voluminous in the infant than in the adult; it increases regularly in size up to five years; increases less up to the time of puberty, and then again rapidly increases in size.

The subjects of arterial hypoplasia are not always of the "infantile type": they are well developed, but are pale, as in chlorosis; the two conditions peculiar to them are *imperfect development of the hair and of the reproductive organs.* The face, armpits, and pubes are smooth, and, in the male, the penis and testicles are incompletely developed.

Such patients in rare instances have been known to die with symptoms of asystole, yet without any lesion discoverable at the autopsy except arterial stenosis and cardiac dilatation. Both Beneke and Virchow have pointed out that subjects of this affection are prone to endocarditis; occasionally albuminuria may exist, and cases have been recorded of associated nephritis. Dr. Lee Dickinson recently showed two specimens of ruptured aneurysms associated with hypoplasia of arteries; and, as he found no degeneration of the vessels, but extreme tenuity of their walls, he attributed the formation of the aneurysms to congenital delicacy of the vessels. Arterial hypoplasia is sometimes associated with hæmophilia; and the hæmorrhagic diathesis may be the explanation of the various extravasations of blood which are found in these cases, but cannot be traced to any aneurysm or ruptured vessel.

The subjects of arterial hypoplasia seldom attain an advanced age; they generally succumb either to asystole, to nephritis, or to some infectious disease; according to Beneke, especially to tuberculosis and typhoid fever.

Acute arteritis.—The older writers, such as Frank and Pinel, describe the diffuse red staining which is found after death in the aorta and large vessels in septic diseases as a general acute arteritis. This, however, was strenuously denied by Laennec, and the opinion arose that acute arteritis does not exist. But, though a rare event, a number of observations have shown that inflammation of the arteries may occur as a complication in local or in general maladies—the former being much the more frequent association.

Local acute arteritis.—Infective inflammation in the neighbourhood of an artery may set up a periarteritis and a subsequent endarteritis; for example, caries of the petrous portion of the temporal bone has been followed by perforation of the carotid artery and death from hæmorrhage. Secondary hæmorrhage is frequently due to infective inflammation of a ligatured artery. In some experiments, which I performed many years ago (not published), I exposed the carotid artery in animals and produced an acute local inflammation by touching the vessel on one side with a nitrate of silver stick; the result was an acute periarteritis at this spot, with a corresponding endarteritis and enormous thickening of the inner coat from proliferation of the subendothelial tissue (*vide* Fig. 5). The proliferation caused rupture of the elastic layer of the intima, and in one case produced an acute aneurysm, probably due to secondary infection of the wound.

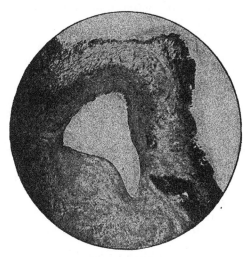

FIG. 5.—Photomicrograph. Experimental arteritis. Section of the carotid artery of a dog showing great thickening of the inner coat at one spot, causing a projection and considerable diminution of the size of the lumen of the vessel. Careful examination shows bright lines running in the media of the healthy part of the arterial wall; these have completely disappeared in the swollen inflamed part. The elastic laminæ have been ruptured by the profuse inflammatory cell proliferation. Just below this spot the coats of the artery gave way and an aneurysm was formed. The acute arteritis was produced by touching the sheath of the artery with lunar caustic. Magnification, 15 diameters.

General acute arteritis.—Crocq *fils*, writing upon experimental arteritis, says there are three questions to answer: (i.) whether a wound itself be capable of bringing about an acute arteritis; (ii.) whether infection be always necessary at the time; (iii.) whether infection afterwards will cause it?

He came to the conclusion, after inoculation with cultures of B. coli and S. pyogenes, that an acute arteritis does not necessarily follow microbial infection; it depends rather upon the nature of the microbe, and on other unknown factors. These results agree with those found in experimental ulcerative endocarditis, which indicate that to produce acute infective arteritis there must be a lesion of the arterial walls and a source of infection which may be brought about in two ways : (a) The microbes may be contained in or carried upon the agent that injures the arterial wall, or (b) microbes circulating in the blood may act upon a previously damaged endarterium or vasa vasorum.

A local infective arteritis may occur in ulcerative endocarditis ; it is not an uncommon cause of aneurysm, and, as first was pointed out by Dr. Osler and Dr. Hughlings Jackson, is almost the invariable cause of cerebral hæmorrhage in young people. I have examined several cases ; and in one of acute aneurysm of the ulnar and posterior tibial arteries, the coats of the aneurysms were attacked by an acute infective inflammation. We can understand that a small particle dislodged from a calcified valve by its rough edges might easily damage the wall of the artery ; and if it carried infection with it, or the blood itself contained infective organisms, it would bring about the very condition which we have seen above to be necessary to produce an acute arteritis experimentally.

General infective arteritis may occur after certain fevers ; for example, after typhoid fever, typhus fever, rheumatic fever, diphtheria, influenza, puerperal fever, and pneumonia. Osler, however, in over 200 recorded cases of typhoid fever, did not meet with a single instance of this complication. The French authors, however, particularly refer to the condition. Legroux has described acute arteritis in articular rheumatism, and Martin in diphtheria

According to Leyden, influenza is more likely to be followed by arteritis than is enteric fever ; such, at any rate, was his experience during the influenza epidemic 1889-90, in which thromboses of the arteries of the lower limbs, only to be explained by an arteritis, frequently occurred.

From some experiments, made by Thérèse, it seems possible that the toxins of the organisms are the direct cause of the arteritis ; for he found that by injecting a filtered culture of streptococcus he could produce the same effect as by injecting the organisms themselves. Acute arteritis has a predilection for the limbs, especially for the lower limbs. Barié found that in eleven out of thirteen cases the lower limbs were attacked, once the hand, once the face ; the posterior tibial was especially liable to it—eight times in eleven. Leyden and Guttmann found the same proportion in influenza, when, in eight cases, the popliteal was affected five times, a femoral artery once, a brachial once, and once a cerebral artery.

Symptoms.—Acute arteritis may come on during the progress of the primary disease or during convalescence. The first symptom is spontaneous localised pain in the limb, exaggerated by movement and pressure. When thrombosis occurs, a hard painful cord can be felt ; and there is enfeeblement and abolition of the pulse, associated with numbness and tingling, followed by anæsthesia, coldness of the skin, and swelling generally unaccompanied by œdema. The local temperature is lowered and the process frequently ends in gangrene, the extent of which varies according to the seat and extent of obstruction [see art. "Thrombosis" in this volume].

Morbid anatomy.—Gelatiniform patches caused by thickening and elevations of the intima, of varying size from a pin's head to a two-shilling piece, are found in the diseased arteries, associated with periarteritis. The patches, examined microscopically, are found to consist of embryonic round cells, spindle and stellate cells arranged in layers; and are associated always with a corresponding area of periarteritis: in fact, it seems highly probable that these varying-sized patches are due primarily to inflammatory changes in the vasa vasorum of the outer coat.

Acute infective aortitis.—A. *Patchy ("en plaques").* B. *Vegetative.* C. *Suppurating.*

A. The first or patchy variety is the commonest, and consists of irregular transparent gelatiniform patches on the inner surface, often stained with hæmoglobin.

B. The second or vegetative is due to a deposit of fibrin on one of the patches, which, as in ulcerative endocarditis, may be a source of acute embolism.

C. The third or suppurating variety is rare, and may be due, as Œttinger supposes, to pyogenetic infection of the vasa vasorum. Pus may then be found between the external or middle coats, and may burst inwards.

In acute aortitis it is only by the complications or accidents which occur that the condition can be surmised; such accidents are acute aneurysm, dissecting aneurysm, rupture with sudden death, and acute infective embolism without obvious valvular disease.

A case of general arteritis, pulmonary and systemic, has been described in a child by Dr. Herbert Hawkins; it was probably the result of congenital syphilis.

Dr. Charlewood Turner has described two cases of ulcerative aortitis—one mycotic, the other septicæmic—in which there were thrombi in the branches of the pulmonary arteries and septicæmia. This condition may be produced by an infective and calcareous aortic valve which, partially broken off at its attachment and striking against the wall of the aorta with every systole, damages the endothelium, and leads to secondary infection of the vessel.

REFERENCES

1. BALLANCE and EDMUNDS. *Ligation in Continuity*, 1891.—2. BARIÉ. "Contribution à l'histoire de l'artérite aigue," *Revue de médecine*, 1884.—3. BROUARDEL. "Études sur variole : lésions vasculaires du cœur et de l'aorte," *Archiv. gén. de méd.* 1874, vol. ii.—4. CHARCOT. *Senile Diseases*, p. 286.—5. CROCQ, *fils.* "Contributions à l'étude expérimentale des artérites infectieuses," *Arch. de méd. expériment.* vol. vi. 1891.—6. GUTTMANN and LEYDEN. *Die Influenze Epidemie*, 1889-90.—7. HAWKINS, H *Path. Soc. Trans.* 1892.—8. LEGROUX. *Soc. méd. des hôp.* 1884.—9. MARTIN. *Revue de méd.* 1881.—10. MOTT. "Cardio-vascular Nutrition, its Relation to Sudden Death," *Practitioner.* 1888. —11. THÉRÈSE. *Thèse de Paris*, 1891.—12. TURNER, F. C. *Path. Soc. Trans.* 1886.

Obliterative arteritis.—This disease was first described by Friedländer, in 1876. It is often accompanied by neuritis, and, before complete obliteration, intermittent claudication of the arteries of the limbs may occur, associated with cyanosis and coldness of the extremities; thus giving rise to a condition resembling that of Raynaud's disease.

The disease is more frequent in men than in women; it affects adults between thirty and sixty. The causes are unknown; it is not associated with any particular diathesis, nor with any acquired disease, such as syphilis, alcoholism, malaria, albuminuria or diabetes. I have, however, recently seen a case of symmetrical gangrene of the lower extremities in a middle-aged man suffering from alcoholic neuritis, the cause of the gangrene being arteritis and thrombosis.

Symptoms.—Like all anatomical modifications of the lumen of the arteries of the limbs which end gradually in occlusion, it may engender various premonitory symptoms long before it culminates in *gangrene.* These symptoms are pain in the limbs frequently occurring in crises, intermittent cyanosis, cramps, coldness, and numbness;—conditions which, transitory at first, afterwards instal themselves permanently. Sooner or later the pulse is no longer felt in the course of the arteries, and the temperature of the part is lowered, indicating the approach of gangrene. Ecchymotic patches appear at one or several points of the extremity of the limb. Eschars arise, and the gangrene, sometimes moist, sometimes dry, spreads with more or less rapidity. The lower limbs are affected more often than the upper, but it may begin in the hands; the affection is frequently, but by no means necessarily, symmetrical. In the amputations that have been practised it has been noticed that the arteries do not bleed, and the wound heals with difficulty unless the amputation have been high above the seat of mortification.

Microscopical examination reveals thickening of the walls of the arteries, due to cellular proliferation of the endarterium and hypertrophy of the middle and external coats; development of vasa vasorum in the middle and external coats, and inflammatory thickening of the small vessels which may have led to complete occlusion. The obliteration of the lumen of the artery may be due to thrombosis or proliferating endarteritis. The coats of the veins may be thickened, but these vessels are not blocked. Dr. Marinesco, to whom I am indebted for the specimen of obliterative endarteritis shown in Fig. 6, found in his case a degeneration of the muscles of the limb whilst the nerves remained unaffected.

Thoma does not agree with Friedländer that there is a special form of obliterative endarteritis; neither does he support the statement of Billroth and Winiwarter that gangrene in both old and young subjects is due to this condition. He considers that these authors have mistaken for it a thrombus replaced by connective tissue occurring in an artery affected with arterio-sclerosis. Certainly the photograph of the specimen supports this view. An interesting paper by Hoegerstedt and Nemmser upon the constriction and closure of large arteries, with an account of three cases, has lately been published in the *Zeitschrift für klinische*

Medicin. The condition is rare. Syphilis in some of the cases appears to have been the principal etiological factor, in others arterio-sclerosis with or without syphilis, and strain. In these cases a number of large arteries of the trunk and limbs have been constricted, and even gradually

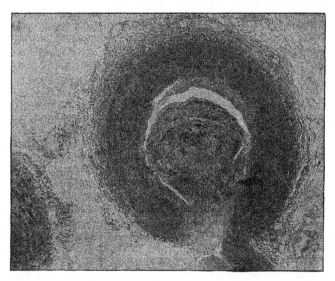

FIG. 6.—Photomicrograph. Section of anterior tibial artery in a case of obliterative endarteritis. This specimen shows the thickening of the inner coat and the existence of a thrombus which extends into a collateral. Really this is an example of arterio-sclerosis producing thrombosis and gangrene. The specimen was kindly given to me by Dr. Marinesco, whose case is referred to in the text. Magnification, 20 diameters.

occluded and converted into fibrous cords. It begins with a thickening of the arterial wall in the form of arterio-sclerosis, or as a syphilitic endarteritis; and it terminates in thrombosis and occlusion. The symptoms are various, according to the arteries affected and the rapidity of the process of occlusion; if it be gradual there is time for the establishment of collateral circulation, and there is no functional defect.

REFERENCES

1. BOILEAU. "Sur le rétrécissement généralisé des artères," *Thèse de Paris,* 1887.—2. BUROW. *Berlin. klin. Wochenschrift,* 1885.—3. DUTIL and LAMY. *Archives de méd. exp.* vol. v. 1893.—4. FRIEDLÄNDER. "Arteritis obliterans," *Cent. f. med. Wiss.* 1876.—5. HEIDENREICH. *La semaine méd.* 1892.—6. HOEGERSTEDT and NEMMSER. "Ueber die krankhafte Verengerung und Verschliessung vom Aortenbogen ausgehender grossen Arterien," *Zeitschrift f. klin. Med.* 1896.—7. JOFFROY and ACHARD. *Archives de méd. exp.* 1889.—8. MARINESCO. "Sur l'Angiomyopathie," *La semaine médicale,* Feb. 1896.—9. RIDEL. *Centralblatt f. Chir.* 1888, p. 554.—10. ROUTIER. *Bulletins de la soc. de chir.* 1887.—11. THOMA. *Text-Book of General Pathology,* vol. i. Translated by Alex. Bruce, M.D., 1896.—12. WIDERMANN. *Beiträge f. klin. Chir.* vol. xi. 1892.—13. WILL. *Berlin. klin. Wochenschrift,* 1886, p. 268.—14. WINIWARTER, VON. *Archiv f. klin. Chirurgie,* vol. xxiii.

Syphilitic arteritis.—*History and Introduction.*—The discovery of the pathology and symptomatology of this affection has been one of the most important advances in modern medicine; many grave nervous diseases are now curable, or amenable to treatment, which were formerly not even diagnosed.

At the end of the seventeenth century both Lancisi and Albertini recognised syphilis as a cause of aneurysm; and Morgagni, in his remarkable work *De sedibus morborum*, describes a necropsy upon a syphilitic patient thus:—"Cor laxum. In una ex arteriæ magnæ valvulis Aruntii corpusculum multo majus quam æquum esset. Sub eoque in ea facie qua valvula valvulas spectabat, membranæ laminæ ex quibus illa fiebat, ad modicum tractum ita sejunctæ, ut quia hiabant specillum immittere inter utramque potuerim. Ipse autem proximus arteriæ truncus albidis intus maculis passim distinctus, nec satis lævis, imo nonnihil inæqualis. Mox autem ad curvaturam *in Aneurysma distentus.*"

In another place he states: "Quod sæpe observavi in aliis cadaveribus, eorum præsertim, qui Syphilide laborarunt et ad *Aneurysma Aortæ* vel ad Pectoris Hydropem sunt dispositi."

Again in the same work he remarks, in describing the autopsy of a syphilitic patient: "Sed in Tenui meninge *arteriarum trunci omnes*— omnesque item earum rami, iique præsertim qui plexum Choroidem versus contendunt, multo erant crassiores æquo et duriores; exsiccatique osseam pluribus in locis naturam ostenderunt. Quinetiam Duram meningem idem ferme in ejus arteriis quæ crassiusculæ ipsæ quoque factæ erant conspectum est." Further on he describes swellings on all the large arteries and their branches, namely, the carotids, subclavians, and even the coronary arteries of the heart.

The investigation of arterial disease in syphilis was allowed to slumber, mainly owing to the teaching of John Hunter, until Dittrich, in 1849, described a case of inflammation and blocking of the right internal carotid and middle cerebral. Ziemssen considers the Danish physician Steenberg the discoverer of the connection of this form of arteritis with syphilis; although before the appearance of his work, in 1860, isolated observations of disease in the larger arteries of the brain had been published by Virchow, Bristow, and others. Wilks was the first author in this country to call attention to syphilitic disease of the arteries, in 1863. He ascribed to syphilis certain nodules found on the cerebral arteries, and also the constricted lumen of these vessels, in a woman aged 38, who, five years previously, had been infected with syphilis, and who died from an apoplectic seizure. In 1868 Professor Clifford Allbutt made a microscopical examination of the vessels, and described *for the first time* the histological changes in a case of "Cerebral Disease in a Syphilitic Patient" in the following words:— "Both the long and cross sections showed great inequality in the thickness of the walls and of the several coats. This change was due to a chronic arteritis with great nuclear and cellular proliferation, and affecting all the coats to some extent, but especially the middle and inner coats. The distinction between the coats was in many places lost." Then again he noted that there was no atheroma. He found also the minutest arteries affected. This important observation did not attract the attention that it deserved, and it was not until 1874 that Heubner published his work upon the microscopical appearances of syphilitic arteritis affecting the cerebral vessels; and this work, so practically important and interesting, may be said to have laid the foundation of our knowledge of the subject. About this time Dr. Julius Mickle published a number of cases of syphilitic arteritis. In 1877 Dr. Barlow demonstrated a similar condition of the cerebral arteries in infants, the subjects of hereditary syphilis.

Although Heubner considered endarteritis invariably primary, yet it is now amply proved that in some cases the disease starts as a periarteritis; and this condition was, according to A. Bruce, first described by Sir John Batty Tuke in 1874. In Allbutt's case, however, there was undoubtedly periarteritis accompanying the endarteritis.

Although syphilis has a special predilection for the cerebral arteries, giving rise to characteristic clinical symptoms, yet other arteries are affected by endarteritis and even periarteritis; but, with the exception of the aorta itself and the coronary arteries, the symptoms presented by arterial disease of the organs due to syphilis are not distinguishable from general syphilitic affection of the organ.

Brain syphilis is an affection of the arteries in one form or another. Even gummata start in the pia-arachnoid around the vessels, although in many instances seemingly situated within the brain substance. It was formerly taught that syphilitic arteritis is usually a late secondary or a tertiary symptom; now most authors concur in believing that it may arise in the early stage of the secondary period, or at any subsequent time. It is now recognised that brain syphilis may and frequently does occur in the first year; indeed the statistics of Hjellmann show that it is most frequent in the first year, and that the numbers diminish with each successive year. Of 30 cases of brain syphilis which I have had under my care, with a sure history of the time of infection, one half occurred within the first four years. Three cases occurred during the first year; four during the second year; five in the third year, and three in the fourth. Pathologically, syphilitic disease of the arteries falls into three groups, but the groups may be associated : (a) obstruction of blood-supply of an organ; (b) irritation; (c) weakening of the arterial walls.

Causes.—A tendency to disease of the cerebral vessels may be hereditary; I have seen two brothers affected at the same time with syphilitic arteritis cerebri. Blows on the head often precede the onset of the disease. Probably, however, the most important cause is neglect of specific treatment. Nearly all authors agree that syphilitic arteritis is much more likely to occur in persons who have not been specifically treated. Toxic influences, such as chronic alcoholism and plumbism, may also be important factors, especially the former. Excesses "in Baccho et in Venere" are often followed by symptoms of arterial disease.

It seems probable also that those blood dyscrasias which raise arterial pressure would tend to internal strain of these vessels, and render them more liable to disease ; especially the aorta and coronary arteries. In the case of the aorta and coronary arteries physical exertion plays a most important part in the symptoms and complications that may arise in connection with syphilitic disease—such as sudden rupture of the aorta, formation of false, dissecting and true aneurysms. I recall very few cases of aneurysm of the aorta in men from whom I had not been able to obtain or detect a specific history. Maclean pointed out that in soldiers the most important cause of aneurysm is syphilis ; and Welch, in 1876, made a number of observations on soldiers, and showed that in 34 cases 17 were undoubtedly syphilitic, and 8 were probably so. He found further, in necropsies on 56, the subjects of syphilis, that 60 per cent had disease of the aorta. Malmesten attributes 80 per cent of aortic aneurysms to syphilis. Likewise a large proportion of cases of aneurysm of the cerebral arteries, and of the large vessels of the body, are of syphilitic origin.

Pathology.—Syphilitic arteritis may affect, simultaneously or successively, a number of arteries of the body ; and in some instances it gives rise to a general affection of the small arteries and arterioles (*vide* Periarteritis nodosa). Again it may be limited to the aorta, or even to the coronary arteries ; but by far the most frequent and important seat of the disease is the brain. The disease falls especially upon the arteries about the base, namely, the vertebrals and the basilar, together with the carotids—the vessels which enter into the formation of the circle of Willis and its branches. The arteries in the Sylvian fissure are very liable to the affection; and on several occasions I have found obliterative endarteritis of the opto-striate branches which enter the island of Reil and the anterior perforated space. Why it should affect these parts of the arterial circulation, and spare the vessels of the hemispheres, has yet received no adequate explanation. It may be that the basal vessels are surrounded with a large quantity of cerebro-spinal fluid which possibly contains the syphilitic toxin. The disease is often bilateral and symmetrical.

Pathological anatomy.—To the naked eye small grayish white opaque nodules or plates are visible in the walls of the vessel; they are firm and of a stiff cartilaginous consistence. The lumen, in cross section, appears narrower, like a half moon; but as the growth proceeds there may be circular constriction of the lumen so as almost to obliterate it (*vide* Fig. 7). In the universal syphilitic arteritis, which is often mistaken for general paralysis of the insane, the small as well as the large arteries are affected. In a case recently examined the small arteries looked like stiff, coarse threads of a dirty white colour ; and on section their walls appeared to be greatly thickened, which accounted for their firmness when rolled between the fingers.

As in the illustration, the vessels are frequently the seat of thrombosis; and eventually they may be changed into firm and solid cylinders : this affection of the intima may be the sole naked-eye appearance of disease; but it may be associated with gummata around the vessels, and gummatous meningitis; or, in the generalised form of syphilitic meningitis, there may be periarteritis and endarteritis affecting all the arteries, great and small (*vide* Fig. 8). Hitherto I have been referring to the vessels of the brain; but I have seen cases of obliterating endarteritis affecting the coronary arteries (*vide* Fig. 9) with or without associated aortitis. Little

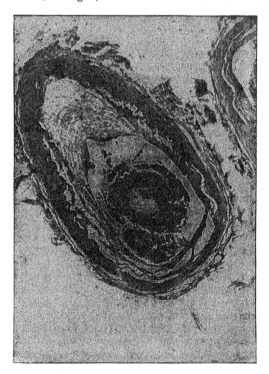

Fig. 7.—Photomicrograph. Syphilitic endarteritis and thrombotic occlusion of the opto-striate branches of the left middle cerebral, producing a defect of speech and right hemiplegia. There was softening of the island of Reil and of the internal capsule and basal ganglia. Patient, aged forty-seven, was certified as a case of general paralysis. Magnification, 50 diameters.

fibrous nodules, caused by a swelling of the intima, obliterated one or both arteries and caused fatty degeneration of the heart. Generally the orifice is so affected; but in one case, a young man who had had syphilis and was suffering with Bright's disease and lead poisoning, the right coronary one inch beyond the orifice was obliterated almost completely.

Out of 50 cases of cardio-vascular disease, which I investigated in the wards and post-mortem room of Charing Cross Hospital, I found three cases of syphilitic coronary stenosis. The appearance of the intima was very much the same as in the cerebral vessels; little fibrous nodular swellings encroached upon the lumen, and in one case to such an extent was the vessel blocked that a large bristle could not be inserted (*vide* Fig. 10). I have also seen most extensive proliferation of the intima in the renal vessels of a syphilitic subject.

It may be asserted, as a general rule, that syphilitic endarteritis is a

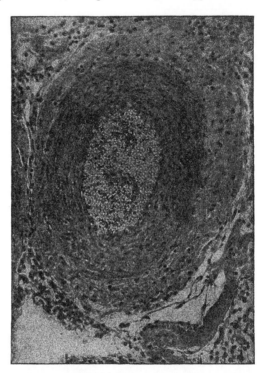

FIG. 8.—Photomicrograph. Cerebro-spinal syphilitic meningitis and periarteritis. The outer and middle coats are infiltrated with leucocytes. The blood in the vessel contains a great excess of leucocytes. The whole of the arteries of the brain and cord were affected; in some situations there was extensive endarteritis, and the whole of the left fossa Sylvii was filled up with a gummatous mass. The case was diagnosed as one of general paralysis of the insane. Magnification, 200 diameters.

distinct process from atheroma. Heubner asserts that the new cell formation of the inner coat always goes on to fibrosis and never undergoes caseation or calcification. Huber argues against this too restricted doctrine of Heubner, and cites a case of a prostitute infected six months before death : at the necropsy extensive endarteritis was found in the aorta, and many of the patches were undergoing caseation and calcification. The observation of Admannson, confirmed by Birch-Hirschfeld, and others, upon the atheromatous changes in the umbilical vessels and

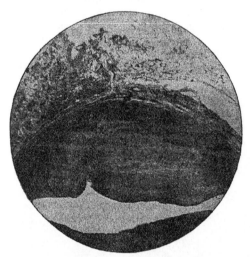

FIG. 9.—Photomicrograph. Endarteritis obliterans of the right coronary one inch from its origin, probably syphilitic, in a man aged twenty-nine the subject of chronic Bright's disease. Lead poisoning. The patient died from cardiac failure. A large thrombus was found in the left ventricle adherent to the apex, also an aneurysm of the abdominal aorta. There was marked fatty degeneration of the right ventricle. Magnification, 20 diameters.

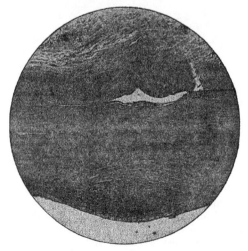

FIG 10.—Photomicrograph. Section of a nodular endarteritis of the left coronary artery. There is no tendency to caseation or calcification. The patient was aged thirty-eight. There was atheroma of the aorta, but little or no affection of the aortic valves. The patient died with obscure symptoms of extreme fatty degeneration of the heart, occasioned by almost complete obliteration of both coronary arteries. Magnification, 75 diameters.

in the arteries of premature fœtuses still-born owing to syphilitic infection from the parents, supports this view; but the rule is nevertheless as Heubner states it.

In several cases of young women with a syphilitic history, who have died in the asylum at Claybury, I have found well-marked general endarteritis cerebri with equally well-marked atheroma of the aorta. Indeed I am beginning to regard atheroma of the aorta in young people as strong presumptive evidence of syphilis.

Microscopical appearances.—The inner coat is greatly thickened by proliferation of the subendothelial layer, so that the elastic lamina will be found separated from the lumen by a great development of newly-formed tissue consisting of spindle and stellate cells; or, in a later stage, of fibrous material. The wall is usually affected unequally, being more thickened on one side than the other; and, when the vessel is cut transversely, the patch of disease is often crescentic in shape. There is very little tendency to degeneration; but as the lesion grows older, it becomes denser, firmer, and cicatricial. Not infrequently the vessel is blocked with a recent or organised thrombus. The elastic coat is sometimes ruptured, sometimes stretched so as to lose its crinkled appearance; and the muscular fibres of the middle coat have often undergone degeneration. The elastic lamina is frequently split; according to Heubner a new elastic lamina may be formed, but this is denied by Cornil. In the case of the aorta and large vessels I have generally found an accompanying peri-arteritis and mesarteritis. The nutrient arteries of the large vessels are greatly thickened, and extensive inflammation is aroused, the vessels being surrounded with leucocytes (*vide* Figs. 11, 12, and 13). In the case of the aorta, the inflamed vessels often penetrate the inner coat, and the inflammation may be so intense that hæmorrhages may occur into the middle and inner coats, as in the case of the aorta figured. With such intense inflammation it can easily be understood how sudden strains may cause a rupture or dilatation of the wall at the diseased spot, and the formation of an aneurysm. As I have already said, there is little or no tendency in the proliferated subendothelial tissue to undergo either caseation or calcification. This rule applies to the cerebral vessels, the most frequent seat of syphilitic disease; but in the case of the aorta it is quite possible that degenerative changes may occur from blocking of the vasa vasorum. Many authors consider that syphilis is a cause of arterio-sclerosis; certainly there is no reason why arterio-sclerosis, a degenerative process, should not be favoured or even induced by the devitalising influence of syphilis.

Hereditary endarteritis syphilitica, described by Barlow, Chiari, Hawkins, and others, presents the same microscopical characters as that of acquired syphilis.

The relation of syphilis to the pathology of aneurysm of the aorta, large vessels, cerebral vessels, and heart will be considered elsewhere.

Symptoms.—The symptoms of syphilitic arteritis may be divided into two categories, (A) obliterative and (B) ectasial arteritis.

A. Obliterative arteritis.—The obliteration may be thrombotic; or there may be occlusion, generally partial, owing to the lateral projection of the proliferated coat.

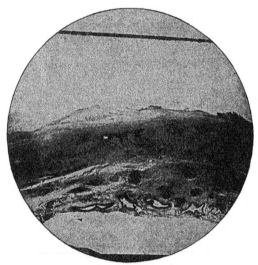

FIG. 11.—Photomicrograph. Periarteritis nodosa. Mœsarteritis and endarteritis of the aorta. The black nodules in the external coat consist of masses of leucocytes ; so also the little black patches in the media. Patient was a man aged forty-seven who died from aortic valvular disease of long standing. Magnification, 10 diameters.

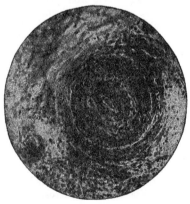

FIG. 12.—Photomicrograph. Endarteritis obliterans of the vasa vasorum of the aorta, from a case of acute syphilitic arteritis with rupture, formation of dissecting aneurysm and death in a man aged thirty-one. Magnification, 150.

B. Ectasial arteritis may be divided into (a) Simple aneurysmal dilatation with the phenomena of irritation or compression of adjacent structures; (b) Aneurysmal dilatation with rupture, ending in cerebral hæmorrhage.

In the first subdivision there may be all possible varieties of hemiplegias, monoplegias, ocular palsies, and aphasia. With complete obliteration a clinical picture may be presented varying with the calibre and seat of the artery. Whereas in partial obliteration the symptoms may be temporary and curable, in complete obliteration it must necessarily be permanent, and in a measure irreparable. The symptoms arising from the ensuing softening of brain substance depend entirely upon the size of the vessel blocked, the situation and area of brain substance supplied by the vessel, and, lastly, upon the possibility of collateral circulation. [For further particulars the reader is referred to the article on "Thrombosis" in this volume.]

Arteritis without accompanying gummatous meningitis, and without

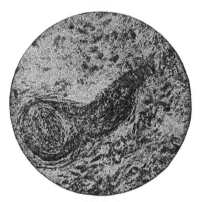

Fig. 13.—Photomicrograph of small nutrient artery of the aorta from a case of chronic Bright's disease, lead poisoning, and (probably) syphilis. Endarteritis obliterans. In the immediate neighbourhood there was nodular atheroma. Examination of sections from this and other cases leads me to believe that the nodular character of the disease in the aorta is due to changes in the vasa vasorum, such as are represented in this and the other photomicrograph. Magnification, 150 diameters.

thrombotic occlusion, may occur ; but it will be gathered from what has been said that a number of vessels of the circle of Willis must be affected before any pronounced symptoms arise; and, according to Heubner, only when two large adjacent branches of the circle of Willis are affected do circulatory disturbances in a hemisphere arise. The result of endarteritis syphilitica of the brain is a disturbance of the circulation of the whole brain, and specially of the hemispheres ; causing, according to the extent of the disease, slight or severe disturbance of the functions of this organ. The result may be psychical disturbances, which Heubner asserts were never absent in the cases observed by himself. These are slowness and difficulty in thinking, loss of decision, weakness of memory (amnesia), apathy, stupor, irritability, various anomalous moods and sleeplessness. These and other allied phenomena can be ascribed to the defective circulation in the hemispheres. It can be understood that if one or more of the large arteries are in great part occluded, considerable variations of the blood-pressure in the hemispheres may result; and this would account for fainting fits and losses of consciousness like true apoplectic seizures.

The transitory character of the early phenomena of syphilitic arteritis (before thrombosis has occurred) is a very important feature. The narrowing of the lumen may be very well marked, but still some blood can get through; or at any rate there is time for collateral circulation to be established, and this is the key to the peculiarities of the symptomatology. As Oppenheim in his valuable work points out, you may have a hemi-paresis lasting perhaps a few minutes, a few hours, or a few days; then it disappears, again to return, and eventually ends in permanent hemiplegia. It may begin with a transitory monoplegia, which gradually extends and affects arm, leg, or face; thus becoming hemiplegic in character, and often associated with aphasia, especially when the hemiplegia is on the right side. Charcot pointed out that one of the most characteristic signs of syphilitic arteritis is aphasia. The transitory trouble in speech may occur several times in the day. There is in other cases temporary word blindness, disordered vision, vertigo, word deafness, and all forms of speech defects, amnesia, alexia, etc. We can easily understand how these losses of function arise: there is a temporary disturbance of the circulation in the various parts of the brain which are concerned with these various functions; but collateral circulation through other vessels supplies the necessary nutrition, and with it the return of function comes back. The experiments of Dr. Leonard Hill throw considerable light upon this subject. He has ligatured both carotid and both vertebral arteries in the dog; the animal is then for some days demented, paretic, and suffers (probably) with psychical blindness. At the end of a week it recovers. He has found the anterior spinal arteries dilated to the size of vertebrals, and these restored the circulation to the hemispheres. The "neurons" had not died from the temporary cutting off of the blood-supply, but they were incapable of exercising their functions. I have examined the brains of these animals microscopically, and I find the cells are for the most part quite normal in structure. If, however, a monkey or cat be used for this experiment, a sufficient collateral circulation is not established soon enough, and the animal usually dies, frequently with convulsions, at the end of twenty-four hours. The cells of the brain in these latter animals exhibit most marked degenerative changes, indicating that recovery would be impossible; and permanent loss of function must have occurred. The gradual obliteration caused by syphilitic endarteritis allows of gradual re-establishment of circulation by collateral branches, and the brain substance is not, therefore, completely deprived of nutrition; the disturbance of circulation is temporary, and the loss of function is also temporary; but, if the disease be not treated, the vessels which allowed of the re-establishment of the circulation become similarly blocked, and then softening of the area of brain supplied by the diseased vessels ensues, and the loss of function is permanent. It is, therefore, of the greatest importance to recognise the disease in the earliest stage—that of the temporary loss of brain function, for it is often very amenable to treatment. Mercurial inunction or injections combined with large doses of iodide of potassium will save a man from softening of the brain, incurable paralysis, and mental failure. Probably the therapeutic action is not so much the opening up of the old obliterated or partially obliterated vessels as the prevention of thrombosis and of the extension of the disease to vessels either little affected or not at all, vessels which are therefore able to maintain the circulation.

Sometimes the patient can describe exactly the onset of the paralysis or aphasia; but usually at the time there was giddiness and dulness of perception, or somnolence, symptoms which sometimes persist even after the paralysis has passed off.

It is much more common to find loss of motor power than loss of sensibility; but various sensory phenomena may occur, such as pain, paræsthesia, hemianæsthesia, hemianopsy, etc. Frequently there is paralysis of cranial nerves, generally associated with hemiplegia. I have recorded a case of complete paralysis of the fifth nerve with enophthalmos and hemiplegia, all on the right side. The most frequent paralysis is some form of *ocular paralysis*, which may be due to a lesion of the nerve or the nucleus. I have recorded a case of paralysis of both third nerves with marked paresis in both lower extremities, and to a less degree in the upper; complete recovery occurred under treatment [*vide* "Disease of Cranial Nerves" in the following volume].

Oppenheim points out that dysarthria is not infrequently met with in association with difficulty of swallowing and bulbar symptoms indicating disease of the basilar or vertebrals. Alternate hemiplegia is another symptom of basilar disease. I have met with various difficulties of speech; namely, a curious drawling staccato speech without any distinct paralysis of the muscles of articulation, due to patchy softening of the hemispheres of a widespread nature.

Mr. Hutchinson relates a case of Anderson's in which, for two years before the onset of severe paralytic symptoms, from occlusion of the basilar, prodroma occurred in the form of headache and psychical disturbances. The disease is apt to be mistaken for general paralysis of the insane, as I have several times seen. In general paralysis, however, the speech defects are not transitory; the tremor is finer, ocular paralysis is rare, Argyll Robertson pupils are very common, and the mental symptoms are usually more marked and more characteristic. Inasmuch as specific treatment is not, as a rule, of much use in general paralysis, but is highly beneficial in syphilitic arteritis, the diagnosis is of the greatest importance. Early treatment decides the prognosis in many cases, and a complete recovery occurs in some. But, as a rule, even under the most favourable circumstances, the patient is not quite the same as before. There is often slight loss of expression in the face, a little slowness and hesitancy in speech, a loss of memory, an inability to undergo mental fatigue, slight weakness of grasp, dragging of the leg or legs, a little spastic rigidity with exaggeration of knee-jerks and clonus. Frequently I have seen patients go on for years apparently well, and then a fresh attack has occurred. [For further particulars and for treatment *vide* articles "Thrombosis" and "Syphilis."]

Syphilitic arteritis affecting the coronary arteries may give rise to severe symptoms of cardiac degeneration.

If, as in the case figured, the arteries are almost completely blocked the heart will undergo acute fatty degeneration from insufficient nutrition. I have seen this occur in several cases. In two of the cases, previously referred to, of coronary obstruction due to syphilis, there was absolutely no valvular lesion. The patients suffered with symptoms of cardiac dilatation ; the pulse was hardly to be felt at the wrist, though, when one hand was placed over the cardiac area, the impulse was forcible, and diffused over a considerable surface ; the other hand upon the pulse detected the fact that many of the beats were not forcible enough to produce a pulse-wave in the radial artery. Such cases are generally rapidly fatal; the patients first complain of breathlessness on exertion without obvious cause, of fainting feelings from cerebral anæmia, especially on assuming the erect posture, of giddiness and vertigo. These cases are of extreme importance from the point of view of life insurance ; as men between twenty and forty, who have had syphilis but who have no signs of valvular disease, may yet exhibit symptoms of cardiac degeneration most difficult to account for. Often there is arrhythmia, and the pulse may sometimes be slow, sometimes quick. Anginal spasms frequently occur.

Syphilitic arteritis followed by thrombosis may affect the branches of the coronary arteries, and cause necrosis of patches of myocardium ; the degenerated tissue may yield, and an aneurysm of the heart result : but more commonly there is a gradual process of coagulation necrosis of the muscles and fibrous substitution, thus accounting for many cases of the so-called fibroid heart of syphilitic origin [*vide* "Diseases of the Heart," vol. v. p. 404].

It is probable that some cases of so-called Raynaud's disease—symmetrical gangrene—are due to syphilitic arteritis.

Hereditary syphilitic arteritis.—The *symptomatology* has a close resemblance to that of the acquired disease of adults; namely, convulsions, headache increased in severity at nights, irritability, paralysis, and speech defects of various kinds. Dr. Barlow states that the result has been sometimes softening, sometimes sclerosis of the brain ; more frequently the latter. If the Rolandic area or the pyramidal system has been affected in any part, descending degeneration of the crossed pyramidal tract occurs, with spastic rigidity of the limbs and contracture ; and he concludes his admirable account, based upon a number of cases, by contrasting the brain disease due to hereditary syphilis with that due to the acquired disease, as follows :—" We find that amentia, in association with eclampsia and spastic limbs, are to be regarded as typical of hereditary syphilis ; hemiplegia, with or without unilateral convulsions, as typical of acquired syphilis in the adult. The morbid anatomy of the former consists mainly of chronic meningitis and endarteritis, with cortical sclerosis and atrophy, whereas the common lesions in acquired syphilis are gummata and softening from arterial disease and thrombosis."

Periarteritis nodosa. — In 1866 Kussmaul and Maier described a hitherto unknown disease which they observed in a tailor who was attacked with Bright's disease and rapid progressive muscular atrophy.

The disease began with diarrhœa, shivers, sweating, and a feeling of numbness in the fingers. The patient was anæmic, but during the progress of the disease the temperature was generally normal, and the heart and the pulse not noticeably changed; the urine was diminished, and contained blood, much albumin, and many epithelial cells and casts. Paralysis began in the index finger and some muscles of thumb, and spread later to the other muscles; there was severe pain in the muscles, both spontaneous and on pressure; parts of the skin were anæsthetic, while others were hyperæsthetic; pains of a colicky nature occurred in the hypochondriac region; there was sometimes constipation, sometimes diarrhœa. Four weeks after admission little nodules, the size of a split pea, were found beneath the skin of the abdomen and chest. At the autopsy little nodular swellings, varying in size from a poppy-seed to a pea, were found on the small arteries of all the muscles, except those of the face, and on most of the subcutaneous arteries. With the exception of the pulmonary, most of the arteries of the body were affected. When examined microscopically, an acute inflammation of the media and adventitia were found.

Four other cases of a somewhat similar character have been described since. Three of these cases have been associated with multiple aneurysms.

Etiology.—Weichselbaum considers this form of arteritis to be of syphilitic origin; von Kahlden does not. The whole course of the disease from the beginning to the fatal end takes from six to twelve weeks; this is not like syphilis. Nor does the localisation suggest this infection, especially the freedom of the cerebral vessels; in fact, though everything points to some general infective agent, nothing has been discovered. The sudden onset of the disease, its rapid course, and the great wasting support this opinion. No micro-organisms have been found in sections, but hitherto no culture preparations have been made.

Symptoms.—The onset of the disease is sudden, with fever and shivers; and its course is soon characterised by progressive marasmus and great anæmia. It is important to observe the absence of a relation between the enormously high pulse frequency and the relatively low temperature during the subsequent course of the disease. Not less characteristic are the violent pains which occur in the most various parts of the body; but they are especially frequent and violent in the hypochondrium, and sometimes are limited to this situation. A rapid progress of the disease to death has been observed in all cases. Enteritis or nephritis generally accompanies the above phenomena; they are probably due to thrombotic occlusion of numerous small arteries, giving rise in the mucous membrane of the intestine to hæmorrhagic infarctions which later lead to ulcers; and in the kidney to multiple ischæmic necrosis. A part of the degenerative change of the renal epithelium may be due to the anæmia; the œdema, which is generally present, may be dependent upon nephritis, anæmia, or the changes in the arteries; or to a combination of these changes. Up till now the case of Kussmaul and Maier is the only one in which nodules were found under the skin during life. Such a symptom, if present, would be of the utmost value in diagnosis. The nervous symptoms are probably due to changes in the arteries supplying the nervous structures of the spinal cord, the spinal ganglia, and the nerves.

Pathological anatomy.—A study of the published cases of this disease show that they must be divided into two classes, distinguished by the presence or absence of syphilis.

A syphilitic nodular periarteritis has been described by Baumgarten, Alex. Bruce, Gilbert, Lion, and Lamy. Really this disease is one of multiple gummata, with general cerebro-spinal, peri- and endarteritis.

Dr. Alex. Bruce divides the cases into three groups :—

(*a*) The outer coat is infiltrated more or less uniformly with round cells, but without any marked tendency to degeneration (*vide* Fig. 8).

(*b*) The outer coat shows a nodular and diffuse cellular infiltration with commencing caseation.

(*c*) The outer coat shows a distinct formation of caseous gummata as well as diffuse periarteritis.

I have observed all these conditions in the same case, and they represent successive stages in the formation of a gumma.

No case has yet been recorded in which a definite periarteritis has been seen more than four years after the primary infection. In fact, the earlier the occurrence of severe cerebral or spinal symptoms following infection the more likely is it to be due to this form of the disease. In a case I recently examined the symptoms appeared within a year of the infection. Gilbert and Lion speak of the symptoms appearing even before the primary stage had passed away.

Symptoms.—The symptoms may be intense headache (worse at night), giddiness, or pains in the head and neck, optic neuritis, vomiting, symptoms of mania, convulsions, unconsciousness, palsies of muscles supplied by cranial nerves, hemiplegia, monoplegia, paraplegia, and aphasia.

Tuberculous arteritis.—This affection is even more specific in its character than the syphilitic affection, because it is possible to recognise the pathogenetic organism in the walls of the vessels. It affects especially the medium-sized and small arteries and arterioles, leaving the large arteries free.

The situations in which tuberculous affection is especially apt to occur are the cerebral arteries, the lobular branches of the pulmonary artery, and the renal arteries.

Specific cerebral arteritis is found in tuberculous meningitis. It starts in most instances in the perivascular lymphatic sheath, and the new formation proceeds from without inwards, invading the middle and inner

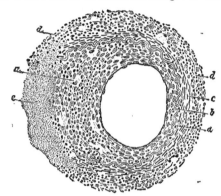

FIG. 14.—Tuberculous arteritis. *a* Intima, a_1 proliferous intima infiltrated with cells and containing tubercle-bacilli ; *b*, inner elastic lamella ; *c*, media ; *d*, proliferous adventitia infiltrated with cells and containing tubercle-bacilli ; *e*, caseous portion of the vessel-wall. (Preparation stained with fuchsin and methylene blue, and mounted in Canada balsam : × 100, but the bacilli have been sketched under a higher magnifying power.)

coats successively. It is especially likely to occur in the middle cerebral and its branches. Damage of the endothelium leads to thrombosis and obliteration of the lumen already considerably constricted, and as a result there is extensive softening of the cerebral substance (*vide* Figs. 14, 15).

Tuberculous lesions of the pulmonary artery belong to the history of excavation in the lungs, and the reader is referred to the article on "Phthisis Pulmonalis" for fuller information. The mechanism is of the same character in all cases; but, according to its seat and distribution, it produces different morbid changes. Along with the peribronchial affection, ending in caseation, there is invasion of the arterioles that accompany the terminal ramifications of the bronchi. In excavation all the tissues are destroyed except the artery and bronchus which are left exposed ; the bronchus, surrounded by the caseous tuberculous material, ulcerates, the artery is at first irritated, and as a result

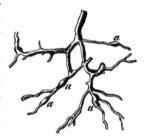

FIG. 15.—Periarteritis nodosa. *a*, Node-like swelling. (Vessels taken from the mesentery of the small intestine : natural size.)

there is proliferation of the inner coat. Thrombosis may occur, or the tuberculous process may invade the wall of the artery on the surface towards the cavity, and soften the coat ; the blood-pressure in the vessel then causes dilatation with formation of an aneurysm of Rasmussen.

In the tuberculous kidney, more especially in the miliary form of the affection, systematised bacillary lesions occur in the course of the radiating arteries. The microbial infection is embolic in origin. The consecutive infective thrombosis can be recognised by the naked eye, and the result is that tracts of caseous material appear along the course of the pyramids of Ferrein; even cones, like infarcts, may be found sometimes (Letulle). Tuberculous arteritis is usually produced by extension of a periarterial focus into the arterial wall; but it may occur primarily from embolic infection, as in the kidney.

To the naked eye the arteries present circumscribed thickenings; at first firm and gray, then friable and yellow. In pulmonary tuberculosis two forms are met with—(a) nodular aneurysmal, (b) obliterating.

Examined microscopically, the walls of the arteries are found infiltrated with round cells, islets of which are found in the adventitia around the vasa vasorum; giant cells may exist. As in syphilis, there is proliferation of the endothelial layer of the intima, and thickening of the same by a new formation consisting of spindle-shaped and stellate cells; the intensity of the inflammation may cause a rupture of the elastic lamina and an incursion of leucocytes in great numbers. The rupture of the elastic lamina with the degeneration and death of the muscular fibres leads to weakening of the wall, and may result in the formation of an aneurysm. Again, as in syphilis, thrombosis or caseation of the granulation tissue may occur; and if the vessel have not been blocked by a thrombus, it often ruptures and so gives rise to hæmorrhage; should rupture not take place, bacillary infection of the blood-stream may occur.

A more favourable termination is fibrous hyperplasia of the adventitia with cicatrisation and occlusion.

Degeneration of the arterial walls.—*Fatty degeneration* is seen principally in the aorta just above the semilunar valves, where in almost all adults will be found opaque whitish spots or lines scarcely if at all elevated; it is not common, however, in the medium-sized arteries, and is, as a rule, of little clinical importance. Fatty degeneration, however, of the small vessels of the brain in general paralysis and in various blood diseases, such as pernicious anæmia, leucocythæmia, scurvy, or purpura, may occasion the symptoms of rupture and hæmorrhage. In the large arteries the process begins with fatty degeneration of the endothelial cells of the intima; these become filled with fat globules which stain black with osmic acid. The endothelium may become detached, and a shallow breach of the surface result; but, as a rule, it leaves the subjacent structures unchanged: yet sometimes there is an extension of the fatty degeneration to the subendothelial layers, and a proliferation of the fixed cells in the neighbourhood, which not infrequently take into their interior the products of fatty disintegration. The tunica media is sometimes the seat of fatty degeneration, the fat granules are seen between the elastic fibres and laminæ, and, when very profuse, the muscular fibres are no longer seen; a disappearance which is due to fatty degeneration of the muscle fibres.

Calcareous degeneration is often associated with fatty changes in the media, especially in the arteries of the lower limbs; it may also be associated with hyaline degeneration or atheroma. Simple calcareous degeneration is a senile change found chiefly in the middle-sized arteries: it affects the muscular fibres of the middle coat, and appears as a band running partly around the vessel, which at the same time is dilated and loses its elasticity; if the change be very far advanced the artery is converted into a tortuous rigid tube (gas-pipe artery). This form of degeneration is frequently followed by gangrene of the lower extremity owing to thrombotic occlusion (*vide* Fig. 24). The calcareous salts are deposited in small glistening granules, which coalesce to form compact plates. Sometimes these calcareous plates may present the appearances of true bone.

In the next section we have to consider a very important and widespread change in the arteries of which the senile condition forms one division.

REFERENCES

Syphilitic Arteritis: 1. ALLBUTT, T. C. "Case of Cerebral Disease in a Syphilitic Patient," *St. George's Hospital Reports*, 1869.—2. BARLOW. *Path. Soc. Trans.* vol. xxviii. —3. BRUCE, ALEX. "Syphilitic Nodose Periarteritis," *Medico-Chir. Soc. Trans.* Edin. 1894.—4. CHARRIER and KLIPPEL. *Revue de médecine exp.* 1894.—5. CORNIL and RANVIER. *Traité d'anatomie pathologique.*—6. DITTRICH. "Der syph. Krankheitsprocessen d. Leber," *Prager Viertelj.* 1849, Bd. xxi. p. 21.—7. GOWERS. *Diseases of the Nervous System.*—8. HEUBNER. *Die luetische Erkrankungen d. Hirnarterien*, Leipzig, 1874.—9. LANCEREAUX. *Dict. encyclopœdique des sciences méd.*—10. LANG. *Vorlesungen über d. Pathologie und Therapie der Syphilis.*—11. MICKLE. *Brit. and Foreign Med.-Chir. Review*, 1875.—12. *Idem. Brit. and Foreign Med. Review*, 1876.—12a. *Idem.* "On Syphilis of the Nervous System," *ibid.* vol. xviii. 1865.—13. MORGAGNI. *De sedibus et causis morborum*, T. ii. p. 369.—14. *Idem.* T. i. p. 297.—15. *Idem.* T. i. p. 296.—16. OPPENHEIM. *Die syphilitische Erkrankungen des Gehirns.*—17. STEENBERG. *Canstatt's Jahresb.* 1861, p. 328.—18. VIRCHOW. *Geschwulste*, Bd. ii. p. 444.—19. WILKS. *Guy's Hospital Reports*, 3rd series, vol. ix. 1865.— 20. WUNDERLICH. *Syphilitic Diseases of the Brain and Spinal Cord.* German Clinical Lectures. Series ii. New Sydenham Soc.—21. VON ZIEMSSEN. *Syphilis of the Nervous System.* Clinical Lectures, German, Author's, 1894. **Tuberculous Arteritis:** 22. CORNIL. "Tuberculosis," *Journal de l'anatomie*, xvi. 1880; and *Pathol. Histology*, London, 1882.— 23. GUARINERI. "Tuberculous Meningitis," *Archiv. p. le scienze med.* vii. 1884.—24. KIENER. "Tuberculosis of Serous Membranes," *Arch. de physiol.* vii. 1880.—25. MARTIN. *Recherches sur le tubercule.* Paris, 1879.—26. MÉNATRIER. "Vascular Lesion in Phthisical Pulmonary Cavities," *Arch. de méd. exp.* ii. 1890.—27. NARSE. *Virchow's Archiv*, cv. 1886.—28. WEIGERT. *Virchow's Archiv*, lxxxviii. 1882. **Periarteritis Nodosa:** 29. EPPINGER. *Pathogenesis d. Aneurysmen.* Berlin, 1887.—30. KUSSMAUL and MAIER. "A Peculiar Arterial Affection," *Deutsche Archiv f. klin. Med.* i.—31. VON KAHLDEN. "Periarteritis Nodosa," *Ziegler's Beiträge*, xi. 1894.—32. FLETCHER. "Periarteritis Nodosa," *Ziegler's Beiträge*, 1892.—33. MEYER, P. "Periarteritis Nodosa," *Virchow's Archiv*, lxxxiv. 1878.—34. WEICHSELBAUM and CHVOSTEK. *Alg. Wien. med. Zeit.* No. 28, 1877.

ARTERIO-SCLEROSIS

Introduction.—The name arterio-sclerosis is applied rather loosely to a thickening of the vessel wall. It includes the obvious naked-eye change in the large arteries, named by some authors atheroma; by others, end-

arteritis deformans.   It includes also arterio-capillary fibrosis, a change
first described by Gull and Sutton, in the walls of the small vessels,
which only becomes obvious on microscopic examination.   Thoma, who
has studied the subject in the most systematic manner, considers it to
be a change of the whole vascular system, which he proposes to name
angio-sclerosis.

Definition.—A local or general thickening of the arterial wall with
loss of elasticity, occasioned mainly by fibrous overgrowth of the tunica
intima, secondary and proportional to weakening of the muscular and
elastic elements of the media.

Etiology.—Old age consists in the set of conditions disposing to
bodily decay ; of these arterio-sclerosis is one of the most obvious manifestations : yet as the hair becomes gray, or falls out, at a comparatively
early age, so the arteries are liable to degeneration in some people early
in life, in others later.

Degeneration of the arteries is one of the most frequent of senile
changes.   All those causes which dispose to bodily decay and early ageing
of the individual will tend towards arterial degeneration.

Certain diatheses favour this process : the chief of · these are gout,
rheumatism, and arthritis ; but apart from these, there appears to be in
some people an hereditary tendency to arterial degeneration.   A number
of diseases of infective nature tend to lower the vitality of the tissues of
the body, including the arteries.   I have already shown that acute
arteritis is apt to follow various infective· diseases ; that scarlet fever, by
its damaging effects on the kidneys and resulting stress, may lead to
permanent strain of the arterial system.   No disease is probably more
productive of arterial degeneration than syphilis, and this in several ways :
(i.) by causing endarteritis of the vasa vasorum, and defective nutrition of the walls of the large arteries ; (ii.) by the devitalising influence
of a toxin, long present in the body, producing anæmia and lowering the
physiological margin of normal metabolism ; so that, in case of injury
or stress of a tissue, the equilibrium is not maintained and degeneration ensues.

Toxic causes of extrinsic origin.—The most important of these are
alcohol and lead.   Dr. Dickinson has shown that people engaged in the
liquor traffic are, on the whole, more liable to arterial degeneration ; and
Dr. Thomas Oliver has shown that renal disease and arterial changes are
induced by lead poisoning [see article "Lead Poisoning," vol. ii. p. 983].
It has long been known that lead may be an important factor in the production of gout, and it is probable that both lead and the toxic agents of
gout cause defective metabolism.

Excess of nitrogenous food is especially injurious to the arterial
system in people leading a sedentary life, and suffering from a gouty
diathesis.   Continuous high pressure in the arteries arises from irritation
of the arterio-capillary system by the products of imperfectly oxidised
nitrogenous waste ; and the increased peripheral resistance leads to compensatory increased force of the heart's action.   At present we know very

little about the injurious effects of leucomaines and ptomaines. It is probable that the former are produced in the body ; the latter may be absorbed from the alimentary canal, and it is conceivable that if they are not destroyed by the liver they are highly injurious.

Occupation.—All causes which tend to increase the force and frequency of the heart's beat will increase the stress on the muscular and elastic structures in the large arteries ; especially if this be accompanied by increase of the peripheral resistance. In particular, occupations involving continuous muscular exertion tend to degeneration of the large arteries ; navvies, blacksmiths, porters, labourers, soldiers are often the subjects of this disease early in life. Important as is the fact that mechanical strain seems of itself competent to produce premature degeneration of the arterial system in a normal healthy man living under healthy conditions, yet, according to Bollinger, horses, oxen, and dogs used for traction purposes, and therefore subject to mechanical strain, do not suffer from atheroma. A Russian, Tschigajew, has studied the mean arterial blood-pressure in Russian peasants while engaged in long and continuous work in the fields during the summer, and while at rest during the winter. During the period of work there was increase of arterial pressure, but this gradually disappeared in the winter. He compared these results with his observations upon labourers in the iron foundries, who work continuously under unhealthy conditions throughout the year ; in the latter class he found permanently high arterial pressure, and thickening of the arteries due to arterio-sclerosis [see "Strain of the Heart," vol. v. pp. 841, 912].

Sex.—Arterio-sclerosis is much more common in men under fifty than in women ; but after the climacteric period it is as common in women as in men ; if not commoner. Men are much more subject, as a rule, to the causes I have already discussed ; and when women are placed under the same conditions they are as liable to arterial degeneration as men. Jusserand has lately pointed out that at Lyons, where a large number of women employed in laborious occupations under unhygienic conditions attend the hospital, the proportion of cases of arterio-sclerosis is larger in the women than in the men. M'Crorie, on examination of the post-mortem records at Glasgow, found that the disease was as frequent in women as in men.

Morbid anatomy and Pathology.—When arterio-sclerosis affects the aorta and its large branches, it is usually named atheroma ; some authors, however, prefer the name endarteritis deformans. Of this there are two varieties—nodosa or circumscripta, and diffusa.

With the naked eye we see oval or circular projections of the inner coat of a more opaque or yellow colour than the surrounding tissue. In the nodular form raised patches, varying in size from a hemp-seed to a shilling, may be seen scattered over the surface of the aorta, especially in the ascending part of the arch, affecting the concave surface rather than the convex ; at the bifurcation of the aorta also they occur ; while between these two situations the atheroma may be absent except around the orifices of the vessels. According to Rokitansky the order of frequency in which other vessels are affected is as follows—splenic, iliac, femoral, coronary, cerebral, uterine, brachial, internal spermatic, common carotid, and hypogastric.   The arteries of the stomach and the mesenteric are but rarely affected, and the pulmonary least of all.   Sach has microscopically examined the arteries in 100 cadavers, and the results of his observations show that in diffuse arterio-sclerosis the arteries of the limbs, especially of the lower limbs, are most frequently affected ; the anterior tibial being the artery most often affected in the body.   The frequency with which the coronaries are affected we can easily understand from their situation, subject as they are to the highest arterial pressure.   The splenic, again, is an artery which must be subject to variable arterial tension ; for during the rhythmical contraction of the muscular tissue of that organ there is a considerable increase of the peripheral resistance.

The relative infrequency of affection of the pulmonary artery, which occurs indeed only under such conditions as involve increased tension of its walls—as, for example, prolonged mitral stenosis—indicates the importance of internal strain as a factor in the degenerative process.

Pepper cites a case in which the pulmonary artery, as a result of prolonged right heart hypertrophy in mitral stenosis, was sclerotic and atheromatous to its minutest subdivisions.   The aorta and the arteries of the systemic circulation were but little affected.   Romberg, however, has described two cases of sclerosis of the pulmonary arteries without valvular disease, and without any marked morbid change in the lungs.   Specially noteworthy is the fact that there was no morbid resistance to the pulmonary circulation.   This is a very rare and peculiar form of disease, and till recently unknown.   There was marked cyanosis, which was not related in a particular degree to congestion.   The right heart was hypertrophied ; probably the disease was congenital.   The lumen of the pulmonary arteries was greatly dilated up to the second division ; that of the smaller arteries notably diminished.   There was marked sclerosis of the intima, the cause of which was not determined.

In the necropsies of the London County Asylums I have been struck by the frequency of arterial degeneration, and with the proportional infrequency of intracerebral hæmorrhage, as compared with my experience and statistics obtained at Charing Cross Hospital.

I have therefore investigated the reports of 300 necropsies made at Claybury Asylum.   Of 160 male cases, the great majority in persons after middle life, there was atheroma of the aorta in 113 ; generally speaking, the disease affected both the aorta and the cerebral vessels. The cerebral vessels were noted as diseased in 60 cases, in 40 markedly so.   In 65 the kidneys showed some degree of interstitial fibrosis, usually not very marked.   The heart was moderately hypertrophied in a few cases, and in only 2 was it much hypertrophied.   Among the 160 cases there were 2 cases of intracerebral hæmorrhage ; one in the cerebellum and one in the usual situation, namely, in the neighbourhood of the basal ganglia.   There were, however, 15 instances of subpial and subarachnoid hæmorrhage in cases of wasting brain disease.   Atheroma was noted in

24 cases out of 86, in people aged 45 or under; 22 of these were the subjects of general paralysis, but out of the 86 cases 60 were general paralytics. Thus it appears that atheroma of the aorta was present in about 1 in 3 cases of general paralysis and 1 in 13 in other cases of men who had died at 45 years of age or under.

Of 140 female necropsies, atheroma of the aorta was observed in 81. Of these, 34 were noted as "marked"; the remainder as "some atheroma." The cerebral vessels were noted as diseased in 49 cases; in 35 marked, in 14 moderate or slight. The kidneys showed moderate interstitial fibrosis in 19, slight in 21, fatty in 9 cases. The heart was moderately hypertrophied in 2 cases, and considerably hypertrophied in 2. There was only 1 case of intracerebral hæmorrhage, and that in an unusual situation, namely, the temporo-sphenoidal lobe.

Three cases of subarachnoid hæmorrhage were noted.

Atheroma of the aorta was noted in 18 cases out of 53 in persons aged 45 or under.

There were 18 cases of general paralysis, and in 10 of these there was atheroma of the aorta; in five cases nodular endarteritis cerebri was discovered on microscopical examination. In one case of atheroma of the aorta no disease of the cerebral arteries was discovered; and there was one case of disease of the cerebral vessels in which the aorta was unaffected. So that more than half the cases among women exhibited arterial disease, just as in the men and without evidence of long previous high arterial pressure; for in none of these cases was there cardiac hypertrophy. The proportion of atheroma in cases other than general paralytic was 1 to 5; in nearly all cases it was slight, and the cerebral vessels were not affected. The modes of death in these cases, in order of frequency, were phthisis, heart disease, epilepsy with "status" or complications, exhaustion from mania, complications arising in mania and melancholia.

Without laying too much stress upon these statistics, for I am not responsible for the notes made with varying degrees of care and discretion, I think they certainly show that my impressions were correct as regards the differences between asylum and hospital experience. The conclusions I think we are warranted in drawing are: (i.) The infrequency of intracerebral hæmorrhage in persons with atheromatous cerebral arteries is probably due to the fact that they have not been the subjects of prolonged high arterial pressure, as shown by the absence of cardiac hypertrophy. (ii.) The interstitial fibrosis of the kidney seldom assumes the degree shown in the small red kidney of chronic Bright's disease. (iii.) Meningeal hæmorrhage is due to rupture of small veins or capillaries. (iv.) The relatively high proportion of atheroma and diseased cerebral vessels in general paralysis, as compared with other diseases, is a distinct point in favour of the view that this disease is due in a majority of instances to syphilis; and this view is supported by some observations made by Dr. Lewis, who has carefully inquired from the patients and their friends into the history of all the male cases admitted into Claybury Asylum in 1897. He has also carefully looked for other evidence in the form of scars, indurated glands, and so on; but of the 200 admissions he found that 70 might be said to have had venereal infection in the form of *hard* or *soft sore*. Of all the cases admitted 24 were general paralytics, in 16 of which there was certain evidence of venereal infection; 3 cases were doubtful in this respect, and in the remainder the evidence was negative. So we may consider that at least two-thirds had had venereal infection. With regard to the soft sore, in many cases it is true syphilis; and, possibly owing to the fact that treatment is not adopted, it is frequently followed later by disease of the nervous system. Hitzig has even suggested that the soft sore has a special toxic action on the nervous system.

The careful microscopical examination which I have made of the cerebral vessels in a large number of people who have died at the age of 45 or under, shows me that, apart from syphilitic brain disease, endarteritis (indistinguishable from syphilitic arteritis) is, relatively to other brain diseases (for example, epilepsy, mania, melancholia, etc.), fairly common in general paralysis. It does not always play a part in the production of symptoms; it does not cause a coarse paralysis until the endarteritis is universal, or some large artery (for example, the basilar, vertebral, middle cerebral, or lenticular striate) is thickened; but I have met with several cases of each of these conditions of vascular occlusion occurring simultaneously with the characteristic cortical changes of general paralysis. Compared with my hospital experience, I find syphilitic arteritis a common condition on the post-mortem table of the asylums; and I am certain that syphilis plays a most important part in the production of many of those organic diseases of the brain which are associated with such mental symptoms as to lead to certification of insanity. (v.) The great proportion of arterial disease among the inmates of asylums is not connected with prolonged high arterial pressure and chronic Bright's disease, but is due to a general degenerative process in which the parenchyma of the kidney takes part. The infrequency of cardiac hypertrophy is probably connected with an infrequency of miliary aneurysms, and, consequently, a proportional infrequency of intracerebral hæmorrhage. (vi.) The frequency of cerebral softening among asylum patients owing to arterial degeneration is most striking.

Councilman, in a recent study of arterio-sclerosis, divides the subject into three varieties—the nodular, the senile, and the diffuse. In the *senile* form he points out that there is atrophy of the liver and kidneys, and that the heart is often small; in one-half of the cases he examined (7 out of 14) there was no hypertrophy. In the *diffuse* form the disease is widespread throughout the aorta and its branches, and in this vessel is often associated with *nodular sclerosis*. The affection occurs in strongly built, middle-aged men. In this class the heart is usually greatly hypertrophied; and when the coronary arteries are involved, as they often are, cardiac dystrophic sclerosis is often associated with it. The kidneys may show extreme sclerosis, but sometimes the organs are increased in size; the capsule is adherent, and the organ is tough. This is a part of a widespread process affecting the arterio-capillary system. To ascertain the relative frequency of atheroma, the reports of 1600 post-mortems made at Charing Cross Hospital were analysed, and of these 380, or nearly one-fourth, were found to exhibit a greater or less degree of atheroma. In these the males were to the females nearly as 3 to 1. Of the remaining 1200 cases there was a large proportion of subjects who had died in infancy and youth, of women, and of cases in which, for some reason or other, complete examination was not made. In 118 cases the atheroma was severe, in 104 moderate, and in the remainder slight. Neglecting the cases in which the reports state that the vessels were slightly affected, we may reckon that there were 222 cases of atheroma. Bollinger, in 1800 necropsies on adults, gives only 136 cases of sclerosis. The difference in the percentage between Bollinger's statistics and mine may probably be explained by the fact that a large number of our male patients, by their occupation and habits, are particularly prone to arterial degeneration. Many are porters at Covent Garden market, dockyard labourers, people engaged at the theatres and in the liquor traffic ; and every year a considerable number are brought in dead or dying by the police.

The subjoined table brings out another important fact in connection with the etiology and pathology of the disease ; namely, the high percentage of granular contracted kidneys and hypertrophy of the heart : thus showing the close association between arterio-sclerosis and chronic Bright's disease.

TABLE showing the connection between atheroma of the vessels, hypertrophy of the heart, and contracted granular kidneys, compiled from examination of 222 cases of atheroma.

	Per Cent.			
	Male.		Female.	
	Severe.	Moderate.	Severe.	Moderate.
Heart alone	24	18	7	5
Kidney alone . . .	22	24	29	45
Heart and kidney . . .	42	40	39	20
Neither heart nor kidney .	12	18	25	30

In these 1600 necropsies there were 60 cases of cerebral hæmorrhage of all kinds ; 30 of these were noted in subjects suffering from granular contracted kidneys and hypertrophied heart. Fagge states that the large majority of cases of cerebral hæmorrhage are associated with granular contracted kidneys and hypertrophied heart. The large percentage of cases in which chronic Bright's disease was associated with atheroma would suggest that the naked-eye change is but a part of the pathological process; and that the microscope would reveal changes in the arterioles and capillaries throughout the body, in many instances localised particularly in the kidneys, which organs, for years past, had been endeavouring to rid the body of the waste products of a defective metabolism. Such a stress on the renal vessels and parenchyma produces in them a degenerative change of a gradually progressive character not limited to these organs, although they show it more particularly. To Gull and Sutton is due the conception of *arterio-sclerosis* as an independent affection, named by them *arterio-capillary fibrosis*. They proved that the red granular contracted kidney of chronic Bright's disease is but a part of a general vascular disease; and their observations were most valuable in demonstrating that what was looked upon as a disease of a single organ was in reality a widespread vascular change throughout the body, secondary to some other process which we now recognise as probably due to defective metabolism. Lancereaux came to the same conclusion, although under his title of *herpetism* his views and observations did not receive in this country the recognition they deserve. He showed, however, that in 61 cases of generalised arterio-sclerosis the associated conditions were—interstitial nephritis, 55; cerebral hæmorrhage or softening, 12; pulmonary emphysema, 21; articular lesions, 14; friability of the bones, 10.

Gull and Sutton showed that of 35 cases of emphysema granular contracted kidney was present in 21; and this quite accords with my own experience. Mahomed made observations on 61 cases of chronic Bright's disease without albuminuria, but with high pressure pulse and cardio-vascular changes. He held that in the red granular contracted kidney the disease was primarily in the vessels generally.

Dr. Dickinson argues that the disease of the kidney is the initial cause of the cardio-vascular change. In 250 cases of granular contracted kidney he found cirrhosis of the liver in 37 instances only. It must be borne in mind, however, that, if excessive internal stress on the vessel wall be the cause of degeneration, then we should not expect the liver to be affected; because we know that, owing to the free anastomosis of the hepatic and portal vascular systems, a rise of internal stress would not readily occur. It might be argued that the 37 cases of cirrhosis were due to alcohol or mechanical congestion. Dickinson says in chronic renal disease there occurs a hypertrophy of the cardio-arterial system which is universal from its origin to its terminations, and affects not only the ventricles and the arterioles, but also the intermediate arteries of every size. He has also shown that in cases of granular contracted kidney abnormal thickening may be demonstrated in the larger as well as in the smaller arteries. His researches show that the aorta, the innominate and the femoral arteries are all increased in the total thickness of their walls, in the thickness of their muscular coat, and in their circumference. He holds, with Bright, that the peripheral resistance is mainly in the capillaries, and opposes the "stop-cock hypothesis" of the late Sir George

Johnson; but he agrees with Johnson that the muscular coat is hypertrophied. A long controversy ensued between Gull and Sutton and Johnson on the causation of the cardiac hypertrophy and high arterial tension. Johnson attributed the thickening of the arterioles to the hypertrophy of the muscular elements; Gull and Sutton to a fibrotic change of arteries and capillaries, beginning usually, but not always, in the kidney. There is truth in both opinions. In the prodromal stages of the disease a spasm of the arterioles is probably brought about by irritation of toxic products, causing contraction of the muscular coat, increased peripheral resistance, and compensatory increased force of the heart's action; whereupon the arterial blood-pressure rises. Thus not only would the heart undergo hypertrophy, but the muscular coat of the arteries also. Professor Allbutt, however, regards this hypertrophy as due not to excessive contraction of the arterioles, which in other diseases, as in Raynaud's disease, does not produce it, but, as in the heart, to a compensation of the dilating pressure.

Sir Wm. Broadbent does not think that the primary obstruction is produced by contraction of the arterioles; he admits that the muscular coat of the arterioles is increased, but that this is secondary to the resistance in the capillaries. Dr. Dickinson points out, in the Baillie lectures, that the capillaries, although containing no muscular fibres, are yet capable of contraction. He admits that, associated with the renal disease, there may be widespread changes in the arterio-capillary system of the whole body, but that the hyaline fibroid change described by Gull and Sutton is secondary to the renal disease.

Thoma made injection experiments upon cadavers with salt solution, observing the times of injection of a given number of litres at a given pressure, when arterio-sclerosis existed, and when it did not. He found it took very much longer to inject the same amount of fluid in the case of sclerosis. Œdema of the lower extremities occurred when only four litres had been injected into a body affected with widespread angio-sclerosis; whereas into the arteries of a body not so affected seventeen litres could be injected before leakage took place. These and other experiments show that when arterio-sclerosis is present the salt solution has to overcome much more resistance in the vessels of the lower extremities, although investigation shows that the lumen of the arteries is not greatly diminished. It may be concluded, therefore, that changes in the permeability of the capillary walls are also present in arterio-sclerosis. Does it not also suggest that the capillary area generally is greatly diminished, probably on account of the fibrotic changes referred to?

Again, the researches of Hoffmann, Runeberg, and other pupils of Thoma prove that the fluid in angio-sclerotic œdema is characterised by a small amount of albumin and low specific gravity, indicating hydræmia of the blood; to this may be attributed the defective metabolism, the abnormal permeability of the capillaries, and the degenerative changes in the muscular and elastic tissues which Rokitansky, Thoma, and most authors believe to be the initial factor in the thickening of the inner coat.

It can easily be understood that a widespread change affecting the capillaries and arterioles may cause an increased peripheral resistance in the circulation which has to be overcome by an increased force of the heart's action, resulting in hypertrophy of the ventricles. These two factors lead to increased stress upon the large arteries, to their eventual distension, laterally and longitudinally, to thickening of their walls, and to tortuosity.

Thoma, by a series of researches, has shown that the thickening of the walls of the arteries, especially of the inner coat, is a process compensatory to the slowing of the current caused by the distension of the vessel. If so, the thickening of the intima may be looked upon rather as a compensatory fibrosis than an endarteritis ; because, as Adami points out, although Thoma speaks of the process as a chronic inflammation, yet he states that a similar process occurs under physiological conditions ; for he and his pupils have shown that a strictly analogous thickening of the intima, due to proliferation of the sub-endothelial layer, occurs at birth in the portions of the aorta between the ductus Botalli and the points of departure of the umbilical arteries, in the uterine arteries after parturition, to a less degree after menstruation, and in the arteries of an amputated limb.

General arterio-capillary fibrosis leads to thickening of the coats of the arteriæ arteriarum ; and I am inclined to believe, from many observations, that frequently degeneration of the media is primarily due to obliteration or obstruction of the vasa vasorum, and consequent defective nutrition of the muscular fibres ; but Adami argues that, if this be so, its influence on the intima is not apparent, for he cannot find evidence that in healthy arteries, or in the earlier stages of arterio-sclerosis, any branches of these vessels pass into the intima. The reply to this argument is—(i.) for what purpose is the elastic lamina fenestrated ? (ii.) no vascular branches pass into the cornea, which consists of layers of branched connective tissue corpuscles quite similar to the sub-endothelial layer of the arteries ; and (iii.) the nodular form of arterio-sclerosis is only to be explained, I think, by supposing that an area of a vessel wall has been damaged by some anatomical imperfection in the blood-supply of the vasa vasorum.

Morbid anatomy.—The process, when it begins by the formation of semi-transparent gelatinous patches, is of the *nodular form.* The patches are scattered about the walls of the aorta and large vessels ; the site of predilection being, as before mentioned, especially related to internal stress. When the process is older the patches are found to be firm, dense, and of cartilaginous consistence. As a rule the endothelial lining of the vessel is intact, and the change is situated in the layer between the endothelium and the elastic lamina ; the older patches are yellowish and opaque, owing to necrobiosis of the deeper layers of the patch where caseation, and frequently calcification, are taking place. When cut into, the former process is recognised by the fatty detritus—something like porridge, or fine meal, as the name atheroma implies—which is seen in the deeper parts. Calcification may be so extensive as to be quite obvious to the naked eye in the form of calcareous plates, producing some resemblance to the hide of a crocodile; or, in the lighter degree, it may only be recognisable by the gritty character of the patch when cut into. If atheromatous material be examined microscopically, crystals of cholesterin, fatty acids, oil globules and disintegrating cells may be observed. Microscopical examination of patches of atheroma will show changes according to the age of the patch; although usually all stages of the disease may be seen, the central portion being the oldest. The endothelial layer is bulged inwards by a great increase in the subendo-thelial layer, the cells of which have undergone proliferation. These cells consist of branched, stellate and fusiform elements, and in the centre they are seen in all stages of necrobiosis; crystals of fatty acids can generally be observed in the deeper and more central portions of a patch.

Examination of the middle coat shows that the muscular fibres present a hyaline swollen appearance, and occasionally the elastic fibres have been found ruptured. Now this would lead to a bulging of the vessel wall were it not for the fact that a proportional compensatory thickening of the inner coat takes place by proliferation of the sub-endothelial layer already referred to. Thoma, by injecting the aorta and large arteries with paraffin wax at a pressure of 160 mm. of mercury (the mean pressure in the aorta), has shown that the paraffin casts are quite smooth, and present none of the irregularities which the nodular plaques would have produced had they not exactly filled up the bulge in the vessel wall produced by the weakened media at the spots where the intima is thickened. Certainly this is a strong argument in favour of the compensatory view.

Why should the proliferated connective tissue cells of the sub-endothelial layer of the intima undergo degeneration in the central parts of the plaque? I look upon it as a process in which the younger and more vigorous cells are able to take up nutriment, while the older, situated in the deeper and more central portions of the patch, perish and undergo fatty degeneration. The process of necrobiosis may extend to the whole patch, and the intima may give way and form an athero-matous ulcer.

Dr. Ainslie Hollis attributes atheroma to an infective process. I think this possible when ulceration occurs.

Diffuse arterio-sclerosis.—This affection occurs especially in men of middle age; it is frequently associated with enlargement of the heart and granular contracted kidney, and corresponds to the cases described by Gull and Sutton as arterio-capillary fibrosis. It begins in the small arteries and capillaries; especially those of the renal cortex, but also in those of the brain and heart. It is very frequently associated with nodular atheroma of the aorta, doubtless due to changes in the vasa vasorum (*vide* Figs. 41, 42). Microscopically the unstriped muscular fibres of the media exhibit hyaline swelling, fatty degeneration, or atrophic changes, so that the muscular elements are often not recognisable; this is especially the case in the small arteries of the kidney, where the wall of the .vessel may appear to consist only of a homogeneous hyaline tissue: sometimes the degenerated atrophied fibres of the media can be made out, but nothing of the elastic lamina, the intima being thickened and represented only by a homogeneous hyaline material with but few nuclei. The capillaries of the glomeruli show this hyaline change especially well, a change which may and frequently does lead to their obliteration (*vide* Figs. 16 and 18). A similar change is found in the vessels of the pia mater (*vide* Fig. 17). The results of these widespread changes are increased resistance to the flow of blood through the capillaries, hyper-

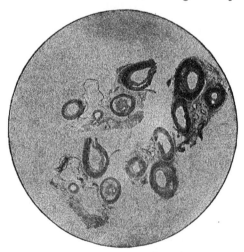

Fig. 16.—Transverse section of the arteries of the kidney from a case of general arterio-sclerosis in a man aged fifty-six. The patient was a soldier and had had syphilis. He suffered from an acute attack of nephritis, with cardiac failure from dystrophic sclerosis. There was dropsy, albuminuria, and a petechial eruption. The arteries were all rigid, tortuous, and atheromatous. The microphotograph shows an obliterative endarteritis of the branches of the renal artery at the hilum of the kidney. Magnification, 6 diameters.

trophy of the left ventricle, dilatation of the larger arteries from degenerative changes in the muscular and elastic tissues of the media, slowing of the circulation, and compensatory proliferation of the subendothelial layer of the inner coat. Disease of the kidneys is always detected if the organs are examined microscopically; but to the naked eye the change is sometimes not so apparent, and may be overlooked; in all cases its degree depends upon the stage of the disease and the mode of death. The red granular contracted kidney is the most characteristic naked-eye appearance. The heart in most cases is greatly hypertrophied, but it is generally tough; if examined microscopically, the muscular fibres are seen to be surrounded by a great excess of fibrous tissue (" Fibro-myocarditis," vol. v. p. 895), and the small arteries and capillaries are thickened and present fibrous hyaline degenerations, generally accompanied by arterio-sclerotic changes in the coronary arteries. Both semilunar and mitral valves may be thickened, opaque and sclerotic.

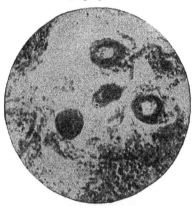

FIG. 17.—Cerebral vessels from a case of arterio-capillary fibrosis. The small vessels of the pia mater show large numbers of leucocytes around. In one vessel the lumen is completely obliterated, in others the walls are much thickened. *Vide* also figure of miliary aneurysms which were obtained from this case. Magnification, 100 diameters.

Sclerosis of the pulmonary artery has already been discussed.

Thoma points out farther that the sclerotic process may affect the veins also—*phlebo-sclerosis.*

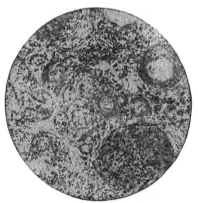

FIG. 18.—Photomicrograph of kidney from a case of arterio-capillary fibrosis. In the centre is a small artery with thickened hyaline walls. The patient was aged forty-eight, and died of cerebral hæmorrhage. The hair vessels are shown in photomicrograph.

The relation of atheroma to aneurysm is of considerable importance and will now be discussed. Of 34 cases of aneurysm of the aorta which occurred in the above-mentioned 1600 post-mortems made at Charing

Cross Hospital, 7 were women, and in nearly all these 34 cases atheroma is recorded. These results correspond very closely with those of Coats and Auld, and of M'Crorie; as will be seen by a comparison of the following table :—

Ages.	Mott.	Coats and Auld.	M'Crorie.
20–30	1	1	1
30–40	10	15	6
40–50	11	10	8
50–60	9	7	7
over 60	3		

In the three schedules there is only one case under thirty, and the majority occur in the two decades between thirty and fifty; this is precisely the period in which atheroma is most frequently met with.

Drs. Coats and Auld came to the conclusion that atheroma is the main cause of aneurysm. They consider that the thickening of the intima, with its subsequent degeneration, is a chronic inflammatory process; that the name Endarteritis deformans of Virchow is therefore correct, and that the changes in the muscular and elastic tissues of the media are brought about by pressure of the degenerated caseous or calcareous intima. I quite agree with them as to the very frequent association of atheroma with aneurysm; but whether the atheroma is an essential or an incidental event is disputable. The arguments of the above authors are that in the great majority of cases of aneurysm atheroma is present; that, like aneurysm, it affects men more than women; that it occurs in the two decades of life when aneurysm is most common. Their view is opposed to that of Eppinger, and in a measure to that of Thoma, who looks upon thickening of the intima as compensatory, and, as one would therefore suppose, rather preventive of aneurysm. Eppinger considers that rupture of the elastic and muscular fibres of the middle coat is the primary cause of ordinary aneurysm, and this may be true of dissecting aneurysm; but it seems a doubtful assertion in respect of sacculated aneurysm: for, apart from Dr. Coats' weighty arguments, Wagner was only able to find microscopic rents in the elastic tissue of the media in high degrees of atheromatous degeneration, and, as suggested by Dr. Coats, these might very well have been brought about by pressure and stretching. Such rents are indicated by the development of fibro-vascular tissue which cicatrises later; and the accepted mesarteritis of Köster appears to Wagner to be generally the result of laceration of the media: yet I feel sure, from my own observations, that in cases of atheroma in the subjects of syphilis a simultaneous periarteritis and mesarteritis may accompany blocking of the vasa vasorum and acute changes in the media (see Fig. 13 and explanation).

Under syphilitic endarteritis I have already referred to the frequency of the association of syphilis and aneurysm, of aneurysm and atheroma, and of syphilis and atheroma. Amongst a large number of necropsies occurring in the London County Asylums I have recently had the opportunity of seeing, occasionally, advanced atheroma of the aorta in conjunction with typical syphilitic endarteritis cerebri in women under thirty, in whom other evidences of syphilis were forthcoming. I cannot but think that an endarteritis obliterans of the vasa vasorum in the neighbourhood of the atheromatous patches is a convincing proof of the effect of syphilis in the production of atheroma of the aorta in comparatively young people, not the subjects of strain (see Figs. 12, 13).

I have already referred to the frequency with which we found granular contracted kidney and cardiac hypertrophy associated with cerebral hæmorrhage. Gull and Sutton made most of their observations on arteriocapillary fibrosis on the vessels of the pia mater. It is rare to find cerebral hæmorrhage in a person under forty who is not the subject of chronic Bright's disease, or of ulcerative endocarditis. Of the 60 cases I have collected, seven were due to intracranial aneurysm, and four of these, all in young subjects, were caused by infective embolism ; the other three were due to atheroma or syphilitic arteritis. Two were due to secondary hæmorrhage from tumours ; in all the remainder some affection of the kidneys was noted. In 80 per cent granular contracted kidney and cardiac hypertrophy were present. In the great majority of the cases the age was over forty-five. The proportion of males to females was 4 to 1. In 48 out of the 60 cases the seat of the affection was in the neighbourhood of the basal ganglia. In four cases the hæmorrhage was meningeal ; in six meningeal and in the hemisphere, in two in the pons Varolii ; in one it was in the cerebellar hemisphere.

Miliary aneurysms.—Atheroma of the larger vessels of the brain has. but an indirect connection with hæmorrhage ; but it is a frequent direct cause of cerebral softening in old people, occasioning in them dementia and paralysis. Still, if the arteries be affected at the base only, it is remarkable how much compensation is possible by collateral circulation. We have already seen that atheroma of the larger vessels is generally associated with arterio-capillary fibrosis; and examination of the small vessels of the brain in cases of cerebral hæmorrhage reveals marked changes in their walls. Charcot and Bouchard, in 77 successive cases of cerebral hæmorrhage, found small aneurysms just visible to the naked eye (measuring from 0·2 mm. to 1 mm. in diameter), which they named miliary aneurysms. They may be found by washing away the brain substance from the vessels, and are more readily seen in the vessels of the pia mater of the convexity ; but, according to Charcot and Bouchard, the order of their frequency in different regions is as follows :—central ganglia, cortex, pons, cerebellum, centrum ovale, middle cerebellar peduncle, crus cerebri, medulla oblongata. This order pretty nearly coincides with the order of frequency of the seat of hæmorrhage. They believe that the aneurysms are the result of a periarteritis. According to Zenker, the primary change is in the inner coat ; but there is no reason to suppose that the process which originates arterio-sclerosis is different in the small arteries of the brain from that of the rest of the body ; it is much more likely that, as Sir William Gowers suggests, the effective element in the change is the loss of the contractile and elastic elements, with resulting fibrous overgrowth of the intima and adventitia. The photographs of the kidney and the cerebral vessels, and the figure of miliary aneurysms well illustrate this point; although the vessels of the brain undoubtedly show evident signs of a periarteritis, as described by Charcot. The aneurysms themselves appear like little red grains on the vessels; sometimes they have a shiny aspect; the colour depends upon the condition of the blood within them. They are sometimes extremely numerous, as many as 100 having been found in one case. It is easily understood how such aneurysms are formed if the muscular and elastic coats are degenerated; the wall of the vessel yields to the pressure of blood, an immature fusiform or sacculated aneurysm takes place, and is liable to rupture at any time (*vide* Fig. 19).

FIG. 19.—Miliary aneurysms (*vide* Fig. 17).

In arterio-sclerosis we have the two factors necessary for the production of aneurysm, namely, weakening of the arterial wall and increase of

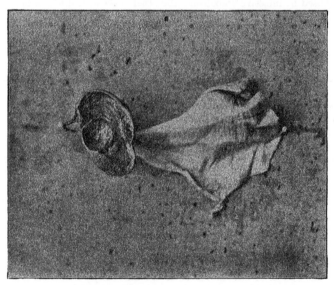

FIG. 20.—Photograph of an aneurysm at the junction of the left internal carotid and posterior communicating; it is attached to a piece of the tentorium. It was the size of a large filbert; the photograph is of half the aneurysm, and shows a round hollow cavity surrounded by a laminated clot. The only symptoms exhibited during life were paralysis of the third nerve on the left side, headache, and outbursts of passion. *Vide* also microphotograph.

blood-pressure. Probably the reason why these aneurysms are found especially in the brain is because of loss of external support, owing to waste of brain substance around; secondly, the arteries are terminal and are derived directly from large trunks.

The relation of cerebral aneurysm to arterio-sclerosis.—I refer now to aneurysm, usually single, varying in size from a pea to a walnut. Primary degeneration of the vessel is an occasional cause in the second half of life (Gowers); this may be a fibroid change or a simple atheroma. Occasionally a simple weakening of the media, rupture of the elastic intima, and formation of an aneurysm may occur. This was so in a patient, a woman aged forty-four, who died suddenly. The photograph (Fig. 20) and photomicrograph (Fig. 21) show, respectively, the aneurysm filled with laminated clot which was seated partly on the posterior communicating, partly on the internal carotid, and a section of the internal carotid just at its bifurcation; several little vesicular swellings were visible on the trunk and its branches in the neighbourhood of the aneurysm, and these, on section and microscopical examination, were found to consist only of the delicate adventitia, the media and intima having been ruptured : this

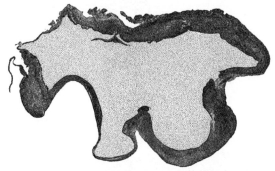

FIG. 21.—Photomicrograph. Transverse section of the internal carotid artery just at its division. At the places where the wall is extremely thin there existed little vesicular dilatations about the size of a large pin's head. As these were close to the sac of the aneurysm, it could not be discovered whether the fatal hæmorrhage had been caused by the rupture of one of them or of the aneurysm itself. Magnification, 10 diameters.

no doubt explains the formation of the aneurysm. Another condition which sometimes gives rise to aneurysm is embolism from the débris of an atheromatous ulcer. This condition, however, is rare. The photograph (Fig. 22) shows an aneurysm at the bifurcation of the middle cerebral artery, obtained from a woman aged thirty-eight, who died from hemiplegia caused by thrombosis extending from this aneurysm back into the middle cerebral trunk. The patient was free from valvular disease, but had general arteriosclerosis. The photograph of the aorta shows recent atheromatous ulcers (Fig. 23). Sections of the aneurysm showed that a calcareous embolus had been driven into the vessel, and set up inflammation followed by dilatation. [For further information concerning cerebral aneurysm see article "Cerebral Hæmorrhage" in the next volume.]

Of the other arteries which are affected by arterio-sclerosis, by far the most important clinically are the coronaries, disease of which may lead to imperfect nutrition and degeneration of the heart. Again, in the vessels of the limbs, as before seen, gangrene, especially of the lower limbs, is prone to come on in old people, owing to arterio-sclerosis of the popliteal and tibial arteries, slowing of the circulation, and thrombosis (Fig. 24). It will be gathered from these remarks on the pathology and the morbid anatomy of arterio-sclerosis that it is a chronic, progressive, and cumulative disease of the whole vascular system, which in different individuals may show a predilection for these particular vessels, or those, according to the various causes, immediate and remote. Many

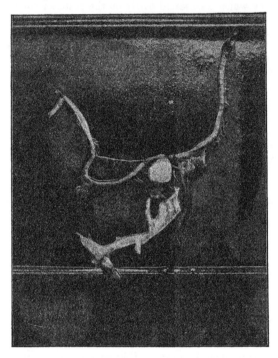

Fig. 22.—Aneurysm of the middle cerebral with thrombosis extending back into the internal carotid. Softening of the central region of the right hemisphere and basal ganglia and left hemiplegia. The aneurysm was produced by impaction of an embolus from the atheromatous ulcer shown in the photograph.

diseases, which we recognise clinically as distinct maladies, are in reality a part of this general progressive change of vessels; namely, chronic Bright's disease, apoplexy, cerebral softening, senile dementia, fibroid heart, and sometimes fatty heart. To sum up: the pathology of arterio-sclerosis is primarily defective metabolism and strain; physiological compensation— that is, increased functional activity of the left ventricle to overcome the increased peripheral resistance in the arterioles and capillaries—ensues and leads to hypertrophy of the muscular structures engaged, and to dilatation of the elastic aorta and large arteries. In the second stage there is thickening of the vessel wall, mainly of the intima, proportional and compensatory to degeneration of the muscular and elastic tissues. In the third stage the compensation process fails, so that should the patient escape the danger of cerebral hæmorrhage he may succumb in the final stage to blocking of his coronary arteries and consequent cardiac failure. Herein the general deficiency of nutrition, which alters the whole metabolism of the body, leads of itself to the failure of the physiological

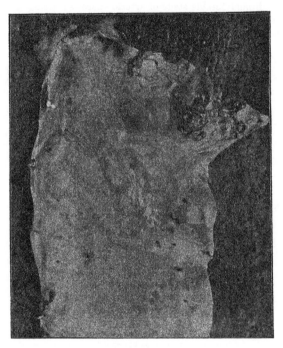

Fig. 23.—Photograph of a portion of the descending aorta and third part of the arch. At the upper part on the right is a patch of ulceration from which portions have been dislodged, that have produced an aneurysm of the right middle cerebral and infarction of the spleen and kidneys. The patient was a woman aged thirty-eight.

compensation which had been set up; and the inefficiently nourished muscular structure of the heart is unable to overcome the resistance in front: dilatation of the left ventricle then follows, and mitral regurgitation, congestion of the lungs (frequently emphysematous), and dropsy, partly cardiac, partly due to changes in the capillary walls and the hydræmic condition of the blood, complete the vicious circle.

Symptomatology.—The clinical history varies in every case according to the organ which suffers most and suffers earliest. If it be admitted that in many instances the disease may and does start in defective

metabolism and altered quality of the blood, and that this is antecedent
to the production of the organic changes in the vessels, and an important
factor in it, then it must also be admitted that there is a stage in which
the disease, if recognised, may be prevented or delayed by prophylactic
measures. Mahomed showed that before the appearance of albumin in
the urine in scarlatinal nephritis there is a rise in blood-pressure (pre-
albuminuric stage). Huchard, Traube, and other authors consider that
there is a prodromal curable stage of arterio-sclerosis ; a stage of toxæmia
causing spasm of the arterio-capillary system, increased peripheral resistance, increased functional activity of the heart, and increased pressure

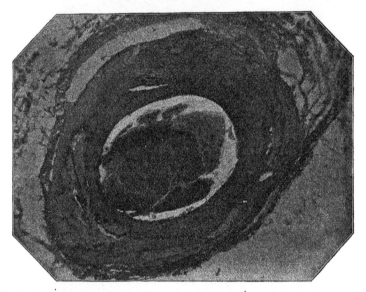

Fig. 24.—Photomicrograph. Anterior tibial artery from a demented patient who suffered from senile
gangrene of the leg. A large calcareous plate can be seen in the middle coat, and the lumen of the
artery is blocked by a recent thrombus.

in the arteries ; but not necessarily changes in the vessel walls. The
toxæmia may produce headache, drowsiness, morning fatigue, and in-
aptitude for work, coldness of the extremities, noises in the ears, migrain-
ous or neuralgic attacks, which, together with the high pressure pulse and
accentuated second sound of the heart occurring in a man of middle age
who lives well, should always suggest premonitory symptoms of arterio-
sclerosis. Dr. Haig asserts that in these cases there is excess of uric acid
in the urine ; it is probable that the toxic agents are many and various,
and arise from defective nitrogenous metabolism ; or possibly, as suggested
by Bouchard, consist of ptomaines and leucomaines absorbed from the
alimentary canal and imperfectly dealt with by the liver.

Under the name senile plethora Professor Allbutt has drawn attention to such irregular and indefinite perturbations of health occurring in persons on the farther side of middle life, the nature of which is indicated by persistent elevations of arterial blood-pressure. This "hyperpiesis," as he names it, may persist for years, especially if untreated; and may never be associated with renal disease, though both maladies may arise, no doubt, from the same or like causes. Dr. Allbutt has watched many individual cases of this kind, over many years, years of more or less persistent ailment, insomnia, cerebral confusion, despondency, and nervousness, but not necessarily of danger to life. Most of these cases, he tells us, are remediable by deobstruent means; and although in all the condition tends to recurrence, yet in the less inveterate each recurrence is less obstinate to treatment and recovery may be anticipated.

When there is sclerosis of the arteries the disease must necessarily be progressive and cumulative; as the vascular degeneration progresses, the nutrition of the body generally and certain organs in particular suffer in their order; not only do the muscular and elastic tissues of the arteries waste, while fibrous tissue takes their place, but the parenchyma of organs and tissues likewise atrophy, and are replaced by fibrous overgrowth: thus the process of decay extends in all directions; and to the symptoms of arterial degeneration are added those of failing or perverted bodily nutrition, with the special symptoms attaching to impaired function of the several organs engaged. Yet, as pointed out by Sir William Gull, certain types of the disease may be constructed. In one case cerebral symptoms, in another cardiac, in another renal symptoms predominate; or again bronchitis and emphysema may first bring the patient to the physician and lead to the recognition of the general character of the disease.

We shall therefore discuss the symptoms under the following headings: (*a*) general nutrition; (*b*) the cardio-vascular symptoms; (*c*) the cerebral; (*d*) the renal; (*e*) the pulmonary.

(*a*) *General nutrition.*—Of this process there are two types: the flabby and corpulent, and the sallow, emaciated and rather cachectic patient with arcus senilis: both are anæmic when the disease is well established, and in both defective metabolism is indicated. The patients frequently complain of dyspepsia, flatulence, and intestinal troubles of various kinds. The anæmic appearance is due in part to deficiency in the number and quality of the red corpuscles, and in part to changes in the walls of the capillaries of the skin.

(*b*) *Cardio-vascular symptoms.*—According to von Basch, dyspnœa is the only criterion of cardiac insufficiency due to arterio-sclerosis, latent or incipient: certainly breathlessness, especially on exertion, is one of the most important subjective features. Syncopal attacks and anginoid pains are likewise indications of their result. The objective symptoms may be manifested in visible tortuous pulsating and rigid temporal and brachial arteries; especially is this noticeable in the emaciated, senile, or prematurely senile patient; but in the corpulent subject the only objective symptom of arterial change may be a high pressure pulse at the wrist, the artery being firm and incompressible, and the pulse wave more evident on firm pressure. The sphygmogram shows a gradual upstroke, no percussion wave and a gradual downstroke in which the dicrotic wave is hardly visible. We can hardly, however, judge by this whether the change be in the arterial wall, or whether it be all due to altered pressure within the vessel. Dr. George Oliver's arteriometer is a very useful instrument for measuring the calibre of the artery, and by it we may ascertain whether the arterial calibre varies with the posture of the patient. Normally, when the patient assumes an erect posture the arterial calibre should be increased, and the blood-pressure increased at the same time. But when arterio-sclerosis is present this change of calibre does not occur; or at any rate the range of variability is diminished in proportion to the rigidity and loss of elasticity of the vessel wall.

"Permanent fixation is not a matter of vaso-motor disturbance, but of organic change." If this be so, we have in Dr. Oliver's instrument a valuable means of deciding whether the stage of arterio-sclerosis is pro-dromal and curable; or whether von Basch is right in asserting that increased arterial blood-pressure is the expression of a vascular change already established.

In the first stages, owing to the increased peripheral resistance, a pure hypertrophy of the left ventricle occurs, and of the right ventricle to a less and variable degree. The area of cardiac dulness is increased, and the impulse is displaced outwards and slightly downward (often this cannot be made out owing to emphysema). There may be reduplication of both first and second sounds; and the latter over the aortic cartilage is accentuated and possibly roughened. This is a physiological com-pensatory process; but, sooner or later, it will fail; and, if other complica-tions do not arise to carry off the patient, he will eventually succumb to cardiac failure thus brought about. Nutrition of the heart substance may be inadequate from many causes; namely, increase of the resistance to be overcome, and participation of the nutrient vessels of the heart in the degenerative process: thus, while the organ has increased work to perform, the quality and quantity of the blood-supply become progressively more impaired, fatty or fibroid degeneration of the myocardium occurs, dilatation of the ventricle ensues, a mitral murmur appears, the veins are mechanically obstructed, the urine is scanty and high-coloured, and dropsy, due partly to cardiac failure, partly to the hydræmic condition of the blood, partly to the altered condition of the vessel walls, encroaches from point to point. Since the whole cardio-vascular system is affected, little can be done beyond temporary alleviation; and the patient generally dies with hypo-static pneumonia. Other cardio-vascular symptoms of a more acute kind may arise; for example, aneurysm of the aorta, affection of the aortic valves by the atheromatous process, or sclerosis of the coronary arteries. In 50 cases of cardio-vascular disease, which I have investigated clinically and pathologically, I met with five cases of severe coronary stenosis uncomplicated with valvular disease, or at any rate not in itself sufficient to produce important symptoms; the substance of the myocardium was the seat of extensive fatty degeneration. Two of the patients died quite suddenly, the cause of death being ascertained after death; in one of the cases coronary disease was suspected during life. One of the most important symptoms of coronary sclerosis is *angina pectoris*, which, as my observations seem to show, occurs especially in cases of increased peripheral resistance, and not in mere stenosis of the coronaries without this increase. In one of the cases referred to, probably syphilitic in origin, these arteries were almost impermeable at their orifices, and yet no anginal symptoms supervened. Slow or arrhythmic pulse is also indicative of coronary arterio-sclerosis. A case has been recorded by Prong in which the pulse-rate was reduced to eight per minute; the autopsy revealed coronary sclerosis. Frey has recorded a case in which the number of pulsations fell to 26; the patient was subject to losses of consciousness preceded by vertigo and followed by general convulsions. At the necropsy stenosis of the coronary arteries and granular kidneys were found.

The following case occurred in my practice, and is very characteristic—a patient, aged sixty-two, subject to fainting fits which last a few minutes, feels giddy on assuming the erect posture, complains of pains in the head, paroxysms of dyspnœa, noises in the ears, occasional attacks of dimness of vision, vomiting, and frequent pains down the left arm. For two months past, he told me, the pulse-rate had not exceeded 24. There was no history of gout, lead, rheumatism or syphilis; the patient looks very ill, is anæmic, cachectic, and emaciated, and presents a well-marked arcus senilis. The heart's impulse is diffuse and indistinctly felt, but the cardiac dulness is not notably increased; the heart's sounds are very irregular and very curious—a lub-dub-dub followed by a pause. The arteries are visible, they are very tortuous and thickened, and can be rolled under the fingers; the pulse is vibratile in character and irregular in force; albuminuria, which was formerly present, has now left him. He had a syncopal attack just before leaving my house.

Thoma lays considerable stress upon angio-sclerotic pain, which he says is generally put down to rheumatism; he supports his argument by the fact of the existence of Pacinian corpuscles on the walls of the vessels, which he has demonstrated.

(c) *Cerebral symptoms.*—I have already spoken of the symptoms of cerebral anæmia in cases of arterio-sclerosis including coronary disease. Grasset, and Rauzier, and Savill also are of opinion that the vertigo may be explained without the cardiac lesion. They attribute the cerebral symptoms to arterio-sclerosis of the vessels of the medulla; and they divide the forms of the vertigo into three types: (i.) Simple vertigo; (ii.) vertigo with epileptiform crises; (iii.) a permanent slow pulse with epileptiform and syncopal attacks (Stokes-Adams disease). Probably several factors take part in producing cerebral anæmia: the loss of elasticity of the cerebral arteries, their partial obliteration, and the weakened action of the heart allow very little compensation in emergency; and a change of posture from sitting to standing, emotion, or other like causes, may suddenly bring about a deprivation of the brain of blood and the onset of the symptoms. Indeed changes in the vessels of the fundus may sometimes be seen with the ophthalmoscope : the retinal vessels seem strangulated or constricted, with diminution of their lumen above and below. The veins are also constricted, especially where they pass over the rigid arteries. Occasionally retinal hæmorrhage may be observed without inflammatory changes. Berheimer advances the opinion that simple optic atrophies in old people may sometimes be the result of arterio-sclerosis : he bases his results on clinical observations and three necropsies. The most important cerebral symptom that occurs in the diffuse form of arterio-sclerosis is due to rupture of miliary aneurysm [vide p. 333 and art. " Cerebral Hæmorrhage " hereafter]. In arterio-sclerosis of the cerebral vessels various psychical disturbances may occur, and seizures of different kinds, even epileptiform, ending in death. Symptoms of focal disease and irritative phenomena following the fits, soon disappear ; but psychical disturbance, marked by apathy, dulness of comprehension, variable temper, delusions, imperfect orientation, weakness of intellect, speech often slow and slurred not monotonous, tremor, hemiplegic phenomena, difference of pupils, or exaggerated reflexes may be present. Grandiose delusions are usually absent. The age of the patients is usually fifty to fifty-five ; the disease runs a course of three to four years, and closely resembles general paralysis (vide Fig. 25).

(d) Renal symptoms supervene in a large number of cases : these are diuresis, urgent in the night, the urine being pale and of low specific gravity, and containing frequently no albumin or but a trace ; uræmic convulsions or spasmodic asthma ; dropsy rarely unless there be complications [vide art. "Bright's Disease," vol. iv.].

(e) The pulmonary symptoms are bronchitis and emphysema, with right heart failure.

Prognosis and Treatment.—The prognosis depends very much upon the stage of the disease ; for in the early period of high arterial pressure very much may be done, by hygienic measures, to prevent and arrest the disease. All conditions which may interfere with the nutrition of the body must be avoided. Mental and bodily strain and excessive business activity should be forbidden. Cold baths, friction, massage and rational daily exercise are to be enjoined.

Diet.—Excess of meat, especially of red meat, is to be avoided. Fish dinners once or twice a week, or even a milk diet, may be recommended in some cases. If there be a gouty tendency, or the disease be of the renal type, this is especially necessary ; as is also the avoidance of certain wines, such as sweet wines, champagnes, and burgundies. Beef tea, meat extracts, and essences, so frequently employed as " supporting measures," should be sparely used or avoided. Certain mineral waters are very useful, for example Carlsbad ; and a course of treatment at one of the many watering-places is very often beneficial—not merely by the drinking of the waters, but by the regular mode of life, diet and exercise. Each patient must be treated, however, according to the nature and relative prominence of the symptoms. It is essential that there should be a regular daily evacuation of the bowels. Spirits should be forbidden, or only allowed in moderate quantity.

If the hyperpiesis of the pulse be very marked, and especially if there be anginal pain, amyl nitrite, trinitrin, or erythrol tetranitrate may be employed. Later, when arterio-sclerosis is well marked, the most useful remedy is sodium or potassium iodide in five to fifteen grain doses three times a day ; the former if the cardiac symptoms are prominent, as it is

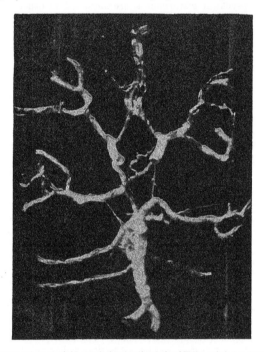

Fig. 25.—Extreme atheroma of the vessels forming the circle of Willis and their principal branches, from a man aged fifty-four suffering from dementia.

less depressing ; it is said to dilate the arteries and to promote nutrition. Some authorities recommend the combination of small doses of liquor arsenicalis with the iodides. When cardiac failure supervenes, and there is incipient regurgitation, we must resort to cardiac tonics, such as digitalis, strophanthus, or spartein; or strychnia and caffeine may be used, especially if œdema of the lungs and dropsy set in. Dr. Sansom recommends the combination of the cardiac tonic with trinitrin or iodides. Ten-minim doses of tincture of digitalis may be given with 1-drop doses of the solution (1 to 100) of nitro-glycerine. Venesection has been employed with success in some cases of cardiac insufficiency with dyspnœa and lividity. It is very desirable to explain to the patient, in the less hopeful cases, that he is suffering from a disease the symptoms of which can only be alleviated, and that alleviation depends almost entirely upon intelligent assistance on his own part in following out implicitly the rules of the physician. The prognosis and treatment of the numerous morbid conditions under which arterio-sclerosis may be manifested, for example, renal disease, lead poisoning, pulmonary fibrosis, and emphysema, cardiac degeneration, aneurysm, cerebral hæmorrhage, migraine, and psychical disturbances, are discussed in other portions of these volumes, and for further information the reader is referred to the special articles upon these subjects.

F. W. Mott.

REFERENCES

1. ADAMI. *Lectures on Fibrosis.*—1a. ALLBUTT, T. C. "Senile Plethora," *Trans. Hunterian Society*, 1895-96.—2. VON BASCH. "Ueber latente Arterio-Sclerose, etc.," *Wiener med. Presse*, Nos. 20, 23, 27, 30 ; 1893.—3. BERHEIMER. "Ueber schweren Veränderung bei hochgrädige Sclerose der Gehirn-Arterien," *Graefe's Archiv*, vol. xxxvii.—4. BOLLINGER. *Pathological Anatomy*, vol. i. p. 28.—5. BREGMAN. "Ein Beitrag zur Angio-Sclerose," *Virchow's Jahrb.* 1891.—6. BROADBENT, Sir WM. *The Pulse.*—7. COATS and AULD. "Endarteritis Deformans and Aneurysm," *Journal of Pathology*, July 1896.—8. COUNCILMAN. *Transactions of Association of American Physicians*, vol. vi.—9. CROCQ, *fils.* "Quelques mots sur l'artério-sclérose," *Gaz. heb. de méd.* Nos. 44, 45 ; 1892.—10. "Discussion on the Relation of Renal Disease to Disturbances of the general Circulation, and to Alterations in the Heart and Blood-vessels," *Intern. Med. Congress*, vol. i. p. 374. London, 1881.—11. DICKINSON, H. "Morbid Effects of Alcohol," *Med.-Chir. Trans.* 1873.—12. DICKINSON. Baillie Lectures. "On the Cardio-vascular Changes of Renal Disease," etc. *Lancet*, July 20, 1895.—13. EPPINGER. *Pathogenesis, Histogenesis u. Aetiologie der Aneurysmen*, 1887.—14. GRASSET and RAUZIER. *Vertige cardio-vasculaire artériel.* —15. GULL and SUTTON. "Arterio-capillary Fibrosis," *Med.-Chir. Transactions*, 1872.—16. HAMPELIN. "Ueber Syphilis u. das Aorten-Aneurysme," *Berl. klin. Wochensch.* Nos. 44, 46, 47 ; 1894.—17. HEGERSTEDT and NEMSER. *Krankhafte Veränderung u. Verschliess.*—18. HELMSTEDTEN. "Du mode de formation des aneurysmes spontanées," *Virch. Jahrb.* Strassburg, 1873.—19. HOFFMANN. "Ueber Aneurysme der basilar Arterien," etc. *Virch. Jahrb.* 1894.—20. HOLLIS. "Ainslie Atheroma," *Journal of Pathology*, 1896.—21. HUCHARD. *Mal. du cœur.*—22. JACOBSOHN. "Ueber die schwere Form der Arterio-Sclerose im central Nerven-System," *Virch. Jahrb.* 1894.—23. JOHNSON, Sir GEORGE. "Relation of Cardio-Vascular Changes to Bright's Disease : a Criticism of Arterio-capillary Fibrosis," *Med.-Chir. Trans.* 1873.—24. VON KÖSTE. "Ueber die Enstehung der spontanen Aneurisme u. die kronische Mesarteritis," *Berlin. klin. Wochensch.* No. 23 ; 1875.—25. LAHN. "Ueber Vascularisation der Media u. Intima bei Endarteritis chronik," *Abth. z. Verh. der Intern. Med. Cong.* Berlin, 1891.—26. LANCEREAUX. *Dictionnaire encyclopédique médicale.*—27. *Idem.* "L'endartérite ou artério-sclérose généralisée," *Arch. gén. du méd.* Jan.-Nov. 1893.—28. LANGHANS. "Anatomy of the Arteries," *Virchow's Archiv*, xxxvi. 1881.—29. LITTEN. "Ueber circumscripte gitterformige Endarteritis," *Deutsche Wochensch.* No. 8, 1889. —30. MACLEAN. *Brit. Med. Jour.* 1876.—31. M'CRORIE, D. "Atheromatous Disease of Arteries," *Glasgow Med. Jour.* vol. xxxviii. 1892.—32. MEIGS. "Chronic Endarteritis and its Clinical and Pathological Effects," *New York Record*, Aug. 24, 1889.—33. DE MUSSY, G. "Étude clinique sur les indurations des artéries," *Arch. gén. de méd.* 1872.—34. PECKLEHARING. "Ueber endothel. Wucherung in Arterien," *Ziegler's Beiträge*, xviii.—35. PRONG. "Stenosis arteriae coronariae cordis," *Virch. Jahrb.* 1893.—36. PUPPE. *Untersuchungen über der Aneurysma der Brust-Aorta.*— —37. ROKITANSKY. *Lehrbuch der Pathologie.*—38. ROMBERG. "Ueber Sclerose der Lungenarterien," *Deutsch. Archiv für klin. Med.* 1891-92.—39. ROY. "On the Elasticity of Arteries," *Journal of Physiology*, iii. 1881.—40. SACHS. "Ueber

Phlebo-Sclerose," *Virch. Jahrb.* 1888.—41. SANSOM. "Diseases of the Blood-Vessels," *Twentieth Century Practice of Medicine*, vol. iv.—42. SAUNDBY. "Hypertrophy of the Vascular System in Granular Degeneration of the Kidney," *Edin. Med. Journ.* Oct. 1896. —42a. SAVILL, T. D. "Arterial Hypermyotrophy," *Brit. Med. Jour.* June 23rd, 1897. —43. STRAUBE. "Ueber die Bedeutung der atheromatosen Arterien-Kranken," Würzburg, *Virch. Jahrb.* 1893. — 44. THOMA. *Pathological Anatomy*, trans. by Dr. Alex. Bruce.—45. *Idem.* "Ueber die Abhändigkeit der Bindegewehe," etc. *Virch. Archiv*, vol. xciii.—46. *Idem.* "Arterial Elasticity," *Lancet*, Nov. 7, 1896. — 47. THOMA and KAEFER. "Ueber die Elasticität gesunden u. kranken Arterien," *Virchow's Archiv*, vol. cxvi.—48. TRAUBE. "Entstehung der Arterio-Sclerose," *Berl. klin. Wochensch.* Nos. 29, 31, 32 ; 1891.—49. TSCHIGAJEW. "The Importance of Muscular Work in the Production of Arterio-sclerosis," *Virch. Jahrb.* 1895.—50. VIRCHOW. *Cellular Pathology.*—51. WELCH. *Trans. Med.-Chir. Soc.* 1876 ; *Lancet*, Nov. 1875.— 52. WILKS and MOXON. *Pathological Anatomy.*

F. W. M.

ANEURYSM OF THE AORTA

Introductory.—It is not intended in this article to discuss at any length the structural characteristics or the pathology of aortic aneurysms, except in so far as these are connected with matters of etiology having a very positive bearing on the prevention and treatment of the disease. The conventional distinctions, which have come down from before the time of Scarpa, between *true* and *false* aneurysms may be regarded now as practically obsolete ; indeed the very application of these names by different authors is often contradictory and positively misleading. Under the more accommodating denomination of *mixed aneurysm* a large number of questionable cases is commonly disposed of ; thus still further confusing the issues supposed to be raised by the first two names. Properly speaking, an aneurysm is a dilatation (ἀνευρύνω) ; and up to the time of Corvisart (1809) the word was applied not only to dilatations of the arteries, but of the heart itself ; the presence of hypertrophy of the ventricles constituting the "active" form of cardiac "aneurysm," while the subordination of this to dilatation was indicated by the term "passive." Laennec and almost all his successors discarded this phraseology—except as regards the comparatively rare instances of sacculated dilatation arising from a ventricle (of which he himself had seen only one instance). For the most part, therefore, he confined the name aneurysm to dilatations of the aorta and other arteries ; and while adopting the current classification, of true and false, did so in a half-hearted way, defending, as it were, the idea of "true" aneurysm against Scarpa, who had indicated the opinion that in all aneurysms there is a solution of continuity in the internal and middle coats ; and that all aneurysms, therefore, currently called such, are "false" according to the more ancient phrase. "An aneurysm," according to Hilton Fagge, "may be defined as a circumscribed tumour containing fluid or solid blood, communicating directly with the canal of an artery, and limited by the tunic which is called the sac." According to this comprehensive definition no aneurysm is more true or more false than another; although the yielding or even destruction of the several coats of the artery may in some degree modify the size and form of the tumour, or its relation to the surrounding parts, and the clinical phenomena observed in the diagnosis. All aneurysms whatever of the aorta, as well as of the minor arteries, involve the idea of abnormal dilatation of a more or less limited area of the vessel; and in almost all that are of any clinical importance, this dilatation presumes a local weakening, mostly accompanied by atrophy of one or more of the vascular coats. To what extent this atrophy may go in a particular instance, and whether it shall affect chiefly one of the coats, or more than one, is determined by circumstances which will presently be considered, but which cannot usually be stated in absolute terms. Even in the smallest and, clinically, the most insignificant pouchings of the inner surface of the aorta,—such as are often found in connection with larger aneurysmal tumours, and occasionally in such numbers as to show various stages of their formation in the same case,—it is impossible to allege that the destructive process is limited to one of the coats. In larger tumours, especially those which are distinctly sacculated, and which communicate with the lumen of the artery by an opening more or less circular, all of the coats may have been destroyed over a considerable area, the tumour adhering to the vertebræ, or to the sternum, eroding these bones, and sometimes perforating them; so that in the one case an external soft and pulsating tumour may appear beneath the skin, and in the other pressure may be exerted on the spinal cord, or its membranes. In the majority of sacculated aneurysms the inner and median coats give way to pressure, or are greatly altered and partly absorbed; and the tumour is circumscribed over a large part of its extent by the outer coat or adventitia only—this coat being often remarkably thickened by a fibrous development. It is extremely rare, if not unknown as regards the systemic arteries, for an aneurysmal pouch to be formed by a protrusion, or hernia (as it has been called), of the inner and middle coats through the outer. But this mode of origin is, on the other hand, often illustrated in those small aneurysmal dilatations of the ramifications of the pulmonary artery in the lungs, which are now well ascertained to be the source of considerable, and sometimes fatal, hæmoptysis in the course of tuberculous disease. In these cases, owing to the gradual breaking up and excavation of the lung tissues around it, support is withdrawn first from the outer wall of the vessel. The adventitia, therefore, is first attacked, and is often much weakened or destroyed; while the two inner coats remain comparatively unaffected, or perhaps nearly normal. But the effect of the continual impact of the blood upon the inner coats is to cause them gradually to yield at the point where they are unsupported by the equable pressure of the outer coat, and of the tissues in the midst of which the vessel normally lies. Thus a hernial protrusion of the two inner coats may be established, or of one of them, through the adventitia. Although, therefore, the description of such cases hardly belongs to the present article, it is most instructive to consider them in connection with the general pathology and etiology of the subject.

In cases of fusiform or globular dilatations in the axis of a considerable artery (the "true aneurysms" of the older writers), there is no reason to suppose that the pathological processes differ essentially from those attending the beginnings of sacculated aneurysms. The coats of the vessel, one or more of them, are in some way or other locally weakened, so as to afford less resistance than the rest of the artery to the distending force of the blood; but the weakening, or it may be the degeneration and atrophy of these coats is so evenly distributed (within the limits of the part affected) that no pouching occurs, but only an all-round increase of the lumen, which is often stationary for considerable periods; especially in persons advanced in life and not subject to great exertion, or in persons enfeebled by disease and not abounding in blood. The peculiarity of such aneurysms, from the clinical point of view, is that they may give rise to no symptoms at all, even when they are known by physical signs to exist. For instance, I have known an aneurysm of this kind in the innominate artery quite palpable to the finger for years in an elderly woman, and yet, so to speak, a mere pathological curiosity; for in the case here referred to it had existed for an indefinite period, and the subject of it was a remarkably healthy old woman, who managed to survive most, if not all of her own children; these having had an hereditary taint of phthisis derived from the father, a member of the medical profession. His widow had learned from him what was the probable nature of the beating in her neck, and thus only it became known to third parties, as she never complained of it, and so far as is known did not die of it; indeed she survived, and was well known to me, till she was close upon eighty years of age.

Closely resembling these cases of fusiform dilatation of the medium-sized arteries are those of general dilatation of the arch of the aorta, in which, without any sacculated formation and presumably with the persistence, if not the integrity, of all the coats of the vessel, there is a great, sometimes an enormous enlargement, most commonly in the ascending or transverse part of the arch, and often involving the origins, at least, of one or more of the arteries springing from the arch; yet without anything that, clinically speaking, can be definitely called a tumour. Such cases are to be recognised, when they can be distinguished at all during life from sacculated aneurysms, chiefly by the absence of the distinctive symptoms attending the latter; these will be enumerated farther on in this article. The reason for alluding to this now is to make the general remark, that it is not at all the so-called *true* aneurysms which furnish the leading facts upon which the diagnosis of the disease, in the case of internal or aortic aneurysms at least, must be held to rest. In the well-known work of Dr. Walshe, and in relation to the arch of the aorta, 28 pages are given to the consideration of "simple and compound lateral sacculations," and barely a single page to "peripheric dilating aneurysms, fusiform and globular"; the last (globular) being so rare that this distinguished observer had only noted a single instance. It is evident, therefore, that "true" aneurysms will have but a small place in the present article; yet they are not without interest, because they illustrate a different form of the effect of the forces producing aneurysm in general, as regards the particular vessels, or portions of vessels, in which they occur.

Dissecting aneurysm.—This is a very peculiar and really most interesting mode of vascular disease, first carefully described by Laennec, who, however, had seen one case only. The inner and partly also the median coats of the vessel (in most cases the aorta near its origin) are torn through by what often resembles, more or less, a clean cut or rent, by which the blood, gaining access to the muscular fibres of the media, opens them out so as to make its way by a kind of burrowing or "dissecting" process among these fibres for considerable distances in the line of the axis of the vessel, the normal lumen of which often remains clear, but is sometimes also obstructed so as to give rise to serious clinical consequences. The abnormal or dissected course of the blood-stream comes to an end in one of two ways: either the outer coat gives way, with the result, usually, of immediate death by hæmorrhage; or the false passage, after pursuing a course it may be of many inches, or from the arch down even to the iliac vessels, enters again the main channel; in the latter case life may be preserved for months, or even for years, under more or less disabling conditions, the true cause of which can rarely be known until after death.

Etiology.—It has already been stated that the localised dilatation which constitutes an aneurysm presumes a local weakening, mostly accompanied by atrophy, of one or more of the coats of the vessel. The other element, which concurs with the above in producing dilatation, is, of course, the intra-vascular pressure acting from within outwards, and, in the case of the aorta especially, increased in a considerable degree at each pulsation of the left ventricle. In the normal condition, notwithstanding the variations in this stress from moment to moment, and its maintenance up to the point of physiological efficiency during a long lifetime, the balance existing between the elastic resistance of the vascular walls (chiefly due to the middle coat) and the forces tending to expansion is wonderfully well preserved; and it is not very uncommon to find persons attaining even advanced age in whom neither the heart, nor any of the greater arteries, has suffered in any appreciable degree. This, if duly considered from the purely physical point of view, is nothing less than wonderful; and the wonder of it will surely increase when we remember how difficult—nay, how impossible—it would be to construct an artificial machine of elastic and distensible materials, which would not only resist indefinitely a constant mean internal pressure acting upon it through the contained liquids, but also a sudden impulse and variable increase of that pressure repeated periodically at the rate of over 100,000 times a day, or, say, 40,000,000 times a year, unceasingly, for all the 70 years of an average healthy human life. It is quite true that this ideal perfection of the human machine is not attained in all cases, even of comparatively healthy persons; but the marvel is that it should ever be attained, or even approached, in any case. In most of the hollow viscera a certain loss of tenacity and physical resilience is experienced as age advances; and in the urinary bladder this is very notably the case, leading to more tardy evacuation, and sometimes, in the later periods of life, to the entire loss of control or of power in it. Yet the strain to which the urinary bladder is subjected, in a moderately well-regulated existence, is as nothing compared to that which inevitably falls upon the heart and arteries in the propulsion and circulation of the blood. The true marvel, it may be repeated, is not that the vascular coats do, in comparatively rare and exceptional instances,[1] yield to that strain so as to incur local or general dilatation, but that they should ever escape this consequence.

So much is clear, even as the expression of mere physical laws, with respect to the subject now before us. The most general expression, perhaps, which can be given to the causation of aneurysm, as a question of physics apart from considerations founded on pathological experience, is the following:—"A local disproportion in the normal balance between the amount of lateral pressure inside the artery and the elastic resistance of the vascular walls, arising either from abnormal increase of the former or diminution of the latter; most frequently, indeed, from both these causes in combination" (1). Yet this leads us but a small way in the investigation of the facts, although it may be accepted as a formula sufficiently comprehensive to include all the essential physical conditions of such aneurysmal dilatation.

When pathological observation is brought to bear on this subject, the first thing to be noticed is the coincidence, in the great majority of cases, of varying degrees of chronic *endarteritis deformans* (Virchow), or, as it is also called, atheromatous degeneration of the intima and media, or of both, with aneurysms in every part of the arterial system, and especially in the aorta. This degeneration, notoriously one of advancing life (*malum senile arteriarum*), is in most cases very pronounced in its characters in the aorta; and as very few cases of aneurysm of this vessel occur altogether without degenerative changes, it is apt to be taken for granted that these invariably precede and dispose to the dilatation. But this conclusion, though plausible, and probably to some extent true, must not be held to satisfy all the conditions of the etiological problem. Sixty years ago (1837), in what is perhaps the most elaborate memoir ever published on the heart and arterial system medically considered, Bizot drew attention, for the first time on a numerical basis, to the age-incidence of the lesions now commonly spoken of as endarteritis, in their various stages as carefully described by him. As regards all these,

---

[1] Professor Coats has found that in 300 consecutive post-mortem examinations, carefully recorded with a special view to this point, the "beginnings of aneurysms," in the shape of slight depressions or pouchings of the coats, were found in 8 cases, 3 of which were cases of sacculated aneurysm."

he pointed out that they "increase considerably in frequency as the subjects examined are older"; and further, that the most advanced stages of the lesions (apart from aneurysm) occur most frequently at the most advanced ages (*loc. cit.* p. 283). In contrast with this very marked age-relation of the lesions commonly supposed to lead up to aneurysm, Bizot does not fail to show (near the end of his long paper, p. 409) that 108 subjects affected with aneurysm (collected indiscriminately from various sources) presented almost as great a number below forty years of age as between that age and seventy; while only four cases out of the whole number were in persons beyond seventy years of age. In another respect also (to be discussed farther on), Bizot may be said to have anticipated by many years more modern observations and opinions, by pointing out that (with certain curious exceptions which he does not attempt to explain) atheromatous lesions of the aorta are, on the whole, nearly equally distributed between the two sexes, while aneurysms very largely predominate in the male sex; and from the whole inquiry into this particular branch of his subject he concludes (p. 411) "that the laws which preside over the development of the arterial lesions (that is, endarteritis) differ in various ways from those which rule the formation of aneurysms, although these are generally and rightly regarded as connected with the other arterial alterations." To complete the account here of what is due to this excellent observer, it is necessary to quote the sentence which follows:—"We must take into account, undoubtedly, the determining causes (of aneurysms), such as blows, falls, violent movements, which have a great influence, and it can thus be understood how women and old men, who are usually less exposed to these, are also much less frequently affected with aneurysms." Confining attention, however, in the meantime to the question of age, one of the most recent pathological manuals states the relation of aneurysm to atheroma in the following terms:—"Aneurysms are most frequent between the ages of thirty and forty. On the other hand, atheroma, although not infrequent between these ages, is much more common after forty. It will thus be seen that aneurysms coincide with the time of life *when the period of greatest bodily vigour overlaps the period of occurrence of atheroma*" (17). In other words, while both aneurysms and atheromatous degenerations are exceedingly rare in youth and early manhood, the order of precedence in advancing life of the two diseases is (or seems to be) rather the converse of what might be expected on the view of the latter being the cause of the former. And the comparison of the infrequency of aneurysms at very advanced ages,—during which time of life atheroma certainly does not tend to diminish, with the occasional, though rare, occurrence, even of sacculated aneurysms, long before atheroma to any considerable extent can be suspected, gives us reason to suspend our judgment on the necessary dependence of dilatation upon previous disease of the vascular walls. That atheroma does dispose to aneurysm it is not possible to doubt; and that in the great majority of cases, at least, an incipient and more or less definitely localised weakening or atrophy of the intima and the media, from this or from some other cause, gives an opening and an occasion to the pouching which forms the first step in a sacculated aneurysm, is too evident to require elaborate proof.

About twenty-eight years ago (1871) a very remarkable paper was published by Professor Clifford Allbutt in the St. George's Hospital Reports, which, though not chiefly devoted to the consideration of aneurysms, can hardly be left out of account in reference to this subject. The general argument of Dr. Allbutt is, that in estimating "the effects of overwork and strain on the heart and great blood-vessels," too little importance has been attached to these factors in the etiology of cardiac disease, not only as secondary and concurrent causes, intensifying the results of previous disease, but as causes tending to the production of, and sometimes demonstrably producing, the very changes of structure which have been supposed to be constitutional in origin. From observations gathered "among a heavily-laden population," Dr. Allbutt was led to conclude that "a large number of heart cases (occur) in young, well-made subjects of healthy build, and previously unaffected by constitutional disease." A similar conclusion, arrived at on quite independent evidence, as regards young men in the prime of life serving in the army, was published by Dr. Myers in 1870, and formed the most important and practical argument in detail of his work on *Diseases of the Heart among Soldiers* (60), quoted and discussed in the article above referred to. Both writers clearly affirm that whether as regards the dangers to the endocardium during comparatively early life, or the degenerative changes of a later period, "strain" is not only a coincident and as it were secondary cause of valvular deformity, or of cardiac dilatation without valve disease, but in many cases the true starting-point of the whole series of these changes. In cases of simple dilatation, with or without compensatory hypertrophy, it is argued that the endocardium suffers sooner or later from the exaggerated and repeated impulses of a heart constantly struggling with a tendency to overloading of the ventricle, and propelling its blood with mechanical over-exertion at each stroke through orifices, or into vessels, the lining membranes of which are not fitted to sustain these abnormal impulses. Sometimes the valves (the aortic chiefly) give way suddenly, and aortic regurgitation is at once established as the result of a single violent effort or accident; but this is comparatively rare. At other times the mitral valve becomes subject to incompetence, "not due to a stretching of the orifice so much as to a deterioration in the muscular and tendinous cords of the valves" (Allbutt). Apart, however, from these incidents, the results of a life spent in "continuous labour, such as hammer work," or with liability to "more sudden strains, like the lifting of weights," is apt to be fraught with disaster to the heart. As long, indeed, as the bodily frame generally is well nourished, and the entire muscular system (including the heart) is developed in proportion to the strain thrown upon it; as long, too, as the lungs are structurally intact, ample in volume, unrestrained in their expansion, and sufficiently active in function to interpose no obstacle to the aeration of the blood, the circulation may not suffer, even from very great exertions, as in rowing competitions. But if severe and laborious exertions and strain are persisted in, either from choice or necessity, when these conditions of physiological counterpoise are not fulfilled, then the heart will suffer; in the first instance functionally (irritability and acceleration), and then, sooner or later, from dilatation first of the right and then of the left ventricle, which may or may not be associated with corresponding hypertrophy.   Dr Allbutt holds (*loc. cit.* p. 27) that, under these circumstances, "chronic inflammation of the aorta and aortic valves" is the usual result of such dilatation, whether compensated partially or not; and that it is often a matter of accident whether the valves give way first or whether the hypertrophied left ventricle, with its superfluity of blood projected at each stroke upon the first part of the aortic arch, leads to disease there.   Such disease, originating really in strain, may take the form either of loss of elasticity and dilatation of the arterial coats in the first instance, or of "points of endoarteritis, with diffuse granular exudation among the fibres of the middle coat," followed by "pouching of the aorta, with consequent or concomitant incompetence of the valves" (*loc. cit.* p. 38). . . . "If, however, one sudden effort be the cause of mischief, we never find pouching of the aorta as a consequence; but we find a crack which may be in the floor of the aorta causing regurgitation, or in the side of it giving rise to saccular aneurysm" (*ibid.* p. 46).

It is difficult to present, within the brief compass now at my disposal, the main argument of a paper at every point replete with particular illustrations, and having many side issues which it is impossible to discuss here. But the reader will easily infer from these extracts the importance of the questions raised by Dr. Allbutt concerning the etiology of aneurysm, and especially of aneurysm in the first part of the aorta.   The author is indeed careful to disclaim any intention of setting aside as of no account the influence of constitutional states.   "In claiming attention for the mechanical origin of aneurysms of the aorta," he writes, p. 49, " I do not thereby deny a like effect to constitutional degeneration."   But he maintains "that we do not pay sufficient attention to the fact that aortic aneurysms, both thoracic and abdominal, do so frequently occur in men who are young and of healthy tissues.   If these patients attribute their disease to a particular strain, the note-taker is as likely as not to set the story aside as immaterial. . . . A sudden strain, however, is not only a cause, but the commonest cause of aortic aneurysm. . . . That on the post-mortem the aorta is found to be atheromatous is no ground for the complacent assumption that the 'atheroma' is antecedent.   On the contrary, the endarteritis is as probably a consequence of the same kind as the diffuse mischief surrounding an injury to any other tissue."

It is now sufficiently obvious that in all this we have to deal with an exceedingly complicated problem; one having at least two aspects, not necessarily contradictory, and as regards either side of which a plausible case can be made out by argument; while in the more exact statement of the etiological problem, so as to comprehend all the results of experience, the difficulties are nearly insuperable. We have already seen that, in respect of age, aneurysm tends to occur at a period of life not inconsiderably anticipating, but at the same time overlapping, the age of the senile degenerations,[1] a fact which tends in favour of Professor Allbutt's hypothesis. A similar confirmation of the view that strenuous bodily effort, to the extent of producing strain, has a good deal to do with the causation of aneurysm, arises from the notoriously much greater frequency of aneurysms of the aorta in the male sex and in certain very laborious occupations peculiar to men; while the predominance of atheroma, on the other hand, even if it be admitted as possible in men, is not nearly so marked nor so extreme. The facts as regards the relative frequency of simple atheroma in the two sexes have already been referred to above, on the excellent authority of Bizot; and a much more recent observer, M'Crorie, relying upon the cases occurring in the Glasgow Royal Infirmary, has arrived at the conclusion that the liability to atheromatous changes in the arteries in the two sexes is about equal. In contrast with this, good authorities, such as Hodgson, have usually placed the predominating incidence of aneurysms in the male sex at eight or nine men to one woman. This applies, however, chiefly to aneurysms of the external vessels. In aneurysms of the cerebral arteries, according to Professor Coats, the disparity of the sexes is by no means apparent. In dissecting aneurysms it has even been affirmed that the female sex predominates; but this is not in accordance with the cases collated by Dr. Peacock, which give 39 males against 30 females. On the other hand, there is a fact not alluded to in Professor Allbutt's memoir, which tends more or less definitely in the contrary direction. The strongly contrasted statements of Hope, affirming the frequent or invariable coincidence of hypertrophy of the left ventricle with aneurysm of the aorta, and of Stokes denying this association (on the presumption in both cases of the latter being the cause, the former the effect), have given rise to a number of more recent observations and statements on the subject; and though it cannot be said that the question has ever been thoroughly and critically dealt with on the basis of a large series of observations carefully recorded *ad hoc*,[2] it must be considered as now tolerably well

---

[1] In a monograph presently to be referred to (18), Drs. Coats and Aula mention some details on this point which, though founded on too small numbers to be absolutely trustworthy as statistics, are nevertheless interesting and suggestive. In his careful researches in the Royal Infirmary of Glasgow, M'Crorie found that in only one case out of twenty-four were the subjects affected with atheroma under forty years of age; while in the Western Infirmary Museum very nearly one-half (16 out of 33 specimens) of the aneurysms of the aorta there collected occurred in cases which, *as they came to a fatal termination before the fortieth year of age*, must probably have had their initiation on the average some years earlier still.

[2] A very recent statement by Dr. Sansom (75) tends to supply the deficiency above noted from the carefully tabulated necropsies of the London Hospital. Among 82 cases of aneurysm of the thoracic aorta, 41 were in such positions that the aortic valves were not implicated; enlargement of the left ventricle was evidenced in only nine, and in three of these there was only slight hypertrophy. In 41 cases in which the aortic valves were involved, hypertrophy and dilatation of the left ventricle were manifested

established that, except in cases of the first part of the arch (in many of which the valves of the heart are also involved) hypertrophy of either ventricle is not in any very notable degree an accompaniment of most aneurysms at the time of the death of the patient; in some cases indeed even a relative atrophy of the whole heart has been found present; and in some of these the aneurysm, though not close to the heart, was of large size and presumably of some considerable duration.[1]

A sufficiently striking example of this fact (but only one out of many) may be mentioned here, because the case has other points of interest, and was minutely and exhaustively examined from the pathological point of view by Dr. Coats, and by myself clinically. A slater, æt. 29, was admitted to the Western Infirmary of Glasgow with an obscure disease, apparently dating approximately from an attack of "lumbago" two years before, for which he had been treated in another hospital, with the result of being dismissed apparently "well." After very careful and repeated examination in the Western Infirmary, the diagnosis was made (correctly) that the patient was affected by some eroding disease of the vertebræ on the left side, involving the left pleura and the base of the lung; but also (incorrectly) that this was most probably an empyema, based upon a more or less septic or infective osteitis. The misleading element here was the temperature, which (a rare exception in aneurysms) was found to be highly febrile throughout, running up to 104·6° F. and with very marked diurnal oscillations.[2] The case ultimately proved fatal, about three weeks after admission, by hæmothorax; and the necropsy revealed an aneurysm of the descending (thoracic) aorta, not very large, projecting against and eroding the bodies of the lower dorsal vertebræ; besides this, the aorta was highly atheromatous in many places, with several incipient aneurysms in the form of small and clinically insignificant pouching of the coats of the artery, and almost complete destruction of the media; so that the wall, even of the smallest pouches, was formed by the intima and adventitia only, with mere vestiges or microscopic islets of the media. No more characteristic case to illustrate the beginnings of aneurysm than this can possibly be imagined.

Now, in this case, apart from its diagnostic interest briefly alluded to above, there are several points worthy of attention from the etiological

in 35. The result of these observations, therefore, is generally in conformity with the statements in the text; but it is still to be desired that the actual weights and averages in the similar group of cases should be placed on record, with due regard in particular cases to the general conformation and muscularity of the body; especially in those cases where the weight approximates to the normal average, or is even small, as in one case presently to be noted in the text of this article. Dr. Sansom further says, "A huge aneurysm may be accompanied by a small heart." Dr. Walshe had already stated that "a very large sac of some years' growth, and situated in that part of the vessel (the arch), may fail to induce the smallest increase in the heart's bulk " (6).

[1] See Hayden, *Diseases of the Heart and Aorta*, 1875. Reference is made to most of the other authorities at pp. 486-488; also pp. 1082, 1083; the subject being fully considered in the light of the author's personal experience.

[2] The very unusual character of the case in this respect led to its being recorded and fully discussed, as to the diagnosis, in a clinical lecture (30). But no adequate explanation of these anomalous temperatures was afforded by the necropsy.

side. The actual aneurysm must in all probability have been one of some standing, if it was (as it appeared to be) the cause of the symptoms designated as "lumbago" two years before. The aorta was much diseased otherwise, and presented, in fact, a pronounced example of the pathological disposition to aneurysm in its most strongly marked form. But with all this complexity of arterial disease the heart weighed only 8 oz., and, though the tissue was pale, its muscular structure and valves appeared to be normal. Evidently the order of events set forth by Professor Allbutt as the usual succession arising from strain is not at all apparent in this instance. And yet, careful inquiry after the patient's death obtained from his relatives the statement of a fact which he had not disclosed during his lifetime ; either during his last illness or during the one that occurred two years before, to which, therefore, we presume that he attached very little importance. While working on the roof of a house at his occupation, and apparently in good health, this comparatively young man had in some way received a severe strain which was followed by orchitis, a strain which therefore may have been, in one sense or another, a cause either of the aneurysmal tumour at first, or of some notable increase in a tumour already existing. Although the injury did not present itself in this light to the patient, it may be at once admitted that in this case strain, as a possible etiological factor, is tolerably well made out. But is it conceivable that this one severe strain, giving to it every possible credit as a cause, could have been responsible for all the multiplied lesions in the arterial system of this man under thirty years of age, who from his daily occupation may easily be supposed to have been liable to occasional, but scarcely to habitual or continuous over-exertion or effort ? To ask this question is at the same time to answer it. It seems impossible to regard the pouching of the coats of the aorta in this case, much less the atheroma which probably determined the pouching, as due primarily to strain ; that is, to the inordinate blood-pressure and increased impulse of a heart which after death was found to weigh only 8 ounces. The utmost that can be conceded to the strain is that the one particular pouch, which actually developed into an aneurysmal tumour of clinical importance, may have been locally determined by the twist or sudden wrench of the body which gave rise to the orchitis. And even so much as this is far from certain, when it is considered that all the pouched parts of the vascular wall, as well as others that were not perceptibly so affected, had so suffered from local destruction by atrophy or rupture of the fibres of the median coat as to have lost altogether their chief element of elastic resistance to the impact of the blood in the distension of the artery. Whatever, therefore, the effect of strain may have been in this case in giving an impetus to the disease, it can hardly be regarded as its starting-point. "Constitutional causes"—an admittedly, but in this instance conveniently vague phrase [1]—must have laid

---

[1] It is to be regretted that in consequence of the erroneous diagnosis in this case, and the urgency of the symptoms during the short time the patient was under observation, no adequate inquiry was made (such as would have been proper in a case supposed to be one

the foundations of this very early occurrence of disease in the intima, which had already extended at so many points to the media, breaking it up so completely as to render the artery quite defenceless even against the ordinary distending forces of the circulation; and all the more, of course, against any particular disturbing cause such as is above indicated.

While, therefore, I am inclined to concur with Professor Allbutt in giving due effect to the statements of aneurysmal patients referring their disease to a particular strain, and while I am in no degree disposed to minimise the importance either of sudden strain or of continuous violent effort in the production of aortic aneurysm or of valvular disease, I also think that a *caveat* must be entered against the too unqualified acceptance of the general statement that "in men who are young and of healthy tissues . . . a sudden strain is not only a cause, but the commonest cause of aortic aneurysm, for in the majority of cases this cause is alleged, it is reasonable, and it stands alone." As the case quoted above shows, it would be possible to err in more than one direction in the inference that, when a sudden strain is either alleged or has existed as a cause, it "stands alone" even in a man much below the age of forty. It may be even then only a secondary link in the chain of causation in which "constitutional causes" of arterial failure have both pre-existed in fact and been of primary importance.[1] I have very carefully inquired into this point for many years past, in cases of aortic aneurysm, where the diagnosis was unquestionable; and in the majority (perhaps even a large proportion) of the cases I have failed to get evidence of such a character as to confirm the above general statement. In not a few cases there is no evidence of such sudden onset at all; but even when such evidence is spontaneously given or elicited by inquiries, it should be remembered that in this as in all other chronic affections, patients are very likely to declare as an obvious and primary cause of their disease what may be only one in a complicated series of causes, and not in reality the starting-point of the disease. Further, what seems to be (according to the patient) the cause of the symptoms may be only the comparatively late increase of an aneurysm long present in a more latent condition; as in a case recorded by Dr. Hayden (*Diseases of the Heart and Aorta*, case 138), where three weeks before death the patient, habitually intemperate and exposed to strain in his ordinary occupation, was suddenly seized, while carrying a heavy load, with pain in his head and difficulty of breathing.

In the estimate of continuous or habitual laborious effort as a cause

---

of vascular disease) into the antecedents of the patient in respect of alcohol, syphilis, and so forth.

[1] May the Editor be permitted to say that after twenty-seven years' more experience he has modified his opinions largely in the direction indicated by his distinguished contributor, as will be seen in his article on Aortic Disease (vol. v. p. 912). At the same time he would still urge, as he urges in the article referred to, that a normal-sized ventricle is consistent with enormous fluctuations of blood-pressure, and is indeed the rule unless the mean pressure of the blood be permanently raised; this, however, as he has endeavoured to show, is not the usual state of things (p. 843).

the difficulties are still greater, of course, than in the case of a sudden and obvious development of symptoms following a strain. It may be held as quite well established that extremely laborious occupations do dispose to aneurysm ; and that the arguments adduced above as to age and sex are valid up to the point of a strong presumption in favour of such causation ; but we must always be cautious in arriving at the conclusion that in an individual case, even of a man presumed to be healthy and not subject to senile degenerations, hard labour has been the only or the primary cause of the disease.

These cautions being premised, however, there are abundant evidences in general medical experience tending to show that sudden violence or strain, even when not directly applied to the thorax, may lay the first foundations of lesions having either the actual character of aneurysm of the aorta, or likely to become such. Take, for example, the following case briefly recorded by Dr. Paul (80), but valuable in the present connection on account of the very precise details. Male, aged 48. On a Monday he was hunting when his horse ran away with him, and he was subjected to severe strain in endeavouring to check the animal, and from the horse jumping with him from a field down into a road at several feet lower level. At this point the horse suddenly stopped, and the rider, without any fall or other sensible injury, was attacked with pain in his chest and a feeling of faintness. He was able to get home without assistance, but continued in a depressed state, with hurried breathing and a pain below the left nipple. Next morning he was much relieved, and the effects of the strain seemed to be passing away. On the Saturday (fifth day after the accident) he was visited by his medical attendant, and described himself as much better ; but while they were chatting together the patient quite suddenly died. The body was that of a well-nourished man, strong and muscular. In the ascending aorta, just above the valves, was a rent about ¾ inch long, through the internal and middle coats. It passed into a space between the middle and external coats filled with blood clot—a dissecting aneurysm, in fact—which had separated the coats on the posterior aspect for about 7 or 8 inches. From this a very small burst had taken place into the pericardium, which was found filled with blood.

In this case there was a very distinct history of an accident involving strain, but not of any local injury or contusion of the thorax apparently adequate to the production of the effects described. A very similar case as regards the lesion in the aorta occurred within my own cognisance, in consultation, in the practice of the late Dr. Macfarlane of Kilmarnock, who sent the parts for preservation to the Museum of the Western Infirmary (series ii. No. 197). In this case, however, the history of an accident involving sudden strain or injury could not be obtained. All that the most careful inquiry elicited was, that the patient was addicted to bouts of heavy drinking, carried to the point of alcoholic coma, from one of which he was just emerging when he was taken ill. He was a middle-aged man of robust constitution and generally healthy appearance, actively engaged in professional business. What happened to him during his intemperate fit (which had led to his being brought home in a state of helpless insensibility) can never be known. Although his occupation did not tend to over-exertion or strain, and nothing had been ever revealed to his regular medical attendant as to any previous illness, I was able to infer, from all the facts communicated to me thirty-four hours before the death of the patient, that some probably aneurysmal condition would be found as the cause of his sudden and nearly fatal collapse, from which, indeed, he partially recovered; he died, however, in a second attack attended by coma and convulsion. The rent in the inner and middle coats of the aorta, half an inch above the valves, was nearly 2 inches long. The heart in both ventricles, and also the arch of the aorta, were more or less dilated. In a case recorded and beautifully figured in the *Chatham Army Museum Reports*, 4th fasciculus (pl. x. fig. 6), London, 1841, a very similar lesion will be found; but here also the history is wanting in detail. In another case, however (fig. 5), portrayed on the same page as the preceding, a very extensive rupture of all the coats of the vessel occurred just above the valves, and yet another rent near the origin of the left subclavian. In the first, the laceration extended "nearly throughout the whole circumference of the vessel; a very narrow slip only of the middle coat connecting them at the posterior part." In this case the history of the injury is very clear; but it does not appear that any bone was injured in the thorax, although "the right os femoris was fractured at its neck." The man, æt. 45, "was found dead in a chalk pit, into which he was supposed to have fallen when intoxicated." A parallel case of internal disaster to the vascular system resembling this one in respect to the manifestly traumatic origin, but at a much earlier age, and therefore removed from all presumptions of atheromatous or other "constitutional" infirmity, is recorded in a footnote (where it has, apparently, escaped the attention of almost all systematic authorities) in the *Transactions of the Edinburgh Medico-Chirurgical Society*, vol. i. 1824, p. 662. The preparation is in the Museum of the Royal College of Surgeons of Edinburgh, and is, I suppose, an unique example of the grave internal injury which may take place from an accident leaving all the external parts intact. "A girl, ten years of age, was run over by a loaded cart. She gave a scream before the wheel passed over her body, but appeared to have died instantly, as she uttered no more sounds. There was scarcely any external injury. Not a single rib was broken, and the only visible evidences of extravasation or of bruises externally were a slight extravasation under the right nipple, and some bruises about the ankles, attributed to the foot of the horse. The internal injuries were confined to the heart, which was extensively lacerated. Both ventricles and both auricles were laid open by the laceration, and the septum was torn to shreds. About one-half of the substance of the heart had burst a way for itself through the pericardium into the right cavity of the thorax, where it was found immersed in a very large quantity of grumous blood, and was still attached to the other part by very small portion near the apex, where the rent had stopped. The urinary bladder was completely contracted."

It is in cases such as the above that the more evident effects of sudden injury on the arterial and vascular systems can be most definitely appreciated; and in the last case, though not one of aneurysm or even of disease (properly speaking) at all, it is especially remarkable that laceration, amounting to ruin and all but complete detachment of the heart, had taken place from an injury, severe, indeed, but not such as to have left any considerable impression on the external walls of the thorax. When death follows suddenly, as in this case, and when the age and other circumstances are such as to minimise or exclude the suspicion of previous disease, the traumatic history stands out clearly enough. Some of the recorded cases of dissecting aneurysm, especially those which after a brief interval open into the pericardium from the first part of the aorta, carry at least a strong presumption of such traumatic origin in the abrupt —often transverse and quite sharp and linear—severance of the inner and partly the middle coat, from which the blood makes its way through the latter, dissecting and separating the layers of muscular fibres for a longer or shorter distance. But even in dissecting aneurysms, thus characterised, the history of injury and strain is often entirely wanting, or by no means so clearly defined as to correspond with the appearances observed after death. The remarkably interesting and valuable summary and tabular statement of eighty cases of dissecting aneurysm collected and analysed by Dr. Peacock, in which, however, the histories of the cases recorded are too often unsatisfactory as regards details, show in a general way that an obviously traumatic cause is the exception, not the rule. Thus in a preparation laid before the Pathological Society of London by Sir S. Wilks (vol. xi. p. 58), and closely resembling in its anatomical details some of those above referred to, it is expressly stated that there was no history of injury or of any severe illness. The internal rent, $2\frac{1}{2}$ inches long, extended almost completely round the vessel, and was joined to another nearer the valves. Moreover, the injury or shock, when it is definitely recorded, often seems to be singularly inadequate to the production of the effect. Thus in one case, noted many years ago by myself (but of which the reference has been mislaid), a powerfully-built young man, presumably in good health, leaped from a wall about 13 feet high into a paved court-yard, alighting on his feet; without any apparent loss of balance. Shortly afterwards, however, he staggered and fainted, and almost immediately died. The heart and vessels were sound in their structure, but a rupture in the first part of the aorta was found, opening into the pericardium, as in several of the preceding cases. In this instance a concussion, which might have been almost deliberately encountered by a young athlete without the slightest misgiving, was, nevertheless, the apparent, and almost certainly the actual, cause of a fatal internal injury. In a remarkable case recorded by Dr. Finlayson (29a) a rupture of the descending aorta took place, seemingly as the result of an accidental injury, which, however, was severe enough to have caused fracture of a rib. The patient returned to his work in two days; but about a fortnight later became breathless, had pain in the left side, and, from nearly this time till his death two months after the injury, continued spitting up blood. In this case there was no aneurysm proper; but it is probable that the inner and middle coats had given way first, after the manner of a dissecting aneurysm as above indicated.

The net result of this rather prolonged discussion is that while it is in a high degree reasonable to affirm that both continuous effort and sudden or violent strain or injury are in a very appreciable degree causes of aneurysm, the question of how far, and at what stage in a particular case these causes have come into operation, is often one of the utmost difficulty and complexity. Reverting to the purely physical argument, as stated earlier in this article, it may justly be held that it would be almost too wonderful for belief were the arteries (and especially the aorta), a series of elastic tubes containing blood, constantly under high pressure—a pressure which is momentarily increased, several thousand times an hour, by each impulse of the left ventricle—to escape damage altogether during a long life of varied activity, not only from sudden and more or less severe accidents, but also from "the thousand natural shocks that flesh is heir to." Where exact observation fails us hitherto is chiefly in interpreting the relation of the cause to the effect as actually observed; especially in cases in which the apparent origin of the disease, or of the symptoms, is not sudden, but where the slowly acting and often repeated results of "strain" may at any stage, or at every stage under observation, have been in operation conjointly with other known predisposing causes of aneurysm—atheroma, syphilis, exhausting or acute diseases, and so forth.

This seems to be the proper place to refer to a most important paper which has come into my hands while engaged in the preceding investigation. In a very elaborate research, conducted almost purely from the pathological point of view jointly by Professor Coats and Dr. Auld (18), and founded on careful and minute microscopical and other observations which it will be impossible to detail here, the connection of *endarteritis deformans* with the distending force of the ventricle as a cause (especially in the aorta), is maintained upon grounds which are all the more striking because the clinical considerations which have been chiefly adduced in the present article have been almost wholly left aside. The origin (according to these observers) of the patches which at a later stage become atheroma, is always in the intima; and is of the nature of a thickening by what is, in essentials, a reduplication of the normal tissue of the intima, and, like it, non-vascular. The effect of this would sometimes appear to be rather a strengthening of the arterial wall in the areas where it occurs; but, on the other hand, this tissue is very prone to degeneration, and chiefly to fatty degeneration, as is often seen in the most exaggerated degree in the cerebral arteries, without any implication of the other tunics. In the aorta, however, these latter almost always tend to become involved; and, in the case of the media, an atrophy or rupture of the muscular fibres is frequently the result; the gaps being filled up with new material which is more or less vascular, but, of course, of inferior capacity of resistance.

The processes by which these secondary results are attained, as regards the media and adventitia, are submitted by the authors to a very exhaustive, but, as above indicated, a purely pathological investigation in detail. "In regard to the causation," they remark (*loc. cit.* pp. 97, 98), "there are two factors to be considered, namely, the weakness of the wall, implied in the fact that the disease is one of senility ; and, secondly, the influence of the blood-pressure." The latter "is capable of a two-fold interpretation. It is calculated when in excess to weaken the wall of the vessel. We have indeed seen reason to believe that, in diseases characterised by hypertrophy of the left ventricle, the exaggerated impulse of the blood is a frequent cause of an early development of atheroma, *as if a premature senility of the arteries were thus producible.* On the other hand, mechanical irritation is a recognised cause of inflammation, and we have to consider to what extent the disease is to be regarded as inflammatory in its nature."

It is not without significance that, according to the authors, atheroma of the pulmonary artery "scarcely occurs except in cases in which the right ventricle is much hypertrophied" (p. 82). Again, in the systemic arteries, atheroma, as a general rule, diminishes in frequency from the arch of the aorta outwards ; the most notable exception among the smaller arteries being the cerebral vessels, "whose walls are less supported from the outside than those of the limbs" (p. 101), and in which both atheroma and aneurysms are relatively frequent. The authors have met with only one case of popliteal aneurysm, which in France, and perhaps also elsewhere, used to be regarded as by far the most frequent of external aneurysms, and attributed to the stretching and other injuries to the artery liable to occur at this point in postillions and others in the course of their occupation. But then, the progress of the railroad, even in France, has nearly superseded the postillion as a necessary part of the human machinery of locomotion. [*Vide* art. "Diseases of the Arteries," p. 321.]

The argument which follows is much too intricate to be here presented in conformity with the limits and the purpose of this article. When, however, weakness of the vascular wall exists, either as a cause or as a consequence of atheroma, "that lesion will be liable to manifest itself in other lesions, both of the intima and of the other coats. A weakened vessel, liable to be stretched beyond its powers of resistance, is apt to undergo partial tears and ruptures of its fibres. This is much more likely in the aorta, where the thickness of the wall is much less in comparison with the calibre, than in the other vessels. . . . An aorta subjected to the stress of a hypertrophied left ventricle, *or exposed to the frequent rises of blood-pressure incident to a strenuous occupation*, is likely to have small injuries to its coats which will lead to inflammatory manifestations in numerous small local centres. These phenomena in the middle and external coats are much less manifest in the smaller vessels" (pp. 100,

101). "The intrusion of the (atheromatous) patch has a most important influence on the middle coat, especially where the thickening is abrupt. It causes, in some cases, rupture of the fibres of that coat, and consequent gaps in the continuity of its proper tissue.. The effect does not limit itself to the media, but is liable to extend to the adventitia. A solid body continually protruded against the wall will have results extending through the wall. These local injuries have an important influence in the causation of aneurysm" (p. 102).

It is not, however, the opinion of the authors that atheroma, or *endarteritis nodosa*, necessarily leads on to any or all of the above results. The thickening which is the primary result of endarteritis may, indeed, in some cases and in some degrees, like the callus of a broken bone, or the fibroid investment of an abscess, be a strengthening, locally and temporarily, of the vascular wall; and this not in the intima only, but also in the other coats. In this instance, as in most others revealed to us by pathology, restorative or compensatory processes go hand in hand with destructive. "In elderly persons the compensation so provided is usually sufficient, but in those who are subjected to severe bodily exertion the case is different. Atheroma and consecutive arteritis are in them pre-eminently defensive processes. It is the weak point in this line of defence which is liable to become the starting-point of an aneurysm" (p. 109). Further, the influence of an emaciating disease, or of an acute disease attended with much constitutional suffering, "may lead to degenerative changes in the media, and may, presumably, render it more liable to atrophy (p. 112). . . . In cases of recovery from severe illness, should the heart be restored to full vigour before the arteries have completely recovered, there may be the opportunity given for the formation of an aneurysm" (p. 115). These propositions are supported by cases examined with great care, to which it is impossible to allude further here.

Finally, the question of syphilis as a cause of arterial disease, and especially of aneurysm of the aorta, must have a few words, although it is not especially insisted on in the very interesting memoir from which I have just quoted. It cannot be regarded as improbable that syphilis should be among the many causes of diminished resistance in the walls of arteries, if we consider it merely as a constitutional disease, influencing almost every organ and tissue in the body, and often leading up to the very circumstances suggested in the preceding paragraph. We know, moreover, from the researches of Allbutt, Heubner, and many others, that in the smaller vessels, especially of the brain, syphilis plays an important part in degenerative changes, which, however, are rather obstructive than aneurysmal. It is not, therefore, antecedently improbable that syphilis, occurring as it does coincidently with the very period of life at which aneurysm chiefly prevails, may rank among its causes, as has often been affirmed, without, perhaps, anything like adequate evidence. Dr. Sansom (75), whose important monograph on the Diseases of the Heart and Blood-vessels has been already referred to, has "observed many cases of aortic aneurysm in which the origin from syphilitic disease of the aorta has been evident." He cites Karl Malmsten of Stockholm as affirming that "in about 80 per cent of the cases collated by himself the existence of syphilis was definitely made out." The latest, and perhaps the most extreme supporter of this view is Professor Drummond of Newcastle (22), who has " found it a good practical rule *not* to diagnose aneurysm, in a doubtful case, in the absence of syphilis." The basis for this rather astonishing doctrine is the further statement that, in the course of observation in a locality where aneurysms are extremely frequent among the labouring population, in an inquiry pursued with special care, and carried on with a view to this point "for many years," he had been led to remark that " no ·indisputable case has come under my notice in which specific disease was awanting, except two or three examples of that interesting condition, acute softening of the arterial wall with aneurysmal bulgings, in malignant endocarditis." Arterial strain through hard work, though admitted as an etiological factor, is by Dr. Drummond relegated to an entirely secondary position, requiring, in the vast majority of instances, to be multiplied by specific arteritis, in order that the product be aneurysm ; and then it is the lesser quantity of the two." [1]

Symptoms ; physical signs ; diagnosis.—There are at least three distinct lines on which the diagnosis of an aneurysm of the aorta may be approached ; and the relative importance and significance of these varies so much in different cases, that it is highly expedient, and even necessary, to give due consideration to each of them in each individual case. For while a pulsating tumour may be as evident a fact to the eye, ear, and touch, as any physical fact can be, and while the diagnosis may thus be as free from difficulty in the case of the aorta as in that of any external artery, it is also true that in many cases it is not so, and that the discovery and recognition of an aortic aneurysm may be one of the most interesting, and also one of the most obscure problems of medical diagnosis. There is reason to think that even the majority of aneurysms are absolutely latent in their early stages. From the first slight pouchings of the endarterium and middle coat to the growth of a tumour which, by its pressure upon important parts, gives rise to very manifest symptoms, or even threatens life directly and obviously from moment to moment, is a progress which may be so gradual and insidious as to excite no attention until the tumour is already patent to eye and hand ; and cannot fail to reveal itself, even to the patient. It is far from uncommon, indeed, for patients to come to the physician on their discovery of an abnormal pulsation somewhere ; and, in the case of the abdominal aorta, at least, such abnormal pulsation, in nine cases out of ten, is not aneurysmal. On the other hand, it is far from uncommon for patient and physician to be utterly misled by the early symptoms when they occur — the more obvious phenomena being dignified with some con-

---

[1] It might perhaps be desirable to inquire, in reference to the statement given above, in what class of cases, being adults and mostly hospital patients, it would be regarded, according to the author, as "indisputable" that "specific disease was awanting." The address itself throws no light upon this.

ventional name that both misses and masks the true diagnosis. It is not too much to say that " neuralgia," " rheumatism," " pleurisy," " pleurodynia," or, in the case of the abdomen, " colic," have diverted attention from many an aortic aneurysm: I have known such cases treated for months under such designations without misgiving, until the appalling nature of the real disease was suddenly revealed by some nearly fatal accident—by the discovery of a pulsating tumour near the surface, or by some new and ominous combination of symptoms. To give only one instance : a physician of some distinction, and of repute in physical diagnosis (now long since dead), was attending an elderly nobleman for what seemed to be a gouty attack associated with " pleurisy." The treatment was apparently successful ; the disease was yielding, the visits became less frequent, and the patient seemed convalescent. The physician, who lived many miles away, took his leave with some such flattering words on his lips. Hardly had he got well on his way homewards when he was recalled to find the patient suddenly dead from profuse hæmoptysis. A small *aneurysm* of the descending aorta had been pressing upon the left bronchus, and had opened into it with immediately fatal effect. It is not intended by this striking instance to throw blame on any one, but it is only too obvious how much misunderstanding might arise out of such a mistake in diagnosis, followed speedily by so tragic an issue. In the interest, therefore, alike of the patient and of the physician, the *early diagnosis of aneurysm* is a point of medical discipline towards which all the faculties of the mind, trained by observation and reflection, ought to be bent. And by the early diagnosis I mean a suspicion or inferential diagnosis, formed perhaps long before the facts either of physical or of general diagnosis are such as to justify expression. Thus we may be saved at least from committing ourselves to a purely conventional and erroneous opinion of the kind above illustrated. I was once summoned by a gentleman well known to me, and whom I had occasionally advised in illness, to the bedside of an eminent man of business in Edinburgh. The case was represented as urgent, the messenger was his brother ; the aid of the family medical attendant, an old and much-respected practitioner, was unobtainable at the time, but he concurred in the application to me. Now another and younger brother of this patient had been for a considerable time under my own care for an unquestionable aortic aneurysm. In the case now before us no such diagnosis or suspicion had arisen ; but the man proved to be exceedingly ill, and in very great pain and suffering, which he had been relieving by large inhalations from a bottle of chloroform secreted under his pillow. The tell-tale fact in this instance was a peculiarity of the pupil of the eye, which will be referred to hereafter. The diagnosis was at once forced by the inquiry, " Is it a case like my brother's ?"— to which the only possible reply was, " Yes, I think so." The death of the patient within twenty-four hours led to an autopsy, at which this diagnosis was fully confirmed : an aneurysm of the aorta, pressing upon and eroding several of the bodies of the vertebræ, was so placed as to compromise the cilio-spinal branches of the sympathetic nerve ; and this (a unique fact in my experience) on both sides.[1]

Now, in the early diagnosis of aortic aneurysm, all the three lines of investigation above referred to may come into play in various degrees ; and their relative importance may vary almost indefinitely with the circumstances of the case. There may be (i.) the *etiological factor* in diagnosis, involving questions of predisposition ; (ii.) the *symptomatic factor*, founded on the active manifestations of illness ; (iii.) *the factor of physical diagnosis* proper, or the objective phenomena indicating tumour ; in which may be included not only the discovery of it as a fact, but also a positive or an inferential diagnosis of its precise position, its interference with adjoining structures, its approximate size and rate of progress, and the probabilities of its future course.

I. *Etiological diagnosis.*—It is not suggested, by placing this first in order, that this line of investigation is either the most important or the most likely to lead to an early recognition of an aortic aneurysm. But, if it be true that the very earliest stages of most internal aneurysms are without appreciable symptoms or physical signs—and it would be hard to deny this in view of what pathology teaches—then it follows that, in a corresponding proportion of cases, the only key to a right diagnosis must be by such etiological presumption. The age, sex, and habit of the patient, the circumstances of his daily life and occupation, the evidence of strain or of more or less serious accident, such as might lead to aneurysm, will all come into consideration, and will have their due weight. To think thus, habitually and almost instinctively, without overdoing it, remembering always that aneurysm of the aorta is relatively rare—this is, perhaps, the high-water mark of a physician's skill in diagnosis. The preceding investigation of the causes of aneurysms in general will, it is hoped, prove serviceable in placing the whole etiological argument in a right point of view, apart from particular cases.

It is commonly said that "a man is just as old as his arteries" ; and this medical saw is peculiarly appropriate and very cogent in its application to the present subject, and to the very period of life at which (as we have seen) the tendency to the formation of an aneurysm may be said especially to prevail. Whether we are to consider over-exertion and strain as the primary causes, or only as the incidents of an "aneurysmal diathesis," it remains true that an atheromatous or other allied condition of the arterial system, if it can be ascertained to exist in the arteries most accessible to observation, may be taken in many cases as the index to that liability. Whatever fallacies may underlie the general presumption that the *arcus senilis* of the cornea implies fatty degeneration elsewhere, or that the usual physiognomical signs of advancing age,—the first gray hairs, or the crow's feet at the corners of the eyes,—carry the presumption of other and more serious internal changes, there needs be no hesitation in affirming that *premature senility* in the arterial system generally carries

---

[1] This case is noticed in connection with that of the brother above referred to in the writer's *Clinical Medicine*, 1862, p. 558.

with it a farther presumption [1] of such changes in the aorta as may dispose it to yield to the immediate causes of aneurysm, and to pouching of its internal and middle coats, with the consequences above referred to. Of course it does not necessarily follow that senile changes in the aorta, or any other artery, must lead to such pouching; and in point of fact it is comparatively rarely that this result occurs in the gradual and simultaneous evolution of the degenerative changes of advancing age. It has been already remarked that *endarteritis deformans* tends in some cases, and in an imperfect way (though always with loss of elasticity), even to strengthen the arterial coats against the initiation of some kinds of aneurysmal lesions. At all events it is chiefly, if not exclusively, when the exciting causes of aneurysm (which are also those of rupture of the coats as above described) are brought into operation, through irregular or abnormal forms of activity, that the relative loss of resistance at some points of an atheromatous vessel exposes it to a more considerable risk of either gradual or sudden yielding to internal pressure, especially if unequally distributed. Now, it is a well-known fact, admirably illustrated in the experience of an iron-master quoted in the paper above referred to, that the merely physical energy of workmen engaged in very strenuous occupations diminishes rapidly after the age of fifty. "Iron-workers, as a rule, are able to hold on to severe work up to about fifty; a few five years longer, but more under fifty than over it. About this time of life they perspire more, the action of the heart seems to fail them, and very soon they have to give place to younger men" (18, p. 27). This is quite in accordance with average or every-day experience. The young man brings his newly-found vigour and physical energy into whatever he has to do, and does it with almost an exuberance of will, and sometimes to his own detriment. If, however, he be sound in body, and sufficiently strong for his work, he learns in most instances to keep within the measure of his ability, and no harm results, even from a very strenuous occupation. The middle-aged or ageing man has learned this lesson even more thoroughly, and has probably also, if skilful and well conducted, risen above the necessity of the severest kinds of labour. When age approaches, therefore, he is prepared to meet it by reducing considerably the tax upon his bodily energies; and as (according to the proverb) a man is "a fool or his own physician at forty," so it may be argued that at fifty most men, by a sure instinct, will have effected a compromise of some kind between their physical powers and their real or fancied necessities. The labourer becomes a foreman, or takes to some kind of less exacting labour, even at a sacrifice of wages; or skill and

---

[1] Professor Coats, from purely pathological data, arrives at the conclusion that atheroma is much more frequent in the aorta, and especially in the arch, than in any of the other arteries with the exception, perhaps, of the coronary and the cerebral vessels; diminishing in frequency, on the whole (with these exceptions) from the larger to the smaller arteries. There may be "advanced atheroma in one set of arteries, with very little in the system generally." On the other hand, atheroma may be "very widespread throughout the body, affecting at intervals almost all the arteries, down to those of comparatively small calibre."—Coats and Auld, (18) pp. 4, 5.

good fortune come into play, and enable the man to secure some of those advantages which come with age and experience. In some occupations, however, the life is very hard, and the chances of such promotion very slight. The dock porter, or the wielder of the heavy hammer, is too often debarred from all the chances that happen to most men of improving his condition—all the more if his habits and his apparent necessities are such as to make him the slave of his work. He must work on till he drops—and he does work on till he drops. It is in such cases that premature senility most readily asserts itself, in the arteries as elsewhere. Such a man may be as old at forty as another man at sixty. Atheroma, among other changes, readily obtains a hold, and still more readily leads up to those further changes in the vessels which have been already insisted on as the beginnings of aneurysm. And this usually comes precisely at the age when the period of a possibly premature invasion of atheroma is over-lapped (as was formerly said) by the age of the greatest bodily vigour, and therefore of continued and strenuous exertion; that is, from thirty or thirty-five to forty-five or fifty years of age.

All these circumstances have to be considered in every case where even the slightest suspicion of incipient aneurysmal disease arises. During youth and adolescence, and in the earlier years of manhood or woman-hood (especially in women), an aneurysm of the aorta is so rare that its occurrence might take even the most experienced and wary of physicians by surprise. But it ought not to be so when the age, the occupation, the evidence — perhaps spontaneously given or perhaps elicited by questions—of particular strains or injuries combine with the physical demonstration of atheroma in the more accessible parts of the arterial system. In such cases it is necessary to assume that (as it is put by Dr. Coats in the paper referred to), "where atheroma exists, it is usually present in the aorta"; and whether a diagnosis of aneurysm is to be founded on this or not, a proclivity to the disease at anyrate is established.

For many years, and long before the introduction of the sphygmo-graph into the methods of physical diagnosis, I have been in the habit of directing the attention of students to the importance of a general survey of the arterial system in respect of the visible and tangible evidences of atheroma. The ordinary, and indeed universal practice of feeling and numbering the pulse at the wrist, although derived from the most remote antiquity, and the subject of numberless learned and special dis-sertations from the times of Galen and Rufus the Ephesian onwards, is too often taught and practised in a perfunctory and thoroughly inadequate fashion. Not a single treatise (I believe) before the present century, or indeed before even its last half or quarter, ever alludes to more than what can be gained by placing one or two fingers in a stationary posi-tion upon one or two points of the vessel, as has been the tradition of physicians in all ages. The proper way of feeling the pulse, however, even as a general rule (and here the living finger has an immense advantage over the sphygmograph), is to cause the finger to travel up and down the artery, taking careful note of the physical condition of this very familiar but often imperfectly explored vessel, its normal or undue resistance at different points, its straight or tortuous course, and the presence or absence of irregularities, varying in degree from slight apparent thickenings here and there, up to calcareous changes occupying the whole circumference and a more or less considerable longitudinal range. When this has been accomplished in the radial artery (which can be easily done without exciting undue attention), the presence or absence of results may lead to an extension of the survey to other arteries ; and, as a rule, should always do so when there is the remotest suspicion of atheroma. The temporal arteries are always within sight and touch ; but information of a valuable kind may often be got by extending the inquiry from the radials on both sides to the brachial and axillary arteries, which, if tortuous and hardened at points, give almost conclusive evidence of the state of the arterial system, and therefore probably of the aorta. Similar evidence is often given by the arteries of the thyroid axis, the *transversalis colli* and *humeri*, which lie in a very superficial position easily to be reached by the exploring finger without arousing anxious suspicions in the mind of the patient. The arteries of the lower extremities may afford still more valuable revelations, and it is often easy to include them in the survey, especially the iliacs and femorals ; but they do not come quite so naturally within the scope of an examination conducted on the above lines, and are therefore more apt to be omitted, in women, or under other circumstances of reserve arising in the pursuit of diagnostic indications. The abdominal aorta, in spare persons with non-resistant abdominal walls, is quite within the range of easy examination ; and a physician is hardly excusable if he neglects habitually, even in the most ordinary cases, a mode of investigation so easily applied. In the practice of many insurance offices a specific statement as to the state of the arteries is rightly insisted on ; and it is to be hoped, therefore, that the early diagnosis of aneurysm, and of any predisposition thereto, may profit by the habit of investigation thus cultivated.

The sphygmograph, and other instrumental aids to diagnosis, may sometimes afford suggestions or premonition of aneurysm, founded on the diagnosis of premature senility of the arteries. But the great variety and often essential differences in the pulse-tracings of atheroma and arterio-sclerosis show that very little secure assistance can be obtained in this way in early and doubtful cases. The typical pulse of high arterial pressure and of rigid arteries, with its somewhat retarded upstroke and broad summit level, on which the tidal wave is grafted, as it were, occasionally even before reaching the summit, while the descending line shows sometimes but little dicrotism, sometimes a dicrotic wave high in the line of descent, is assuredly not to be relied upon ; it occurs under many circumstances where no reasonable suspicion of aneurysm can arise. When indeed the instrument is applied to a rigid part of the vessel, it will usually demonstrate the fact by the increased pressure required to bring out the maximum of pulsation, and the difficulty of obliterating the pulse by still increased pressure; but these facts are also easily ascertained by the finger, together with much that is more instructive. Dr. George Oliver, however, has recently invented instruments called by him the *arteriometer* and the *high-pressure gauge*. The former, by registering on an index the distance traversed between the very slightest pressure which will procure an impulse at all, to the degree which completely obliterates the impulse, is intended to determine the calibre of the artery examined under different circumstances. Dr. Oliver finds that in health the calibre of the arteries is constantly varying, within physiological limits, especially according to posture; the variations following a definite law or order. These physiological variations are much restricted, of course, when the coats of the artery are rigid or inflexible from disease. "Another valuable piece of evidence, as shown by the instrument, is a persistent reduction of the normal calibre of the artery. Under normal conditions the maximum calibre of the radial artery in man varies from 2 to 2·5 mm., and in women from 1·8 to 2·3 mm. Organic reduction of this calibre is met with in arteriosclerosis, in syphilis, and in chronic gout. The conjunction of invariability of calibre in various postures, and reduction of calibre below the normal, is important evidence of a lasting morbid condition which leads strongly to the diagnosis of the diseases mentioned" (Sansom, 75, p. 537). Further evidence, however, is required of the suitability of these methods.

II. *Symptomatic diagnosis.*—It has not been possible to exclude this branch of the diagnosis of aneurysm of the aorta from what has been said already, because symptoms may be said, in one sense or another, to be concerned in, if not to occupy, the whole field of the manifestations of every disease. The importance of this part of the inquiry, however, especially in the case of the early symptoms—those which may occur considerably in advance of the facts cognisable by physical diagnosis—is so great that a special heading devoted to this point seems alike necessary and expedient from the strictly practical point of view. Aneurysm of the aorta, in many or in most cases latent as regards its beginnings, comes into the ken of the medical observer only through facts or symptoms which, in the first instance, are communicated to him by the patient, and on which the skilled physician founds a tentative diagnosis (or it may be only a guess) as a guide for further inquiries. And in this case the importance of happy guessing (as the late Dr. John Brown called it, following an Aristotelian precedent) is such that it often constitutes the only effective suggestion for a matured diagnosis, if it cannot really be raised to a higher rank. At all events it will not be disputed that the physician who uses suggestions of this kind to good effect, but at the same time without too confidently yielding to first impressions, is in a much more favourable position than one who allows himself to be misled by merely conventional phrases, as indicated in a previous part of this article.

1. *Pain* is a feature of aneurysmal disease which, though it may be sometimes wanting, and, when present, indefinitely various in character and in degree, ought always to put the physician on his guard. In the majority of cases of abdominal aneurysm, and in not a few of thoracic, pain is the first, the most notable, and often the most enduring symptom of the whole group. Nothing, however, can be more variable in different cases than the character and the continuity of the pain. In some it is comparatively slight, accidental, and easily yielding to treatment; in others, it is the predominating feature in the case, and the persistence and severity of it appear more than any other to threaten the life and disturb the comfort and nightly rest of the patient. It has been noticed, moreover, by observers that aneurysmal pain is apparently of two distinct kinds: the one acute, paroxysmal, subject to great remissions and exacerbations; the other, more or less constant, dull and gnawing, and more accurately localised, thus corresponding in all probability with erosion of the osseous structures (mainly the bodies of the vertebræ or the sternum) with which the aneurysm may be in contact. The former kind of pain is attributed to pressure on sensory nerves; the latter, to destructive action of the extending tumour upon more solid and fixed parts, especially, as stated, the bones. It is not quite certain that these two kinds of pain can always be distinguished and referred to their respective sources quite accurately; but it is necessary to have both of them in view in investigating a supposed aneurysm. Paroxysmal pain is, undoubtedly, a most suggestive fact, even when its locality and its attributes fail to point to particular nerves. We have seen that in some dissecting aneurysms, even without tumour properly so called, the rending or otherwise yielding of the coats of the vessel was accompanied by severe pain; which afterwards became much less, and at the moment of the fatal crisis may even have been entirely absent. It is therefore antecedently probable that, in a certain proportion of those cases at least in which the progress of an aneurysm of the aorta (otherwise latent) has been initiated or accelerated by strain, initial pain of this kind, the character and situation of which will be determined by the position of the tumour, will be reported. The pain, however, is sometimes so involved in the history of a local injury that, unless supported by other facts, it will almost certainly be set down to some other cause. It is in cases of this kind that the etiological diagnosis, already adverted to, comes into prominence as affording, not indeed the assurance of aneurysm, but the most suggestive hints towards a secure diagnosis. The slater already referred to (p. 354) might very easily have been suspected of something more than "lumbago," had it been established that at the time of his accidental strain he was the subject of a highly atheromatous condition of the arterial system.

In thoracic aneurysms the pains are apt not only to affect the precordial region, or to spring from it, but to extend sharply or indefinitely into the neck; and even into the face, the shoulders, and down one or both arms. The late Dr. Ross of Manchester (73, p. 604) regarded these peripheral (that is, not obviously visceral) pains as due to irritation "conducted to the portion of the spinal cord from which the viscus derived its splanchnic nerve, and thence spread in the gray matter of the posterior horns, whence by the law of eccentric projection it was referred to the termination of the somatic nerves derived from the segment of the cord." This, in the case of the heart, would mean especially the first and second dorsal segments; for Mackenzie and Head have since affirmed (55) that in aortic disease the pain is referred along the first, second, third, and fourth dorsal areas; while in angina pectoris it may even extend as low as the ninth dorsal, and is always accompanied by pain in certain cervical areas also. In some instances these peripheral pains may obscure the more centric pains, or seem even to inhibit them; so that the latter are apt to escape attention. I myself (31, p. 37) have particularly referred to one such case of very long duration, with (in the end) very manifest evidences of erosion of the bones, in which "there had been pains shooting down both arms to the finger-tips and round the body at the level of the armpits, more or less constantly for eleven years, and this almost apart from any symptoms that could be noted as cardiac or respiratory during that lengthened period." In not a few instances in which the diagnosis from other facts is well established, aneurysm of the arch of the aorta leads to symptoms closely resembling typical angina pectoris; and, as in angina pectoris proper, the pain and numbness of the left arm are sometimes such as to obscure the precordial sensation. In other instances, pain quite definitely referred to the heart may precede the overt diagnosis of aneurysm by so long a period as to raise a doubt whether it has really had such origin;[1] although the signs of the disease as actually existing are unmistakable. Again, there may be very little complaint of cardiac pain, but only of pains evidently due to the eroding action and pressure of the tumour upon bones and nerve-trunks; or there may be but little localised pain of the latter kind, or even in some cases no pain at all, even where the tumour is seen and felt to have made its way through the sternum. The varieties of pain are indeed incalculable; and yet its suggestiveness as a symptom can never be overlooked in any case, or at least ought not to be. Dr. Walshe (85, p. 488) remarks that in thoracic aneurysm pain is the chief factor in inducing emaciation, by no means a constant fact in aneurysmal cases. "From the analysis of seventeen cases of aneurysm of the arch," he writes, "the inference clearly flows, that the presence or absence of pain of serious character is the real element in determining or warding off early emaciation."

In abdominal aneurysms the significance and real importance of pain

---

[1] *International Clinics, loc. cit.* p. 36. The first alarm of disease in the case here referred to arose from pain reputed as cardiac sixteen years before the patient was admitted to hospital with an evident aneurysm of the arch, projecting in the jugular fossa, and attended at the time of admission by *intermittent* pain, very distinctly cardiac in character and situation. This pain, together with some irregularities in the action of the heart, were apparently the chief early symptoms of the disease, and had led to his being advised, sixteen years before, to give up his occupation (a stonemason).

as a symptom is even greater than in thoracic; and this remark applies with peculiar force to those tumours of the upper part of the abdominal aorta, sometimes involving its branches also, which originate immediately below or between the crura of the diaphragm. In such cases pain, of a peculiarly intense and wearing character, is rarely absent; and, by the unrest and the emaciation which attend it, often conduces largely to the exhaustion and death of the patient. All observers have concurred in this opinion; though perhaps attention was first drawn to the fact by a classical case recorded in great detail by Dr. Beatty, and in subsequent communications by Dr. Law. The latter writer attributes to Dr. Beatty not only priority, but claims for him also that he gave a new impulse to the diagnosis of aneurysm, which Andral had fully acknowledged by copying the details of Dr. Beatty's case into an edition of Laennec's work. The twofold character of the pain, partly more enduring and partly paroxysmal, is fully discussed; the latter being likened to the pain in lead colic. *Mutatis mutandis*, this description will apply to aneurysmal pains generally, whether in the thorax or the abdomen; but in the latter it is to be remarked that the character of the physical diagnosis, often excessively obscure, gives to the pains a pre-eminent, almost a paramount importance.

A very remarkable, perhaps almost an unique instance of the *absence of pain* during a considerable part of the history and progress of an abdominal aneurysm of large size, and easily verified by physical signs, is recorded in *International Clinics* (31, p. 37 *et seq.*) During many months of close observation and treatment, this patient (Jas. G. æt. 52, miner) could scarcely be brought to admit the existence of any pain, or indeed any inconvenience at all, from a large and expansive tumour which was adjudged, indeed, to be in process of healing, but which seemed to have been of very slow growth; the early symptoms (including the pain) having been all attributed to "the stomach." In this case, however, the aneurysm occupied the lower section of the abdominal aorta, where the nervous implications are, of course, much less intricate than in the upper parts.

Both in thoracic and abdominal aneurysms, in which pain predominates, and in which the diagnosis may be otherwise obscure, a. kind of therapeutic test may be applied with probable advantage. It is in these cases that iodide of potassium is not only, as a rule, well borne in large doses, but, in conjunction with general measures to be afterwards discussed, exercises the most striking and sometimes the most immediate relief as regards the pain. Ninety grains or more in the twenty-four hours can sometimes be tolerated for months together; not only without iodism or any other ill results, but with the most clear conviction on the part of the patient that he owes his exemption from severe symptoms mainly to the remedy. It is not, perhaps, quite certain that such a result can occur only in aneurysm; but, so far as my observation extends, it is in aneurysmal cases chiefly that so striking and so convincing a therapeutic success, as regards this single symptom, has been achieved.

On the whole, and as the final summary of this part of the symptomatic diagnosis, the following sentence from the paper above referred
to (p. 35) may be taken as embodying briefly my own views as
addressed to clinical students :—"It is a good practical rule, that whenever you encounter in your experience a case of obstinate or frequently
recurring pain, such as might, constructively, be due to pressure upon
nerves or upon solid parts, and such as is not fairly in accordance with
some disease known to exist in the organs of the thorax or abdomen,
the suspicion, at least, of an aneurysm ought in all cases to arise."

2. *Cardiac collapse, syncope, palpitation, etc.*—In a very considerable
proportion of aortic aneurysms, as we have seen above, the heart remains
unaffected both as to structure and function ; and this even when the
tumour may be of very large size. Indeed, except in so far as the heart
participates in the etiological derangements of function which go to make up
the complex of the antecedents, there is no good evidence, strictly speaking,
that cardiac symptoms are more characteristic of aneurysm than of any
other disease not appertaining to the thorax in the first instance. In
abdominal aneurysms, in particular, cardiac symptoms are quite exceptional, and usually point to separate and independent disease of the
heart itself. But when the first part of the arch is concerned, so that
either the aortic valvular structures are implicated, or the coronary
arteries are the seat of coincident disease, every kind of cardiac symptom
characteristic of these states may also concur with, and in some cases
may be apparently even the first evidences of an aneurysm which at
a later period becomes evident to physical diagnosis, or is only revealed
after death ; which is in such cases not rarely sudden. Indeed there is
little to distinguish some cases of aneurysm of this kind from cases
of fatal angina pectoris commonly so called, and not of aneurysmal
origin. In one of my own cases (31) a distinctly cardiac diagnosis had
been formulated on medical grounds so long as sixteen years before ;
and yet, although the symptoms had always remained (when present)
definitely cardiac in character, they yielded so completely at this late date
to hospital treatment as to become absolutely quiescent while the case remained under observation. In a few cases, however, cardiac failure or
irregularity of action, syncope, or the very peculiar and indescribable sense
of impending death which enters so largely into the conception of angina
pectoris, may (even without a corresponding degree of pain) appear to be
among the earliest symptoms of aneurysm ; yet this is exceptional, and
very probably indicates not only a sac arising very close to the heart
(and therefore likely to burst into the pericardium), but also a more or less
sudden rupture of the coats, as in dissecting aneurysms ; an event very well
illustrated in the case of the accident during hunting above referred to
(p. 357). It seems reasonable to infer that in cases pathologically similar
to this, even when not obviously connected with a particular injury or
shock, failure of cardiac action in some of its manifestations may be the
first symptom of the giving way of the internal and middle coats ; unless
it be too slowly and gradually effected to give rise to symptoms at all.

3. *Respiratory symptoms; cough, dyspnœa, laryngeal phenomena.*—The symptoms in this group are much more complex, and more important in the diagnosis of aneurysm, than those in the preceding group; but they are also more involved in the physical diagnosis proper, which will be treated of farther on. At present we are chiefly concerned with those which rank among the early symptoms, or give the first warnings of aneurysmal disease.

Amongst all these early respiratory symptoms *cough* is perhaps one of the most frequent and easily appreciable, if not the most distinctive. It is true that cough, in itself, as a mere clinical fact and apart from its special characters, is not only one of the commonest, but also one of the least significant of symptoms—significant only of a certain amount of irritation, however produced, communicated to the afferent nerves of the respiratory tract. And yet cough is · sometimes so distinctive of aneurysm of the aortic arch, that a fair and reasonable guess, if not a diagnosis, might proceed upon this symptom alone; as will appear when this subject is more particularly discussed farther on. A phenomenon of this degree of importance requires, however, careful discrimination; and a diagnosis thus made is not by any means to be taken as mere cleverness, or an example of lucky guessing, but as a deliberate recognition of physiological facts and principles which, in not a few instances as I shall show, may lead up to a secure and well-founded inferential diagnosis.

One distinguishing peculiarity (though by no means the most distinctive) of all or almost all respiratory symptoms in aneurysm runs on lines parallel to that of the pain. The most characteristic respiratory disturbances in aortic aneurysm arise from the pressure of the expanding sac, not so much on solid organs or bony structures as on nerves. Hence the *paroxysmal* character. of these symptoms—a fact noted, as regards aneurysmal disease, ever since the time of Morgagni. A cough out of all proportion to the apparent catarrh, or expectoration; a dyspnœa which is at one moment extreme, and very shortly thereafter much relieved, or absent, may reasonably suggest aneurysm; and, if accompanied at times by pains of the character described above, may almost constitute a diagnosis. But this conclusion will follow with yet greater probability if the cough and the dyspnœa be laryngeal in type; that is, so marked and so characterised as to suggest either spasm or paralysis of the muscles whose special function it is to open or to close the glottis.

The reasonable basis of evidence, which leads to the statement just made, lies in the knowledge of the fact, revealed by pathological anatomy, that many aneurysms of the arch are so placed as to involve, and sometimes to implicate destructively, the recurrent laryngeal nerve [1] on one or the other side (usually the left); and of the corresponding facts,

---

[1] Legallois, and after him Dr. John Reid (professor in St. Andrews) (70), were the first to determine experimentally the significance of cases of this kind, the clinical and pathological records of which can be traced back to Morgagni, and even earlier. Dr. Todd (79) was probably the first to detect atrophy of the laryngeal muscles on the side on which the recurrent nerve had undergone compression. Other references are given in the present writer's *Clinical Medicine*, 1862, p. 461.

that in some of these cases the laryngeal muscles suffer atrophy on one side, while in others, even without apparent atrophy, the laryngoscope shows an unilateral lesion of function in these muscles. Leaving the latter method of investigation out of consideration for the present, it may be affirmed that long before the laryngoscope was brought into use these facts had been well ascertained; and the diagnosis of aneurysm as emerging from the presence of laryngeal symptoms with an unaltered laryngeal mucous membrane was fairly well understood. To ascertain, as far as possible, this last and most important negative fact, I lay hold of the tongue and draw it forward; then I introduce the finger of the right hand at the left corner of the patient's mouth, thus gaining the advantage of proximity to the point to be investigated; then I push the finger rapidly over the epiglottis, and hook this back, as it were, on the finger until the finger-tip has been guided down to the arytenoid cartilages, and made to travel all over the adjacent mucous membrane as far as it can reach, so as to detect, if possible, any abnormal thickening or roughness such as to betray an inflammatory or ulcerative lesion.[1] There is no real difficulty in this exploration when the method of it has once been practically learned; and, although it has been reduced in importance by the beautiful mechanism of the laryngeal mirror, it ought still to remain available for cases of urgency, when perhaps laryngoscopy may be out of the question. The practical conclusion to be thus arrived at (and confirmed if possible by laryngoscopy) is that, when the laryngeal mucous membrane is intact, symptoms at all resembling those of laryngeal disease are almost sure to arise from intrathoracic tumour, often otherwise impossible of detection, pressing upon one or other of the laryngeal nerves (usually the left recurrent), and sometimes implicating also the vagus; the great majority of such tumours, again, being aneurysms of the arch, or in some cases (but more rarely) of the innominate and right subclavian arteries.

The cases which, in general practice, may thus superficially most resemble or be confounded with aneurysms interfering with laryngeal innervation, will be mostly such as in prelaryngoscopic days would have been named chronic or acute laryngitis; including a great number and variety of ulcerative or other lesions arising from tubercle, syphilis, and in some cases mere inflammation or malignant growths within the larynx. The diagnosis of these cases has, of course, been so much facilitated, and rendered more precise by the use of the laryngoscope, that the following remarks must be taken as merely applying to the first suspicions or provisional diagnosis of disease of this kind; which, how-

---

[1] The method here referred to was adopted before the first visit of Czermak to this country had revealed to me the value and importance of laryngeal examination as applied to such cases; one of which, read to the Medico-Chirurgical Society of Edinburgh on 18th June, 1857, had attracted much attention owing to the difficulties of the diagnosis, and the performance of tracheotomy to relieve suffocation. In the course of Czermak's visit to Edinburgh (being the first occasion, I believe, when the use of instrumental laryngeal diagnosis was publicly set forth in Scotland) I was able to submit to him a test case, in which the eminent inventor of the laryngoscope demonstrated the immobility of the muscles on one side of the glottis.

ever, are often of extreme importance, both as regards the immediate relief of the patient and the credit of the physician. To mistake an intrathoracic tumour for laryngitis, or the spasm that attends such disease for croup or other disease directly implicating the glottis in structural change, is an error that has probably occurred much more frequently than it has been recorded, and which may now be regarded as virtually impossible, when time is given for a full and complete estimate of the facts.

(a) The most dangerous of all the symptoms thus occurring is sudden and *paroxysmal dyspnœa, attended by stridor,* sometimes with the inspiration only, at other times with both inspiration and expiration; but most commonly with the former. Such attacks are often present when the cause of them is quite manifest, such as a pulsating tumour either presenting itself externally, or easily recognised by the most superficial examination. But it not infrequently happens also that such an attack of dyspnœa is the very first indication, either to the patient or to any one else, of disease involving danger, or otherwise differing in character from current ailments. To arrive at a just conclusion under such circumstances is obviously of the highest importance; and justifies us in placing this symptom in the front rank among the early indications of aneurysm of the aorta.[1] The dyspnœa is sometimes so extreme, moreover, that no laryngoscopic or other examination in detail can be attempted at first; and the presumptive diagnosis must be based only upon the manifest facts considered in urgency, and with a view to prognosis and treatment. When, however, a laryngoscopic examination, and other means of careful physical diagnosis, can be brought deliberately to bear on the problem, the difficulties will be found in most cases to disappear. In particular it may be confidently affirmed that *unilateral paralysis or inaction of the glottic muscles* (often maintaining what is called the "cadaveric position"), in the absence of visible lesion otherwise, is an almost conclusive sign of thoracic tumour, aneurysmal or other, implicating the laryngeal nerves.

The peculiar importance of laryngeal stridor with dyspnœa is not merely diagnostic. For when this symptom is once ascertained to be present in a well-marked form, it may also be said largely to govern the prognosis. In not a few cases the paroxysmal increase of this symptom induces fatal or nearly fatal consequences at a period when no other facts reveal the presence of organic disease; and when also, from the small size and deep situation of the aneurysm, physical signs proper may be entirely wanting. It has already been remarked that tracheotomy has repeatedly been performed under such circumstances (but usually with very unsatisfactory results) for the relief of the more obvious symptoms.

---

[1] *Clin. Med.,* Cases I. II. and III. in the chapter on Aneurysm are specially referred to as illustrating the difficulties experienced (in the absence of laryngoscopy, however) in arriving at a true diagnosis in some cases of this kind. See also (22), where the diagnosis, although correctly made (here also apart from laryngoscopy), involved the eminent physician concerned in a most vexatious lawsuit; thus strongly confirming the remarks made above.

(*b*) Next in importance to laryngeal dyspnœa with stridor may be placed *cough with some peculiarity of intonation or character* to distinguish it from the almost infinite varieties of symptomatic cough attending the progress of acute or chronic pulmonary disease. Here, as in previous instances, it may be merely a greatly exaggerated and highly paroxysmal symptom, one which in degree or kind may be considered relatively abnormal. But in other cases the cough itself is so remarkable, that even the least observant person cannot fail to mark it, or indeed be greatly disturbed and impressed by it, as by a fact of no ordinary significance. "In some cases" (see lecture above referred to, *International Clinics*, 1894, vol. iv. p. 45) "you may even make a very good guess at an aneurysm if the patient is within earshot, and you have not even seen him or known about his case otherwise, though I by no means advise you to be satisfied with so guessing." It is difficult to characterise, or to express accurately in words, all the varieties of cough which may thus arrest attention. "Hoarse, clanging, laryngeal," are phrases employed by one of the most acute diagnosticians (Walshe, *op. cit.* p. 491) in writing on this subject; and no doubt the association of a peculiarly noisy or "brassy" cough, with even a very slight or moderate degree of the laryngeal stridor noticed above, is a fact that usually carries great significance. But a still more remarkable quality of the aneurysmal cough in some cases has been too little noticed by most authors, and derives its chief significance from the fact that (apart from cases of very great alteration or destruction of the larynx) it is essentially a paralytic phenomenon. The cough in such cases is imperfect, that is, deficient in the sharply explosive element which indicates with the utmost precision to the ear the first act of a strictly normal cough—the forcible closure of the glottis. It is a cough with imperfectly or only partially closed glottis, and as such takes on a perfectly distinctive character to the ear, apart altogether from its special intonation or qualities in other respects. Dr. Wyllie, who has given to this variety the name of *bovine cough*, explains it by the observation that the forcible—as compared with the ordinary or vocal—closure of the glottis is accomplished by bringing into operation the false vocal cords, which, with the ventricles of Morgagni, "constitute a valve, with cusp facing downwards, which is fitted, when the edges of the false cords are brought into apposition, to oppose the exit of air." The cow, he adds, "has no false vocal cords or ventricles of Morgagni; its cough is therefore a long loud grunt or a wheeze, without a proper initiatory explosion." However this may be, there is no doubt of the fact that in the human subject and in aneurysmal cases, paralysis of the adductors of the glottis is often most clearly revealed by a cough of this kind, even when there is no alteration of the voice such as to attract attention. And a cough with imperfectly closed glottis, when found in association with even the slightest degree of stridor or dyspnœa as aforesaid, is as nearly absolutely distinctive of thoracic tumour or aneurysm as anything apart from its patent physical signs can possibly be.

(c) Although, as above indicated, the *voice* may be unaffected, or comparatively little altered, when, owing to pressure on the laryngeal nerves, some of the more dangerous or more striking phenomena above mentioned are present, yet alterations of the speaking voice play a not inconsiderable part in the pressure symptoms of aneurysm. Dr. Walshe (p. 491) has summarised these alterations in a single sentence, in words that cannot be improved upon: " The speaking voice may be husky, muffled, cracked, and hoarse, or simply weakened, or tremulous and variable in pitch, or actually lowered in register." Some of these varieties he attributes to "chronic laryngitis," itself the result of pressure, or to œdema of the glottis from venous stasis; but all of them, even to complete aphonia, may no doubt be due to uncomplicated paralysis of the vocal cords. According to Dr. Newman, "the voice becomes altered in pitch, impure, and wanting in tone, and on straining to speak loudly readily breaks into a falsetto." Cases have occurred to the present writer as well as to Dr. Newman (in the paper above referred to) in which aphonia in one or other degree has been absolutely the first symptom of what has afterwards proved to be aneurysmal pressure on the recurrent; and in one case, recently under observation, this condition had continued unchanged for many months, with paralysis of the left vocal cord practically complete. Clinical experience, however, teaches that alterations of the speaking voice alone, apart from some of the other symptomatic phenomena above referred to, are not usually due to the pressure of a tumour; and therefore facts of this order, although not by any means unimportant, are of secondary importance in the early diagnosis of aneurysm of the aorta. Taken in connection with the preceding data, however, they form a distinct portion of the clinical picture which, often at a very early date, and long before physical signs (in the ordinary sense of the words) can be recognised, may lead to an inferential diagnosis with something like scientific precision.

It will be convenient, at this stage, to interpose a few remarks on the entire group of phenomena here discussed, with special reference to the more modern doctrines of laryngeal innervation. This subject has been most elaborately considered in the fourth volume of this work (p. 841 *et seq.*, "Laryngeal Neuroses ") by two very distinguished experts ; and as regards the bearings of laryngoscopy, and of experimental physiology, on the intricate questions involved, Sir Felix Semon (one of the two) has enunciated a law, as being applicable generally to paralytic lesions arising from pressure on the recurrents, namely, "that in all progressive organic lesions of the centres or trunks of the motor laryngeal nerves, the abductors of the vocal cords succumb much earlier than the adductors" (p. 843). He further affirms that while paralysis of the adductors (occurring primarily or alone) "is almost invariably bilateral, and due to functional disorders," unilateral paralysis of the abductors, on the other hand, almost always indicates organic disease, and is thus of the greatest possible importance in the diagnosis of the earliest stages of pressure on the corresponding recurrent nerve. It is maintained, moreover, that in this early stage of strictly unilateral abductor paralysis there are not necessarily any vocal or respiratory symptoms, or even functional disturbances, such as to give rise to practical inconvenience. Such unilateral abductor paralysis, therefore, can only, in the first instance, be detected by the laryngoscope, the use of which, therefore, is strongly advocated as a routine in all cases where even the most remote presumption can arise of a thoracic tumour; or of anything, whether centric or peripheral in its relation to the nervous system, which may implicate the motor nerves of the larynx (p. 853). The importance of these statements need not be questioned, inasmuch as they rest upon independent and detailed clinical investigation, and are generally in accord with what has been stated above. The absolute universality of the "law," and the hypothesis on which it rests, may be held to be to a certain extent an open question ; but in respect of aneurysm and its diagnosis we may accept the position that the earliest phenomenon which will present itself on a laryngoscopic examination, as indicating pressure on the recurrent, will be an over-adduction or at least permanent adduction of one vocal cord, which "remains fixed in the median line, that is, in the position of phonation" (p. 853). It might be expected that such a position of the cord in inspiration would lead to more or less of embarrassment of the breathing ; but when the opposite cord is freely movable, we have good evidence that this is not necessarily the case ; that if difficulty of inspiration occurs under such circumstances at all, it is usually during exertion only. Bilateral abductor paralysis, if approximately complete, is a much more formidable condition ; the chink of the glottis then remains permanently in the position of phonation, with great impediment to the free access of air in inspiration, and a corresponding amount of stridor ; but bilateral abductor paralysis from pressure on the recurrents is rare, and is usually incomplete, so that the difficulty may not be so extreme as is here indicated, and may be felt chiefly during exertion. There seems to be no doubt at all, therefore, that, considered merely from the point of view of paralysis, aneurysmal pressure on the recurrent laryngeal is scarcely adequate to the production of those extremely violent, suffocative, and highly paroxysmal attacks, attended with marked stridor, and apt to be suddenly fatal, which have been described in the present article. It seems impossible, then, to avoid the conclusion that these exquisitely paroxysmal attacks are due not so much to abductor paralysis as to spasm of the adductors (as in laryngismus stridulus) arising indirectly from reflex irritation through the vagus. It is well established, indeed, by experiments, from the time of Professor John Reid downwards (70), that irritation of the proximal or afferent fibres of the cut vagus in the neck will produce bilateral spasm attended with such suffocative paroxysms ; and the fact that such spasms usually occur in connection with pressure on the trachea, whereby its lumen is permanently encroached on more or less, while the extreme and paroxysmal phenomena, including the stridor, are quite evidently laryngeal, is in harmony with this view of reflex irritation ; which is also adopted by Dr. David Newman in the important paper already referred to. Moreover, one of the most extreme cases of such suffocative spasms ever personally witnessed by myself, was carefully examined for evidences of aneurysmal pressure, with negative results. The patient recovered from these repeated paroxysms, and did not die from dyspnœa, but from simple exhaustion; the necropsy revealed, as the cause of the symptoms, a very extensive, but also extremely chronic, probably syphilitic, ulceration near the bifurcation of the trachea; the upper two-thirds of which, together with the larynx and mucous membrane of the glottis, were perfectly normal (*Glasgow Medical Journal*, June 1890, p. 463). In contrast with this case, I have recently had the opportunity of observing (*Western Infirmary of Glasgow, Pathological Reports*, No. 538) a sarcomatous growth involving the mediastinum and right lung, in which the main bronchus leading to the latter was nearly, if not completely occluded; and flat nodules of the growth were found in the mucosa of the lower trachea; but in this case without any evidence either of spasm or of laryngeal paralysis.

The late Sir George Johnson believed that he had obtained evidence in support of the "theory that a long-continued irritation of the trunk of one vagus may, through its afferent fibres, so disturb the common centre of the two vagi as to cause either bilateral spasm or bilateral palsy of the laryngeal muscles" (48). As regards bilateral spasm, this position is quite unassailable, and is in accordance with experimental evidence; but as regards palsy on the opposite side from the irritation it is different. "Broadbent's law," which is referred to by Sir G. Johnson as corroborating this surmise, would in fact have precisely the opposite effect. Broadbent's law is concerned with explaining (and does very perfectly explain) the exemption from paralysis of muscles which, normally, act always together on the two sides, when there is a centric unilateral lesion which otherwise might be expected to give rise to unilateral paralysis. To make this law cover the case supposed, of a paralysis reflected from the seat of a peripheral unilateral lesion so as to give rise to bilateral paralysis, is altogether at variance with the principle involved; and probably not supported by any precise clinical or experimental evidence.

4. *Hæmorrhage*, especially in the form of hæmoptysis, is undoubtedly one of the symptomatic phenomena of aneurysm of the aorta entitled to separate consideration; both because it may be (though as a rule it is not) among the earliest symptoms, and because, when occurring at any period in the course of the disease (where the diagnosis is not otherwise evident), it may be easily mistaken for the much more frequent hæmoptysis of tubercular phthisis, or for that of cardiac valve disease. The not infrequent and always very impressive fact of a fatal hæmorrhage from an aneurysmal sac (with sudden death) tends rather to obscure the real value of hæmorrhage as a symptom; because when presented in this light it is, however striking as a fact, of comparatively small diagnostic importance. If a man drops down in the street, of whom nothing otherwise is known, and dies within a few minutes or seconds, the probabilities are greatly in favour of its being a case of aneurysm

fatal through profuse internal hæmorrhage. But this is hardly a diagnosis; it is rather a mere guess or presumption, founded upon probabilities only, and of no value at all as regards the individual patient. Had the previous history of such a person been accurately known, it might probably have been ascertained that the fatal hæmorrhage was not by any means the first; and it is to these earlier, often much earlier, attacks that attention ought chiefly to be directed, in order that this symptom may assume its proper rank as a warning of the disease. Cases have been recorded in which the first known or considerable hæmoptysis in aneurysm had occurred months, or even years, before the fatal result (see case of J. B. farther on); and the fatal result, even after several attacks of this kind (as in the well-known case of the great surgeon, Robert Liston), may not be due to hæmorrhage at all. A state even of entire quiescence in the more urgent symptoms of aneurysmal disease may follow a profuse—almost fatal—hæmoptysis. More commonly minor discharges of blood are repeated at intervals during what remains of life after a more considerable bleeding.

The pathological explanation of these facts is now fairly well understood. The progress of an aneurysmal sac is almost constantly attended by a deposit of fibrin on its walls internally; by preference in those parts of the sac more remote from the active blood-current. It seems at least probable that a chemical ferment arising from the white blood corpuscles or leucocytes, thrown aside from the current and cohering in masses to the altered wall of the vessel, is the active principle in determining this coagulation. At all events the decolourised fibrin is usually deposited in successive layers, of which the outer one adheres closely to the inner wall of the aneurysm; the others form concentrically inwards towards the blood-current, or, in a sacculated aneurysm with a well-marked opening from the vessel, towards that opening. The thickness and firm consistence of these fibrinous concretions is often such as to present very marked indications of a spontaneous healing process, whereby the pressure outwards of the blood in the sac is in part resisted, and the weakened vascular walls are protected from rupture. In rare cases an obliteration of the aneurysmal sac may thus take place, and a complete cure be established. And in many more cases the obstacle to a very sudden rupture through a considerable opening is such that when rupture ultimately takes place toward a mucous membrane, or a cutaneous surface, not only is the opening relatively small, but the flow of blood, impeded by coagula newly formed or of long standing, is also much less profuse than might have been expected, and may even be a mere oozing, or succession of oozings, filtered through these obstructions. The accompanying woodcut (Fig. 26) from the author's *Clinical Medicine*, p. 525, shows the appearances observed in a case of this kind, in which this interesting process is depicted in its nascent stages; the actual opening in the tracheal mucous membrane being of merely pinhole size, and "surrounded by five or six minute papillary eminences, with pale apices, on a congested membrane," any one of which might presumably have given way as soon almost as the one which actually led to the hæmorrhage; the bleeding in this case, moreover, was not fatal, but had been taking place "in small quantities for some time before the fatal event" by suffocation. Cases such as this (and they are by no means very infrequent) form most interesting object-lessons to set against the current impression so widely diffused, that the "bursting of a blood-vessel" is the cause invariably and inevitably of sudden death.

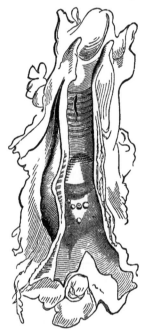

Fig. 26.—Pinhole perforation of aneurysm in a mucous membrane.

The facts, as clinically observed in aneurysmal hæmoptysis, are often obscured by the want of exact evidence whether the smaller losses of blood come from the interior of the sac, or from some accidental pulmonary congestion which may presumably have arisen from pressure on the veins, or on the lung itself. But when (as in Mr. Liston's case) a very considerable hæmorrhage is succeeded by a period of quiescence, and death takes place five months later, with slight discharges of blood during the interval (July to December 1847), it is impossible to avoid the conclusions that a rupture of the sac took place in the first instance, and healed up again more or less completely. Mr. Liston's case was perhaps the first in which, owing to the celebrity of the subject of it, and the wide circulation given to the leading facts in medical journals, the conclusion was brought home to the medical profession generally that the "bursting of a blood-vessel" in aneurysm is not necessarily or immediately fatal. A careful survey, however, of the laborious collections of Crisp and Sibson, made by myself in 1859, afforded "only nine, or perhaps ten, instances in which an interval of a month or more existed between (aneurysmal) hæmoptysis and death; and in very few of these was there an interval nearly so long as in Mr. Liston's case between a considerable bleeding and the fatal event" (loc. cit. p. 515). The case of J. B., therefore, above referred to, was not unwarrantably regarded as being probably unique, and was discussed with proportionate fulness.

In this case the leading facts as regards the hæmoptysis, very succinctly stated, are as follows :—

The patient, J. B., who was 40 years old at the time of his death, had in all probability been the subject of his fatal disease for ten years, although no accurate diagnosis of aneurysm was made till about six years before his death. Five years before death, while giving evidence in a court of justice, a very sudden and large gush of pure blood occurred, causing him to faint ; and this was renewed an hour or two later in his own house. After these two severe attacks the hæmorrhage subsided ; and although the physical signs of a large aneurysm were quite apparent, and the probability, therefore, of a rupture into the air-passages was fully considered, his health improved so much after a long period of enforced rest, along with a variety of medical treatment, that he was allowed to take gentle exercise, and ultimately even to handle a light fishing-rod to some good effect for three successive summers, without any appreciable injury, and with a fair amount of enjoyment of life. "But in the midst of this improved state of health he continued occasionally to bring up a more or less tinged expectoration—sometimes rusty, sometimes purple, almost never of anything approaching pure blood." Although the progress of the disease (as indicated by the physical signs) was slow, there was a gradual extension of the tumour so as to invade the left lung, of which the sounds became more and more impaired. Ultimately emaciation, dyspnœa, and laryngeal phenomena, with occasional dysphagia and angina-like pains, marked the transition to a much more urgent condition ; in the midst of which the respiration of the left lung was completely suppressed, and percussion became dull all over the left side. "He frequently brought up blood more copiously than he had done since the first attack of hæmoptysis, but never in large quantity or pure." At last, "a small gush of blood, probably not exceeding eight or ten ounces, occurred, which terminated life by suffocation in a few minutes." The necropsy, carefully performed in view of these facts, showed a very large aneurysm of the descending aorta, resting on the vertebræ and on the thoracic wall above, adherent over a considerable space to the left lung, and opening very freely into the left bronchus and trachea. "The left bronchus is stretched over the sac, and *has its posterior wall absorbed throughout its whole length.* The sac is filled with firm coagulum, *which is freely exposed to view from the interior of the bronchus.* Exactly at the bifurcation of the trachea there exists another opening into the sac ; it is not larger than will admit a probe, and *from its smooth rounded edges has evidently been a long time present. This opening, too, rests upon a firm, solid, laminated clot.*"—(*Clin. Med.* p. 513.)

In this case it is impossible to doubt that the first very serious hæmoptysis indicated a rupture from the aneurysmal sac into the air-passages (perhaps at the bifurcation of the trachea, as above stated) ; and that in the subsequent progress of the case this opening very nearly healed up ; the accumulation of laminated fibrin behind the opening effectually resisting the blood-pressure at the original site of rupture, even while the gradual ulcerative absorption of the wall of the left bronchus was at once disabling the left lung entirely, and at the same time opening up new channels for minor hæmorrhages, the last of which proved fatal by closing up, temporarily, the bronchus of the opposite, or relatively sound, lung. It is thus amply demonstrated that for nearly five years (four years and eight months) from the first "bursting of a blood-vessel" in a case of aortic aneurysm, reparative and ulcerative processes may go on side by side, without any loss of blood so considerable as to be in itself dangerous or even urgent.

Parallel instances are not wanting of rupture of aneurysms into other mucous cavities, or on the cutaneous surface of the body.   Two of these last, published many years ago and never seriously questioned, are referred to in the article from which the foregoing case is extracted (p. 517).   In one of these an aneurysm of the arch and of the innominate artery burst externally opposite the cartilage of the third rib, giving rise to a very large flow of blood, described to the local surgeon as "somewhat larger than a quill."   Strange to say, the patient, "nothing alarmed, got hold of a bowl and held it at arm's length to receive the red arch which he supposed was the contents of a 'bloody boil,' pressing the tumour with his chin to effect a more speedy clearance.   After about a pint of blood had gushed out, he fainted and the bleeding stopped." He died of typhus fever about four months afterwards without any new bleeding.

In the other case communicated by Dr. Neligan to Dr. Stokes, a ship-carpenter, æt. 56, was considered to have all the signs and symptoms of an aneurysm of the aorta opening externally about the second rib on the right side in front.   "For more than a year," it is reported, "the tumour discharged at intervals, sometimes copiously and in a continuous stream, a quantity of blood sufficient to cause alarm, and occasionally arrested with difficulty."   After one of these hæmorrhages (which occurred under Dr. Neligan's own observation) "the tumour diminished considerably in size, and became much more dense, losing the fluctuating character it previously had."   Three weeks after another and much less copious hæmorrhage the patient left the hospital, "stating that he felt quite well." The further progress of this case is not described, but enough is stated to give emphasis to the lesson taught by the above case of J. B.   Most persons who have had a long experience of aneurysmal cases, and especially in hospital, must have seen several in which the tumour had made so much way towards the surface, even in some cases softening and becoming fluctuant, as to render it extremely probable that at any time a fatal rupture might take place.   On the other hand, my own experience (possibly exceptional) is that in over forty years' service as a hospital physician, with probably a larger share than common of cases of internal aneurysm, an actual rupture on the surface of the body has been among the rarest of incidents; and a rupture directly fatal by hæmorrhage has not yet occurred. A case of this rare issue, however, of very recent occurrence, is referred to farther on, in the section on treatment.

Ruptures of abdominal aneurysms on the gastric or intestinal surface are much more rare than the opening of thoracic aneurysms into the air-passages, and are probably still more rarely survived for any considerable time.   But in one instance, at least, I have recorded (Clin. Medicine, p. 495) an aneurysm of the superior mesenteric artery, which had apparently given rise to repeated attacks of hæmatemesis, in their clinical features closely simulating a case of gastric ulcer opening into a considerable vessel; especially as the age and social condition of the patient (female servant, æt. 16) accorded much better with this diagnosis than with that of aneurysm. After several nearly fatal attacks of this kind, the patient made an apparent recovery, but continued dyspeptic, and ultimately died very suddenly from a rupture of the aneurysm into the peritoneal cavity. The earlier lesion was discovered to have been an opening into the duodenum, which had almost healed up, but presented still " a very small ecchymosed spot, perforated in the centre by a minute opening, into which a moderately fine probe could be passed for a line or two, but was there arrested." The rupture into the peritoneum, of much greater size and evidently torn edges, was in the immediate neighbourhood.

When aneurysmal hæmorrhage takes place into serous cavities it is extremely rare for death to be long delayed. But even in such a case days (at least) may intervene, and the hæmorrhage take place at intervals; so that in one case, already referred to, the gradual filling up of one pleura with blood was mistaken for an empyema. In another case it was strongly suspected (*Clin. Med.* p. 517) that what appeared to be an inflammatory effusion (hæmorrhagic pericarditis) was really a hæmorrhage (aneurysmal); the blood having been churned about in the course of the movements of the heart so as to decolourise its fibrin. Even some of the cases of dissecting aneurysm, already referred to as opening into the pericardium, lend themselves more easily to the view of a succession of hæmorrhages than of a single gush of blood fatal at once. But it is difficult in such cases to place the facts in this respect beyond question.

In cases of aneurysmal hæmoptysis (to which the majority of observations refer) it has been established (*Clin. Med.* p. 520) that hæmorrhages short of a directly fatal result may take place for weeks or for months in the form of—" 1st, A frothy bronchitic sputum streaked with blood; 2nd, A rusty sputum very like that of pneumonia, but usually more abundant, more frothy, and less viscid; 3rd, A deeply-dyed purple or brownish purple sputum, like the so-called 'prune-juice' expectoration, closely resembling that of pulmonary hæmorrhagic condensation from valvular disease of the heart; 4th, Any of the preceding, alternating with small discharges of pure, unmixed, but generally imperfectly coagulated blood." When such hæmorrhagic sputa approximate to the characters observed in pulmonary condensations, it is legitimate to infer that such condensations exist; and it is probably quite impossible, in some cases at least, to distinguish the aneurysmal from other forms of such condensations: but it is desirable none the less to have it clearly in view that such changes may be due to an aneurysm pressing on a main bronchus. The pulmonary alterations thence arising may vary almost indefinitely from recent condensations, with partial lobular collapse of the lung (and giving the impression as if blood had been pumped backwards into it through the bronchus), and infiltrations of older standing, "nodulated and dense, some violet-coloured, others of a sandstone gray tint." In other cases, also, softening and ulceration of the tissues of the lung take place, leading up to a true bronchial and aneurysmal phthisis, of course non-tuberculous. Some of these changes are well illustrated in two woodcuts (*Clin. Med.* pp. 482, 483) from a case in which, although no very considerable hæmorrhage ever took place, the sputum from first to last under observation was blood-stained to a high degree, and the left lung was found to be

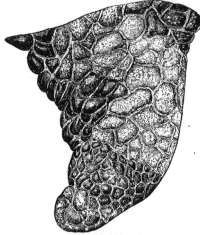

completely condensed, with evidently · lobularly disposed lesions throughout. The left bronchus was incorporated with the sac of an aneurysm, and had its posterior wall deficient for about an inch ; its calibre was almost completely occupied at this point by a firm, gray coagulum of blood which projected out of the aneurysmal sac. Fig. 27 shows the surface of the lung in this very remarkable case, with the lobular condensations above referred to, strongly indicated by the interlobular septa, and evidently puffed out with partly purple-coloured and recent, partly decolourised and older, blood conveyed from the bronchus. Fig. 28 shows the same lung in section, with strings of tough, blood-stained mucus

FIG. 27.—Surface of left lung in case of W. G., showing lobular condensation, from old and recent hæmorrhage into left bronchus. The differences of colour and of prominence of the lobules are due to the differences of date of the hæmorrhagic condensation ; the older hæmorrhage being nearly decolourised, and in part absorbed, or converted into a puriform matter, which is seen at points forming small abscesses below the surface.

emerging from some of the larger bronchial divisions.

The diagnostic indications arising from these facts will be discussed farther on in connection with the physical diagnosis.

5. *Dysphagia.*—This, as an incidental symptom of aneurysm of the aorta, is far from unimportant ; but its importance is rarely so great as to place it in the first rank of diagnostic symptoms. Dysphagia may arise either from the direct pressure of the sac on the œsophagus, or from pressure on the pneumogastric nerves or their œsophageal branches. In either case it will be chiefly aneurysms of the descending aorta that will give rise to this symptom. When such an aneurysm is not otherwise revealed or suspected (and it is very easy to conceive of such a case), the whole of the symptoms present may be those of stricture of the œsophagus, and instruments may be employed, perhaps with disastrous results. It is well known to some of the older members of the medical profession in London [1] that one of the most consummate surgeons of the last generation had been so unfortunate, when exploring a case of this kind, as to plunge an œsophageal sound into the sac of an aneurysm lying close to and compressing the œsophagus, with the result that the patient died immediately in the consulting-room. Another case, which might have had a similar issue, will be found referred to in a footnote at p. 559 of the author's *Clinical Medicine.*

[1] The writer learned the facts from the late Sir Spencer Wells.

In the preceding list of symptoms, those only are included which most frequently present themselves as part of an early diagnosis, before the physical signs and consideration of the whole history of the case have established its true character as one of arterial disease. The more incidental symptoms arising in the progress of aneurysms of some standing, as from pressure on or perforation of veins, and the like, will be discussed later.

III. *Physical diagnosis.*—Under this head will be considered all those objective facts which, occurring manifestly in the course of internal aneurysms, or elicited by percussion, auscultation, and so forth, apart from

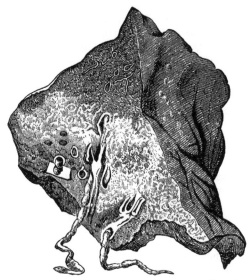

FIG. 28.—Section of lung, the surface of which is shown in Fig. 27. The varieties of colour and the bronchial abscesses are less clearly defined. The bronchi are seen to be full of blood in different stages of alteration.

any statements made by the patient, or any suggestive history of symptoms such as is alluded to above, may reveal to the physician the existence of the disease. It is needless to insist on the great importance of this aspect of diagnosis, as tending to precision and, in some cases, to the only well-assured evidence of the truth.

An aneurysm in an external, and still more in a very superficial vessel, like the femoral or the carotid artery, is usually more easily recognised by its physical characters than by any symptoms it may incidentally give rise to. A tumour lying superficially, and yet close to an artery, and deriving a pulsation from it, is a fact not easily overlooked; and the patient himself goes in search of medical advice, in many cases with a tolerably clear idea of what is wrong with him. It is still necessary, however, to raise the question whether the tumour be aneurysmal, or one only deriving pulsation from the artery indirectly;

and surgeons of the most unquestionable skill and experience have been misled in this diagnosis. But when the aneurysm arises from a deeply-seated vessel, or one included in a bony cavity like the thorax, the diagnosis is much more difficult, and is often inferential. For not only may there be no tumour externally appearing, or even recognised by physical signs, but a tumour may occur without sensible pulsation on the one hand, and pulsation without tumour on the other; furthermore, a pulsating tumour is not necessarily aneurysmal. The diagnosis is to be made on the same principles as apply to an external aneurysm, wherever it can be made at all.

The arch of the aorta does not anywhere (unless it be close to the sternal insertion of the second right cartilage) immediately underlie the thoracic wall; but a very moderate degree of dilatation will, under certain circumstances, give rise to undue pulsation, which can be appreciated by the hand placed over the manubrium, or by a finger in the jugular fossa. Such abnormal conditions may or may not be, strictly speaking, aneurysmal; but they must be investigated by every means of physical diagnosis, and compared with all the inferences from history and symptoms to which reference has already been made under the previous sections of this article.

A sense of undue pulsation of the aorta, however, may arise only as part of a more generalised phenomenon, namely, an increased pulsation throughout the arterial system; or (to confine the remark within limits) in all the more considerable systemic arteries of the neck and extremities, as in the well-known "water-hammer pulse" or "pulse of unfilled arteries" of aortic regurgitation. Such a condition, if unattended by evidence of tumour or of well-marked dilatation of some particular aspect of the arch or of the vessels immediately arising from it, is entirely without significance in relation to the present subject. But it is otherwise when the sense of undue pulsation is localised strictly; where, for example, it extends to one sterno-clavicular articulation and not to the other; or where it can be felt in the jugular fossa as conveying a more or less abnormal resistance to the finger, mounting upwards with each impulse, and so placed as to indicate the arch and the innominate artery on the right side, or the arch and the left carotid on the left side of the mesial line. And when, in addition to these signs or independent of them, there is a decidedly abnormal state of the percussion in or near the manubrium sterni, within limits which can be exactly defined,—more especially if the abnormally dull percussion corresponds in its area with that of an abnormal impulse to the hand, or a visible heave of the thoracic wall at each ventricular pulsation,—the diagnosis of aneurysm is fairly well confirmed. However, we shall still keep in view that a glandular or other tumour occupying the mediastinum, and deriving impulse from the aorta, may give rise to physical signs all but indistinguishable from those of an aneurysm,—a distinction only to be made, if at all, by the most careful and refined judgment on all the facts of the case, including the history as above.

As in the majority of cases of aneurysm of the arch the impulse is more freely carried to the right, and that aspect of the vessel is not only thus very frequently involved in dilatation, but when so involved is nearest the surface, it is not surprising that dulness on percussion should be, "as a rule, most easily and completely detected to the right of the sternum, and in connection with the ascending portion of the arch and its angle on the right side" (Walshe, p. 483). But this cannot be taken as a rule without many exceptions; an aneurysm may underlie the manubrium sterni so as to be precisely divided (as regards its dull percussion) by the mesial line, or so as to extend equally to either side ; and the prominence, and still more the impulse, may not be most marked on the side which has most of the dull percussion. But when these three facts coincide, or nearly so, tumour or prominence, expansive pulsation, and limited dull percussion, the site of all of them being the manubrium or near it, and no present evidence otherwise of glandular enlargement, an aneurysm of the arch may be assumed to exist, with a high degree of probability almost amounting to practical certainty.

The percussion in these cases should be very carefully conducted, the heart being first mapped out with as much precision as possible, especially as regards its basic margin. If this be normal, or at (say) the level of the fourth rib, then any substernal or manubrial dulness which can be clearly defined as separate from this must be taken as of great significance, even when it does not present either of the two other signs above referred to. The dulness arising from a sacculated aneurysm may extend quite up to the sternal notch (in which case it will usually be associated with abnormal pulsation or resistance in the jugular fossa), or it may fall short of this and present a somewhat pear-shaped area, diminishing downwards so as, even when it touches the cardiac dull area, to be quite obviously distinct from it, being separated by a comparatively narrow neck. Or again, the dulness may in some cases (where the aneurysm is close to the heart) be quite inseparable from the cardiac area, and only distinguished as a separate fact by the prominence, or abnormal impulse or sounds communicated to it. Sometimes, but on the whole rather rarely, no abnormal dulness at all can be detected by light percussion, while a stronger stroke gives a sense of something abnormal, including an apparent increase of deep resistance. Such "deep percussion," however, is subject to many fallacies, and is rarely to be relied upon apart from other facts. Dr. Walshe has indicated (p. 131) that, "by careful percussion in the course of the arch, a sac as large as a good-sized walnut may be discovered if it lie anywhere between the second right interspace and the left border of the sternum." If the aneurysm, however, extends backwards or downwards, or to any considerable degree leftwards from the above position, it will be correspondingly difficult of detection by percussion alone.

In regard to the pulsation, as discovered in different localities in connection with aneurysmal sacs, Dr. Sansom (75, p. 499) affirms that in 25 out of 32 cases (about 80 per cent) it existed to the right of the sternum, the site of greatest individual frequency being the second right inter-space; while in a still large number the site was either not very precise, or "in various sites from the sixth rib below to the right clavicle above"; there being "in one case only a central pulsation of the sternum rising into the neck." It is always of importance to ascertain, when possible, if the pulsation correspond with a general expansile movement of the tumour; this, when of some considerable size and prominence, may usually be best perceived by the hand and eye together; the former being employed so as to grasp the swelling from side to side, as well as to determine the forward impulse; the latter being placed so as to catch the tumour in profile, looking sideways along the surface rather than directly down upon it. The light should be carefully managed; and sometimes half-lights, or even shadows, thrown on the surface will reveal more than the most direct and strong illumination. Pieces of paper or card bent at an angle, and with one end attached to the surface, while the other is free and acts as an indicator recording and magnifying the expansile movement, may be employed at different points of the tumour; or two stethoscopes (Sansom) "may be held applied by their chest pieces, and their divergence demonstrated" (this, however, will only apply to considerable prominences). Fagge and Pye Smith recommend that a piece of adhesive plaster, with a slit cut down its centre, should be applied over the tumour; "if this be narrowly watched, the slit will be seen to widen at each expansile pulsation." It should be kept in mind, however, that even in very large and prominent aneurysmal tumours, expansile pulsation may be shown with great difficulty, or not at all, owing to the occupation of the exposed part of the sac with dense masses of fibrin. And the amount of pulsation may increase or diminish indefinitely, while the case is under observation.

The impulse communicated to an aneurysmal sac is of course repeated at each stroke of the heart, and may usually be taken as roughly cor-responding in time with the ventricular systole. In strict accuracy, however, the aneurysmal impulse is not ventricular-systolic, but rather arterial-diastolic in rhythm, that is, just perceptibly (in some cases), but as a rule very slightly, postponed to the ventricular impulse, as indicated by the pulse of the heart. Theoretically, indeed, the pulse of an aneurysmal sac ought to be momentarily retarded, even as compared with the arterial diastole in the vessel from which it springs; but it is not easy, nor is it usually necessary to make any practical use of distinctions so fine-drawn as this. The impulse is rarely punctate, and it usually gives the im-pression of being more or less diffused over the whole exposed prominence (if any) corresponding with the sac; it has a broadly heaving character, and is therefore more easily appreciated by the whole hand than by the finger; and it becomes more evident when considerable counter-pressure is made (which must, however, be cautiously attempted in some cases). A sense of vibration, sometimes prolonged, and amounting to a jarring thrill ("sufficient almost to tickle the hand," as Walshe says), may accompany the impulse, or may even be present when the impulse is very slight; this phenomenon, however, is very inconstant and apt to vary in the same case, from causes very imperfectly known. A second impulse, or rather vibratory jog, alternating with the first, and coinciding in time closely with the second sound of the heart, may follow each heave of the sac, and may in some cases be an even more startling sensation to the hand than the other. This (often called diastolic) shock is really determined by the recoil of the column of blood which has been propelled into the aneurysm during the cardiac systole, and is closely associated with the exaggeration and alteration of the second sound presently to be described. It is not a true "impulse," although, from the difficulty of finding a good descriptive name, it is apt to be so called.

Aneurysmal sounds and murmurs.—Each of the phenomena above described may be attended with a sound bearing some relation to a normal cardiac sound; though as a rule exceeding it in intensity, as well as distinguished from it by position and character. Or there may be murmur as well as sound, and the murmur heard may resemble or may differ from a valvular murmur. Often, in aneurysms arising very near the heart, the aortic valves are actually implicated; or are the seat of independent disease or insufficiency. Further, the aneurysm may actually be one of the valve itself, that is, a pouching towards the ventricle of one or other sigmoid segment; or it may be partly of the valvular segment and partly of the insertion close to the sinuses of Valsalva, or involving them. An aneurysm so situated (small in size as a rule, and of course altogether out of the range of physical diagnosis otherwise) may have ruptured backwards into the ventricle; and this may give rise to well-marked aortic insufficiency without any evidences at the autopsy of primary endocardial vegetations at the edge of the segment. A diagnosis in such cases as to the real cause of the murmur may be impossible, or only possible through collateral considerations. But when murmurs, one or more, are either confined to the seat of prominence (or of dull percussion) quite outside the cardiac area, or when they are so manifestly louder there, or so altered in quality as to carry home to the ear the conviction that they arise in the sac of an aneurysm, they are usually to be interpreted accordingly. The physical theory of aneurysmal murmurs is by no means so well defined as always to allow of their causes being clearly inferred from their clinical characters; and the varying statements and opinions even of good authorities are far from convincing. In all probability a relatively small orifice of communication between the artery and the sac disposes to murmur; and something must also be due to the state of the margins of such an opening, the angle at which the blood-current is propelled through it, and the force and volume of the current going to expand the sac or by its recoil carried back from it into the vessel. Certain it is that the mere frequency of murmurs has been exaggerated; and that in about half the cases (Douglas Powell) of sacculated aneurysm no murmur of any kind is audible. In a large proportion of the cases, however, in which a murmur can be detected, it coincides with the expansion of the sac, and is then the audible counterpart of the vibratile fremitus already described. In a much smaller proportion of cases (apart from those in which the aortic valves are involved) there is a murmur both with the expansion and the recoil of the sac. In a still smaller proportion the recoil only is accompanied by murmur. Aneurysmal murmurs, especially such as coincide with the expansion of the sac, are often not only of great intensity, but of a very peculiar quality (described by Walshe as "roaring"), and suggestive of the waves of sound being reflected and intensified in a large cavity; this may occur without any very unusual impetus, or any increase of the sounds in other respects.

Among the almost innumerable alterations that have been described under this head is a very intense, highly accentuated and deep-toned booming, ring'ng, or clanging second sound, obviously due to the exaggerated recoil of the blood on the aortic valves, modified in some way by the presence either of a sacculated aneurysm or of a dilated arch (Begbie). Although the precise acoustic significance of this sign is not even yet fully determined, and it is certainly not pathognomonic of sacculated aneurysm, it is, when well marked, always a fact of importance as tending to that diagnosis. The phenomenon occurs, of course, only when the valves are fairly competent; but there may be coincident hypertrophy of the left ventricle.

Dr. Sansom (75, p. 500) has indicated, as a fact within his experience, that a systolic aneurysmal murmur, otherwise inaudible or very feebly heard, may be conveyed loudly to the ear of an observer through the column of air in the trachea, " by causing the patient to place within his mouth the small chest-piece of the binaural stethoscope, and to close his lips over it." This observation, if further confirmed, may be of very great importance, as it might give evidence of aneurysms in positions in which the physical signs are otherwise wanting or extremely obscure. In order, however, to avoid erroneous interpretations it will be necessary to distinguish, if possible, between murmurs so conveyed and the curious phenomenon described in 1859 by Dr. Thorburn of Manchester, and afterwards (1862) by Dr. Radcliffe Hall under the name of "pulse-breath," when the cardiac pulsations become definitely audible through the air expired (the mouth being held open); and even, as in a case published by Dr. Finlayson (29), at a distance of two to three feet. Dr. Sansom's method does not appear to have been employed in any of the cases recorded by these observers; but in the very careful commentary attached to Dr. Finlayson's case it will appear that "pulse-breath" is not so much related to aneurysm as to air-filled cavities of considerable size, either within the lung or from pneumothorax, so placed as to act as resonators in transmitting the cardiac sounds to the air in the trachea and upper air-passages. It would even appear probable that in healthy subjects, under certain circumstances, a minor degree of the phenomenon in question may sometimes be observed.

Displacement of the trachea or upper air-passages; Tracheal tugging.— When an aneurysm arises from the transverse portion of the arch, in such a position that its pressure is in the first instance backwards or downwards, it may not reveal itself by any of the physical signs hitherto noticed, but, on the other hand, may impinge upon or compress the trachea or the left—or even, in some rare cases, the right—bronchus, so as to give rise to evidences of displacement. In most instances, even when of small or very moderate size, such sacculated aneurysms will also be revealed by symptoms—that is, by dyspnœa, cough, or both, having some of the peculiarities of character remarked upon in a previous section of this article. Even when not very amenable to mere physical diagnosis, therefore, such aneurysms are not often latent in the sense of being wholly unsuspected; and the chief value of physical diagnosis is clearly and unmistakably to confirm a suspicion derived from a combination of symptoms which might otherwise pass under some other more or less erroneous designation. In all such cases the critical examination of the jugular fossa, anterior and posterior mediastinum, and of both lungs is imperative, and should proceed upon a combined use of all the most improved methods of inspection, mensuration, percussion, auscultation, and the like, employed comparatively over every part of the chest at which information can be gained. The slightest lateral deviation of the trachea, for example, at its lower part, as compared with a line drawn from the pomum Adami to the precise middle of the suprasternal notch, is a sign of the most signal importance, and in general easy of recognition; while of less easy recognition, but still of very manifest account, will be a displacement of the trachea directly backwards, giving rise to an inordinate depth of the trachea in the jugular fossa; even if there should be no lateral deviation, and no sense of a pulsating tumour felt on deep palpation from above. If either of these signs concur with even the least well-defined abnormality or dull percussion in the sternal region in front, or in the dorsal region close to the spine behind; or if the respiratory murmur is of a peculiarly harsh and blowing quality over some such limited area in the immediate neighbourhood of the air-passages, the diagnosis of pressure, most probably from an aneurysm, will inevitably follow; and the situation and extent of the tumour, whether deeper or more superficial, will be very accurately suggested in general by the direction of the deviation or the localisation of the signs in other respects. *Diminished mobility of the trachea*, in the act of swallowing, as compared with its normal upward and downward movement, is also to be kept in view, and, with more or less displacement, may amount to proof of pressure, and probably of adhesion of its anterior or lateral walls to some abnormal growth within the chest. To this order of phenomena belongs the very remarkable sign commonly called tracheal tugging, as first shortly described (though not under that name) in a letter in the *Lancet* by Major Oliver (64); and afterwards made the subject of a much more extended investigation by Drs. Ross and Macdonell, of M'Gill College, Montreal. These observations, with the very suggestive further researches of Dr. Ewart of St. George's Hospital (25) and Dr. Grimsdale, may be briefly summarised as follows :—

Tracheal tugging is to be carefully distinguished from the mere pulsatile movement which the trachea, as well as all the adjacent structures in
the neck, may sometimes seem to derive from the normal or more or less
exaggerated pulses of the carotid arteries in certain cases and positions.
The true tracheal tugging is a distinct sense of traction downwards,
accompanying each beat of the heart, when steady though moderate
traction upwards is made by the fingers pressing up the cricoid cartilage
in such a way as gently to draw the windpipe (as it were) upwards in
the neck, though only to such an extent as to make manifest the sign
referred to.   Dr. Ewart, who seems to have given much attention to the
details of the method, recommends that the patient should be seated in
a chair, with his head somewhat thrown back and steadied against the
breast of the observer (standing behind the chair).   "The tips of both
index fingers are then inserted under the cricoid cartilage, which is
gently raised by them."   This method is not only less troublesome to
the patient (in whom an increase of dyspnœa might in some cases be
determined by any more rough handling), but it is as regards the result
to be obtained "almost too delicate"—a slight amount of pulsatile
traction being felt by the observer in a certain proportion even of normal
cases.   When, however, "tracheal tugging" is distinctly abnormal in
degree, the probabilities are very great in favour of its revealing an
aneurysm; and as it seems to be established that aneurysm, when confined to the ascending part of the arch, does not produce this sign,
the aneurysm will implicate the transverse part of the arch, and in
all probability will be so placed as to bear downwards upon the left
bronchus from the postero-inferior aspect of the vessel.   At all events
the sac will in such cases be placed so as to involve the bifurcation of the
trachea and one or other bronchus; and as it is precisely in this situation
that a small or very moderate-sized tumour may most readily escape
other means of physical diagnosis, the importance of this sign when
clearly established seems to be especially great as a guide to an early
diagnosis.   For the reason already alleged, however, it will be prudent
to abstain from attaching too great a significance to the more slight or
indefinite degrees of tugging in cases in which corroborative symptoms
are not present at all.   It may be that, as Dr. Ewart suggests (25,
p. 598), "the slight tugging discovered in healthy persons may have its
origin in the pulsation of the pulmonary artery," which lies closer even
than the aorta to the trachea under normal circumstances.   What is
clearly established is that this quasi-normal phenomenon takes place
chiefly under two conditions, namely, (i.) cardio-vascular excitement, and
(ii.) forcible inspiration, which in all probability acts by depressing the
air-passages as a whole, and thus bringing them into closer relations with
the vessels.   It is also said to occur more readily " in people with full
chests and prominent infraclavicular regions " (Grimsdale, p. 106); and
in one case, at least, of emphysema and bronchitis it was found present
to a degree that might easily have led to a fallacy in diagnosis.   On
the other hand, it is much less apt to occur in phthisis and in mitral

disease than even in health. On the whole it does not appear possible, in the meantime, to place entire confidence in this sign; yet Dr. Ewart is still disposed to regard it as important in its more pronounced forms, although far from being pathognomonic, as at first supposed by Oliver and Macdonell. Its chief value will probably be as an early guide to the position of the tumour in cases where one or two suspicious symptoms have already made it most likely that an aneurysm exists, but where, apart from this sign, physical diagnosis fails to reveal anything distinctive.

Deficiency or other alterations of respiratory murmur resulting from pressure.—When an aneurysm is so placed as not to give rise to any of the above physical signs, its existence may sometimes be inferred from some well-marked alteration of the pulmonary sounds, such as to amount to positive evidence that the access of air through one or other division of the greater bronchial tubes has been shut off, or locally interfered with. In the majority of such cases it is the left bronchus which is obstructed, and an impairment to a notable extent of the respiratory murmur of the left lung or of one or other of its lobes may, even in the absence of all other physical changes (or perhaps it would be more correct to say all the more because of such absence), become a very suggestive sign of tumour compressing either the lung itself directly or the bronchus leading to it. In the former case (compression of lung directly) the symptoms may not be very considerable, or they may indefinitely resemble those of pneumonia or of pleurisy ; but when the bronchus is compressed there are frequently asthmatic symptoms of a highly paroxysmal character, although they may not be characterised by any of those peculiarities above described as due to pressure on the laryngeal nerves or on the trachea. Cough may also be present, harsh and paroxysmal, though without any special laryngeal quality. As it is quite possible for a relatively small aneurysm, springing from the first part of the descending aorta, to give rise to most of these symptoms, and as the deep position of such a tumour makes it difficult or impossible to arrive at any other than an inferential diagnosis, it must be admitted that a correct opinion can only be formed, if at all, from a very careful consideration of all the facts. If, however, hæmorrhage has occurred (even though not in very considerable amount), and if it can be affirmed that there is no evidence otherwise of cardiac, tuberculous, or syphilitic disease ; and if, further, the obstruction or compression of the bronchus has taken place somewhat suddenly, in a case already under observation for symptoms not otherwise definable, the great probability of aneurysm as a cause of them should never be lost sight of.

Dr. D. Drummond has indicated that in certain cases of aneurysm of the aorta, in which the sac is so placed as to influence the currents of air in the trachea, a rhythmic blowing sound, synchronous with the action of the heart, can be heard on placing the stethoscope over the trachea externally. It is not yet quite certain what amount of practical importance attaches to this sign, which may be identical in character and origin with the phenomenon of "pulse-breath," already indicated, or with Dr. Sansom's sign of an audible rhythmic murmur communicated through the air in the mouth by the lips of the patient closing over the chestpiece of the stethoscope.[1]

Pressure-signs (or signs of local obstruction) connected with the arterial system.—When an aneurysm is placed so as to cause obstruction either to the current or to the impulse of the blood, not in the aorta itself but in one or more of its leading branches, very important and sometimes conclusive evidence of the fact may be obtained from a careful comparative observation of the pulses in the radials, the humerals, subclavians, and carotid arteries of each side ; care being taken, of course, that merely anatomical differences (as, for example, from an abnormal distribution of any of these vessels) are excluded as far as possible. The sphygmograph, as well as the ordinary tactile manipulation of the pulses, may here be brought into play ; but it is important to remark that small and ill-defined differences between the radial pulses on the two sides are not to be relied upon, unless it can be clearly established that they are constant, and have come into existence during the period of observation, and along with the appearance of other symptoms or physical signs suggestive of aneurysm. When, indeed, during the course of observation of the case, a more or less well-marked relative weakening of the pulse occurs on one side, and is found to be constant or on the increase, especially if it affect both the carotid and the subclavian, and is to be traced down from these vessels to their furthest ramifications on the side affected, the inference is usually plain enough. An aneurysm of the arch or (if on the right side) of the innominate artery may by its position either have directly obstructed these vessels, or, by the secondary formation of fibrinous layers within the sac, may have led to their becoming gradually sealed up against the impulse of the blood. The pulse-wave in such cases may be wholly obliterated, or it may be greatly diminished in magnitude, and retarded in time, so as to lead not only to difference in volume, but also to a want of synchronism in the two radial pulses. The sphygmographic expression of this difference is that while the pulse on the unaffected side retains all its normal characters— including the abrupt upstroke, with its acute apex, the tidal and dicrotic wave following in the line of descent—all of these appearances are either wanting or greatly modified in the sphygmogram of the affected side. Here the upstroke is a very gradual rise to a flat or obtuse apex ; there is no tidal wave, and rarely any trace of dicrotism. Much experience, however, is required in the use of the instrument, and a familiarity with all the modifications that may be produced by accidental causes in judging of the minor modifications ; and, in all cases, it is well to examine carefully the entire arterial system within range of the finger, and this repeatedly at intervals, in order to get security, as far as possible, against sources of fallacy such as are referred to above. Further, Dr. Bramwell has pointed out that even when one or more aneurysms, involving the arteries of the neck and upper extremities, are "filled with firm clots,

---

[1] This sign may be present in cases of large non-saccular atheromatous dilatation of the arch.—ED.

through which a straight narrow channel for the blood remains," there may yet be no abnormal characters of the sphygmogram, and the pulse-tracings from the two radials may be almost identical.

Modifications in the arterial pulses, not so definite as the above, may be produced by a very large aneurysm, or general dilatation of the arch, without any marked difference between the two sides, in consequence of loss of the elastic resistance of the vascular coats; the wave consequent on the ventricular systole is thus expended on the blood in the first part of the vessel, from which it is feebly propagated into the divisions. And a large aneurysm in the thoracic or upper abdominal aorta may so intercept the pulse-wave as to lead to its being feebly felt, or not felt at all, in the arteries of the lower extremities. Cases have even been recorded, where an aneurysm pretty low down in the course of the aorta has been practically cured by one higher up; the force and impulse of the blood-stream having been so much checked by the latter as to promote firm coagulation and entire cessation of the pulsation originally present in the former. [Bennett (9), referred to in the section on treatment, p. 426.]

Pressure - signs connected with the venous system. — It has been remarked by several authors that aneurysms are less apt to give rise to obstruction of the veins of the thorax, or to pressure on them, than are malignant or glandular tumours. This remark is probably correct; but still there is a small minority of aneurysmal cases in which by obstructive pressure on the auricle, vena cava superior, or innominate veins, disorders of the circulation may arise to tell their own tale concerning the seat of obstruction. In a very much smaller number of cases, the aneurysmal sac opens spontaneously into some other part of the vascular system, or into a great vein, causing what, in the case of a limb, would be called a varicose aneurysm, marked, in some cases, by a sudden aggravation or modification of the symptoms. Obstruction of the vein in such cases may be followed by thrombus, extending to some of the external branches which may be found more or less rigid; or, the development of a collateral venous circulation may lead to great enlargement of the superficial veins of the neck, thorax, and abdomen. According to Dr. Bristowe, even a complete obstruction of the superior cava may occur without immediately fatal result; the circulation being diverted into collateral channels, and large tortuous veins becoming apparent between the axilla and the groin, forming a junction with the external iliac vein. The most characteristic result, however, of obstructive pressure on the vena cava superior is dropsy of the upper part of the body, including one or both upper extremities; and often extreme puffiness of the face with livid discoloration, venous engorgement, and a brawny collar-like distension of the integument of the neck; in some cases also exophthalmos takes place on one or on both sides. Dr. Sansom suggests that "if the obstruction be above the azygos vein, the lividity and œdema are confined to the head and arms; if it be below the point of entrance of the azygos, the chest will share in the congestion." If one or other innominate vein be specially involved, the external lesion may be limited to the corresponding side. If under such circumstances the aneurysm should open into the vena cava, there may be a quite sudden increase of cyanosis, accompanied by a sense of something giving way; which, however (as in a case recorded by myself (33)), may not be referred to the actual seat of the lesion, and may be entirely unaccompanied by pain, though with a sense of faintness or collapse. This may even be one of the earliest symptoms of serious organic disease, and may either be preceded or succeeded by the swelling. The clinical picture thus afforded of cyanosis, venous congestion or, it may be, marked pulsation, and dropsy of the upper part of the body, with dyspnœa and cough which (as compared with the cyanosis) may even be insignificant, is one which leads up almost certainly to the diagnosis of aneurysm, or of some other tumour implicating the superior cava. And in such cases the fatal issue may occur, without any of the other complications previously adverted to, from cerebral oppression (as in apoplexy) with its usual accompaniment of stertorous breathing, easily distinguishable from the stridor caused by pressure on the trachea or the recurrent laryngeal nerve.[1] But in such extremely rare cases details are often wanting, or are not recorded with such exactness and fulness of knowledge as to make them available for general inferences. The conditions as to the presence of murmurs indicating communication of an intrathoracic aneurysm with a vein have been very variously stated. In some cases (as in the two just referred to) there may be either no appreciable murmur, or the murmurs may not be in any way characteristic. In others there are both murmur and well-marked thrill. Observations of varicose aneurysm and aneurysmal varix in external parts (especially at the bend of the arm) have furnished details of importance as regards the much less frequent class of cases now under consideration. "If a lateral communication exist in any part of the body between a contiguous artery and vein," writes Dr. Walshe (p. 147), "so as to permit the current from the former to enter the latter, a murmur of whizzing or whirring character, and essentially intermittent, results, mingled with a continuous sound specially engendered in the vein." Continuity of the murmur, therefore, such as to give it more or less resemblance to the well-known venous hum or *bruit-de-diable*, even while receiving an impetus of intensity from the cardiac pulsation, is probably distinctive of an internal, as of an external varicose aneurysm. "If there

[1] This phenomenon, independently observed by the author (33) and Dr. Ewart (26), in two cases closely resembling each other, was made the subject of supplementary remarks by the latter (27), which, although not perhaps conclusive, are well worthy of consideration. In Dr. Ewart's case blood-letting was performed to relieve the symptoms; and, although the fact is not mentioned in the report, Dr. Ewart was led, two years later, during the discussion on another case (28), to mention that "the blood escaped from the opened vein in jets, as from an artery"—a fact of which, he says, he "did not recognise the full significance at the time, but felt that it was a point of much importance." Dr. Ewart was also strongly inclined to think (retrospectively) that "the colour of the blood spirting from the vein was brighter than appeared consistent with the degree of cyanosis." Although this remark does not appear in the original report by Dr. Sisley, it is probably one that should not be overlooked.

be a loud continuous murmur," says Dr. Sansom, "manifesting increase of loudness with each cardiac systole, accompanied by thrill, but heard independently of the normal sounds of the heart, and only over those parts where the aorta is in close relations with a great venous trunk, this must be considered as evidence of a communication between artery and vein—*a varicose aneurysm of the aorta*. If the maximum of such sound be about the second (right) intercostal space, it is probable that there is a communication between the aorta and the superior vena cava or with the right auricle. If the maximum be on the corresponding part of the left side of the sternum, it may be that the aorta has opened into the pulmonary artery or upper part of right ventricle."

In what is probably the most recent case of communication with the superior cava, brought by Dr. Ord before the Pathological Society of London on Feb. 17, 1891, and discussed at length by several members at that meeting (65), the abnormal sound is described as "a long continuous humming murmur, never ceasing, but varying in intensity, more sonorous during systole, fainter during diastole, conducted into the neck, and heard over the whole right side of the chest posteriorly." In this case the aneurysm originated about two inches above the aortic valves, and contained very little clot. It was about the size of an orange, and opened into the superior cava by a perforation about half an inch in length. All the conditions, therefore, were favourable for the production of murmur in the highest possible degree ; and two cases of Dr. Bristowe's are referred to as having presented exactly similar conditions, which had also been observed and compared by more than one of the parties to the discussion. Dr. Hadden suggested (Dr. Ord concurring) that "such murmurs had been known to occur in very vascular sarcomata " ; to which, it may be added (as involving a possible fallacy in diagnosis), that the enlarged thyroid gland in exophthalmic goitre is occasionally the seat of them.

Certainly one of the rarest cases on record, if not absolutely unique, is one which occurred in the Sta. Maria Hospital at Florence, in the clinic of Professor Colzi ; and is only too briefly narrated in the *British Medical Journal* by the late Dr. Wilson of Florence (89), who invited attention to it in the hope (but apparently in vain) of discovering some parallel case. A man, aged 37, received a stiletto wound immediately under the left clavicle, which (as was afterwards shown) must have perforated the innominate vein and the arch of the aorta at the same moment, and led to profuse hæmorrhage and insensibility at the time of the occurrence. He was confined to bed for a month, the wound, however, healing by first intention. Four months afterwards the left side of the face and the left arm were observed to swell. Two years later a dark red discoloration of the same parts took place, and the superficial veins of the supraclavicular region and upper thorax became distended and pulsatile. There was also exophthalmos (non-pulsatile). On applying the hand over the dilated veins a vibratory thrill, characteristic of varicose aneurysm, was noticed, and a corresponding murmur was heard, and could be traced along the course of the left internal jugular, the axillary, and the left brachial veins, and on the cranial bones along the course of the sinuses. Eleven years after the injury symptoms of jugular thrombosis took place, followed in a few days by apoplexy and death. The post-mortem examination revealed the following extremely interesting details, which the author of this article has been enabled to state with more fulness than in Dr. Wilson's brief report, owing to the kindness of Dr. Coldstream, who has transmitted an extract from Professor Colzi's own narrative (19), with some remarks of the professor thereon :—There was found acute cerebral œdema; the left innominate vein was dilated, and formed a large cavity like an orange, which communicated by an aperture of about seven millimetres length with the arch of the aorta, the aperture being between the origin of the innominate and the left carotid artery. In the regions of the internal jugular and axillary veins (in the face, neck, and arm of the left side) were noted the ordinary alterations of varicose aneurysm.

Professor Colzi urged the importance of the case as proving how, with a wound of the arch of the aorta, a patient had been able to live for eleven years. The case, as one of traumatic arterio-venous aneurysm between the left innominate vein and the arch of the aorta, is unique in literature. Colzi believes that the continuance of life after the lesion of these vessels, in this case, was due to the fact that each vessel was wounded at the same moment. The mechanism, he supposes, may be stated as follows :—The entrance wound was above, and small, corresponding to the cartilage of the first rib, oblique in direction. Necessarily the instrument, before reaching the aorta, had first to pass through the innominate vein; then, in withdrawing the weapon, the blood of the aorta was precipitated into the left innominate vein. This vessel being suddenly dilated, it is probable that a loss of parallelism between the external wound and its deep extremity took place, thus proving an obstacle to the passage of the blood (to the surface); while, on the other hand, the blood from the wounded aorta found a way of exit by the innominate vein to the right side of the heart, and thence, by the pulmonary circulation, back again to the left heart. The sternum, the thick connective tissue of the anterior mediastinum, the swelling-up of the innominate vein itself, tended to block up the space, and to cause the loss of parallelism referred to; while the difference of the pressure between the aorta and the innominate vein allowed the easy passage of blood from the former to the latter; thus the escape of the blood (of the aorta) to the right side of the heart prevented a more serious hæmorrhage. Along with the arterial rupture an intravenous auto-infusion took place at the same time.

Pressure-signs connected with the pupil, or otherwise indicating interference with the sympathetic, or with the nerves proceeding from the ciliospinal region of the cord.—It is now very nearly 170 years since attention was first drawn by Pourfour du Petit to the results of certain experiments on the vagus and sympathetic nerves in the neck of the dog; from which he drew the startling inference that "the intercostal (sympathetic) nerves furnish branches which convey the spirits into the eyes." Although these experiments were exactly on the same lines as those which have attracted so much more notice during the present century, they do not appear to have had much influence in their own day either on physiology or pathology; and, although confirmed in some measure by other observers, it remained for Dr. John Reid, in the course of his experimental investigations on the vagus nerve (1828), to make it clear that the ocular phenomena referred to (persistent contraction of the pupil, ptosis, redness of the conjunctiva, etc.) were due to the interrupted nervous communication through the sympathetic nerve; other supposed causes being excluded by a careful experimental induction (70). Dr. Reid has also the credit of having first adverted to a possible pathological and diagnostic significance of these facts, inasmuch as he refers to a case described in the *Medical Gazette* (71), where "the right carotid, the vagus, and surrounding parts are described as being enveloped in a large morbid (cancerous) tumour; and where, consequently, the sympathetic could hardly be supposed to escape." In this case "the pupil of that side is described as becoming smaller in the course of the disease." Valentin, from further experiments, and from a consideration of the whole arrangement of the nerves involved, concluded that the pupil derives its motor nervous supply from two sources—the nerves which act on the radiating fibres being derived from the spinal system, through the sympathetic ganglion and nerve in the neck; while those which supply the circular fibres are conveyed through the inferior branch of the motor oculi nerve. Budge and Waller subsequently showed that the nervous filaments which pass from the spinal cord to the sympathetic, and are thus conducted upwards to join the ophthalmic branch of the fifth (after it has passed through the Gasserian ganglion), are derived chiefly from the anterior roots of the two lowest cervical and the six uppermost dorsal nerves; and to the corresponding portion of the spinal cord itself (as the origin of these nerves) they accordingly gave the name of the *cilio-spinal region*. Further experiments showed that lesions of the spinal cord in this region produce all the effects on the pupil hitherto attributed to section of the sympathetic in the neck; and, in regard to the condition of the pupil, that myosis, as the result of a destructive lesion, and occasionally dilatation of the pupil as the result of irritation of these nervous connections, might arise from a cause operating either on the spinal cord and the nerves arising from it in this region, or on the sympathetic, from the lower cervical ganglion upwards. The myosis thus arising was interpreted as the result of withdrawal of nervous influence from the radiating fibres, whereby the pupil was left under the action of the circular fibres, more or less without antagonism. It had already been observed by Trousseau, and also by Romberg, that myosis is a clinical feature (though not a constant one) of certain spinal affections, notably of locomotor ataxy or tabes dorsalis; but this remark seems to have been made without any clear relation to a physiological explanation; and Dr. Argyll Robertson, writing in 1869, with all the details of the innervation fully in view, expresses surprise that "so comparatively few cases of spinal affection have been recorded in which this symptom (myosis) has been observed." It is remarkable, indeed, that several even of the experimentalists who followed in the wake of Pourfour du Petit seem to have failed to observe the myosis, or even have denied its occurrence after section of the sympathetic,—a fact, however, which is now too clearly ascertained to admit of any doubt. It would almost seem that, except in connection with poisoning by opium,[1] myosis had scarcely attracted the attention of clinical observers at all; and it is therefore the less surprising that a quite casual observation by Dr. Walshe, made in 1853 (85, p. 496), was probably the first instance actually placed on record of this symptom in connection with aneurysm. Previously to this, however, Dr. MacDonnell of Montreal had observed (1850) a case of malignant tumour, producing pressure on the sympathetic, in connection with contracted pupil, ptosis, and epistaxis, all on the same side with the malignant growth. In 1854, the author of this article placed before the Medico-Chirurgical Society of Edinburgh a patient affected with aneurysm projecting into the neck, and accompanied by contraction of the pupil on the affected side. The experimental data from Pourfour du Petit downwards were referred to, and a discussion took place, whereby, during the life of the patient, the case was brought under careful consideration with reference to the whole range of the physiological facts; the details being afterwards published, with the necropsy and some further remarks, in August 1855 (Clin. Med. p. 526). Dr. MacDonnell's case, above referred to, was first published in the Montreal Medical Chronicle, June 1858, under the suggestive title, "Contraction of the Pupil, a Symptom of Intrathoracic Tumours"; and upon the basis of the information thus obtained, and of other cases furnished by Drs. Gairdner, Williamson, Banks, and others, Dr. John Ogle prepared for the Medical and Chirurgical Society of London a most elaborate paper (63), which may still be consulted with advantage as the most accessible review of the whole subject up to the date of its publication (1858). Dr. Ogle, besides presenting a large body of evidence as regards spinal myosis, has also been able to produce cases tending to show that relative dilatation of the pupil may (as in experiments on the sympathetic) result for a time from irritation of the same nerves; the further compression or destruction of which may lead to the more permanent symptom of myosis.

In 1869, Dr. Argyll Robertson subjected the whole subject of what may now be called *spinal myosis* to a very careful inquiry (72) founded on five newly-observed cases; none of which, however, was of aneurysm or tumour. Apart from the rather intricate physiological questions connected with the new investigation, the discovery of the law of what is

---

[1] Even the myosis of opium-poisoning, important as it is from the medico-legal point of view, appears, according to Dr. Ogle (63, p. 438), never to have been definitely referred to till 1818, and then only in a single case, which, moreover, remained almost unnoticed for several years afterwards.

now commonly called the "Argyll-Robertson pupil" has a very definite bearing upon the present subject.[1] It is found that in spinal myosis generally, while the further contraction of the pupils during accommodation of the· eye to near objects (and also in response to Calabar bean), continues to be observed, the influence of light on the pupil is, as a rule, wholly lost. The retina continues active, but the reflexes between the retina and the pupil are suspended or abolished; being dependent (as Dr. Robertson believes) on the integrity of the cilio-spinal communications passing through the ciliary ganglion. The effect of atropine on the pupil in spinal myosis, on the other hand, although in no instance lost, is considerably retarded, and the dilatation resulting is never so complete as in a normal eye. These observations, so far as atropine is concerned, are exactly in accordance with those made by myself, in 1854, in the case of aneurysm above referred to. Calabar bean was not at that time in use as a myositic, and possibly there may be some want of precision in the statements about the light reflexes; it appears, however, that "the dilatation of the left (the myotic pupil), even in deep shadow, was very slight" (*Clin. Med.* pp. 530, 531). There need, therefore, be little hesitation in affirming that the "Argyll-Robertson pupil" will be found to be as characteristic of the cases depending on intra-thoracic or aneurysmal tumours as it is of the other forms of spinal myosis.

Dr. Seaton Reid has published a case which seems to show that an aneurysm arising even below the diaphragm, and therefore beyond the recognised cilio-spinal region of the cord, may give rise to spinal myosis (Walshe, 85, p. 522). But many more details would be required to carry conviction on this point, unless it can be shown to be in accord with physiological experience.

In applying these well-ascertained principles to the diagnosis of individual cases, it is important to remark further that relative dilatation of the pupil, and sometimes dilatation alternating with or succeeded by contraction, have been recorded in several cases by Dr. Ogle and others as concurring with, or caused by the interference of aneurysmal or other tumours with the nervous structures in the neck. This phenomenon is explained as being in accordance with the results of galvanic or other stimulation of the sympathetic nerve; the experiments of Brown-Sequard, Bernard, and others having shown that in animals a certain amount of dilatation follows (less, however, according to H. Müller, than that produced by belladonna) when galvanism is applied either to the upper

---

[1] Dr. Robertson's own statement as to the cases of spinal myosis above referred to, is that "in all of them there was marked contraction of the pupil, which differed from myosis due to other causes, in that the pupil was insensible to light, but contracted still further during the act of accommodation for near objects, while strong solutions of atropine only induced a medium dilatation of the pupil." The physiological questions, which cannot be dealt with here, will be found admirably and compendiously discussed in the *Lancet*, vol. i. 1870, p. 126 ; and in a letter by Dr. Robertson in the same volume, p. 211. The essential facts, whatever their theoretical explanation, do not appear to be involved in any dispute.

portion of the nerve after section, or to the entire nerve in the neck (see Ogle, 63, p. 408, and compare p. 421 *et seq.*). It seems, however, not always to be quite clear that in these cases the dilatation observed was due to the cause assigned; and, as the experiments in question lead to the inference that such dilatation is always a more or less temporary condition, it is safe to affirm that myosis, having the characters above referred to and not subject to variation under a lengthened observation, is a fact of far greater value and importance in the diagnosis of aneurysm than such an amount of dilatation as is here presupposed. For in spinal myosis the pupil does not dilate at all appreciably when the influence of light is withdrawn; although it is influenced to a certain extent both by belladonna and Calabar bean in opposite directions. It usually maintains a nearly fixed diameter of about $\frac{1}{12}$ in., and is in marked contrast with the mobile and presumably normal pupil of the opposite side. And the influence of belladonna upon it, whether given internally or in the form of a solution of atropine locally employed, is always much less than on the sound and mobile iris; and is also delayed in time as compared with the other. There is considerable risk of fallacy if these details are not carefully attended to; or if a physiological difference in the size of the two pupils at any given time is allowed to suggest the idea of aneurysmal pressure. I have even been led to figure, as an exemplary case (*Clin. Med.* p. 557), one which, although so puzzling otherwise in the physical diagnosis as to be quite exceptional, proved, in fact, not to be a case of aneurysm or tumour at all! Relative or complete immobility of one pupil, however, under varying conditions of light, when associated with such diminution in size as to be clearly abnormal, will very certainly indicate spinal myosis if the opposite pupil be normal in all respects.

It can only be in the most extremely rare cases of aneurysm that the lesion referred to will be bilateral. In one case, however (already referred to in this article, p. 364), it appeared to me that a diagnosis to this effect was justified by the necropsy. The case is briefly recorded (*Clin. Med.* p. 558), and was noticed still more briefly, in Dr. Ogle's paper (*loc. cit.* p. 415, note 3). It would perhaps be possible, even now, to raise a doubt whether opium may not (though the fact was strongly denied) have had to do with the myosis in this case. But at all events the diagnosis, made under circumstances of great difficulty, proved absolutely correct.

"*Clubbing*" *of finger-ends* in aneurysm of the aorta.—This is a rather rare incident, but has been observed by myself, as present unilaterally, in one or two instances in which the pressure of the tumour was exercised chiefly towards the corresponding side; probably with implication of the subclavian artery and its surroundings. Sir Thomas Smith has placed on record a case of this kind, in which the right axillary artery was the seat of an aneurysm which pressed probably both on the vein and nerves, causing pain and numbness in the arm and hand; "the arm generally was not swollen, but the fingers were œdematous and very markedly clubbed, those on the opposite hand being quite natural; the radial pulse was unaffected." The remarks appended to this case are well worthy of consideration, but do not seem to offer a final solution to the questions raised. It is, however, a fact, giving to this case an additional importance, that after ligature of the subclavian artery (although the patient only lived twenty days, dying of pyæmia) the clubbing of the fingers was "almost entirely removed."

Diagnosis.—The *diagnosis of locality* in thoracic aneurysm, complicated as it appears to be and necessarily is, according to the preceding considerations, may be fairly summed up in the following six propositions; here only somewhat modified and expanded from the form in which I submitted them thirty-five years ago (*Clinical Medicine*, p. 552), and since then constantly tried by continually repeated practical tests in individual cases, namely :—

(i.) That aneurysm of the aorta, when accompanied by symptoms more or less closely resembling angina pectoris, more especially if it have influenced the volume and the functional activity of the heart in a notable degree (as in producing hypertrophy, cardiac irregularity, palpitation, cardiac collapse, etc.), is probably situate in the ascending portion of the arch, and near the cardiac plexus of nerves. Such aneurysms may or may not be of a size and character to give positive physical signs to auscultation and percussion, apart from those of the cardiac hypertrophy and valvular disease with which they are very commonly associated. The natural course of such aneurysms is to rupture into the pericardium ; or to compress, perhaps open into, one or other auricle, or the pulmonary artery. A sudden increase of cyanosis to a remarkable extent might indicate such a change in the condition of an aneurysm already known or suspected to be present; while dropsy more or less suddenly occurring in the upper part of the body would indicate obstruction of the vena cava superior. Opening into the pericardium is not always followed (as is popularly supposed) by absolutely sudden and immediate death, but probably always by symptoms of severe collapse ; death following at an interval measured by hours.

(ii.) That aneurysm of the aorta, when attended by laryngeal or tracheal symptoms (imperfect closure of the glottis, changes in the character of the voice or cough, stridor in inspiration, or any combination of these), is likely to be so placed as to involve the right, or much more commonly the left, recurrent nerve. Stridor during inspiration, however (and in a less degree or not at all, during expiration), is even more decidedly a symptom of pressure on the trachea, or perhaps on the vagus trunk) ; and is often, like other forms of disordered innervation, highly paroxysmal. The peculiar significance of all these symptoms in diagnosis is that they are most apt to arise with aneurysms of no great size, and so deeply seated as otherwise to be entirely beyond the range of physical diagnosis (unless from the single, but on this account very important, sign of tracheal tugging). When arising on the posterior and inferior aspect of the arch, an aneurysm may even cause death by laryngeal or tracheal suffocation before it is large enough to give rise to any physical signs. But the use of the laryngoscope in such cases will usually detect unilateral paralysis of the glottic muscles, with a stationary and cadaveric, or otherwise highly adducted position of the corresponding vocal cord (commonly, of course the left). It is probably, if not always, to be expected that, in such unilateral paralysis arising from pressure, the abductor muscles will succumb considerably in advance of the adductors; paralysis in the first instance of the latter being almost always bilateral, and often functional (as in hysterical aphonia). Spasm of the adductors (from reflex irritation) is probably almost always bilateral and not so easily verifiable as paralysis; being, however, in various degrees the real source of some of the most dangerous of the conditions above referred to.

(iii.) That aneurysm, characterised chiefly by symptoms of bronchial asthma and orthopnœa, often with severe paroxysms of coughing, and expectoration which may be of little significance, though it may be in other cases bloodstained in every degree, can with great probability be inferred to be so placed as to exercise pressure on one bronchus (usually the left), or on the bifurcation of the trachea, inclining to one or other branch; and this inference will follow almost certainly from the symptoms alone, if the phenomena mentioned under the last heading as indicating laryngeal or tracheal disturbance, are wanting. The aneurysm in such cases may be wholly overlooked until it presents itself under the apparent symptomatic guise of spasmodic asthma, pleurisy, or pneumonia, as the case may be. Being situate in the commencement of the descending portion of the arch, and in contact mostly with the left bronchus, it may very easily escape physical diagnosis altogether; but, on the other hand, evidences of restricted access of air to the whole of one lung, or to some definite portion or lobe of it, sometimes also with dull percussion, will usually confirm the inferences to be drawn from the symptoms.

(iv.) That aneurysm, producing a permanent and well-marked contraction (spinal myosis),—or perhaps in rare instances some degree of much less permanent dilatation—of the pupil on one side (excessively rarely on both sides), may be expected to arise from the upper and back part of the arch or its primary branches; the sac projecting backwards so as to implicate the sympathetic trunk or its ganglia, and in most instances also the vertebræ (lower cervical and upper dorsal), so as to intercept the nervous communications passing from the spinal cord in these regions to the sympathetic.

(v.) That dysphagia (rarely a primary symptom in aneurysm, but not rarely associated with some of the preceding) indicates pressure either on the œsophagus directly or on the pneumogastric nerve, and a corresponding situation of the tumour, which in this case also may entirely elude physical diagnosis proper.

(vi.) Aneurysms which come within the range of physical diagnosis may or may not be attended by any of the preceding symptoms. The great majority of such aneurysms arise from the upper and anterior aspects of the arch, projecting upwards (towards the jugular fossa and supraclavicular spaces), or forwards (towards the manubrium sterni and costal cartilages). The diagnosis of such aneurysms is usually easy and comparatively secure ; for the existence of a pulsating tumour, or a dull percussion at the manubrium with alterations of the cardiac sounds over it, at once raises and almost solves the questions at issue. But it is worth while to remark that it is only in the positions above defined that an aneurysm of the arch can be expected to attain sufficient bulk to be easily discoverable by physical diagnosis proper, without involving important internal structures, and leading to very marked functional disturbance. The enormous size attained by some aneurysms arising from the anterior and upper aspect of the arch without any pressure symptoms (except as regards the bones) is indeed very remarkable. When the posterior and inferior aspects of the arch are involved, such large tumours cannot possibly occur without serious complications of the various kinds described above. The absence of such complications, therefore, may lead to more exact inferences as to the confines of the tumour; while the presence of them, or of some of them, may in some instances give rise to a strong suspicion, if not to an absolute certainty, of the presence of more than one aneurysm in the particular case. In the descending aorta, at a point so far down as to keep clear of any relations with the airpassages and their nerves, aneurysms may also attain a large size without any very striking symptomatic manifestations. In most of these cases, however, the vertebræ are eroded, and the peculiar gnawing pains will excite a suspicion which may be corroborated by very careful percussion on either side of the spine posteriorly. In a few instances such considerable aneurysms of the descending aorta will make their way to the surface in the form of a pulsating tumour, eroding and displacing the heads and angles of two or three of the ribs ; and in a not inconsiderable number of cases the spinal canal is invaded through the eroded vertebral column, pressure occurring on the cord, with paraplegia as the result. In all these cases pain must be looked upon as the dominating and often the guiding symptom in diagnosis. (A remarkably misleading instance of high temperatures associated with such pains, giving rise to a suspicion of spinal caries with septic empyema, is alluded to above, p. 354.)

In abdominal aneurysms the same rules of diagnosis will usually apply as to aneurysms of the descending aorta within the thorax. But here physical diagnosis comes more forward ; and the modes of functional interference are both more complex and more obscure than is the case in thoracic tumours. The subject of pain, usually the leading symptom in such cases, has already been pretty fully discussed in the preceding pages. The almost infinite varieties of functional disturbance, — that is, of nutrition, digestion, innervation, and so forth,—can only be adequately dealt with by the application of much care and attention to all the facts of the individual case (*vide* next article).

The application of the X rays to the diagnosis of internal aneurysms.—I am able to appeal on this subject to one who was probably the earliest in date to apply this method of examination to the thoracic viscera—Dr. John Macintyre of Glasgow, whose excellent work in all that concerns the X rays gives to his statements an importance in the estimate of future probabilities not easily attainable otherwise. Dr. Macintyre writes as follows :—

"The Röntgen rays have lately been used as a means of discovering lesions of the thoracic viscera. The subject has been approached from two standpoints : (a) the photographic, and (b) direct vision by means of the fluorescent screen. For the most part in this country potassium-platino-cyanide or barium-platino-cyanide salt has been used; while in America calcium-tungstate has been largely employed. Further, owing to the physical conditions, the most successful results have so far been obtained by direct vision.

"The results obtained are due to the difference in density of the thoracic structures, enabling us to distinguish soft tissues, such as the heart, the large blood-vessels, etc., from the less dense lungs, which offer comparatively little resistance to the rays. All these again are easily distinguished from the still denser surrounding osseous boundaries. The diagnosis of pathological conditions in the thorax by means of the X rays depends upon the fact that, we have been able, to a very considerable extent, to see or to photograph shadows of the normal viscera with sufficient accuracy to allow of comparison between these and deviations from the normal. Among such deviations, we may see pulsation in shadows clearly not cardiac, and so detect an aneurysm. In March 1896 I was able, by means of the fluorescent screen, and afterward by photography, to detect the greater part of the thoracic organs with distinctness sufficient to demonstrate pulsation in the normal cardiac area ; and shortly afterwards abnormal signs were made out. From time to time since then I have distinctly seen pulsation in cases of thoracic aneurysm ; and while, like others, I admit that examination by the Röntgen rays must now be considered an addition to our methods of diagnosis, in none of my cases could I say the lesion could not have been detected by other means.

"Dr. Campbell Thomson, who gives his experience and some results of tracing the outline of cardiac aneurysm and aneurysm of the first part of the aorta (78), says, that in some cases a doubtful condition may be made clear, and in others diagnosis still further confirmed. Dr. Walsh quotes a case of Dr. Coupland's of doubtful deep aneurysm in the chest, and claims that the evidence obtained by means of the fluorescent screen 'converted a doubtful into a certain diagnosis.' Dr. Francis H. Williams states that he has examined with the fluoroscope and taken radiographs of one subclavian and several thoracic aneurysms. He also says, 'It is obvious that aneurysms of the thoracic aorta can sometimes be detected earlier by X ray examination than in any other way.' In obscure thoracic cases, where an aneurysm of certain portions of the aorta is suspected but does not exist, it may probably be excluded by an X ray examination.

"It is clear from the above, firstly, that by the use of the Röntgen rays thoracic aneurysms have been detected; secondly, that this mode of investigation may now be fairly regarded as an additional aid to diagnosis; and, lastly, that with greater experience and improvements in methods better results may be expected in the future."

Prognosis of aneurysm of the aorta.—There is nò need formally to declare that this must always be grave, inasmuch as the partially healing processes to which allusion has already been made (see p. 381) are rarely of such completeness as to enable the pouched and weakened vascular coats to withstand permanently the pressure and impulse of the blood-current distending the sac from within, and considerably reinforced at each stroke of the heart. When, as in the case of the aorta, the dilated portion of the vessel is mostly beyond the reach of such effective control as, in external arteries, is applied by the Hunterian and other operations, there is little to be expected, ordinarily, in the way of a radical cure. All that can be relied upon under such conditions, in the way of natural forces tending to stay the course of the disease, is the formation in sacculated aneurysms of such concentric layers of fibrinous clot as may strengthen considerably the walls of the vessel at the points where they are most seriously damaged, and thus form a protecting barrier against the ever-recurring impetus which, as a rule, tends towards still further expansion. In rare cases it is well established that a practical cure (or a lengthened arrest of progress amounting to a cure as regards the symptoms) has occurred; and if—as is not very infrequent—the patient die of some other disease, the processes of repair then being ascertained in the dead body while the symptoms had been in abeyance some time before death, it may be said, as the French surgeon is reported to have said of his patient dying after an operation, "Messieurs, il est mort—guéri!" But such incidents, although deserving of careful study and consideration, can hardly be said much to diminish the gravity of the prognosis in any individual case of well-established aneurysmal tumour arising near the centre of the circulation. Whatever in such cases can reasonably be done to diminish the pressure of the arterial blood and the shocks arising from the ever-recurring cardiac impulse, or to favour such stagnation of the currents in the sac as may admit of its walls becoming lined with fibrin in layers, is undoubtedly in the direction of a natural cure; as will appear in the remarks to follow on treatment. Meanwhile, it is to be affirmed that, while the popular judgment probably errs in attaching to most cases of aneurysm the awful prognosis of very sudden death, and especially death by hæmorrhage or "rupture of a blood-vessel," the publicity which has been given, and rightly given, to a few exceptional cases of actual or apparent cure in aortic aneurysms may have tended to inspire hopes which are too often doomed to disappointment.

It is quite certain, however, that the absolute risk of very sudden death by rupture in aneurysms of the aorta has been popularly, and perhaps also medically, over-estimated; owing to the influence on the imagination of numerous cases of this form of fatal issue continually emerging in coroner's courts, and often sensationally recorded in the public prints. A few cases of this kind, widely known and much talked about, are noted as representative instances; from which it is very easy to generalise, inaccurately, that when a man has an aneurysm of the aorta, it is all but certain that he will ere long drop down in the street, or perish with the like startling and tragic suddenness. In point of fact, as every hospital physician of some standing knows by experience, this is by no means the case; and it would probably be an error to say that even the majority of deaths from aneurysm are thus sudden or unexpected. In thirty-two cases of fatal rupture of intrathoracic aneurysms, of which a brief but valuable synopsis has been recently published by Dr. Kelynack, he affirms that death was usually sudden, "in many instances practically instantaneous." But six of the thirty-two were the subjects of coroners' inquests, not even deaths in the Manchester Royal Infirmary, on the returns of which (4593 miscellaneous autopsies) the statements in question are based. In a private letter Dr. Kelynack states, that he has "notes of a large number of cases in which death occurred from other causes than rupture;" and this no doubt accords with the general experience. The mean age of the thirty-two patients who died by rupture was forty years; all but two were men. The ascending and transverse portions of the arch were the seats of the lesion in very nearly three-fourths of the cases; the remaining nine cases were in the descending portions of the thoracic aorta. In twenty-two cases the rupture was either into the pericardium or the pleural cavities (most frequently, of course, the left). In other cases it was into the œsophagus, or the air-passages; in three cases externally, in one into the superior vena cava. The exact numbers are too small to have much importance; but it is probable that the proportion of ruptures into the pericardium is higher than it would have been but for the coroners' inquest cases; and the same bias may account for a somewhat larger proportion of cases of aneurysm in the first part of the arch than would otherwise have appeared. The relatively small number of the cases of rupture into the air-passages is certainly not in accordance with my experience, or at least with my personal impressions of the facts as I have witnessed them; on the other hand, it is notable that even the small proportion of three cases rupturing with fatal results externally is in excess of my hospital experience, as also that of Dr. Kelynack himself, who, in the letter above quoted, adds, "I have never seen a case of aortic aneurysm actually rupture externally, although not a few on the point of so doing."

On the whole, then, the prognosis of aortic aneurysm, gloomy as it unquestionably must remain, is perhaps at no time quite so bad or so immediately hopeless as it is often represented. An aneurysm of large size, and apparently tending rapidly towards the surface, and at the same time softening and apparently pointing so as to resemble an abscess, may still become consolidated and recede when external rupture has been looked for from day to day. A rupture into the air-passages, as already remarked (p. 381), may precede the fatal event by weeks or months, or in rare instances by years; and the patient may even enjoy a fair measure of passably good health in the interval. Even the most frightful and urgent paroxysms of dyspnœa with stridor, threatening immediate suffocation and raising the question of tracheotomy by way of relief as a forlorn hope, may sometimes be allayed to a very remarkable degree; and the death, when it occurs, may not be obviously due at all to suffocation. And although instances of positive cure—in the popular sense of the word— are few and far between, the histories of not a few cases lead to the inference that the period from the first pouching of the vascular coats to the final and fatal result may be an interval of many years, during a considerable portion of which symptoms may be in abeyance, and the progress of the disease either exceedingly slow or altogether suspended by means of the natural processes of repair already signified. It is stated (Sansom, 75, p. 514) that " Sir William Broadbent has observed patients who remained well for ten years; Dr. Ord. has mentioned a similar fact. Hayden said that the duration of life in aneurysm of the abdominal aorta is from fifteen days to eleven years." A case of great interest from this point of view, as well as on account of the treatment, has been placed on record by Dr. Gibson of Edinburgh. The general conditions of life in this case were by no means favourable, and the aneurysm, afterwards shown on autopsy to have arisen " from the convex aspect of the ascending portion of the arch," must prob- ably have been in existence for a not inconsiderable time before it was discovered. Yet this man, 39 years of age, and a lamp- lighter by occupation, had his life prolonged for twelve years from the period of the first observation, spending only a few months in all in hospital under strict conditions of regimen and medicinal treatment; while at other times he "undertook the duties of the keeper of one of the Edinburgh monuments, which involved his ascending sometimes fifty times a day to a height of almost 200 feet." I have witnessed cases the history of which implied the probability of a like, or even a longer duration; but in none of them was the fact so clearly demonstrated as in this case. It is, however, on the basis of such cases, carefully studied, and duly considered in reference to treatment, that all remedial agents worthy of the name must be used and tested in the cure of the disease.

Treatment.—It will be well, in the first instance, to direct attention to the proposals and experiments that have been made towards what may be termed a radical cure of aneurysm of the aorta, as opposed to the more gradual and, so to speak, more unambitious aids to the natural healing processes which have already been adverted to under the headings both of diagnosis and prognosis. Most of the means which have been adopted or proposed with the former object in view have, of course, proceeded more or less on the lines of the results obtained by surgeons in dealing with the arteries of the extremities; and many of them are associated with operative procedures belonging rather to surgery proper than to medicine.

Deligation of the abdominal aorta was performed, as is well known, by Sir Astley Cooper (14), in the case of an aneurysm involving the left common iliac artery, and threatening immediate death by hæmorrhage. The operation in this case was avowedly a last resort, after unsuccessful attempts had been made to deal with the hæmorrhage locally; the patient survived for forty hours. In a subsequent case, recorded by Mr. James, death followed on the night of the operation. Among four or five later cases one patient is said to have survived for ten days; and this fact, together with the much more successful results of ligature of the aorta in the lower animals, seems to go some way towards establishing that, theoretically, the operation is a practicable one, and might, as regards the immediate results, be survived long enough to allow of a bare chance of the cure of an aneurysm under very favourable circumstances; or might be proposed under circumstances of such immediate danger as to justify almost any "forlorn hope." Most persons, however, will probably agree with Mr. Holmes, that "the natural repugnance of surgeons to perform great operations which cannot be expected to succeed, will either banish this altogether from practice, or restrict it to a very few exceptional cases," most of them aneurysms, or injuries, not of the aorta but of the iliac arteries. In aneurysm of the aorta itself the operation could probably only be thought of as a distal one, and the chances of real success are thereby incalculably diminished. It is evident, indeed, that the sudden diversion of the arterial blood from so large a section of the body as the two lower extremities and the pelvis, would inevitably, at least for the time being, cause an increased impetus towards the aneurysmal sac through the non-occluded section of the aorta and its branches above; and even the establishment of a collateral circulation, while absolutely essential to success, would not be unattended in some cases by the danger of an increased determination of blood, for a time, through the aneurysm itself.

Distal operations by ligature.—In all but an exceedingly small proportion of abdominal aneurysms, and in all thoracic aneurysms of the aorta, deligation of vessels can only be performed, if at all, on the principle of distal occlusion; that is, on the rather slender chance that an obstruction more or less complete to the exit of blood from the sac by a simultaneous or successive deligation of vessels leading out of it or beyond it may give rise to a temporary stagnation, such as may allow of the reparative forces, which are presumably at work even without such interference, being brought more effectively into play for the consolidation and ultimate obliteration of the sac. Perhaps the most considerable success claimed in this direction in the case of vessels implicating the arch of the aorta is that of Mr. Barwell, who reports a case of distal operation for an innominate aneurysm, possibly involving also the arch; it was treated by simultaneous deligation of the carotid and subclavian arteries. In five other operations more or less resembling this one,—two of them, however, being innominate cases only, the others probably involving the arch,— success is claimed in all but the first, which was for "a very large aorto-innominate aneurysm." Mr. Christopher Heath has performed this double operation on a patient who survived for four years; the case being at the time one of doubtful diagnosis, but after death shown to be aortic aneurysm. In other cases the results were much less satisfactory, death following the operation in some of them within a few hours. Ligature of the left carotid alone has sometimes appeared to be success-ful; but on the whole, from a careful and comprehensive view of the whole subject,· the chances of a permanently good result in these operations do not appear to be much greater than are sometimes obtained in the spontaneous arrest, for a time at least, of aneurysmal tumours without surgical interference.

Compression of the abdominal aorta has been employed with a degree of apparent success which demands notice, although the cases to which it is applicable are comparatively few. As, however, more than seventy-five per cent (133 out of 177 cases, according to Sibson) of aneurysms involving the aorta below the diaphragm arise very high up, in the region of the cœliac axis or of the superior mesenteric artery, it is impossible to suppose that proximal pressure can ever become a recognised means of cure in any but a small minority of cases; those, namely, which are only a few inches above the bifurcation, and which allow of an effectually controlling pressure being exercised by the hand, or by a tourniquet, in the region interposed between the giving off of the renal arteries and the tumour. Above this region the aorta lies too deep, and too much involved with important structures, to allow of the hope of its being ever successfully subjected to compression.

The possibility, however, of thus dealing with an aneurysm low down in the abdominal aorta was first demonstrated in the well-known and now classical case submitted to the Medico-Chirurgical Society of London in 1864 by Mr. Charles Moore and Dr. Wm. Murray of Newcastle (59)— the latter of whom may be said both to have suggested the treatment and to have been its chief promoter; first in this paper and later in a little volume published in 1871. Having ascertained, in the first instance, that by firm pressure with the hand in this case above the tumour, the pulsa-tions in the aneurysmal sac could be effectually controlled, it occurred to Dr. Murray that, by first placing the patient under chloroform so as to make tolerance possible, and then using mechanical pressure by a tourniquet so carefully adjusted as to secure the complete interruption of the circulation in the sac for some hours at a time, it might be practicable safely to bring about rapid coagulation in such a way as to lead at once to obliteration of the sac, and so by a single operation, as it were, to cure the disease completely. "The principle," he adds (59, *b*, p. 11), "on which the rapid cure rests is clearly the complete stagnation of a mass of blood in the aneurysm until it coagulates." To this "rapid method" as contrasted with the "old method," which in the hands of Bellingham and other Irish authorities had been extensively employed in external aneurysms, and in which the cure "lasted on an average five-and-twenty days "—Dr. Murray attaches great importance. He regards "the sudden and complete consolidation of an *internal* aneurysm" as "an entirely new fact in medical science," and looks forward to its being "no uncommon result" when chloroform is employed, and pressure used in the method indicated. In this case the pressure was applied on two occasions at an interval of three days. On the first occasion of two hours' compression difficulties were experienced, and the results as regards the aneurysm were not important; but it is recorded that the patient passed no urine for nearly thirty hours. On the second occasion five hours were occupied by the pressure, but it was during the last hour only that complete control of the pulsations in the tumour was obtained. This result was evidently of the nature of a surprise. "To my astonishment the tumour had now become perfectly pulseless, and every indication of pulsation in the aorta below it had disappeared." It is certainly very remarkable that the consolidation of the tumour seems to have gone on quite steadily from this moment; and that even the very next day there was "no pulsation in the tumour, which is now perfectly station-ary, hard, resistent, and lessened in size" (p. 20). The pulse in the femoral arteries was also gone; but the secretion of urine was in this instance uninterrupted, or was quickly re-established. The details are very interesting, but cannot be further cited here. They show that a complete cure was obtained; certainly not without some rather severe symptoms, but probably with the minimum amount of danger or in-convenience consistent with the method. It is not, however, irrelevant to remark here that the patient (who had remained well and fit for work in the interval) contracted a second aneurysm near the cœliac axis,[1] of which he died suddenly some years later. The necropsy revealed the complete consolidation of the first aneurysm, which was converted into a fibrous mass; a great shrinking in the trunk of the inferior mesenteric artery ("dwindled to the size of the radial artery") which arose out of this obliterated aneurysmal sac; the enormous enlargement, on the other hand, of the superior mesenteric ("as large as the aorta"), and a corresponding increase of size in all the vessels entering into the very highly-developed collateral circulation which had been established through the epigastrics, internal mammary, intercostals, and circumflex iliac arteries outside the abdomen, and the hepatic, colica media and sinistra, and hæmorrhoidal arteries, etc.

This is undoubtedly a most interesting, if also a very rare case, and merits all the wide notice it has received. But, although the principles and the practice involved in it are alike well worthy of consideration,

---

[1] Although the author evidently regards this fact as having no direct connection with the operation, it is possible to entertain the question whether the changes in the vessel higher up, which resulted in the aneurysm that proved fatal in the second instance, may not have also been in part involved in the cure of the first tumour; as in a case of the late Professor Bennett, to be noted afterwards, p. 426.

it does not appear that the anticipations of Dr. Murray (as to such rapid cures becoming "no uncommon result" of further prosecution of his method) have been borne out. During the thirty-three years that have elapsed Dr. Murray himself has not contributed any more facts in detail to the history of the subject; although two such cures are attributed by him to Dr. Heath of Newcastle, but without any such precise narrative, even as regards the main incidents, as to allow of its being stated positively whether these were cases of aortic aneurysm or not. In one of the two cases, thus briefly and informally glanced at rather than recorded, it is stated (59, *b, c*) that "consolidation was distinctly observed to occur within twenty minutes,' previously to which, however, "pressure had been kept up irregularly for about ten hours, when the patient fainted under the chloroform." This attempt having been entirely without result as regards the tumour, "the patient was urged to bear a final attempt without chloroform." "To our amazement," it is added, "when at the end of twenty minutes he declared that he could bear the pressure no longer, we found the aneurysm had become solid and had ceased to beat." It is thus apparent that in both the cases in which Dr. Murray was chiefly concerned, the successful result came as a surprise, after a series of abortive attempts, some of which were almost attended by disaster. It is greatly to be desired that Dr. Murray would even now attempt a complete, and a reasoned account of the whole of the Newcastle experience up to the present date. We know from other sources that aneurysm is a relatively common disease in Newcastle; and Dr. Philipson, writing in 1878, had the singular good fortune of being able to present three successive cases of abdominal aortic aneurysm of which two were cured. Of these two, however, one was treated, without any attempt at local interference, by iodide of potassium; and, in the other, the kind of arterial compression employed differed very considerably (and apparently with intention on Dr. Philipson's part) from that advocated by Dr. Murray. Dr. Philipson's experience is summed up in the following brief sentence:—"The conclusion deducible from this consideration is that aneurysmal tumours of the lower portion of the abdominal aorta may be successfully treated by arterial compression on the cardiac side of the aneurysm, but that the method is a dangerous one, and should not be employed until the constitutional treatment has failed; and that, if arterial compression be employed, it should be moderate and prolonged, rather than complete and of short duration." In these words Dr. Philipson cannot but have had in view some experience which may not have been placed upon record, but which must be taken as very materially qualifying the more sanguine expectations entertained by Dr. Murray in 1871 (see chap. v. of his treatise), with respect to the ease and security of the "rapid method" of proximal pressure; in regard to which Dr. Murray not only leaves us to infer perfect safety, but "that it has not failed in any one instance" (p. 43).

Apart from the Newcastle experience, I am not aware of more

than two cases in which compression of the abdominal aorta appears to have been successfully practised for aneurysm of this vessel.[1] One of these was recorded in the *Med. Chirurg. Transactions of London* by Dr. Moxon and Mr. Durham in 1872; the other by Dr. Greenhow in the succeeding year. Both cases are remarkably interesting as regards the details, and the results in the end appear to have been satisfactory; but no one can peruse the carefully elaborated reports of these cases, showing the difficulties and not inconsiderable risks encountered during the progress of the treatment, without perceiving that, as regards the ease and simplicity, and above all the safety, claimed on behalf of the "rapid cure" by Dr. Murray, they are the reverse of reassuring. Dr. Greenhow, in reference to his own case, states that "the pulsation in the aneurysm continued for a considerable number of days after the last application of pressure to the aorta." In Dr. Moxon and Mr. Durham's case "pulsation in the aneurysm continued for a month"—the ultimate issue of the case being equally favourable. "It would now appear certain," Dr. Greenhow adds, "that the process of cure in these cases, by coagulation of blood in the sac of the aneurysm, is not necessarily a rapid process, but may go on so slowly that the passage of blood through the aneurysm may not cease for many days, nor in some cases until after the lapse of weeks."

It is not necessary, perhaps not even expedient, to pass any critical judgment on these various observations concerning the cure of abdominal aneurysms by compression. The statement, as above, of the few instances on record in which the details are adequately given, and the rather ominous negative fact that, notwithstanding the length of time that these proposals have been before the medical profession, successes have not multiplied, and confidence has not apparently increased, may be regarded as representing, as far as may be, the present state of opinion. It is not desirable to impose any undue restraint upon the enterprise of future observers, when confronted with dangerous, and too often incurable, disease; but it is at least legitimate to put on record the serious inquiry whether, after all, the risks encountered from the operative interference proposed may not be even greater than those of the disease itself which, as we have seen, is occasionally, if not very frequently, cured spontaneously; and certainly is not rarely suspended in its progress for considerable periods.

[1] In 1874 Mr. Holmes published (44) a table of all the cases he could then find, "in which rapid pressure had been applied with a view of curing aneurysms at a single sitting —an attempt which, in many of them, was repeated at subsequent sittings with varying success." Six cases are regarded as probably or certainly aortic; of these, three were successful; two were fatal, and in the sixth the attempt was abandoned before fatal injury had been inflicted. In ten the aneurysm was iliac, or ilio-femoral; seven were cured. In the other three the attempt failed, and all the patients died after ligature of the vessels, which in one case was the aorta."

"The dangers which are incidental to the compression of the arteries of the belly are, first, those attending prolonged anæsthesia; secondly, the risk of peritonitis from irritation of the peritoneum either covering the bowels or the mesentery; and, thirdly, contusion of the pancreas, kidney, or other viscera. The operation is both a difficult and a very dangerous one."

It appears sufficiently evident from these facts that the future of compression, possible in a very small proportion of abdominal aneurysms, is still undetermined; and will probably depend more on the ultimate judgment of surgical experts in respect of the results obtained in other arterial trunks, than on further attempts upon the abdominal aorta. Still, it is well to know that such cures have been obtained; and even if we have to admit that the "rapid cure"—in Dr. Murray's sense of the word—can only be expected as an extremely rare and exceptional, not to say incalculable, piece of good fortune, it may still be held that when the pulsations in the sac can be adequately and completely controlled by the hand compressing the aorta below the origin of the renal arteries (so as not to incur the risk of suppression of urine), the "rapid cure" may, with due precautions, be still attempted occasionally. Lister's tourniquet will be the most suitable instrument for effecting compression in such cases. There will remain, however, cases, more or less numerous, in which the "old method" of Bellingham and others may be used with advantage; and in all probability the opinion of Dr. Philipson, above cited, will be found not far from the truth.

Introduction of foreign bodies into the sac—Filipuncture.—This name has been applied (perhaps not very happily) to "a new method of procuring the consolidation of fibrin in certain incurable aneurysms"—announced by Mr. Charles Hewitt Moore in 1864. The patient, on whom this daring attempt was made, was under the care of Dr. Murchison; and although the latter eminent physician does not appear to have had much share in the arguments on behalf of the·proposal, it may well be that the joint publication even of an unsuccessful result under such auspices may have tended to give more currency to the method than it can be considered to deserve upon its merits—unless upon the very unsafe principle of "melius anceps remedium quam nullum." The argument on which this method is advocated by Mr. Moore, although ingeniously stated, is a rather crude one; inasmuch as it assumes that the mere increase of the coagulation of fibrin within an aneurysmal sac (apart altogether from the vital or physiological conditions under which the coagulation takes place) constitutes a genuine imitation of the natural processes of cure. The stratified deposits on the inside of the sac are regarded by Mr. Moore (as they are by every one else) in the light of a natural process making for cure; but they are (he says) insufficient for this purpose, inasmuch as, although the supply of fibrin in the blood is ample, "there is nothing on which it can settle except the wall; but any quantity which may collect on it (the inner lining of the sac) is almost invariably insufficient to resist the expansive force of the arterial current. In the centre of the aneurysm there is, meanwhile, a space full of blood, with fibrin ready to consolidate upon any apt material. . . . Therefore (it is necessary) to extend the surface on which fibrin may coagulate." The fallacy here is in the assumption that, provided a sufficient quantity of fibrin is coagulated, it is of no consequence, or at least of minor consequence, where and how the separation of the fibrin occurs. Accordingly, the practical course suggested is to introduce from without into the sac some foreign body, giving a large and complicated surface, to induce the coagulation and to attract the fibrin when separated. The "innocuousness" of metallic wire when used for sutures suggested it to Mr. Moore as the most suitable material for this purpose; and accordingly no less than twenty-eight yards of fine iron wire were introduced into the aneurysm in Dr. Murchison's case through a fine canula—the expectation being that "the wire would remain in the aneurysm, enveloped in clot, and be harmless." The operation occupied an hour, and presented no unforeseen difficulties; the immediate results are reported as favourable; but in less than twenty-four hours there were ominous symptoms of disaster, both local and general, portending inflammation of the sac, with rigors; and the patient died within five days after the operation, with all the evidences of septic or pyæmic infection. The case is very fully and faithfully reported, along with the necropsy; but, notwithstanding the attempt to extract from it some hope for the future of the operation, it seems rather surprising that it should have been ever repeated. Yet filipuncture, with various modifications in detail, has been adopted as a method of treatment in aneurysms both at home and abroad,—horse-hair, carbolised catgut, and other substances, having been employed as materials more likely than metals to be absorbed, or to remain innocuously, after the insertion has fulfilled its object; antiseptic precautions also being rigidly insisted upon. On the other hand, so much as seventy-four feet of silver wire were introduced in one case by Mr. Hulke. Baccelli advocated the use of watch-springs of several millimetres in breadth, and from 20 to 40 centimetres in length, to be projected into the sac and left there; but in the course of discussion M. Verneuil stated that among 34 cases known to have been treated by filipuncture, 30 had proved fatal within a year after the operation. The general opinion of the French Academy was unfavourable to it. M. Loreta, however, has recorded a case of aneurysm of the abdominal aorta in which, after laparotomy had been performed, seventy-two yards of silvered copper wire were inserted into the sac, with the result, apparently, of a very considerable consolidation and reduction in bulk. The author claims a cure, but the patient died on the ninety-second day after the operation from sudden rupture of the sac. This is perhaps the nearest approach to success after filipuncture that has been obtained.

Less dangerous than filipuncture, but also in all probability even less effective as ordinarily performed, is the introduction of needles into the sac of an aneurysm temporarily, so as to form centres for the coagulation of fibrin from the circulating blood. To this process allusion will be made later. Meanwhile, it may suffice to refer to Holmes (42) for many interesting details both as to this method and also as to the injection of liquid coagulating agents into the sac; a proceeding repeatedly attempted, without much success, in external aneurysms, but assuredly much more fraught with danger, and less likely to be successful in aortic aneurysms, than in those of the lesser trunks.

Galvano-puncture or electrolysis.—This method, first adopted by Benjamin Phillips in 1832, but owing its later reputation chiefly to Pétrequin, and Ciniselli (15, 16), has been, in recent times, specially recommended in aortic aneurysms; or in those altogether beyond the reach of other surgical procedures. A striking case of Ciniselli's, where a considerable aneurysm of the ascending aorta, projecting on the right side, and rapidly increasing, was arrested, and after ten weeks apparently cured, will be found in abstract in Holmes' *System of Surgery;* wherein also a very complete account is given of Ciniselli's method, with all details down to 1883. The method has obtained support chiefly in Italy; but in this country more recently Althaus, John Duncan, and M'Call Anderson have advocated it, and have claimed more or less successful results. In a case recorded by Dr. Anderson in a woman, aged 46, several operations were performed, the aneurysm being of the aorta and of considerable size. A progressive improvement was noted, and seven months later the external tumour was reduced to about a quarter of its former size, and was felt to be solid and only slightly pulsating. On the other hand, there are not wanting cases in which the electro-puncture of aneurysms was followed almost immediately by consequences which must act as a warning. Two such cases are briefly referred to by Dr. Sansom: in each of these the operation was performed by men of the most special qualifications and experience in electrical procedure; in each case great pain was experienced during the operation, and arterial blood spurted freely from the punctures; cellulitis supervened, and the patients succumbed within a few days. Probably the cases were not very favourable ones, the aneurysms having approached the surface, and being presumably not far removed, any way, from a fatal result. But Dr. Sansom has placed it on record as regards his own case, that —"It was my conviction that the patient's suffering was increased by the operation, and that the policy of non-interference would have been better." My own rather small experience is somewhat to the same effect. In three successive cases of large aneurysms nearing the surface (admittedly more or less progressive, and therefore not favourable for the operation) electrolysis was determined on as a last resort, and after consultation; care being taken that all the precautions and all the special experience and skill available were employed in the details of the manipulations. The result was that in all these three cases, occurring within a brief period, there was inflammatory action and ultimately leakage of blood, to a greater or less degree, at the points of puncture; and although these patients cannot be said to have absolutely died from hæmorrhage, they are still the only instances which I can recall to memory for a long series of years of actual rupture externally in aortic aneurysm. [Another case of external rupture, which proved fatal, has occurred to me since this was written, and will be mentioned p. 429.] The preparations are in the museum of the Glasgow Western Infirmary, and I feel bound to add that, like Dr. Sansom, I derived so little encouragement from the actual observation of these cases that I have never again recommended electro-puncture in aortic aneurysm. At the same time, it is only right to record that in 41 cases, treated and classified by Ciniselli, he freely admits that in those which projected beyond the thorax, or had eroded the bones and projected externally, little or no benefit resulted from electro-puncture as performed by him: " The aneurysms that give the best results are those that are entirely endothoracic, lateral (sacculated), of small or moderate size, and free from vessels arising out of the sac, or from valvular lesions ; that these beneficial effects are still appreciable where the aneurysm is partly lateral and partly cylindrical, if the dilata-tion of the whole artery is not great ; that they are merely transitory in the cylindrical form, or in those that are mainly cylindrical, or those which, though lateral, are of very large size ; and that no benefit can be anticipated in those which have increased to such an extent as to erode the bones and project through the thorax." The difficulty of applying these principles in advance is perhaps not inconsiderable ; but Ciniselli claims that in the cases belonging to the first order (22 out of 41) " all derived benefit in the form of diminution or disappearance of neuralgic pain, mitigation of dyspnœa, more regularity of circulation, power of lying on the opposite side to the aneurysm, restoration of calm-ness, sleep, general comfort, strength, and power of taking exercise. The tumour also became more solid and the pulsation less expansive. This amelioration was maintained in more than half the cases for a time varying from one to four years ; and was still continuing in two, operated on one four years, the other two years, before the report." In a much more extensive series of recorded cases treated by electrolysis Petit reckons that 68 out of 114 were improved. There are some differences as to procedure, more particularly as to whether the inserted needles should be connected only with the anode (or positive pole), or with both the anode and cathode in succession, as recommended by Ciniselli. But on all such purely surgical details the reader must be invited to refer to the authors here cited.

Professor Macewen's method—The production of white thrombi in organic connection with the inner wall of the aneurysm.—The following remarks, upon a method which may be considered as still in its infancy com-pared with some of those already mentioned, will be found, nevertheless, of great interest, as probably throwing a new light on the causes of failure, and thus pointing the way to better results which, so far as they are attainable, will apply to aortic as well as to other aneurysms, in respect of their principle. [It is perhaps only right to say here that I do not pretend to any personal experience of this method, but I have examined in Professor Macewen's private museum all the preparations to be here-after referred to.]

In an inaugural address by Professor Macewen, a method is pro-posed for the treatment of aneurysm which, while as yet no absolute and unqualified success can be claimed for it in the case of internal aneurysms, is founded nevertheless on principles applicable in a measure to them as well as to external tumours. Professor Macewen objects to most of the surgical methods hitherto adopted for promoting coagulation, that the thrombi thus produced—as, for example, in electrolysis or filipuncture, —are not formed in accordance with the natural laws of the healing process in aneurysms as known to us. A clot, which is formed after the manner of the crystallisation of salts around a nucleus in a saturated solution, is always more or less of a mere physico-chemical precipitate, and is not constituted to undergo those vital changes which adapt it for the permanent occlusion of an aneurysmal sac. Even when it is, as it must be, largely composed of fibrin, it is of fibrin loosely compacted, largely saturated with serum, and enclosing red corpuscles with a small proportion of leucocytes; formed, moreover, in a position having no relations with the wall of the vessel or of the aneurysm, and therefore lying like a foreign body in the midst of the blood current. Such a clot is, in short, essentially a "red thrombus"; and it is argued with great force that a thrombus so formed is not suitable for organisation, so as to permanently occlude or obliterate the sac. "As the fibrin contracts serum is exuded, the mass diminishes in bulk and, though at the outset it may have filled the sac, thereby producing occlusion, yet, owing to this shrinking, the blood stream may be re-established, especially when the walls of the aneurysm are not collapsible." The tendency of a "red thrombus, which is simply a mass devoid of vitality," is to undergo one of several changes, almost all of which are, as regards the permanent and safe occlusion of the aneurysmal sac, alike unfavourable, and some dangerous; either by way of embolisms or of septic infections, the result of red or yellow softening of the imperfectly vitalised thrombus, transmitted to distant parts. The alternative proposed is to proceed by "inducing the formation of white thrombi within the sac"—in contact with its wall, and tending to become incorporated with its structure, as occurs in the natural processes of spontaneous healing. Even in the "successful stray cases" which have given rise to a "half-hearted belief" in some of the lines of treatment before referred to, Dr. Macewen argues that the cure has really been accomplished not so much by the organisation of the "red thrombi" formed at the anode of the electric needle, or around the steel wire, horsehair, or other foreign body introduced into the sac, as by the more physiological process of irritation of the wall of the latter, determining the accretion to it of white thrombi, thus "setting up a reparative inflammatory process." The object of the new operation is to favour such a natural process of repair by simple means, without incurring the risks and the disadvantages of the formation of red thrombi at all. This process is necessarily slow and gradual; indeed, the slower the more sure it is in its result. "Leucocytes, derived partly from the vessel wall, but mainly by segregation from the blood stream, become firmly adherent to the vessel. When this process has been initiated it tends to grow by superimposed accretions, so that a parietal thrombus may proceed till complete occlusion occurs. . . . The white thrombus is prone to undergo replacement by vascularised fibrous tissue, the granular fibrin originally deposited being absorbed, and taking no share in the new formation." It might even be possible to suppose—as an "ideal result"—that an aneurysmal sac might thus be obliterated, while the lumen of the vessel was preserved, and a new endothelium was formed. But, as a general rule, the end to be looked to is the complete obliteration alike of the sac and of the artery. In the young, and with arterial walls as yet little degenerated, the reparative process goes on more rapidly; in the opposite case much more slowly. But in all cases it may be held that "the introduction of foreign bodies into the sac of an aneurysm in which the blood is freely circulating with the object of forming red thrombi, is not the most certain way of producing occlusion of the vessel. White thrombi are more suitable for permanent occlusion under such circumstances."

The surgical details of the operation proposed and the precautions necessary cannot be fully stated here. Dr. Macewen's first attempt in this direction was made in 1875, and is noticed in the *Glasgow Medical Journal* for 1876, and the *Lancet* for 1877. One or more pins, carefully rendered aseptic, are introduced into the sac and passed through the cavity, so that the point, or points, "just touch and no more" the opposite wall. "Then one of two methods may be employed—either to move the pin over the surface of the inner wall so as to irritate its surface, or to allow the impulse of the blood-current playing on the very thin pin to effect the same object. . . . The irritation ought to be just sufficient to set up reparative exudation, and must not exceed this. . . . After acting for ten minutes at one part the point of the pin, without being removed from the sac, ought to be shifted to another spot, and so on until the greater portion of the internal surface opposite to the point of entrance has been touched. This ought to be done in a methodical manner. The punctures from without may be made at one or at several points, as may be necessary to reach in detail the greater part of the surface. It is probable that a few hours only would be sufficient to effect all that is necessary from one insertion; but in no case ought a pin to remain in the sac for more than forty-eight hours. A retention of them for twenty-four or thirty-six hours seems to produce a greater effect than for a shorter period of time. Thickening of the coats of the aneurysm is usually to be discovered early, but not always. There is probably no immediate diminution of the eccentric impulse, and it may be days, or occasionally even weeks, before any tangible change can be made out. But a slow consolidation, especially in the deeper parts of the sac, is nevertheless going on, and every separate point at which irritation has taken place becomes a centre for the formation of thrombi, which tend to become gradually organised in layers. The natural process of repair is thus powerfully aided without its essential character being interfered with, or even, it may be, traversed, as in all proceedings tending to the formation of red thrombi. And this remark applies not only to electrolysis, etc., but to some apparently simpler proceedings, in which pins have been inserted with the view of directly arresting the circulation of blood through coagulation around their extremities while remaining within the sac."

Four cases are narrated. In the first of these a large aortic aneurysm, far advanced, and threatening death through repeated attacks of dyspnœa—one of which proved fatal a month after the treatment began—can only be considered as laying a foundation for the study of details, as revealed both during life and at the necropsy. A considerable amount of consolidation, however, took place, and hopes were entertained of still greater progress at the time of the fatal result, which was sudden, and had no connection with the proceedings employed. In the second case a very large femoral aneurysm, extending to the external iliac and measuring five inches in diameter, was completely cured. The patient died thirteen months afterwards from carcinoma of the tongue; and the necropsy disclosed no fewer than three aneurysms : namely (*a*), the one treated, completely obliterated and converted into "dense vascularised fibrous tissue"; (*b*) a small aneurysm of the opposite femoral, still pervious, and occupied by a red stratified thrombus, easily detached from the vessel wall; (*c*) a large aneurysm of the descending aortic arch. Both of these latter aneurysms were probably in a state of latency owing to the great exhaustion produced by the fatal disease; but they show the more strongly on that account the unfavourable conditions under which the cure was accomplished in the one sac subjected to treatment. The third case was an aneurysm of the abdominal aorta, presenting in the epigastric region, evidently of large size, and of a character and position which would have been a bar to any other kind of treatment beyond constitutional remedies. After only three applications of the operative treatment within a month, the tumour had greatly diminished, and the patient insisted on going back to his work. He remained in seeming good health two years and a half afterwards. The fourth and last case was one of intra-thoracic aneurysm, probably of left subclavian, accompanied by great swelling, pain, numbness, and loss of power in the left arm, treated by induction of white thrombi within the sac; the result being an apparent cure, with complete consolidation of the aneurysm, and restoration of function in the arm.

Professor Macewen allows me to add to the record of this last case as follows :—"September 1897.—This patient is still living, is constantly at work, and the aneurysm has entirely disappeared, so that the cure may now be regarded as absolute." Records of a number of cases of cure of aneurysm by this method reported in the medical journals have been shown to me.

Medical curative methods—Albertini and Valsalva.—The treatment of aneurysms, and especially of internal aneurysms, by constitutional methods has always been regarded as proceeding more or less on the lines of favouring, as much as possible, the natural processes of cure already adverted to. The pathology of aortic aneurysms came very gradually out of obscurity; and even in the time of Morgagni (1762) was far from being well understood. But it is to the unwritten precept of Valsalva, reported to us by Morgagni, that we owe the first reasoned attempt at a cure of this kind, which in one case, as there recorded, appears to have been successfully carried out; the patient having died afterwards of another disease, when the aneurysm was found shrunk and "callous." The essence of the treatment, now commonly called Valsalva's, as first reported to Morgagni by his friend Albertini, was to detain the patient very strictly in bed for forty days, and during this period to subject him to repeated bleedings, while at the same time the diet and drink were carefully ordered so that the daily allowance, administered in three or four meals, should never be such as to fill up the blood-vessels. "He made it a custom," says Morgagni, "to diminish the quantity of meat and drink more and more every day till it was brought down to half a pound of pudding in the morning, and in the evening half that quantity, and nothing else except water, and this also within a certain weight. After he had sufficiently reduced the patient by this method so that, by reason of weakness, he could scarcely raise his hand from the bed in which he lay, the quantity of aliment was increased again by degrees till the necessary strength returned, so as to allow of rising up." It is suggested that the pulsation in the aneurysm can be arrested entirely by this method; but even should the arrest not be quite complete at first, the disease may still be in course of cure, if. the patient will continue to submit to a modified and strict, but not quite so severe, regimen for some time to come. The difficulty in carrying out this treatment effectively, as stated by Morgagni (no doubt on the basis of Valsalva's experience, as well as his own), is that "there will be many to whom this method of cure may seem much more insufferable than the disease itself; especially at the only time when it can be of use (the beginnings of the aneurysm), when the inconveniences actually felt are slight, so that patients are easily led to delay until continual and grievous suffering, or even impending death itself, can no longer be avoided by any remedy whatever." The discussion that follows is very interesting; and may perhaps admit of the inference that failures of Valsalva's method were already well known in Morgagni's time, but were attributed (as failures usually are) to the remedy not having been adopted in time. But another inference follows even more clearly from this long discussion by the great pathologist of the seventeenth century, and from the cases submitted in illustration; namely, that, with all his respect (amounting almost to veneration) for Valsalva, Morgagni himself seems to have used the method very tentatively, and with no inconsiderable misgiving. For in one case of doubtful diagnosis, which is narrated at length, he gave a qualified opinion that under the whole circumstances venesection should not be omitted, "because we believed that, if it were of no advantage, it could be of no injury, inasmuch as he [the nobleman in question] was a man of firm strength, of a good habit of body, and had a good complexion for his youth. Moreover, as it was then the spring-time, blood-letting could be in no respect injurious, and would be particularly useful." The patient was enjoined to observe the effect on himself of the first blood-letting, and to have it repeated "before the end of the spring," only if he was convinced that it was of service to him ; a strict regimen (but not statedly that of Valsalva) being at the same time observed. This opinion of Morgagni, along with another senior physician's, was probably communicated in writing to the ordinary medical advisers, and was acted on to the extent (very limited, according to the ideas of that period) of taking upon one occasion eight ounces and on another six ounces of blood, "and no more." On this last occasion, however, "this nobleman immediately cried out that the surgeon had killed him," and fell into a succession of fainting fits, in the midst of which he died. Morgagni believed that the death was due not to the remedy, but to the internal rupture of the aneurysm; and he enters fully into the means which he adopted to protect the reputation of the surgeons in attendance, which had been popularly assailed. He regrets that there was no necropsy, but arrives at the general conclusion that this case "ought to be a caution to all practitioners not to compel patients to submit to any remedy to which they are utterly averse, especially in obscure diseases, whether the remedy is of great importance or has only the appearance of being so."

It would seem from these contemporary statements, which have been too often passed over in later references to the method of Valsalva, that its success, even according to its early advocates, was far from being well established ; this, too, at a time when blood-letting was largely and unhesitatingly practised in all acute diseases, and when the use of a precautionary or hygienic blood-letting "in the spring-time" in plethoric or robust subjects was still in complete accord with popular as well as medical opinion. What is chiefly surprising under these circumstances is that there are not many more well-authenticated instances of cure, or apparent cure, recorded under this method. Even the single case above referred to, and said to be confirmed by necropsy, (the only one, be it said, that is clearly attributed to Valsalva himself) has not escaped criticism. And if the evidence in this case be not conclusive, it is assuredly not strengthened by the instance of the "young nun" coupled with it by Morgagni, on the testimony of Stancario, in which a cure is claimed for Valsalva's method under circumstances which could hardly have seemed to deserve the notice taken of them but for Morgagni's courteous recognition of the worth and credibility of his informant. Indeed, it remains doubtful, even now, if there is a single case of well-authenticated cure of an aneurysm by Valsalva's treatment in all that has reached us from Morgagni's time in the records of the eighteenth century. Still, as a theoretically reasonable method (though admittedly difficult of execution) it continued to hold its own in virtue of the great names under which it was at first propounded ; and it was more or less supported during the present century by such authors as Corvisart, Laennec, Chomel, and others. Some of these (as Chomel and Pelletau) advocated much larger blood-lettings than probably would have been recommended by Valsalva, and at longer intervals ; others, again, among whom Hope in this country may be enumerated, were in favour of small and more frequently repeated losses of blood. Within my own recollection the only deliberate attempt to follow in the footsteps of Valsalva that has come to my knowledge is that recorded by the late Professor Hughes Bennett who treated two cases in Edinburgh, one of which is recorded in great detail, while the other is more briefly alluded to (9). In both these cases relief to certain symptoms is said to have followed the bleedings, which in the first case were large and frequently repeated; the treatment being carried on over two years and a half, and regulated in detail according to the symptoms : the relief was (it is said) "so evident as to strike all who witnessed it, and to cause the patient continually to request that he might be bled." The case is a most instructive one, for there were in fact two aneurysms, one abdominal and one thoracic; the former of which only was known to exist during life. This one appeared to have undergone consolidation to a marked extent, and was supposed (not unnaturally) to be yielding to the treatment; while the other and much larger thoracic aneurysm was pursuing a fatal course in advance, and by its enormous size (absorbing and diffusing the cardiac impulse) it may very probably have caused in a great measure the diminished pulsation and the consolidation within the smaller sac. It is sufficiently obvious, from the account given of this case, that the circumstances were far too complicated to make much for evidence of efficacy of the Valsalva treatment (as indeed Bennett himself admits). The other case was treated apparently more exactly after Valsalva's instruction for forty days, at the end of which time the patient "walked out of the house, with little assistance, to the nearest cab-stand, and left the city." Evidently neither of these cases can be claimed as a cure of aortic aneurysm, in the ordinary sense of the word. The patients in both cases were refractory; and there is reason to believe that the one who was longest under treatment poisoned himself wilfully at last by swallowing a liniment of aconite. While fully recognising the benefits of the treatment, therefore, in the way of temporarily relieving symptoms, Dr. Bennett, as the result of his experience, maintains that Valsalva's treatment cannot be fully carried out in hospital, "or indeed in any circumstances, without a degree of surveillance which it would be very difficult to obtain."

The Bellingham and Tufnell treatment.—This method, which has enjoyed considerable reputation under the latter of the two names given above, may be regarded as a modification of the Albertini-Valsalva method in accordance with the views of the present century, and with the experience gained by the Irish surgeons of the treatment of external aneurysms by compression. The principles of the method were first clearly stated in a paper (8) read before the Surgical Society of Ireland in 1852 by Dr. Bellingham, upon two very remarkable cases, the first of which had been carefully watched for three years, and the second for a shorter time. Dr. Bellingham died before he was able to make any further contribution to the subject; but Mr. Tufnell, who was associated with him in these early efforts, continued to employ the method "with such a degree of success [he records] as I believe has been unprecedented under any other mode previously attempted." Mr. Tufnell's small monograph published in 1875 refers to eleven cases, in most of which the evidence of arrest in the progress of the disease, if not of complete cure, is well made out; and, with Dr. Bellingham's two cases already referred to, it forms a very notable contribution to the therapeutics of aneurysm as the result of over twenty years' experience. One of the cases recorded by Tufnell is not, indeed, an aneurysm of the aorta, but of the popliteal artery; it is, however, not the least remarkable of the series, inasmuch as the military surgeon who furnished the facts to Mr. Tufnell claims to have cured the disease "by rest and restricted diet in twelve days," without any surgical interference whatever; the case having been under observation for three years at the time of the record. "What surgeon a few years ago," adds Mr. Tufnell, "would have believed that popliteal aneurysm could have been so cured? Yet, so it is."

The principles of the method are admirably stated by Dr. Bellingham in connection with a brief historic retrospect extending from Valsalva downwards. He altogether repudiates (unless in "a very few cases") the use of blood-letting as a part of the treatment; seeing that it tends to defibrinate the blood, to cause anæmia, and at the same time, by unduly exhausting the patient, to quicken the circulation. The true indications to be followed are: (i.) To diminish the distending force of the blood from within (and above all, to diminish the frequency as much as possible of the heart's beats); (ii.) To favour the deposition of fibrine on the walls of the sac; (iii.) To maintain this process until the sac is filled up, and thus obliterated; (iv.) To bring about these results without deteriorating the quality of the blood, or diminishing too much the patient's strength. The whole of these indications are confessedly based upon the knowledge of the modes in which the spontaneous cure of aneurysm is occasionally brought about; and, in addition, upon direct observation of the effects of compression in external aneurysms, whereby the distending force of the blood is controlled, and the quantity of blood transmitted through the sac is greatly diminished. "In external aneurysm these objects can be effected by compressing the artery upon the cardiac side; in aneurysm of the aorta we can only effect them indirectly by acting upon the general circulation."

Hence the paramount importance of *rest*. "As exercise has the effect of quickening the heart's action, and rest has the opposite effect, and tends to quiet the circulation, absolute rest of body and mind are indispensable as preliminaries." Mr. Tufnell, who insists not less than his predecessor upon rest as of primary importance, calculates that if by merely maintaining the horizontal position the number of pulsations can be reduced by thirty in the minute, this will correspond with a diminution in the number of cardiac impulses amounting to no less than 43,200 in twenty-four hours. In any case the diminished number of the beats is, when exercise of the limbs and muscles is withdrawn, accompanied by a diminution also in the force of the individual beats. So that on every ground the recumbent position for a long period, and as little disturbance as possible, even for the most pressing bodily wants, is even a more essential part of the method presently under consideration than in that attributed to Valsalva. But the use of frequent venesections carried to the point of absolute prostration is objected to, by both Bellingham and Tufnell, as being really opposed to the end in view.

The length of time during which recumbency is to be maintained is variously stated. Bellingham only indicates that the patient should be "confined to bed during a portion, at least, of the period that the treatment (dietetic) lasts." Tufnell, on the other hand, insists on "two months or ten weeks at least, and this period to be passed without the patient, if possible, sitting even once erect." (Dr. George Balfour has even gone much further than this, and has insisted on recumbency being maintained for many months.) All the arrangements of detail must be accommodated to this primary necessity. A "light, cheerful, and airy room ; a special attendant, always at hand to offer such aid as the patient may require ; to read, to converse with, or amuse him, are insisted on. The bed must be constructed and arranged so that the evacuations can be withdrawn without disturbance. Upon the bedstead must be placed two hair mattresses, one upon the other, both full and elastic. Upon these (in proper site to receive the sacrum and hips) a large water cushion properly but not over-filled ; upon this, a double blanket sewn at the corners and sides to the lower mattress, and upon the blanket a fine linen sheet similarly attached, to prevent all wrinkling in the bed and disturbance of the sheet ; another linen sheet (folded as after a lithotomy operation) laid transversely to receive the buttocks, and to be drawn from beneath them from time to time. On this bed, when once comfortably settled, the individual must be content to lie without changing his position further than to turn from side to side, or occasionally round upon his face, should such movement give relief to the dorsal pain, as it sometimes will" (Tufnell).

The rest of this treatment is mainly dietetic. Bellingham, indeed, discountenances almost all the medicinal remedies that had been in use up to his time. "I am neither an advocate for bleeding nor purgatives (except occasionally if required), nor for diuretics or digitalis, or for any of the other medicines which have been used in this disease, with the exception of opium, and this only when sleep is prevented by pain." Tufnell is not quite so rigid ; but there is nothing in his remarks to counteract the above principle ; and it must be sufficiently obvious that disturbing remedies of any kind are opposed to the primary condition so much insisted on. The dietetic treatment and the whole regimen, according to Bellingham, "consists in limiting the patients for a given period to the smallest quantity of fluid possible ; in diminishing considerably, likewise, the solid aliment ; in confining the patient at the same time to bed, and endeavouring to maintain the mind in as tranquil a state as possible. . . . I do not think we shall be able to effect much unless precise directions are laid down. I would limit the patient to three meals a day, the morning and evening meal to consist of two ounces of liquid and the same of solid nutriment; the midday meal of from two to four ounces of liquid, with from two to four ounces of solid. The liquid may consist of milk or tea, the solid of bread; and at the midday meal, of bread and meat in equal quantities. No deviation from this dietary should be permitted, and it must be persevered in for a fixed period—six weeks or a month at least, when it may gradually be improved." Tufnell's dietary varies a little in detail, and is perhaps a little less exacting, but the principle is the same. " For breakfast, two ounces of white bread and butter, with two ounces of cocoa or milk. For dinner, three ounces of broiled or boiled meat, with three ounces of potatoes or bread, and four ounces of water or light claret. For supper, two ounces of bread and butter, and two ounces of milk or tea, making in the aggregate ten ounces of solid and eight of fluid food in the twenty-four hours, *and no more.*" He adds in a note, however, that in some irritable constitutions this restriction of diet cannot be tolerated, and must be relaxed. Thirst, if severely felt, is to be met by " holding a pebble in the mouth to favour the secretion of saliva, or by sucking from time to time a small portion of ice."

Summary of medical treatment—Iodide of potassium.—In what remains to be stated here concerning the medical and medicinal treatment of aortic aneurysm, I shall not occupy space with details which, however important, may be reasonably regarded as the application of general medical and therapeutic knowledge to particular circumstances incidentally arising, not in aneurysm only, but in many other forms of disease also. The relief of pain; the control of conditions evidently spasmodic, such as are referred to above; the remedies for cardiac collapse or failure occurring in particular cases; even the treatment of pulmonary engorgement or impending asphyxia, of cyanosis, of localised dropsies, and so forth, do not in any essential particular differ from the course of treatment needed under like circumstances of various origin. All that is special in the application to aneurysm will be easily enough inferred from the general statement that, while we are dealing with a too generally fatal, and often incurable, organic disease, the physician who has carefully adverted to the natural processes of cure, and who has had personal experience of more or less favourable changes occurring even in the most unpromising cases, will be in a position to use these and other palliative resources with the greatest amount of intelligence, and, within certain limits, of hope for a good result. Even as I write these lines a case has proved fatal in the Western Infirmary of Glasgow, of which it may fairly be said that the marvel is, not that the patient has succumbed, but that she was able to survive so long, and to pass through so many phases of betterment and relapse, under what in a pathological sense appear to have been the most adverse possible conditions. In this case (Eliz. Y., æt. 43, Ward VI. Journal L. 1898) the aneurysm occupied a large area in the front of the arch, the orifice between the artery and the sac being such as would easily have passed a small orange. The whole of the thoracic aorta was a mass of atheroma ; and so numerous were the points at which tumour had appeared externally in the progress of the case, that the suggestion arose — supported considerably by the symptoms — that a plurality of tumours, some of which might very probably have been beyond the arch, might have existed. Pulsating tumour, however, was detected in the front of the thorax more than four years before the patient's death by external hæmorrhage ; and the absolute duration of the disease must have been indefinitely longer than this. Without going into details, it may be stated in general terms that on two or three occasions during the above period well-marked subsidence and induration of the portions of the aneurysm most directly under observation had undoubtedly taken place; and a tumour at one time extending upwards in the neck so as greatly to hamper the movements of the head, and described as being $4\frac{1}{2}$ inches in diameter, and as extending almost to the angle of the jaw, receded so much as to be hardly observed in the neck at all. At one time, too, the pulsation even in the part of the vast tumour which had eroded the manubrium sterni is described as having been barely perceptible ; and the relief from the cruel and agonising sufferings experienced in the earlier part of the history was so great, that she had absolutely been able (I presume without a medical examination) to enrol herself in a well-known benefit or insurance society as an average or healthy life. The autopsy showed that, notwithstanding the constant and very direct impulses which must have been going on from a by no means greatly weakened heart through an aperture in the vessel of enormous size even in proportion to the tumour, two-thirds of the latter were occupied by thrombi, in some places, it is true, rather loosely compacted, but in others firm and stratified, with suggestion of most persistent efforts at spontaneous healing. And although both rest and dieting, with iodide of potassium, had been employed in the long course of the treatment, it was not easy, in view of the details, to ascribe to any of these, or to all of them together, more than a very subordinate influence in bringing about these results. The case, as regards the mode of its fatal termination, belongs, as already said, to the very great rarities of my personal experience ; on the other hand, the subsidence and relative solidification of aneurysmal tumours when very near the point of rupture externally has been not infrequently observed.

There is, however, one internal remedy which demands attention in respect of the claims made for it of being something more than a palliative, and even, as regards aneurysm, something of the nature of a specific. Iodide of potassium, widely employed in aneurysms of the aorta of late years, mainly through the strenuous advocacy of Dr.

George W. Balfour, has so far fulfilled expectation that few intelligent practitioners for the last quarter of a century have felt justified in neglecting it; and my own experience very fully supports what has been said of it on the side of its practical benefits. According to the very complete and instructive history given by Dr. Balfour in the third edition, just published, of his well-known work, Graves, Nélaton, and Chuckerbutty of Calcutta had been separately and independently led, almost by accident, to observe that in certain painful affections, reputed to be muscular or nervous in origin, relief in a quite remarkable degree appeared to follow the administration of this drug; and also that even the pains of aneurysm might in some cases be so relieved, without any danger or even serious disadvantage from the toxic effects of the remedy. With Dr. Balfour himself the first suggestion of the remedy was in like manner accidental, from its having been prescribed on one occasion for a rheumatic affection, but in a man having a large aortic aneurysm, who obtained unexpected relief from the symptomatic pains of this disease. It is due to Dr. Balfour, however, to state that in working out experimentally the inferences from this happy experience, he has succeeded in establishing much that is of the highest therapeutic importance; even if it should appear that the principle of the treatment is not so clear and undeniable as is the fact of its very great superiority in kind to the *farrago remediorum* employed more or less empirically in aneurysm, as in most other diseases hard to cure. In the first three cases in hospital elaborately recorded by Dr. Balfour, the remedy was employed in doses varying from 60 to 90 grs. a day; and it was only in one of the three that these large quantities had to be temporarily suspended on account of iodism. It is consistent also with my experience that a marked toleration of the remedy often exists in the very cases in which it gives the most relief; and that 30 grs. three times a day will be easily borne for months together without intermission, and with the most striking relief to the symptoms; sometimes also, but not always, with positive diminution in the bulk of very large tumours. At the same time, it is not to be denied that there is in some cases less easy tolerance of the drug; and Dr. Balfour's later experience—even apart from his theory—has led him to use the iodide in a more tentative manner. The patient is to be kept in bed for a few days at the beginning without further treatment, in order to obtain an accurate note of the habitual pulse-rate; and then 10 grs. of potassium iodide are to be given every eight hours. "If the pulse-rate remains unchanged, the dose of the iodide may be increased in a few days up to 15 or more grains every eight hours, raising it by one grain in each dose until the pulse-rate begins to rise. It is but rarely that we can increase the dose to fifteen grains without raising the pulse-rate; indeed it is common enough not to be able to increase the dose beyond ten grains without this taking place. Should the pulse-rate rise the iodide is stopped for one or two days, and then we go back to the highest dose that did not raise the pulse, and continue with that dose. When the iodide has been given in this way the success attained has been quite remarkable; the cessation of pain, the lessening of the pulsation, and the general improvement have been so marked and so rapid as to leave no doubt that this is the true method of administration" (p. 469). Dr. Balfour further says, that in all his experience he has only twice encountered complete intolerance of the iodide. In one of these cases, in which a " copious herpetic eruption—so-called hydroa " —constantly followed the administration, the action of the iodide on the disease (aneurysm) " was markedly ameliorative ;" as, indeed, it seemed to be in the other case also, in which, however, " the very smallest dose gave rise to rapid pulse and to severe neuralgic pains in the abdomen " (p. 471).[1]

As regards the mode of the remedial action, Dr. Balfour has been led to adopt a view differing essentially from that of Chuckerbutty, Roberts, and others; namely, that, through some unknown action of potassium iodide directly on the blood, it favours the coagulation of fibrin, and so conduces to the formation of thrombi in the sac. No such action, he says, has been proved; on the other hand, in more than one of the cases in which the apparent solidification and the diminished pulsation of the sac were most evident, it was demonstrated that no thrombi, but only post-mortem clots, existed. As a matter of fact, therefore, the solidification in these cases could not have been due to coagulation within the sac, but must have been owing to an action of the remedy on the walls of the aneurysm. Here, again, no direct influence of the iodide on the tissues composing the wall can be proved; but an indirect action may possibly be admitted, if, as is said to be experimentally established (Bogolepoff), " one of the chief actions of potassium iodide is to lower the blood tension uniformly throughout the body by dilating the arterioles, the heart's action being at the same time diminished in force" (4, p. 468). The most probable explanation, therefore, according to Balfour, of the therapeutic power of the iodide is to be found in the fact that by lowering the cardiac and vascular tension it arrests or greatly modifies the dilatation of the sac at each stroke of the heart, and thereby brings into operation again

---

[1] In the last edition (1898) of Professor Whitla's *Pharmacy, Materia Medica, and Therapeutics*, p. 345, I find the following suggestion as regards chloride of calcium, a remedy not hitherto in use, so far as I am aware, in the treatment of aneurysm, and not known to me till the text of this article was in type :—" It markedly increases for a time the coagulability of the blood, and Dr. Wright has administered it in doses of 15 to 30 grs., with the view of causing coagulation of the blood in aneurysmal sacs. In one case treated at Netley for abdominal aneurysm by this method, and afterwards, at Dr. Wright's suggestion, treated upon the same plan by the writer, great improvement occurred ; and when the patient was discharged from hospital, pulsation had almost entirely disappeared, and the tumour had very markedly diminished in size." The paper here referred to (by Professor Wright of Netley) on the clinical determination of the coagulability of the blood by a new and simple method, and on the effect of lime salts on the time of coagulation, is a most ingenious one, and will be found in the *British Med. Journal*, 1893, vol. ii. p. 223. More recently still, and after the proofs of this article had been finally corrected, a cure of abdominal aneurysm is said to have been obtained by the continuous administration of *proto-nuclein*. See the *New York Medical Journal* for September 1898.

the "natural elasticity of the arterial coats," which "contract the sac temporarily, and by and by this contraction is strengthened and made permanent by the hypertrophy of these coats, and mainly of the *adventitia*" (4, p. 438).

Whatever view may be taken of the cogency of these arguments (which should be read in connection with the whole of the details presented), I fully believe that we have in iodide of potassium a remedy which ought to be carefully and deliberately employed in most, if not in all, cases of aneurysm of the aorta, in aid of the other and occasionally spontaneous healing processes already discussed. I fear it must also be admitted that, after all is done, the treatment will only too often disappoint expectation; while, on the other hand, the surprising instances of arrest for long periods, and even of apparent cure occasionally, tend to keep up hope even at the worst. The future treatment of this formidable disease, therefore, will probably consist in some combination of these various methods: complete rest, in the great majority of cases, for a period at least of weeks; with some modification of the diet in the Bellingham-Tufnell direction, but not such as to produce great suffering or seriously to weaken the patient; careful avoidance of alcoholic drinks as a rule; regulation of the bowels, but only so far as to avoid constipation and straining; and, in general, the use of palliatives for symptoms incidentally arising, and especially for very severe pain, dyspnœa (spasmodic or continuous), and hæmorrhage. To deal with these means in detail would lead us far beyond the possibilities of this article, already prolonged in excess of the limits originally assigned to it.

The very latest alleged cure of aneurysm by medical means, one which has been the subject of frequent discussions in the Académie de médecine since these pages were corrected finally for the press, is that advocated by Lancereaux and Paulesco: "Treatment of aneurysms in general, and of aneurysm of the aorta in particular, by subcutaneous injections of a gelatinous solution." Under the circumstances above stated, the following detailed references only can be inserted here: *Bulletin de l'académie de médecine*, 1897, vol. xxxvii. p. 784; and 1898, vol. xl. pp. 241, 313, 336, 353, 419, 426, 577.

W. T. GAIRDNER.

REFERENCES

1. ALLBUTT, T. CLIFFORD. *St. George's Hospital Reports*, 1871, vol. v. p. 49.—2. ANDERSON, M'CALL. *Clinical Medicine*, 1877.—3. BACCELLI. *Acad. de méd. Paris*, Jan. 28, 1878.—4. BALFOUR, G. W. *Clinical Lectures on Diseases of the Heart and Aorta*, 3rd edit. 1898, Lecture 17.—5. BARWELL. *Med.-Chir. Trans.*, vol. lxviii. p. 133.—6. BEATTY. *Dublin Hospital Reports*, vol. vi. 1830.—7. BEGBIE, WARBURTON. *Edin. Med. Journ.* June 1863.—8. BELLINGHAM, O'BRYEN. "On the Curative Treatment of Aneurysm of the Aorta, with Cases," *Dublin Medical Press*, vol. xxvii. p. 81.—9. BENNETT, J. H. *Principles and Practice of Medicine*, 5th edit. 1849, p. 626.—10. BIZOT. *Mémoires de la société médicale d'observation*, tome i. 1837.—11. BRAMWELL. *Diseases of Heart and Thoracic Aorta*, 1884, p. 285.—12. BRISTOWE. *Theory and Practice of Medicine.*—13. BROWNE, OSWALD. *Thesis for M.D. Cantab.*, 1897.—14. CHARCOT and BALL. *Dict. des sciences médicales*, v. p. 561.—

15. CINISELLI. *Gazette des hôpitaux*, 1868.—16. *Idem. L'elettrolisi e le sue applicazioni terapeutiche*, 1880.—17. COATS. *Manual of Pathology*, 3rd edit. 1895, p. 484.—18. COATS and AULD. *Journal of Pathology and Bacteriology*, July 1896.—19. COLZI. *Lo sperimentale*, Feb. 1, 1895.—20. COOPER, Sir ASTLEY. *Surgical Essays*, vol. i. p. 128.—21. DAVIDSON. *Lancet*, vol. ii. 1891, p. 1436 ; vol. i. 1892, p. 435.—22. DRUMMOND, D. *British Medical Journal*, 1893, Aug. 5, p. 299.—23. *Edin. Med. Journal*, June 1878, p. 1076.—24. *Edin. Monthly Journal of Medical Science* (remarks by Mr. Syme in discussion Med.-Chir. Soc. of Edinburgh, including a written statement by Mr. Ramsay, surgeon at Broughty Ferry), vol. x. p. 89.—25. EWART. *British Medical Journal*, 1892, vol. i. p. 596.—26. *Idem. Lancet*, June 15 and 22, 1889. — 27. *Idem. Lancet*, Aug. 17, 1889.—28. *Idem. Lancet*, 1891, vol. i. p. 429.—29. FINLAYSON. *British Medical Journal*, 3rd March 1883, p. 403.—29a. *Idem. Glasgow Medical Journal*, April 1896, p. 298. — 30. GAIRDNER. *The Clinical Journal*, 1892, vol. i. p. 97 ; vol. vi. p. 235.—31. *Idem.* "The Early Symptoms of Aneurysm of the Aorta, as anticipating Physical Diagnosis," *International Clinics*, 1894, vol. iv. p. 34. Philadelphia.—32. *Idem. Clinical Medicine : Observations recorded at the Bedside, with Commentaries*, pp. 455-477, 509. Edinburgh, 1862.—33. *Idem. Lancet*, vol. i. 1889, p. 1233.—34. *Idem. Lancet*, June 15 and 22, 1889.—35. *Idem. Monthly Journal of Medical Science*, Jan. 1855, p. 71 ; *Edin. Medical Journal*, Aug. 1855, p. 143 ; *Clinical Medicine*, 1862, pp. 526, 554.—36. *Idem. Trans. Royal Med. and Chir. Soc.* vol. xlii. p. 189.—37. *Idem. Glasgow Medical Journal*, 1890, p. 463.—38. GIBSON. *International Clinics*, 1896-97, vol. ii. p. 52.—39. GRIMSDALE. *Practitioner*, vol. xlviii. p. 96.—39a. HAYDEN. *Diseases of the Heart and Aorta*, 1875.—40. HEATH, CHRISTOPHER. *Lancet*, Jan. 25, 1867.—41. HODGSON. *Treatise on the Disease of Arteries and Veins, containing the Pathology and Treatment of Aneurysm, etc.* London, 1815.—42. HOLMES. *System of Surgery*, 3rd edit. 1883, vol. iii. p. 147.—43. *Idem.* Vol. iii. p. 118, *et seq.*—44. *Idem.* Vol. iii. p. 145.—45. *Idem.* Vol. iii. pp. 80-82.—46. *Idem. Lancet*, Oct. 10, 1874. —47. *Idem. System of Surgery*, iii. 76-79.—48. JOHNSON, Sir GEORGE. *Med.-Chir. Trans.* vol. lviii. p. 38.—49. KELYNACK. *Lancet*, July 1897.—50. LAW. *Dublin Journal of Medical Science*, 1842, vol. xxi. p. 450 ; 1844, vol. xxv.—51. LÉPINE. "Traitement des aneurysmes par la méthode de Moore," *Semaine médicale*, 1887, p. 213.—52. M'CRORIE. "Atheromatous Disease of Arteries," *Glasgow Medical Journal*, 1892. —53. MACEWEN, Prof. *Lancet*, 1890, vol. ii. p. 1086.—54. MACINTYRE, JOHN. *Lancet*, 23rd May 1896.—55. MACKENZIE and HEAD. *Brain*, vol. xvi.—56. *Med.-Chir. Soc. of Glasgow*, 6th Dec. 1895.—57. MOORE, CHARLES HEWITT. *Med.-Chir. Trans.* 1864, vol. xlvii.—58. MORGAGNI. "De Sedibus et Causis Morborum per Anatomen indagatis," *Epist.* xvii. 30, 31.—59. MURRAY, WM. (*a*) "An Account of a Case of Aneurysm of the Abdominal Aorta, which was cured by Compression of that Artery immediately above the Tumour by the rapid method ;" communicated by the late Charles H. Moore, F.R.C.S. ; read 24th May 1864, *Med.-Chir. Trans.* 1864. (*b*) "The rapid Cure of Aneurysm by Pressure, illustrated by the Case of Mark Wilson, cured of Aneurysm of the Abdominal Aorta in the year 1864," (*c*) *Brit. Med. Jour.* 5th October 1867 ; where also two cases (not of aortic or abdominal aneurysms, however) by Dr. Mapother are reported to the British Medical Association meeting in Dublin, together with an interesting discussion on the subject, in which Mr. Collis, Mr. Earnest Hart, Dr. Geoghegan, and others took part. — 60. MYERS, A. B. R. *Diseases of the Heart among Soldiers.* — 61. NELIGAN. *Diseases of Heart and Aorta*, p. 582.—62. NEWMAN. "A Lecture on some Points in relation to the Diagnostic Significance and Therapeutic Indications of Laryngeal Symptoms resulting from Pressure of Aneurysms upon the Vagus and Recurrent Laryngeal Nerves," *Brit. Med. Jour.* July 2, 1887. [A later communication to the meeting of the Brit. Med. Assoc. Edin., will be found in the *Glas. Med. Jour.*, August 1898.—63. OGLE, JOHN. *Trans. Med. and Chir. Soc. Lond.* 1858, vol. xli. p. 397.—64. OLIVER. *Lancet*, vol. ii. 1878, p. 406.—65. ORD. *Lancet*, vol. i. 1891, p. 429.—66. PEACOCK. *Path. Trans.* vol. xiv. p. 87.—67. PÉTREQUIN. *Comptes Rendus*, 1845.—68. PHILIPSON. *Brit. Med. Jour.* 1878, vol. i. p. 331.—69. POURFOUR DU PETIT. *Histoire de l'academie royale des sciences*, an 1727. — 70. REID, Prof. JOHN. *Edin. Med. and Surg. Journ.* vol. xlix. p. 132 ; vol. lii. p. 36.—71. *Idem. Medical Gazette*, September 29, 1838.—72. ROBERTSON, ARGYLL. *Edin. Med. Journ.* vol. xiv. p. 696 ; vol. xv. p. 487.—73. ROSS. *Lancet*, 1891, vol. i.—74. ROSS and MACDONNELL. *Lancet*, vol. i. 1891, pp. 535, 650.—75. SANSOM. *Twentieth Century*

Practice of Medicine, vol. iv. pp. 490, 492.—76. *Idem. Diagnosis of Diseases of the Heart and Thoracic Aorta*, 1892, p. 249.—76a. SEMON. In the present work, vol. iv. p. 841.—77. SMITH, Sir THOMAS. *Path. Trans.* vol. xxiii. p. 74.—78. THOMSON, CAMPBELL. *Lancet*, 10th Oct. and 12th Dec. 1896.—79. TODD. *Lancet*, June 1841, p. 400.—80. PAUL. *Trans. Path. Soc. Lond.* vol. xxxvii. p. 173. — 81. WILKS. *Trans. Path. Soc. Lond.* vol. xvi. p. 77 (woodcut at p. 78).—82. *Trans. Path.* vol. xxi. p. 132.—83. TUFNELL, JOLLIFFE. *The Successful Treatment of Internal Aneurysm by Consolidation of the Contents of the Sac.* London, 1875.—84. VOGT, P. "Aneurysma," *Real-Encyclopädie der gesammten Heilkunde*, vol. i. p. 295.—85. WALSHE, W. H. *Diseases of Heart*, 4th edit.—86. WALSH. *The Röntgen Rays in Medical Work*, 1897, p. 105.—87. WILLIAMS, CHAS. J. B. *The Case of the late Earl of St. Maur.* Lond. 1870.—88. WILLIAMS, FRANCIS H. *Trans. Assoc. of American Physicians*, 1897, vol. xxii. p. 330.—89. WILSON. *British Medical Journal*, 1895, vol. ii. p. 184.—90. WYLLIE. *Edin. Hospital Reports*, vol. i. p. 67.

W. T. G.

ANEURYSMS OF ARTERIES IN THE ABDOMEN

Aneurysms of the limbs come into the domain of surgery and are not considered here ; aneurysms of the pulmonary, coronary, and cerebral vessels are described elsewhere. Aneurysms of the branches of the abdominal aorta are comparatively rare and require but a brief description.

ANEURYSM OF THE BRANCHES OF THE CŒLIAC AXIS.—As already mentioned, the occurrence of an aneurysm of the abdominal aorta close to the origin of the cœliac axis, or involving it, is by no means un-frequent ; but aneurysms on the branches of the cœliac axis are very uncommon.

ANEURYSMS OF THE HEPATIC ARTERY have been recorded in about twenty-six instances, but examination of Metropolitan and other museums would increase the number of published cases ; thus there is a large hepatic aneurysm, the size of a cocoa-nut, in the Museum of Surgeons' Hall, Edinburgh, and another the size of a turkey's egg in the Museum of St. George's Hospital.

These aneurysms may be due to septic embolism ; and from the comparatively unsupported condition of the visceral arteries in the abdominal cavity, simple non-infective embolism is more likely to be followed by aneurysm in them than in other situations ; except, perhaps, in the circle of Willis, where the arteries lie on a yielding water-bed, the subarachnoid space. Injury has been noted as a cause of hepatic aneurysm ; thus Mester's patient was kicked in the abdomen by a horse.

A very interesting specimen of an aneurysm, the size of a walnut, was found by the late Dr. Pearson Irvine inside an abscess in the left lobe of the liver; here the aneurysm was produced by inflammation and ulceration of the outer coats of the artery in the same way that aneurysms are formed in vomicæ during the course of pulmonary tuberculosis. Intrahepatic aneurysms have, however, attracted very little attention, and are indeed very rarely seen.

In most cases of hepatic aneurysm there is no evidence of embolism or traumatism; and yet these factors seem more probable than mere chronic endarteritis, for the small superficial arteries in other parts of the body, such as the radial or temporal, though badly supported and frequently atheromatous, rarely undergo aneurysmal dilatation, save from embolism or injury. Perhaps in some instances the cause of the embolus, such as a calcareous plate from the aorta, has been overlooked, or has passed away before the patient's death. Still in many instances no antecedent condition, except endarteritis, is recorded.

Symptoms of hepatic aneurysm.—Pain is nearly always present, and may be taken for that of biliary colic; in fact "pseudo-biliary" colic may be due to the pressure of the aneurysm on the bile-ducts.

Jaundice, from pressure on the bile-ducts, very frequently occurs, though the jaundice may be slight and not appear until late in the course of the disease.

Aneurysm and new growth on the portal fissure behave, in a miniature fashion, just as the corresponding lesions in the anterior mediastinum with regard to the adjacent venous trunks. Aortic aneurysm rarely causes pressure symptoms on the superior vena cava, while mediastinal growth frequently does. In the same way aneurysm of the hepatic artery, though it may push the portal vein aside, does not obliterate it or give rise to ascites.

Hepatic aneurysm may perforate into the peritoneum and give rise to fatal collapse. Usually it ruptures into some part of the bile-ducts, and the blood thus poured out passes into the alimentary canal and may be vomited, or more often passed by the bowel alone; repeated leakage and hæmorrhages may occur before a fatal one. Rupture of the aneurysm may take place into the hepatic or common bile-ducts, the gall-bladder, colon, and possibly stomach.

A pulsating tremor may be felt in the epigastrium, but this is most likely to be regarded as an abdominal aortic aneurysm, which may also press on the common bile-duct, producing jaundice, and by perforating into the duodenum give rise to melæna.

Aneurysm of the hepatic artery, as in a case recorded by Ledieu, may obstruct the circulation in its branches. Osler refers to a remarkable case, in which aneurysm of the hepatic artery was associated with multiple hepatic abscesses.

Diagnosis is very difficult. Most of the cases have been regarded as examples of duodenal ulcer or cholelithiasis, while, as mentioned above, an aneurysm of the aorta in this region may resemble an aneurysm of the hepatic artery.

ANEURYSMS OF THE SPLENIC ARTERY are rare; rather less than twenty have been put on record. The artery is one that is véry prone to atheroma, and small aneurysms may occur on it, and, giving rise to no symptoms, be found accidentally at the autopsy. The larger ones may rupture into the stomach, into the transverse colon, or into the peritoneal cavity. Osler's case, in which the colon was perforated by the aneurysm, simulated a gastric ulcer.

ANEURYSMS OF THE CORONARIA VENTRICULI ARTERY, or of the other arteries supplying the stomach, like aneurysms of the other branches of the cœliac axis, are very rare; about ten have been published.

They may be due to embolism or to arterial disease. Sir R. Douglas Powell described an aneurysm the size of a pea situated on the floor of a gastric ulcer; the coats of the artery elsewhere were healthy, and the production of the aneurysm was evidently analogous to the formation of aneurysms on the branches of the pulmonary artery in tuberculous vomicæ; the aneurysm being due to ulceration and weakening of its outer coats. It is certainly remarkable that aneurysms are not more frequent in gastric and duodenal ulcers. Some slight dilatation may possibly occur before erosion becomes complete, more often indeed than is supposed.

Of the recorded cases most of the examples are independent of gastric ulcer, in which case they give rise to no signs, and to indefinite symptoms, if to any. In a case recorded by Villard, the aneurysm communicated by a small channel with the stomach; but the ulceration of the mucous membrane was secondary to the aneurysm, not its cause.

ANEURYSMS OF THE SUPERIOR MESENTERIC ARTERY occur, as far as recorded cases go, with about the same frequency as aneurysms of the several branches of the cœliac axis; I have collected about twenty-two examples.

The superior mesenteric artery is badly supported, and is therefore more likely, when non-infective embolism occurs, to dilate and become aneurysmal than arteries that are better embedded and supported in firm tissues. Embolism was found to be the cause of several of the recorded aneurysms of the superior mesenteric artery; and Dr. J. W. Ogle draws attention to an analogous condition in animals,—aneurysm of the mesenteric artery as a result of impaction of worms (strongyli).

Not only septic and benign embolism, but traumatism, atheroma, and syphilis may be invoked as possible causes in some cases. In the rare condition of periarteritis nodosa the ill-supported mesenteric vessels are notably affected (Morley Fletcher).

The aneurysm may be situated either in the main trunk of the superior mesenteric artery at or near its origin, or on some of its numerous peripheral branches.

When the aneurysm is situated near the origin of the artery from the aorta it may exert pressure on the bile-duct and give rise to jaundice, as in Dr. J. A. Wilson's case; or it may press on the renal arteries. Dr. B. Yeo met with a remarkable example of uræmia from compression of both the renal arteries by an aneurysm of the superior mesenteric artery.

When the aneurysm is on the peripheral branches it is more likely to be due to embolism than to other causes. It gives rise to pain as do aneurysms involving the trunk of the vessel, and may rupture into the mesentery, or into the general cavity of the peritoneum. Aneurysms of the superior mesenteric artery may be palpable through the abdominal wall.

Aneurysm is extremely rare on the inferior mesenteric artery. A case was described by the late Dr. Peacock.

ANEURYSMS OF THE RENAL ARTERIES may be due to atheroma, trauma, or embolism. Osler speaks of small aneurysms of the renal artery as not being very uncommon.

An aneurysm involving the whole trunk of the renal artery may so interfere with the blood-supply as to lead to a condition like that of arterio-sclerotic atrophy of the kidney; an infective aneurysm may lead to necrosis of the kidney. .

By rupture a renal aneurysm may lead to extensive retro-peritoneal hæmorrhage around the kidney.

H. D. ROLLESTON.

REFERENCES

1. CATON. *Trans. Clinical Soc. London,* vol. xix. p. 275 (Hepatic Aneurysm).— 2. FLETCHER, H. M. *Beitr. z. path. Anat. u. z. allg. Path.,* Jena, 1892, Bd. xi. S. 323.—3. IRVINE, P. *Trans. Path. Soc. London,* vol. xxix. p. 128.—4. LEDIEU. *Journ. de Bord.,* Mars 1856; quoted by Frerichs, "Diseases of the Liver," vol. ii. p. 378.—5. MESTER. *Zeitschrift f. klin. Med.* 1895, Bd. xxviii. S. 93. This paper refers to twenty cases.—6. OGLE, J. W. *Trans. Path. Soc. London,* vol. viii. p. 168.—7. OSLER. *Principles of Medicine,* edit. iii. p. 787.—8. PEACOCK. *Trans. Path. Soc. London,* vol. xii. p. 73.—9. POWELL, R. D. *Trans. Path. Soc. London,* vol. xxix. p. 133.—10. WILSON, J. A. *Trans. Med. Chir. Soc. London,* vol. xxiv. p. 221.—11. VILLARD. *Bull. soc. anat. Paris,* vol. xliii. p. 7; 1867.—12. YEO, B. *Trans. Path. Soc. London,* vol. xxviii. p. 94.

H. D. R.

DISEASES OF THE LYMPHATIC VESSELS

THE diseases of the lymphatic glands have been treated incidentally in other articles, and reference may be made here to Scrofula (vol. iv.), Hodgkin's Disease (vol. iv.), Syphilis (vol. ii.), Glandular Fever (vol. ii.)

Acute adenitis is so essentially a surgical affection that it has not been thought advisable to devote a special article to it in a *System of Medicine;* but, at the risk of some apparent inconsistency, a brief sketch of lymphangitis has been introduced.

Lymphangitis. — By lymphangitis, or angioleucitis, is understood inflammation of the walls of the lymphatic vessels. It is practically always associated with inflammation of the tissues immediately surrounding the vessels — peri-lymphangitis — and with inflammation of the corresponding lymphatic glands.

It is best studied clinically in the superficial forms which attack the skin and subcutaneous tissues; but it also attacks the deeper structures and the viscera, and plays there a part in the extension of inflammatory and suppurative processes. It is probable that in some cases of suppurative nephritis and pylephlebitic abscesses in the liver, lymphangitis is more important than is generally recognised; especially when the primary source of infection is at a distance, as in the bladder or appendix; and when there is no manifest continuity of inflammation in the ureter or portal vein.

Lymphangitis may be acute, chronic, or recurrent.

Acute lymphangitis is the best recognised form, and will be described below. **Chronic lymphangitis** is commonly seen in tuberculosis affecting internal organs; but it occurs in other specific diseases, such as syphilis; while recurrent lymphangitis, like erysipelas, is prone to arise in parts damaged by a previous attack. Thus lymphangitis readily occurs on slight provocation in areas affected with elephantiasis; and also tends to supervene where the lymphatic vessels are dilated, as in macroglossia and in some lymphangiomata; for example, in cystic lymphangioma of the neck.

Lymphangitis is not a specific disease, and thus differs from erysipelas, which it resembles in many other ways. It has been shown that lymphangitis may be due to S. pyogenes aureus, S. pyogenes, and the closely-related S. erysipelatosus; and filarial and malarial lymphangitis have been described. It is moreover an accompaniment of many specific diseases, both acute and chronic. The lymphatic vessels are in such intimate communication with the spaces and interstices of the tissues that any poison or micro-organisms in these situations readily pass into the lymphatics; in this way lymphangitis may spread from an abscess or a phlebitis. The lymphatic vessels may, however, be found full of micro-organisms without their walls being inflamed.

It is hardly necessary to enumerate the various methods by which micro-organisms and septic products can gain an entry into the lymphatics. The skin may seem intact, and the orifice by which the infection entered may not be visible. On the other hand, it may start from the abraded surface in skin affections; or from pricks, leech bites, and so forth. Thus severe lymphangitis may rapidly follow in a person who has made a necropsy on a septic case, who had either no manifest breach of cutaneous surface or only some slight abrasion near the nails. As putrefaction of the dead body advances the risk and danger of infection from it diminishes. In the present day, when the subjects for dissection are carefully injected and preserved, lymphangitis is rarely set up by dissection wounds.

Besides a low or impaired state of nutrition, previous local injury and disease, there are some general factors which dispose to the incidence of lymphangitis; such as alcoholism, gout, and chronic renal disease. The frequency of various secondary infections in renal disease is well known, and the occurrence of lymphangitis is another example of this.

The lymphatic system being better developed and apparently more susceptible early in life, lymphangitis will, other things being equal, be more likely to occur then.

Trauma without any breach of surface only gives rise to lymphangitis when the resistance of the affected parts has been reduced by some pre-existing disease. This is the case, as has already been mentioned, in elephantiasis and macroglossia. In this connection the possibility of micro-organisms having remained latent in the tissues until stirred up to fresh activity must be borne in mind.

From recent observations on fatal cases of burns, made by Bardeen, it appears that inflammatory and degenerative changes in the lymphatic vessels and glands are due to poisonous bodies reaching them by means of the blood-stream. In other words, infection from within must be reckoned with as a cause of lymphangitis.

Acute lymphangitis.—Acute superficial lymphangitis may come on a few hours after infection, and rapidly spread with the production of severe constitutional symptoms; or, on the other hand, it may have a long period of incubation, and not appear until the wound has healed through which the infective agent presumably was introduced.

Signs and symptoms.—Lymphangitis may attack either the lymphatic capillaries (reticular lymphangitis) or the larger trunks; usually these two conditions are combined.

When the smaller vessels are affected there is redness and swelling, and the condition may resemble erythema. If the inflammation be of sufficient intensity, a certain amount of œdema of the skin may be superadded.

The trunks may be affected without the reticular form of lymphangitis being visible; and may then appear as red streaks meandering from the point of infection towards the nearest lymphatic glands. The red lines may be irregular, and not manifest in the whole course of the lymphatic vessels. The redness is broader than the lymphatic trunk, the extension being due to peri-lymphangitis. If there be much infiltration the lines may be palpable as cords under the skin.

The glands soon become painful and swollen from adenitis.

The *symptoms* are—(i.) local:—pain in various degrees is usually present in the affected region; it is increased on movement, and is accompanied by some tenderness on pressure: and (ii.) the general constitutional disturbance accompanying the febrile state—malaise, headache, thirst, loss of appetite, and shivering. The symptoms vary, of course, with the degree of the infective process, and in marked cases may be extremely severe.

Morbid anatomy.—The intima of the vessel becomes swollen, and at the same time the endothelial cells proliferate, undergo degenerative changes, and are thrown off; and the walls become swollen by infiltration with small cells. By extension peri-lymphangitis is set up, the tissues immediately around being occupied with leucocytes. The contents of the vessel first become turbid, and then coagulation leads to thrombosis. When suppuration occurs the clot in the vessel breaks up, and the other changes are intensified; pus being found both inside and outside the vessel, as well as in its walls.

Results.—In slight cases resolution rapidly occurs; commonly after a week to ten days the inflammation passes away, the thrombus inside the vessel is absorbed, and the exudation in the immediate neighbourhood is removed. But the glands do not subside so soon, and chronic adenitis may be left behind. Desquamation of the skin may occur, as in erysipelas; but the scales are not so large.

In other cases organisation of the thrombus and of the inflammatory products may occur, and give rise to chronic lymphangitis and sclerosis of the lymphatic trunks. This may lead farther to thickening of the subcutaneous tissues and a condition of elephantiasis.

In severe cases of lymphangitis suppuration and numerous abscesses may occur, which of course require free incision. There is then danger of septicæmia, or even of pyæmia.

The prognosis depends largely on the form of lymphangitis, on the occurrence of suppuration, and on the state of the health, antecedents, and resistance of the patient.

The diagnosis of lymphangitis is generally easy. In its slighter forms it must be distinguished from erythema. From erysipelas, its course in the line of the lymphatics and the absence of a definite margin differentiate it. From superficial phlebitis the absence of the blocked vein will distinguish it.

Treatment.—The original wound, if there be one, should be carefully disinfected and treated antiseptically. The part should be kept at rest and, if it be a limb, should be raised. An application of equal parts of extract of belladonna and glycerine to the area of lymphangitis usually gives relief. Lead lotion may be applied to reduce the pain. Hot poppy fomentations may also be tried. Antiseptic lotions, and baths containing carbolic acid, or other antiseptics, have recently been employed with success; dressings of perchloride of mercury, 1 in 1000, have also been recommended. Salzwedel has obtained extremely good results from the application of dressings containing alcohol (95 per cent) to parts attacked with lymphangitis.

If suppuration occurs incisions are of course required as soon as practicable.

For the œdema and thickening left behind, massage and the application of pressure by means of bandages may be employed.

The general health must be sustained by fresh air; and removal from depressing surroundings is desirable. Good diet and tonics, such as iron and quinine, should form part of the treatment.

Tuberculous lymphangitis forms an essential part of the spread of local tuberculosis, and can be well studied in the peritoneum in the cases of tuberculous enteritis.

In the skin it is comparatively seldom seen, and, curiously enough, is rare in connection with tuberculous glands in the neck. It is sometimes seen, however, on the extremities, and usually follows local inoculation ; it has then a special tendency to produce local abscesses in the course of the lymphatics. These have been thought to depend on secondary infection with pyogenetic microbes, and to be favoured by the fact that the lymphatic vessels of the limb, before any glands are reached, are larger than elsewhere on the skin, and the flow through them slower. The glands are liable to be affected, and the infection may become generalised. Various forms of tuberculous lymphangitis have been described by the French school.

In the course of *syphilis* the lymphatic vessels leading from the primary sore to the amygdaloid glands may form hard cords.

The affection of the *lymphatics in glanders* is described in the special article in the second volume (p. 514).

Obstruction of the thoracic duct.—The extreme freedom of the anastomotic communications of the lymphatic vessels forming the tributaries of the thoracic duct, and the fact that the lymphatic system is not a closed scheme of vessels but is in continuity with the interstices of the tissues, must be taken into account in considering the subject of obstruction of the thoracic duct. It is remarkable how frequently all signs of it are absent, when, from the presence of tumours, aneurysms, or dense adhesions, it might naturally be expected. In addition to the compensatory efforts on the part of collateral lymphatic anastomoses some complementary absorption is accomplished by the venous channels ; and it is highly probable, therefore, that concomitant venous obstruction plays an important part in the production of dilated lymphatics and œdema. Obstruction may take place in any part of the course of the thoracic duct ; but the effects are more often noticed when the interference with the flow of its contents is near the termination of the duct on the outer side of the left internal jugular vein, at its junction with the subclavian vein. This may be due partly to the greater frequency of tumour and other causes leading to obstruction in this situation ; partly to the consolidation of the duct here into a single trunk, and partly, again, to the greater difficulty of a compensatory collateral circulation between the parts of the duct above and below the obstruction, than in the case of obstruction lower down. Tumours or inflammatory formations in the superior mediastinum, that press on the thoracic duct, would be likely to interfere with those lymphatic trunks in the anterior mediastinum which convey lymph from the peritoneal cavity, and eventually open into the thoracic duct or right lymphatic duct.

Causes of obstruction to the thoracic duct.—Mediastinal growths—especially those in the anterior mediastinum, or enlarged glands from tuberculous, lymphadenomatous, or malignant infection, may compress the duct from without. The results of past inflammatory processes, cicatricial adhesions, may have the same effect, but rarely do.

Aneurysm of the aorta is an extremely rare cause of obstruction of the thoracic duct. The gradual increase of the size of the sac, and the absence of any infiltration, probably allow a collateral circulation to develop itself.

Sir S. Wilks mentions an exceptional case of exophthalmic goitre in which the enlarged thyroid gland passed deeply into the thorax, and was thought, by pressure on the duct, to account for the extreme emaciation.

Thrombosis of the left innominate vein has been recorded by Ormerod and Sidney Martin as a cause of obstruction of the thoracic duct. This lesion, though by no means excessively rare, necessarily obstructs the outflow of lymph from the duct; and, unless free anastomosis with the right lymphatic duct is established, the effects of backward pressure in the lymphatic system must follow. If the thrombosis extend into the duct itself these results would be rendered more marked.

In tricuspid incompetence backward pressure has, in a few isolated cases, led to lymphatic stagnation in the thoracic duct. Here, again, it is possible that thrombosis in the duct might have occurred, and so given rise to obstruction.

Changes in the walls of the duct, whether infiltration with new growth, tubercle, or inflammatory products, may cause obstruction. Congenital stenosis has been suggested, and, if it occurs at all, is best explained as the result of some inflammation early in life.

Considering that tubercle and carcinoma travel by the lymphatics the infrequency with which infiltration of the walls of the duct with these formations have been demonstrated is remarkable.

As regards obstruction due to causes inside the lumen, thrombosis and backward pressure have already been referred to. Thrombosis after injury and rupture may be due to extravasation of blood, whereby obstruction below the rupture is produced.

In filarial disease the duct is probably obstructed by the parent worms (*vide* vol. ii. p. 1079).

It is possible that emboli of new growth might block up the lumen of the duct; this was not unlikely in a case recorded by Dr. Turney.

The results of obstruction to the flow of lymph through the thoracic duct, like those of the backward pressure in the venous system, are widespread. Lymphatic stagnation leads to dilatation and opening up of collateral circulation; if for any cause this fail to compensate, transudation, leakage, and, from rupture of its tributaries or even of the thoracic duct or receptaculum, free escape of lymph will follow.

The dilatation of the lymphatics, or lymphangiectasis, may be very diffuse, and its occurrence in different parts of the body and its relation to lymphangioma will be referred to later.

Elephantiasis is discussed elsewhere under the chapters on filarial disease (vol. ii.) and diseases of the skin (see vol. vii.) Chylous ascites, and conditions resembling it, will be described in the following section.

Chylous ascites.—Chylous ascites is due to the escape of chyle into the peritoneal cavity, whether from transudation of chyle through distended lacteals or from rupture of the thoracic duct, of the larger lymphatic trunks, of varicose lymph vessels, or of lymphangiomata.

There is an allied form of ascites in which the fluid contains fat globules, and thus resembles chylous ascites; but there is no evidence that it comes from the lymphatic system. This condition, to which further reference will be made, may be called *chyliform or fatty ascites* (p. 447), in contradistinction to true chylous ascites. In yet another variety of ascites the naked-eye appearances resemble those in the former groups; but analysis shows that there is no fat, or only a trace, and that the milkiness is due to the presence of albumin: such cases are described as milky, non-fatty ascites (p. 448).

Between these three kinds of ascites a good deal of confusion exists, and cases examined with the naked eye only may belong to any one of them. It must be admitted that the distinction between chylous and chyliform ascites may be difficult, but it is not of much practical importance.

True chylous ascites.—The *fluid* has a specific gravity, varying from 1015-1020, though it may slightly transgress these limits. It is alkaline in reaction and only in exceptional instances neutral. The fluid resists putrefactive changes for a long time, and is usually devoid of smell; though occasionally the odour of foods taken by the mouth may become apparent. It does not clot spontaneously on standing, and thus differs from the urine in chyluria, which owes its coagulating power largely to admixture with blood; but it separates into layers, the uppermost being creamy from the supernatant fat and readily soluble in ether. The milkiness and opalescence are due to the presence of minutely divided fat; the emulsion being much finer than in chyliform or fatty ascites wherein distinct globules of oil are seen. The quantity of fat varies in different cases, and under different conditions in the same individual; if the diet contain much fatty food the amount in the peritoneal effusion will be enhanced: thus Strauss, in a patient fed on butter, noticed a considerable increase in the percentage of fat in the chylous ascitic fluid, and was able to recognise in it the fat given by the mouth. On an average fat is present to the extent of 1 per cent, while in chyle it is 0·9 per cent.

The percentage of albumin varies very considerably: in Sidney Martin's case it was 4·46; in Hoppe-Seyler's 3·66 per cent; in Gillespie's 3·2 per cent; and in two analyses quoted by Halliburton 28·78 per cent, and 21·08 per cent respectively. If peritonitis be present the increased exudation would lead to a higher percentage. Admixture with peritoneal fluid and lymph from other sources render the constitution of the fluid in true chylous ascites different from that of chyle.

Sugar, which is generally present in lymph, and consequently in chyle, and in peritoneal fluid, may be, but is not constantly, found in true chylous

ascites. It has been thought that its presence, in the absence of glycosuria, would differentiate true chylous from chyliform ascites ; but this
criterion can hardly be of much value, for sugar may occur in other peritoneal exudations ; while, on analysis of the chylous fluid in the abdomen
in Strauss's case of chylous ascites with definite perforations on the
lymphatic trunks of the mesentery, no sugar was found. Again, in fatty
or non-chylous ascites, where much cell metabolism has taken place with
discharge of the contents of the cells into the peritoneal fluid, copper-
reducing substances would probably be readily produced.

The causes of chylous ascites.—Obstruction to the flow of lymph in any
part of the course of the thoracic duct or right lymphatic duct naturally
tends to produce increased pressure in the lymphatic vessels behind the
obstruction, and dilatation of them ; this may be followed by the opening
up of a collateral circulation, so that the lymph eventually enters the
general circulation ; or, on the other hand, if this means of compensation
fail, the pressure in the obstructed lymph channels may lead to leakage
by transudation into the peritoneal cavity or tissues around ; or even to a
grosser lesion, such as rupture or perforation of the thoracic duct or its
tributaries. The stomata of the thin-walled lymphatic vessels offer a
ready means by which free transudation can take place ; and the consequent outpouring may be compared to the hæmatemesis of chronic
gastric congestion in hepatic cirrhosis.

In considering the causes of chylous ascites seriatim the various ways
in which the thoracic duct may be obstructed in the different parts of its
course must be first borne in mind. These have already been referred to,
and need not be rehearsed again (*vide* Obstruction of the thoracic duct,
p. 442). When the receptaculum chyli is involved the thoracic duct
above may be quite healthy, and lymph may then pass into it by anastomotic channels, and no chylous ascites be induced.

The thoracic duct and the receptaculum chyli are liable to be
pressed upon or directly involved by malignant growths or other
formations in their immediate neighbourhood. But although chylous,
and especially chyliform, ascites is often associated with malignant
disease of the peritoneum, the association of new growth involving the
thoracic duct and chylous ascites, probable as it might seem at first
sight, has been comparatively seldom established. Schramn describes
such a case, but refers to five recorded examples of malignant growths
involving the thoracic duct without chylous ascites. Troisier met with
three similar examples of new growth ; in one there was no ascites, and
in the other two the ascites was not chylous or chyliform. Senator, however, describes a woman, aged forty-seven, with malignant disease of the
ovaries and secondary growths in the mesenteric glands and thoracic duct,
who had milky effusions into the peritoneum and pleuræ ; and a similar
case had previously been recorded by Leydhecker. Other cases have been
observed, in which a fatty peritoneal effusion has been associated with
malignant disease of the receptaculum chyli ; but it appears that out of
eleven cases of malignant disease involving the thoracic duct or

receptaculum chyli true chylous ascites was absent in eight. So either the duct remained pervious, which seems rather improbable, or a compensatory collateral circulation was developed. In cases of filariasis, where the parent worms probably obstruct the lower part of the thoracic duct, chylous ascites is much less frequent than the other well-known manifestations of the disease (*vide* volume ii. p. 1074). How often it has occurred it is difficult to make out, as the recognition of filarial disease is comparatively recent, and chylous ascites under any conditions is rare.

Traumatic rupture of the thoracic duct is a very rare accident; in Quincke's case, in a man run over by a cart, chylous effusions into the right pleura and peritoneum followed; the division of the duct by a stab appears to have been recorded in very few cases.

Wilhelm has recorded what may have been a rupture during the paroxysms of whooping-cough in an infant six months old. Busey refers to a case in which primary rupture of the thoracic duct was attributed to vomiting; and three in which muscular effort was the reputed cause. Injury and rupture in the intrathoracic portion of the thoracic duct, by leading to hæmorrhage and thrombosis inside the duct, may produce obstruction to the flow of lymph from the abdomen. Rupture of the thoracic duct below the point of obstruction has been more often assumed than demonstrated in cases of chylous ascites. In Cayley's case, where the obstruction was at the entrance into the jugular vein, the receptaculum chyli was ruptured; and, in addition to chylous ascites, a large effusion of lymph took place behind the peritoneum. In Whitla's well-known case the middle third of the thoracic duct was obstructed by tuberculous infiltration, and the receptaculum chyli had ruptured. In 27 cases of chylous ascites, collected by Busey, rupture was found 11 times; this includes secondary rupture from obstruction as well as primary rupture from traumatism and so forth.

Malignant disease involving the aortic or mesenteric glands may produce dilatation of the lymphatics. In Strauss's case rupture of two lymphatic trunks on the anterior surface of the mesentery gave rise to chylous ascites. But the point of escape of the chyle is, generally speaking, difficult to find; and in many cases the chylous effusion is presumably a general oozing or transudation. Dilatation of the chyle vessels is by no means always present when chylous ascites and malignant intra-abdominal disease coexist; but this does not prove that escape of chyle has not occurred, for the obstruction may involve small vessels which have subsequently emptied themselves into the peritoneal cavity, and so are no longer apparent or prominent at the autopsy. On the other hand, the milky effusion in malignant disease of the peritoneum may be chyliform or fatty, rather than due to an escape of real chyle. This point will be discussed later; but it may be pointed out in passing that it is often very difficult to gather from the records whether the effusion in any individual instance contained small fatty particles (chyle) or larger globules derived from changes in suspended cells—the mere presence of fat being enough to lead to the effusion being called chylous. Malignant disease of the abdomen appears to be the most frequent cause or concomitant of chylous ascites ; thus in 33 cases, collected by Treigny, it was responsible for 10.

Chronic peritonitis, by contracting widely on the smaller lymphatic trunks and producing a change in their walls, might conceivably give rise to transudation of their contents, or even to minute ruptures. In a woman, aged 67, from whose abdomen during life a milky effusion containing a fine emulsion of fat was removed on several occasions, well-marked chronic peritonitis was found at the autopsy, together with a few nodules of secondary growth ; it is interesting to note that at the autopsy the ascitic effusion had lost its chylous character and was serous (F. J. Smith).

In some cases of chronic peritonitis, and especially in tuberculous peritonitis, it appears probable that the ascitic effusion was chyliform or fatty rather than true chylous ascites ; the fat being derived from degenerate leucocytes, and not poured out of the chyle vessels.

In a few cases chylous ascites has been referred to the backward pressure of heart lesions leading to thrombosis of the jugular vein into which the thoracic duct opens (Ormerod, Sidney Martin) ; to thrombosis of lymph in the thoracic duct from stagnation without venous thrombosis (Oppolzer), or merely to the mechanical effects of lymphatic stagnation (Rokitansky). It has also been described in rare instances in hepatic cirrhosis. In Merklin's case of atrophic cirrhosis chylous ascites followed a fall ; and thus suggests the possibility of laceration of lymphatic vessels, though this was not made out at the autopsy. In other examples, as was certainly the case in one instance that came under my observation, the milky effusion was perhaps not truly chylous, but a chyliform or a milky non-chylous ascites. In exceptional instances rupture of a chylous mesenteric cyst may lead to chylous ascites.

Fatty or chyliform ascites.—Closely resembling chylous ascites in appearance, and in the presence of suspended fat, but differing from it in that (*a*) the fat is present in larger globules or inside degenerating cells ; and (*b*) that this fat is not derived from the chyle vessels or thoracic duct, is the form of milky ascites called by Quincke chyliform or fatty ascites.

Since fat is the common feature of them both considerable confusion has arisen ; and it is often difficult to be certain from the recorded cases with which variety we are concerned. In 68 cases, collected by Bargebuhr, 48 appeared to be true chylous and 20 fatty ascites ; and Edwards, in 92 cases, tabulates 64 as true chylous, and the remaining 28 as chyliform ascites. They may both arise under the same conditions—that is in chronic peritonitis and intra-abdominal malignant disease ; though it appears that under these conditions the chyliform ascites is the more frequent. As, however, they are with difficulty separated from each other, and inasmuch as no account of true chylous ascites would be complete without a reference to this closely allied form, a brief description of chyliform ascites is given here, although it is not due to disease of the lymphatic vessels.

Resembling true chylous ascitic fluid to the naked eye, it differs from it microscopically in the size of the oil globules, which are large and not finely-divided, as in the emulsion seen in true chylous ascites. The oil globules may be found enclosed in cells in which they are first formed, and from which they are discharged later, as the result of further degenerative and destructive processes. These appearances were well seen in a case of Dr. Whipham's, in which fatty or chyliform ascites was tapped during life, and found at the autopsy to be associated with carcinoma of the gall-bladder, with numerous growths both in the liver (which weighed 15 lbs.), and in the glands around the receptaculum chyli.

In cases of multiple intra-abdominal growth the chyliform ascites may be due to fatty degeneration of the constituent cells of the growth, which are freely discharged into the peritoneal cavity, or to degeneration changes in leucocytes. Corselli and Frisco suggest that in malignant disease of the peritoneum toxic bodies are produced by the growth, which induce fatty degeneration in the cells in the ascitic fluid, and so lead to fatty ascites. A similar hypothesis would explain the fatty ascites sometimes associated with tuberculous peritonitis, wherein the leucocytes in the ascitic effusion under the influence of the tuberculous toxin undergo necrosis and caseation.

In cases of chronic peritonitis—and here it may be mentioned that Letulle and others have insisted on the causal relation between chronic peritonitis and chyliform ascites, the fatty material may be derived from degenerative processes occurring either in leucocytes and fibrin, or in proliferated endothelial cells desquamated from the peritoneum. Guéneau de Mussey had previously expressed much the same opinion when he said that milky pleural effusion is the result of slow modifications occurring in previously formed collections of pus; the leucocytes disappearing and disintegrating into granular and fatty débris. In oily, fatty, or chyliform effusion there is no manifest obstruction in the lymphatic or chyliferous vessels. The distinction between the truly chylous and the fatty or chyliform ascites is of little practical importance. When after several tappings the originally clear fluid becomes milky, the change is due to degenerative changes in the suspended cells; such cases of chyliform ascites may occur in the course of heart disease.

Prof. Osler (24) considers that some cases of chyliform ascites may be due to a milk diet and permanent lipæmia, such as is present in young animals, and in diabetics. Lactescent blood serum, which may either be fatty as in lipæmia, or limpid, will be mentioned in the next paragraph.

Milky non-chylous (non-fatty) ascites.—This form of milky ascites has comparatively recently been distinguished from chylous and chyliform ascites. The ascitic fluid is milky and to the naked eye resembles that of the two preceding groups; but neither microscopically nor chemically does it show any fatty constituents. It differs from true chylous ascites also in not separating into layers when allowed to stand. The fluid is alkaline, has no tendency to putrefy, and retains its characters when filtered.   Its opalescence is not due to bacteria, for it may be quite sterile, but to some albuminous body produced by the degenerative changes in cells suspended in an ascitic effusion.   Lion considered this proteid body to be allied to casein, and to one of the glycoproteids.   He refers to six cases of opalescent ascites, from which by analysis Hammersten obtained muco-albumin.   It may be found in cases of malignant disease of the peritoneum, when the cells of the growth have been said, to supply the milky constituent.   It may occur, however, without the presence of any growth, and then is possibly due to changes in suspended leucocytes or desquamated endothelial cells of the peritoneum.

In cases of repeated tapping the later effusions may be milky, although the earlier ones were quite clear.   In such instances the production of the milky ascites resembles that put forward to explain fatty or chyliform ascites, in that it is a degenerative change in cells suspended in the effusion; the difference being that in chyliform ascites fat is produced, while in non-fatty milky ascites the product is albuminous.

In what has been said thus far, the production of milky non-fatty ascites has been explained as a local change.   It may, however, be but a manifestation of a lactescent condition of the blood serum generally. Milky blood serum may be of two kinds:—(a) fatty, the condition of lipæmia seen in diabetes mellitus, which occasionally occurs in other persons; this condition, especially when the patient is on a milk diet, may produce chyliform or fatty ascites: (b) limpid, this may be physiological in some persons after a heavy meal; or it may be pathological, and is then, according to Castaigne, especially associated with epithelial change in the kidney.   The presence of limpid liquor sanguinis may account for some cases of milky non-fatty ascites.

The signs, whether of chylous, chyliform, or milky non-chylous ascites, are those of ordinary ascites, from which it cannot be distinguished, unless there be some cutaneous lymphangiectasis, until the abdomen is tapped and the milky fluid drawn off.   Microscopical examination will then be required to decide whether it is chylous, fatty, or non-fatty milky ascites.

The onset may be sudden or gradual; and, after tapping, the fluid, when there is leakage from rupture of the lymphatic trunks, tends to reaccumulate rapidly.   In such cases very large amounts may be removed within a few months.   When there is transudation of chyle without any breach of continuity of the lymphatic vessels the effusion is less, and it does not reaccumulate in the same way.

Symptoms.—Increasing weakness and debility, from the continued loss of chyle and partial starvation, naturally follow.   But well-marked emaciation is prevented, probably in several ways: some absorption of fatty material from the intestine through the portal vein probably occurs normally, and in these circumstances may be increased.   The establishment of a collateral circulation, and the possibility that some reabsorption from the peritoneal cavity may take place through the lymphatic vessels which pass up through the anterior mediastinum and open into the thoracic duct above the obstruction, or into the right lymphatic duct, are other factors that must be taken into account. Moreover, there may be signs of chylous effusions into one or both pleuræ, and œdema of the legs may occur late in the course of the case.

The symptoms of whatsoever primary cause gave rise to the lymphatic obstruction may, of course, be the most prominent features of the case ; and in chyliform ascites the symptoms may be even less definite, inasmuch as the results of the primary disease are more likely to be in evidence.

Diagnosis depends on the removal of the characteristic fluid and its microscopic examination. The existence, in rare instances, of dilated lymphatics or fistulæ on the exterior of the body would, of course, suggest that a concomitant ascites is chylous.

An increase in the proportion of fatty materials in the effusion in response to fatty food given by the mouth (Strauss's sign) would be corroborative evidence.

The distinction of true chylous, chyliform, fatty or oily ascites, and non fatty milky ascites has been sufficiently discussed already.

Prognosis.—Most, but not all, cases of chylous and chyliform ascites prove fatal. This not so much because of the character of the effusion, though the impairment of nutrition from interference with the entrance of chyle into the general circulation may be considerable, as from the primary cause, often malignant disease, to which it is due ; of 53 cases tabulated by Busey, 33 ended in death. The prognosis would, for this reason, be better in the rare traumatic cases ; but rupture of the thoracic duct or receptaculum chyli is formidable on account of the very free escape of chyle.

Treatment chiefly consists in the maintenance of the patient's strength on general principles, and in the mitigation of symptoms as they arise. If dyspnœa or distension occur, tapping should be performed ; but this of course increases the drain and loss of chyle, and in true chylous ascites should not be adopted unless necessary. In chyliform and non-fatty milky ascites this objection does not hold.

Chylous and chyliform pleural effusions.—These are comparable to similar conditions in the peritoneal cavity. The occurrence of true chylothorax has been comparatively seldom recorded. Busey mentions ten instances, and a few have been described since the date of his paper.

It is due to traumatic rupture, or to obstruction of the thoracic duct in the thoracic part of its course, in about an equal number of cases. It may be bilateral or unilateral. Sometimes, when unilateral, there is a limpid effusion on the other side. In Dr. Turney's case the effusion was chylous in the right pleura, and fatty or chyliform on the left. In a majority of the cases chylous ascites was present as well.

Chyliform or fatty pleural effusion may occur, and probably is not infrequent ; it is due to much the same causes as chyliform ascites, but especially to chronic pleurisy. It is probable that non-fatty milky pleural effusions also occur.

The signs, symptoms, and treatment are the same as those of simple pleural effusion (*vide* article in vol. v. p. 349 on Diseases of the Pleura, where chylous pleural effusion is referred to).

Chylocele or chylous effusion into the tunica vaginalis testis, which occurs in filarial disease, has been met with without any evidence of this affection (Shattock).

Lymphangiectasis and Lymphangioma. — Those tumours are analogous to ordinary hæmangioma, but are composed of lymphatic vessels or spaces. According to their structure and formation a classification of three varieties is generally described; but, as will be seen later, this is a convenient rather than a rigid division of these tumours, for two or all three of the different forms may co-exist in the same growth.

1. *Simple lymphangioma* is formed by dilatation of pre-existing lymphatics, and is due to some obstruction to the removal of lymph from the affected part. Subsequently the interstitial tissue between the dilated vessels becomes increased in amount; this is lymphangiectasis or lymphatic varix, which is not a tumour or neoplasm in the usual acceptance of the term. Although, whenever lymphangiectasis occurs, there is probably some obstruction to the removal of lymph it cannot always be demonstrated; and in such cases the word lymphangioma is sometimes employed. Some transient inflammation of the part may give rise to fibrosis, sufficient to compress the efferent lymphatic vessels, without leaving any more tangible impress of its occurrence. Thus dilatation of the lymphatic vessels of the tongue has been known to follow erysipelas of adjacent parts, just as elephantiasis of the limbs is a sequel of the same inflammatory process.

Allchin and Hebb have described a remarkable case of lymphangiectasis of the small intestine in which the mesenteric glands were also varicose, but no definite obstruction was forthcoming. A similar condition is sometimes seen in undoubted obstruction of the thoracic duct, and has been found associated with chylous ascites. The symptoms of lymphangiectasis of the intestine, so far as they are recognised, are vomiting and exhausting diarrhœa.

Elephantiasis due to filarial disease has already been described (vol. ii. p. 1080), and other such effects of lymphatic obstruction will be dealt with among the diseases of the skin. Lymph scrotum and varicose lymphatic glands on the groin may follow obstruction other than that of filarial disease; but in other respects the condition is the same and does not require a separate description.

Dilatation of the lymphatic vessels of the lung is sometimes due to pressure at the root of the lung; and in such cases the branching and dilated lymphatics are well seen under the visceral pleura.

Cripps and Berry have described two remarkable cases of numerous cysts of various sizes, and with clear contents, in the great omentum. In both instances there were a few peritoneal adhesions, and the possibility of their being dilated lymphatics due to obstruction was raised. Small lymphatic varicosities may occur on the peritoneum ; an exaggeration of this condition may give rise to mesenteric cysts (*vide* p. 456).

In Dr. R. Crawfurd's case of floating liver, where jaundice was due to torsion of the bile-duct, the intrahepatic lymphatic vessels were much dilated.

In a case of diabetic lipæmia I have seen the lymphatic vessels around the cœliac axis and in the portal fissure markedly distended with chyle.

These examples serve to illustrate the occurrence of lymphangiectasis ; and it may be noted that simple dilatation of the lymph channels occurs also in cases of cavernous and cystic lymphangioma.

2. *Cavernous lymphangioma.*—This is analogous to cavernous angioma, and is due to the formation of new lymphatic vessels, which in the first instance arise as solid cords formed of endothelial cells proliferating from the inside of lymphatic vessels. These cords unite with others, and then become hollowed out so as to form lymph channels,—homoplastic formation. It is therefore a farther stage of a simple lymphangioma, and may be compared with the transformation of a simple into a cavernous angioma.

The interstitial tissue between the lymph spaces, as the result of the constant pressure to which it is subjected by the growth, usually under-goes atrophy and tends to disappear to a greater or less extent. It may, however, contain a certain amount of fat in addition to fibrous and areolar tissue, and show young connective cells, leucocytic infiltration, and blood-vessels. Stiles regards the presence of smooth muscular fibres in the walls of the lymph spaces as a means of distinguishing cavernous lymph-angioma from lymphangiectasis. The contents of the spaces are clear and resemble lymph ; when they occur in the abdomen or in its immediate neighbourhood they may contain chyle (chylangioma).

Another (heteroplastic) mode of origin of lymphangioma has been described by Wegner, in which the new formation of lymphatic channels takes place independently of pre-existing vessels. Granulation tissue first develops and then lymphatic spaces are formed inside it. This mode of origin, though it has been generally accepted, is difficult to prove by histological examination.

Lymphangioma circumscriptum cutis, the so-called "Lupus lymphaticus," is an example of a cavernous angioma ; it will be described under new growths of the skin.

Cavernous lymphangioma, or lymphatic nævus, is often associated with lymphangiectasis or with cystic lymphangioma ; these combinations may be seen in macroglossia and congenital serous cysts of the neck.

The distinction between cavernous and cystic lymphangioma is rather one of degree than of kind.

Cystic lymphangioma may be met with in various parts of the body. Usually these growths are subcutaneous ; but they may be deeply situated, for example, on the peritoneum or among the abdominal viscera. In the neck, where they are frequently found, they may have deep connections, and travel along the intermuscular processes of cervical fascia. They may occur on the limbs, giving rise to macromelia ; on the trunk, in the neighbourhood of the sacrum; on the tongue, and, more rarely, on the face. Their structure is on the same lines as that of cavernous lymphangioma; but the spaces are larger and form cysts of varying sizes, which, except in their endothelial lining, no longer resemble lymphatic vessels.

The cysts may be separate, or they may communicate with each other; and, by destruction of the intervening walls, a multilocular cyst may be transformed into a unilocular cyst. Except for the projection of intracystic buds the interior of the cysts is smooth; though when inflammation has supervened their lining may become granular and rough.

The fluid in the cysts is clear, alkaline in reaction, and contains albumin, and salts, chiefly NaCl; but, when the cysts have been inflamed, it may be mixed with blood in various stages of retrogression, and contain cholesterin or pus. The contents of the cysts may present widely different characters in parts of the same tumour.

The tissue between the cysts may be of various kinds,—fibrous tissue; fat; sarcomatous tissue; blood - vessels, sometimes numerous; smooth muscular tissue; elastic fibres, and nerves. The presence of blood-vessels, which may project in the form of buds into the cysts, has in the past given rise to the opinion that these congenital serous cysts are derived, by obstructive and other changes, from ordinary hæmangioma and not primarily from lymphatic vessels. It is true that cystic formations containing lymph are sometimes found in the middle of erectile tumours; but this can be explained by supposing that, from the first, such tumours are composed both of lymphatics and of blood-vessels. On the whole this surmise appears less likely to be true than the alternative that these congenital serous cysts are cystic lymphangiomata. Although they cannot be absolutely proved to be lymphatic in origin, the facts (a) that they are often associated and sometimes anatomically connected with other congenital defects of the lymphatic system, such as macroglossia and macrocheilia; and (b), that they are in communication with the lymphatic trunks, are in favour of these congenital serous cysts being regarded as lymphangioma.

The number of blood-vessels in a cystic lymphangioma may increase in number, so that the tumour might eventually be regarded as a combination of hæmangioma and of lymphangioma. In other cases the interstitial fat increases in amount, so that the tumour may be said to undergo transformation into a lipoma, and so to be cured. When aspirated, blood is often poured out; and Mr. D'Arcy Power considers that the fibrous growths, sometimes seen after numerous tappings, may be due to changes taking place in this extravasation.

Like other kinds of lymphangioma the cystic form is extremely prone to recurrent attacks of inflammation; this fact must be borne in mind in connection with their operative treatment. Inflammation may follow mere aspiration; and though this may, and in rare cases does, lead to rapid and almost spontaneous cure, it may be the cause of severe and fatal suppuration.

Cystic lymphangiomata may remain stationary, and in some instances have been known to undergo spontaneous involution; on the other hand they may grow rapidly.

In most cases they are congenital in origin, by some authors they are said always to be so.

In many instances, as has been already pointed out, a cystic lymphangioma is combined with the other two forms, simple and cavernous lymphangioma.

The more dangerous situations for cystic lymphangioma are on the neck and in the sacro-perineal region.

When superficial, lymphangioma may give rise to lymphorrhagia, a condition which, from its inconvenience, may require surgical interference; but otherwise, unless excessive, it is not of any great importance.

The treatment of lymphangioma is entirely surgical; pressure may be applied so as to empty the contents into the adjacent lymphatics and lead to consolidation. Puncture is often employed, and may be frequently repeated; electrolysis again may be tried, but under modern antiseptic precautions excision is probably the most successful, and certainly the most trustworthy form of treatment.

Lymphangioma must be diagnosed from nævus, from fatty tumour, and, when occurring on the extremities, from local giant growth. When lymphangiomata project through the inguinal rings they may be mistaken for hernia.

Macroglossia.—Although congenital enlargement of the tongue may be due to other factors, it depends in the great majority of the cases on dilatation of the lymphatics and coexisting hyperplasia of the surrounding connective-tissue elements. The condition, it is true, may arise in later life as the result of lymphatic obstruction; thus Robin and Laredde refer to dilatation of the lingual lymphatics following erysipelas; but, generally speaking, it is congenital. It may remain latent or comparatively stationary for a time, and then increase in size, gradually or suddenly.

Various forms of lymphangioma are met with, and frequently the simple and cavernous varieties are combined in the same specimen; more rarely the cystic form is present as well.

The tongue in the condition of lymphangiectasis, or simple lymphangioma, is covered with minute cysts extending into the papillæ. In other cases there may be a localised cavernous lymphangioma exactly comparable to an ordinary cavernous hæmangioma. Usually, in well-marked examples of macroglossia, there is a combination of lymphangiectasis and the cavernous lymphangioma, the later having supervened on the simpler condition.

Inflammation is readily induced in the tongue affected with macroglossia, and the attacks are apt to recur on very slight provocation; though the individual attacks are usually of but slight intensity, eventually they lead to very considerable enlargement of the organ. The attacks of inflammation induce small cell infiltration around the lymphatic spaces, and tend to exaggerate the elephantoid condition of the tongue, which may reach huge dimensions, and even touch the sternum.

In well-marked cases the substance of the tongue is widely excavated by lymphatic spaces; in the slighter cases, previously referred to, the surface of the tongue may be affected almost exclusively.

Treatment should first be applied in the form of pressure, either directly to the tongue by an elastic band, or, indirectly, by keeping the mouth closed (except during meals) by a bandage or some other appropriate means, whereby the tongue is compressed against the hard palate. If this fail, or if the tongue be so enlarged already that it projects from the mouth, a wedge-shaped piece of it should be removed.

Macrocheilia is a similar condition to macroglossia, with which it may be associated. It attacks the lips, by preference the upper lip; and has been known to be unilateral, or to occupy both lips.

Mr. Arbuthnot Lane successfully treated a marked case of macrocheilia affecting both lips by electrolysis, and considers this plan preferable to excision of part of the lip.

Congenital serous cysts of the neck.—Hydrocele of the neck. Cystic hygroma of the neck. Cystic lymphangioma of the neck.

These cysts form a distinct group; they are congenital in origin, and occur in the seat of election of congenital serous cysts, that is in the neck. As mentioned already, under the heading of cystic lymphangioma, it has been suggested that these congenital serous cysts are derived from hæmangiomata by a process of obliteration of their vascular connections and the establishment of a secondary communication between the blood-vessels thus isolated and the lymphatic system. But the connection of the congenital serous cysts with the lymphatic system, and their occasional association with other kinds of lymphangioma, such as macroglossia and macrocheilia, make it probable that they are lymphangioma from the first. In the case of congenital serous cysts on the neck, two other sources of origin—the salivary glands and the intercarotid gland—have been suggested, but on no sufficient basis of fact. For, as a rule, these cysts are quite independent of the salivary glands; and, even when invaded, the glands appear otherwise healthy: in addition to this the congenital cysts are lined by endothelium, and not by epithelium, as they should be if derived from the salivary glands.

Cystic lymphangioma of the neck must be distinguished from the cysts which arise from the branchial cysts, and which are lined by epithelium derived from the fore-gut. These cysts are lined by columnar or by squamous epithelium, and have usually been spoken of as mucoid or dermoid cysts; but, as Mr. Shattock has shown, these terms are not very suitable, and in this instance might with advantage be replaced by the name mucosal cysts. Carcinoma may develop in the remains of the branchial clefts—branchogenous carcinoma—and a cystic tumour may result. This rare and acquired condition must be also distinguished from the congenital cysts of the neck now under consideration.

The cystic lymphangiomata usually occupy the anterior or lateral surfaces of the neck, and are rarely seen on the back. They may be unilateral or occur on both sides; when in the median line they tend to extend into both anterior triangles. They vary much in size; the unilateral are smaller, but the median may extend from the jaw to the sternum, and then resemble the appearances seen in diffuse lipoma.

They have been divided into multilocular, and simple or unilocular cysts; but there is no fundamental difference between them, for the former by destruction of the septa of its constituent cysts may tend to become unilocular, and processes or diverticula may pass off from a unilocular cyst. Differences, however, exist from the point of view of their clinical aspects and treatment. The unilocular cysts, according to Lannelongue and Achard, are found almost exclusively anteriorly, and on the left side of the neck; but the compound or multilocular cysts have no such limitations.

These cysts tend to burrow and extend under the cervical fascia between the muscles of the neck, to which they become adherent, and often travel down along the sheath of the subclavian vessels into the axilla; they have been known to travel into the mediastinum. This tendency to burrow deeply and to become adherent to muscles, vessels, and nerves is important; for an attempt at removal may reveal a far wider extension of the cyst than was at first apparent.

The cystic and cavernous forms of lymphangioma are often found united in the cysts of the neck.

The other features of congenital cysts of the neck have been referred to under the previous heading of cystic lymphangioma.

Mesenteric cysts.—Mesenteric cysts of any kind are rare. Moyniham in a recent paper has collected 100 cases.

Some mesenteric cysts, but by no means all, may be due to dilatation of lymphatic vessels and to lymphangiomatous growth. Dilated lymphatics, and less commonly cavernous and cystic lymphangiomata, may, however, occur in the peritoneal cavity without producing any of the signs or symptoms of a mesenteric cyst.

The mesenteric cysts that may be referred to as lymphatic in origin are the chylous cysts and some of the serous cysts. Both varieties may be either unilocular or multilocular. They may owe their origin to dilatation of part of a lymphatic vessel, due to obstruction probably of an inflammatory nature. When a chylous cyst is produced communication with the lacteals is preserved; but, in order to make a lymphatic origin applicable to serous cysts, we must suppose that the lymph from this source is excluded. Some of the cysts situated near the spine have been attributed to dilatation of the receptaculum chyli; another explanation is that the cysts are due to degenerative changes and to dilatation in the lymphatic glands of the mesentery. In some of these cysts the remains of lymphoid tissue have been described, but this appearance is capable of another explanation, namely, that it is the leucocytic infiltration of a cavernous lymphangioma. The origin of cysts in the mesentery in dilatation of lymphatic glands is, however, rendered highly probable by the analogy of varicose lymphatic glands on the groin in filarial disease.

It is said that hæmorrhage may take place into a cyst previously containing serum, and the cyst will then imitate the sanguineous cysts due to traumatism. This, however, is not the place to consider the other varieties of mesenteric cysts, namely, the sanguineous, the dermoid, the hydatid, and those said to owe their origin to the remains of the Wolffian body.

The clinical signs of mesenteric cysts are summarised by Moyniham as being—

(i.) Prominence of a fluctuating, generally spherical tumour near the umbilicus.

(ii.) Great mobility, especially in the transverse direction, and the possibility of rotation round a central axis.

(iii.) The presence of a zone of resonance around the cyst, and a belt of resonance across it.

The symptoms may be either (*a*) chronic, of the nature of colicky pain due to interference with the intestine and gastro-intestinal disturbance, the presence of a tumour distinguishing the case from one of simple gastro-enteritis; or (*b*) those of acute intestinal obstruction.

Malignant growths in lymphatic vessels.—In the various forms of carcinoma, except rodent ulcer, early and often extensive infiltration of the lymphatic vessels occurs. The carcinomatous infection travels along the lymphatic vessels in the direction of the blood stream; but there is some evidence to show that in certain cases it may also spread against the lymph stream (55). In sarcoma, on the other hand, lymphatic infection is the exception; though it is the rule in primary sarcomatous growths of the testes and of lymphatic structures: in the latter, indeed, the growth may be said to be already inside the lymphatic system; as a good example of this case sarcoma of the tonsil may be cited. Primary sarcoma may occur in lymphatic glands, and, structurally, may be either round or spindle-celled. Growth of this kind should not be called lympho-sarcoma, merely because it originates in lymphatic glands, but lymphatic gland sarcoma. The term lympho-sarcoma is a structural term, and should be confined to a growth composed of small round cells with a delicate reticulum. It may occur in pre-existing lymphatic structures, though it by no means always does. In exceptional cases sarcoma in other parts of the body may lead to lymphatic infection. This is true of melanotic sarcoma, and in some cases where the skin is involved.

Whether sarcoma arises primarily in the lymphatic vessels apart from lymphatic glands and serous membranes is, from the comparatively small size of the thoracic duct and other lymphatic vessels, a very difficult point to investigate, and one about which there is no certain knowledge. Such an origin may be conjectured in the case of some of the aberrant growths, called endothelioma, found in connection with the pleura or peritoneum; but the proof is wanting.

H. D. ROLLESTON.

REFERENCES

Lymphangitis : 1. BARDEEN. *Journal of Experimental Medicine*, New York, Sept. 1897.—2. DUPLAY and RECLU. *Traité de chirurgie*, tome i. p. 646.—3. EVE. "Tuberculous Lymphangitis," *Trans. Clin. Soc.* vol. xxviii. p. 25.—4. WALZWEDEL. *Berlin. klin. Wochen.* 1896, Nos. 46, 47. **Obstruction of the Thoracic Duct, Chylous and Chyliform Effusions :** 5. ACHARD. *Bull. soc. méd. des hôp.* 1896.—6. APERT. *Bull. Soc. anat. de Paris*, 1897, p. 187.—7. BARGEBUHR. *Deutsch. Arch. f. klin. Med.* li.—8. BUSEY. *American Journal of the Medical Sciences*, 1889, July–Dec. p. 575 ; new series, vol. xcviii.—9. CASTAIGNE. *Arch. gén. de méd.* 1897, June, p. 666.—10. CAYLEY. *Trans. Path. Soc. Lond.* vol. xvii. p. 163.—11. CHARCOT, BRISSAUD. *Traité de médecine*, vol. v.—12. CORSELLI and FRISCO. *Riforma med.* Roma, 1897, p. 278.—13. DAWSON. *Twentieth Century Practice of Medicine*, vol. iv.—14. EDWARDS. *Medicine*, Detroit, Aug. 1895. Quoted by Gillespie, *Edin. Med. Journal*, 1897, p. 807. —15. GILLESPIE. *Edinburgh Medical Journal*, Dec. 1897.—16. HALLIBURTON. *Textbook of Chemical Physiology and Pathology*, 1891.—17. LETULLE. *Rev. de méd.*, Paris, 1884, tome iv. p. 722.—18. LEYDHECKER. *Virchow's Archiv*, Bd. cxxxiv.—19. LION. *Arch. de méd. expér. et d'anat. path.* vol. v. p. 826.—20. MARTIN, S. *Trans. Path. Soc.* vol. xlii. p. 93.—21. MERKLEN. *Medical Week*, 1897, p. 253.—22. OPPOLZER. *Allg. Wien. med. Zeit.* 1861, p. 149.—23. ORMEROD. *Trans. Path. Soc.* vol. xix. p. 199.—24. OSLER. *Principles and Practice of Medicine*, edition ii. p. 509.—25. QUINCKE. *Deutsches Arch. f. klin. Med.* xvi. 1875, p. 121.—26. ROKITANSKY. *Lehrb. der path. Anat.* 3rd ed. 1865, vol. ii. p. 388.—27. SCHRAMN. *Berlin. klin. Woch.* Oct. 26, 1896, No. 43.—28. SENATOR. *Charité-Annalen*, Jahrg. xx. —29. SHATTOCK. *Trans. Path. Soc.* vol. xxxv. p. 250.—30. SMITH, F. J. *Trans. Path. Soc. Lond.* vol. xlii. p. 100.—31. STRAUSS. *Arch. de physiol. et de path.* vii. 367.—32. TREIGNY. *Journ. des practiciens*, Jan. 22, 1898.—33. TROISIER. *La médecine moderne*, Oct. 13, 1897 ; and *La presse médicale*, May 21, 1898.—34. TURNEY. *Trans. Path. Soc.* vol. xliv. p. 1.—35. WHITLA. *Brit. Med. Journ.* 1885, vol. i. p. 1089.—36. WHYTE and GILLESPIE. *Edinburgh Medical Journal*, Dec. 1897, p. 551.—37. WILHELM. *Gaz. hebd. de méd. et de chirurg.* May 21, 1875, p. 332, No. 21.—38. WILKS. *Path. Anatomy*, p. 184, edition 1889. **Lymphangiomata :** 39. ALLCHIN and HEBB. *Trans. Path. Soc. Lond.* vol. xlvi. p. 221.—40. BERRY, J. *Trans. Path. Soc. Lond.* vol. xlviii. p. 105.—41. BUTLIN. *Diseases of the Tongue*, 1885.—42. CRAWFURD, R. *Lancet*, 1897, vol. ii.—43. CRIPPS, H. *Trans. Path. Soc. Lond.* vol. xlvii. p. 85.—44. DAWSON. "Diseases of Lymphatic Vessels," *Twentieth Century Practice of Medicine*, vol. iv. p. 641.—45. LANE, W. A. *Trans. Clin. Soc. London*, vol. xxvi. p. 223.—46. LANNELONGUE and ACHARD. *Traité des kystes congénitaux*, p. 279.—47. MOYNIHAM. *Annals of Surgery*, July 1897, with bibliography of Mesenteric Cysts.—48. POWER, D'A. *Brit. Med. Journ.* 1897, vol. ii. p. 1633.—49. QUENU. *Traité de chirurgie ;* DUPLAY and RECLU. Article "Lymphangioma," tome i. p. 498. —50. ROBIN and LAREDDE. *Arch. de méd. expérimentale et d'anat. path.* 1896, p. 459.—51. SHATTOCK. *Trans. Path. Soc. Lond.* vol. xlviii. p. 254.—52. STILES. *Edinburgh Hospital Reports*, vol. i. p. 520.—53. TREVES. "Malignant Cysts of the Neck," *Trans. Path. Soc. Lond.* vol. xxxviii. p. 360.—54. WEGNER. *Archiv f. klin. Chir.* 1876, Bd. xx. S. 641.—55. WHITE. *Philadelphia Medical Journal*, vol. i. p. 847, May 7, 1898.

H. D. R.

DISEASES OF MUSCLES. TROPHONEUROSES

MYOSITIS

MYOTONIA CONGENITA (THOMSEN'S DISEASE)

IDIOPATHIC MUSCULAR ATROPHY AND HYPERTROPHY

FACIAL HEMIATROPHY AND HEMI-HYPERTROPHY

GENERAL PATHOLOGY OF THE NERVOUS SYSTEM

TREMOR, "TENDON-PHENOMENON," AND SPASM

TROPHONEUROSES—

NEUROTROPHIC DISEASES OF BONES AND JOINTS

NEUROTROPHIC DISEASES OF SOFT TISSUES

ADIPOSIS DOLOROSA

RAYNAUD'S DISEASE

ERYTHROMELALGIA

MYOSITIS

THE inflammatory conditions of muscles may be grouped under the following heads :—

A. Primary affections of the muscle. (*a*) Acute polymyositis. (*b*) Myositis due to trauma and to direct extension from an inflammatory focus. (*c*) Myositis due to the invasion of the muscle by trichina.

B. Secondary affections of the muscle in the course of· some acute or chronic disease; the resulting condition may be either general or local, parenchymatous or interstitial, suppurative or non-suppurative : (*a*) myositis occurring in the course of the specific fevers, such as typhoid, typhus, small-pox, and so forth ; (*b*) infective myositis occurring in pyæmia, puerperal fever, ulcerative endocarditis, glanders, infected wounds, actinomycosis, erysipelas, and gonorrhœa ; (*c*) syphilitic myositis—(α) diffuse syphilitic myositis, (β) muscle gumma.

C. Myositis ossificans.

New growths are omitted altogether as they belong to the sphere of surgery.

A. **Primary affections of the muscles.**—(*a*) *Acute polymyositis.*—The characteristics of this disease, known also under the names Dermato-myositis and Pseudo-trichinosis, have been defined during the last ten years.

In 1887 Unverricht, Hepp, and Wagner all described cases of this nature, Hepp's case being published under the title of Pseudo-trichinosis. Strümpell, in 1891, described another case, with autopsy, and summed up the leading features of the disease. Since that date several cases have been reported with autopsy.

Causation.—The cause of the disease is obscure ; two hypotheses have been suggested—first, that the disease is due to a toxin ; secondly, that it is due to an animal parasite of the group gregarinæ ; but neither of these hypotheses has been proved. It is possible that some of the cases described under the above heading may have been due to trichina (Wagner's case) ; such cases should obviously be excluded from this group (see vol. ii. p. 1048). Careful examination of the muscles has given a negative result, both bacteriologically and as regards trichina.

The suggestion that the condition is due to a toxin derived from the ingesta would be supported by the cases observed by Senator and Kell; for in the case reported by the former the disease followed the eating of some stale crabs, and in the latter the ingestion of a fish, by which three persons were said to have been infected, and of whom one died. In Senator's case the disease did not appear till some time after the eating of the crabs; whereas in Kell's cases it manifested itself within a few hours, though the cases were not simultaneous; the case in which it first showed itself proved fatal.

The suggestion that the disease is due to a gregarine is based on the occurrence in the lower animals of myositis due to a protozoon, a sporozoon of the group gregarinæ; and it is also stated that Virchow has observed in a hog affected with gregarinal myositis a skin lesion very similar to that seen in the acute polymyositis of man. In this connection, however, the researches of Pluymers on the sarcosporidies may be of interest as showing how small may be the irritation to which they may give rise.

The disease has occurred in the course of diabetes, pulmonary phthisis, tuberculous disease of the intestines; and, after injury to the tongue. Myositis due to syphilis should not be classed under this heading.

There is no evidence to show that the disease is contagious, save possibly that which is brought forward by Lewy; and the nature of his cases may well be called in question.

Pathology.—Almost any or all the muscles of the body may be affected; but the masseters and the ocular muscles usually escape. The muscular tissue is swollen and of a yellowish-white colour, and appears covered with brownish-red patches. Hæmorrhages can be seen in the muscle. Sometimes the most striking condition of the muscle is its soft, friable condition. The microscopical examination shows both a parenchymatous and interstitial inflammatory condition of the muscle, and it may be either focal or diffuse. The muscle fibres are swollen and granular, and for the most part have lost their striation; often they show a hyaline or waxy degeneration; vacuoles are present, but there is no proof that fatty degeneration occurs. Increase of round cells between the fibres is always present, and hæmorrhages can be seen in this situation. From a digest of the various cases, Pfeiffer comes to the conclusion that the disease is primarily an affection of the connective tissue, and that the muscle fibres become affected secondarily. The heart muscle was involved in one case. The brain, spinal cord, and the peripheral nerves show no change. There is often a pneumonic condition of the lungs. The spleen is enlarged and soft.

Age and sex.—Out of 11 cases, collected by Pfeiffer, 4 were women and 7 were men. The youngest described case occurred in a patient aged seventeen, and the oldest in a man aged seventy. No case has been reported in children.

Symptoms.—The disease is characterised by swelling of the extremities due to an inflammatory œdema of the subcutaneous tissue and the muscles, attended by acute pain and rigidity of the muscles, great tenderness on pressure, and an erythematous rash, resembling erysipelas, situated over the affected muscles.

The onset of the disease is gradual, with malaise, weakness, loss of appetite, headache, and sometimes vomiting. There is usually a moderate rise of temperature but no rigor; and the local symptoms manifest themselves later, with acute pain, of a cramp-like character, and tenderness, beginning usually in the legs or arms. At the beginning of the illness the pain is not generally so severe that the limbs cannot be moved; later, however, the least movement causes so much pain that the patient lies helpless in bed. Other muscles of the body may become affected—the diaphragm, the intercostals, and the muscles of deglutition—so that the patient has great difficulty in speaking and swallowing. The tongue and the muscles of the eye are reported to have been affected in some cases. Sensation is perfectly preserved, and the nerves are not tender on pressure. The joints are unaffected. The knee-jerks are generally present, though the swollen condition of the limb and the pain caused by percussion may give rise to some difficulty in obtaining them. The electrical reactions in this stage of the disease, when tested, have been found normal. Stomatitis and throat affections may occur either early or late in the disease. The urine is generally normal, but it may contain some albumen. The spleen is commonly enlarged. The course of the disease tends in the slighter cases to complete recovery after a duration of some weeks; in one case recovery took place in twelve days (Plehn). In the severer forms recovery is often protracted; atrophy of the muscles follows the subsidence of the inflammation; electrical changes are found in the muscles; and marked pigmentation of the skin may be permanent.

The severest cases end in death, from affection of the muscles of respiration, or from secondary affections of the lungs, bronchitis, or pneumonia.

That slighter forms of the disease exist which do not correspond in all particulars with the disease as above described, is obvious from examination of the reported cases. The diagnosis of such cases will always be called in question, for it is almost impossible to distinguish them from syphilitic or infective myositis, or from slighter cases of trichinosis.

Diagnosis.—The disease, as above described, has certain definite features, namely, a gradual onset, attended by inflammatory swelling of the muscles, together with redness and swelling of the skin and subcutaneous tissue situated over the involved muscles, extreme tenderness, but no loss of sensation. It is necessary, therefore, to distinguish this disease from—

(i.) Trichinosis. The presence of initial digestive disturbance and of considerable œdema of the face and eyelids early in the disease would point to infection by trichina; but the only certain test is the search for the trichinæ in the motions, or in an excised portion of the muscle.

(ii.) Neuro-myositis, in which the primary lesion is nervous. The more marked paralysis, the anæsthesia, the earlier and more rapid atrophy, the loss of knee-jerk, together with other evidence of nerve lesion and the absence of the characteristic skin affection, would point to a primary nerve lesion.

(iii.) Infective myositis. The presence of a focus of infection, and the positive bacteriological result on examination of the muscles, would distinguish this from acute polymyositis.

(iv.) The condition has also to be distinguished from syphilitic myositis.

Prognosis, both with regard to the immediate recovery and also with regard to the subsequent effects of the disease, is by no means good. The disease in its severer forms is very fatal. In its less severe form it may lead to considerable muscular atrophy, and even in the slighter cases recovery may be prolonged.

The immediate treatment can only be directed to the relief of pain, the removal from the body of the source of irritation, and the nutrition of the patient. Later the treatment will be directed to the bronchitis and pneumonia, and, as far as possible, to the prevention of the atrophy of the muscles.

(b) Myositis due to trauma and to direct extension from an inflammatory focus requires only to be mentioned as forming one of the primary affections of muscle, but needs no detailed description here.

(c) Myositis due to trichina will be found fully dealt with in the second volume of this System (p. 1048).

B. **Secondary affections of muscles.**—(a) *Myositis due to the specific fevers.* — The changes occurring in muscle during the course of the specific fevers should rather be regarded as degeneration than as inflammation ; these changes have been found especially in the course of typhoid fever, and they give rise to a dull pale fish-like appearance of the muscle. On microscopical examination the fibres are seen to be swollen and hyaline in appearance, the transverse striation having disappeared ; this process usually affects some of the fibres only, the others retaining their striation. When suppuration takes place in the muscle it has been shown that the abscesses contain streptococci, staphylococci, and other micro-organisms ; they are therefore due to infection, and belong to the following class :—

(b) *Infective myositis.*—This may be due to infection in pyæmia, puerperal fever, ulcerative endocarditis, glanders, actinomycosis ; or from an infected wound or boil. The disease is often attended with rigors, the local muscular symptoms being often masked by the general symptoms. The disease frequently ends fatally.

The muscles in cases of this nature have a dirty-red colour, and on pressure a grayish-red fluid exudes. On microscopical examination of the muscle the transverse striation is seen to be lost, and there is an increase of the intermuscular cells—and, in suitably stained specimens—streptococci can be seen in the muscular tissue. The occurrence of actual abscesses in the muscle would seem to depend on the length of time that the disease has existed ; in some cases in which the general infection has been very acute no abscesses have been found in the muscles, whereas in the longer standing cases numerous abscesses occur.

The bacteriological examination of the muscle and of the pus shows the presence of streptococci; these, however, are not always present in great numbers in the muscle; and such a case, in which the micro-organism escaped detection in the muscle, and in which the source of infection was not obvious (viz. the ear, etc.), might well pass for a case of polymyositis so long as suppuration did not occur.

The occurrence of rigors and the affection of the joints, together with the difference in the character of the skin affection, should distinguish it from polymyositis.

Myositis due to gonorrhœal infection is dealt with in the article on "Gonorrhœal Rheumatism," in the third volume of this System.

(c) *Syphilitic myositis.*—Two forms are described—(a) Diffuse syphilitic myositis; (β) Gumma of the muscle.

(a) Pathology.—Diffuse syphilitic myositis is in its first stage attended by swelling of the muscle, with deposit of a plastic material between the muscle fibres; in the later stages this material undergoes fibrous change, and atrophy of the muscle fibres takes place. According to Lewin the diffuse form of myositis occurs early in the disease, generally between the second and ninth month after infection. Of the cases collected by him 50 per cent occurred during the first year after infection. The microscopical appearances described are :—dilatation of the vessels, exudation of granular cells, and at the same time proliferation of the muscle nuclei, the cells lying in part between the primitive bundles, in part within the bundles. Furthermore, an increase of the interstitial connective tissue takes place, and the individual fibres and the muscle bundles become separated from one another; lastly, the muscle fibres themselves become opaque and their contents granular; the striation of the fibre disappears. Some fibres, however, undergo simple atrophy, and then the striation is preserved even in the smallest fibres.

Symptoms.—The disease is gradual in its onset, starting with pain (generally worse at night) in one or more muscles, attended with redness of the skin and some tenderness on pressure. The temperature is often slightly raised. After a few days or weeks other muscles may become affected. The muscle feels hard and brawny, there is diminished power, and a contracted position of the limb may be present according to the muscle affected. The biceps muscle would seem to be more commonly affected than any other. Neumann, in a series of 11 cases, found the biceps muscle affected eight times. Recovery is slow, and is often attended with considerable atrophy of the muscle or the muscles affected.

(β) Gumma of muscle.—This condition, according to Lewin, occurs later in the disease than the foregoing change, in some cases as late as twenty-one years after infection. It is attended by little pain; the patient notices a hard swelling in the muscle which is not tender on pressure though some pain is caused in the muscle when it is put into action. The lesion is sometimes symmetrical; out of 7 cases collected by Eger it was symmetrical in 3. In some cases the presence of the tumour may give rise to very little disturbance of function in the muscle.

C. **Myositis ossificans.**—Some mention of this disease should perhaps be made here ; for although it has been regarded as an inflammatory condition, yet other observers have regarded it in the light of a new growth. It would seem to occur as the result of very slight injury, giving rise to painful swellings in the muscle, in which ossification takes place, with the formation of knobbed and branching fragments of osseous tissue. These osseous masses may either lie free in the muscle or be attached to the bones. The most frequent seat of onset is in the muscles of the neck, back, and thorax; and it gradually extends to other muscles of the body, so that in the course of years the body becomes absolutely rigid. The disease frequently starts in youth, and sometimes in quite young children.

The formation of the new bone always takes place in the connective tissue, the atrophy of the muscle fibres being secondary.

Fred. E. Batten.

REFERENCES

Acute polymyositis : 1. HERRICK. *Amer. Jour. Med. Sci.* 1896, vol. cxi. p. 414.— 2. KELL. *Jour. Amer. Med. Ass.* Chicago, 1896, vol. xxvi. p. 967.—3. V. KORNILOW. *Deutsch. Zeit. f. Nervenheilk.* 1897, Bd. ix. S. 119.—4. PFEIFFER. *Centralblatt für allg. Path. u. path. Anat.* 1896, Bd. vii. S. 81.—5. PLUYMERS. *Arch. de méd. expér. et d'anat. path.* Paris, 1896, tome viii. p. 761.—6. STRÜMPELL. *Deutsche Zeit. für Nervenheil.* 1891, Bd. i. S. 479. A full bibliography will be found under 1, 4, and 6. **Infective myositis :** 7. BOISSON. *Arch. d. méd. et phar. mil.* 1895, tome xxv. p. 122. — 8. DUPLAY. *Union méd.* Paris, 1895, tome lix. p. 601.—9. FRAENKEL. *Deutsch. med. Woch.* 1894, Bd. xx. p. 193.—10. HAYEN. *Dict. encyclo. des sci. méd.* 1876, vol. x. p. 728.—11. NEUMANN. *Deutsche med. Woch.* 1895, Bd. xxi. p. 386.—12. PHILLIPS. *Brit. Med. Jour.* 1886, vol. ii. p. 1215.—13. SCRIBA. *Deutsche Zeit. f. Chir.* 1885, Bd. xxii. p. 497.—14. TREVES. *Clinical Soc. Trans.* 1887, vol. xx. p. 80 —15. WAETZOLD. *Zeit. f. klin. Med.* 1893, Bd. xxii. p. 600.—16. WALTHER. *Deutsche Zeit. f. Chir.* 1887, Bd. xxv. p. 260.—17. WINCKEL. *Gynäkolog. Centralblatt,* 1878, Bd. ii. p. 145.—18. ZEIGLER. *Pathological Anatomy.* **Syphilitic myositis :** 19. EGER. *Deutsche med. Woch.* 1896, Bd. xxii. S. 565.—20. HERRICK. *Amer. Jour. Med. Sci.* 1896, vol. cxi. S. 414.—21. LEWIN. *Charité-Annalen,* 1891, Bd. xvi. p. 753.—22. NEUMANN. *Viertel. f. Dermat. u. Syphilis,* 1888, Bd. xx. p. 19.—23. Idem. *Allg. Wien. med. Zeit.* 1896, Bd. xli. pp. 267-279. — 24. WILKS and MOXON. *Pathological Anatomy,* p. 99. **Myositis ossificans :** 25. LEXER. *Centralblatt f. Pathologie,* 1896, Bd. vii. p. 929. — 26. PINCUS. *Deutsche Zeit. f. Chir.* 1897, Bd. xliv. p. 179.— 27. ZIEGLER. *Pathological Anatomy.*

F. E. B.

MYOTONIA CONGENITA

SYNONYM.—*Thomsen's disease*

Definitions.—Thomsen's disease is a malady the chief feature of which is that upon the execution of any voluntary movement the muscles brought into play remain contracted for some seconds.

History.—It is usually said that Sir Charles Bell first described this disorder; but he gave it no name, and I think that any one reading his description will agree that it is extremely doubtful whether the cases which he described were really examples of Thomsen's disease. Two cases were referred to by Benedikt in 1864; but it was the publication, in 1876, by Dr. Thomsen, a Danish physician, of a description of the disease as it existed in himself that first directed attention to it. Since then several cases have been published; but the disorder is excessively rare; indeed, it is probable that Thomsen's disease is the rarest in medicine. In 1890, when I collected all the cases that had then been published, and showed one at the Medical Society, an account of which is published in the *Guy's Hospital Reports* (vol. xlvi.), only one case had been shown at the Medical Societies of Great Britain or mentioned in our medical journals; namely, that exhibited by Dr. Buzzard at the Neurological Society in 1887. It was described by him in the *Lancet* of that year. At the same time that I brought my case before the Medical Society Dr Herschell showed two brothers suffering from the disorder. It appears to be equally rare in all countries. Cases have been recorded in Germany, France, Italy, Russia, Sweden, America, and England.

Causes.—No cause for Thomsen's disease has been discovered. One or two cases have been set down to fright; but in the great majority there is no evidence of this, and frights of some sort or another are so common that their influence, if any, is indeterminable.

Heredity.—In nearly all the cases recorded the disorder existed in several relatives of the patient—generally in one of the parents, and in the patient's brothers, sisters, and children. This is so marked a feature that it must be regarded as one of the characteristics of the disease. Several of Thomsen's relatives were affected with it, and my patient's father and sister and two of his father's cousins had suffered from it.

Some authors have been inclined to lay stress upon the fact that other neuroses have been present in the same family. Many of Thomsen's ancestors suffered from mental weakness; nevertheless, as it is so often expressly stated that there was no neurotic history, I do not think that a family history of neuroses has much bearing on the matter. The patient himself is rarely of neurotic habit.

Age.—When the patients first come under observation they are usually about twenty years old; mine was nineteen. Generally they

either say they have had the disease as long as they can remember, or
that it came on in childhood, when they first noticed that they could not
take part in games because of the stiffness of the muscles.

Sex.—It is much commoner in males than in females. In fact, few of
the described cases have occurred in women, although it is often stated
that some female relative of the patient is suffering from it.

Symptoms.—*Peculiarity of movement.*—This only occurs in voluntary
movements, and consists in the fact that the contraction of the muscle
which the patient wills to move is slower than normal, and that, because it
relaxes gradually and very slowly, it remains for some seconds more or
less contracted ; this contraction is so strong that the antagonistic muscles
cannot overcome it. If a certain voluntary movement is repeated several
times the patient begins to execute each movement before the preceding
contraction had completely relaxed, and thus his difficulty as regards the
stiffness gradually becomes less and less in each movement. Walking is
very commonly affected ; for example, if the patient be standing still and
set out to walk, he puts forward one leg rather slowly, it then remains
stiff for a few seconds ; the next time it is moved the stiffness is of shorter
duration, and he soon walks quite comfortably even for miles ; but if
he trip against a stone, and thus bring into play some new muscular
combination, the muscles newly engaged become stiff, and he may fall
down. Flexion of the fingers usually illustrates the peculiarity of the
disease very well ; thus, in my patient it is obvious that the flexor muscles
contract more slowly than normal ; they appear to remain completely
contracted for from one to three seconds, and then they are not
completely relaxed, for if he is told to unclose the hand as quickly as
possible it is often between seven and ten seconds before the extensors
completely overcome the flexors ; as they do so, first the metacarpo-
phalangeal joints become slowly extended, then the middle phalangeal, and
finally the terminal phalangeal joints. If flexion be repeated as rapidly
as possible the second contraction obviously succeeds more rapidly than the
first, the third more rapidly than the second ; and after about half a dozen
contractions the action appears quite normal ; yet even then myographic
tracings show that many contractions take place before they become quite
regular. The difficulty is the same whatever muscles are affected, and
different patients find different movements particularly difficult. Thus
my patient, who is a carpenter, finds it difficult to saw, for he cannot start
easily, and, when his sawing has become even and free, if he stop to rest
the difficulty reappears directly he begins again. He cannot turn his
head, nor extend his thighs, nor put out his tongue, nor contract his
facial muscles properly. If he is told to open and shut his mouth it is
some few seconds before the masseter and internal pterygoid can overcome
the contraction of the depressors of the jaw ; but after two or three
movements the opening and closing of the mouth become easy. His
father finds going up and down stairs particularly difficult. Other
patients have noticed the difficulty in dancing and drilling ; indeed,
the difficulty of which the patient chiefly complains is almost always

connected with some movement of the extremities. Occasionally the stiffness is much more marked during the second movement than during the first. These peculiar arrests appear to be affected neither by cold, by direction of the attention to them, by mental excitement, by time of day, by alcohol, by meals, nor by temperature; but sometimes if the patient be fatigued the peculiarity is especially prominent.

Such a defect in the acts of swallowing, respiration, micturition, defæcation, and parturition has never been recorded; but with these exceptions the stiffness may be observed in any movement executed by voluntary muscles. The muscles of the arms and legs are most commonly implicated; the legs, perhaps, a little oftener than the arms. The muscles of the trunk, as shown in stooping, and those of the head and neck, are often affected; so also are those of the face and of mastication. Some of the rarest muscles to be implicated are those of deglutition, the ocular muscles—affection of which gives rise to squint and diplopia—and the laryngeal muscles, which may have been disordered in some cases in which a difficulty of speech was observed; but difficulty of breathing has never occurred. The interossei often escape; my patient can write very well although his long flexors are badly affected. The superficial and deep reflexes are normal. Usually the grasp, as tested with the dynamometer, is, if anything, below the normal standard; this is especially noteworthy, as in these patients the muscles usually look bulky. There are no sensory disturbances, and the optic discs are healthy.

Electrical reactions.—These, which are characteristic of the disease, have been collectively named by Erb the "myotonic reaction." They are as follows: (i.) The motor nerves show no increase of irritability to mechanical stimuli; (ii.) To the faradic current the motor nerves are quantitatively normal, but if the current be strong the contraction produced on closing the circuit lasts much longer than it does in health; (iii.) To the galvanic current the motor nerves are quantitatively normal; but here also if the current be strong the contraction lasts longer than in health; (iv.) Mechanical stimuli applied to the muscles, as by hitting them, induce contractions more easily than in health; these contractions often last from five to thirty seconds; (v.) The faradic current applied directly to the muscles, if strong, sets up a contraction which lasts from five to thirty seconds; (vi.) When the galvanic current is applied directly to the muscle K.C.C. and A.C.C. are equally easy to obtain; while in health, as is well known, K.C.C. is more readily elicited than A.C.C. In Thomsen's disease even with weak currents the contraction lasts longer than in health; with strong currents it lasts some seconds and relaxes very slowly. With the stabile application well-formed wave-like contractions are seen to proceed slowly from the cathode to the anode.

Many observers have confirmed these observations of Erb; but it is quite exceptional for all the points of his "myotonic reaction" to be observed in the same case. Thus in my patient points ii., iii., v., and vi. correspond to Erb's description, except that I, like many observers, cannot obtain the wave-like contractions he describes as following the stabile application of the galvanic current. On the other hand, I am easily able, by rolling the ulnar nerve of my patient under my fingers, to make the muscles supplied by it contract; although I found by repeated observation that in healthy persons this is not easy to do. The contraction and relaxation are both prolonged, but I cannot make the patient's muscles contract when I hit them. Thus I have failed to make Erb's first and fourth points.

Myographic tracings. — Some French observers took myographic tracings of the movements; I did the same, and the tracings obtained will be found in the Guy's Hospital Reports, vol. xlvi. They show in detail the peculiarities of the muscular contraction; for instance, a tracing was taken of the contraction of the flexors of the forearm when the patient opened and shut his hand as fast as he could. The first contraction was very slow, and the muscles took four seconds to reach their maximum contraction. This remained for fully a second, and then relaxation began; but the second contraction started 6·15 seconds after the beginning of the first, and therefore well before relaxation was complete. Like the first, it was slow and remained at its maximum a short time, but from the beginning of the second contraction to the beginning of the third was only 4·1 seconds: the second was not so powerful as the first. The interval between the subsequent contractions gradually became shorter and their intensity feebler and feebler until the ninth contraction, when the amplitude became greater; and from then to the twenty-third the interval between the contractions became gradually less, and for the most part the amplitude increased. After this the contractions were regular, frequent, and ample; and from the beginning of one to the beginning of the next was 1·3 seconds. The first few movements often showed slight irregularity of tracing both in contraction and relaxation.

Tracings, therefore, teach us graphically, not only what is evident when the movement is watched, but also that it is a long while before contraction and relaxation are normal; that, after the first one or two, contraction is feeble for a time; and that the early contractions and relaxations are often a little irregular.

Tracings were also taken showing the result of a single contraction of the extensors of the forearm induced by the galvanic current. The rise occupied ·09 of a second, the fall or relaxation occupied ·5 of a second; while in a contraction of my own extensors obtained under precisely similar conditions the rise occupied ·06 of a second, and the fall ·15· These figures show very well that in Thomsen's disease the contraction and relaxation, but especially the relaxation, are much prolonged. In other experiments a tetanising current was used; and here again it was shown that both contraction and relaxation, but especially relaxation, were much longer than in health. I made many experiments to determine the length of the latent period, because Blumeau and one or two other experimenters have stated that in Thomsen's disease it is prolonged; I always found, however, that it was of the same length as that of a healthy person.

Duration.—So far as is known the disease never passes off; on the other hand it has never been the cause of death. The stiffness usually becomes a little worse at puberty.

Histology.—A necropsy has only once been performed upon a case of this disease, and this is recorded by Déjerine and Sottas. Their patient, a man aged 37, died of acute nephritis. They could not by the most careful examination find anything abnormal in the brain, spinal cord, or peripheral nerves. Their examination of the muscles confirms in every particular the description given by Erb, Nearonow, myself, and others, all of whom took a piece from the affected muscles during life. My patient willingly consented, and under chloroform a small piece was cut out of the flexors of the left forearm. The most important abnormality of the muscle in Thomsen's disease is the great width of the muscular fibres. Those of my patient were from $\frac{1}{150}$ to $\frac{1}{300}$ of an inch wide. The normal width of the fibres of the voluntary muscles of the limbs is, according to Quain, from $\frac{1}{400}$ to $\frac{1}{750}$ of an inch; and I controlled the examination by some normal fibres from the flexors of an adult forearm, and found them to vary between $\frac{1}{350}$ and $\frac{1}{1000}$ of an inch in width. Thus we see that in Thomsen's disease the fibres are quite double the width of those in the normal state; indeed, cases have been described in which they were four times as wide. The transverse striation is always very feebly marked, the border of the fibre is slightly and irregularly curved, and the nuclei of the sarcolemma are increased in number. Some observers have described an increase of the connective tissue between the fibres. If present at all, it was very slight in Déjerine and Sottas' case, and in mine. Erb has figured and described large vacuoles in the fibres, but no other observer has seen them.

Pathology.—The occurrence of the disease in several members of the same family, and the fact that it is nearly always first detected in childhood, shows that it is congenital; and it would appear that each individual affected is from his birth faultily constructed, so that some of his muscular fibres all through his life grow abnormally, and in consequence of this abnormal growth contract in an abnormal manner. This is more in harmony with what we know of other diseases than to believe, as Déjerine and Sottas apparently do, that the abnormal contraction of the muscle leads to its abnormal growth. All who have written on the subject agree that it is a disease solely of the muscular system.

In any discussion on the pathology of the disease, it must always be borne in mind that the peculiar contractions are exactly the same as those which may be induced in animals which have been poisoned by veratria; as may be readily seen by comparing the curves I obtained with those in a text-book of Physiology. Ringer and Sainsbury found that if phosphate of soda be given to an animal and the sciatic nerve then stimulated, contractions like those of Thomsen's disease are produced; and this even if curare had been previously injected. Hence it appears that the Thomsen-like contractions are due to the action of phosphate of soda on the muscular fibres themselves.

Treatment.—No treatment that has been employed has had any good effect. Thomsen thought he was better the more active his life. The sister of Dr. Herschell's patient said the disease lessened after she was married.

W. HALE WHITE.

REFERENCES

1. BELL, CHARLES. *The Nervous System of the Human Body*, 1st ed. p. cl. and iv. 1830.—2. BENEDIKT. *Nervenpathologie und Electrotherapie*, 1st ed. 1864.—3. ERB. *Die Thomsen'sche Krankheit (Myotonia congenita)*. Leipzig, 1886.—4. *Idem.* "Ueber die Thomsen'sche Krankheit (Myotonia congenita)," *Deutsches Arch. f. klin. Medicin*, Bd. xlv. S. 529.—5. BUZZARD. *Lancet*, 14th May 1887.—6. GOWERS. *Diseases of the Nervous System*, vol. i. 2nd ed.—7. BALLET and MARIE. "Spasme musculaire au début des mouvements volontaires," *Archives de neurologie*, January 1883.—8. RINGER and SAINSBURY. *Lancet*, pp. 767, 816, 860 ; 1884.—9. THOMSEN, Dr. "Tonische Krampfe in willkürlich beweglichen Muskeln in Folge von ererbter psychischer Disposition," *Archiv fur Psychiatrie*, 1876, Bd. vi. S. 702.—10. *Idem. Centralblatt f. Nervenkrankheiten*, 1885, S. 193.—11. BLUMEAU. *Neurolog. Centralblatt*, 1889, p. 679.—12. NEARONOW. *Neurolog. Centralblatt*, 1889, S. 239.—13. DÉJERINE and SOTTAS. "Sur un cas de maladie de Thomsen, suivi d'autopsie," *Revue de médecine*, 1895, xv. p. 241.—14. WHITE, W. HALE. "On Thomsen's Disease," *Guy's Hospital Reports*, vol. xlvi. 1889.

W. H. W.

IDIOPATHIC MUSCULAR ATROPHY AND HYPERTROPHY

SYNONYM.—*Primary progressive myopathy, progressive muscular dystrophy* (Erb).

Definition.—Under the name of idiopathic muscular atrophy is comprised a group of cases which, though for some time confused with atrophies of muscles due to lesions in the spinal cord, are now considered to be due to lesions of the muscular substance itself, the cord not being affected. Clinically they are distinguished by atrophy and hypertrophy of muscles, which differ in their grouping from that obtained in the progressive muscular atrophy due to disease of the anterior cornua of the spinal cord. Etiologically they are characterised by occurrence in several members of one family of the same or of a subsequent generation. In all these cases the muscles themselves are at fault, and though the changes do not usually occur for a few or, it may be, for several years after birth, the disease is essentially congenital.

As the changes in the muscles may, on the one hand, be in the muscular tissue leading to atrophy, and, on the other hand, in the connective tissue leading to hypertrophy, the comprehensive name progressive muscular dystrophy is more applicable to the members of this group generally than the name atrophy. In this group are included several varieties which will be described separately ; but as these varieties agree in being due to changes in the muscles, apart from the central nervous system, they can all be included under the general name.

History.—The first cases described were those now known as pseudo-hypertrophic paralysis, of which instances were described by Sir Charles Bell (in 1830) and by Partridge (1847). Meryon, who gave a very accurate description of four boys in one family affected by atrophy with contractures, published in 1852 (21) an account of a necropsy, in which he states that the spinal cord and nerves were carefully examined microscopically, and not the slightest trace of disease was detected in the ganglion cells of the gray matter and the anterior roots; the only structural change observed was in the muscular fibres, which were broken down and converted into oil globules and granular matter; of these changes he gave drawings. Meryon, in 1852, called the disease a granular and fatty degeneration of voluntary muscles. In 1853 Little referred to two exemplary cases of pseudo-hypertrophic paralysis, which he observed in 1847 in two brothers with enlarged calves, talipes equinus, lordosis on standing, cyphosis on sitting, and atrophy of the upper arms with large deltoids; at the necropsy the gastrocnemii were found large and fatty with only traces of muscle tissue; but no mention is made of the spinal cord. In 1855 Duchenne (8) published cases of progressive muscular atrophy in adults and children, and described some of these cases in adults as beginning in the trunk muscles or shoulder, and in the latter as affecting the facial muscles, and especially the orbicularis oris; but he ascribed them to lesions of the cord. Duchenne, in 1855 (9), speaking on "atrophie musculaire graisseuse," and on an autopsy of a case by Cruveilhier, refers to Meryon's case, the figures illustrating which, Duchenne says, have a great similarity with the features he has seen in cases of "atrophie musculaire graisseuse," and he dismisses the matter with the opinion that Meryon's case was one of a "muscular affection commencing in infancy, of which I state that I have seen a good number, and which I will call Paralysie atrophique graisseuse de l'enfance," a disease which, from his description on p. 839 (*loc. cit.*), was evidently infantile paralysis.

Meryon, in 1864 (22), describes an autopsy made on a second case in 1859, in which he states that not a trace of disease was found in the central nervous system, also that these cases may be recognised by the absence of any symptom of central disturbance, and that they are not the same as simple muscular atrophy, but are due to lesions of the muscles only. He says, "M. Duchenne has referred my first case to a category of disease which he designs as nervous in character, resulting from some antecedent febrile affection, and terminating in rapid recovery or in degeneration into fat of the affected muscles, and he calls this 'Atrophie graisseuse de l'enfance,' . . . but my cases have nothing in common with these." Meryon further showed the hereditary nature of his cases; and also stated that in one family there was an uncommon increase of the gastrocnemii. He further states, "I am induced to believe in an idiopathic disease of the muscles, dependent perhaps on defective nutrition. Spontaneous twitchings are not apt to occur."

In 1865 Eulenberg and Cohnheim described and examined a case after death, and found no changes in the spinal cord, and in 1871 this condition was confirmed by Charcot in a case of Duchenne's.

From these extracts it is evident that Meryon, in 1852, was the first observer to attribute these cases to idiopathic diseases of the muscles. This is all the more important as the first description of these cases has been ascribed to Duchenne, who, in 1861 (10), described them under the name of Paraplegie congenitale cerebrale hypertrophique; it was not until 1868 that he recognised the malady as independent of all alteration of the nervous system, and gave it the name of pseudo-hypertrophic paralysis. Duchenne laid great stress on the hypertrophy of the muscles, which was not a prominent feature of Meryon's cases. Adams, in 1868, published several cases; and in 1876 Leyden put into a separate class certain muscular atrophies which occur in families, and called them "hereditary."

In 1882 Erb (11) described a form of muscular atrophy occurring in young people, in whom the muscles did not give the reaction of degeneration to electrical testing, and this form he qualified as "juvenile."

Landouzy and Déjerine, in 1884, published a note, with one necropsy, on cases after the so-called facio-scapulo-humeral type, in which the spinal cord and peripheral nerves were exempt, but where there was a simple atrophy of the muscle fibres; and they distinguished between these cases, which they called "Myopathie atrophique progressive" of childhood, and the "Atrophie progressive myelopathique" of adults, in which the cord is involved. In 1885 these authors published a full paper on their cases.

In 1884, two months after the above, Erb (12) published a full account of the juvenile form of muscular atrophy.

The best account in this country of pseudo-hypertrophic paralysis is the monograph by Sir W. Gowers.

There are, therefore, three principal groups to be described:—

    I. Pseudo-hypertrophic muscular paralysis.
    II. The juvenile form of progressive muscular atrophy.
    III. The facio-scapulo-humeral form.

Besides these there are intermediate forms which are not sufficiently uniform to be grouped in another class.

Of the second group the earliest record that I can find of any case is that of a man named Seurat, who was exhibited in London in 1825 as the "Living Skeleton"; from the drawings of this man given in Hone's Everyday Book, and from the description of the case, I have no doubt that his case was a form of juvenile muscular atrophy. The patient was healthy till the age of ten years, when the muscles began to waste; and at the time of the description, when he was twenty-eight years old, the wasting especially affected the muscles of the trunk, humerus, and femur, a distribution which, as will be seen later, is characteristic of these cases.

I. Pseudo-hypertrophic paralysis (Myo-sclerotic paralysis).

Etiology.—*Age.*—Pseudo-hypertrophic paralysis is essentially a disease of childhood. In some cases the child has never walked properly; in others the child is quite well till four or five years old; or the onset may be delayed till the ninth or tenth year; or again, in a few cases, till puberty.

Sex.—Boys are very much more often attacked than girls. This is in marked contrast to the cases of the juvenile type which attacks both sexes about equally.

Heredity.—The disease is peculiar in attacking several members of the same family. In Meryon's cases, quoted above, all the four boys of one family were attacked, while the six girls escaped. But although the women of a family escape they are able to transmit the disease to their sons, and cases are on record in which the disease has been transmitted by the female side to the third generation (Gowers). The disease does not seem to be induced or affected by social surroundings.

Symptoms. — The increased size of the muscles is not usually observed by the friends; this is probably due to the fact that a uniform enlargement of the muscles is considered as a mark of strength, while atrophy is associated with paralysis; thus, it is unusual for the patient to be brought at an early stage for advice on account of the large size of the muscles.

The first symptom which the parents notice is the frequency and readiness with which the child falls down, and the difficulty that it has in getting on to its feet again; as the friends will say "the least touch makes the child fall." Another early observation is the difficulty in going upstairs.

Associated with this weakness is an alteration in the size of the muscles of the limbs and trunk. The alteration is either in the direction of hypertrophy or of atrophy, and it is remarkable that certain muscles have a tendency to hypertrophy and others to atrophy; although some muscles are said to hypertrophy at first and to atrophy later, the condition which the muscle assumes at first is frequently maintained throughout.

Of the muscles which enlarge, the calf muscles, the gastrocnemius and soleus especially are thus affected. They may at first be only harder than natural, but frequently they enlarge very much, as in the case of a boy aged twelve years, in whom the calf measured 14½ inches (Gowers); they assume a peculiar shape, the posterior border of the calf presenting an elliptical shape, so that the most prominent point of the convex curve is over the middle of the calf, whereas in true muscular hypertrophy the calves are flatter. The weakness of these muscles can be demonstrated by the inability of the patient to stand on tip-toes, whereby it is made evident that the increased size is not due to increase of muscular tissue.

The anterior tibials are said to be increased in some cases, but this is certainly unusual. Of the other muscles of the lower limb, the extensors of the knee and the gluteus maximus are especially enlarged. Of the extensors of the knee the vastus externus is perhaps the most commonly enlarged, and it is characterised by causing an abrupt projection just above the knee. The glutei are uniformly enlarged and hard to the touch. The flexors of the knee, and the flexors and adductors of the hip-joint are usually atrophied. The erector spinæ is in some cases hypertrophied, in others atrophied.

In the shoulder the hypertrophied muscles are the deltoid and the supra- and infra-spinati, which are nearly always enlarged ; the deltoid is very much enlarged, and if it be felt during relaxation, by passively supporting the arm at right angles to the trunk, it will be found harder than natural. The condition of the supra-spinatus, from its being covered by the trapezius, is more difficult to ascertain ; but the infra-spinatus stands out prominently as a hard mass.

Of the muscles which are wasted, the lower half of the pectoralis major arising from the sternum and the latissimus dorsi are almost invariably affected ; the absence of the former is well shown by making the patient advance both arms horizontally forwards, when on pressing the hands together the upper fibres alone of the pectoralis major will be seen to contract, and the sharp lower border of these fibres will be felt passing to the upper end of the sternum. Absence of the latissimus dorsi and pectoralis major (lower half) can also be shown by making the patient adduct the humerus, previously raised to the horizontal line, against resistance, when no muscle will be seen going from the humerus towards the pelvic brim, and the teres muscles will stand out. The trapezius, rhomboids and serratus magnus are usually not affected, though the last may be wasted.

In the arm the triceps is usually hypertrophied, presenting a convex outline which is very characteristic, while the biceps is atrophied.

In the hand and forearm the muscles usually escape, but the extensors of the wrist and fingers are sometimes slightly enlarged, and the supinator longus may be atrophied or enlarged. The intrinsic muscles of the hand nearly always escape ; but examples of hypertrophy have been observed by Sachs, and enlargement of the abductor indicis by Taylor.

The muscles of the face and neck are not affected as a rule, but in a few cases the tongue and masseters have been enlarged.

The weakness of the muscles gives rise to a peculiar attitude and gait. While sitting down nothing peculiar is noticed ; but when the patient is told to stand up, especially from a low seat, he finds considerable difficulty in doing so. This is due in great measure to weakness of the extensors of the hips and of the knees. Also, in getting up from the supine position on the ground certain actions are performed which are quite characteristic. Instead of assuming the sitting position, the patient rotates the whole trunk by means of pressure with the arms on the ground, so as to get on to one side ; he then flexes the hips, drawing up the knees under the abdomen, and is enabled by rotating the trunk round the knees as a fixed point to get on to his hands and knees "on all-fours" ; he next extends the knees by throwing the head well down between the arms, so as to bring the centre of gravity as much forwards from the hips as possible. When the knees are extended he keeps the feet fixed, travels back on his hands, and then suddenly transfers one hand from the ground to his knee and then the other hand; now he has to extend the hip, and this he does by transferring each hand in turn to a higher point along the thigh till, by suddenly throwing the shoulders back he can extend the hip and get the trunk into the erect posture, shifting his centre of gravity backwards. In standing the patient keeps his feet wide apart to insure a broad basis, and in walking he has a peculiar "waddle," throwing the shoulders from side to side ; this action is to enable the feet to clear the ground, and it is particularly noticed when there is paralysis of the anterior tibial muscles and of the flexors of the hips. Another symptom observed, if there is weakness of the extensors of the knee, is that the knee comes forward in advance of the foot, the leg being swung into the extended position before receiving the weight of the body.

Another important deformity is that of the spine, which changes its curves in the standing and sitting positions; on standing there is frequently marked lordosis, the concavity being most in the lumbar region, with a marked compensatory· convex curve of the cervical and upper dorsal region, so that a plumb-line hung from the most prominent point of this upper curve would fall an inch or more behind the gluteal region ; on sitting down, these curves either disappear altogether or the spine forms one curve with its concavity forwards (cyphosis). The causes which produce these curves are discussed farther on, as well as the deformity of the scapula produced by paralysis of its muscles.

Besides the above deformities, which are due to paralysis of the muscles, there is another which is due to the contracture of certain muscles, and notably of those of the calf (producing talipes equinus); this contracture occurs rather early in the disease, and appears to be due to the gradual shortening of the fibrous tissue of the muscle, which in these cases is much hypertrophied, and consequently it takes place only in the muscles which are enlarged.

The electrical reactions of the muscles are very important, especially from a diagnostic point of view. At first there is no alteration, but, as the muscles whether in atrophy or hypertrophy become weaker, the amount of contraction both to faradic and galvanic currents diminishes. This is owing to the fact that only those fibrils can contract which still retain their muscular qualities. As the disease progresses, the strength of the currents has to be increased until, finally, when there is no more muscular tissue left, the muscle ceases to respond to either current. There is never, however, what is known as the reaction of degeneration, namely, a slow, deliberate contraction to the constant current, and a readier response to the anode closing of the circuit than to the cathode closing (Erb).

The persistence of the knee-jerk depends upon the state of the extensor quadriceps cruris. It has been said that the knee-jerk is increased in the early stages of the disease, but I have never yet seen such a case. As the extensor cruris becomes more involved and weaker, the knee-jerk diminishes and is finally abolished; it probably varies directly as the integrity of the vastus internus, for Professor Sherrington has shown that the presence of the knee-jerk in the monkey depends entirely on the integrity of this part of the extensor quadriceps. Ankle clonus is never obtained.

The superficial reflexes, such as the plantar, are obtained as long as there are any muscles to respond to the sensory stimulus.

Another symptom, which separates these cases from progressive spinal muscular atrophy, is the complete absence of muscular fibrillar contractions, which are never observed.

Sensation for all kinds of stimulation is always intact.

The sphincters are not affected except perhaps at the very end of the disease.

The degree to which the muscles are hypertrophied or atrophied varies very much, and in some cases atrophy so predominates that hypertrophy exists to a slight degree or not at all.

II. THE JUVENILE FORM OF PROGRESSIVE MUSCULAR ATROPHY, to which Erb first directed attention, differs from the preceding in that the muscles are usually atrophied, not hypertrophied; and that the onset of the disease is much later in life. It will be described nnder the next type.

III. THE FACIAL SCAPULO-HUMERAL FORM OF LANDOUZY AND DÉJERINE is probably the same disease as the juvenile form, but the face muscles also are affected. It is advisable, therefore, to describe the groups together under the name *Idiopathic muscular atrophy, or Progressive myopathy.*

The hereditary nature of the disease is markedly present not only in one generation, but running through several. In one instance 24 cases were distributed through five generations (Barsickow). Still, in many cases no other members of the family are found to be affected.

The sexes are about equally affected, a point of distinction from pseudo-hypertrophic paralysis.

According to Erb's account of his cases in 1882 and 1884, the disease attacks children or young people about the time of puberty; always beginning before the twentieth year. The muscles first affected are those of the shoulder girdle and of the upper arm; and the list includes the pectorales major and minor, trapezius, latissimus dorsi, biceps, brachialis anticus, supinator longus, triceps, and later the thigh muscles, and the anterior tibial muscles and peronei. The face is not affected, and the forearm muscles, with the exception of the supinator longus, escape.

The account given of their cases by Landouzy and Déjerine in 1884 is, that they were described by Duchenne (8) originally under the name of progressive muscular atrophy of childhood, but were confused by him with cases of spinal cord origin; the authors consider them to be myopathic as opposed to the myelopathic progressive muscular atrophy of adults. The disease begins most often in infancy, and in the face; it may, however, begin in youth, in adult, or in advanced age.

When it begins in the face the orbiculares palpebrarum and oris are the first to be attacked, and thus arises a peculiar physiognomy, which gives to the face when at rest a sanctimonious expression (facies béat) : the lips are prominent, and the forehead smooth as ivory ; the eyeballs are apparently prominent, and on movement of the face a retraction of the angles of the mouth without elevation of the upper lip produces a curious, sad expression, the immobility of the features contrasting with the animation of the eyes.

After the face, the atrophy nearly always attacks next the upper limbs, and especially the muscles about the shoulders and arms ; hence the name " facio-scapulo-humeral " palsy.

The muscles which escape are the supra- and infra-spinati, the subscapularis, the flexors of the wrist and fingers, and the muscles of the eyes, mastication, swallowing, and speech. The muscles are atrophied from the beginning, and there is no hypertrophy.

Fibrillar contractions of the muscles are absent, and idio-muscular contraction disappears or is much diminished. Electrical contraction, to both currents, is modified quantitatively ; the normal formula is diminished, but it is not inverted ; that is to say, there is no reaction of degeneration. As a rule the tendon reflexes do not disappear till the muscles are very much atrophied.

In youth and adult life the disease is said to be rarer than in childhood, and does not always begin with the face ; it may start in the upper limbs, or even in the lower limbs, and the face may or may not be affected later.

The lesion consists of an atrophic myositis with a very slight amount of sclerosis.

According to Landouzy and Déjerine, their facio-scapulo-humeral form is quite distinct from the juvenile form of muscular atrophy of Erb. They state that their disease more often begins in the face than not ; that in progressive atrophy of myelopathic or spinal cord origin the face is never affected, and that atrophy of the muscles of the face is the only clinical character by which one can distinguish the disease at once.

The cases in this country evidently differ from those met with in France. In the first place, I would say that Erb's juvenile form of muscular atrophy is very much more common than the facial scapulo-humeral ; that the latter form begins more frequently about puberty than at an earlier age ; and that the statement that affection of the face is diagnostic of the myopathic disease can hardly be maintained. When contrasted with cases of progressive muscular atrophy of spinal origin in which bulbar paralysis affects the facial muscles, we observe that the spinal character is shown by a peculiar association of certain muscles of the face. The cases which I have seen in this country appear to be instances of Erb's juvenile form of atrophy with the facial symptoms added ; and the changes consist in atrophy of the muscles without hypertrophy.

In Erb's juvenile form, the biceps, triceps, and supinator longus are the first to be affected ; in a short time the pectoralis major and latissimus dorsi are wasted; the serratus magnus is usually paralysed; and, as the deltoids, along with the supra- and infra-spinati, are often preserved, the scapulæ project very much at their posterior border when the arms are held out in front by the patient. The trapezius is especially liable to be affected along its whole breadth, including the highest clavicular fibres, whereby the slope of the neck to the shoulders is altered—a condition which is very characteristic of myopathies; and sometimes the sterno-mastoids are wasted : the forearm, with the exception of the supinator longus, escapes; and so also do the hand muscles, except in some cases, of which I have seen one where the face was also affected.

The back and trunk muscles are frequently much affected, and give rise to the following deformities of the spine :—(i.) When on standing up there is marked lordosis, so that a plumb-line let fall from the most prominent point of the dorsal spine, hangs several inches behind the sacrum; whereas on sitting down the lordosis disappears, or is transformed into cyphosis; here the erector spinæ muscles are at fault. (ii.) When with extreme lordosis the sacrum projects back so much that the plumb-line does not fall without the sacrum, it will be found that the pelvis is tilted forwards; and in addition to weakness of the erector spinæ there is weakness of the glutei : in this case the lordosis disappears on sitting down. (iii.) When the former condition of lordosis does not disappear on sitting down, there is superadded weakness of the recti abdominis muscles, which are unable to keep up traction on the thorax from the pelvis in front to flex the spine, and to prevent the abdominal wall from projecting forwards. The trunk in these extreme cases assumes a swan-like appearance, and the walk is very like the waddle of that bird. In the lower limbs, besides the glutei, the adductors and the flexors of the hip are often weak, and especially the quadriceps extensor cruris, which may be much wasted; below the knee the anterior tibial muscles suffer occasionally.

'In the facio-scapulo-humeral groups the orbicularis palpebrarum is wasted, and so weak that the patient cannot completely close the eyelids, and soap gets into the eyes in washing the face. The eyelids can be opened with the slightest pressure of the finger, and there is no power of "screwing-up" the eye by the outer fibres of the orbicularis. The levator anguli oris and the orbicularis oris are paralysed, so that there is no power to elevate the upper lip, or to purse up the lips as in whistling. In connection with the affection of these muscles of the face, it is important to note that the muscles of the eyeball escape, and also that the tongue is not involved. As there is reason to believe that the orbicularis palpebrarum gets its nerve-supply through the facial nerve from the 3rd nucleus (Mendel), and the orbicularis oris from the hypoglossal nucleus (Gowers), the fact of the ocular muscles and the tongue not being affected with the orbiculares palpebrarum and oris, would be strong evidence, in determining the diagnosis of any case, against the lesion being in the pons or medulla.

In a case of the facio-scapulo-humeral type, lately under my care, all the muscles of the face were affected except the zygomatici and the corrugator supercilii; the following muscles were absent, or very much atrophied :—the sterno-mastoids, trapezii (except the median horizontal part), deltoids, supinator longus, biceps, triceps, latissimus dorsi, serratus magnus, thenar muscles, first dorsal interossei ; recti abdominis, erectores spinæ; glutei, abductors of the hip, extensors of the knee, and peronei. The supra- and infra-spinati were well marked and perhaps slightly hypertrophied.

In both these forms, as in pseudo-hypertrophic paralysis, there are no fibrillar contractions of the muscles ; the electrical reactions to both forms of current become less, but there is never any reaction of degeneration ; the knee-jerks are retained as long as there are any muscle fibres left in the vastus internus to respond, and then only are they lost. Sensation is never lost, and the sphincters are not affected.

Besides these three symptom groups there are many intermediate forms ; for instance, cases occur in children with all the symptoms of pseudo-hypertrophic paralysis, but without any hypertrophy. On the other hand, cases of myopathy occur in adults in whom some of the muscles are hypertrophied ; but at present they are not sufficiently marked to justify a separate classification.

The course of these diseases is very slow and gradual, but the degree, to which the atrophy reaches in extent and severity, differs in the several groups, and this difference seems to depend on the age at which the disease begins. Pseudo-hypertrophic paralysis is the most fatal form, and in this country it certainly begins at a younger age than the other forms of the malady ; it is remarkable that those rare cases which begin in adult life, and present hypertrophy of some of the muscles, do not run the unfavourable course that cases of ordinary pseudo-hypertrophic paralysis do.

Cases of Erb's juvenile form run a more favourable course than the ordinary pseudo-hypertrophic paralysis, and the atrophy progresses to a certain degree and then often remains stationary ; cases are met with in adults which have not materially altered for eighteen or more years. Also in the case of the facio-humeral series the course depends much on whether the disease began in childhood or after puberty ; as in the latter case the patient may live many years.

The course and duration of pseudo-hypertrophic paralysis vary much in different cases ; and the disease may be divided into two stages, which are separated by the moment when the patient is no longer able to walk. After this time, which may occur when the disease has lasted a few years, the patient rapidly gets worse. It is not usual for the patient to die from the disease itself, yet if he gets a slight attack of bronchitis or pneumonia, the respiratory muscles are so weak that he succumbs to the pulmonary disease : it is unusual for these patients to live over the twentieth year.

Pathology.—The morbid changes are entirely confined to the muscles ; no changes have been found in the spinal cord, the spinal roots, or the peripheral nerves, except in one case (7) where the cord was normal except at the last dorsal segment, where was found an area of granular disintegration in the intermediate substance on each side ; but the cells of the anterior cornua have never been atrophied.

The muscles are found after death either to be very wasted, or, if they have been enlarged, to have diminished to about the normal size. They are paler than natural, and in extreme cases, when cut across, give the appearance of a fatty tumour without any trace of muscle.

When examined under the microscope the muscle fibres, when moderately affected, are diminished in size and numbers, and are separated by fat cells and by bands of fibrous tissue. The relative amount of fat and fibrous tissue differs in different muscles. The change in the muscle is primarily interstitial, and consists of an overgrowth of fat and nucleated fibrous tissue between the muscle fibres, and secondarily in the muscle fibres, which become narrow and irregular in shape. The transverse striation is at first preserved; but it becomes more faint, and finally disappears, and the muscle undergoes a granular degeneration. Rarely the muscle fibres show fatty degeneration, a longitudinal striation or fissuring, vitreous (waxy) degeneration or vacuolation (Gowers). According to Duchenne, the sheaths of the sarcolemma appear to contain fat cells which are really derived from the surrounding connective tissue, and which otherwise differ from the fatty granular condition characteristic of fatty degeneration of muscle; and the interstitial connective tissue is not produced by fibroid degeneration of the muscle.

The fibres have been removed for examination during life by incision by Billroth, or by a harpoon invented by Duchenne; and some of the muscle fibres so removed have been found actually larger than normal (Gowers). It seems, therefore, that the enlargement of the muscle may be due to actual hypertrophy of the muscle fibres as well as to the overgrowth of fat. The change in the muscle does not affect all the fibres at the same time, so that some fibres may be hypertrophied and others may have passed on to the next stage of atrophy. On the other hand, according to Erb (13), the changes are primarily in the muscular substance itself, those in the interstitial tissue being secondary, so that the muscle fibres hypertrophy, their nuclei increase, they are enlarged and subdivision occurs. Soon the muscle fibres atrophy and disappear, and this is attended by increase of the connective tissue with proliferation of nuclei. In this tissue fat appears, and on this depends whether the muscle is atrophied or hypertrophied.

From the changes found after death, it is evident that this disease in its three forms must be looked upon as an idiopathic disease of the muscles, and independent of any changes in the spinal cord or nerves; as was first pointed out by Meryon in 1852: though in his cases the hypertrophy of the muscles was not a prominent feature, and was not pointed out by him.

Erb, however, considers that his juvenile form is not a pure myopathy, but depends on the nervous system; so that, whereas progressive spinal muscular atrophy would be an anatomical disturbance of trophic centres in the cord, his form would be a functional disturbance in the cord.

The difference in the condition assumed by the muscles, that is hypertrophy or atrophy, seems to be due to the amount of fat and fibrous tissue respectively. Those muscles in which the changes are in the direction of formation of fat are the enlarged muscles, and are liable subsequently to atrophy; those in which fibrous changes occur become hard and diminish in size; while in a third group, such as the lower half of the pectoralis major and the latissimus dorsi, the muscles seem to waste and disappear without formation of fat or fibrous tissue. It is difficult to explain why the muscles should behave in this way; but from the hereditary nature of the disease, and from its tendency to attack several members of the same family, it seems that the disposition of the muscles to undergo this fibrous and fatty overgrowth is inherited.

The reason why certain muscles should be singled out by this disease has been given by Babinski and Onanoff, who explain it by the relative times of development of the different muscles. Thus, in examining a five months' fœtus, they ascertained that the muscles which were the most developed included the supinator longus, the serratus magnus, latissimus dorsi, rhomboids, middle and lower part of trapezius, orbicularis oris, quadriceps extensor cruris, tibialis anterior, and, to a less degree, the deltoid, biceps, triceps, infra-spinatus, sub-scapularis, crural muscles; whilst the hand muscles were least developed. As the muscles ranked first are those which are particularly affected in myopathies, the authors conclude that the muscles which are the first to be developed are the first to undergo degeneration in these diseases.

In the hypertrophied muscles the blood-vessels, arteries, and veins are said to be increased and surrounded by foci of embryonal cells. An endarteritis is thus produced which causes a narrowing or blocking of the vessels (Babes).

The intra-muscular nerves have been found intact by most observers (Blocq and Marinesco), but slight changes have been found by Fürstner and by Babes, and especially in the end muscle plate. Changes in the axis-cylinders of the peripheral nerves have been found in places by Gombault, especially near the muscles; these structures had completely disappeared, but the cells of the anterior horns were healthy. The muscle-spindles are not altered (Batten).

The cause of the changes in the muscles has been ascribed by Babes to the changes in the vessels described above, on which their diminished nutrition ensues.

Diagnosis.—This has to be made from diseases of the gray matter of the spinal cord, as progressive muscular atrophy, subacute poliomyelitis, and syringomyelia; from diseases of the anterior roots; from diseases of the peripheral nerves.

The characteristic symptoms of myopathies are:—1. the gradual onset; 2. the distribution and grouping of the affected muscles, which do not conform to a spinal cord or a peripheral nerve type; 3. absence of any fibrillar contractions; 4. absence of the reaction of degeneration to electrical testing; 5. absence of any form of altered sensation.

The distribution and grouping of the affected muscles is the most important symptom, and, as will be seen presently, this distribution is completely at variance with what is found in undoubted spinal cases.

The grouping of the muscles of the upper arm and shoulder, which is characteristic of disease of the anterior horns in the cervical enlargement, or of the anterior roots coming from them, is as follows :—the deltoid, supra-spinatus, infra-spinatus, clavicular part of the pectoralis major, biceps, brachialis anticus, and supinator longus, are involved together as one group—which is probably supplied by the 5th cervical root; the latissimus dorsi, sternal part of pectoralis major, and triceps form another group—which is probably supplied by the 6th cervical root.

Some years ago, before the juvenile form of muscular atrophy was satisfactorily proved to be an idiopathic disease of the muscles, I made lists of the muscles affected in this disease, and in pseudo-hypertrophic paralysis, and found that the grouping does not correspond to that found in undoubted diseases of the spinal cord. For instance, in pseudo-hypertrophic paralysis the deltoid and triceps are hypertrophied, while the biceps, latissimus dorsi, and sternal half of the pectoralis major are wasted; and in the juvenile form the biceps, triceps, and supinator longus are wasted, while the deltoid, supra- and infra-spinati are preserved. Hence muscles which, in spinal cord diseases, are grouped together in a common fate, are here dissociated and follow the behaviour of muscles belonging to other spinal groups. In the same way, in the type of Landouzy and Déjerine, as already pointed out, the association between the orbicularis oris and the muscles of the tongue, and between the orbicularis palpebrarum and the external muscles of the eye, which is characteristic of nuclear lesions, is not found; hence in this form of myopathy, the orbicularis oris and the orbicularis palpebrarum are affected while the muscles of the tongue and of the eyeball are quite free. The grouping of the muscles implicated is of the greatest value in making a diagnosis in doubtful cases; and it has not perhaps been credited with the importance it deserves.

The presence of hypertrophy, associated with weakness, is a certain sign of myopathy ; but, as it is frequently absent, the other symptoms are of more importance.

Prognosis.—As stated above, pseudo-hypertrophic paralysis is the most fatal, the patient usually dying from some pulmonary complication before reaching twenty years of age ; while the facio-scapulo-humeral type and Erb's juvenile form may be consistent with life for many years.

Compared with other diseases the prognosis in the two last forms is much better than in progressive spinal muscular atrophy, but not so good as in subacute poliomyelitis.

As regards the muscles, those which have been attacked never recover; but in the two last forms the disease usually reaches a certain point and then becomes stationary ; and in this case the patient may continue for many years without any further deterioration.

Treatment.—As the disease is probably due to a congenital defect in the muscles themselves, it is difficult for therapeutics to have much effect.

The most important means are to keep the patient warm, and to be very careful, especially in the later stages, that he does not take cold, or get any pulmonary attack.

The muscles should be exercised both passively and actively: passively, by means of massage to the affected muscles, manipulation of the joints to prevent contracture, and by faradising the affected muscles; actively, by getting the patient to perform certain movements every day short of fatigue. He should be encouraged to walk as long as possible, as it has been observed that the subjects of pseudo-hypertrophic paralysis always get rapidly worse when they cease to be able to walk. For this purpose it is advisable to recommend tenotomy when the contracture of the calf muscles is sufficient to prevent walking, and when at the same time the other muscles of the leg are capable of the appropriate movements. No drug has been found to arrest the disease; the best treatment is to keep up the health and strength by tonics and cod-liver oil; the phosphate of iron, arsenic, phosphorus, and strychnine may also be given to improve the general condition, but they are not known to have any specific action upon the affected muscles.

CHARLES E. BEEVOR.

REFERENCES

1. ADAMS, W. *Path. Trans.* 1868.—2. BABINSKI and ONANOFF. *Soc. de biologie,* Feb. 11, 1888.—3. BATTEN. *Brain,* 1897.—4. BELL, Sir CHARLES. *Nervous System,* 2nd edit. 1830, p. 160.—5. BLOCQ and MARINESCO. *Arch. de neurol.* 1893, xxv.— 6. CHARCOT. *Soc. de biologie,* Oct. 1871.—7. CLARKE, LOCKHART, and GOWERS. *Med. Chir. Trans.* vol. lvii. p. 247.—8. DUCHENNE. *L'électrisation localisée,* 1st edit. 1855.—9. *Idem. Loc. cit.* p. 555.—10. *Idem. L'électrisation local.* 2nd edit. 1861; *Archives générales de méd.* 1868.—11. ERB. *Handbuch der Electrotherapie,* p. 389, 1882. —12. *Idem. Deutsches Arch. f. klin. Med.* March 1884.—13. *Idem. Progressive Musc. Dystrophy,* New Sydenham Soc. 1894.—14. EULENBERG and COHNHEIM. *Berlin. klin. Wochenschr.* No. 50, 1865.—15. FÜRSTNER. *Verein der Neurol. u. Alienist. Süd-Ost-Deutschlands,* June 1893.—16. GOMBAULT. *Arch. expériment. de méd.* 1889, p. 633.—17. GOWERS. *Pseud-Hypertroph. Paral.* 1879.—18. LANDOUZY and DÉJERINE. *Acad. des sciences,* Jan. 1884; and *Rev. de méd.* 1885.—19. LEYDEN. *Klin. d. Rückenmark-Krankh.* 1876, Band ii. 525.—20. LITTLE. *On the Deformities of the Human Frame,* 1853, p. 14, note.—21. MERYON. *Med. Chir. Trans.* vol. xxxv. p. 73, 1852.—22. *Idem. On Paralysis,* p. 210, 1864.—23. PARTRIDGE. *Med. Times and Gazette,* 1847, p. 244.—24. TAYLOR. *Trans. Clin. Soc.* 1891.

C. E. B.

FACIAL HEMIATROPHY AND HEMIHYPERTROPHY

SYNONYMS.—*Hemiatrophia facialis progressiva; Umschriebene Gesichtschwund; Hémiatrophie faciale.*

Introduction.—This is a relatively rare disease, only about one hundred cases having thus far been recorded. The characteristic changes begin more commonly before puberty than after it; no true instance of this condition having occurred after thirty years of age. The disease is commoner in women than in men.

In a few cases a direct heredity has been traced, while various exciting causes have been suggested. In some cases it is doubtful how far acute infectious disease, such as scarlet fever, measles, typhoid fever or erysipelas, and such morbid conditions as tonsillitis, influenza, and abscess in the neighbourhood of the ear may have been the direct excitant; but in others some injury has been noted shortly before the onset of the disease.

It may be fairly stated that in the majority of cases no obvious cause is to be found.

Symptoms.—The first symptom is usually the appearance upon the cheek, chin, or forehead of a white, or whitish-yellow, spot or patch. Originally somewhat ill-defined and limited in size, this patch gradually · increases; in some instances by the agglomeration of other similar spots. The skin over this area assumes a parchment-like appearance, in many cases being distinctly "glossy"; and, if the disease begin on the cheek, a well-marked depression under the malar bone, due to atrophy of the subcutaneous fat, readily attracts attention. The rapidity and extent of the change varies in different cases; in some, the affection is limited to one part of the face, the commonest site being the cheek and adjoining parts; in this case one side presents a curious shrunken appearance, the atrophy being limited by the middle line.

In addition to the alterations in the true skin the subcutaneous fat is largely affected; so that in the centre of the patch this tissue is conspicuously absent.

Should the change involve the eyebrows, or hairy parts of the face, these are observed to change colour; and in some cases the hair thins and falls out. Sweating and other cutaneous secretions are lessened on the atrophied side, although this is not without exceptions.

Microscopically the epidermis has not been found definitely affected; but the skin papillæ are atrophied, and there is a general thinning of the connective tissues, and atrophy of the subcutaneous fat.

These are the earlier and characteristic changes of facial hemiatrophy—the disease beginning in the skin and subcutaneous fatty tissue. The shrinking in size of the bones and muscles, to be discussed presently, are later changes. Möbius has pointed out that in the cases in which a lesion of the cervical sympathetic nerve has caused a false appearance of hemiatrophy the skin and fat are not atrophied.

The facial muscles in old-standing cases are thinned from atrophy and absorption of fat; but they do not show any degenerative change, nor any paralysis of movement volitionally or in emotion, except in so far as the sclerous condition of the skin acts as an impediment. Functionally they are unaffected, giving no degenerative electrical reaction. The faradic excitability of the muscles of the atrophied side is often increased; but this arises from the lessened resistance to the current owing to the disappearance of the subcutaneous fat.

From similar causes hemiatrophy of the tongue has been noted in some cases; but this atrophy is not the muscular change which occurs in true lingual hemiatrophy from lesion of the hypoglossal nerve or nucleus; the reactions of the lingual muscles are not altered.

The bones of the face become shrunken, the change affecting the frontal, malar, and the upper and lower maxillary to an equal extent. The osseous atrophy is greatest in those cases in which the change began before or at puberty, but is not confined to them.

The nasal cartilages usually share in the general atrophy; the ear is least affected.

Common sensation is not abolished, nor is the sense of taste in those cases in which there is concomitant atrophy of the tongue.

Various *associated symptoms* have been described,—for example, neuralgic pains over the area of trigeminal distribution; twitching of the facial muscles; and evidence of affection of the cervical sympathetic nerve.

Fromhold-Treu, for purposes of description and classification, has distinguished the following varieties: (*a*) complete unilateral cases; (*b*) incomplete unilateral cases. Most instances belong to this variety in the early stages, but some have been recorded in which the disease was apparently limited to special parts; for example, Gulland's case, where the atrophy was limited to the first division of the trigeminus (*Edin. Hosp. Reports*, vol. i. p. 384), and Bärwinkel's case, where the atrophy was limited to the second division. (*c*) Bilateral cases. (*d*) Cases with implication of other parts of the body; for example, the cases of Virchow-Mendel, and of Hutchinson (*Archives of Surgery*, July 1891, p. 44).

The **differential diagnosis** is to be made from several other conditions; but there is little difficulty in recognising the true facial hemiatrophy, when it is borne in mind that the essential change lies in atrophy of the *cutis vera* and subcutaneous connective and fatty tissues. The conditions which bear a superficial resemblance to this disease are: (*a*) congenital facial atrophy and other asymmetry; (*b*) facial asymmetry in infantile hemiplegia; (*c*) facial and trigeminal palsy with muscular atrophy; (*d*) palsy of the cervical sympathetic nerve.

Pathology.—There are five cases on record in which a necropsy has been made, but in only one of these (the case of Virchow-Mendel) has the pathological condition been fully described. This was a pure case of old-standing facial hemiatrophy. The trigeminal nerve showed microscopically the pathological appearances of a proliferating interstitial neuritis; the facial nerve was normal. The principal changes discovered in the central nervous axis were atrophy of the so-called descending trigeminal root and of the cells of the *substantia ferruginea pontis*.

Mendel's contention is that the facial hemiatrophy is brought about by the interstitial neuritis; while the atrophy of the descending trigeminal root supports Merkel's view that this is the "trophic" root of the fifth nerve. But it is still doubtful how far the cutaneous condition is directly due to the nerve lesion. It is difficult to understand how the alleged "trophic" fibres of the fifth nerve could be affected so extensively without some simultaneous implication of the sensory fibres which experiment has shown to form the whole of the sensory division of this nerve; and it will be shown elsewhere (art. "Cranial Nerves," p. 752) that the so-called "trophic" root of Merkel does not contain trophic but motor fibres. A careful reading of Mendel's paper brings out the fact that, notwithstanding the existence of the interstitial neuritis, most of the trigeminal nerve fibres were normal; it appears, therefore, more logical to regard the nervous and cutaneous lesions as arising from one and the same cause, and not as cause and effect.

The older views upon the causation of facial hemiatrophy may be now disregarded, for they are based, not upon actual pathological facts, but upon speculative considerations. Hence it is scarcely necessary to do more than refer to the "trophoneurosis" of Romberg; the "vasomotor" surmise of Stilling; and that of "sympathetic affection" propounded by Seeligmuller and others. The view most in harmony with all the facts seems to point to an arrest of development during the growing period, or towards the end of it. What the cause of this arrest may be is doubtful; according to Hutchinson, it arises from a morphœa of the fifth cranial nerve. That the arrested development occurs over the area of distribution of the trigeminus on one side, does not imply a direct trophic influence of the nerve upon the affected structures, but merely that the peripheral distribution of the nerve guides the process of nutrition; for it is well known that patches of morphœa and scleroderma, and even the vesicular rash of herpes, do not necessarily correspond directly to any known peripheral branch or branches, but to certain segments of the central nervous axis (Head).

Little need be said regarding **prognosis**. In the majority of cases the atrophic process is progressive, although in some it has been spontaneously arrested; the disease has no tendency to shorten life. The atrophy in the large majority of cases is confined to the face, commonly to one side of it; and in a few rare instances to a portion of one side.

The **treatment** lies in the administration of general and nervine tonics and in local applications to the skin of the face. Of the former may be mentioned quinine, iron, arsenic, and strychnine; of the latter are gentle massage, carefully regulated facial gymnastics, and the application of electricity, preferably the constant current.

FACIAL HEMIHYPERTROPHY.—Scattered throughout medical records are a few rare cases of what may be regarded as the converse of facial hemiatrophy, namely, unilateral facial hypertrophy. Some of the cases are of congenital nature; but in others the disease appears to have begun shortly before puberty. The change, which consists in an increased growth of the tissues of the affected region, involves not only the bones but also the soft parts. Thus the skin over the forehead, cheek, and chin is rough, coarse, and thickened—a change which equally affects the hair and sebaceous follicles. The bony enlargements are specially noticed on the forehead, supra-orbital ridge, and malar prominence.

In two cases in which the skull was examined after death (Hutchinson, Thomson) the bony overgrowth consisted of a general osseous hypertrophy with the addition of broad based exostoses, large and small, limited exactly to one side of the skull, face, and jaws. Similar changes were noted on the palate, basilar process, and sphenoid bone. These exostoses were not limited to the external surface, for in places they were also observed projecting into the cranial cavity. The osseous change is of the nature of a true hypertrophy; for, in addition to the points already noted, there were found enlargement of the cancellated structure, distension of the natural sinuses, and of the vascular and nervous canals (Thomson).

Even less can be said of the cause of this hypertrophic condition than has been stated with regard to hemiatrophy. In the recorded cases the change has been limited to the area of distribution of the fifth cranial nerve. But there is as much difficulty in accepting the view that such hypertrophy is due to an exalted "trophic" influence of this nerve, as in believing that the conversely atrophic condition arises from a diminished "trophic" influence. In the latter instance the change is one of arrested development, and not of retrogression from a normal standard; while in the former it appears to be an evolutionary development of a precocious nature during the growing period, rather than a pathological overgrowth.

WILLIAM ALDREN TURNER.

REFERENCES

Mention is made only of those works in which the whole subject is considered; reference to individual cases is to be found in most of them; while some special references are given in the text.
Hemiatrophy: 1. PARRY. Collected writings, 1825, vol. i. p. 478.—2. ROMBERG. *Klinische Ergebnisse*, Berlin, 1846, p. 75.—3. BÄRWINKEL. *Arch. d. Heilkünde*, 1868, ix. p. 151. — 4. EULENBERG. "Gesichtatrophie," *Handbook*, 1875, xii. p. 54. —5. LEWIN. *Charité-Annalen*, 1884, p. 619.—6. MILLS. Pepper's *System of Medicine*, vol. v. p. 693.—7. FROMHOLD-TREU. *Die Hemiatrophia facialis progressiva.* Diss. Inaug. Dorpat. 1893.—8. MÖBIUS. "Der umschriebene Gesichtschwund," *Spec. Path. und Therap.* 1895. Wien.—9. BRAMWELL. *Atlas of Clinical Medicine*, 1892, vol. i. p. 97. **Post-mortem records in**: 10. PISSLING. *Zeitsch. d. ges. Wiener Aerzte*, 1852. p. 496.—11. JOLLY and RECKLINGHAUSEN. *Archiv f. Psych.* 1872, iii. p. 711.—12. HOMÉN. *Neurol. Centralbl.* 1890, ix. No. 13.—13. GRAFF. Referred to by Fromhold-Treu, *op. sup. cit.*—14. MENDEL. *Neurol. Centralbl.* vii. No. 14. **Hemihypertrophy**: 15. HUTCHINSON, J. *Illustrated Med. News*, 1889, p. 82.—16. ALEXIS THOMSON. *Trans. Med.-Chi. Soc. Edin.* vol. x. p. 3.—17. D. W. MONTGOMERY. *Med. News*, July 1893.

W. A. T.

GENERAL PATHOLOGY OF THE NERVOUS SYSTEM

IN order that this article may be intelligible to readers who are unfamiliar with the most recent discoveries in the physiology of the nervous system, it is desirable to begin by setting these forth as succinctly as possible in a few preliminary paragraphs.

The Neuron.—The modern conception of the neuron is that of a variously contoured protoplasmic centrum—the cell body, enclosing a nucleus of relatively large size, and a well-defined nucleolus. From the cell body, or from a protoplasmic extension of the cell (neuro-dendron), the nerve process or *axon* is given off. This axon may be naked, and terminate in free arborisations more or less complicated; or, becoming ensheathed, it may be continuous with a medullated nerve fibre, to end in like manner. The nucleated nerve-cell, its naked or ensheathed axon and terminal arborisation constitute the essential elements of the neuron.

A further development, however, seldom absent, is seen in certain protoplasmic extensions from the cell body, which are subject to repeated division and subdivision, and are often plume-like in arrangement: these are *the dendrons*. The dendrons are possessed of numerous minute lateral projections, gemmules, spines, or "thorns" as they have been variously called; these processes possibly subserve the purpose of a more intimate connection betwixt them and the terminal arborisations of axons and collaterals. They strongly suggest the function of vibrissæ, and, together with the dendrons, are probably to be regarded as an apparatus for the collection of impressions brought from a wide area to the nerve cell. In adendritic cells the cell body itself receives such stimuli. The dendritic processes are regarded as functioning towards the cell (cellulipetal); the axons away from the cell (cellulifugal); the former being recipient organs, the latter distributive, and conveying nerve impulses so aroused to distal nerve cells or peripheral organs—muscle, vessel, or gland. Golgi taught that the dendrons have a vegetative part to play, being, as he conceived, nutritive radicles of the nerve cell in close connection with the vascular and lymphatic apparatus.

The *axon* is subject to great variety of distribution; thus, in the case of the pyramidal cells of the cortex, the axon may divide into a projection fibre and a commissural fibre (callosal), after having given off several collaterals in its course; and these callosal fibres may terminate in arborisations around nerve cells in the opposite hemisphere. In certain cortical regions it may divide and subdivide, ramifying over an extensive tract (Golgi's sensory cells); or again, as in the cerebellum and cornu ammonis, it may form a rich plexiform distribution around neighbouring cells (basket cells, etc.) The nerve cell may be possessed not of one but of several axons; and such axons are not one and indivisible to their

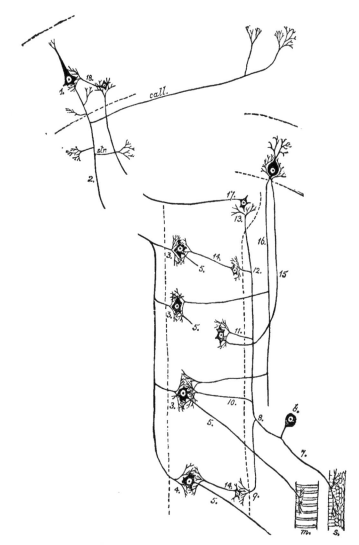

PLATE I.—Diagram illustrating the Neuronic System.

1, Nerve-cell of cortex cerebri ; 2, its axon ; 3, 4, its collaterals ending in arborisations around cells of anterior cornu ; *call*., collateral passing as a callosal fibre to cortex of opposite hemisphere ; *str*., collateral passing to corpus striatum ; 5, axon of cornu-cell ending in muscular fibre (*m*) ; 6, cell of one of the spinal ganglia ; 7, branch of axon after bifurcation forming arborisation over a sensory surface ; 8, central branch distributing terminal arborisations to cells of posterior horn (9) ; of anterior horn (10) ; of Clarke's column (11), and posterior columns of the bulb (13) ; 14, axon of cells of posterior horn distributed to motor cells ; 15, fibre of ascending cerebellar tract passing up to cell of cerebellum ; 16, axon of latter supplying cells of anterior horn ; 17, axon of cell of bulb passing through fillet to small cortical cell in cortex ; 18, axon of latter forming arborisation around large cell of cerebral cortex.

To face p. 490.

termini, as formerly taught, but usually give off several lateral branches or collaterals, which also terminate in free arborisations like the axon itself.

Just as these terminal arborisations do not anastomose, neither do the dendrons; so that the neuron from the ultimate termini of its axon and collaterals, to the remotest dendritic twig, is an anatomical unit, structurally independent of surrounding nerve cells.

Thus the complete conception of the neuron embraces the nerve cell, its dendritic branches, its axon, naked or medullated, its collaterals, and the terminal arborisations of both. By their ultimate divisions the axons and collaterals of one cell embrace the dendrons and the body of another nerve cell; thus chains of neurons are formed, which in the cerebro-spinal system increase in complexity from the cord to medulla, and thence to the brain cortex. In no case, however, is actual organic continuity supposed to be established thereby.

The cell body consists of a structureless achromatic substance (interfilar mass of Flemming, ground substance, cytolymph or enchylema) supporting a fine reticular meshwork of fibres—the *cytoreticulum* or spongioplasm (filar mass of Flemming). The cytoreticulum appears to be identical with the fine fibrils traced by Max Schultze from the protoplasmic processes into the body of the cell. There is great doubt whether these fibrils are all projected into the axis-cylinder process, or whether they completely traverse the cell; there is reason for the belief that many end or originate in the cytoplasm, or are even connected with the nucleus itself. Indeed, van Beneden and Klein teach that the nuclear membrane is formed by a condensation of the general reticulum of cell and nucleus. The fibres of the cytoreticulum are usually regarded as the lines along which nervous impulses travel. In the mesh-like intervals between these fibres lie the peculiar chromophil bodies of Nissl, so readily stained by his methylene-blue method.

The nucleus, or karyoplasm, also shows a reticulum of exceedingly fine fibrils, probably connected with the cytoreticulum, and floating in the karyolymph. Amongst these fibrils are scattered the chromatin particles —often grouped in a coarser network, stained deeply by basic dyes. These chromatin particles are almost certainly identical with nuclein; the greater the proportion of nucleic acid in the latter the more highly phosphorised is the chromatin; and the more deeply stained by basic dye. Recent research would certainly indicate that the chromatin (nuclein) in some manner regulates the synthetic metabolism of the cell (Wilson); thus, in most cells during the phase of vegetative activity, the chromatin appropriates albumin, growing in bulk but losing its staining capacity; whilst, during reproductive stages, the albumin is separated, and the chromatin, having now a higher percentage of nucleic acid, stains intensely. Physiological experimentation on unicellular organisms teaches us the same fact; namely, that the nucleus is essential to the absorption of food and the growth of the cytoplasm, whilst the chromatin is chiefly, if not solely, concerned in the exercise of such control over cell nutrition.

Formerly the protoplasmic processes of the cerebral cortex were considered to be in part terminal within the gray matter of the brain (terminal plexuses); inosculating, in part, with corresponding branches from other units (intercellular plexuses). The free terminal arborescences were regarded as embracing the possibilities for further differentiations of structure, corresponding possibly to more elaborate evolution of mental or sentient activity; and this may still hold good. The intercellular plexuses, as the organised or integrated tracts, the less alterable and established relationships betwixt cell and cell, are now regarded as a free dendritic ramification. Furthermore, there arose from the former view the conception of consolidated cell groupings, structurally united again with distal cell groupings, for functional co-operation. The cell groupings of course exist, but each unit or neuron comprising a group is organically independent of its fellow, yet functionally co-operative; since the collaterals of its axon place it in dynamic relationship with the various cells of that group, and also of distal groups. Hence we may still truthfully speak of functionally consolidated cell groupings.

The more elaborate the dendritic expansions, the more elaborate the psychic or neural activity; the greater the latency period, and, with this prolongation of the time element, the more vivid the conscious states accompanying the excitation of these dendritic nerve tracts by terminal arborisations. The cell itself was conceived as the dynamic centre not only for nutritive and reproductive activities, but also as the source of nervous energy in the form of the so-called nerve current. When we consider the extreme caution and reserve of Max Schultze as to the absence of any centric origin for the ultimate fibrils from the cytoplastic substance itself, the assumption that the nerve cell can no longer be regarded as the centre of nervous energy or of psychic activity, as lately asserted by some, appears to be a hasty and unwarrantable generalisation. On this point Apathy's elaborate work may be consulted with advantage.

Again, the rising potential of the cell may be traced to nutritional rhythm; whilst the application of the appropriate stimulus or the termination of a nutritional cycle would necessarily lead to discharge along lines of least resistance.

Passing to *the pathological indications* of these facts, we find, first, that the morphological unity of the neuron and the doctrine of contiguity rather than continuity of related neurons, favour a strict limitation of degenerative changes, arising in a nerve chain, to the individual neuron affected. Thus in motor neurons, where the trophic centre (*i.e.* the cell); or the axon emerging from it, is affected to a minor degree, we get a primary parenchymatous degeneration. Should the lesion, however, be destructive of the cell, or the axon be severed, the more active or Wallerian degeneration ensues—in both instances confined to the neuron affected.

In like manner focal lesions of the motor cortex, medulla, or cord lead to a secondary parenchymatous degeneration, which exhibits the same tendency to systemic limitation. In the next place, the cell being the trophic centre of the emergent axon, the distal parts of the latter or terminal arborisations will suffer first when such trophic influence is arrested.

Similarly, tabes dorsalis affords us an illustration of the degeneration of a sensory neuron formed by the ganglion cell of the posterior root, the peripheral sensory root, and the centripetal fibre in the posterior column of the cord.

Lesions of the motor axons, whether by section, electric, chemical, or thermal irritation, issue in so-called chromatolysis—the chromophil granules are diffused towards the periphery of the cell, the nucleus becomes eccentric, but no implication of the achromatin network is observed. Such changes are not to be regarded as of much import, since they are transient, the cell returning to its normal in the course of some two or three months (Marinesco, van Gehuchten).

This restitution of the chromophil granules, however, does not occur in the ganglion cells on the spinal roots after section of the peripheral sensory nerves : here the nerve cells concerned show a notable degree of chromatolysis, and eventually disappear altogether. In like manner, section of the cellulipetal process of all peripheral sensory neurons leads to destructive chromatolysis and disappearance of the cell; a fact explained by van Gehuchten as due to the cutting off of trophic influence exerted upon the cell by peripheral stimuli.

Although Golgi's view of the nutritive functions of dendrites is now almost universally discarded, yet, as recipient agencies conveying stimuli to the nerve cell, we may plausibly regard them as having a trophic influence upon the latter ; and, since their ultimate fibrils are brought into intimate relationship with the protoplasm immediately surrounding the nucleus (karyopetal sphere), the latter, as already remarked, probably regulates and controls such influence.

In certain cortical affections, especially in general paralysis, these dendrons are peculiarly exposed to lesion ; and this may largely account for the grave changes found in the cytoplasm. In fatty degeneration of the nerve cells also these dendrons suffer seriously, but here the primary change is within the nerve cell; the dendrons suffer secondarily. Formerly, we used to speak of the breaking down of the intercellular plexus—the fact still remains that the lateral and basal dendritic expansions from the cortical cells, which are intimately interblended, though not in organic continuity, are largely degenerated and broken down in certain forms of insanity, and long prior to destruction of the cell itself. It is an interesting question, to which no reply can at present be given, whether the contact of the dendrites of different cells influences the currents aroused in them by the axons ; or whether this contact is simply conducive to a spread of discharge from cell to cell ? It is a rather significant fact that in certain nervous territories the cell arrangements distinctly favour this contact of dendrons, whereas in others few such facilities are afforded.

System diseases.—By this term we mean the exclusive implication of nerve tracts having a community of function—of certain links in the chain of neurons which extend from the periphery to the brain cortex, or conversely. These neuron chains have two main levels—a cortico-spinal and a peripheral, each of which has its sensory and motor links. Any one of these neuron links may be the site of degeneration; or any combination of such system degenerations may exist (Combined system diseases).

Diseases of the higher level motor neurons would include—(a) Primary lateral sclerosis or spastic spinal paralysis; (b) Secondary or descending lateral sclerosis from focal lesions.

Diseases of the motor neurons of the lower level would include—(c) Acute anterior poliomyelitis; (d) Chronic anterior poliomyelitis or progressive muscular atrophy; (e) Progressive bulbar paralysis.

Diseases of the sensory neurons would embrace—(f) Posterior spinal sclerosis or tabes dorsalis; (g) Sclerosis of the columns of Goll or of Burdach separately; (h) Sclerosis of the direct cerebellar tract.

Combined system diseases would embrace—(i) Postero-lateral sclerosis or ataxic paraplegia; (j) Sclerosis of posterior, lateral, and direct cerebellar tracts or Friedreich's disease (hereditary ataxia).

Etiological considerations.—The chief indication of a system disease of the neuron is its intrinsic nervous origin — the primary change originates in the nervous element. The main factor in determining this incidence in many cases is probably hereditary tendency; a neuropathic history is often forthcoming, as for example in Friedreich's disease. The incidence of the attack upon the particular neuron chain is probably due in many cases to the selective capacity shown by certain nerve centres and tracts for certain toxic agents; thus the syphilitic poison is especially prone to attack the sensory spinal neuron (tabes dorsalis); in general paralysis, which many believe to be of toxic origin, the lateral and more rarely the posterior columns are concerned; alcohol involves the peripheral nerve trunks in a multiple neuritis.

In explaining the simultaneous implication of posterior and lateral columns we must not forget that the terminal arborisations of the crossed pyramidal fibres, as well as those of the collaterals of the sensory neurons, both engage the dendrites of the motor neuron; and probably by this means establish a community of morbid liability.

Before considering in detail the more important morbid processes whereby the nervous tissues suffer, a few remarks may not be out of place with respect to certain intrinsic qualities more or less peculiar to these tissues, which act as determining factors and regulate the incidence of their diseases.

Neuropathic inheritance.—The nervous system is subject to the law or mode of inheritance, whereby is entailed upon it what we call a neuropathic tendency. However unexplained and mysterious be the operations of this process, we are constantly led to recognise its influence; and to admit epilepsy, alcoholism, syphilis, chorea, and insanity as factors in the evolution of pathological states in the offspring.

Differentiated function.—The exquisite elaboration of the principle of the physiological division of labour betokened by the differentiation of medullated strands and centres, together with the operation of the Wallerian law, bestows on certain affections of the nervous system a characteristic limitation, resulting in the so-called *system diseases;* such as ordinary ascending and descending lateral sclerosis, the implication of cornual and analogous centres of the bulbar nuclei, the poliomyelopathies, or the mixed system diseases where two or more systems are associated in the morbid process. In all these alike, the more strict the systemic limitation the more exclusively is the affection a simple parenchymatous one in origin; the more diffuse, the more reason is there to regard it as of interstitial origin.

Trophic influence.—The nutrition of a medullated nerve-fibre is dependent upon (*a*) its continuity with the cell from which it emerges; (*b*) the functional activity of the cell and conductibility of the fibre; (*c*) the functional activity of the cell units constituting the medullated segments of the nerve-tube. The functional activity of the cell, therefore, embraces, according to modern views, a certain trophic influence upon the nerve-fibre, and the cell itself is spoken of as its trophic centre. It may, perhaps, be nearer the truth to regard the nutrition of the individual units which have coalesced in the formation of the nerve-tube as being regulated by the nerve current emanating from the "trophic" centre.

Where the nerve-tube suffers from atrophy or degeneration, one or other of the following causes are mostly found :—(*a*) disuse, as in amputation of limbs or as a result of central paralysis; (*β*) nutritional changes in the cell induced by certain poisons, or other agency interfering with normal metabolism; (*γ*) destructive implication of the cell or severance of the fibre from its trophic centre by section, pressure, inflammatory reaction, and so forth; (*δ*) over-stimulation or functional over-strain.

That very rapid changes in nutrition of nerve-cells may readily be induced is proved by Ehrlich's and Brieger's experiments, where compression of the aorta in the rabbit produced, in the course of one hour, necrosis of the gray matter and cells of the spinal cord. Nissl also has lately shown that well-marked structural changes can be produced in the nerve-cells of the spinal cord by alcohol, strychnine, morphia, lead, phosphorus, and arsenic. Even if no visible lesion affect the nerve centres, or peripheral nerves, an early rise in irritability of muscle or nerve to galvanic or faradaic stimulation may indicate altered nutrition. In chorea this increased nerve and muscle irritability has been noted by Benedikt, Rosenthal, and Gowers; and the latter attributes the affection to an altered nutrition of the motor cells of the cortex due to a blood toxin, allied to or identical with that of rheumatism, acting in predisposed subjects at the adolescent epoch of life. The motor nerve-cells are regarded as regulating the nutrition of the muscles which they supply; the integrity of the cornual cells thus being essential to the nutrition of the muscles of the trunk and limbs. It matters not that the cortico-spinal or central link be sclerosed throughout, as in lateral sclerosis; no nutritive change need be apparent in the cornual cells, their efferent fibres, or in the muscles they supply. Again, in Friedreich's disease, or hereditary ataxic paraplegia, both the posterior and lateral columns of the cord are blocked by sclerosis, the former as much so as in tabes; yet, since in the large proportion of cases the cornual cells are intact, no muscular atrophy ensues. Muscular atrophy, therefore, as dependent upon neural influence, has its origin in profound nutritional changes in the trophic motor cells, or their efferent fibres; and this holds good for the whole series of spinal and cranial nerves. In like manner the sensory fibres of the cord have as their trophic centres the ganglia on the posterior roots; severed from these cells the sensory roots degenerate upwards and downwards in their course through the cord, their collaterals succumbing to the same change.

Selective capacity of nervous tissues.—The special affinity betrayed by tissues, nervous and non-nervous, for various chemical compounds, toxic or otherwise, is a most notable endowment. Some agencies, such as chloral, trional, and other hypnotics, directly depress the cerebral cortex; others, like cocaine when locally applied, affect sensory nerve trunks, the sensory tracts of the cord, and even the cortex itself. A large group of vegetable alkaloids, such as conine, curara, nicotin, paralyse the muscle end-plates of the motor nerves—an effect also produced by snake venom, as well as by neurine and choline, which are closely allied to the powerful poison muscarine. On the other hand, physostigmine paralyses the cord, leaving the brain and nerves practically intact. Again, certain mineral poisons — bisulphide of carbon, arsenic, and lead—induce paralysis by the establishment of polyneuritis; whilst the prolonged use of alcohol may be followed by a multiple neuritis, resembling in every way secondary parenchymatous and interstitial forms of neuritis. Tissue metabolism is also profoundly affected through the agency of curara. Lastly, numerous bacterial products exhibit the same selective operation in the mode of their attack; the toxins of tetanus and hydrophobia exhaust themselves upon the ganglionic cells of the central nervous system, whilst the diphtheria toxin sets up a parenchymatous degeneration of peripheral nerves, sensory and motor, followed by muscular degeneration [*vide* art. "Diphtheria," vol. ii. p. 741].

Reflected influence.—The transference of a peripheral irritation through the medium of the sensory mechanism of the cord may result in inhibitory, paralytic, or modifying influences on certain spinal centres, which in their turn regulate the nutrition or functional activity of distal parts; thus is explained the very rapid muscular atrophy of painful joint diseases. Illustrating the same influence, we have the paraplegia associated with chronic renal, vesical, or bowel disease, in which, although occasionally any ascending neuritis has issued in secondary myelitis, it seems probable that the result is often a purely reflex functional disturbance.

Tissue degradation from disuse.—The vital capacity of a tissue is in inverse proportion to the amount of its connective framework. This is well exemplified in normal and pathological conditions of the muscular system; but still more strikingly is this law displayed in the degeneration of the nervous system, central and peripheral. Why function should be so intimately bound up with the development of connective tissue it may be difficult to explain; but some light is cast upon the question by the fact that inflammatory activity in these tissues is always associated with active transudation and diapedesis, the leucocytes playing the chief part in removal of waste products; whilst in times of waning activity (senile and degenerative states generally) the fixed tissue elements play the more prominent part in removal and assimilation of tissue débris. The decline in functional activity no longer demands the same activity in circulation, transudation and diapedesis; and the fixed cells of the tissue to a great extent appear to supplant in its office the vagrant leucocyte. The proliferation of these elements and their eventual fibrillation result in the various degrees of sclerosis so characteristic of degraded tissue. Chronic insanity and senile brain decay afford striking instances of such connective replacement; the changes noted in the nerves, and especially the posterior roots of amputated limbs, are of this character; and so likewise the Wallerian degeneration of nerves severed from their trophic cells (vol. i. p. 182).

Atrophy.—Strictly speaking, atrophy is a quantitative and not a qualitative change—a diminution in size or number of elements without obvious qualitative variation (degeneration). It is doubtful whether in this sense we can speak of atrophy of the nervous tissues despite the force of a priori views and analogy; even if pure atrophy occur in these tissues it must be difficult to prove. We therefore imply by atrophy of the central nervous organs wasting of structure associated with qualitative change in nutrition, almost invariably fatty or granular in nature. We must exclude such apparent atrophies as are seen in the brain of children defective in development or epileptic; the reduction in size of a hemisphere of cerebrum or cerebellum (hypoplasia); the attenuation of a cluster of convolutions (microgyria), or again the condition of microcephalus: all these are instances of congenital arrest in development. Atrophy of the brain may be general or local; the former is best illustrated by senile atrophy. Every tissue cell has its limit of growth, functional activity, and decay; the nerve-cell is no exception to this rule. Apart from the degenerative tendencies and shortening of existence due to over-stimulation or other injurious agency, there is the tendency to physiological senescence, which may also be prematurely initiated. With failing vigour in the cell metabolism there is associated a qualitative change in nutrition due to defective oxidation, respiratory impairment, deficient oxyhæmoglobin, loss of cardiac energy; all of which are causes of fatty atrophy. In states of inanition nerve tissue is the last to suffer, and then to a minimum degree; hence the diminished aliment which old age supplies does not explain the extensive atrophy which occurs in the nervous centres; in fact, the qualitative or degenerative change is the chief agent in this decay.   In general paralysis the atrophic state of brain is often extreme ; but here again the qualitative changes in nutrition are all important and due to inflammatory reaction [*vide* subsequent art. "General Paralysis"]. In it, as well as in chronic insanity, a tendency is observed to limitation of the wasting to certain definite areas of the cerebrum.

Inflammation.—Inflammation of the nervous tissues, just as in other localities, is in every sense a reaction to injury or irritation, and tends towards reparative ends.   In so complex a tissue as the brain, the extent to which the several constituents participate in the morbid process admits of great variation, according to the character of the injury or irritation causing the reaction.   In certain cases, far the more numerous, the vascular tissues assume the leading part ; at other times the connective element may present predominating change ; and yet again, with comparatively slight vascular reaction, the medullated fibres of the nervous centres may chiefly suffer : such variations depend upon the nature of the irritant and the acuteness or chronicity of the inflammatory reaction aroused.

Certain anatomical facts explain the peculiar features assumed by inflammatory processes in the brain : thus the tendency to strict limitation (except where the surface is involved) is to a certain extent due to the terminal character of the vascular supply; both cortical and ganglionic arteries being terminal vessels, as long since indicated by Duret.   In like manner we are aware that no communication exists betwixt central and cortical vessels ; here again a further limitation is imposed.   So also in the very special character of its connective element we find a further explanation of the restraint upon the spread of the inflammatory process —the lymph-connective system playing a much more active part than the connective tissues of other organs, being phagocytic in functional endowment, and opposing thereby the tendency to inflammatory encroachment. In the next place, the medullated nerve-fibre has long been known to afford great resistance to inflammatory reaction, traumatism excepted ; nor can we definitely state, even now, whether certain changes in the nerve-cell are really inflammatory or simply degenerative in nature.   Degenerative changes of a parenchymatous nature, implicating the dendrites or terminal arborisations, cannot be assumed to spread beyond their own immediate regional distribution ; since recent research appears definitely to indicate no actual continuity with neighbouring fibre systems—all connection with adjacent or distant cells being simply one of contiguity.   On the other hand, implication of a nerve-cell itself, as the trophic centre for its emergent axon, gravely affects the nutrition of the latter, and reflects distal disturbances.

As regards the brain, it may be affirmed with certainty that a primary or idiopathic cerebritis is not at present recognised.   Inflammation of the nerve centres is most frequently due to violence, as from a blow ; sabre-cut ; fractured skull ; or the laceration of the brain substance so often accompanying concussion : it may arise, secondarily, around a hæmorrhage or blood-clot in the neighbourhood of new growths or foreign bodies ; and frequently from diseased bone, as in caries of the ethmoid and petrous portion of the temporal bones ; from poisons circulating in the blood stream, or from the toxins of micro-organisms in acute infectious diseases, such as diphtheria and erysipelas ; and, as a suppurative form, in pyæmic implication.

The primary condition appears in all cases to be that of a vascular dilatation, followed by diapedesis and leucocytal invasion.   This stage is well seen in all chronic inflammations, such as the chronic meningo-cerebritis of general paralysis, the wandering cells being found in every stage of their amœboid career, from their passage through the vessel's walls into the perivascular spaces around to their permeation of the brain tissue beyond.   The more active form of cerebritis, "acute red softening" of early authors, is too abrupt in its course to offer facilities for favourable observation ; although here also great leucocytal infiltrations occur around the vessels, and rapid disintegration of nerve tissue proceeds.   In the less acute and chronic forms the crowding of the leucocytes is not confined to the perivascular sheath ; but they tend especially to surround the nerve-cells and the lymph cavity in which these cells are placed.

These leucocytes have a large nucleus readily and deeply stained, possess granular contents, are distinctly amœboid, and probably crowd around the nerve elements by virtue of a positive chemiotaxis.   The second stage is a very notable one, and consists in great development of the lymph connective system.   The fixed cells of the cerebro-spinal system are almost certainly mesoblastic in origin, their vascular processes being invariably attached to a nucleated protoplast on the walls of the vessel. These cells, with much protoplasm and a feebly stained nucleus, become now enormously enlarged, multiply by division, and, by fresh accessions from the vessel's walls, and from their inclusion of granules and deeply stained protoplasmic particles (which may be partially digested leucocytes), they play the part of phagocytes to the disintegrating tissues around.

In the cord the changes apparent in inflammatory activity are identical; the spider-cells play a similar part, the changes in the medullated nerve fibres embracing the increase of protoplasm, segmentation of myeline, multiplication of the nuclei along the sheath, and enlargement of the axis-cylinders.   Why does the spider-cell exhibit this unusual activity in certain morbid states ?   A definite answer cannot at present be given to this question ; but it is a suggestive fact that its appearance in this aggressive form dates from the phase of fatty degeneration of the nervous centres in general paralysis, senile brain atrophy, and chronic alcoholic insanity ; it therefore seems to bear some relationship to the period of defective oxygenation.

Parenchymatous degeneration.—The medullated tracts of the cord in particular are subject to a neural atrophy or degeneration, which appears at times to be purely primary, in so far that the trophic centres of the cerebrum may not be implicated, although the pyramidal tracts are sclerosed ; at other times the change is evidently secondary to cortical lesion, or to focal injuries along the motor strands. This latter is what is usually known as descending sclerosis; and we have the former illustrated on the sensory side in ascending sclerosis of the posterior columns, such as is productive of certain forms of tabes. The change is often referred to as a parenchymatous myelitis: it is doubtful whether the name myelitis is correct here—the histological features being much more in accord with a degenerative atrophic process than with genuine inflammation. In general paralysis the descending change so often seen in the lateral columns cannot be traced up into the crura; and although it evidently depends upon cortical degenerations, the appearance is like that of primary systematised sclerosis—a fine sclerous change accompanying the nerve atrophy. On the other hand, in system degenerations resulting from focal destruction of the motor area of the brain, for example in embolic plugging, syphilitic gummata, and the like, the change is much more marked in the vascular and connective elements; and an interstitial myelitis is aroused, with coarse sclerotic induration very dissimilar to the former affection.

Simple primary parenchymatous degeneration of the nerve-tracts is the result of grave nutritional anomalies of their trophic centres: the nerve-cell is not destroyed, nor is its axis-cylinder severed, but the trophic influence transmitted along the emergent fibres from the cell is profoundly modified. Where more complete destruction occurs, we have more acute change in the nerve-fibres and surrounding tissues, and the change approximates to a genuine inflammatory reaction rather than a simple degenerative one. Impaired nutrition of their trophic cells is naturally revealed in the terminal arborisations of the medullated nerve-fibres; these, being farthest removed from the trophic centres, fail in their nutrition first, and a slowly progressive degeneration of these terminal systems ensues; the change steadily making its way upwards along the nerve. Where the nutrition of the motor cells of the cortex is impaired, we get simple parenchymatous degeneration of the lateral columns and direct pyramidal tracts of the cord, not traceable upwards through the pyramids and the crura; where it involves the lowest level, or the motor cells of the anterior cornua, the motor nerves degenerate, and the muscles supplied by their fibres also undergo atrophy. This impairment of central nutrition may be induced during the progress of general paralysis of the insane; or by toxic agencies such as alcohol or the toxins which produce ergotism and pellagra [vide art. "Grain Poisoning," vol. ii. p. 792]. In the latter disease Tuczek describes a pigmentary atrophy of the cells of the anterior cornua, and of the spinal and sympathetic ganglia, as associated with the degenerative changes in the lateral and, occasionally, in the posterior columns of the cord.

In tabes dorsalis it has been conclusively shown that a similar parenchymatous degeneration occurs not infrequently in the peripheral extremities of the spinal nerves; the sensory fibres are exclusively involved, the degeneration, beginning in the sensory filaments of the skin and muscle, becoming less and less obvious as we approach the cord.

Here, then, is a further illustration of simple atrophy of the sensory fibres at their distal end, farthest away from the trophic cells, and unaccompanied by vascular reaction [*vide* art. "Nutrition," vol. i. p. 181]. We now know that degeneration of the peripheral sensory nerves, or of their roots, will issue in genuine tabetic symptoms without any implication of the posterior columns ; or, again, that the latter or cerebrospinal link may be exclusively involved, when like symptoms occur. As an instance of the former may be quoted the so-called alcoholic ataxia or alcoholic pseudo-tabes appearing in certain forms of multiple neuritis.

Nuclear degenerations.—A primary and symmetrical implication of the nuclear cells of the bulb, especially the motor nuclei in its lower half, is followed by a parenchymatous degeneration of their emergent fibres, constituting progressive bulbar paralysis, the glosso-labio-laryngeal paralysis of Duchenne. A like degeneration occasionally affects the central link of fibres passing upwards to the cortex: in fact, Kahler and Pick have traced the course of the degeneration past the crura, and observed atrophy of the convolutions in the Rolandic area. Of similar nature is that degeneration of the central link of the bulbar nuclei, associated with symmetrical lesions of the cortex, basal ganglia, or white matter of the hemispheres, resulting from softenings, hæmorrhage, or sclerosis ; and in particular of the outer segment of the lenticular nucleus, issuing in the acute forms of paralysis known as pseudo-bulbar paralysis or bulbar paralysis of cerebral origin. Similar changes from degeneration of the motor cells of the anterior horn of the cord are developed in their motor nerve-fibres, and usually of the pyramidal tract up as high as the cortex, resulting in so-called progressive muscular atrophy. In all these affections the atrophy of nerve-fibres and the surrounding sclerosis reproduce in all particulars the parenchymatous degeneration of ordinary primary lateral sclerosis of the cord.

Secondary parenchymatous degeneration. — This change is best exemplified in descending sclerosis of the cord following in the wake of destructive lesions such as transverse myelitis, softenings, hæmorrhage into cord, medulla, or brain, along any section of the cortico-spinal link. The changes induced differ considerably from those which characterise the primary forms of degeneration. The process is a far more active one, and resembles in every particular that which follows section of a nerve, and which has long been known as Wallerian degeneration ; namely, increase of protoplasm around the nuclei of the nerve sheath, increase in size and number of the latter, segmentation of myeline, interruption of the axis-cylinder, and eventual removal of the products of degeneration by leucocytes and connective-tissue cells. There is in all these cases notable vascular dilatation, leucocytal infiltration of the perineural sheath and surrounding connective, together with many compound granule cells. In fact, the process is so active in nature as to suggest to some that it would be more appropriately regarded as a parenchymatous myelitis than as a simple degeneration. In later stages spider-cells are found profusely scattered in all such tracts of sclerosis, especially surrounding the degenerating nerve-fibres. Multiple neuritis and the nuclear lesions or poliomyelopathies already referred to, are often the starting-points of such secondary degenerations.

Invasive or Interstitial inflammations.—In notable contrast with the forms of parenchymatous degeneration are the invasive inflammations ; the interstitial forms of neuritis, myelitis, and cerebritis. In these diseases the sclerous invasion, which is the more characteristic feature of the affection, spreads inwards to the nerve elements, directly causing their inflammation and atrophy. The growth starts from the interstitial connective tissue, from the membranes (meningo-myelitis or cerebritis), or from the vascular walls. In all alike the inflammatory reaction is a very marked feature ; the vessels are distended, their coats thickened, small hæmorrhages may occur, the perivascular nuclei are greatly multiplied, leucocytal infiltrations appear; and here also the spider-cells play a remarkable part, being both numerous and large in size. Illustrations of this invasive inflammatory sclerosis are afforded by the chronic meningo-cerebritis resulting in general paralysis of the insane; by chronic alcoholism; chronic myelitis and meningo-myelitis, and again by disseminate sclerosis and polyneuritis.

An important feature of the invasive forms of sclerosis is the diffused and multiple character of the lesions ; the system forms of disease, when complicating the invasive form, being usually secondary to the injuries inflicted by the latter. The multiple character of nerve affections may be taken as strong evidence of its infective or toxic origin; and, in accordance with this view, the more frequent etiological relations are those of alcoholism, syphilis, rheumatism and diphtheria : leprous polyneuritis is a further illustration of this connection. A difficulty arises in attempting to explain the immunity of the spinal cord and its ganglionic cells in alcoholic polyneuritis; why should the toxic effect stop short at the peripheral nerves ? The possible association with rheumatism and the exposed position of the nerve may explain this ; the site may be determined by over-strain, pressure, traumatism, or cold. In general paralysis the invasion is always from the pial surface and vascular tracts ; in certain forms, simulating tabes, the initiation seems also meningeal and vascular ; and undoubtedly there are many intermediate forms of spinal affection which lie between the genuine degenerative form of true tabes and the inflammatory or invasive form. As regards the evidence of toxic origin afforded by the multiple character of the nerve lesions, this feature forms an important element in the diagnosis of syphilis of the cranial nerves; and Mr. Jonathan Hutchinson has suggested a specific origin for the ophthalmoplegia interna which arises apparently from disease of the ciliary ganglion.

Focal sclerosis.—Wholly distinct from systemic and diffuse invasive lesions is focal sclerosis, where minute islets of connective growth occur throughout the medullated tracts—less frequently in the gray matter of the brain and cord, and peripheral nerves—both spinal and cranial. Minute foci of irritation appear to determine this growth at random in the most diversified tracts of the nervous system, often in close contiguity to blood-vessels, whose walls are thickened and nuclei proliferated, whilst spider cells are profusely scattered around. The points of sclerosis may be infinitely small, revealed only to microscopic vision; but to naked-eye observation they usually vary in size from a pin's head to several centimetres in diameter, are firm in consistence, well defined, and of a salmon tint. A most important feature, first indicated by Charcot, is the escape of the axis-cylinder, although the medullated tubes may undergo very considerable atrophy : this fact probably explains the absence of ascending and descending changes. From its erratic, haphazard distribution, its relation to the blood-vessels, its resemblance to certain syphilitic forms of chronic myelitis, and its frequency in chronic alcoholism, we regard this disease as probably toxic in origin.

This morbid process especially characterises the disease known as multiple or disseminate sclerosis; and it is a frequent accompaniment of chronic ،insanity, especially of general paralysis and of chronic alcoholism.

Colloid and Miliary degenerations.—Next in importance to the connective-tissue changes in insanity is the degeneration of medullated nerve-fibre tracts, known as colloid and miliary degeneration. The term colloid carries with it a faulty implication; for the material has nothing in common with the colloid matter found in degenerative changes undergone by new growths, and thè like. The change essentially consists in the appearance of numerous spheroidal, ovoid or pyriform bodies, at times aggregated in clusters, more usually scattered along a linear course corresponding to a medullated nerve-fibre. These bodies are perfectly translucent, colourless, and homogeneous, show no concentric rings, and are not affected by iodine and sulphuric acid. For some time they were regarded as products of connective-tissue cells; we now know them to originate solely from the medullated sheath. Their size varies considerably : the smaller vary from $6\,\mu$ to $12\,\mu$, the larger up to $40\,\mu$; and, as these latter are often elliptical or pyriform, some of them attain the dimensions of $50\,\mu$ by $40\,\mu$. They are found abundantly in the tangential belt of medullated fibres in the peripheral layer of the cortex; far less frequently in the intra-cortical arciform stripes; in great abundance, again, in the white matter of the brain, right up to the gyral radiations of medulla, although the gray matter is almost entirely devoid of them : in the pons and medulla, again, these bodies are not only frequent and numerous, but of great dimensions, and in the spinal cord the lateral columns are peculiarly prone to this form of degeneration. One feature of their disposition is that they never obtrude themselves into the gray matter of the cortex, ganglia, nuclei, or central gray matter of the cord, except where this is traversed by medullated fibres.

When the large-sized bodies found in the bulb and pons are the subject of examination, they are seen in most cases to form a constituent part of the medullated tube; forming indeed large ovoid swellings along its course, into which the stained axis-cylinder can often be traced; and it is this connection which prevents their falling out or being picked out from the tissue, as is the case with the miliary patches to be described later.　Colloid bodies appear to result from a segmentation of medulla, and usually have one or more nucleated cells in contact with them, which resemble the phagocytes of the brain.　Later these morbid bodies become clouded and granular, and may eventually coalesce with similar bodies in their neighbourhood to form large multiloculated masses which show also many spider-cells whose processes permeate the structure of the mass now known as a miliary patch.　The size of these resulting patches is such that in reflected light they may be seen by the naked eye; but the individual colloid bodies require microscopic vision for their detection.

The whole process is one of most chronic character, and differs thus from the more acute change which results when the fibre is severed by section from its trophic cell.　In what the difference in reaction consists we cannot as yet say.

Miliary patches are best studied in the coarse medullated columns of the cord, although they are at times abundantly scattered through the selective sites of colloid degeneration.　Cross sections of the pyramidal tracts will exhibit them as irregular, minute, colourless bodies, from $20\,\mu$ to $50\,\mu$ in diameter, within a deeply-stained area of sclerotic tissue; and they may in chrome specimens be readily picked out of the tissue. Longitudinal sections show them as multilobulated masses pervading the columns along the course of the large medullated nerve-fibres, to the extent of perhaps $200\,\mu$ in length, by about $70\,\mu$ in breadth, and surrounded on all sides by moniliform nerve-fibres, especially by diseased fibres largely varicose which enter the mass at one end, and leave it at the other in a similar condition: or, again, as axis-cylinders swollen and devoid of medulla, or showing segmentation and colloid change. Clear, translucent, and homogeneous at first, later they become clouded, and have a pearly, frosted aspect; the contents become granular, and a large number of spider-cells encroach upon them, crowding also into the sclerosed tissue around.　At this stage few if any axis-cylinders pass through the mass, apparently interrupted; they either terminate at its borders, or are diverted and pressed aside, as are the neighbouring structures, by the apparent density of the morbid material.　A striking feature is the almost invariable presence of a large blood-vessel in close contiguity to the patch, often passing through its structure.　The vascular tunics are thickened, their nuclei proliferating abundantly, hæmatoidin granules are found in the sheath, and leucocytal infiltration with granule cells around indicate the site as one of inflammatory reaction.　The nerve tubuli in the sclerosed area around the patch are atrophied, or entirely absent.

What, then, is the probable explanation of these morbid patches? Are they indicative of a primary sclerosis? are they the results of a focal degenerative change? or again, do they indicate a true parenchymatous neuritis?　We can by no means entertain the first of these assumptions; and as regards the second, it must be borne in mind that the condition seems always associated with the colloid change of nerve-tracts, forming indeed a late, though non-essential feature in this degenerative process. On the other hand, we have every indication here of a strongly irritative process—engorged blood-vessels, thickened vascular walls, proliferating nuclei, leucocytal accumulation, distinct implication of medullated tubuli, large development of spider-cells, and, lastly, an encroaching sclerotic change in the tissue around.   In fact, we have every reason for regarding this change as an accident in the course of colloid degeneration (as it by no means invariably accompanies this change), and as possibly induced by the spread of a chronic inflammatory process to the vascular walls of the large branch which is always in close proximity to the patch. The more essential links in the chain of morbid events appear to be :— (i.) a chronic degenerative change (colloid) in the medullated tracts due to disease probably of an irritative character in their trophic cells ; (ii.) a tendency to focal irritation at certain points along the course of these degenerated tracts, arousing genuine inflammatory reaction (parenchymatous), in which the vascular channels participate, and so on ; (iii.) leading ultimately to destruction of the nerve-fibres involved, and to an encroaching sclerosis in the tissue around.

Chronic alcoholism is peculiarly apt to produce both forms of lesion ; and it is in these cases that we more frequently find colloid passing into the more acute miliary change.   In general paralysis, again, colloid degeneration is frequent ; and it is significant that miliary patches chiefly prevail where alcoholic excess has played a notable part as a cause.   Usually such areas of irritation lie along the lateral columns of the cord at the site of a descending sclerosis.   Again, the acute process which ushers in senile insanity affords further illustration of colloid change in nerve-centres.

Fatty degeneration.—The origin and storage of fat in the system and its appearance within the cell elements in genuine fatty atrophy have received careful attention at the hands of pathologists.   One fact ever stood out prominently—that all tissues, whatever their constitution, are liable to an intrinsic change, under certain conditions, physiological or pathological.   The solitary exception, if such there be, was that of the nervous tissues ; and Cohnheim long maintained that nerve structures were unique in this respect, expressing considerable doubt as to the possibility of lecithin being converted in the organism into fat.   This position can no longer be maintained ; we have the strongest evidence of the formation of fatty granules within the nerve-cells of the cortex and the medullated sheath of nerves—granules which have undoubtedly taken the place of the proteid of the cell itself.   Ziegler indicates how ganglion cells disintegrate with fatty degeneration in ischæmic conditions of brain. Miescher's observations prove that lecithin, which is closely allied to fats, and may be regarded as a glycero-phosphate of neurin, as well as nucleins arise synthetically within the tissues of the body, as shown in the ova of salmon, from the splitting up of the proteids with the fats of the muscles.   So as regards the splitting of the proteid molecule into fat, Hofman's experiments on the growth of eggs of Musca vomitoria on blood, and Bauer's experiments on phosphorus poisoning, are conclusive. In the latter the nitrogen output was doubled, whilst the elimination of carbonic acid and the absorption of oxygen were diminished one-half. Histochemical examination of degenerating medullated nerve-fibres sufficiently testifies to a granular change of undoubtedly fatty nature ; and Marchi's method of examination depends for its success upon the presence of fat in the nerve elements, as indicated by the reaction of the osmic acid. Moreover, Dr. Mott, in his estimate of the amount of phosphorus in the degenerated tracts, has added strong evidence in favour of the convertibility of lecithins into fats [*vide* art. "Nutrition," vol. i. p. 189].

The conditions influencing fatty degeneration of the nerve elements are identical with those which induce similar changes in other tissues— the restriction of the blood current to the part ; a reduced oxygen value of the red blood corpuscles, as occasioned by carbon monoxide, antimony, arsenic, or mineral acids, and possibly from the same cause by phosphorus ; or the same failure in the tissue cells as occurs in senility and after castration. These factors, together with failure in proteid replacement, explain the conditions favouring fatty deposition and degeneration. The synthetic transformations which occur in the passage of the great proteid molecule of the tissues and the lecithin compounds into fat, and subsequently into carbonic acid and water, are still very obscure.

Fatty degeneration of the nerve-cell is revealed by a somewhat altered, swollen contour—the cell tends to assume a more spheroidal outline ; its protoplasm becomes obscured by granular contents most of which are highly refractile ; whilst the cell protoplasm takes up carmine or aniline stains far less vigorously than in health. In unstained preparations the outline of the cell can scarcely be recognised ; and we simply see clusters of granules, assuming closely the form of an ordinary nerve-cell, some pyramidal others more spherical. The nucleus is often displaced by the advancing change ; the lateral processes dwindle down and disappear ; the apex process disintegrates, so that the dendritic portion of the cell has nearly gone before the axon is gravely affected. The latter persists long in a swollen and prominent state, whilst the cell itself gradually breaks down into a little heap of granules—pigmentary and fatty in constitution. That phosphorus poisoning induces fatty degeneration in the nerve-cells of the brain, as it does in other organs, has been conclusively shown in a case, recorded by Elkins and Middlemas, in which the nuclei of the nerve-cells also participated in the fatty change. When treated with osmic acid the greater proportion remains unstained ; but upon the addition of acetic acid the granule groups are seen to enclose a sort of nucleus of much finer granules stained black by the osmium, and certainly of fatty constitution. On the addition of liquor potassæ these dark granules disappear, leaving the pigmented granules unaffected ; evidently the central portion of the pigment granules had undergone a fatty change. The neighbouring vessels are usually but not invariably atheromatous, their perivascular channels full of fat granules and débris with much blood pigment. The lymph-connective elements (spider-cells), containing similar granules, crowd upon the sheaths of the blood-vessels, especially along the course of disintegrating medullated fibres. The latter have undergone a notable varicosity—the segmentation of their medulla resulting in large colourless and lustrous moniliform bodies, unstained, and connected by a narrow stained neck representing the axis-cylinder; in fact, a colloid degeneration has ensued here. In later stages, with disappearance of the segmented medulla, the spider-cell itself is found disintegrated, and a dense meshwork of its felted fibres permanently replaces the former highly-organised tissues.

At first sight this destructive implication of the dendrons might appear confirmatory of Golgi's doctrine that these processes have especially a nutritive function to fulfil; and that, when these nutritive radicles break down, nutrition of the cell becomes so lowered as to lead to fatty atrophy. This, however, is not the case; the change in the nerve-cell appears to be always primary, and the secondary implication of the dendron follows only upon severe affection of the cell protoplasm. Moreover, there is no reason for assuming so close a connection betwixt these dendrites and the lymph-connective and vascular systems as was affirmed by Golgi.

Pigmentary degeneration.—Pigment is a normal constituent of the nerve-cell throughout extensive tracts of the cerebro-spinal system. In the motor cells it is found in the form of bright golden-yellow, amorphous granules, usually occupying the basal extremity of the cell and clearly defined from the cell protoplasm. Its amount would appear to bear some definite relationship to the functional activity of the cell, since not only is it increased in adult life, but is notably present in such nervous affections as are marked by mental and motorial excitement; for example, epileptic insanity, alcoholic insanity, general paralysis, senile mania, chorea, and hydrophobia. So constant is its excess in these affections that its absence or great limitation in other diseases at once suggests failing vigour in the functional manifestations of the nerve elements.

Whenever pigment exists in abnormal amount in the nerve-cells the contents stain deeply, another indication of functional hyperactivity. In hydrophobia this is most notable. The mass of pigment itself is unaffected by the usual stains, remaining either a bright yellow or a dusky brown-yellow; and its encroachment upon the cell contents is evidenced by the passage through the mass of the protoplasmic processes of the cell up to the point where they join the retracting but healthier protoplasm, whilst the part in immediate contact with the pigmented mass often resembles a deep stained sclerosed barrier betwixt the two. Such pigmented collections do not appear to contain iron, as they are not darkened by ammonium sulphide; they are also unaffected by ether, alcohol, caustic alkalies, and fuming nitric acid; they are, moreover, distinctly darkened by osmic acid, indicating the existence of a fatty admixture in the form of still more minute granules betwixt the larger amorphous granules of pigment. The nerve-cell is altered in contour, is more swollen, pyriform, or globose, its nucleus eccentric, flattened, or angular, and often pigmented; whilst its dendrons dwindle to mere threads, traced but a short distance from the cell, evidently degenerate and broken down. As in fatty change, the last portion to persist is the axis-cylinder. The neighbouring vessels are dilated, their perivascular sheaths contain hæmatoidin crystals, whilst leucocytes are scattered through the brain tissue enclosing pigmentary and fatty granules. Eventually the cell loses its dusky brown or fuscous hue, and a further transformation ensues in which fatty globules appear, a pale yellow or colourless aspect replacing the coarser changes of the earlier stage.

Whence is derived the pigment found in the cell? There can be little doubt but that it is derived from the disintegration of red blood corpuscles which have been extravasated, or have passed through the walls of the vessels in states of vascular engorgement. The colouring matter gradually passes out from the free red globules, and gives origin to hæmatoidin crystals and granular pigment; whilst other red globules are enclosed by the colourless lymph corpuscles, and in their interior disintegrate into granular pigment.

This is what occurs in all blood extravasations whatever their site, and pigment-carrying cells are found abundantly in the neighbourhood of necrotic tissue. The nutrition of the nerve-cells appears profoundly modified by the excess of free hæmoglobin in its neighbourhood; and the replacement of the used-up nucleo-albumins of the cell appear to be largely derived from the splitting-up of the hæmoglobin. The subsequent change is one of fatty disintegration—the ultimate removal of pigment being a very slow and prolonged process. We are not concerned here with a mere increase of the physiological pigment of the nerve-cell; as before indicated, in all cells which have a very special part to play, such as nerve-cells of the special sense organs, pigment is found. In morbid states, however, the pigment would appear to be derived direct from decomposed hæmoglobin mixed with the food-stuffs supplied to the nerve-cell, which replaces the normal constituent in just the same manner that fat replaces the proteid of the cell in fatty atrophy: moreover such pigment seems directly to induce the irritative changes subsequently seen in the cell [*vide* art. "Nutrition," vol. i. p. 197].

Vacuolation of nerve-cells.—This change consists in the appearance of one or more colourless, highly refractile bodies, more or less spheroidal in contour, displacing the cell protoplasm, which is usually in a state of granular degeneration. Occasionally the cell is full of such bodies; in other cases the contents have been absorbed or escaped, leaving a genuine vacuole retaining its original form exactly. Vacuolation of the nerve-cell is peculiarly frequent in senile brain atrophy and in chronic alcoholism; it is often well seen in the motor-cells of the chord.

A similar degeneration affects the nuclei of the nerve-cell in chronic alcoholism and in epilepsy. In the latter it appears peculiarly located in the small cells of the second layer of the cortex. It has also been noted in cases of concussion ; both Miles and Macpherson give instructive cases of the traumatic factor in vacuolation.

W. BEVAN LEWIS.

REFERENCES

1. BUNGE. *Physiological and Pathological Chemistry*, 1890. — 2. BUZZARD. *Diseases of the Nervous System*, 1882.—3. CHARCOT. *Diseases of the Nervous System, Lectures on Senile Diseases, Localisation of Cerebral and Spinal Diseases*, Sydenham Soc. Trans.—4. COHNHEIM. *Lectures on General Pathology*, Sydenham Soc. Trans.— 5. CORNIL and RANVIER. *Manual of Pathological Histology*, 1882. — 6. RAMON Y. CAJAL. *Les nouvelles idées sur la structure du système Nerveux*, 1894. — 7. GOWERS. *Diseases of the Nervous System*, 1888.—8. HAMILTON. *Text-book of Pathology*, vols. i. and ii. 1894.—9. WOODHEAD. *Journal of Pathology and Bacteriology.*—10. SUTTON. *Introduction to General Pathology.* — 11. HACK TUKE. *Dictionary of Psychological Medicine.*—12. ZIEGLER. *Special Pathological Anatomy*, Sections 1 to 8 ; trans. by Macalister and Cattell, 1896.—13. *Brain: A Journal of Neurology*, Vols. i. to xix. —14. *Journal of Mental Science*, 1880 to 1897.—15. *La cellule*, t. vii. to xii.—16. *Journal of Comparative Neurology*, 1893 to 1897.—17. *Berl. klin. Wochenschr.*—18. *Archiv für Psychiatrie.* — 19. *Allgemeine Zeitschr. f. Psychiatrie.* — 20. *Archiv f. path. Anatomie und Physiol.* (Virchow).—21. *Brit. and For. Medico-Chirurgical Review.*—22. *Neurol. Centralbl.* 1893 to 1897.—23. *Medico-Chirurgical Transactions.* **Special Articles :**—24. ANDRIEZEN. "Newer Aspects of the Pathology of Insanity," *Brain*, 1894, and *Journ. of Mental Science*, 1894.—24a. APATHY. "Das leitende Element des Nervensystems," *Mitth. aus d. zoolog. Stat. Neap.* Bd. xii. 4.—25. BEADLES. "Degenerative Lesions of the Arterial System in the Insane," *Journ. Mental Science*, January 1895.—26. BERKLEY. "Hyaline Degeneration," *Brain*, vol. xii. 1890.—27. "Finer Anatomy of the Cerebrum," *Brain*, vol. xvii. 1894.—28. "Experimental Lesions produced by Ricin on the Cortical Nerve-Cells," *Neurol. Centralbl.* 11, 1897.—29. BOEDEKER. "Anatomische Befunde bei Dementia Paralytica," *Neurol. Centralbl.* 1897.—30. BOULAY. "Pseudo-bulbar Paralysis " (good bibliography), *Brain*, vols. xiv. to xxxi.—31. BULLOCH. "Hyaline Degeneration of the Spinal Cord," *Brain*, vol. xv. 1892.—32. CAJAL. "Sur la structure de l'écorce cérébrale de quelques mammifères," *La cellule*, t. vii. 1891.—33. CAMPBELL. *Journ. Pathol. and Bacteriology*, February 1894 ; also vol. ii. 1894, "On Vacuolation of Nerve-Cells and Toxæmia."—34. COLELLA. "Sur les altérations histologiques de l'écorce cérébrale dans quelques maladies mentales," *Archives italiennes de biologie*, 1894, p. 216.—35. COLLINS. "Contributions to the Pathology of Epilepsy," *Brain*, vol. xix. 1896.—36. COLMAN. "Pseudo-Bulbar Paralysis," *Brain*, vol. xvii. 1894. — 37. EICHHORST. " Pathology of Alcoholic Paralysis," *Virchow's Archiv*, Bd. cxxix. Heft 1.—38. FISCHER. "Sclerosis of Cornu Ammonis in Epilepsy," *Neurol. Centralbl.* 1893.—39. FRIEDEBERG. "Acute Compression of the Cord," *Neurol. Centralbl.* 1893.—40. VAN GEHUCHTEN. "La structure des centres nerveux : la moelle épinière et le cervelet," *La cellule*, t. vii. 1891, xi. 1895, and xii. 1897.—41. GOMBAULT. "Neuritis and Wallerian Degeneration,' *Arch. de neurol.* 1880.—42. GOODALL. "Spider or Scavenger-cell of the Brain," *Journ. Path. and Bact.* vol. ii. 1894. — 43. GRIFFITHS. "Fatty Degeneration and Atrophy," *Journ. Path. and Bact.* vol. iii. 1895.—44. HANDFORD. "Peripheral Neuritis " (digest), *Brain*, vol. xii. p. 163.—45. HAMILTON. *Microscopical Journ.* vol. xv. 1875 — 46. HILL. "The Chrome Silver Method," *Brain*, 1896. — 47. JULIUSBURGER. "Bemerkungen zur Pathologie der Ganglienzelle," *Neurol. Centralbl.* No. 9, 1896.—48. KESTEVEN. *Brit. and For. Medico-Chir. Rev.* vol. xlviii. 1869. — 49. KLIPPEL and AZOULAY. "Des lésions histologiques de la paralysie générale, étudiées d'après la méthode de Golgi," *Arch. de neurol.* 1894.— 50. KNAGGS and BROWN. "Diffuse Encephalitis," *Brain*, 1893. — 51. KOSTJURIN. "Senile Changes in Cerebral Cortex," *Wiener medic. Jahrbuch*, 1886, Heft 2.—52. LAMY. "Syphilitic Meningo-myelitis," *Neurol. Centralbl.* 1893. — 53. LANGLEY. "Recent Observations on Degeneration and on Nerve Tracts in the Spinal Cord " (critical digest), *Brain*, vol. ii. 1886.—54. LAPINSKY. "Zur Frage über den Zustand der kleinen Capillaren der Gehirnrinde bei Arteriosclerose der grossen Gefässe, ' *Neurol. Centralbl.* No. 20, 1896.—55. MACPHERSON. "Vacuolation of Nerve-Cell Nuclei in

Cerebral Concussion," *Lancet*, May 1892.—56. MARINESCO. "Théorie des Neurones : Application au progressus de dégénérescence et d'atrophie dans le système nerveux," *Presse médicale*, 1895.—57. *Idem*. "Pathologie générale de la cellule nerveuse : lésions secondaires et primitives " (abstract), *Neurol. Centralbl.* No. 11, 1897.—58. MARTIN, Is. "Contribution à l'étude de la structure interne de la moelle épinière chez le poulet et chez la truite," *La cellule*, 1895, t. xi.—59. MARTIN, SIDNEY. "Multiple Neuritis," *Jour. Path. and Bact.* vol. i. 1893.—60. MEYER. "Diphtheritic Paralysis," *Virchow's Archiv*, Bd. lviii. Heft 2.—61. MICKLE. "Syphilis of the Nervous System," *Brain*, vol. xviii. 1895 ; "On General Paralysis " (critical digest), *Brain*, vol. xvii. 1894.—62. MILES. "Effects of Blows over different parts of the Cranium," *Labor. Rep. Roy. Coll. Phys. Edin.*—63. "Mechanism of Brain Injuries," *Brain*, vol. xv. 1892.—64. "Colloid, Miliary, and Pigmentary Changes in Cerebral Traumatism," *Journ. Path. and Bact.* May 1892.—65. MOTT. "Amyotrophic Lateral Sclerosis," *Brain*, vol. xviii. 1895.—66. "Ascending Degenerations resulting from Lesions of the Spinal Cord in Monkeys," *Brain*, vol. xv. 1892.—67. NISSL. "Ueber die Nomenclatur in der Nerven-zellen-anatomie und ihre nächsten Ziele," *Neurol. Centralbl.* No. 3, 1895 ; 68. "On Karyokinesis in the Central Nervous System," *Neurol. Centralbl.* p. 94, 1894.—68a. "Kritische Fragen der Nervenzellen-anatomie," *Neurol. Centralbl.* No. 4, 1896.—69. OBERMEIER. "Zur pathologischen Anatomie der Hirnsyphilis," *Deutsche Zeitschrift für Nervenheilkunde*, No. 3, 1892.—70. ORMEROD. "Friedreich's Disease," *Brain*, vol. xi. p. 406.—71. PICK. "Rückenmarks-Krankheiten."—72. PRYCE. "Diabetic Neuritis," *Brain*, Aug. 1893. —73. REYNOLDS. "On Changes in the Nervous System after Amputation of Limbs " (good bibliography), *Brain*, vol. ix. p. 494.—74. ROBERTSON. "Pathology of Subdural Membranes" (good bibliography), *Journ. Path. and Bact.* vol. iv. 1896.—75. ROSS. "Labio-glosso-pharyngeal Paralysis of Cerebral Origin," *Brain*, vol. v. p. 145. 76. RUTHERFORD and BATTY TUKE. "Miliary Sclerosis," *Edin. Med. Journ.* Sept. 1868.—77. RUXTON and GOODALL. "On Certain Microscopical Changes in the Nerves of the Limbs in General Paralysis of the Insane," *Brain*, vol. xv. 1892.—78. SARBO. "Rückenmarksveränderungen nach zeitweiliger Verschliessung der Bauchaorta," *Neurol. Centralbl.* No. 15, 1895.—79. SCHAFER. "The Nerve-Cell considered as the Basis of Neurology," *Brain*, vol. xvi. 1893 ; also Section "Neurology " in Quain's *Anatomy* (last edition).—80. SCHAFFER. "Ueber Nervenzellenveränderungen während der Inanition," *Neurol. Centralbl.* No. 18, 1897.—81. SHAW. "Aprosexia in Children," *Practitioner*, July 1890.—82. SHERRINGTON. "Bilateral Secondary Degeneration from Unilateral Lesions of Cortex," *Brain*, vol. viii. 1886.—83. "Bilateral Degeneration of Pyramidal Tracts from Unilateral Cortical Lesions," *Brit. Med. Journ.* 1890, vol. i. p. 14.—84. SKAE. "Vacuolation of Nerve-Cell Nuclei in Cortex," *Brit. Med. Journ.* May 1894.—85. TUKE, BATTY. "Colloid, Pigmentary, and Granular Degeneration," *Brit. and For. Med.-Chir. Rev.* July 1873.—86. "The Insanity of Over-exertion," *Morison Lectures*, 1894.—87. VAS. "Changes in Alcoholic and Nicotine Poisoning," *Neurol. Centralbl.* 1894.—88. WELLS. "Post-mortem Nerve Changes," *Journ. Path. and Bact.* vol. iii. 1895.—89. WESTPHAL. "General Paralysis and Disease of the Posterior Columns, *Berlin. klin. Wochenschr.* i. 1881, and *Arch. f. Psych.* vol. xii.—90. WHITWELL. "Vacuolation of Nerve-Cell Nuclei," *Brain*, vol. xii. 1890.—91. WIGLESWORTH. "Pachymeningitis Interna Hæmorrhagica," *Brain*, vol. xv. 1892.

W. B. L.

TREMOR, "TENDON-PHENOMENON," AND SPASM

I. PHYSIOLOGICAL SECTION

THE physiological basis of "spasm," of "tremor," and of the so-called "tendon reflexes" is a compound reaction from two integrated tissues of the body—the nervous and the muscular. Discrimination between the two factors of composition must be attempted even in the briefest sketch of the subject. The nervous factor will be considered first.

Nerve.—*The neuron as a transmitter.*—The discharging and conducting elements of the nervous system are its neurons (ganglion cells), and only they. Each neuron is an eminently excitable cell. The functional waves of change, which it is the office of the nervous system to elaborate and distribute, move along nothing else than a concatenation of neurons. As would be expected in links of a chain, the length of each neuron lies parallel with the direction of transmission of force. At its one end each neuron is an eminently receptive cell, and easy of access by vibrations impinging on its environment : each neuron is throughout from end to end an eminently conductive cell ; that is, it readily propagates a change once started in it. Since one end is receptive and the rest of the cell conductive, the waves of change always travel through the neuron from the receptive end. By powerful artificial means a "change" can be initiated in parts of the neuron remote from the specially receptive end ; the "change" is then found to be propagated in all directions along the neuron ; but under natural circumstances the "change" is always excited at the receptive end only ; hence the sense of propagation is never reversed. The "changes" or "impulses," therefore, circulate in one direction only along the nervous system. This is what has been called by James the "law of forward direction." If the outgoing end of the neuron is turned toward extrinsic—that is, not nervous—tissues, the neuron is *efferent;* if its outgoing end is turned away from extrinsic tissues, the neuron is *afferent.*

Nervous impulses.—Of the "change" or "nervous impulse" inducible in and propagated by the neuron it can be said that it is probably molecular (not chemical), and in quantity almost immeasurably small. Its duration at any one point of the neuron is brief (for example, $\frac{1}{1000}$ sec.) It travels wavelike along the neuron at a speed of some 30 metres a second, and extends about 10 millimetres on either side of its crest. Some of the neurons in man are 4 to 5 feet long ; the duration of the change in them may therefore occupy a large fraction of a second. In the pieces of neurons usually employed for physico-physiological study the wave of disturbance ("nervous impulse") is propagated without alteration in height, length, or speed. But in being propagated along a chain of neurons the "impulse" is profoundly and variously modified. At what points in the chain modification takes place is not with certainty known. It may occur in each neuron at that part whence the stem and other branches of the cell diverge, in fact, at that part which contains the nucleus and is often called "cell body" in contradistinction to "cell branch." An alleged slackening of speed of nerve-impulses through the vagus ganglion is the main datum for this view, which is on the other hand discouraged by the histological fact of unaltered continuity of the primitive fibrils of the neuraxon across the "cell body."

. *The linkage of neurons.*—A feature of the concatenation of neurons more probably explicative of modification and delay of nerve impulses is the *synapse*. The successive neurons of the chain do not actually unite, but, although closely juxtaposed, are links retaining separate entity. They are anatomically discontinuous, physiologically continuous. In view of recent histological evidence the doctrine of their conjunction by anastomosis of terminal filaments has been rejected; in its place points of approximation across varying distances occupied by intercellular substance are held to constitute the linkage, such places of linkage of neurons being called "synapses." The reaction of a neuron to excitation is in nature explosive; the relation between stimulus applied to the neuron and change induced in it, is as between a releasing force and a released one. The wave of disturbance evoked in the initial neuron of a chain when transmitted to its outgoing end becomes releasing force for an explosion in neurons next succeeding. The amount of action will depend partly upon the ease with which the disturbance in neuron A can act across the interval between neuron A and neuron B. In other words, the nature of the synapse, and conditions obtaining at it, must to some extent control the conduction along a chain of neurons. Relatively slight exhibition of contractility by the stem or branches of the neuron will greatly affect the width of intercellular gap at the synapse. Slight retraction of this or that cell branch may afford to the neuron isolation from this or that of its neighbours; on the other hand, protrusion may procure greater facility of communication. The inhibitions of hypnosis may be referable to withdrawal of circumcellular arborisations. Observations by the microscope lend some support to such conjectures.

In the intercellular gap at the synapse between neuron and neuron, not merely the width, but the nature of the ground substance filling it must be apt for the propagation of molecular change across it. In some tissues it is their ground substance which endows them with their functional importance : in the nervous system the properties of that which is the medium of the synapse cannot be negligible. That the direction of nerve impulses is not reversible along the neural chains may be a function of the nature of the synapse. The synapse is likely enough a bridge open to traffic from neuron A to neuron B, but barred to passage in the opposite sense. It is probable that by these synapses the circuits of the nervous system (Hall's "diastaltic arcs") are as securely valved against regurgitation as is the cardio-vascular itself; conditioning the Bell-Magendie law, and other series.

Variability of reaction.—It was stated above that in transit along a chain of neurons nervous impulses may be much modified. Their augmentation or suppression (inhibition), their wide diffusion (for example, in the case of strychnia), or their concentration into a few focal paths, may variously occur. The greater the number of synapses the more variable, the less predicable, the ultimate effect. The reactions which occur along neuron chains of few links only are characterised by "monotony": such are the "simple reflexes." The reactions which employ long chains, traversing many synapses, are immensely variable; so much so as to simulate the reactions termed "volitional." It is a cardinal feature in the architecture of the nervous system that the longest chains all include cerebral—many of them also cerebellar—neurons and synapses. Hence by removal of the cerebrum the longest concatenations are all broken—although multitudinous shorter ones remain. Accordingly we then find manifold nervous reactions still possible, but all broadly characterised by machine-like uniformity in repetition.

Latency of reaction.—The nervous impulse being a moving, wave-like disturbance, the longer the neural chain the longer, other things being equal, the *time* which the impulse will take to pass from the initial to the farther end. This time—the reaction period—has for many chains been measured; it is found to increase with greater complexity of the chain far more than with the mere distance of travel in the chain. This increase of "reaction period" seems chiefly proportioned to the number of links—that is, of synapses—in the chain. The "reaction time" for one and the same circuit varies somewhat; but, apart from this, each additional synapse seems to involve marked additional delay in the transmission of the nervous impulse.

Spread of reaction.—The *distribution* of nervous impulses is obviously dependent on the topographical relations of the neurons and of their stems and branches. Hence in the nervous system minute anatomy yields much information about paths of nervous conduction. Other things equal, the nearer together any two neurons lie the more likely the existence of connections between them. But exceptions to this statement are very numerous. Thus, certain cerebral neurons near the upper end of the Rolandic fissure are more closely connected with certain in the spinal lumbar region than with any in the thoracic or cervical regions. A rule with far fewer exceptions is the following:—each neuron at its "ingoing" end is branched, so that it presents not one but hundreds of points of access; at its "outgoing" end also it is branched, so that it discharges not merely upon one but upon several (perhaps some hundreds of) other neurons; and these rules hold also for the peripheral neurons, connected as they are at one end with non-nervous tissues; thus the motor neuron discharges upon many muscle fibres. From this rule there results "spread" —the almost universal concomitant of the march of impulses. It is only by synapses that "spread" takes place: the wave of change sweeping within a neuron does not induce waves of change in other neurons even close alongside it (J. Müller's law of isolated conduction), unless by transit across the synapses at its outgoing ends.

Rhythmic discharge.—An important feature of the *discharge* of the neuron is that it tends to be recurrent; that is, the explosion evoked even by a momentary stimulus tends to be repeated fewer or more times. It has been questioned whether one single and sole explosion is ever given by a neuron in reply to excitation applied to it physiologically, that is, *via* a synapse; but such does seem to have been recorded (Wundt). The prolonged steady action of muscles which characterises "willed" movements is unobtainable by continuous application of any artificial stimulus; but it is imperfectly imitable by rapidly intermitting certain kinds of artificial excitation. Hence, it is argued, the prolonged natural discharges of neurons underlying willed and natural movements are probably of intermittent nature. The hypothesis is supported by abundant evidence of rhythmic activity in muscular and sensifacient cells. The rhythm of the discharge in neurons must vary much, even in the same cell, from time to time. It seems to be slowest when the neuron is fatigued. It ranges probably from 50 per sec. to 5 per sec. We do not know how the discharges from the individual neurons composing a nerve-centre are co-ordinated in time. To consider a concrete case: the spinal motor neurons innervating the flexor brevis pollicis are some 200 in number; they lie scattered through at least three segments of the cord, the last cervical and the two highest thoracic; each of them on entering the muscle throws out a leash of some 30 filaments bearing each a terminal arborisation applied to the receptive motor plate of a column of muscle cells. It is obvious that the maintenance of willed or other "natural" contraction of the muscle, on the hypothesis of intermittent discharge by neurons, presupposes co-ordination in the time of discharge of the individual neurons. The discharging may take place by platoon firing, or by company firing, or by desultory rank firing. On this much discussed point it can only be said that the general opinion is in favour of platoon firing; the existence of a certain tremor in "natural" movements supporting such a view, and the failure to obtain "secondary tetanus" from "natural" movements not precluding it.

Tonus of nerve.—The wave of change (nervous impulse) induced in a neuron by advent of a stimulus is, after all, only a sudden augmentation of an activity continuous within the neuron—a sudden accentuation of one (the disintegrative) phase of the metabolism inherent and inseparable from its life. The nervous impulse is, so to say, the sudden transient glow of an ember continuously black-hot. The continuous lesser "change," or stream of changes, sets through the neuron, and is distributed by it to other neurons in the same direction and by the same synapses as are its nerve impulses. This gentle continuous activity of the neuron is designated its "tonus": in its effect (for example, upon muscle) it appears perfectly continuous; it may, however, be in reality intermittent. Its origin is uncertain. In part it seems to be autochthonous, an inner stimulation of the cell itself, by itself, in result of its own metabolism; but it is chiefly referable to mild continual excitation applied to the neuron by other neurons, similarly possessed of tonus, and so placed in the

neural chain as to discharge upon it.   In tracing the tonus of neurons to
its source, one is always led link by link against the current of nerve force—
so to say, "up stream"—to the first beginnings of the chains of neurons in
the sensifacient surfaces of the body.   From these, in the eye, ear, skin, and
other sensory surfaces, tonus, constantly initiated, is constantly conducted
into the nervous system *via* the great efferent neurons, the fundamental
links of the whole concatenation of the system.   The amount of tonus may
be varied in several ways.   Thus, the tonus of the motor neurons of the
spinal cord is much lessened by breaking the neurons of the afferent spinal
nerve roots, the tonus of which latter normally plays upon the former.
Chloroform depresses, strychnia augments neural tonus ; venosity temporarily exalts and then depresses.   It would appear that a certain degree of
spinal tonus in the motor neurons is necessary for their appropriate response to the mandates of volition ; when the anterior horn cells have been
deprived of spinal tonus, extreme deficiency in certain willed movements
immediately results (Mott and Sherrington).   And to the tonus of the
spinal motor neurons that of cerebral and cerebellar neurons contribute :
the cerebral tonus certainly descends mainly from the Rolandic region of
the cortex of the heteronymous hemisphere ; the cerebellar mainly from
its homonymous hemisphere, partly in an indirect manner by way of the
cerebral hemisphere of the crossed side, partly probably in a less indirect
manner through Deiter's nucleus (Mott, Ferrier, and Turner).   In like
manner the tonus of cerebral and cerebellar neurons is the outcome of
an interaction of various factors, partly autocthonous, partly of extrinsic,
probably especially of spinal origin.   Further discussion of tonus is,
however, inadmissible here.

Muscle.—We now turn to the muscular element in neuro-muscular reactions. The contractions of muscle fibres, like the "impulses" of neurons, are
explosive settings free of energy ; but they involve relatively huge quantities of material and easily measurable chemical changes.   As said above,
continuous application of artificial stimuli fails to elicit any continuous
contraction of muscle ; but by rapidly repeating a momentary stimulus
contraction, apparently continuous, can be kept up for a while.   This
experimental "tetanus" is proved to be really a fusion of simple, brief
"spasms," each due to a single explosion in the contractile cells.   The
spasm of contraction started in a muscle fibre travels wave-like along it,
as does the "impulse" along a neuron ; but it occupies ten times as
great a longitudinal extent, moves ten times more slowly, and consequently is at any one point a hundred times more prolonged.   Muscular
contractions, although the indices of nerve discharge most accessible to
us, are therefore very coarse indices only.   Thus in physiological tetanus
the simple spasms fuse to a prolonged and apparently continuous one, but
the exciting cause is, we know, abruptly discontinuous in kind.   Again,
the intensity of contraction is but an uncertain guide to the intensity
of nerve discharge ; the force of an explosion depends less on the size of
the spark applied than on the amount of explosive material in store ; in

the heart muscle the amount of explosion does not depend at all on the strength of the stimulus applied.

Tonus of muscle.—The "tonus" of muscle, like that of nerve, is of twofold origin. One element in it is "peripheral," intramuscular, autochthonous; exemplary of that tonus resident in all living tissue, vegetal and animal. To this is superadded a tonus of central source contributed from the continual glow of excitement in the spinal motor neuron, whose outgoing end plays upon the muscle cells, whose ingoing end is played upon by other neurons, spinal, cerebral, and cerebellar. The autochthonous component of muscular tonus is increased by venosity of blood-supply, by mechanical tension applied to the muscle fibres, by certain drugs, such, for example, as veratria, or digitalis, and so forth. The neural component of muscular tonus has been discussed above.

Under the conditions of the experiments performed in the laboratory, long-continued spasms, such as constitute "rigidities" at all comparable with those coming under the notice of the clinician, are hardly ever seen. I have, however, recently discovered that if, in the cat and rabbit, the hemispheres be removed—including the basal ganglia—there ensues in a few minutes a condition of steady extreme extension of the elbow and knee and ankle joints, with retraction of the neck and elevation of the tail. So forcible is this extension that the animal can be placed erect on the four feet; and it requires considerable force to flex the knees and elbows. This extensor spasm may last for several days; it is at first unaccompanied by any perceptible tremor; it can be inhibited by excitation of appropriate sensory nerves; section of the sensory spinal roots causes it immediately to be relaxed in the limb in which the sensory roots are severed. Semi-section of the cord abolishes it below the place of semi-section on the same side. Semi-section of the bulb above the decussation of the pyramidal tracts abolishes it on the same side as the semi-section. It appears therefore to result from an uncrossed influence arising somewhere above the lower end of the fourth ventricle and below the cerebral hemispheres. This condition I have called "decerebrate rigidity." It is the most eminently tonic spasm that can be produced by experiment.

The bearing upon "spasm," "tremor," and the so-called "tendon reflexes" of the neuro-muscular functions above outlined appears at present disappointingly remote. Whether, for instance, chronic spasm is based on long-continued intermittent neural discharge like that underlying physiological "tetanus," or on excessive tonus of motor neurons remains obscure. Yet it appears admissible to think that to the physiological qualities of neurons, to their receptivity, conduction, explosive discharge, and tonus—exalted, depressed, or inco-ordinately connected—the abnormal phenomena are referable.

Tremor in willed movements.—The muscular contractions which execute willed movements are themselves found, when examined minutely, to be often slightly tremulant. The rate of tremor varies from 40 per sec., down to 8 per sec., according to circumstances, the quicker rates being more usual in short, sharp movements. The briefest willed contraction endures about $\frac{1}{3}$ of a sec., its myogram indicating a tetanus of four or five fused simple contractions (Kronecher and Stanley Hall). The briefest eye-wink takes about ·308 sec.; of this time the depressing of the eye occupies about ·091 sec. (Garten). The briefest willed flexion (for example, of a finger) lasts no longer than $\frac{1}{14}$ sec.; the briefest willed movement is therefore much shorter than the briefest willed contraction; this result is attained by the cutting short of the movement set up by one group of muscles (for example, flexors) by after-coming innervation of the antagonistic group (for example, extensors). The limit set to the frequency of repetition of the same one movement seems to be 11 per sec. Schumann No. 8 piano quartette Scherzo requires rhythmic movement of the hand 8 times per sec. A simple syllable (la) can be repeated about 11 times a sec. The jaw can be depressed as frequently as 7 times per sec.; at the ankle, however, such frequency is impossible.

Experimental irritation contracture.—A form of chronic spasm which is of interest in relation to the tremor of willed movements is the so-called " irritation contracture " observable in the monkey (but not in other laboratory animals) subjected to lesions trespassing on the Rolandic cortex or its subjacent pyramidal path. This chronic contraction super-venes usually on septic mischief complicating a lesion which involves a part only of the Rolandic area. Though a persistent spasm, it is slightly tremulant, with a fibrillar tremor, and is at times a distinct clonus. The muscles affected belong to groups the cortical centres for which have not been included in the lesion, at least not wholly. It is probably due to chemical irritation of cortical neurons near the wound.

Experimental paralytic contracture.—A different kind of experimental " contracture," probably rather of the nature of exaggerated " tonus " than allied to muscular " tetanus," follows in the monkey (but not in other laboratory animals) upon total or very large ablations of the Rolandic cortex. It has nothing to do with mere trauma, and usually begins about a month after the healing of the wound. It is hardly, if at all, tremulant. It is a phenomenon whose onset is hastened by want of exercise of the paretic limb. The limb becomes permanently flexed at elbow or knee, the shoulder or hip being adducted, the ankle flexed. If the animal be encouraged to use the paretic limb freely and in roomy surroundings, or if passive gymnastics are practised, this form of contracture may be indefinitely postponed, and in early stages arrested. The fibres of the affected muscles degenerate after a time; the degeneration affects the stretched extensors more than the contracted flexors; the atrophy is a result of the inactivity. The reason why other laboratory animals do not manifest this contracture is probably because the necessary intensity of paresis cannot be induced in them by brain lesions. A similar " con-tracture " generally ensues in the hind limbs of the monkey after total severance of the spinal cord in the thoracic region (Sherrington).

The *tendon phenomena* are clearly and inseparably connected with " tonus."

The knee-jerk.—It is to the "neural" element in muscle tonus that the tendon phenomena is intimately associated. The earliest studied of these phenomena, the knee-jerk, may serve as an example of the class. It is a simple spasm (that is, a contraction due to a single explosion) of part of the quadriceps extensor muscle, usually elicited by a tap or other brief mechanical stimulus applied to the muscle fibres mediately through tendon. The contraction is a direct reply to a stimulus applied more or less mediately. The reply is obtainable only from muscle fibres possessed of their "neural" tonus. Of the factors summed in the tonus of the motor neuron, only some appear favourable to the occurrence of the jerk; indeed, the cerebral component restrains the jerk, which is more easily obtained when cerebral neurons have been interrupted, or when cerebral tonus is diverted from the "jerk" neurons to other neurons—for example on "reinforcement" by clasping the hands (Jendrassik). Also unfavourable to development of the "jerk" is that factor of the tonus of the motor neuron traceable to afferent neurons coming up from the hamstring muscles, the antagonists of the quadriceps (Sherrington). Hence a favourable posture of the limb to elicit the jerk is one insuring relaxation of the hamstring muscles (for example, when the leg hangs crossed over the other). Conversely, an element of the neural tonus very adjuvant to the "jerk" is that developed *via* the afferent neurons passing between the quadriceps itself and its motor neurons in the lumbar cord : in fact, this latter component of the tonus seems, as regards the jerk, essential; for severance of the sensory spinal root concerned in it permanently abolishes the jerk, even although the tonus derived from other spinal segments and from cerebrum and cerebellum remain uninterrupted. Transection of the spinal cord above the lumbar enlargement depresses the knee-jerk for a time : in the cat and dog and rabbit for a few minutes only, in the monkey usually for a much longer period, often for several days. Strychnia occasionally restores the jerk temporarily, even after section of the sensory nerve roots ; and it is to be remembered that the spasms of strychnia are considered to be reflex. Compression of the abdominal aorta depriving the spinal-cord of blood-supply at first exalts, later depresses and abolishes the knee-jerk (Prévost.) Chemical anæsthesia rapidly abolishes the knee-jerk. Depriving the peripheral structures themselves of blood—for example, by application of an Esmarch bandage—abolishes the jerk much more slowly; for example, after twenty minutes (Sternberg). Loss of blood causes the jerk to become more brisk (Prus). That increase of the cerebral, cerebellar, and even of distant spinal discharge upon the motor neurons of the "jerk" should antagonise the development of the reaction is probably due to a consequent blocking out of the reflex influence of the local afferent neurons from the motor neurons in question. Under abnormally favourable conditions, the muscular reply, even in response to a single tap, is not a single but a multiple spasm (Adamkiewicz, and others) ; more so still when the mechanical stimulation is prolonged, for example, by depressing the patella (or in calf muscles by depressing the heel) : a "clonus" then results. The knee-jerk is sometimes spoken of as a "tendon reflex"; no other reflex factor is, however, among the conditions essential for the jerk than the local spinal tonus above mentioned. The brevity of the time (Westphal, Burkhardt, Waller) necessary for the calling forth of the reaction,—that is, the shortness of interval between the tap and the beginning of the resultant spasm,—excludes the possibility of reflex development. So also with the jaw-jerk. The knee-jerk time, according to Waller's latest measurements, is 0·008 sec.; it must be due therefore to direct excitation. The fact that its myogram shows it to be a simple twitch (Eulenburg, MacWilliam) is therefore what ought to be expected. The time of the crossed knee-jerk is five times as long (Burkhardt) as of the uncrossed. The crossed knee-jerk may be truly reflex.

A little experience in observations on the knee-jerk imparts a notion of what is to be understood by an average strength of the jerk; just as the average volume and pressure of the pulse are recognised. By this means it is found that wide departures are met with in perfectly healthy individuals, and are recognisable without recourse to such refined methods of measurement as have been employed by Bowditch and Warren, and by Lombard. As a general rule a knee-jerk is "improved" by a preliminary knee-jerk; that is, its latent period is shortened (Brissaud), and the excursion of the movement is amplified (Heller, Meyer). In badly-nourished, weakly persons the first tap on the patellar tendon may be ineffectual, and the best jerk responsive to the sixth, seventh, or eighth tap of a repeated series (Schreiber). The same is true of ankle clonus. Similarly taps on the tendon too light to elicit a jerk at all when applied at intervals of 5-10 seconds, will ultimately elicit it. (Jarisch and Schiff under v. Basch.)

In sleep the knee-jerk becomes depressed, even to complete abeyance when sleep is deep.

After a certain number of knee-jerks have been elicited the individual jerks become smaller; this seems due to fatigue. Extreme bodily fatigue diminishes the knee-jerk (Lombard), and occasionally abolishes it for a while; the phenomenon returns after rest (Muhr, Jendrassik, Eisenlohr, Sternberg, de Renzi). Fatigue of the extensor muscles of the knee, without general fatigue, has been found by Sternberg and Orchanski to diminish the jerk. Rubbing of the skin of the leg and thigh is an effectual way of increasing the knee-jerk in weakly persons; and it may be thus revealed where at first trial it seemed to be wanting (Schreiber, Weir Mitchell, and Lewis). Similarly a cold bath can increase it (Beevor, Dünges, Sternberg); indeed the bath is a more effectual means than any other.

Bowditch and Warren have investigated the time-relations between the moment of application of various accessory stimuli and the incidence of the effect upon the jerk. The accessory stimuli used were cool draughts of air upon the skin or mucous membranes. The maximal amount of increase—of positive reinforcement—of the jerk occurred when the tap on the tendon followed the accessory stimuli at one to

three-tenths of a second interval.   In most persons the accessory
stimulus not merely increased the jerk, but, subsequent to the increase,
diminished it; in other words, the stimulus was favourable to the development of a jerk in response to taps delivered within half a second after its
own occurrence, but acted unfavourably to the development of jerks responsive to taps delivered in the second half of the succeeding second.
The accessory stimulus ceases to have influence, either positive or
negative, after lapse of 1·7 sec. to 2·5 sec.   Westphal noted that when
ankle clonus has disappeared after an epileptiform seizure a pin-prick
of the plantar skin will restore it.   Mitchell and Lewis found the knee-
jerk increased immediately after a magnesium light had been flashed on
the eye.   Sternberg recommends the sound of a clapping of the hands
as a useful reinforcement just before eliciting the jerk.   In 1885
Jendrassik discovered that the execution of a willed ·movement by
the arm renders the knee-jerk for the time being more brisk—"rein-
forces" it.   This is well carried out by asking the patient whose hand
holds that of a bystander to grip it forcibly, at which moment the
knee-jerk is to be elicited.   This seems the converse of the fact that for
the obtaining of the jerk it is essential that the patient should let his
lower limb "go," in other words, take off his attention from it and let it
hang slack.   Wundt and Münsterberg argue that a slight degree of
contraction of muscles is the physiological substratum of all attention.
It is certain that the turning of the attention to the performance of
some movement by the arm assists to insure that looseness and freedom
from tension in the thigh muscles which is essential for the provocation
of the jerk.   The motor cells when preoccupied under cerebral influence
appear incapable of the jerk.   To remove attention and cerebral influence
from the jerk muscles it is a good plan to tell the patient to fix his gaze
on some mark, for example, upon the ceiling, or, in the case of young
children, to examine the jerk when the child is feeding; for instance,
when taking the breast.

From the above it is seen that at least four modes of reinforcing the
knee-jerk are of easy application: (i.) repetition of the tap upon the
tendon; (ii.) rubbing of the skin of the limb itself, or still better the
use of a cold bath; (iii.) some stimulus through the special senses,
such as by a loud clapping of the hands; (iv.) willed movement of the
arm.   The importance of these devices for increasing the jerk is well
shown by the fact that Eulenburg concluded from his examination of
338 healthy children prior to the coming into use of the reinforcements
that the knee-jerk was absent in 16 of them; whereas Pelizæus and
Remak found later, with use of the reinforcements, that the knee-jerk
was present in every one of 2403 healthy children examined in succession.
The knee-jerk is very brisk in infants and young children; ankle clonus
and a clonic knee-jerk are said to occur in a large proportion of healthy
children (Faragó).   Möbius states that the knee-jerk is frequently
absent in old people of normal health.   Sternberg, on the other hand,
using the devices for reinforcement, not known at the time of Möbius,

found that the research knee-jerk is hardly ever, if ever, really absent in healthy people, even although some of those examined by him were over ninety years of age. The first effect of general fatigue is to increase the knee-jerk; the ultimate effect, if the fatigue be severe, is to diminish it; sexual excess tends at first to exaggerate the knee-jerk. In winter the knee-jerk is not obtainable in the frog; but in the breeding season it is present. In sleep, as I have said, the jerk is diminished, and in deep sleep quite abolished. I found this so also in puppies in which the spinal cord had been severed in the mid-thoracic region. In these animals I found the jerk less brisk during digestion of a heavy meal than after a day's abstinence.

The influence of the cerebrum on the jerk is seen in the exaggerated knee-jerk obtained in "decerebrate rigidity," and the regularity of time reaction noted in Rosenheim's experiments. Ziehen has noted the increase of jerk following extirpation of a cortical centre; Adamkiewicz the increase of jerk under gradually increasing cerebral compression. It has been noted that after decapitation in man (executed criminals) the knee-jerk continues obtainable for a minute or more. Regarding any effect of removal of portions of the cerebellum upon the knee-jerk the evidence is not concordant.

True deep reflexes.—Although the above "jerks" are not reflexes, true reflexes can be elicited by mechanical stimuli applied to tendons, fasciæ, periosteum, etc. A smart tap on any accessible tendon generally evokes a responsive spasm in one or more adjacent muscles. Certain bone surfaces are similarly very dependably "reflexogenous." Thus: the inner femoral condyle and the inner malleolus for the adductors of the thigh; the front of the tibia for the quadriceps; the front of the heel or ball of the hallux, also the shin, for the gastrocnemius; the outer edge of the foot for tibialis posticus; the styloid of the radius for the biceps, less frequently the triceps as well; the wrist end of the ulna for the triceps, less regularly the biceps; the humeral condyles, olecranon, or acromion for the biceps and triceps; the crista scapulæ for the deltoid.

Addendum.—The subjoined data may be of service in connection with the above :—

One "simple discharge" of a frog's gastrocnemius gives an electro-motive force of ·08 volt.

The branches of the stem process (neuraxon) of a neuron may offer a cross-section 347,000 times greater than that of the parent stem (malaptererus).

Latent period of direct muscular contraction, $\frac{1}{100}$ sec.

„   „   tendon phenomenon, $\frac{1}{100}$ sec. Jaw-jerk, $\frac{2}{100}$ sec.

„   „   direct muscular contraction recorded by same method as that employed for tendon phenomenon, $\frac{1}{100}$ sec.

„   „   simple reflex contraction, $\frac{3}{100}$ sec.

Reaction time to touch, $\frac{14}{100}$ sec.

„   „   sight, $\frac{18}{100}$ sec.

The arc followed by the reflex spinal tonus on which the knee-jerk is dependent

is contained (in man) (a) in the nerve trunk of the quadriceps extensor
cruris (except rectus femoris), especially in the nerve of the crureus and
vastus medialis ; (β) in the sensory roots of the 4th and 3rd lumbar
nerves (especially of the 4th) ; (γ) in the motor roots of the same nerves.
The lateral halves of the cord can be split by a median incision without
interfering with the arc of the knee-jerk.
Frequency of ankle clonus is 7-9 per sec.

EXPERIMENTAL DATA CONCERNING "TENDON-PHENOMENA"

KNEE-JERK—

Reaction time for knee-jerk (rabbit)	.	·01	sec.	Waller, 1890.
"	"	"	(man)	. ·025 "	Eulenburg, 1879.
"	"	"	(man)	. ·03 "	Waller, 1881.
"	for conjunctival reflex	.	·05 "	Exner, 1874.
"	for crossed knee-jerk	.	·06 "	Burckhardt, 1877.

Muscles involved in the jerk (Sherrington, 1892)—
    Vastus internus and crureus chiefly, vastus externus slightly, rectus
    femoris not at all.
Dependent on a reflex arc, of which—

    I. The *sensory path* is composed by—
        1. Peripheral part—sensory fibres in the nerve of the vastus
        internus and crureus muscles (Sherrington).
        2. Spinal part — sensory fibres in the 5th (chiefly) and 4th
        lumbar nerves of monkey (the 4th and 3rd lumbar roots of
        man).

    II. The *motor path* is composed by—
        1. Peripheral part—motor fibres in the nerve of the vastus
        internus and crureus muscles (chiefly), and of the vastus
        externus (slightly).
        2. Spinal part—the 5th (chiefly) and 4th (slightly) motor lumbar
        nerve root, monkey (4th and 3rd lumbar, man).

    III. The *central* part—
        Chiefly 5th lumbar and slightly 4th lumbar segment in monkey
        (that is, in man, 4th and 3rd lumbar segments).

In the monkey (Sherrington), splitting the lumbar cord lengthwise along the
    median plane does not abolish the knee-jerk.   Transection above the 4th
    lumbar segment usually depresses the jerk for a short time, occasionally
    suppressing it for a week or more, sometimes not suppressing it at all, even
    for a few minutes.
Excitation, mechanical or otherwise, of the flexor muscles of the knee, for
    example, by stretching, massage, etc., temporarily depresses and even
    abolishes the reaction.   Similarly excitation of the central end of the
    nerve supplying the hamstring muscles temporarily depresses or even
    extinguishes the jerk.   Kneeling or stretching the fore tibial muscles
    has a similar but much less marked effect.   Excitation of the skin or of
    cutaneous nerves appears to have much less effect.

The graphic record of a knee-jerk shows that it lasts one-tenth of a second, and gives on the myographion a curve identical with that of a simple muscle twitch (Eulenburg, 1879).

ANKLE CLONUS—

8-10 movements per sec. Waller, 1882.

JAW-JERK—

Reaction time ·02 sec. De Watteville, 1885.

C. S. SHERRINGTON.

REFERENCES

1. ADAMKIEWICZ. *Zeitschrift f. klin. Medicin,* iii. p. 450.—2. BEEVOR, C. "On the Condition of the Knee-Jerk, Ankle-Clonus, and Plantar-Reflex after Epileptic Fits," *Brain,* vol. v. p. 56.—3. BOWDITCH and WARREN. *Journal of Physiology,* xi. 1890.—4. BRISSAUD. *Recherches anatomo-pathologiques et physiologiques sur la contracture,* Paris, 1880 ; *Archives de neurologie,* 1890, xix. p. 1.—5. BUZNS, L. *Neurol. Centralbl.* 1893, p. 28.—6. BURCKHARDT. *Festschrift an Albrecht v. Haller,* Bern, 1877.—7. DÜNGES. "Ueber das Verhalten der Sehnenreflexe bei Abkühlung der Körperoberflache." Dissert. Bonn. 1889.—8. EISENLOHR. *Festschrift f. Eröffn. d. neuen allg. Krankenhauses z. Hamburg,* Eppendorf, 1889 ; *Deutsche med. Woch.* 1890, p. 841 ; *Deutsche med. Woch.* 1892, p. 1105. — 9. EULENBURG, A. *Zeitschrift f. klin. Med.* iv. 179 ; *Deutsche med. Woch.* 1881, p. 181 ; *Neurol. Centralbl.* 1882.— 10. FARAGO, J. *Archiv f. Kinderheilkunde,* 1887, viii. 385.—11. FERRIER, D. *Brain,* 1894.—12. FERRIER, D., and TURNER, W. ALDREN. *Philosoph. Transactions Royal Society,* 1895.—13. GARTEN, S. *Pflüger's Archiv f. Physiol.* vol. lxxi. 1898. —14. HELLER, J. "Zur diagnost. Messung des Kniephänomens," *Berlin. klin. Woch.* 1886, 903.—15. JAMES, W. *Principles of Psychology,* vols. i. and ii. London, 1891.—16. JARISCH, A., and SCHIFF, E. *Med. Jahrbuch. d. Gesellsch. d. Aerzte.* Wien, 1882, p. 261 (v. Basch's laboratory).—17. JENDRASSIK, E. "Beiträge für Lehre v. den Sehnenreflexen," *Deutsches Archiv f. klin. Medicin,* xxxiii. 177 ; "Zur Untersuchungsmethode des Kniephänomens," *Neurolog. Centralbl.* 1885, p. 412 ; "Ueber die Localisation der Reflexe," *Budapest Orvosi Hétilap,* 1886, 1161.—18. KRIES, V. *Archiv für Physiologie,* 1888.—19. KRONECHER and STANLEY HALL. *Archiv für Physiologie,* 1879.—20. LOMBARD. *Journal of Physiology,* x. p. 122 ; *Archiv für Physiologie,* 1889, supplement volume, p. 292. — 21. MACWILLIAM. *Centralbl. f. d. med. Wissensch.* 1887, p. 627.—22. MEYER, G. "Untersuchungen über das Kniephänomen," *Berlin. klin. Woch.* 1888, p. 23.—23. MITCHELL, WEIR, and LEWIS. "Physiological Studies of the Knee-jerk and of the Reaction of Muscles under Mechanical and other Excitants," *Medical News,* Feb. 13, 1886. —24. MÖBIUS, P. J. *Centralbl. f. Nervenheilk.* 1883, p. 217.—25. MOTT and SHERRINGTON. *Proceedings Royal Society,* 1895.—26. MUHR. *Psychiatrisches Centralblatt,* 1878.—27. MÜLLER, J. *Elements of Physiology,* vols. i. and ii. Baly-translation, London, 1830.—28. MUNK, H. *Sitzungsb. der Berlin. Akad.*—29. ORCHANSKI. *Wratsch,* 1884, No. 31.—30. PELIZOEUS. *Archiv f. Psych. u. Nervenkrankh.* xiv. 402 ; *Neurolog. Centralbl.* 1886, p. 50.—31. PRÉVOST. *Rev. méd. de la Suisse Romande,* 1881.—32. PRÉVOST and WALLER. *Rev. méd. de la Suisse Romande,* 1881.—33. REMAK, E. *Archiv f. Psych. u. Nervenkrankh.* v. 555, xiv. 167, xvii. 240 ; *Deutsche med. Woch.* 1889, p. 250 ; *Berlin. klin. Woch.* 1890, p. 349.—34. RENZI, DE. *Rivista clinica e terapeutica,* 1888, 7.—35. ROSENHEIM, T. *Archiv f. Psych. u. Nervenkrankh.* xv. p. 184, and xviii. p. 782.—36. RUSSELL, J. R. *Proc. Roy. Soc.* 1894.—37. SALOMONSEN. *Nederl. Tijdschr.* 1890, No. ii.—38. SCHREIBER, J. *Archiv f. exper. Path. u. Pharmakol.* vol. xviii. p. 270 ; *Deutsches Archiv f. klin. Med.* 1884, xxxv. 254.—39. SCHULTZE, F., and FÜRBRINGER, P. *Centralbl. f. d. med. Wissensch.* 1875, p. 929.—40. SCHWARTZ, A. *Arch. f. Psych. u. Nervenkrankh.* xiii. 621.—41. SEELIGMÜLLER. *Centralbl. f. Chirurgie,* 1878, p. 281.—42. SHARKEY, S. J. Gulstonian Lectures on "Spasm in Chronic Nerve Disease," *Lancet,* 1886, pp. 531, 576,

623.—43. SHERRINGTON. *Philos. Transactions; Proc. Roy. Soc.* Nov. 1896; *Proc. Roy. Soc.* 1893.—44. SPITZKA, E. C. *American Journ. of Neurol. and Psychiat.* 1883, August.—45. STERNBERG. "Sehnenreflexe bei Ermüdung" *Centralblatt für Physiologie*, 1887, p. 81; *Sitzungsber. d. k.-k. Akad. d. Wissensch. in Wien*, 1891, vol. c. Part iii. p. 251.—46. *Idem. Die Sehnenreflexe*, Vienna, 1893.—47. STRÜMPELL, A. and MÖBIUS, P. J. *Münchener med. Wochenschr.* 1886, p. 601.—48. WALLER. *Lancet*, 1881; *Brain*, vol. iii. p. 179; *Journal of Physiology*, vol. ii. p. 384, 1890.— 49. WESTPHAL, C. "Ueber Erkrankungen des Ruckenmarks," *Virchow's Archiv*, xxxix.; "Bewegungserschein. an gelähmten Gliedern," *Archiv f. Psychiatrie u. Nervenkrankheiten*, v. 803, x. 243, x. 294, xii. 798, xiv. 87, xv. 731, xvii. 547, xviii. 628.— 50. WUNDT. W. *Unters. f. Mechan. d. Nerv. u. Nervencent.* 1876.—51. ZIEHEN, TH. "Die diagnostische Bedeutung der Steigerung des Kniephänomens u. des Fuss-clonus," *Correspondenz-Blätter des allg. ärztl. Vereines von Thüringen*, 1889, No. 1, also previously, 1887.

C. S. S.

II. CLINICAL AND PATHOLOGICAL SECTION

TREMOR.—Tremor is a condition in which the normal, voluntary, continuous, muscular contraction is broken up into a series of minor contractions, which are more or less effectual in attaining the end desired; it may also occur independently of any willed movement, and it may be regularly recurrent, as in paralysis agitans; or irregular, as in alcoholic tremor.

When we call to mind that a muscular contraction is the result of a number of nerve impulses, which follow one another so closely as to fuse almost into one, it is natural to suppose that tremor may be due to conditions which diminish the rate with which these waves succeed each other, and so produce a series of muscular contractions instead of a single one. This supposition is supported by the fact that normal voluntary movements are slightly tremulous, and that fatigue of a neuron makes its discharge less rapid. From this point of view, therefore, tremor may be looked upon as an early stage in the "dissolution" of nerve energy, which, if progressive, would lead to paralysis; and this is seen to be the case in such diseases as alcoholic and other poisonings, and in general paralysis of the insane.

I have recorded several cases in which a slowly-growing tuberculous mass involved the internal capsules; in these cases tremor was the early symptom, which gradually gave way to paralysis as the disease advanced (*Spasm in Chronic Nerve-disease*, Gulstonian Lectures, 1886).

Remembering the complexity of the anatomy and physiology of the nervous system, we are not surprised to find that this disintegration of nerve impulses travelling towards muscles may result from disease in various situations. While we recognise therefore the great defects in our knowledge of the finer changes which take place in the nerve elements in health and disease, we may take the following as a provisional and rough classification of the conditions which produce tremor:—

1. Deficient or otherwise altered activity of nerve cells.
2. Inhibition of the action of lower cells by higher.

3. Impediments to conduction.
    (a) Owing to disease of the conducting nerve fibres.
    (b) Owing to disease in the synapses, or in the interstitial
        tissues about them.

    1. Deficient or otherwise altered activity of nerve cells.—It is probable that tremor does not result from changes in muscles alone, but rather from altered conditions of the nerve centres and fibres which call them into action. Even the " fibrillary tremors" of progressive muscular atrophy are due to the slow degenerative changes going on in the anterior cornua of the spinal cord. In the case of voluntary muscles, in which alone we have any experience of tremor, the nerve path is a very long one: originating in the " motor centres" of the cortex, it passes down in the pyramidal tracts—direct and crossed—to form connections with the cells in the anterior cornua of the spinal cord; and thence it is continued by the efferent anterior roots to its termination in the muscles.

    In certain states of general debility, after long illnesses for example, the enfeebled activity of the whole nervous system is evident, and expresses itself on the motor side in tremulous action of the muscles. A very similar condition is seen in old age, when the lowered vigour of the nervous system is due to the natural diminution in the energy of the metabolic processes which is observable in all the organs of the body.

    Between the tremor of healthy old age and that of paralysis agitans there is but a difference of degree. In normal old age the tremor is elicited only when voluntary actions are attempted; but in paralysis agitans the steady flow of nerve energy which passes along the motor tracts, and produces healthy " tone," is also slowed to such a degree that continuous and rapid tremors are produced independently of volitional effort. If a patient suffering from this disease be asked to perform some voluntary act, the additional nerve energy thus evoked may steady the muscles in action. I have seen a man the movements of whose hands were exceedingly tremulous, who nevertheless could still call forth momentarily steady action sufficient for the purpose of shooting rabbits.

    Certain poisons, such as alcohol or mercury, act upon the nerve tissue in such a manner as to give rise to uncertain and tremulous action of muscles. By what means they interfere with the rapid and regular succession of nerve waves is not precisely known.

    In general paralysis, a disease which depends upon a slow degeneration, often accompanied by inflammation, of the cortical centres of the brain, tremor is usually a very marked symptom; and depends upon an altered condition of the nerve cells and fibres, and of the interstitial tissue which surrounds them.

    2. Inhibition of action of nerve cells producing tremor.—It is a well-known fact that certain nerves act in an inhibitory manner upon muscles; moderate irritation of the vagus, for instance, slows the contractions of the heart, and violent stimulation of it may paralyse that organ. But it is also a matter of ordinary observation that disturbances in certain regions of the brain inhibit the action of other regions. Emotions, such as fear and fright, may completely paralyse voluntary muscular actions; and when less intense we see them produce a condition in which, though voluntary movements are performed, they are accompanied by muscular tremor.

It is not improbable that in the numerous cases of chorea which originate in fright, emotional inhibition gives rise to the disorderly muscular action; while those cases which are intimately associated with rheumatism are the result of the action of the rheumatic poison (whatever this may be) upon the central nervous system.

3. **Impediments to conduction.**—(*a*) *Disease of nerve fibres* is not a common cause of tremor; for generally speaking the alteration in the fibres is sufficient to give rise to paralysis. The diseases classed under the head of peripheral neuritis present, as a rule, symptoms of loss of power pure and simple. But tremors are sometimes seen in the earlier stages of alcoholic neuritis; for example, long after the period when they could be attributed to a more general alcoholic intoxication.

(*b*) *Tremors due to alteration in interstitial tissues.*—There are certain symptoms of nerve disease which appear to owe their presence to an alteration of the connective tissues which surround the nerve elements themselves; unless, indeed, it be held that all such interstitial diseases are secondary to pathological changes in the more active constituents of the nervous system. The importance now attached by physiologists to the conduction of nerve impulses across the synapses may necessitate a much more careful consideration of pathological alterations occurring in their neighbourhood. Disseminate sclerosis is an example of disease attacking the interstitial tissues and giving rise to tremulous muscular action. It appears as if the presence of this abnormal condition around the nerves produced a difficulty in the transmission of nerve impulses along the tract affected, without absolutely stopping them. Hence what should be one steady continuous muscular act is subdivided into a succession of jerky or tremulous movements in the desired direction.

Now that it has been shown that the neuraxon of one cell does not communicate directly with another nerve cell, but breaks up into fine fibrillæ about the arborisations of that cell, so that the nerve impulse has to cross the interstitial matter between them, it is quite possible that alterations in and about the synapses may prove to be the causes of some varieties of tremor. In general paralysis of the insane the tremor may be due, to a considerable extent, to the alteration in the substance which links, while it also separates, the nerve constituents of the cortex.

The cerebellum, as a great co-ordinator of muscular actions, might be expected, when diseased, to give rise to tremulous and irregular movements: and so it does; though mainly, if not only, when the central lobe is affected.

We cannot at present be said to possess a scientific knowledge of the pathology of tremor, and the little which I venture to write upon the subject must be taken as in the main speculative.

Kinds of tremor.—From a clinical point of view tremors may be divided into two classes—(A) "Intention tremors," and (B) "Passive tremors."

A. Intention tremors—that is to say, tremors which are produced or, if not produced, are at least exaggerated by voluntary movement.

Disseminate sclerosis affords the most characteristic representative of this class. In this disease no tremor at all exists until the patient attempts some voluntary act, such as raising a glass to his lips. Instead of a steady continuous movement of the arm in the desired direction, a discontinuous jerky movement occurs, the jerks being roughly speaking in the direction of the willed movement. The jerks generally increase in rapidity and diminish in amplitude as the goal is neared. Nystagmus also illustrates well this variety of tremor.

In general paralysis and in Graves' disease the tremors are much finer, but likewise require voluntary action to evoke them. In the former disease they are irregular, and produce a halting and interrupted action of the muscles in action, as is seen in the slow blurred speech of the general paralytic.

In Graves' disease the tremor is very fine and vibratory, and does not materially interfere with muscular action.

Mercurial tremor may be constant, but it is increased by voluntary effort.

B. Passive tremors—tremors which are independent of voluntary movement.

The most typical example of this class is paralysis agitans. In this disease regular, continuous, fine oscillations are always present, except during sleep.

Authors vary considerably in the estimated rate of these various tremors.

Charcot gives   3 – 6   per sec. for paralysis agitans.
Peterson   „   3·7 – 5·6   „   „   „
Gowers   „   4·8 – 7   „   „   „
Peterson   „   7·9 – 8·1   „   for the earlier stages of disseminated sclerosis.
   „   „   4·6 – 6·3   „   for later stages.
Charcot   „   8·9 or more per sec. for Basedow's disease and for alcoholic tremors.

The pathological conditions giving rise to the various tremors which have been mentioned are for the most part tangible anatomical changes in the nervous system, as, for example, in disseminate sclerosis and general paralysis; or they consist in the presence of poisons, such as mercury, lead, or alcohol, which may finally bring about anatomical alterations. But every form of tremulous movement which has been mentioned may occur in the condition known as hysteria: that is to say, disorders of function, which are often transient and destitute as yet of any demonstrated anatomical basis, may closely simulate tremors which are the result of clearly proved pathological changes in nerve structures. It is only by a careful consideration of the accompanying circumstances, and of the other symptoms which attend the cases, that a diagnosis between the two classes can be arrived at.

THE TENDON REFLEXES IN DISEASE.—Authors are not yet agreed whether the normal "tendon reflex" is a true reflex or the direct contraction of muscle due to tapping its tendon : the great majority of them, however, believe that it is not a true reflex (*vide* p. 519). Inasmuch as in either case a healthy condition of the muscle, as well as of its afferent and efferent nerves and of the spinal centres with which they are connected, is essential to its production, its clinical importance depends upon the evidence which it affords respecting the state of these structures. Disease of any one of them causes alteration in the "jerk."

Probably all muscles may contract when their tendons are suddenly "tapped," but only certain selected muscles are examined in this way by the clinician : hence the terms "elbow-jerk," "wrist-jerk," "tendo-Achillis-jerk," "jaw-jerk," and, most important of all, "knee-jerk." So rarely is the latter absent in normal individuals, that its presence in health may be taken as constant (*vide* p. 521).

What is the normal "knee-jerk," or "patellar reflex"—to take this as a representative of this class of phenomena? The reply must be that there is no normal mean in the muscular response to the tap upon the tendon which is found in all healthy persons. There are healthy people in whom it is feeble and difficult to obtain ; and there are others, apparently in no better or worse condition of health, in whom it is very brisk. More than this, even in the same individual the "jerk" varies more or less with conditions which can hardly be called departures from health, if indeed they can be estimated at all. This, however, holds true with regard to all the functions of the body ; they all vary in health within certain limits : and the clinical difficulty of distinguishing healthy from unhealthy conditions in their early stages depends mainly upon this fact.

All one can say is that, as a rule, in normal individuals the "jerk" is a single one, and follows quickly upon the tap on the tendon ; but the extent of the "jerk" is variable. Where it appears to be absent at first, it may often be brought out by so-called "reinforcement" (*vide* p. 520).

Many sensory stimuli increase the knee-jerk by increasing the tone of the muscles in general ; for instance, touching the skin with cold or hot objects, pinching the skin, directing a bright light upon the eye or a loud sound upon the ear : in fact a continuous, though variable, stream of tone-producing energy flows in at all the sensory organs (*vide* p. 520).

It is not, therefore, a matter for wonder that even in healthy people the tendon reflexes are very variable in degree. In disease they may be altered either in the direction of decrease or increase.

Diminution and disappearance of the "jerk."—It has already been said that, whether the knee-jerk be a true reflex or not, a healthy condition of the nerve and muscle constituents of the reflex arc are essential to its production. When any one of these constituents is diseased the knee-jerk becomes modified, and nearly always either diminished or absent.

(a) *Disease of afferent nerves.*—It has been shown experimentally that great diminution in the jerk follows section of the afferent spinal nerve: and the lesion in tabes dorsalis is situated in the course of the afferent nerves which have entered the posterior spinal root; consequently the knee-jerk is absent in this disease, owing to the loss of muscular tone produced by the lesion. But in ataxic paraplegia, where to the usual lesion present in tabes is added disease of the lateral columns, the knee-jerk is not absent and may be exaggerated. The probable explanation of this is that, while the disease in the course of the afferent nerve lowers tonus, disease of the pyramidal tract increases it; and this increase more than compensates the diminution due to the lesion in the posterior root fibres.

In the majority of cases of alcoholic, diphtheritic, and other forms of peripheral neuritis the disease affects both motor and sensory nerves alike; so that in addition to pain and anæsthesia there is also motor weakness. But in some instances there appears to be no motor weakness, and yet the knee-jerk may be absent. This is probably due to affection of the sensory nerves, on the integrity of which tonus depends; a tap then upon the tendon of the atonic muscles fails to produce the jerk. The tendon reflex is a very sensitive indicator of muscular tone, and it often remains absent for a long time after patients appear to have recovered from sensory and motor paralysis.

Sternberg (*Die Sehnenreflexe und ihre Bedeutung*, 1893) states that the reflex in neuritis may be increased, probably by irritation of the sensory nerves: this condition I have never met with.

(b) *Disease of the efferent nerve.*—Peripheral neuritis is due to a very large number of causes, principally poisons of one kind or another—microbic, metallic, alcoholic, gaseous. If they affect the efferent nerve of the reflex arc upon which any of the tendon reflexes depends, the jerk disappears. The poisons of diphtheria and alcohol are well-known examples of this function. In some general diseases, such as diabetes, which lead to great debility, the jerk disappears; sometimes owing to the presence of peripheral neuritis, often, probably, to loss of muscular tone, independently of neuritis.

(c) *Disease of the cells in the anterior cornua of the spinal cord.*—This is not an uncommon cause of loss of the knee-jerk. In infantile paralysis, and in the similar disease which is sometimes met with in adults, the jerk is absent. In paraplegia due to myelitis the knee-jerk may be exaggerated or it may be absent. When that portion of the cord is affected from which the third and fourth lumbar nerves issue, it is absent; when the disease is above these lumbar centres, it is exaggerated, owing to diminution of the inhibitory action of the pyramidal tract fibres.

In progressive muscular atrophy, which is due to very slow degeneration of the cells in the anterior cornua, the jerks gradually disappear as the muscles get more and more wasted.

(d) *Disease of the muscle on which the jerk depends.*—Gross disease of the muscle would, of course, produce loss of the jerk; but this hardly occurs primarily: it is almost always due to affections of the spinal centre which is connected with its motor nerve, or of the nerve itself. Pseudo-hypertrophic paralysis and other forms of idiopathic muscular atrophy are, however, exceptions to this rule, as they are diseases of the muscles, and not of the nerves which supply them; in them the jerk disappears gradually as the muscles disappear.

In conditions of extreme general wasting and feebleness the tendon reflex may disappear. This is probably due partly to the feeble condition of the muscle, and partly to that of the nerves connected with it.

In traumatic rupture or complete disorganisation of the spinal cord above the lumbar enlargement the knee-jerk disappears, and may remain permanently absent, or reappear after some time. Why this happens is not clear. If the result were due to shock, the "jerk" should return much sooner than it does. Moreover, when myelitis, or pressure on the spinal cord by tumours, produces complete anæsthesia and complete paraplegia, the knee-jerk does not disappear, but is usually exaggerated. Sternberg asserts from actual observation that in sudden decapitation in man, and in clean division of the cord in animals, the knee-jerks do not disappear: and he argues that their absence in certain traumatic cases is due to the grossness of the lesion, which crushes the cord and irritates the inhibitory pyramidal tracts.

In relation to this question it must be remembered that the condition of muscle which is best adapted to the production of this tendon reflex, is one intermediate between atony and spasm. Either of the latter conditions will prevent the jerk. In many cases of paraplegia due to lesions above the lumbar centres there is a gradual development of spasm and permanent rigidity of the muscles of the leg; and this rigidity alone renders it impossible to elicit the knee-jerk.

In sudden lesions of the brain producing coma, such, for instance, as hæmorrhage, if the coma be profound the tendon reflexes are absent; if it be not so profound they are present, and even exaggerated on the side opposite to that on which the hæmorrhage has occurred. The explanation of this again is not very evident.

Increase of the jerks.—It is very doubtful whether increase of the tendon reflexes ever occurs from a primary affection of the afferent or efferent nerve of the reflex arc, or from alterations in the muscles. And the same may be said in regard to the spinal centre with which these nerves are connected. The only exception which must be made to this statement is that certain poisons, such as strychnine, produce temporary increase of these phenomena. Strychnine is said to do this by its action on the afferent nerves.

Increase of the tendon reflexes is nevertheless very commonly met with, and in the great majority of cases depends upon diseases of the pyramidal tracts. The normal effect of these tracts upon the spinal centres upon which the jerks depend, is to restrain their activity ; thus when they are divided or diseased the tendon reflexes are increased. As the pyramidal tracts arise in the "motor regions" of the cortex and traverse the internal capsules, the corona cerebri, the pons, medulla, and spinal cord, it is clear that a great number of pathological conditions affecting the brain and cord will be accompanied by increased activity of the "jerks." In hemiplegia, due to whatever cause, this is the case. In inflammation, tumours, and like diseases of the cervical and dorsal region of the spinal cord, they are likewise increased.

Each pyramidal tract divides ; a smaller portion of its fibres descend in the anterior column of its own side, the greater number occupy the lateral column of the opposite side. In unilateral brain lesions, therefore, there is generally an increase of the knee-jerk on both sides, the increase being greater on the side opposite to the lesion. The division of the pyramidal tract above is liable to great variations, so that most if not all the fibres may cross, or most if not all may be direct ; consequently the phenomena of disease vary likewise. If, however, it can be shown that all the fibres of the pyramidal tract cross, either in the medulla oblongata or later in the cord below, then the bilateral increase of the tendon reflexes, owing to a unilateral lesion, must depend upon some connection between the fibres on one side and the anterior cornual cells on both sides.

In the subjects of neurasthenia, whose whole nervous system seems to be in a feeble condition, the tendon reflexes are, as a rule, increased. This may be due to the cerebral centres and their efferent pyramidal tracts, as the most highly developed parts of the nervous system, suffering out of proportion to the rest ; thus their inhibitory influence over the lower spinal centres is lessened, and the tendon reflexes thereby exaggerated. In some of the cases referred to, however, the tendon reflexes are diminished ; possibly owing to the neurasthenic condition affecting the centres in the cord as well as those in the brain.

There are a certain number of cases in which the tendon reflexes are diminished or absent, although the reflex arcs are healthy and the disease situated in the central nervous system above them. Such a case I have lately seen, in which violent pain in the head, vomiting, optic neuritis, and mental dulness, lasting for some months, indicated the presence of a cerebral tumour. There was no paralysis, motor or sensory. The knee-jerks could not be elicited. The explanation of such cases, which occur from time to time, and of cases of cerebellar disease, in which the tendon reflexes may be normal, diminished, absent, or exaggerated, cannot at present be given. Sternberg suggests that slight degrees of irritation of the pyramidal tract fibres may increase their inhibitory influence and prevent the tendon phenomena; but in the case quoted above there was no evidence of any irritation producing increased tone, which under such circumstances we should have expected. We know that the general muscular tone of the body depends largely on in-going sensory stimuli of all kinds, which flood the nervous system with energy; these may come from sensory organs, but they also originate from active intellectual and emotional operations. It is quite possible that at present we underrate these influences, and that the stoppage of such stimuli, owing to disease of certain portions of the nervous system, may depress or extinguish the tendon phenomena—just as division of afferent nerves in the cord has been experimentally shown to do.

Clonus.—As already remarked, when the inhibitory influence of the pyramidal tract has been diminished by disease, increased tone is produced in the spinal centres below the lesion, and the tendon reflexes are exaggerated. In a later stage, when the lesion in the course of the pyramidal tract has very seriously damaged the fibres, rigidity of the limbs sets in. But there is an intermediate stage in which clonus appears, and usually multiple "jerk"; that is to say, when the patella tendon is tapped, instead of one knee-jerk several may occur in succession. In healthy persons placed in such a position that the patella tendon is slack, no contraction of muscle follows sudden depression of that bone. But when "tone" is increased, sudden muscular contraction is produced. If "tone" be still more increased stretching the patella tendon, by sudden depression of the bone, results in a series of muscular contractions. The same occurs when by sudden flexure of the foot the tendo Achillis is stretched. This phenomenon is called clonus. While simple exaggeration of the knee-jerk informs us that the tone of the muscle is heightened, clonus means that "tone" has been still further increased; and in most cases it is owing to increasing paralysis of the pyramidal tract fibres. Hence we look for clonus at a later stage of all those affections of the brain and spinal cord, already referred to, which produce increased "jerks." Just as one speaks of the "knee-jerk," "tendo Achillis jerk," "jaw-jerk," "wrist-jerk," and so forth, so we use the corresponding terms "knee clonus," "foot clonus," "jaw clonus," "wrist clonus," and the like.

It happens occasionally that ankle clonus is present and the knee-jerk absent in the same case. This association is due to a lesion which destroys the lumbar centres on which the integrity of the knee-jerk depends, and at the same time interferes with the fibres of the pyramidal tracts which control the lower centres presiding over the nerves connected with the tendo Achillis and its muscle.

SPASM.—By spasm is meant excessive muscular contraction; and, in the case of those muscles which are under the control of the will, excessive contraction is that which occurs in defiance of the will; or which, although beginning as a voluntary act, transgresses the limits which the will would impose upon it.

Where involuntary muscles are concerned the definition of "excessive" is more difficult. When the muscles of the intestine, for instance, make spasmodic efforts to drive along the contents of the bowel through a portion which has been narrowed by disease, so far from the muscular action being excessive, it may be insufficient for the purpose. In such a case, and in others of a similar kind, it can only be said that spasm is muscular contraction which exceeds that which occurs in conditions of health, and in the course of the normal physiological processes.

Muscular spasm is, for the most part, a nerve phenomenon ; though it probably occurs sometimes from causes acting directly on the muscular fibres. "Cramp," for instance, may sometimes be due to the circulation in the muscles of poisons originating in deranged digestive processes, or in abnormal metabolic changes in other parts ; or perhaps inflammation of the fibrous sheath of the muscle itself may produce it. Still it may be accepted that the nervous system is responsible, as a rule, for the occurrence of spasm in muscles.

Some cases of distortion of limbs appear at first sight to be due to muscular spasm, when in reality they are not so. Take, for example, the claw-hand in progressive muscular atrophy : here atrophy of the interossei muscles occurs, and, the opponents continuing to act normally, hyperextension of the proximal and flexion of the peripheral phalanges of the fingers occurs. But there is in reality no overaction or spasm on the part of the extensors : equilibrium is overthrown by atrophy of their antagonists ; hence the distortion.

Another instance of a similar kind is found in the disease called "pachymeningitis cervicalis," where the distortion varies according to the position of the disease in the cervical region. If that part be diseased from which the median and ulnar nerves emanate, the muscles supplied by .the intact musculo-spiral produce that form of distortion in which the wrist is extended ; while, if the upper half of the cervical region be the seat of the disease, the muscles innervated by the median and ulnar nerves produce quite a different condition, one in which the wrist is flexed.

Looking at the subject from a clinical point of view, the following varieties of spasm may be observed.

Kinds of spasm.—1. *Tonic spasm or contraction.*—This is a constant, steady contraction of the muscles involved, varying from a condition of slightly increased tone up to one of extreme rigidity. It is well seen in the later stages of hemiplegia due to whatever cause ; and in cases of paraplegia where the pyramidal tracts are partially cut off by disease from the spinal centres below. It also occurs in cases of "primary lateral sclerosis," and in "porencephaly," where large defects occur in the cerebral hemispheres, either as congenital malformations or as the result of early disease. The "motor centres" in the cortex of the brain and the pyramidal tracts which descend from them through the cord are the agents which give rise to contracture. Slight interference with the healthy condition of these nerve-structures results in the loosening of the reins which inhibit the spinal centres; and increase in "tendon reflexes" is the first evidence given of the change. A little more disease of these tracts, and "clonus" is seen; and, finally, in grosser disease we get "contracture."

2. *Clonic or intermittent spasm*, the second clinical variety, is that in which the muscular contraction is not continuous, but intermittent. Periods of action are succeeded by periods of inaction. The spasm may recur at regular or at irregular intervals, and with every degree of rapidity. These conditions are illustrated in chorea, spasmodic wry-neck, facial spasm, and in many varieties of hysterical or functional spasm.

The causes underlying many cases of clonic spasm are very obscure. But the well-known pathological conditions which produce hemiplegia are not infrequently followed by clonic spasm in the paralysed muscles; thus conditions of athetosis or post-hemiplegic movements of various kinds result.

3. *Tonic and clonic muscular contractions.*—In a third variety of spasm these conditions are combined. This is well exemplified in many cases of congenital defects, or diseases of portions of the hemispheres occurring in early life, which give rise to a porencephalic condition. In them there is a certain amount of persistent rigidity of muscle, combined with frequently recurring movements. The latter are sometimes extremely violent, and may be quite uncontrollable.

If the subject of spasm be looked at more from the pathological point of view, it must be confessed that our knowledge is very defective, and that many instances of this condition are at present quite inexplicable. A review, however, of the possible, probable, and well-known conditions giving rise to spasm may be useful.

Spasm as a symptom—1. *Spasm in relation with the pyramidal tracts.*— The connection which exists between disease in the course of the pyramidal tract and spastic conditions of the limbs is very frequently exemplified at the bedside. In a large proportion of cases of softening of the brain, whether due to embolism or thrombosis of arteries, and in cases of cerebral hæmorrhage with hemiplegia or monoplegia, contracture often supervenes in the limbs,—if they remain permanently paralysed. This is usually more marked in the arm than in the leg, and, the flexor muscles being more powerful than the extensors, more or less flexion at the joints results. This is accompanied by increased tendon reflexes, and often by clonus. The removal of cerebral inhibition from the spinal centres increases the action of the cells in the anterior columns on the muscles which they innervate; this is curiously illustrated in certain rare cases which have been recorded, in which after its extinction in tabes dorsalis the knee-jerk has reappeared on the supervention of an attack of hemiplegia.

The same effect is observed in cases of ataxic paraplegia in which, in spite of the presence of disease of the posterior columns, the knee-jerk is exaggerated ; the removal of the inhibitory influence of the pyramidal tract more than compensating the diminution of the nerve energy which under healthy conditions reaches the anterior cells through the posterior root fibres.

Congenital defects in the pyramidal tract have the same influence on the centres below ; and the spastic condition present in the weakened limbs under such circumstances is strong evidence in favour of the explanation which has been adopted as regards the spasm which follows upon diseases of this tract ; namely, that it is due to removal of the inhibitory influence of the pyramidal tract. Disease of the cortical "motor centres" in the brain produces the same results.

Occasionally the spasm is bilateral although the lesion of the pyramidal tract is unilateral. This is probably explained by the more equal division of the tract at its decussation in the medulla oblongata, so that there are more "direct" and less "crossed" fibres than usual ; or, if all the pyramidal tract fibres decussate either in the medulla oblongata or in the cord below, the tract fibres of each side must be connected with the anterior cornua on both sides.

In most of the ordinary cases of hemiplegia, though there is not bilateral spasm, there is bilateral increase of the tendon reflexes.

When the lesion interfering with the pyramidal tract fibres is in the cord, as in cases of transverse myelitis and primary softening in the dorsal regions, bilateral spasm of the legs occurs.

When spasm accompanies the presence of tumours of the cerebellum, it is probably not due directly to the cerebellar disease, but to the pressure which the tumour exerts on the pons and medulla below.

Contracture, or fixed spasm, is a comparatively frequent result of cerebral lesions which permanently interrupt the nerve-impulses proceeding from the cortex along the pyramidal tract. But, in addition, mobile spasms have been observed in great variety, either after hemiplegia or independently of it. Sometimes they attend voluntary movements only, sometimes they are involuntary and continuous ; but in all of them the retention of a large amount of voluntary control over the affected limbs is a striking feature. In addition to the mobile spasm there is often a certain degree of fixed spasm, though a marked degree of the latter·would be incompatible with the development of the former. The names athetosis, post-hemiplegic chorea, post-hemiplegic inco-ordination, and the like are applied to these conditions.

The lesion in such cases has been found in a variety of positions—in the cortex, in the optic thalami, in the corpora striata, and so forth. A case lately seen by myself suggested a lesion of the crus cerebri. The patient was a girl of twenty who, since the age of eight years, had suffered from violent irregular spasm of her left arm. She had in addition paralysis of the right 3rd nerve, and almost complete atrophy of the right optic nerve.

All the varietes of mobile spasm seem to result from a mixture, in varying proportions, of paralysis, spasm, and irritation ; and their develop ment depends upon lesions which interfere with the functions of the motor centres and fibres, but which do not interrupt them completely. In cases where a tumour presses upon the cortex of the brain, or upon the cord, recurring attacks of spasm often precede the continuous rigid contracture which finally sets in. This is probably due to fluctuating conditions of the circulation within the growth which alter its size and consequently its pressure from time to time.

2. *Spasm due to disease of efferent spinal nerves.*—In the description which has been given of contracture the active agency in its production has been attributed to the spinal centres; removal of the inhibitory influence of the pyramidal tract induces overaction in them, and spasm, of the muscles which they innervate, results. But does disease of the spinal centre, or of its afferent or efferent nerve, produce spasm? Disease of the motor nerves is far from an unusual occurrence; musculo-spiral paralysis, for instance, is often seen in quite early stages of spinal disease, but muscular spasm is not one of the symptoms. In chronic poisoning by lead and alcohol various nerve symptoms are met with, including paralysis, and even muscular rigidity; but the latter is due to the contraction of the unopposed healthy muscles, and is not produced directly by the diseased nerves. In inflammation of the sciatic nerve twitchings and sudden cramp may be experienced: but they are very transient phenomena. The implication of motor or mixed nerves in a growth gives rise to similar symptoms, in addition to great pain; but well-marked spasm scarcely occurs. Clonic spasm is not infrequently seen in the late stages of facial paralysis, when there is shortening of the muscle from atrophy; the spasm is then due to irritation of the nerves and muscle fibres which have survived the process of destruction.

The attacks of spasm which occur in spinal meningitis are probably reflex in origin, and not due to direct irritation of motor nerves.

The pathology of tetany is doubtful, but there is no good reason for supposing that it has any connection with irritation of motor nerves (*vide* art. "Tetany" in the next volume).

It would appear, therefore, that while occasional spasm may occur in peripheral nerve disease, from direct irritation of motor filaments, and may even now and then be permanent, it is quite exceptional to find it amongst the marked phenomena in such cases.

3. *Spasm in relation to disease of the afferent nerve and its centre.*—How far spasm is produced in a reflex way is an exceedingly difficult question. Cases of general convulsions, as well as of local spasm, are frequently explained in this way, and yet the explanations are so incapable of proof that the arguments adduced in favour of such an origin often carry very little conviction. Many such cases occur where some sensory nerve is the seat of severe pain; or where a diseased part is painful to move. A good example of the former class is spasm of the muscles of the face accompanying facial neuralgia; of the latter, rigidity of muscles surrounding a painful joint. But the most ordinary method of expressing pain is by over-action of the facial muscles, while the ordinary way of preventing

pain in joint-disease is by keeping the joint still, and opposing attempts at movement by contraction of muscles which prevent it; and it is often very difficult to decide how far the muscular action is voluntary, how far involuntary and reflex.

No one who observes the great variety in the degree of muscular contraction produced by similar stimuli applied to different individuals, can be surprised at finding evidence that persistent spasm may sometimes occur as the product of a reflex act; or that a stimulus which produces no motor result in one person, gives rise to definite muscular contractions in another not equally healthy. Thus in hemiplegia accompanied by descending sclerosis in the lateral columns deep reflexes are much more brisk than they were before the hemiplegia occurred; and even contractures previously existing may be suddenly increased by comparatively slight injuries. If this increased reflex excitability be due to the hyperphysio-logical activity of spinal centres which have been freed from cerebral control, similar disorders of nerve centres rather than of nerve fibres are probably the most fruitful causes of reflex spasm. Hence it is scarcely too much to say that the injury or disease which supplies the stimulus to the sensory nerve in such cases, though apparently the principal agent in the production of spasm, is really so only from a limited point of view. Were the nerve centre in a healthy and stable condition, muscular spasm would not occur. Thus in tetanus it is the hyperactive condition of the nerve centres produced by the specific toxin that gives rise to the muscular spasm.

In speaking, therefore, of reflex spasm resulting from irritation of afferent nerves the nerve centre must be considered at the same time; for it is questionable how far stimuli applied to afferent nerves could produce muscular spasm if the centres were healthy.

Reflex spasm no doubt occurs, but how frequently it does so, and how far the afferent or efferent nerves, or the nerve centres take the leading part in its production, are points which it is difficult to decide. A good instance of reflex spasm is recorded by Mr. Clutton (*St. Thomas's Hospital Reports*, vol. x. p. 64). A boy, aged fourteen, had been bitten in the face by a dog eighteen months previously. The spot had been painless until a month before his appearence at the Hospital; but since that time he had suffered from constant shooting pains in the neck, which always started from the scar. At the same time that the pain was felt the angle of the mouth was drawn outwards, and the skin of the neck was wrinkled by the platysma. The whole side of the neck and face blushed, and then became bathed in perspiration. This succession of symptoms recurred every time the scar was pinched. Butyl-chloral-hydrate in five-grain doses twice a day cured the affection.

Weir Mitchell in his work on *Injuries of Nerves* gives instances of reflex spasm: and similar phenomena are often referred to intestinal, uterine, or other irritation; but not always with sufficient reason.

Children are specially prone to convulsions and spasm; and it is interesting to remember that in them the pyramidal tracts, the great controllers of reflex muscular contraction, are for a long time incompletely developed. In the brain afferent and efferent nerves and nerve centres are so closely packed together that it is quite impossible in many cases of spasm of cerebral origin to say which of these takes the leading part in the disturbance.

4. *Spasmodic muscular contractions which appear to have the same explanations as tendon-reflexes.*—Muscles contract when they are put on the stretch by their opponents; and the interaction of the two sets of muscles has the effect of controlling and steadying movements which might otherwise be jerky and uncertain. But a tendon may be overstretched and spasm may result. A medical man took a vehicle in order to drive to a house where he was going to stay for a while. The driver put him down 2½ miles from his destination and drove off. The doctor had a heavy bag and had to carry it himself. For four days after this he suffered from constant contraction of the triceps muscle of his right arm whenever he flexed the latter. Such a case represents a very small departure from the normal, but it suggests an explanation of more troublesome affections; such, for instance, as the following :—A girl, aged nineteen, had her wrist sprained and bent backwards five years before she was seen by me. She had been obliged to carry her arm in a sling for some weeks. Ever since then she had suffered without intermission from "twitching in the arm and palm of the hand." The general power of the arm was found on examination to be unimpaired; but there were spasmodic contractions of the palmaris longus, which occurred with perfect regularity ninety times in the minute. In such instances it is probable that the spinal centres are in an unstable condition, as such continued rhythmic spasm after a sprain is quite exceptional. Every one is familiar with the ankle clonus which is sometimes set up in healthy people when sitting with the toes on the ground and the heels a little raised. If the clonus be once started it may be difficult to stop it by an effort of the will, unless the position of the leg be altered. This is probably a physiological representative of a certain class of muscular spasms which have assumed pathological dimensions.

Functional spasm.—The spasmodic affections which have already been considered owe their origin directly or indirectly to some gross tangible disease. But there are many cases in which this is not so, and where the most careful pathological examination by skilled observers reveals nothing. Nor is the spasm under such conditions necessarily short-lived: on the contrary, it may last for months or years. Fine anatomical alterations, no doubt, occur in the nerve structures involved, but we know not what they are. The similarity which exists between the two classes of cases, not only in the manner in which the muscular spasm shows itself but also in its distribution, indicates that the same parts of the nervous system are involved in gross disease and in functional. Clinically the diagnosis between them rests not so much on differences in the character of the muscular spasm, as on considerations of age, sex, the circumstances under which they originated, and the sensory and other phenomena which accompany them.   It has been seen what an important part the pyramidal tract, and the centres in the cortex from which it emanates, play in the production of spasm due to gross disease.   In most cases it is defective transmission of nervous energy along this tract which indirectly produces spasm by the resulting over-activity of the spinal centres.   If, therefore, there were evidence of a similar condition of feebleness on the part of the brain, and of the fibres which travel from it along the cord in functional cases, this would explain the origin of a number of cases of functional spasm. The frequency with which total or partial hemianæsthesia occurs in these cases, involving all the senses, shows that there is deficient nerve power, or neurasthenia, of the whole brain ; and great increase of the deep reflexes or even clonus points to the absence of the normal inhibitory power of the pyramidal tract.   In cases of hysterical hemianæsthesia, without any marked loss of power or muscular spasm, it may be shown that motor power is really deficient on the side affected.   In one such instance the right arm could only reach forty-five on the dynamometer scale, while the left reached fifty, the right being the anæsthetic side.   Although the striking phenomena, sensory and motor, may appear in these cases to be unilateral, careful examination shows that they are really bilateral, but more marked on one side than on the other.   So that it may be asserted that there is a general deficiency of nervous energy in the brain as a whole, although one side or even smaller portions of the organ may be specially affected. And this probably accounts for defects in sensation and in movement, and for the spasm which exists in many of these cases—phenomena which simulate closely those of gross disease of the same parts.   The diminished energy in the cells of the motor area of the cortex, and the consequent diminution in the inhibitory or steadying action of the fibres proceeding from them to the spinal motor centres, may be looked upon as the important factor in the production of hysterical paralysis and spasm.   This feebleness may extend to the centres in the cord as well, and give rise to the absence of knee-jerk and flaccid paralysis—conditions which are not infrequent in functional disease.   In some cases, in fact, there may be deficient nerve power from one end of the nervous system to the other ; either generally distributed, or more marked in some centres and nerve tracts than in others.   A girl of sixteen, for instance, lost the use of her left hand for eighteen months.   She was a strong healthy girl and free from evident hysterical tendencies.   The affection began with swelling and blueness of the fingers, such as is seen in chilblains; the hand was cold and numb, had a swollen, puffy look, and was completely paralysed.   She recovered suddenly after the application of a blister to the wrist, and then lost power in the left leg, which also suddenly got well.

The so-called "Professional hyperkineses" (writer's cramp, histrionic spasm, pianist's cramp, telegraphist's cramp, etc.) admit of a similar explanation : but in them the diminished power in the voluntary motor tract is due to exhaustion from overwork.   All the conditions of spasm which occur in cases of gross lesions of the nervous system may be found,

more or less accurately reproduced, in functional cases.   Exaggeration of
the "tendon-phenomena" plays an important part in some of the latter
class, just as it has been shown to do in the former.   A healthy
girl, æt. sixteen, who had never had an illness, and who had no
evident neurotic peculiarities, went out for a row on the Thames with
some friends in the summer of 1885.   She rowed without interruption
for five hours, a very unusual effort.   About an hour after returning
home her arms "began to twitch," and the movements continued unin-
terruptedly until I saw her in the following December.   Both arms were
then the seat of similar and synchronous movements, occurring regularly
about 160 times a minute.   They consisted of rapid elevation and retraction of the arm at the shoulder, partial flexion at the elbow, and slight
extension at the wrist: in fact, they bore a very marked resemblance to
the movements of the hands and arms in rowing, the extreme rapidity of
the "stroke" making up for the limited extent of the movements.   In
these rhythmical spasms the slight stretching of the tendons of one set of
muscles, produced by the action of their opponents, makes them contract,
and they in their turn bring the latter into play.

The condition of the nervous system which gives rise to functional
spasm is very ill-defined in its nature; it is, as far as one can judge, a
diminution in the nervous energy which specially affects, or is more pronounced in, the higher centres.   Hysterical people are those who produce
a limited supply of such energy, probably on account of some inherited or
acquired anatomical and physiological peculiarities.   But the standard
of health in different individuals at different times is as variable in the
nervous system as it is in other organs; and there are many patients
who suffer from muscular spasm, and other symptoms of functional nerve
disease, who, under more favourable conditions of life, would have remained free from them; while there are others who look almost with
scorn upon such sufferers, and who, nevertheless, if subjected to hardship
involving stress and strain upon their nervous system, might themselves
fall into the category of "hysterical" patients.

It will no doubt have been observed that in the course of the remarks
which have been made on "tendon reflexes" and on "spasm," little or no
reference has been made to the cerebellum.   And this is an intentional
omission; for I have failed in obtaining at the bedside precise information as to the effect of diseases of this organ upon the phenomena in
question.   It may be that the cerebellum plays an important part in the
production of spasm and in the modification of the tendon reflexes; but
the evidence that this is so does not at present appear to be decisive.   It
is, therefore, thought advisable simply to quote Dr. Hughlings Jackson's
views on the matter.   In the first Hughlings Jackson lecture, which this
eminent neurologist delivered before the Neurological Society on 8th
December 1897, the following remarks are to be found:—

"I have now to restate an old hypothesis on dynamical relations of
the two sub-systems by intermediation of motor centres of the lowest
level.   Speaking very roughly, and neglecting some parts of the body,

the cerebellum represents movements of the skeletal muscles in the order trunk, leg, arm, preponderatingly extensor-wise; the cerebrum represents movements of the same muscles in the order arm, leg, trunk, preponderatingly flexor-wise. It is also supposed that impulses from motor centres of the higher levels of each sub-system continuously act upon the motor centres of the lowest level; that the impulses from each set of higher levels antagonise or inhibit one another in different degrees upon different lowest motor centres; that the degree with which the cerebral and the cerebellar impulses antagonise one another is the same as the order of the degree of their different representations of movements of muscles of the body. In accordance with this hypothesis the rigidity in the common cerebral paralysis, hemiplegia, results because cerebral influence being taken off the lowest motor centres as the cerebrum represents movements in the order arm, leg, trunk, cerebellar influence upon those lowest motor centres is no longer antagonised; there is cerebellar 'influx' into the parts which the cerebrum has abandoned.

" It was asserted against this hypothesis that upon complete transverse lesion of the spinal cord above the lumbar enlargement—both cerebral and cerebellar influence being excluded from motor centres below the lesion—the legs are rigid and the knee-jerks exaggerated. But a few years ago Dr. Charlton Bastian brought forward cases showing that upon total transverse lesion of the spinal cord above the lumbar enlargement the legs are flaccid and the knee-jerks absent. His conclusions are, I think, adopted by most neurologists in this country; they have been confirmed by Bowlby, Thorburn, and Bruns (of Hanover). I have several times stated the objections which may be brought against the theory of cerebral and cerebellar influx, some of which I admit to be serious.

" There is another way of considering the hypothesis of relations of the cerebral and cerebellar sub-systems to one another by their having the lowest level in common; we may compare and contrast certain cerebral and certain cerebellar maladies with one another as being Complementary Inverses (corresponding opposites). The best marked Complementary Inverse is a case of extensive cerebellar paralysis (trunk, legs, arms), and rigidity as the corresponding opposite of the double hemiplegia (arms, legs, trunk), and rigidity of an advanced case of paralysis agitans; in the former the attitude is opisthotonic, in the latter slightly emprosthotonic. There is another very important Complementary Inverse; in some cases of tumour of the middle lobe of the cerebellum there are tetanus-like seizures. They, being paroxysmal, are obviously of different nature from the persisting cerebellar paralysis with rigidity just mentioned as certainly as an epileptiform paroxysm (I mean the epilepsy described by Bravais, 1827) is of different nature from hemiplegia with rigidity. These tetanus-like seizures depend, I suppose, on occasional excessive discharges beginning in some part of the cerebellum; such paroxysms are, speaking generally, the Complementary Inverse of epileptiform or epileptic seizures from sudden occasional excessive discharges beginning in a part of the cerebral cortex. I used to think that drawing back of the neck was especially a cerebellar symptom. Dr. Buzzard has, however, published a case of retraction of the head from tumour of one temporo-sphenoidal lobe. Tetanus-like seizures occur in cases of glioma of the pons. I have pointed out that when there is cerebellar tumour such seizures may be said to be owing to pressure on the adjacent corpora quadrigemina or subjacent medulla. Those who adopt the pressure hypothesis have, in some cases of tumour of the middle lobe of the cerebellum, three things to account for: (1) cerebellar paralysis, (2) cerebellar paralysis with rigidity, and (3) tetanus-like seizures."

SPASM OF INVOLUNTARY MUSCLES.—In defining the meaning of spasm at the beginning of this article I said :—

"By spasm is meant excessive muscular contraction ; and in the case of those muscles which are under the control of the will, excessive contraction is that which occurs in defiance of the will ; or which, although beginning as a voluntary act, transgresses the limits which the will would impose upon it. Where involuntary muscles are concerned the definition of excessive is more difficult. When the muscles of the intestine, for instance, make spasmodic efforts to drive along the contents of the bowel through a portion which has been narrowed by disease, so far from the muscular action being excessive, it may be insufficient for the purpose. In such a case, and in others of a similar kind, it can only be said that spasm is muscular contraction which exceeds that which occurs in conditions of health, and in the course of the normal physiological processes."

Under ordinary circumstances, between meals, intestinal peristalsis goes on slowly and continuously, as a result of the automatic action of the nerve cells and fibres which are found in the wall of the bowel. When food passes along the gut the movements are increased reflexly ; and irritating substances may give rise to acute spasm on the part of the muscular coats, while chronic obstruction will give rise to chronic spasm with frequently recurring paroxysms of increased severity. Persistent spasm of this kind produces marked muscular hypertrophy, and the wall of the bowel increases in thickness. Such cases may be looked upon as instances of functional spasm. Most cases of visceral spasm are probably of the functional variety : but the "visceral crises" of locomotor ataxy must be ascribed to gross nerve lesions. The vomiting produced by tumours and other diseases of the brain is another instance of spasm due to a gross lesion ; but the exact way in which the vomiting is brought about is uncertain.

Functional spasm of the muscles of the oesophagus gives rise to temporary stricture of this tube which may disappear after a bougie has been passed once, or oftener. Cramp of the muscles of the limbs may occur in gouty patients, owing probably to the circulation of uric acid : and similar paroxysms of muscular spasm may no doubt affect involuntary muscles. The sphincter ani is occasionally in such subjects the seat of the most painful spasm. Not only in the gastro-intestinal canal does spasm occur, but probably wherever involuntary muscles are found in the body.

The vascular system, for instance, affords us examples. Ergot taken internally, or subcutaneously administered, produces contraction of the muscular coat of the arteries, and even gangrene may result therefrom. In Raynaud's disease spasmodic contraction of the arteries occurs in the stage of "local syncope," and may produce gangrene. Attacks of megrim are often accompanied by evident contraction of the temporal artery, which, as the attack subsides, again becomes softer and larger. There is reason to think that in this disease a similar condition of vascular spasm is present in other organs too; for during and somewhat preceding the attacks the urine may be much diminished; and then, as soon as the attack goes off, flow freely again. The inability of the stomach during the attack to digest, or even to absorb fluids which may be present, and the sudden recovery of its power as soon as the attack subsides, are probably due to vascular spasm.

Again in the respiratory system the muscles may overact. The paroxysms of asthma are accompanied by a narrowing of the smaller bronchial tubes which gives rise to diminished entry of air into the lung and to numberless rhonchi.

In hysteria intense adductor spasm of the vocal chords sometimes occurs, giving rise to dyspnœa and stridor. Even the diaphragm is not exempt from spasm. A very neurotic woman, aged thirty-seven, had for eleven years suffered from periodical attacks in which loud, squelching and churning noises were produced within the abdomen audible at a distance from her. On close examination it was seen that the abdominal movements were produced by jerky, spasmodic descents of the diaphragm, and hiccough often accompanied them. There was no evidence of gastro-intestinal distension, and no pain. The woman also suffered from attacks of asthma.

Paroxysms of renal and hepatic colic are probably largely due to the spasmodic contractions of the bile-ducts and gall bladder in the one case, and of the ureter in the other, which are induced by the presence of a calculus.

The same occurs in the case of the urinary bladder when a calculus, enlarged prostate, stricture, or other pathological condition interferes with the easy flow of urine from it.

The uterus, too, another of the hollow muscular organs, may often be the seat of spasm, produced either by local conditions or by the circulation of poisons, such as ergot, through its substance.

The ovaries contain muscular tissue, and it is possible that paroxysmal contractions of this may be responsible for some of the pains and other disturbances which affect these organs.

It appears, therefore, from what has been said, that spasm is not confined to voluntary muscles, but may occur wherever muscle of any kind is found.   If the pathology of spasm in voluntary muscle is often obscure, and difficult to explain, it is frequently no less obscure in cases of visceral spasm.   But it may be asserted, probably with truth, that in the latter case, as a rule, the pathology is more simple, the overaction of the muscles being often produced by local causes, and then generally reflex in character.

SEYMOUR J. SHARKEY

TROPHONEUROSES

NEUROTROPHIC AFFECTIONS OF BONES AND JOINTS

Introductory.—The conception of trophic centres which control the nutrition of the bones and joints was formulated by J. K. Mitchell, as far back as the year 1831, in an article on the occurrence of arthropathies as sequels of disease or injury of the spine. Mitchell even made the daring suggestion that the articular lesion in acute rheumatism might be the effect of changes in the nervous centres. These hypotheses met with no general acceptance at the time, yet their survival in the minds of the few was shown during the next thirty years by occasional records in medical literature of arthropathies following various affections of the brain and spinal cord. But curiously enough it was not till the year 1868 that attention was directed by Charcot to the trophic lesions of locomotor ataxy. The first case in this country was reported by Clifford Allbutt in the following year.

Charcot's observations established once for all the existence of the joint disease which bears his name, and on which so large a part of our knowledge of nervous arthropathies depends. His work indeed was so complete that little remained for subsequent observers except to offer explanations, and to fill up details. The power of his name secured him a respectful hearing at once, and, in France at all events, a ready acquiescence; but elsewhere, and particularly in Germany, his views met with the most strenuous opposition, an opposition indeed which is not even yet silenced. Virchow, Volkmann, and Strümpell, for example, were among the leaders of scientific thought who contested the correctness of Charcot's deductions; and so great was their influence that for ten or fifteen years after, while records of Charcot's disease were abounding in France and fairly common in England, in Germany their scarcity was remarkable.

Weir Mitchell's description of spontaneous fractures in tabes, published in 1873, formed an addition to our knowledge of hardly less importance than Charcot's of 1868. This was followed at a very short interval by further observations from Charcot, who early saw the intimate relation between the changes in the bones which lead to spontaneous fracture and those which form the basis of affections of joints. It was some years, however, before this connection received wide recognition, and during this period the osteopathies failed to attract the universal interest which had been so rapidly given to the arthropathies. But since then the history of the two affections has become inseparable, and justly so. During the eighties the increasing number of records in every literature gives evidence of interest in both aspects of the disease which, already growing, received an additional impetus in the latter half of the decade or the recognition of similar changes in syringomyelia.

For many reasons the affections of bones and joints which, though not peculiar to tabes, are characteristic of it, dominate the whole field of trophic action. Their close connection with a disease which possesses so definite a morbid anatomy, the comparative frequency of their occurrence, and, lastly, their own characters, claim for them a position above that of all other trophoneuroses. The first and main part of the present article will therefore be devoted to a description of tabetic osteopathies and arthropathies; these will be taken as the chief types of such affections, and will therefore be used to some extent as a standard of comparison in dealing with others.

PART I. TROPHIC LESIONS IN TABES. — **A. Osteopathies.** — In the majority of cases the occurrence of a spontaneous fracture gives the first clinical evidence of the osseous lesion; but not infrequently pain is referred to the spot for long periods of time before the bone actually gives way (Pitres et Vaillard). The observation has been repeatedly made that the lightning pains are especially severe in the limb afterwards to be the seat of a spontaneous fracture.

Osteopathies, and consequently spontaneous fractures, occur most frequently in the long bones, particularly in those of the lower extremities; but they may affect any part of the skeleton. Where the short bones are involved, as in the case of the vertebræ and tarsus, the condition is so complex and characteristic, in consequence of changes in the connecting articulations, as to require a description apart from both osteopathies and arthropathies. Under any circumstances fractures are most frequently met with in limbs already the seat of arthropathies; and tend to occur in that part of the bone which enters into relation with an affected joint.

Spontaneous fracture.—This may be spontaneous in the strictest sense of the word, as when the lesion passes altogether unnoticed or is discovered by accident; but more commonly it is precipitated by some slight muscular effort or mechanical strain. How slight this may be is shown by the fact that the mere act of turning over in bed has sufficed. In one case fracture of the humerus occurred while the patient was pulling on his boot; and in several cases the femur has been broken by the exertion of walking.

The most conspicuous feature of these fractures, after their spontaneity, is their complete painlessness. So absolute is this that, unless the injury be such as to render locomotion a physical impossibility, the patient will continue to get about on the broken limb without the least suspicion of what has occurred. Apart from this insensibility the fracture presents no special features ; though it is stated that the amount of displacement of bones and of swelling of soft parts is usually excessive. The process of repair sets in with at least the usual rapidity ; but exceptions to this rule have been described (Rivington) in which little or no attempt at union took place. The amount of callus is nearly always abnormally great ; and, even if allowance be made for the rough treatment incidental on the painlessness of the parts, it is still in excess of what is formed under other conditions. Occasionally a union which has been effected under the shelter of an enormous mass of callus again gives way, without any apparent cause except the absorption of the new material. In a large proportion of cases the fractures are multiple ; and there is a distinct tendency for the same bone to suffer repeatedly.

B. Arthropathies. — Arthropathies may occur at any stage of tabes, and not infrequently are the first serious indication of the malady. Even in the affected limb anæsthesia of the joint may be the only sign of nervous change ; and this may be present without involving cutaneous sensation. As a rule, however, a careful examination will reveal more definite signs of the spinal disease.

In something like 75 per cent of the cases the joints affected belong to the lower extremities. Thus out of 268 tabetic arthropathies collected by Chipault, 207 were in the lower limbs ; of these 120 affected the knee, and 57 the hip. It has been noticed that, when the lesion affects the articulations of the upper limbs, it is in the late stage, when the tabetic change has spread to the cervical region of the cord. With the exception of those of the feet, which constitute a special group and will be considered under a separate heading, the smaller articulations are but rarely affected. In the list of 268 arthropathies just quoted the wrist joint figures three times ; the finger joints twice, and the temporomaxillary articulation once. Frequently the arthropathies are multiple, and then most commonly symmetrical. A joint which has been damaged in any way shows a special proclivity to attack ; as in the case of old fracture of wrist recorded by Chipault, or the dislocation of hip mentioned by Virchow. As in tuberculous arthritis, slight injuries may precipitate an attack ; though the possibility of intra-capsular fracture must then be taken into account.

Premonitory symptoms.—In the large majority of cases these are completely absent ; but several records show that the onset of the arthropathy may be preceded by pain referred to the articulation. This may either be of the nature of lightning pain, or may assume a rheumatic character, varying with changes in the weather. In one instance this prodromal symptom had lasted for twenty-three years (Tournier) ; in another for thirty.

Onset.—Reference has already been made to the fact that an arthropathy may be immediately preceded by an injury of so trivial a nature that under ordinary conditions it would be utterly inadequate to produce any serious result. Very frequently even this slight traumatic factor is absent, and the joint affection appears as a bolt from the blue. The patient wakes up in the morning and finds that one knee is much swollen ; or, as he is walking in the street, his leg suddenly gives way under him (Marie).

But even more remarkable than the suddenness of onset is the utter painlessness of the condition. In consequence of this absence of pain the amount of disability produced by the grossest disease of joints may be almost incredibly small ; as for example in the case of arthropathy of knee mentioned by Strümpell, in which the patient continued to shoot for a whole season on foot until dislocation occurred. Painlessness may be regarded then as all but pathognomonic of this form of nervous arthropathy ; exceptions to this rule have been recorded (Fort), but they are few in number ; and even in them the pain was transient, and present only at the outset. In these cases it may probably be regarded as analogous to anæsthesia dolorosa.

Clinical condition. — In the first stage the joint is distended with fluid, often to a degree rarely reached in any other form of disease. In many cases the effusion is not limited to the articulation itself, or even to the surrounding tissues, but infiltrates the whole limb. In either event the result is to produce a characteristic solid œdema which does not pit on pressure, and the extent of which varies within the widest limits. From the condition of extreme distension the skin over the affected area is white and shining, while the subcutaneous veins become correspondingly prominent. On palpation nothing abnormal in the joint may be felt ; but, if the swelling be less extreme than has been described, it is often possible to elicit crepitus ; or to detect the presence of loose bodies, and even of irregular fragments of bone within the articular cavity. Both active and passive movements may be freely carried on without causing the patient the least inconvenience ; and already an abnormal degree of mobility may be apparent.

In this the first stage all joints present to a great extent a similar condition ; but with the absorption of the intra-articular effusion and the subcutaneous œdema—a process which may occupy a period of either weeks or months—and the evolution of the second stage, a notable difference between the various articulations becomes obvious. The morbid process in nervous arthropathies may be considered as made up of two opposing factors, both acting on the osseous elements of the joint : the one leads to rarefaction and absorption of the bone, the other to hypertrophy or overgrowth. It is a curious fact that the relative activity of these opposing forces varies with the nature of the articulation. In the ball-and-socket joints, such as the hip and shoulder, the atrophic factor predominates ; while in the hinge joints, such as the knee and elbow, overgrowth carries the day.

In the hip-joint type the atrophic process leads to a rapid destruction of the head, neck, and even of the trochanteric region of the femur ; and displacement is the common result. There is some compensatory formation of osteophytic deposits at the margin of the acetabulum and about the trochanters ; but as a rule these are of no great size or extent, and they may be completely absent.

On the other. hand, when the disease affects the knee or elbow, the outgrowths of bone, particularly about the head of the tibia and patella, are commonly so extensive as to constitute the most prominent clinical feature. Atrophy, however, does occur ; but, affecting as it does the femoral condyles and central part of the tibia, is masked by the presence of outlying bony deposits. At a' late period the articulation may become immovably fixed by osseous anchylosis ; but more frequently it falls into the other extreme of abnormal mobility.

It must not be supposed that in every case the condition of the joint steadily deteriorates until destruction is complete. The effusion may subside and leave little obvious change behind ; though it is seldom that the laxity of the capsule which results from its over-distension is not the cause of some impairment of function. Unfortunately, even in what appear to be favourable conditions, a relapse is only too likely to occur ; and the final state of an articulation which seemed at one time to be returning to health may be no better than that of the worst type of the disease ; whether it take the form of anchylosis or of flail joint.

C. Osteo-arthropathies.—*Vertebral lesions.*—The precise nature of these has been the subject of much discussion, though their symptomatology has been clearly established by the observations of Krönig and others. These trophic lesions of the vertebral column are extremely rare when compared with those of other bones and joints in tabes. For example, they do not appear in Chipault's collection of 268 tabetic arthropathies. A remarkable fact, which may be gathered from the somewhat scanty observations on record, is the special liability of the lumbar portion of the spine. The two chief characteristics of the other tabetic trophoneuroses—painlessness and apparent causelessness—are equally pronounced in this special form. In one case a marked angular curvature appeared suddenly, and without obvious cause ; in others fracture of the spinal column took place on a slight slip in walking, or in coming down stairs. In all alike pain was absent, and interference with the power of locomotion very slight. In one of these patients, the fracture being in the lumbar region, the fragments could be slid one over the other without pain. The displacement may be so considerable that the patient notices the projection of the luxated portion into the abdomen as a palpable tumour. Still, in spite of such gross deformity, symptoms of pressure on the spinal cord rarely if ever occur.

The tabetic foot.—The first case was described and the patient shown by Mr. H. W. Page at the International Congress in London in 1881. In 1883 Charcot recorded his first observation, coupled with an inexplicable claim for priority. As in the case of the vertebral changes, it may be ranked either among the arthropathies or osteopathies ; but these considerations are reserved for the section dealing with its pathology.

The tabetic foot occurs with unusual frequency in the early stage of tabes and even in the preataxic period. Its onset is commonly abrupt, and nearly always unaccompanied by pain. If seen in the early stage, the only obvious change may consist in an abnormal swelling of the back of the foot (Marie); but, as a rule, the characteristic deformity is fully established before the patient comes under medical observation. The foot has then acquired a most distinctive quadrate or truncated appearance, which has been aptly likened to the artificial deformity of the Chinese lady; the arch has completely disappeared, and the toes look as if they took their rise immediately from the tarsus; the explanation of this is that the metatarsus may be dislocated either above or below the proximal part of the foot. The malleoli are generally much thickened, and, in consequence of the collapse of the calcaneum, often rest on the ground. The ankle joint may show a characteristic arthropathy, and thickening may extend some distance up the bones of the leg. The soft tissues of the foot are the seat of a hard œdema, and the skin is often distinctly hypertrophied. On manipulation bony crepitus is elicited, which is often so distinct and diffuse that the foot may feel like a mere bag of bones. Frequently, though by no means always, these processes are accompanied or preceded by perforating ulcer, the presence of which, by means of secondary infection, may be the cause of necrotic changes in the metatarsus or phalanges.

A second variety of trophic foot may be recognised, in which the osseous changes appear to depend entirely on the presence of a perforating ulcer with its attendant infections. The necrotic process begins at the base of the ulcer, and steadily extends, until in the course of years perhaps, a large portion of the skeleton has been exfoliated; the resulting condition strongly resembles that of the pure tabetic foot. This should, however, still be regarded as a complicated tropho-neurosis of the subcutaneous or cutaneous rather than of the osseous tissues (p. 572).

Morbid anatomy.—A. *Changes in the bones.*—Even to the naked eye the bones may be obviously diseased; the surface has a worm-eaten appearance, and shows the openings of channels of considerable size communicating with the medullary cavity. But side by side with these indications of absorption may be seen evidence of deposits of fresh tissue; these are either localised, in the form of osteophytes which may attain to the proportions of a tumour, or are spread, as a more or less irregular layer of new bone, over the adjacent portion of the shaft (von Kahlden, Rotter). It is doubtful, however, if these osteophytic changes occur to any extent in the absence of fracture or other source of irritation. A cross section shows, in the large majority of cases, marked enlargement of the medullary cavity at the expense of the compact tissue, which may have almost disappeared. This extension of the central canal also takes place longitudinally, so as to replace to some extent the cancellous tissue of the epiphysis.

The microscopic appearances are those of a rarefactive ostitis ; the Haversian canals throughout are dilated, and the pits in their walls show the ravages of the osteoclasts by which the process of absorption is being carried on. But even before absorption has begun the picro-carmine reaction shows that decalcification is taking place ; and this change may be so extreme that the bone becomes soft enough to be cut with a knife. The medullary tissue is also the seat of well-marked changes ; briefly these consist in a tendency to embryonic reversion on the one hand and to fatty degeneration on the other.

Chemical analysis (Regnard) shows a most striking deviation from normal bone, consisting in a reduction of the inorganic elements of the structure from 66 per cent to 24 per cent ; and in an increase of the organic constituents from 33 per cent to 76 per cent. The loss of inorganic matter falls mainly on the phosphates, the proportion of which sinks from 50 per cent to 10 per cent ; while on the organic side the ratio of fat rises to 37 per cent.

Finally Pitres and Vaillard, and other observers subsequently, have found degeneration of the nutrient nerve of the affected bone.

Such then are the changes in the osseous structure which lead to spontaneous fracture : they may affect the whole of the skeleton ; they may involve the one bone in its entirety ; or they may be limited to the precise spot at which the fracture has occurred, or is about to occur. The few cases of apparently spontaneous fracture in which examination has failed to reveal these changes in the bone (Schultze) might more accurately be described as fractures from muscular action ; such fractures may occur in the healthy subject, and the liability must be vastly increased by the presence of ataxy or analgesia, or of both these defects in combination.

B. *Changes in the joints.*—Before entering upon a description of the morbid anatomy of the arthropathies, it may be stated, both for the sake of emphasis and to avoid repetition, that the osseous changes which have been detailed as essentially constituting an osteopathy are present in the bones entering into the formation of diseased joints. The special characteristics of an arthropathy, under whichsoever type it may happen to fall, are added to or superimposed upon those of an osteopathy.

There is reason to believe that even in the absence of an obvious arthropathy the joints of tabetics may be the seat of marked change. Jürgens examined apparently healthy joints ; and, in those of larger size, found dilatation of the capsule with elongation of the ligaments, which was often considerable. He further noticed hyperæmia of the synovial membrane and other soft structures, which he attributed to vaso-motor disturbance of central origin. The laxity of capsule described by Jürgens will go some way to explain the remarkable capacity for rapid and extreme distension which is displayed from the outset by the tabétic joint : it may also favour the operation of the traumatic influences which so often provide the exciting cause of the outbreak ; but whether its importance is to be rated at a higher level than this is a matter for doubt.

Pathological observations during the earliest stage of an arthropathy, that is, during the period of effusion, are rare. The fluid may be sanguineous, but is, as a rule, clear and of the nature of synovia. The joint capsule has been found distended, softened, and at times almost destroyed. Hyperæmia of the synovial membrane with villous hypertrophy is a common feature, as is also softening or even destruction of the articular cartilage; foreign bodies are almost constantly present, and may either have been detached from the synovial fringes or result from an intra-articular fracture.

In discussing the fully-established disease from the anatomical point of view, the clinical division into a hypertrophic and an atrophic form may conveniently be retained. It will be remembered that the former represents the affection of the knee and elbow, the latter that of the hip and shoulder; and, moreover, that the form has no relation either to the severity or the duration of the disease.

(a) Hypertrophic form.—Outside the capsule there is a strong tendency to the formation of bony deposits : these may occur simply as marginal osteophytes about the articulation; or they may extend into the tendons and muscles surrounding the joint, and form masses so considerable as to suggest an ossifying myositis (von Kahlden, Thompson). The capsule itself may undergo partial or complete ossification; or, on the other hand, may disappear by coalescence with the neighbouring soft structures.

Within the joint the ends of the bones are greatly and irregularly enlarged by osteophytes; the articular cartilage has disappeared in large part, and the bone so exposed has a porous, spongy appearance : occasionally, but this is exceptional, it is sclerosed and eburnated, as in rheumatoid arthritis. Intra-capsular fracture is a common event, the fragments remaining as foreign bodies within the joint. Not infrequently, however, a more or less complete bony union results between the opposed surfaces, and the final condition is one of anchylosis in place of the common flail joint. In most cases the synovial membrane is the seat of profuse villous overgrowth; and as a result the cavity may contain hundreds of melon-seed bodies which have become detached. But though the prevailing note is hypertrophy, still the activity of the opposite process can be recognised in the wearing away of parts of the articulation.

(b) Atrophic form.—In the neighbourhood of the hip and shoulder joints the tendency to the formation of bony deposits is comparatively slight, though indications of it may appear. Within the articulation it is altogether absent. The synovial membrane and other soft structures have completely disappeared; the dislocated femur or humerus has lost all its normal characteristics in the process of atrophy, and strongly resembles the drumstick to which Charcot compared it. Similar changes are found in the acetabulum, which is flattened out and has the same porous appearance which is noticed about the femur. In many instances the rarefactive process has extended far beyond its margins, and has involved a considerable portion of the iliac bone.

C. Vertebral lesions.—It is difficult to say whether these should be ranked as osteopathies or arthropathies; without continuing a barren discussion we may adopt the term osteo-arthropathy which has been suggested, and has the advantage of implying no hypothesis. The pathological evidence is scanty, and consists mainly of the cases recorded by Charcot, and later by Pitres and Vaillard. In the patient observed by the latter the vertebral column became slowly deformed without any local pain; later there were formed around the spinous and transverse processes of the affected vertebræ "veritable osseous tumours accessible to palpation." At the necropsy the first lumbar vertebra was found to be almost totally destroyed: the second was remarkable from the development of osteophytes which covered its body and transverse processes, and led to a very considerable enlargement. The bodies of all the lumbar vertebræ and of the last five dorsal were covered with osteophytic deposits. No reference is made to the state of the articulations. The condition described corresponds very closely to that found clinically by Krönig.

D. *The tabetic foot.*—It is impossible to give any systematic account of the pathological processes which result in this deformity; for, in spite of the comparative uniformity of the clinical product, their variety is infinite. Where perforating ulcer coexists it may be necessary to distinguish the changes which take place in the anterior part of the foot from those which affect the posterior. In such cases it is only in the posterior part that trophic lesions can be studied in their purity; while in the region of the metatarsus and phalanges such changes, if existent, are hopelessly complicated by the presence of others due to the introduction of infection from without. Disease of the ankle joint forms no integral part of the tabetic foot, though in a large proportion of cases it coexists with it. It tends to assume the hypertrophic rather than the atrophic form; both tibia and fibula (including the malleoli) being thickly overlaid with periosteal deposits. At the same time, the cavity of the articulation commonly extends, at the expense of its smaller neighbours, until most of the tarsal joints may be included within it (Targett). In the foot, however, atrophic processes predominate: all the bones are light, porous, and prone to fracture; the smaller ones either disappear altogether or remain as unrecognisable fragments, while the larger, and of these the calcaneum is the most frequent sufferer, collapse under the weight they have to support. The articular surfaces are eroded or, less frequently, connected by new bone. Displacements are almost invariable, the most prevalent form being a dislocation of the anterior part of the foot, including the metatarsus either above or below the tarsus. To this the curious squat shape of the foot is largely due.

In the metatarsal region, particularly when the trophic ulcer governs the situation, the bony structures are often completely lost; having undergone necrosis and been thrown off, or otherwise removed, through the wound. By the same process the metatarso-phalangeal joint is disintegrated, and one or more of the phalanges may have disappeared. At the farther limits of the area exposed to infection signs of osteoplastic peri-

ostitis are often evident; though elsewhere they may be conspicuous by
their absence.

Trophic changes have hitherto been described as they occur in locomotor ataxy. They are not limited to this disease, however, and a short
consideration of their occurrence under other circumstances therefore
becomes necessary.

TROPHIC LESIONS IN SYRINGOMYELIA.—The bone and joint lesions in
syringomyelia are practically identical with those in tabes; such differences as do exist are to be found rather in the frequency with which they
occur, and the parts of the skeleton which they affect, than in any
anatomical peculiarity. In the first place, their relative frequency is
considerably greater in syringomyelia than in tabes; in the latter disease
the proportion of cases which present joint or bone lesions is not more
than 3 per cent or 4 per cent; in the former the lowest estimate
would place it at 10 per cent (Sokoloff), the highest at 40 per cent,
or even more (Schlesinger). Again, whereas in tabes the lower extremities, as compared with the upper, are affected in at least 75 per cent,
in syringomyelia the proportion is reversed; the incidence being in about
80 per cent of the cases on the bones and joints of the upper limbs. Out
of 97 syringomyelic arthropathies, collected by Schlesinger, 29 involved
the shoulder joint, 24 the elbow, and 18 the wrist.

In tabes the trophic lesions show a striking tendency both to multiplicity and symmetry; in syringomyelia, on the other hand, while there
is an even greater tendency than in tabes to multiplicity, that to symmetry
is lost. The anatomical distinctions are slight; in syringomyelia the joint
affections are believed to be more chronic, and to show a stronger leaning
towards hypertrophy, than in tabes. The shaft of a neighbouring bone
may show extensive periosteal deposit to a degree rarely seen in the latter
disease. In syringomyelia, again, necrosis of affected bones is a common
event; and though this may be explained to a great extent by the presence
of trophic ulcers which, as in the tabetic foot, allow of secondary infection,
still cases occur in which this explanation does not apply. In a patient
of my own with typical "pieds tabétiques" of syringomyelic origin, bony
sequestra had been thrown off from both feet over a space of six years;
but perforating ulcer existed on the one side only. Another patient at
present under observation is a good example of the length to which these
necrotic processes may go: for the past fifty years she has been parting
with the bones of both feet piecemeal, with comparatively little pain, until
now the extremities look as if a clumsy Syme's amputation had been performed on both sides. Skiagrams show that the posterior part of the os
calcis and fragments of the astragalus are the only parts left of the skeleton
of the foot. Both tibia and fibula are much rarefied, and for their lower
fourth are covered with periosteal deposits. The case is in all probability
one of syringomyelia; though the ordinary dissociation of sensation is
absent.

Skiagrams of a syringomyelic arthropathy of the wrist in another patient, now under observation, show well-marked erosion of the central part of the radial articular surface, with peripheral periosteal deposits which extend some distance up the shaft. Immediately beneath the eroded surface the head of the radius is irregularly sclerosed and rarefied. The styloid process of both bones of the forearm is considerably enlarged. The changes described extend up the shaft for a distance of about two inches, so far as the radius is concerned; the ulna is healthy with the exception of the head. The carpal bones are somewhat displaced, but not perceptibly altered in structure. One or two small outgrowths are visible on the shafts of metacarpals and phalanges, but in other respects the bones are healthy.

Much discussion has arisen on the occurrence of vertebral lesions in syringomyelia, the arguments centering round the nature of the scoliosis which is so common. Roth found degeneration of the erector spinæ muscles in one case, and maintained that the deformity was paralytic. His views have received some support (Londe and Perrey), but most authors have decided in favour of a trophic origin (Schlesinger, Bruhl, Morvan, and others). In my opinion the question is not ripe for settlement: on the one hand it may be argued that such de-formity is not uncommon in other chronic diseases, as in acromegaly or osteitis deformans, where a connection with the nervous system is im-probable; and that where undoubted trophic lesions of vertebræ exist, as in tabes, the condition is altogether dissimilar to that found in syringo-myelia: on the other hand, except on the hypothesis of a trophic affec-tion, it is difficult to explain the acute accession of the deformity which sometimes takes place. A young woman, aged twenty-one, now under my care with definite symptoms of syringomyelia, manifested the characteristic curve to a most marked degree in the space of a few weeks. At the same time she complained of pain and stiffness in the part of the back affected. There was no tenderness of the spine, and no indication of any intercurrent disease. The only part of the muscular system which shows any sign of wasting or weakness is the intrinsic musculature of the hand. The general nutrition is perfect, and the patient is still pursuing her ordinary avocations.

It must be remembered that syringomyelia sometimes results from an injury, and rarely may follow an acute myelitis (Schlesinger); such a sequence of events may account for the syringomyelic or tabetic form of arthropathy under what appear to be independent morbid conditions.

TROPHIC LESION IN DEMENTIA PARALYTICA.—Fragility of bones lead-ing to spontaneous fracture is comparatively frequent; and the occurrence of arthropathies has been recorded, though the event is rare (Shaw, Lloyd, and others). These forms of nervous disease are, however, so often associated with the lesions of tabes that the fact loses most of its signifi-cance; and the trophic troubles, especially when they involve the joints, must be regarded as pertaining to the tabetic rather than to the paralytic element. Moreover, in general paralysis, as in other forms of chronic insanity, an atrophic change in the bones may occur which we are not justified in attributing to a trophic or direct nervous origin. Its explanation is to be sought rather in a general lowering of nutrition than in a derangement of nervous control in the part affected. In dementia paralytica, then, these apparent trophic changes must be scrutinised with extreme care, when they will be found to fall roughly into two classes: (a) those which are truly trophic but really tabetic; and (b) those which are not trophic but dependent on a lowering of nutrition which the bones suffer in common with the rest of the body.

The changes in the bones which have been described in this relation would appear to be those of pure atrophy with its associated decalcification; they involve the ribs with especial frequency, but may affect the whole skeleton from the skull downwards. The fractures are often extremely numerous (Ogle, Crichton Browne, Neumann, Gudden). No general rules can be laid down which will decide the pathology of every case; except perhaps that if arthropathies coexist the probabilities are strongly in favour of a neuropathic origin.

IN LEPROSY the bone changes need even more discrimination than those in general paralysis. They may be divided into three classes: (i.) pure atrophy, such as is met with after section of a peripheral nerve; (ii.) a form of atrophy which results from the invasion of the medulla by leprous granulomatous tissue (Sawtschenko); and (iii.) necrosis in connection with septic infection from ulcerative lesions of the superficial tissues. The allegation of a true Charcot's arthropathy in leprosy has been the subject of much discussion; it is denied by some writers (Chipault, Londe, and Perrey) and maintained by others (Hansen and Looft). On the whole, the weight of evidence is in favour of the presence of the change in this disease. Hansen says (p. 76):—

"Professor Heiberg has described a foot which resembles the pied tabétique. According to Heiberg a characteristic of these leprous trophoneurotic joint affections is swelling and laxness of the capsule of the joint, and wearing away and atrophy of the ends of the bones, or periostitis ossificans, and hypertrophy of the ends of the bones, which is especially seen in the tarsal and metatarsal joints. We have been able to confirm these results of Heiberg, and have also seen, in such an ankle, growth of the synovial membrane with villous projections; the capsule of the ankle joint was loose and lax, the talus smooth and oblique, and the cartilage worn away; and marked outward subluxation of the foot was present."

This statement can leave no doubt that typical trophic affections of the joints do occur in leprosy; a point of considerable importance, for it is the one disease of peripheral nerves in which they are found. In all probability this exceptional position is to be explained by the chronicity of the nerve lesion; which is hardly equalled in any other form of peripheral neuritis, but finds a close parallel in the slowly-progressing tabetic change in the cord.

There are then three diseases in which the characteristic combination of bone with joint lesions of trophic origin may be found; they are tabes, syringomyelia, and leprosy. Their occurrence is so rare in leprosy, and the parent disease is of such subordinate importance in this country, that further discussion of the causes of arthropathies will be confined to the purely spinal degenerations.

PATHOGENY.—Before discussing the origin of the changes in Charcot's disease a short reference must be made to the various and divergent explanations which have been offered, mainly from German sources, in substitution of the trophic hypothesis. Two of these can be dismissed in a few words; they are Strümpell's hypothesis of a syphilitic and Volkmann's of a traumatic arthritis. So long as the lesion was recognised in tabes only, with the almost invariable syphilitic antecedents of that disease, Strümpell's suggestion may have caused some hesitation; but with the recognition of precisely similar lesions in syringomyelia, with which syphilis has nothing to do, the hesitation disappeared. Volkmann's suggestion rested on the assumption that the affection of joints occurs especially in the later stages of tabes, when the ataxy is most extreme and injuries more likely to be received. It is now acknowledged that the joint lesions are limited to no period of the disease; indeed, if they have a preference it is for the earlier stages of the malady. Moreover, their presence in syringomyelia, a disease in which ataxy is commonly absent, dealt a final blow to the belief in their traumatic origin.

But Virchow's claims for the identity of Charcot's disease with arthritis deformans deserve a fuller consideration. The clinical differences are so gross that they need hardly be mentioned; but it must be confessed that the morbid anatomy shows remarkable similarity in the two conditions; undoubtedly, in the earlier stage at all events, definite distinction may not be possible (Virchow, Targett, and others). Every attempt to establish an absolutely pathognomonic feature has failed, though a tiro need find no difficulty in distinguishing a typical specimen of Charcot's joint from one of arthritis deformans. The differences at first sight seem of cumulative rather than of specific value; of degree rather than of kind.

Virchow has shown that the morbid process in arthritis deformans originates in the articular cartilage. We have seen that, with regard to the trophic lesions which we are now considering, there are reasons for believing that the primary lesion is seated rather in the bone; and that the change in the cartilage is secondary. It can hardly be a mere coincidence that in the two diseases, tabes and syringomyelia, which practically constitute the sphere of trophic arthropathies, the osteopathies should form an almost equally prominent feature; or that the bone and joint lesions should, in a large proportion of cases, show themselves in the same individuals, in the same limb, and even in the same part of the limb. We have already seen that the alterations in the structure of the bone, which lead to spontaneous fracture, occur in the epiphysis as well as in the diaphysis; and many examinations have proved their presence in the bony structures of an affected joint (Marie), an observation which may be confirmed in any pathological museum. It is, indeed, to the presence of this change that some of the most characteristic features of arthropathy, the rapid and excessive wearing away of the articular extremities and the consequent dislocations, are due. There is much to be said for the view which has been advanced, and strongly supported, that in some cases an arthropathy is simply a spontaneous fracture of the epiphysis (Rotter, Weizsacker, and others); the absolutely sudden onset of the joint mischief, its occurrence after a slight trauma, and the detection of fragments of bone within the articulation at an early stage, are all strongly suggestive of intra-capsular fracture as the immediate cause (Tournier, Westphal). In two cases the head of the tibia in an arthropathic knee, which had been resected, was found to be the seat of multiple fractures (Rotter); in others the fluid effused without warning into a joint has been proved to consist of blood (Brissaud). Still spontaneous fracture cannot be considered an invariable or even perhaps a common cause of arthropathies; for those of gradual onset, and also probably for some others, another explanation must be found: stated in brief, it is that the rarefactive process in the epiphysis extends to the auricular cartilage and undermines it. Ziegler suggests this, though as a minor occurrence, in arthritis deformans; and he illustrates its advance side by side with the changes proceeding from above. The cartilage undermined in this way shows proliferation of its cells, and undergoes erosion as in arthritis deformans; while the exposed bone may either develop compensatory change in the form of eburnation or, under other circumstances, may simply undergo destruction. The rough similarity between the final results in the two cases becomes easily explicable if we suppose that the vicious circle is, *mutatis mutandis*, the same in both; though in one the disease takes the cartilage as its starting-point, in the other the bone. The tabetic foot is, by almost universal agreement, a combination of osteopathy and arthropathy; the latter being secondary to the former. Is it probable that an arthropathy should start in one part of the body from the bone and from the cartilage in another?

Our conclusion then is that, in spite of the superficial resemblance, arthritis deformans and Charcot's disease of joints are fundamentally different, even in their anatomy. If this be accepted, the case both for the specificity of the latter affection, and, by implication, for its neurotic origin, may be regarded as complete; and we may proceed to discuss its relations with the nervous system.

What are the paths by which the supposed controlling nervous influence is conveyed? Little consideration is necessary to show that it is the sensory tract which must be concerned. In all the three diseases, which in the preceding pages have been credited with arthropathies and osteopathies, the lesion is mainly on the sensory side.

It has already been made clear that, so far as the joints themselves are concerned, the common nervous factor is absence of pain; whether the primary disease be tabes or syringomyelia. The dissociation of sensation which constitutes the main and sometimes the only symptom of the latter disease still further simplifies the problem by allowing the elimination of the paths of tactile and muscular sense, the implication of which in tabes confuses the issues. In syringomyelia, again, the ground is still further narrowed; for the sensory defect may even be limited to the articular structures concerned, as in a case already quoted. By this process of exclusion it may be taken as proved that the fibres concerned with nutrition either accompany or are identical with those which conduct impressions of pain and temperature. Whether these latter are separate or distinct there is at present little evidence to show; the fact that the joint surfaces in health are sensitive both to thermal and painful impressions suggests that the same fibre subserves both functions; for it is difficult to see the use of a separate thermal apparatus for these parts.

What level of the sensory tract is responsible for the joint lesion, and what is the mechanism by which it acts? The conception of a controlling centre in the medulla (Buzzard) must be rejected; the fact that the trophic lesions always occur in the territory which corresponds to the level of the nervous disease is conclusive. Thus in tabes, where the lumbar enlargement is specially involved, the trophic lesions are almost limited to the lower limbs; in syringomyelia where the cervical part of the cord is affected their distribution is as distinctly confined to the upper. There can be no doubt that if such a centre or centres exist in the cord they must be distributed throughout its whole length.

But, before proceeding farther in the discussion of the position of a trophic centre, it will be well to ascertain in what part of the nervous system the actual lesion, which appears to be potent in the production of trophic changes, is found. Is it in the spinal cord, the nerve roots, or the peripheral nerves? In tabes the conditions are too complex to give a reply; for the disease involves all three structures. By several observers the perversion has been ascribed to the peripheral nerves in tabes on the ground of changes in the nutrient nerve of the joint òr bone (Pitres and Carrière, Heydenreich and Liouville, and others); but their position became untenable on the discovery of identical articular and osseous trophoneuroses in syringomyelia where nerve and root lesions are commonly absent. It is true that even here neuritis has been described; but it is inconceivable, considering the nature of the disease, that it should have been anything more than a secondary degeneration. There can be no doubt then that, in syringomyelia at all events, the interference with the nutritive control of the joints is due to the lesion which specially affects the posterior gray matter of the cord; and by a fair analogy the similar trophic changes which occur in tabes may be attributed to the degeneration of the spinal cord rather than to that of the peripheral nerves, or nerve roots. But, even if a decision were possible, present views of pathology have robbed the question of much of its interest; it is, to say the least, a matter for doubt whether the site of the lesion in peripheral neuritis, except of course in the case of mechanical interference, differs from that in poliomyelitis. Both may alike be regarded as affections of the whole neuron, and such differences as exist are attributable to variations in the nature rather than in the position of the lesion. It has already been suggested, on a previous page, that the occurrence of arthropathies in leprosy, as in tabes, may be due to the unique chronicity of the leprous change in the nerves. We may conclude therefore that, granted certain favouring conditions, the same result may occur from disease of any part of the lower sensory tract.

Little is known with certainty of the processes and means of trophic influences, but several possible alternatives may be recognised. The first consists in the existence of special trophic fibres which conduct peripherally, and the sole duty of which is to regulate the processes of nutrition. No discussion of so far-reaching a topic can be entered into here; but, as regards the bones and joints at all events, it may be stated that the existence of such fibres is purely speculative, and if any less speculative explanation can be found it should be preferred.

The second possibility lies in the paralysis or irritation of vaso-motor fibres or centres. In support of it several observations pointing to a hyperæmia of the affected joints might be cited; but it must be owned, on the other hand, that their condition, so far as vascularity is concerned, is so utterly variable that no argument can be based upon it. Certainly, in the large majority of cases, there is no evidence either of vaso-motor paralysis or of irritation, to any marked degree. The complexity of the resulting lesion offers a still greater difficulty in the way of accepting such a view. Attention has already been called to the fact that the change in the tissues affected can be considered neither as atrophy nor hyperplasia, but as a combination of the two in varying proportions; to produce this result the irritation or paralysis, whichever it may be, must be supposed to act at the same time in diametrically opposite directions. This fact stands out in marked contrast with the effects of interference with vaso-motor action as they are met with in other conditions in which, according as the centres are irritated or paralysed, either hyperæmia with hyperplasia or anæmia with atrophy may occur; but not the two together.

The third suggestion, which was originally made by Marinesco and confirmed by Brissaud, is to the effect that the sensory fibres which supply the articulation form the afferent path of a reflex arc, the efferent portion of which is provided by nerves having a vaso-motor function. Marinesco supposes that these sensory nerves are continually transmitting impulses to the vaso-motor centre, keeping it, so to speak, in a state of tonus. In accordance with the demands so made the nutrition of each particular tract is maintained by means of the blood-supply which is regulated by efferent vaso-motor fibres. In the absence of these warning messages from the joint or bone the blood-supply becomes inadequate, and atrophy ensues. That part of the hypothesis which postulates the maintenance of nutrition by means of reflex action, initiated by the sensory fibres of the joint, certainly appears worthy of provisional acceptance; at all events it has some claim to an anatomical basis. In the posterior root there is a bundle of efferent fibres, the function of which is unknown, but which may well form the outward part of the arc. It has been proved, too, by Raymond and Onanoff's experiments, that reflex action, though of a different kind, is actually originated from articular surfaces. A traumatic arthropathy was produced in both knees of a rabbit, and in addition the posterior root was divided on the one side: on the side on which the root had been divided no muscular atrophy occurred, yet on the other it appeared as usual. It would seem that the efferent part of this reflex arc would be concerned with the vaso-motor supply of the muscles rather than their actual nutrition; for, how-ever marked the wasting, no reaction of degeneration is found in such arthritic atrophy. But here our agreement with Marinesco must cease. To account for the hyperplastic element, which still remains unexplained, he proceeds to argue for a sort of compensatory process; basing the hypothesis on some experiments of Bizzozero, he supposes the preserva-tion of a certain proportion of the afferent fibres from the joint, in consequence of which the areas subject to their control receive the nutri-tive material which, but for the destruction of its nerve-supply, would have gone to a neighbouring territory. For the pseudo-compensatory action which he postulates there seems to be no evidence, whether clini-cal or pathological. If it took place an inverse relation between the amount of atrophy and hyperplasia would surely be perceptible; but this is not the case. Moreover the degree of atrophy in the articular tissues should be proportional to the severity of the spinal mischief; but no such relation can be detected.

Granting the existence of Marinesco's reflex arc for nutritive pur-poses, something more is necessary to explain the mingled character of an osteoarthropathy, to show why the lesion should partake both of atrophy and of overgrowth. It will be remembered that on a previous page attention was called to the fact that the predominance of the one or the other of these two factors depends not upon the nature or stage of the spinal disease, but upon the anatomical character of the articulation. Generally speaking, the ball-and-socket joints assume the atrophic form, the hinge joints the hypertrophic. To this statement, a second may be added, namely, that atrophy tends to occur at the centre of the articula-tion, hypertrophy at the periphery. These facts are mentioned here in order to lay stress upon the important part played by mechanical condi-tions, quite apart from nervous influence. Of the two factors atrophy would appear to be the more fundamental, especially if it be reduced to its simplest element, that of interstitial rarefaction, and the gross change of form regarded as a mere accident.

In the tabetic foot, and in the bones which become the seat of spontaneous fracture, this rarefactive change may be seen in its purity; while in the most hypertrophic arthropathy it is rarely if ever absent. It should be considered as especially the trophic lesion; the direct con-sequence of the non-transmission to the nervous centres of the demands for nutritive material. When the bone in which it is progressing happens to form part of an articulation it succumbs to the strains thrown upon it, and to the friction entailed by the movements of the joint; to alterations in structure are now added changes in form. In consequence of the loss of the normal articular surface irritative processes are set up which, if the conditions be favourable, result on the one hand in overgrowth of the synovial membrane, and on the other in hyperplasia of the cartilage and bone at the periphery. As in arthritis deformans, it seems probable that this peripheral hyperplasia is due partly to the conveyance of irritation, partly to the comparative exemption of that part of the joint from pressure. This process it is which constitutes the variable element in nervous arthropathies: in the hip joint where the articular head of the femur is completely embraced by the acetabulum, and where in consequence pressure and friction are evenly distributed over every part, whether central or circumferential, it is practically absent. In the knee the mutual adaptation of the articular surfaces is much less accurate, and varies in degree with the movements of the joint; it is most imperfect about the margin of the head of the tibia which, even during the active use of the articulation, may lie almost or altogether without the zone of pressure. Consequently that part of the articular cartilage and bone becomes the seat of active hyperplastic processes; while the femoral condyles and the central part of the tibial head may be undergoing an equally pronounced atrophy.

The hyperplastic element in a nervous arthropathy may then be considered as of primarily local origin. If it be argued that these indications of reaction to irritative influences and capacity for reparative processes are incompatible with the loss of nervous control many facts can be adduced to refute such a supposition. Union takes place, with the formation of an exuberant callus, in a bone which has undergone spontaneous fracture from nervous atrophy; to borrow an analogy from cutaneous lesions, the trophic corn exists side by side with the perforating ulcer; and the perforating ulcer itself heals readily when it is placed under favourable influences.

But a belief in the local origin of the hyperplastic process need not entail a denial of a nervous factor which may modify the result. Though in their general outline the changes resemble those met with in arthritis deformans, still, as has been already noted, they differ very materially in their extent. In both tabetic and syringomyelic arthropathy an amount of overgrowth is found which may attain the proportions of actual tumour formation, and which is not met with in any other disease; it is possible that this difference of degree is the result of morbid nervous influences, and represents what might be called an ataxy of reaction.

That a difference in the extent of a morbid process may be sufficient to indicate its neurotic origin is seen in the case of hyperpyrexia as compared with pyrexia. Nor is this surprising; the nervous system should be regarded as regulating tissue processes, not as originating them: and when nervous influence is deranged its evidence would be found, not in the occurrence of new pathological conditions, but in the modification or exaggeration of old ones.

Whether in the case in question the supposed nervous derangement be of a paralytic or an irritative nature it is difficult to decide with certainty. There are some reasons for supposing it to be irritative. Some years ago Dr. Buzzard drew attention to the frequency of various visceral crises in cases of tabetic arthropathy. In spite of subsequent contradictions this may now be regarded as the truth, though not the whole truth. There is no doubt that the patients who suffer from what Brissaud calls the sensory form of tabes are especially liable to arthropathies. By the sensory form of the disease is meant that in which irritative symptoms on the sensory side predominate, such as lightning pains and the various crises, while the degree of ataxy may be trivial. Brissaud goes so far as to say that he has never seen an arthropathy in a case of pure motor tabes. In syringomyelia, again, the patients who manifest arthropathies are frequently those who have pain. It is a striking fact, too, that in Friedreich's disease, with the absence of the irritative sensory phenomena of tabes, trophic lesions also cease to appear.

Our conclusions may be summarised as follows :—

1. The fundamental change in both arthropathies and osteopathies is an eccentric atrophy of bone.

2. This is a true trophic lesion resulting from disease of afferent fibres which normally 'form part of a reflex arc by which the local nutrition is regulated.

3. The hyperplastic element in arthropathies is primarily of local origin; but the changes so initiated are modified by a derangement of nervous influences which is probably of an irritative nature.

PART II.—It is impossible to enter upon a description of the trophic lesions other than those which have already been considered, without a strong sense of the difficulty and uncertainty of the subject. The osteo-arthropathies of tabes and syringomyelia are, as we have seen, peculiarly characteristic in themselves, and the spinal diseases with which they are connected are hardly less so : those which follow are to a large extent indistinguishable from other and ordinary affections; and their claims to a nervous parentage extend to every portion of the cerebro-spinal system. One of the chief difficulties in estimating the justice of these claims lies in the fact that almost without exception they are associated with paralysis; and that, as regards the bones at least, the morbid change is identical with that which occurs from disuse alone. It is equally impossible to distinguish the changes which occur in the joints of a paralysed limb from those which may result from an ordinary rheumatic affection. Neither of these difficulties, it is hardly necessary to say, is to be regarded as insuperable, or as excluding a neurotic source for the changes in bones and joints; but together they certainly call for a rigorous investigation in each individual case. In this somewhat chaotic group the lesions which follow injuries or disease of the peripheral nerves stand on the firmest basis, and, taken in this order, will be dealt with first.

TROPHIC AFFECTIONS FOLLOWING LESIONS OF PERIPHERAL NERVES.—
The clinical importance of the changes in the bones which undoubtedly
occur is very slight; owing to the associated paralysis, spontaneous
fracture is hardly ever seen, and subjective indications are completely
absent. The osseous atrophy alters the texture rather than the form of
the bone, and is therefore beyond the ken of the clinician.

Arthritis is a rare occurrence, and is found almost exclusively in
surgical affections; not in those in which the nerve is actually divided,
but where it is compressed or otherwise irritated; as, for example, by a
mass of callus or a tumour. In the classical case recorded by Packard,
arthropathies of the knee and foot followed compression of the sciatic
nerve by a tumour. Chipault found a destructive arthritis of the
elbow in a patient whose brachial plexus was compressed by the callus
formed in connection with a broken clavicle. These, and a few similar
cases, form exceptions to the rule that neurotic arthropathies affect the
small joints of the hand and foot rather than the larger articulations.
Opinions show some divergence as to the character of the articular
lesions, and much more as to their frequency. Chipault, for example,
maintains that changes in the joints are an almost constant result of
injuries to peripheral nerves; most writers, however, though holding
different views as to their nature, agree as to their comparative rarity.
Weir Mitchell describes such joints (which he regards as not uncommon)
as follows :—" We may then have one articulation—and if only one, a
large one—involved; or perhaps all the joints of a finger, or every joint
of a hand, or of the entire limb may suffer. The swelling is never very
great, the redness usually slight, and the tenderness on touch or motion
exquisite. This condition of things remains with little change during
weeks or months, and then slowly declines, leaving the joints stiff,
enlarged, and somewhat sensitive, especially as to movement. A small
proportion of such cases find ready relief; but in many of them the
resultant anchylosis proves utterly unconquerable, so that it is vain to
try to restore mobility by manipulation or splints."

Mr. Bowlby, on the other hand, considers such cases rare; he
has never seen any so acute or painful. The articular lesions which
he has met with are of a more chronic and less severe kind; in his
experience at a period of from one to six weeks after an injury (to the
nerve) the joints will usually be found somewhat stiff but not painful.
Occasionally, however, there is pain, tenderness and swelling. The
terminal condition is one of fibrous anchylosis. Bowlby compares the
whole process to that of chronic rheumatism.

The anatomical changes are—in the first stage; effusion into the
synovial cavity with hyperæmia of the synovial membrane: in the
second, dryness of the synovial cavity, adhesion of the synovial pouches,
and shortening with infiltration of the capsule and the surrounding
structures: in the last stage the condition is one of pseudo-anchylosis
progressive contraction of the capsule, muscles and ligaments which
embrace the joint. In rare cases true fibrous anchylosis may take

place from the extension of the synovial membrane over the surface of the cartilage, with fibrous metaplasia of this structure; but this, when it does occur, is found only after prolonged periods. Almost without exception the bone and cartilage remain unaltered until they have become affected by disuse. The simple fixation of the joint, then, is mainly of peri-articular origin, and undoubtedly may be explained by the effects of disuse alone; but as regards the causation of the subacute synovitis or arthritis observed in an early stage a dogmatic opinion is less ready. They are absolutely indistinguishable from those produced by an ordinary subacute rheumatism; and considering the frequent occurrence of this disease, or congeries of diseases, the danger of mistaking the *post hoc* for the *propter hoc* is considerable. In a case of injury to the ulnar nerve, which came under my own observation, severe pains were complained of in the joints of the affected hand; and it appeared as if a trophic arthritis were in progress: but the appearance of the symptoms on the corresponding articulations of the opposite side soon disproved the direct connection of the articular with the neurotic lesion.

From their peculiar liability to disease it would seem that the joints, even in the normal subject, constitute an area of less resistance; and it is probable that the impairment of the local nutrition in consequence of the injury to the nerve, or more directly as a result of the loss of function which that injury involves, will intensify this lack of resisting power. When we consider the every-day occurrence of injuries to peripheral nerves the sequel of articular changes must be regarded as rare; while in ordinary toxic neuritis it is even more so, if indeed it ever occurs. While then the fact is fully accepted that such a sequence of events may take place, a certain amount of scepticism seems to be called for before the direct causal nexus between two lesions which constantly occur independently can be admitted. At first sight there is no improbability in the supposition that injuries to peripheral nerves can and do set up a trophic arthritis, and there are many facts which go to prove it; yet the frequency of the coincidence is not sufficient in itself to carry conviction; and in the individual case the possibility of other than nervous causes must be carefully considered.

Experimental section of nerves in animals has repeatedly confirmed the existence of the osseous atrophy which has been found under similar conditions in the human subject (Ogle and others); though there is some dispute whether the change results in lengthening or in shortening of the bone (Nasse, Ghillini, Schiff). On the other hand, great difficulty has been found in the artificial production of arthropathies; as Talamon suggests, this is probably due to the fact that for the production of an arthropathy, not division but prolonged irritation of a nerve is necessary; a condition difficult to provide, and still more difficult to maintain.

Trophic affections following lesions of the spinal cord (exclusive of tabes and syringomyelia).—(*a*) **Of Bones.**—Atrophy is a common event, but may nearly always be accounted for by the effects of prolonged disuse. From the associated paralysis it can rarely reveal itself by spontaneous fracture; though some examples of this are on record (Rivington): in some cases it would appear that the change in the bone was the direct result of the nerve lesion, for the limbs in which spontaneous fracture occurred, though not under the influence of the will, were in a state of active spasm, and their general nutrition was excellent. Reparative processes in the bones below the level of a destructive lesion of the cord generally proceed with as much energy as under normal conditions (Rivington). Dr. Ogle, however, has reported four cases in which fractures below the level of a fracture of spine showed no signs of union, while those above united with average readiness.

One lesion of the cord—anterior poliomyelitis—calls for special attention; most pronounced atrophic changes in bones occur in association with that form of it which underlies the disease known as infantile paralysis. It was long thought that this afforded convincing proof that the seat of the trophic centre for the skeleton lay in the anterior horns; under the influence of this belief Charcot sought in these structures for the explanation of the osseous lesions in tabes. The fact that osseous lesions do not occur in the progressive muscular atrophy form of anterior poliomyelitis practically negatives the surmise that the changes which take place in infancy are due to the loss of a specific trophic influence. They undoubtedly depend upon the practical destruction of the muscles at an early stage of growth; the bone, deprived of the normal stimulus which it should receive from the stress and strain of its muscular attachments and starved of its blood-supply by the lack of muscular action, fails to develop.

(*b*) **Of Joints.**—In 1831 J. K. Mitchell recorded instances of arthropathies following Pott's disease of spine; and in 1858 Gull published a similar series. In 1859 Magnier described the same sequel in acute myelitis; and other writers have followed him: it is quite possible, however, that in these cases the joint suffered from infection by the same organism which set up the inflammation in the cord. It will be seen that in the large majority of cases the primary affection of the spinal cord consists either in an injury, such as a stab, or in compression. Examples may be found of the occurrence of arthropathies in progressive muscular atrophy (Prautois and Etienne), or in amyotrophic lateral sclerosis; but they are among the rarities of medicine and, unless the report is quite recent, are valueless on account of the probable confusion with syringomyelia.

The distribution of the articular lesions differs from that which occurs as a sequence of injuries to peripheral nerves in that the larger joints are attacked in preference to the smaller. The character of the arthritis is not essentially different, though there is perhaps a greater tendency to free effusion of fluid. It may take the form of a subacute inflammation with pain and redness, as in rheumatism; or a painless hydrarthrosis may set in to which attention is attracted only by accident. Rarely, as in Riedel's case, actual destruction of the joint occurs; it is interesting to note that the patient in question was still able to walk about, an unusual occurrence in these spinal cord arthropathies. Eight days after the injury—a stab between the first and second lumbar vertebræ—the knee joint is said to have been disorganised. Another exceptional instance is that recorded by Alexandrini, where a fracture of the cervical spine was followed by a hæmorrhagic effusion into all the joints on the paralysed right side. In a case of fracture of the tenth dorsal vertebra, observed by Chipault, both knees and ankles were distended on the fifth day with a considerable amount of aseptic fluid; the ligaments were stretched and the cartilage eroded, but there was no osseous change.

TROPHIC AFFECTIONS FOLLOWING LESIONS OF THE BRAIN.—(*a*) **Of Bones.**—The somewhat frequent occurrence in the insane of fragilitas ossium, leading to spontaneous fracture, has already been mentioned with special reference to dementia paralytica. It is not, however, confined to any particular form of insanity; and, as already stated, is included in the group of trophic lesions with a considerable degree of doubt. There is every reason to believe that the bones share in the degradation of nutrition which is common to every form of chronic mental disease; and, though this may be described as itself a trophic lesion, it is in so general a sense that the phrase ceases to have any meaning. In epilepsy, a disease closely akin to insanity, Vazelle has described a similar series of changes. In the paralysis resulting from various focal diseases of the brain spontaneous fracture has frequently been met with; but not until the limbs had become atrophied from prolonged disuse.

(*b*) **Of Joints.**—The first mention of the occurrence of arthritis in hemiplegia is to be found in an article by Scott Alison in the *Lancet* for 1847. Charcot reported several cases in 1868; Hitzig several more in 1869; and since then there have been scattered publications on the same subject.

Neither the nature, the position, nor the severity of the cerebral disease appears to be a determining factor in the production of arthropathics; so little influence has the amount of paralysis that in one case, reported by Koschewnikow, aphasia was the only paralytic symptom present. Hitzig remarks that the arthropathy frequently affects the less paralysed limb; and that the slighter forms of hemiplegia are more liable to it than the more severe. With regard ·to the former of these observations, it is remarkable that the shoulder is the articulation almost invariably affected; whereas in hemiplegia the arm, as a rule, shows more paralysis than the leg. In all Hitzig's seven cases there were signs of vaso-motor disturbance in the shape of increase of local temperature and œdema. The arthropathy never occurred before the fourth week, and seemed often to be precipitated by the patient leaving his bed. The implicated joints were excessively tender, and on manipulation loud crepitus was heard. Hitzig ascribes the arthritis to local causes, mainly to the paralytic subluxation of the head of the humerus; and compares it to the changes set up by prolonged fixation of a limb.

A more recent writer (Koschewnikow) makes the startling statement that six out of nine hemiplegics under his care manifest arthritis ; in their distribution and character the articular lesions were similar to those recorded by Charcot and Hitzig.

In the few autopsies which have been made (Charcot, Hitzig, Koschewnikow) the morbid changes have always been those of acute or subacute synovitis. Effusion has commonly been absent, and the synovial membrane has shown villous overgrowth and hyperæmia. The peripheral nerves and nerve roots have been found healthy.

Etiology.—Little remains to be said on this point save to notice the atmosphere of doubt by which the hypothesis of an immediate nervous origin for these articular lesions is surrounded. The complete absence of any sort of relation between the characters of the brain affection and the occurrence of an arthropathy seems almost to disprove a direct causal connection. The majority of the patients are at an advanced period of life, when the joints are particularly liable to degenerative changes under any condition which entails disuse or even impairment of function. Disuse implies diminished blood-supply, and in consequence the already impoverished tissue suffers in its nutrition still further. The improbabilities of an interpretation based on the existence of a cerebral nutritive centre are obvious ; a trophic centre which is co-extensive with the whole brain condemns itself.

Space will permit but a passing reference to the possibilities of neurotrophic disturbance in certain diseases mostly of obscure pathology. Osteomalacia seems sometimes hardly compatible with any other than a nervous origin. It has been found in association with syringomyelia, possibly as a trophic symptom of that disease (Moses) ; and may occur in connection with forms of insanity (Crichton Browne).

The osseous changes of osteitis deformans have been connected with degenerations of the spinal cord, but on grounds which seem to be insufficient (Marinesco and Gilles de la Tourette, Leopold Levi) ; the same claim has been made for acromegaly ; and in fact for most of the diseases with the pathology of which we are unacquainted. It is useless to deal further with mere speculations.

H. G. TURNEY.

REFERENCES

1. ALLBUTT, T. CLIFFORD. *St. George's Hosp. Reports*, 1869.—2. BOWLBY. *Injuries and Diseases of Nerves*, 1895, p. 52.—3. BRISSAUD. *Nouv. icon. de la Salpêtrière*, 1894, p. 209.—4. BROWNE, CRICHTON. *Annual Report of the West Riding Lunatic Asylum* for 1871.—5. BRUHL. Essay on Syringomyelia, *Trans. New Sydenham Soc.* 1897.—6. BUZZARD. *Lancet*, vol. i. 1893, p. 473.—7. CHARCOT, J. M. "Sur quelques arthopathies qui paraissent dépendre d'une lésion du cerveau et de la mœlle épinière," *Arch. de phys.* 1868, p. 160.—8. *Idem. Gaz. des hôp.* 1885, No, 12.—9. *Idem. Op. cit.* ref. 2, p. 396.—10. CHARCOT and FÉRÉ. *Arch. de neurologie*, 1883, t. vi. p. 305.—11. *Idem. Progrès méd.* t. xi. 1883, p. 606.—12. CHIPAULT. *Traité de chirurgie, le Dentu et Delbet*, Paris, 1896. t. iii. p. 458.—13. *Idem.* "Complications nerveuses des fractures de la clavicule," *Nouv. icon.*

de la Salpêt. 1894.—14. *Idem.* "Les arthropathies au point de vu chirurgicale," *ibid.* p. 299.—15. FORT. *Thèse de Paris,* 1891.—16. GHILLINI. *Revue d'orthopédie,* 1897, No. 5, p. 325.—17. GUDDEN. *Arch. f. Psych.* Bd. ii. 1870.—18. GULL. *Guy's Hosp. Reports,* 1858, p. 206.—19. HANSEN and LOOFT. *Leprosy in its Clinical and Pathological Aspects.* Trans. by Norman Walker. p. 76.—20. HEYDENREICH and LIOUVILLE. *Bull. de la soc. anat.* 1874, p. 256.—21. HITZIG. *Virchow's Archiv,* Bd. xlviii. S. 345.—22. JÜRGENS. *Berl. klin. Woch.* 1886, S. 851.—23. VON KAHLDEN. *Virchow's Archiv,* Bd. cix. S. 318.—24. *Idem. Op. cit.*—25 KOSCHEWNIKOW. *Arch. f. Psych.* 1892, Bd. xxiv. S. 534.—26. KRÖNIG. *Zeitsch. f. klin. Med.* Bd. xiv. 1888.—27. LEVI. *Nouv. icon. de la Salpêt.* 1897, No. 5, p. 113.—28. LONDE and PERREY. *Nouv. icon. de la Salpêtrière,* 1894, p. 232.—29. *Idem. Op. cit.*—30. MAGNIER. *Moniteur des sci. méd.* 1859.—31. MARIE. "Lectures on Diseases of the Spinal Cord," *Trans. New Sydenham Soc.* 1895, p. 211.—32. *Idem. Op. cit.* p. 217.—33. MARINESCO. *Revue neurologique,* 1894, p. 409.—34. MARINESCO and G. DE LA TOURETTE. *Soc. méd. des hôp.* 1895, June.—35. MITCHELL, J. K. *Amer. Journal of Med. Sci.* 1831, vol. viii. p. 55.—36. MORVAN. *Gaz. hebdom.* 1889.—37. MOSES. *Berl. klin. Woch.* 1883, S. 762. 38. NASSE. *Arch. f. Physiol.* Bd. xx. 1880, S 361.—39. NEUMANN. Diss. *Ueber die Knochenbrüche bei Geisteskranken,* Berlin, 1883.—40. OGLE. *St. George's Hosp. Reports,* vol. vi. 1871-72.—41. *Idem. Op. cit.*—42. PACKARD. *Path. Soc. of Philad.* Oct. 1863 (quoted by W. Mitchell).—43. PITRES and VAILLARD. *Revue de médecine,* 1886, p. 562. 44. *Idem. Op. cit.*—45. *Idem. Soc. de biologie,* 1885, p. 679.—46. PITRES and CARRIÈRE. *Arch. clin. de Bordeaux,* 1896, p. 493.—47. PRAUTOIS and ETIENNE. *Rev. de méd.* 1894, t. xiv. p. 300.—48. REGNARD. *Comptes rendus de l'acad. de sc.* 1879.— 49. RIVINGTON. "Fracture of Long Bones from Slight Causes," *Medico-Chi. Trans.* vol. lxxvi. 1893.—50. *Idem. Op. cit.* p. 180.—51. ROTTER. *Archiv f. klin. Chir.* Bd. xxxvi. 1887, S. 1 *et seq.*—52. *Idem. Loc. cit.*—53. SAWTSCHENKO. Zeigler's *Beiträge,* Bd. ix. 1891.—54. SCHLESINGER. *Syringomyelia,* 1895.—55. SCHULTZE. *Virchow's Archiv,* Bd. xii.—56. SHAW. "Arthropathies in G. P." *Arch. of Med.* New York, 1883.—57. SOKOLOFF. *Arthropathies syringomyéliques,* 1891.—58. STRÜMPELL. *Lehrbuch der speciell. Pathologie,* 1892, Bd. ii. Th. 1, S. 239.—59. TALAMON. *Revue mensuelle,* 1878.— 60. TARGETT. *Trans. Path. Soc. London,* vol. xlviii. p. 288. —61. *Idem. Clin. Soc. Trans.* 1894, vol xxvii. p. 215.—62. THOMPSON. *Edinburgh Hosp. Reports,* 1894, p. 590.—63. TOURNIER. *Revue de médecine,* 1897, p 221.— 64. *Idem. Op. cit.*—65. VAZELLE. *Thèse de Paris,* 1894-95.—66. VIRCHOW. *Berl. klin. Woch.* 1886, Nos. 48, 49, 50.—67. WEIR, MITCHELL. "The Influence of Rest on Locomotor Ataxy." *Amer. Journ. Med. Sci.* July 1873, p. 113.—68. *Idem. Injuries of Nerves.* Philadelphia, 1872.—69. WEIZSÄCKER. *Beiträge zur klin. Chir.* 1887, Bd. iii.—70. WESTPHAL. *Berl. klin. Woch.* No. 29, 1881.—71. ZIEGLER. *Special Path. Anatomy,* Eng. transl. 8th ed. vol. i. p. 272.

H. G. T.

NEUROTROPHIC DISEASES OF SOFT TISSUES

THE nervous system in the normal condition is concerned in adjusting the actions of the body, and ultimately its cellular elements, to the external forces that are constantly playing upon it. The external play of forces may range within considerable limits without straining the powers of internal adjustment; and within these limits they promote the active function of the cellular elements concerned, and thereby maintain and promote the health of the body. But when these limits are exceeded injury or disease must result. As long as a person remains in health his powers of adjustment are prompt in action, from inherited instinct and acquired habit. But with the supervention of nerve disease external forces are no longer estimated at their true value, accurate internal adjustment fails, and thus the road is open to the encroachment of disease.

In the instance of the peripheral sensory nerves, when from any cause they are abnormally irritated, there is a perversion of sensation ; the skin becomes too sensitive, and stimuli that should excite only to healthy action become irritant, and cause pruritus, soreness, or pain. When, from injury or disease, the sensory nerves are destroyed,—as, for example, when the nerve-supply of the foot is experimentally severed in animals,—the insensitive part is no longer able to estimate the forces brought to bear upon it, and becomes in consequence peculiarly liable to disease ; and when the peripheral sensory nerves are degenerated, as in tabes dorsalis, similar trophic lesions may result (*vide* p. 546).

Irritation of nerves, when excessive, will cause the appearance of eruptions, even when the part is protected from external irritation ; but it is difficult to exclude all sources of irritation from a part that is over-sensitive to simple contacts and changes of temperature. When the irritation is chronic, slow changes take place in the structure of the tissues ; which become evident in the altered texture and pigmentation of the skin, in alteration of the epidermal appendages, and in softening of fibrous, cartilaginous, and osseous tissues. Of the changes in the deeper tissues there is proof in the readiness with which joints are sprained and bones are broken with the use of little force.

Tissues deprived of their normal innervation not only become subject to injury in an unwonted degree from mechanical and physico-chemical forces, but they lose also their power of resistance to micro-organisms. Microbes obtain access more readily than before to the cellular tissues, and even penetrate to the deeper structures ; they enter the joints more frequently than is the case in diffuse inflammation where the nerves are intact, and set up suppurative arthritis. Seeing that the insensitive skin is more than usually liable to breach of surface, attacks of diffuse inflammation are of frequent recurrence in such cases. These repeated erysipelatous attacks cause a blocking of the lymphatics, retention of lymph, and consequent hypertrophy of the part,—thus producing a condition of spurious elephantiasis, a state of limb which is favourable to the development of an ichthyotic condition of skin. Areas of hypertrophied papillæ are formed under adherent scales of epidermis and whatever may adhere to them upon the skin of those who habitually neglect the use of soap and water. They may be found on the back, beneath the hanging breasts of fat persons, and in other situations favourable to the retention of warmth and moisture. Areas of such enlarged papillæ, sometimes very extensive, are to be found especially on the limbs of persons suffering from chronic ulcers of the leg. The epidermis, dirty and soddened by the discharges, sometimes presents papillæ projecting like thickly set spines, some of which break off and bleed when the thick encrusting layer of epidermis is detached ; especially in those cases in which the foot is enlarged by solid œdema : finally, the formation of ichthyotic patches is favoured by faulty innervation. Thus three contributory causes of ichthyotic skin may act simultaneously in persons who are the subjects of peripheral nerve degeneration; namely, moist unwashed skin, chronic œdema, and degeneration of associated nerves. The part most favourably situated for the occurrence of these lesions is the foot and leg.

Peripheral sensory trophoneuroses.—Of the trophoneuroses muscular atrophy, the arthropathies are described elsewhere. (See previous art. on Neurotrophic Bone Disease.)

Erythema may follow neuralgia of the fifth nerve, and is frequently seen in the parts supplied by a nerve that has been injured. It may be irregularly distributed in blotches, which sometimes have the appearance of chilblains.

Glossy skin is most frequently found after wounds which have injured the nerves of the part affected; but it may also occur after destructive inflammation or injury, and it generally appears during the period of cicatrisation. The skin is smooth, red and shining, almost free from wrinkles, and devoid of hair. Sometimes it is blotched with patches like chilblains. When affecting the hand the fingers may taper towards their extremities. There are generally tenderness; pain, especially on movement, which extends up the limb; and often subcutaneous œdema.

Urticaria is sometimes of nervous origin, and has been seen to accompany the lightning pains of ataxia.

Eczema may be the direct result of nerve-irritation, and may appear on a part protected from external irritation. It may be papular or vesicular, and the vesicles may be large or small. The vesicles have been seen, accompanied by neuralgic pains, upon the area of distribution of an injured nerve. Eczema, often inveterate, is readily excited on parts subjected to nerve-degeneration. Iodine painted on the part, for instance, or even any simple dressing that tends to retain the perspiration, may set it up; and when so easily excited it proves difficult to remove.

Herpes is a common result of nerve irritation, inflammation, or compression; it is treated fully hereafter ("Diseases of the Skin").

Pemphigus may form rapidly over the area of an injured nerve; and bullæ are sometimes seen upon the backs of the hands and fingers in the last stage of general paralysis of the insane; the parts upon which they appear being devoid of sensation. In such cases the nerves have been found very extensively degenerated.

Ichthyosis may appear locally as the result of nerve degeneration, and may cover a definite area; or the papillæ are found in lines parallel to the nerve-distribution. A congenital form, ichthyosis hystrix, consists of patches arranged in a manner determined by the direction of the nerves, and is confined strictly to one-half of the body. It is accompanied by defective mental development.

Pigmentary changes, that is, irregular distributions of pigment in the skin. Well-defined areas of abnormally white skin are surrounded by parts of a deeper pigmentation than is normal, which is deepest in the neighbourhood of the blanched areas. In some pigmentary diseases

of the skin the parts devoid of colouring matter are arranged in a manner
suggestive of nerve influence, and may correspond closely in distribution
with the cutaneous nerves.   (See Vitiligo, Morphœa, in a later volume.)
In vitiligo degeneration of the nerves supplying the part has been
observed by Leloir.

Epidermal changes.—The epidermis, nails, and hair may each and all
be affected.   The hairs turn white, hypertrophy, become stumpy and
brittle, or fall out.   The nails may be rapidly shed, or a purple discoloration of them, due to effusion of blood between the matrix and nail,
precedes a slower separation.   They may come away from their bed
by progressive detachment from the free edge backwards.   The change
most often seen is a slow alteration in their texture, in which they lose
their gloss, become of a yellow or yellowish brown colour, ridged transversely, curved laterally and longitudinally, and brittle.   Complete
division of nerves gives rise, in a certain proportion of cases, to transverse
ridging of the nails.   The same transverse ridges may be induced by a
severe illness in which the nerves are not particularly involved.   These
changes may extend, beyond the area supplied by an injured nerve, to
other nails ; this may be due to the gravity of a concomitant illness, or
to a neuritis spreading up the injured nerve and involving others.

The epidermis, on parts most pressed upon, hypertrophies and forms
callosities and corns, which may become the source of a series of troubles.
They are usually found of very large size on the sole of the foot, either
on the ball of the great toe or farther outwards ; often in both situations :
but they may occur at any point of pressure, and have been met with on
the hands, where they may give rise to the same series of mischievous
results, presently to be given in detail.   Owing to pressure, the corns,
which are generally large and deep, cause atrophy of the true skin lying
beneath the core, and a sort of bursa is formed between it and the cutis,
which at this spot loses the power of forming epidermis ; while the papillæ
immediately around hypertrophy, and the cuticle is abnormally thick and
abundant.   The contents of the bursal cavity, often sanguineous from
injury inflicted by the hard core of the corn upon the delicate parts
beneath, may be forced by pressure through the softer layers of epidermis, and appear as a bulla at one side, which will burst, and open the
way to suppuration by the admission of micro-organisms.   Pus is apt to
form in the bursa, however, without the formation of such a visible
opening, and, being unable to escape, burrows deeply into the sole of the
foot, and may appear some distance away—often between the toes or on
the dorsum pedis.   If the corn be cut and the bursal sac opened, the part
remaining in this condition is then known as *perforating ulcer*.   This, in
its fully established condition, is a deep, ragged-looking ulcer, surrounded
by a heaped-up ring of epidermis.   A probe from the bottom of it may
be made to penetrate a sinus, which may lead in any direction ; and
sometimes carious or necrosed bone is found.   The discharge is fœtid,
and the foot may be bathed in a cold sweat.   There may or may not be
direct evidence of loss of sensation in the skin ; but, when there is not,

the patient, by the pressure he can bear upon the part, may still betray a deficient sense of pain. For instance, one man was unaware of the existence of suppuration beneath a corn on the sole of his foot, and did not realise that inflammation was present until the dorsum pedis became red and swollen at a point where the pus was appearing; yet when tested his sensation appeared normal. Yet there is generally pain, which may be considerable, especially when the core of the corn presses deeply; and there is a history of shooting pains in the limb at some former period. The recorded cases of perforating ulcer in man did not warrant the description of an acute perforating ulcer; but the following case, now under my care, is a notable one. The skin at the two points of greatest pressure in each foot, the ball and heel, when first seen, presented ulcers of the normal skin; these perforated deeply, but there was no ring of thickened epidermis. One big toe joint was perforated. The evidences of nervous disease in this case are anæsthesia of the ends of both big toes, and auditory hallucinations.

When the ulcer is placed under favourable conditions, provided there be no disease of bone, it heals readily. It is closed by the rapid ingrowth of the epidermis from all sides, the long papillary processes of which give a ragged appearance to its edges. Meeting in the middle, they coalesce and obliterate all signs of the opening. The central mass then dries, and, shrinking away from the surrounding ring of epidermis, cracks, and thus forms a fissure two or three lines in depth, often circular. This, however, does not endure any length of time, as the quickly growing epidermis pressing inwards again closes it; and the corn tends to form a conical projection. If this central mass be cut out a cavity is found beneath it; and its under surface is ragged from the interlacing of the epidermal papillæ. The base of the cavity presents a smooth blue glistening surface devoid of epidermal formation. Suppuration is likely to recur in this bursal sac; and this, together with the rapid epidermal formation, leads to rapid changes in the appearance of the part.

Perforating ulcer, especially after some years' duration, may be found associated with other evidences of nerve-degeneration; and this, together with the results of inflammation, brings about the following appearances :— the skin may be pigmented, or may present an ichthyotic condition, and the nails and hairs may exhibit changes already described : the shape of the foot may be altered, bossy prominences, due to a condition of the nature of tabetic arthropathy, deforming the tarsus : a phalangeal, tarsal, or ankle joint may be suppurating, or a toe absent through a like condition at some former time. The foot is sometimes shortened from loss of bone by caries or necrosis of the tarsus and metatarsus, a result most commonly found in leprosy; or it may be enlarged from repeated diffuse inflammation and resultant chronic œdema.

Besides these local appearances there is frequently evidence of nerve-disease elsewhere in association with it. Perforating ulcer has been observed in locomotor ataxia, Friedreich's disease, general paralysis of the insane, compression of nerves or spinal cord by tumours, peripheral nerve degeneration following neuritis due to alcohol, diabetes, and leprosy ; also after injuries of nerves or spinal cord, and in spina bifida, in which the peripheral nerves were implicated before finally quitting the spinal canal.   In all these various diseases and injuries a common factor, peripheral nerve degeneration, is the condition which, if it do not actively excite the skin lesion that ultimately leads to perforating ulcer, passively permits it through deficient innervation.   In some cases of perforating ulcer the only nerve disease discovered has been degeneration only of the ends of the nerve in the neighbourhood of the ulcer ; and, as this is also found to exist in the case of ordinary corns, it is probable that some cases of perforating ulcer are purely of local origin.

Suppurating corns on the toes of those who are the subjects of peripheral nerve degeneration have a like origin ; and they also may be attended by destructive arthritis, the pus penetrating the joint before it has excited sufficient attention to lead to its evacuation.   The presence of such a condition is in itself enough to arouse suspicion as to the integrity of the nerves ; and not infrequently the sufferer presents unmistakable signs of a failing nervous system.   It has been seen several times in an early stage of general paralysis.

The skin may atrophy, including its papillæ, hair follicles and glandular structures.

Facial hemiatrophy is a peculiar condition in which all the tissues of one-half of the face are wasted, the bones included.   The superior maxilla is most markedly affected.   It generally comes on before the age of twenty.   In one of the very few cases that have been examined after death the fifth nerve was degenerated in all its branches as the result of inflammation of its trunk (see special article, p. 485).

Bedsores, in which faulty nervous conditions are evident, occur especially in injuries and diseases of the spinal cord in which considerable destruction has taken place, especially of the gray matter.   In the last stage of spastic paralysis acute bedsores suddenly come on in those who have been bed-ridden for months and not nursed with great care and skill.   Every part pressed upon in turn becomes purple, so that within two or three days the buttocks, sacrum, and hips may be in a state of incipient gangrene.   Pressure on any part in such cases tends to induce sloughing ; for instance, when the contracted lower limbs press upon one another the femoral artery may thus become exposed and the tibia laid bare.   Bedsores observed very rarely in cerebral lesions, such as hæmorrhage, occur on the buttock of the paralysed side, rather than over the sacrum.   This situation is determined, in many cases at any rate, by the lying of the paralytic upon that side, as he always tends to do ; but the weighty opinion of Charcot must be recorded that some such cases are more exclusively of trophoneurotic origin.   .

Acute bedsores may occur in other than nervous diseases in which there is great feebleness and prostration.   The bullæ which appear upon the heels and elsewhere, to which a nervous origin has been attributed, are of frequent occurrence in the old and feeble ; and depend upon the degree in which the gangrene has affected the skin. If this be not destroyed in its whole thickness bullæ appear; but if it be gangrenous throughout the sphacelus becomes black, dry, and hard; bullæ appearing at its edges.

Painless whitlow affects the fingers of patients suffering from peripheral nerve disease of the upper extremities; and when the ungual phalanx is destroyed a permanent scar and deformity is left. The whitlow is often sub-cuticular, and may give rise to ulceration which progressively destroys a considerable portion of the tissues of the tip of the finger.

Gangrene may be determined by the failure of innervation; thus it occurs sometimes in diabetes, and where the blood supply is in part cut off. When the brachial artery is occluded, and the ulnar nerve severed at the same time, gangrene will occur more readily in the area of distribution of this nerve. Indeed, acute neuritis may alone be the cause of gangrene.

Functional disturbances.—The perspiration in cases of trophic nerve affection of the skin may be excessive, or it may be diminished. When the skin is pale and cold it is sometimes bathed in a profuse perspiration, as in rheumatoid arthritis. All glands are under nervous control, a perversion of which may lead to abnormal abundance or deficiency of secretion; but little is known of the effect of the nerves upon the glandular organs of the skin other than the sudorific.

Pathology.—Mental shock may turn the hair white, and it has been followed also by pigmentary changes in the skin itself. Reflex action has also produced such effects as effusion into joints and affections of the skin. But very little is definitely known of peripheral lesions due to cerebral disease or to reflex action. The conditions here dealt with are due to a perversion or loss of the normal innervation of a part, either through irritation of a nerve in some part of its course from its proximal distribution in the spinal cord to its peripheral terminations; or to more or less impairment or loss of nerve function through injury or disease of the nerve or of the spinal cord at its seat of origin. Many of the conditions found in peripheral nerve degeneration that have been detailed above are not the result of nerve influence, but are due to the absence of it. Apart from external irritation, the effect of lost innervation is atrophic in character; but where the play of external forces is permitted hypertrophies sometimes result, as is the case in the formation of perforating ulcer with its ring of overgrown epidermis in animals whose sciatic nerve has been experimentally cut across; and it is probable that hypertrophy of the skin papillæ has a like origin. When, in addition to the loss of innervation and the injurious action of external forces, there is decreased resistance in the tissues themselves, in consequence of a general dyscrasia or other internal cause, the way is open to an increased activity of the injurious processes; as in the example given above of gangrene following neuritis in diabetes.

Treatment.—As, when there is a perversion of normal innervation, injury is likely to follow external irritation or the incidence of even

normal mechanical or other forces, special care is needed to protect the
affected parts.   In irritation an over-sensitive skin would prompt to this ;
· but in the absence of normal sensation the patient is exposed to many risks
of which insensitive parts can afford no warning.   These parts need to be
economised in their use, and to be protected from wear and tear as much
as possible.   The parts most exposed, generally the lower limbs and
especially the feet, may be relieved of pressure and jar by suitable boots,
thick felt beneath the soles, a knee prop when one foot is affected,
or crutches.   Blisters, excoriations, and corns should be guarded against ;
and scrupulous cleanliness is needed to avoid microbic invasion.   When
joints or bones are invaded, surgical interference may become necessary ;
but amputation is to be regarded as a last resort, for the stump is
likely to become affected in its turn.   A stronger exception must be
made to the removal of toe joints, which often recover under treatment
by antiseptic foot-baths.

JOHN HOPKINS.

REFERENCES

1. BOWLBY. *Injuries and Diseases of Nerves,* chap. v. "Trophic Changes caused
by Nerve Injury."—2. COHNHEIM. " Lectures on General Pathology," *Pathology of Nutrition,* vol. ii. New Sydenham Society.—3. DUPLAY and MORAT. *Arch. gén. d. méd.* vi.
serie, tom. xxi. 1873.—4. LELOIR. *Twentieth Century Practice of Medicine,* vol. v. art.
"Dermatoneuroses."—5. PITRES and VAILLARD. *Arch. d. Physiol.* v. 1885, p. 208.—
6. SAVORY and BUTLIN. *Trans. Medico-Chir. Soc.* 1879, vol. lxii. pp. 273, 384.—
7. SCHWIMMER. Ziemssen's *Handbook,* art. "Special Path." xiv.

J. H.

ADIPOSIS DOLOROSA

By·the kindness of Dr. Dercum I was enabled to see and to examine in
Philadelphia the case upon which his first description of this disease
was founded.   I also saw a second and more recent case in his wards.
The first case, in a woman of some 55 years of age, presented clearly
enough the group of signs and symptoms described by the author ; the
other case was less far advanced, but plainly of the same kind.

I was satisfied that the condition is sufficiently definite and peculiar
to need a separate description, and a name.

As defined by Dercum (4), adiposis dolorosa is a disorder characterised
by irregular, sometimes symmetrical, deposits of fatty masses in various
portions of the body, preceded by or attended with pain.   It appears
at about middle life or later ; and the larger number of cases reported
have occurred in women.   In some there has been an alcoholic history,
in others a syphilitic history ; in others again rheumatism has been an
antecedent factor ; and it is said that bodily injury may be a provocative

agency. Nothing more definite, however, can be said of the causes. The principal manifestation is the presence of masses of fatty tissue of variable size, sometimes exceedingly large, variously distributed upon the trunk and the extremities, and the seat of pain, sometimes spontaneous sometimes induced by pressure or manipulation. The affection may set in with pain of neuritic character; and the swelling may undergo increase of size in paroxysms attended with exacerbations of pain. The new fatty tissue often has a boggy, soft, at times pultaceous and worm-like feel; or harder, slippery, fatty tumours may be rolled under the hand. Face, hands, and feet are not invaded. In some cases sensibility is impaired. The skin exhibits no obvious change. Hæmorrhages from mucous surfaces have been observed in some cases. The disease is essentially chronic, with a tendency to be progressive in course. The morbid anatomy consists, so far as is known, in an increase of fatty and connective tissue, with degenerative changes in nerves. The thyroid gland has been found indurated and calcareous. The disorder differs from other forms of obesity in its partial and lumpy distribution, in the presence of pains, and sometimes of impaired sensibility; and from myxœdema in the freedom of face, hands, and feet, and in the absence of the pronounced mental and trophic manifestations of this disease. In treatment good results have been attributed to the use of thyroid extract and of massage. A few cases have been put on record by other observers.

EDITOR.

REFERENCES[1]

1. COLLINS. "Adiposis Dolorosa," art. in *Text-book on Nerv. Diseases* by American authors. Ed. Dercum. Phil. 1895.—2. DERCUM. *University Med. Mag.* Dec. 1888. —3. *Idem. Amer. Jour. of Med. Sci.* 1892.—4. *Idem. Twentieth Century Practice*, vol. xi. p. 554.—5. ESHNER. "Case of Adiposis Dolorosa," *Phil. Med. Jour.* Oct. 8, 1898. —6. EWALD. *Berl. klin. Woch.* Jan. 21, 1895.—7. HENRY. *Journal of Nervous and Mental Diseases*, March 1891.—8. SPILLER. *Medical News*, Feb. 26, 1898.

ED.

RAYNAUD'S DISEASE

Local syncope; Local asphyxia; Symmetrical gangrene.

Definition.—Raynaud's disease comprehends three clinical groups of cases; namely, local syncope, local asphyxia, and symmetrical gangrene; and these three groups have the following features in common, namely :—(a) a temporary but recurrent morbid alteration in the blood-supply, and in the consequent nutrition of the extremities, and in some instances also of certain internal structures; (b) circulatory and nutritive

[1] To Eshner I am indebted for this list of references.—ED.

VOL. VI   2 P

changes generally affecting similar parts on the two sides, though the changes are not necessarily equal in extent on both, and, exceptionally, the final manifestation may even be unilateral; (c) a spasmodic and recurrent contraction of the arterioles—as is generally maintained—supplying the parts concerned and causing the morbid changes. It is presumed that there is no primary organic change in the walls or lumen of the blood-vessels adequate to explain these results.

Historical note.—Maurice Raynaud published his thesis on local asphyxial and symmetrical gangrene of the extremities in 1862; and his final contribution on this subject appeared in the first volume of the *Archives de médecine* for 1874.

Before Raynaud's time there had been a frank recognition of many cases of spontaneous gangrene in which no tangible occlusion of blood-vessels, either from thrombosis or embolism, could be established; obscure examples, arising as complications of typhoid and other exanthems, and in various morbid blood states like diabetes, had been recorded, and suggestions had even been made that lesions of the nervous system might play a part in the causation of some of these cases. But Raynaud gathered together observations on simple phenomena like "dead fingers;" on cases of recurring attacks of paroxysmal blueness of the extremities; and, finally, on examples of limited benign forms of superficial gangrene in all of which symmetry was a marked feature. He showed how these three groups of symptoms were associated, and that the gangrene was often the final outcome of the other two. His contention was that the one feature common and essential to these three morbid states is a spasmodic and frequently recurrent contraction of the walls of the arterioles supplying the extremities concerned. Since the publication of Raynaud's final contribution, there have been several additions to knowledge more or less cognate to his subject; and in some directions new researches, especially on peripheral neuritis, may somewhat modify the interpretation of some of the cases which he would have included : on the other hand, certain observations have widened the scope of his original contention. It would appear best in this article to summarise the views of Raynaud, as originally stated by him, and then to show how far they require modification. The physiological basis on which it may be said that Raynaud's disease rests is the change which takes place on the surface of the body, and especially at its extremities, as the result of temporary exposure to cold. Local syncope has its analogue in the condition of simple pallor which is the result of contraction of all the surface vessels concerned, and which leaves the superficial tissues exsanguine. In the temporary blueness or cyanosis of the surface, which may also result from exposure to cold, there is contraction of the arteries with partial venous stasis—and this is the analogue of local asphyxia.

In both these conditions we assume the contraction of the vessels to be a reflex act ; the result of a sensory excitation of the cutaneous nerves, and an efferent impulse from the vaso-motor centre in the cord determining contraction of the walls of the arterioles. The nearest analogue to the symmetrical gangrene with which we are concerned is frost-bite, in which a limited death of end structures is the result of prolonged or rapid exposure to severe cold, whereby the blood-supply is suddenly arrested.

LOCAL SYNCOPE.—The simplest form of this morbid state is the phenomenon commonly known as "dead fingers." In such an attack complete pallor of corresponding fingers of the two hands occurs rather suddenly. The index, or little finger, of each hand may be solely affected; or more than one finger of each hand may suffer: when this is the case the invasion of the other fingers may be either contemporaneous or progressive; and if progressive the same order is generally maintained. Much less commonly the whole hands up to the wrists, or indeed the lower part of each forearm also become involved.

The toes and feet may suffer likewise; either separately, or contemporaneously with the upper extremities.

In the mild cases there is only slight discomfort in connection with the attack, namely, during the pallid stage, a little pain which is compared to cramp; but the chief complaint is of a slight difficulty in the performance of small movements. The patient may be unable to grasp, or sew, or pick up small objects; and in like manner some slight difficulty may be experienced in straightening the toes. The extemities look thin and tapering, and the finger-tips are occasionally wrinkled, as in the algid stage of cholera. The surface temperature is lowered and there is generally some modification of sensation. Of these modifications analgesia is most common; but the tactile sense is blunted, although the difference between heat and cold is still appreciable. The radial pulse is frequently unaltered, but in some recorded cases it became small and scarcely perceptible; it is in the small arteries and arterioles, as a rule, that the important alteration occurs; that there is temporary abeyance of the blood current is shown by the fact that, in severe cases, no bleeding ensues when punctures of the affected extremity are made with a lancet.

The duration of the attack varies between wide limits; it may last but a few minutes, or, in severe cases, several hours. In the mild cases there is little to mark the end of the attack beyond the return to normal temperature, colour, mobility, and bulk of the extremity concerned; but in the severe cases the reaction is attended with burning pain. The arterial pulsations become very manifest (especially if the pulse has been feeble in the pallid stage), the extremities become hot, and the skin of a dull red colour. There is then great intolerance of pressure and a craving for cold applications or exposure to cold air. During the reaction stage perspiration sometimes occurs on parts of the extremities affected.

Recurrence of the attacks of local syncope is often very regular. Thus in the simplest form of "dead fingers" the subject of the complaint expects the familiar phenomenon before, during, or after the morning bath; and it only vanishes with the morning meal.

More severe forms of the affection, which disable for a time and render the sufferer a virtual invalid, often occur in a cycle of two or three months' duration; during which period an attack may set in regularly at a given hour in the day. So striking is this periodicity that the suggestion of malarial origin is not surprising. But it is noteworthy, during one of these cycles, that there is not only a recurrence at the same hour, but also a daily increase in the number and severity of the attacks; then a gradual diminution in number down to a vanishing point, when immunity returns for a varying interval.

It is astonishing how little constitutional disturbance may accompany these attacks, except some degree of exhaustion dependent on the pain and, in bad cases, on the sleeplessness. The general nutrition often suffers remarkably little.

Local syncope is more common in the colder than in the warmer months of the year. Attacks, mild or severe, are often precipitated by exposure to cold air or cold water; but in one of the cycles of the severe form of the affection the most insignificant difference—as, for example, to pass from one room to the other—may determine an attack; and the occurrence of a chilly day in the middle of warm weather may start a cycle of attacks. Yet lowering of the surrounding temperature is but one of the determining factors: a certain number of those who suffer from the malady in its mild form experience it, with or without a general feeling of chilliness, during the period which succeeds the taking of a full meal. Such persons are often the subjects of slow digestion; nevertheless the liability to mild attacks of this kind is quite compatible with considerable bodily vigour and endurance.

Raynaud was inclined to lay stress on the neurotic side of local syncope; and it is undoubted that the severe forms are more commonly met with in women than in men, and especially in those who manifest hysterical phenomena. Certain recorded cases appear to have been initiated by a violent emotion, and others by traumatism in a way precisely analogous with what occurs in some functional paralyses. Amongst the multiform manifestations of neurasthenia attacks of local syncope are by no means uncommon.

In one case the malady supervened on a condition of exhaustion after severe diarrhœa and prolonged "nursing." Mental distress or fag have also been recorded as antecedents. There is no very obvious relation to menstruation, though in some cases the attacks have coincided with amenorrhœa. In one case a woman found her liability to attacks of local syncope completely disappear with the commencements of her successive pregnancies. Although generally symmetrical, there are rare cases in which local syncope is predominantly, and, perhaps, exclusively one-sided; a notable example of this kind is recorded by Graves. Even in such cases, however, if care be taken to observe the attack throughout, a lesser degree of the affection on the side apparently healthy may often be found, either preceding or succeeding the chief manifestation.

The ultimate prognosis of the mild cases is not grave. The affection is regarded by the person subject to it as a sort of habit of the circulation which he accepts or ignores. As already stated, moderately severe cases with their neurotic accompaniments often go through a cycle with gradual increase in frequency and severity of the paroxysms, and then subside and ultimately disappear. But there are rare cases of local syncope in which the paroxysms gradually tend to lengthen, till at last, though there are exacerbations, there is scarcely any true interval; these cases sometimes end in terminal gangrene. Such cases will be considered hereafter, and likewise the treatment of local syncope in general.

LOCAL ASPHYXIA.—Local asphyxia, in common with local syncope, has these characters—that it is an affection of the extremities of the body; that the attacks are paroxysmal and recurrent; and that there is symmetry in the parts attacked. Raynaud was inclined indeed to regard it as a later stage of local syncope. An attack may begin, after exposure to cold water or cold air, with pallor of the affected extremities; but this initial pallor is frequently of very short duration, so short that the observer may fail to see it, the first really striking feature being the sudden appearance of duskiness of the skin of the affected parts.

A simple characteristic case which affects both hands and forearms affords the best opportunity of watching a paroxysm from beginning to end. There are a good many variations in the series; but either the whole hand becomes dusky, or certain fingers are picked out, the colour change beginning at the tips and advancing proximally. The march of the paroxysm may be from finger to finger; then gradually the hand becomes invaded up to the wrist and, with lessening severity, along the greater part of the forearm up to the elbow, but rarely above it. The fingers of both hands may be affected simultaneously, though not to an equal degree. Sometimes one hand becomes affected first, and a definite interval of time elapses before the attack begins in the other. The colour varies within considerable limits; purplish red, slate blue, indigo, and the colour of blue-black ink are tints which are often noted.

The nails become extremely dark from the subjacent colour change in the matrix; and, when individual fingers are picked out, the contrast with those not affected is very striking.

Simultaneously the affected parts become extremely cold to the touch. In one of Raynaud's cases there was a difference of fifteen degrees between the temperature of the palm and that of the axilla. The pain is, as a rule, much more severe than that of local syncope, and often makes the patient moan or scream. Throughout a prolonged attack there are decided remissions and exacerbations, suggesting alternating and varying spasms of vessels with varying effect on nerve endings. Pressure of any kind is often unbearable. The tactile sense is diminished, but, on account of the pain and restlessness, it is very difficult to test it. There may be analgesia to a superficial pin-prick, but by a deep prick pain is elicited. There is recognition of the difference between heat and cold, and cold is often preferred to heat. The patient may be unable to grasp small bodies, such as a pin; and there is some temporary difficulty in the performance of the finger movements. The veins on the back of the hand, wrist, and forearm show marked distension as the general blueness of the surface increases up to its maximum; and a curious livid marbling along the sides of the veins is often to be seen on the proximal side of the limit of the deep coloration. In one case, which I observed during the march of the paroxysm, portions of the veins on the back of the hand become quite moniliform; that is to say, there was an alternation of small dark swellings with narrow, almost colourless, intervals between them. Whilst under observation the dark swellings gradually altered their position along the course of the veins, pointing to a varying contraction of the walls of these vessels. As with local syncope, the radial pulse may remain unchanged during the attack, or may become smaller in volume; if the subsequent reaction be severe the pulse then becomes full. In some cases during the paroxysm a slight tumefaction of the fingers and of the back of the hand occurs, which is in fact a slight degree of œdema.

The area of temporary whiteness of skin, which can always be produced by firm pressure on the hand, remains obvious during the paroxysm for a much longer time than normal; showing the excessive slowness of capillary reaction.

As in attacks of local syncope, there may be a sudden outbreak of moisture over the whole hand near the end of the attack. The duration of a paroxysm may be from one to six or seven hours.

The subsidence of the paroxysm may be sudden; more commonly it is gradual. The finger first affected generally leads the way in the return to normal colour; but the change may start on the back of the hand instead of on the finger-tips. Islands of less deep blue appear, gradually unite, and by degrees replace the dark area; but there are often curious remissions in this process, blue and red areas appearing alternately. Ultimately the whole extremity becomes deep red, and for a varying time feels quite hot; sometimes the radial pulse becomes full. One finger-tip may remain blue for a time when the rest of the hand is red; but the œdema may continue for a couple of hours, or for half a day, after the paroxysm is over. This, however, is exceptional; the early return to the normal state is the rule. The temperature in the mouth is often unaltered during a paroxysm; but subsequently a very slight pyrexia may ensue. In a protracted case (that of a woman aged 45) under my own care the mouth temperature during an attack was sometimes normal; sometimes 97·6° F.; rarely a little above normal (99° F.). In the evening after an attack, and sometimes next day, the temperature occasionally rose to 100° or 101° F.

In rare cases a little desquamation over the extremities of the digits occurs for a few days after a severe attack. During the colder months a paroxysm of the kind described may be induced, in one who is subject to such attacks, by going out of doors, or by putting the hands into cold water. But it may also be precipitated by some emotional disturbance; in one case it occurred after a fright, and simultaneously with the sudden arrest of the menstrual flow. It may occur during convalescence after parturition, especially if the patient have been poorly fed or badly nourished. An attack of choleraic diarrhœa may determine it. As with local syncope, the attacks sometimes come in cycles; and, during a cycle, passage from one room into another, in which the temperature is a little lower, seems sometimes to induce an attack. Again, in summer weather a sudden drop of temperature seems likewise, in a predisposed person, to determine an attack. But when a cycle is established the attacks are apt to begin at the same hour for several successive days, independently of any obvious determining cause. Also, they gradually increase in frequency or duration, or both, so that several occur in the same day; then by degrees the attacks become less frequent and less severe, till they come to a vanishing point; and once more the patient has immunity for a longer or shorter interval.

In those who are liable to attacks of local asphyxia there is considerable variation both as to frequency and duration. A single solitary attack may occur, or a cycle may last for a few days, or for a week, or for two months. The more severe cycles last from two months up to ten months; but in them, as well as in some of the shorter cases, symmetrical gangrene frequently occurs, a condition which will be discussed separately. The foregoing may be taken as the description of the simplest form of local asphyxia as it affects the upper limbs; but it is to be noted that other parts may be affected in like manner. Thus the lower limbs are affected at least as often as the upper, and corresponding toes are often picked out; the local asphyxia sometimes extends to the heels, above each ankle, or even up to the knees. The alteration of sensation is not so marked in the feet as in the hands. Occasionally during the attack the patient is unable to recognise the nature of the surface on which he stands; or, when the attack is fairly established, even to stand at all; in one case, however, under my own care, some impending attacks were warded off by prolonged and vigorous walks. In some instances all four extremities suffer, either simultaneously or in succession. Raynaud has pointed out that in persons who suffer from attacks not always of identical distribution, if all four extremities are affected the incidence is not so severe on any one of them as when two only are concerned, or one only. Also (as in local syncope), though symmetry is observed, there is sometimes great inequality in the incidence of the affection on the two sides; so that at certain stages it may be described as unilateral.

The helix of the ear may suffer, either simultaneously with the feet or hands or, in some cases, without the invasion of these members. In rare cases the nose is affected. The zygomatic regions may also suffer, and occasionally the nates and the front of the thighs. When the areas of local asphyxia in the same individual are multiple some of them may be almost painless.

Reddish purple, round, or oval areas on the limbs sometimes appear in proximity to the sites of the local asphyxia. They may be raised and painful, presenting some resemblance to erythema papulatum or erythema nodosum; but they sometimes affect the deeper layers of the skin also, present no obvious elevation, and give rise to no pain. The latter form is persistent for many weeks, and leaves curious pigmented patches behind it. It is more common in the cases which go on to gangrene; occasionally indeed these "*tachetées*" (as they have been called by French writers) become themselves the site of a limited gangrene, as in one of Dr. Southey's cases. Possibly the cases described by Dr. Cavafy as symmetrical congestive mottling may be milder examples of the same condition.

With respect to deeper structures the occasional occurrence of slight œdema has already been mentioned. This œdema may continue for half a day after the subsidence of the paroxysm.

Raynaud observes that in some of his cases there was fibrous ankylosis of terminal phalangeal articulations, and some thickening along the processes of the palmar fascia, which persisted between the paroxysms but ultimately vanished with the other signs of the disease. I have notes of a case in which the same association and the same sequence occurred.

SYMMETRICAL GANGRENE. — Raynaud described local syncope, local asphyxia, and symmetrical gangrene as three successive stages of the same malady. In a broad way this series may be accepted, but it requires a little qualification: for, in some cases, gangrene supervenes upon attacks of recurring cyanosis of the extremities; in others the dominant character is local syncope, in which the fingers are subject to paroxysms of pallor, bloodlessness, and pain; and by degrees these conditions become almost constant, the digits assuming a more and more parchment-like and tapering appearance, and gangrene supervening rather suddenly, without any definite intermediate attacks of local asphyxia (vide Fig. 29). In both forms the glacial coldness of the extremities becomes very pronounced and continuous, and the pain is almost unbearable. Small bullæ may form first on one extremity, then on another; the bulla breaks and gives exit to a little blood-stained fluid; it then collapses, and a small black epidermic layer covers the area which becomes gangrenous. The process is generally definitive in the sense that the extent of the gangrene is limited, or nearly limited, by the boundary of the small area on which the bulla forms. The blackened epidermic layer forms the top of a hard, thickened eschar, around which arises a zone of ulceration which leads to the gradual separation of a sequestrum of skin. The bed of the nail is often involved, and the nail separates, either wholly or in part; and a new nail grows which may be somewhat deformed. Though the

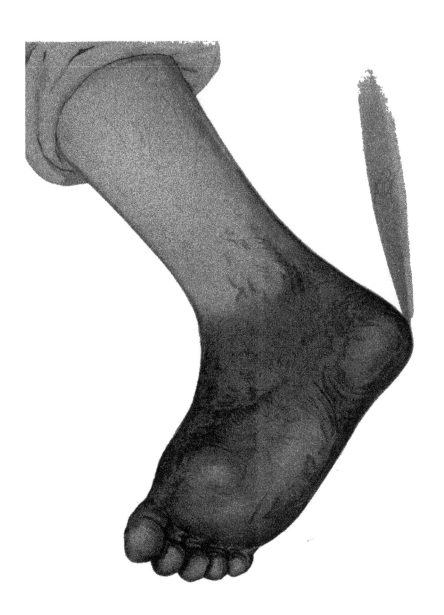

PLATE I.

Foot in case of Raynaud's disease. Drawing made during attack of local asphyxia.

Girl aged 5 years. Attacks began when 3½ years old in the month of February. She had been carried out in somebody's arms, and was wearing at the time woollen stockings and boots. When brought in to the house complained of cold. The feet were blue and the blueness extended up to the ankles ; it lasted for seven hours.

She vomited, but nothing else remarkable was observed. Next day she played as usual. From this time she was liable to repeated attacks in the winter after exposure, but also in the house if she sat about much. The attacks did not occur whilst the child was in bed.

In a typical seizure one foot becomes suddenly blue, beginning at the toes, extending to the ankle. The veins on the dorsum and lower part of the leg are slightly distended. Both feet suffer, but to an unequal degree, one foot being attacked a little later than the other. Both feet are stone cold. In other attacks the hands and forearms are affected as well as the feet.

Distension of the veins of the dorsum of the hand and of the forearm is very marked. In one attack varying contraction of the veins was obvious to the naked eye. Dark knotty swellings appeared with almost colourless intervals between them. The knotty swellings altered their position along the course of the veins during the progress of the paroxysm.

During the paroxysms the radial pulse is only just perceptible. Between the attacks there is no indication of any alteration of the arteries whatever. The pain begins with the onset of the blueness. During the earlier and middle stages of the attack, the child screams when the hand or foot is touched. During the later stage she is often lethargic. When the attack is subsiding, mottled areas of less intense blueness become manifest in the middle of the dorsum of the hand and foot ; successive digits become less blue ; ultimately the extremity becomes pink and to the observer's hand feels hotter than natural. The attacks observed in hospital were seldom longer than two hours' duration ; occasionally they lasted only half an hour. The body temperature (axilla and rectum) was normal in some of the attacks, but rose a little in the evening and on the next day (100° F. and 101·2°). Hæmoglobinuria was not present. The child was observed during several winters. No sign of vascular or nerve disorder appeared. She derived great benefit from galvanic treatment during the paroxysms.

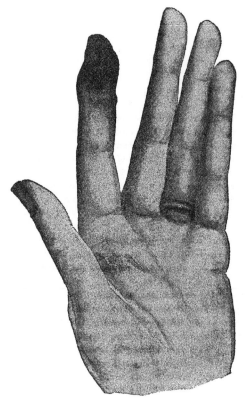

FIG. 29.

Symmetrical gangrene of tip of both index fingers following attacks of local syncope.

The patient was a delicate lady in poor circumstances who had suffered much trouble. When first seen in May 1885 she was 44 years old. The only point of importance in her history was that fourteen years previously she had lived in Mauritius for four years, and suffered severely from ague. During the last thirteen years she had lived at an English seaside place, and there was no evidence that she had had any distinct malarial attack.

During the previous winter she had suffered from dead fingers on rising, some fingers being worse than others. At these times she had the usual clumsiness of local syncope and was unable to close her fingers. Later on in the day she could sew, knit, and play the piano as usual. The tip of the tongue and the lips felt numbed during cold weather, and in a cold wind she complained that her lips became so stiff that she could hardly speak.

She was a pale, pinched, poorly-nourished woman with some pigmentation of the face. The lips, nose, and ears were thin and waxy looking, and the finger ends tapering, · pale, and cold with a very slight blue tint at the extremities.

There were no gross vascular signs, and no signs of peripheral or central nervous disease. The viscera were normal and the urine was natural. In the beginning of December she appeared again, having been comfortable during the summer, but with the onset of the cold weather her symptoms had returned in an aggravated form. The fingers as before were thin, pale, and tapering, and very slight contraction was beginning to appear at the terminal joints. The extremity of the left index finger was in a state of gangrene. Two-thirds of the palmar surface between the tip and the normal transverse groove were black and mummified, and on the dorsal surface a groove was forming round the nail, but only the distal half of the matrix was black. The gangrene was almost dry and was free from any smell of decomposition. (The drawing was made a fortnight later when the granulating margin of the line of demarcation had become obvious.) There was no anæsthesia except at the extreme tip. The slight atrophy of the hand was general, there was no picking out of any group of muscles.

The radial arteries were well and equally felt ; they were not at all tortuous and did not roll under the finger. They were perhaps small, but the patient was a small woman and had small limbs.

The right hand resembled the left in every respect except the gangrene ; but this began to threaten, sixteen days subsequently, in an identically similar spot on the tip of the right index finger. The progress of the gangrene was like that of the left finger. Although by the end of two months the pain had ceased, six months had elapsed before the cicatrisation was complete. There was no separation of bone, and the ultimate appearance of the fingers was as though the extreme tips had been cut off with a knife, leaving, however, the proximal half of the matrix of the nail, so that a small nail was reproduced.

Although the gangrene had not been averted, the patient's general nutrition, as well as the nutrition of her extremities, had been greatly improved by galvanism, shampooing, Turkish baths, rest, and nourishing food. She continued these remedies with gradually lessening zeal, and got through the next winter without any recurrence of gangrene. But next spring she showed some thin scaly areas over all the projecting points of her upper extremities, and the hands felt cold, dry, and a little stiff and horny. Dry scaly areas appeared also on the margins of the ears, and now the chest walls began to show the hidebound condition of scleroderma. This gradually increased, and next year she died.

The details of her last illness were not obtained beyond that she became progressively marasmic.

gangrenous process may extend down to the bone it is quite exceptional for any necrosis of the bone to take place. The scar which is left after complete cicatrisation may indeed be very small, but the tip of the affected finger remains tapering in form.

In some cases the process is even more benign than that which has been described. No bulla forms, but the extremity shows a gradual mummification, and a small blackened area slowly separates by a quiet ulceration, leaving exceedingly little deformity.

The process of gangrene may affect several finger-tips, or only a single finger-tip on the two hands. The affection may be either simultaneous or successive.

When the toes are affected the lesions are often confined to the plantar surface, and the separation of the sequestrum of skin is more quickly effected than in the fingers; the nails frequently escape, and the toes do not present the tapering shape which is so characteristic of the affection of the fingers. Some months subsequently, on examining the plantar surface of toes which have been attacked with this form of gangrene, the only abnormalities found are small white scars, such as might have resulted from cutting away a small slice of the true skin.

Raynaud speaks of the nose and external ears being threatened, but he had not seen mortification of these parts. A definite loss of the substance of some part of the margin of the helix occurred, several times, in two cases of local asphyxia which were under my own care. One of these is delineated in the accompanying figure (Fig. 30).

Besides the benign cases which have been described, there are others, of which Raynaud quotes exceptional examples, in which the spontaneous gangrene affects larger portions of the extremities, as far up, indeed, as the wrists or the ankles, or even the knees.

Diagnosis of the foregoing diseases.—From the pallor of chlorosis local syncope is distinguished by its being a local and paroxysmal rather than a general and persistent condition.

Local asphyxia cannot be distinguished from the effect produced in a solitary instance by frost-bite or exposure to extreme cold. We are rather concerned with a recurrent paroxysmal habit of the circulation, the phenomena of which are often determined by an insignificant lowering of temperature, or even by a mere emotional disturbance. From the signs in the extremities which characterise a case of congenital heart disease it is easy to distinguish those which belong to local asphyxia; the blueness of the extremities in a case of morbus cæruleus is an exaggeration of the general cyanotic colour of the body; but, moreover, there is marked clubbing or bulbous condition of the finger ends, the toes, and the nose. In local asphyxia there is no general blueness; the lips and tongue are remarkably free from this change of colour; the finger ends are either tapering or, in rare cases, the seat of a temporary œdema, and they are seldom clubbed, or but slightly so: furthermore, the intermittency of the blueness of the

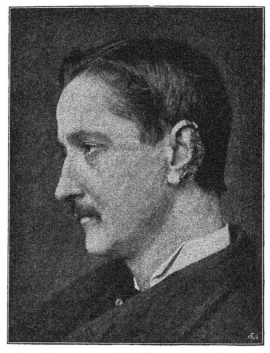

FIG. 30.

Ear of a man, aged 30, who was the subject of Raynaud's disease with recurrent attacks of symmetrical gangrene. On the helix, antihelix, and in the fossa between them, there is a surface to a considerable extent black and gangrenous, with a sharp cut edge and a few scanty granulations from which there is some bleeding. The other ear is not so severely attacked, but shows signs of past loss of substance and a recent thin black edge of gangrene and some indolent granulations. There is some patchy pigmentation of the cheeks.

The man had lived at the Cape for a few years, and "whilst working his way up country" had suffered for three weeks from what was considered a malarial illness. In December 1885 he came home by long sea route, and when sailing round Cape Horn he felt the cold severely, and suffered from burning pain at the edge of both ears. Then a black spot appeared which was followed by some loss of substance. Every winter since then he has been liable to burning attacks, followed ultimately by black areas of gangrene on the edge of each ear.

His vulnerable time is from November to April. Since his return to England he has had three attacks of what is assumed to be ague with definite shivers; each attack has lasted two days. Otherwise his health has been good. He says that on some occasions he has passed dark urine. That which was examined at the time of one of the gangrenous attacks showed no trace of hæmoglobin or of albumin.

The edge of the spleen could not be felt.

extremities is characteristic. When Raynaud's first observations were published peripheral neuritis had not been studied with the complete methods of pathological and clinical research which have subsequently been brought to bear upon it; but Raynaud pointed out that the anæsthesia and the paresis of local asphyxia are too transient to be the outcome of primary and permanent changes of nerve trunks and their branches; and that the pains of local asphyxia and of its later phase, symmetrical gangrene, are not propagated along recognised nerve paths. Local asphyxia is often confounded with chilblains; but in the latter the more or less circumscribed areas of dull red colour are generally situated at some little distance from the very ends of the digits affected; they are somewhat swollen, they present some degree of actual inflammatory exudation, and, although they come and go, their duration is not paroxysmal: in all these respects they differ from areas of local asphyxia. Symmetrical gangrene, in its proneness to mummification, resembles some of the quiet forms of senile gangrene; but it differs in several ways. (i.) As to distribution: senile gangrene is limited to a single limb, or, if it affect more than one limb, the lesions are successive in order. The lower limbs are more frequently affected than the upper; while in symmetrical gangrene, as the name indicates, corresponding extremities are attacked simultaneously, and the upper limbs quite as commonly as the lower. (ii.) As to extent: symmetrical gangrene is typically limited to the skin and the sub-cutaneous structures, whilst senile gangrene is generally more profound, either affecting a whole toe or a great part of the foot. (iii.) As to progress: symmetrical gangrene is more definite than senile gangrene. It frequently attacks the extremities of several toes on both sides at once, or after a short interval; these become superficially gangrenous in isolated spots, and the gangrene does not extend beyond the areas at first invaded. Senile gangrene, on the other hand, tends to be serpiginous; it begins at a single point, and spreads to an in-determinate extent. (iv.) As to the state of the arteries: in senile gangrene there are generally indications of atheroma; the vessels which supply the limb are cord-like, and often the arterial pulsation in them is much diminished, or even obliterated. In symmetrical gangrene of Raynaud's type no alteration of the arterial walls can be detected, and the arterial pulsations are generally quite distinct. (v.) As to the age of the patient: in symmetrical gangrene many of the cases have occurred in quite young persons, even in children, subjects in whom the factor of arterial degeneration, in the ordinary sense, does not arise.

In respect to the embolic origin of certain cases of gangrene it may be pointed out that such cases differ from Raynaud's disease in that they are rarely symmetrical, and that a source of emboli may be found either in damaged cardiac valves or in cardiac thrombi. Nevertheless Raynaud, amongst rare contributory causes of symmetrical gangrene, admits valvular defects, and congenital narrowing of the aorta and of the systemic arteries. I have had under my own care one example in a child, the subject of cardiac disease with great enfeeblement of systemic circulation, in whom local asphyxia and limited symmetrical gangrene of fingers of Raynaud's type appeared, and in whom the autopsy failed to yield evidence of embolic obstruction; such cases are, however, very rare.

Phlebitis, when it leads to gangrene, gives rise to the moist form of this lesion; and not to the limited symmetrical manifestations with which we are now concerned.

As a rule, it may be taken that there is no naked-eye change in the heart or large vessels to explain the phenomena of the symmetrical gangrene of Raynaud's form.

In diabetic gangrene we have either a lesion which is primarily traumatic or inflammatory, and which runs on to acute rapid necrosis; or one in which premature arterial change, or trophic nerve disturbance, plays an important part.

Raynaud's disease bears a strong resemblance to ergotism. Although we have a large mass of detailed statement concerning the toxic effects of ergot in the way of gangrene, yet the anatomical descriptions of the arteries in fatal cases are singularly meagre. Raynaud made several attempts to estimate the effects of toxic doses of ergot on some of the lower animals, but failed to obtain any results in the least comparable with the form of symmetrical gangrene with which we are concerned. In two of his clinical cases rye flour had been used for a time in the diet, but there was no evidence that the rye was infected. Another case was that of a woman who was confined in November, and in February began to suffer from local asphyxia, which was ultimately succeeded by gangrene of the finger-tips; this patient had taken a gramme and a half of ergot during her labour, but the interval between this and the appearance of the symptoms of local asphyxia was surely too long for us to suppose that the drug had played any part in their production. In the other cases ergot, as a possible factor, could be excluded with tolerable confidence.

Nosological affinities.—The most interesting of the later observations lead to a wider conception of the morbid processes concerned, and first amongst these comes Raynaud's own discovery that occasional *temporary alterations in the fundus oculi* alternate or coincide with manifestations of local asphyxia in the extremities.

In his last memoir Raynaud relates the case of a man, aged fifty-nine, with no relevant antecedent, except intermittent fever thirty-five years previously, who in the month of December began to suffer from local asphyxia of the fingers of one hand, and in the next month of the fingers of the other hand; then the feet were affected, and then disturbances of vision set in: when he came under observation he had very cold hands and indurations of the flexor tendons; and he exhibited intermittent attacks of local asphyxia on going out into the air or on bathing his hands in cold water. The feet were affected likewise, but less severely. The heart was normal, the radial pulse and the pulse in the posterior tibials and arteries of the feet were perfectly perceptible, and the arteries were not indurated. The eyesight was good in both eyes during the attack; but during the period which followed, and whilst the fingers were returning to their normal colour, the sight, especially that of the left eye, became dimmed—to recover, however, at the onset of a new attack. Ophthalmoscopic examination of the left eye during a period of reaction,—that is to say, when the cyanotic colour of the extremities was at its minimum,—showed that "the central artery of the retina and its branches had very clear contours, and that they were definitely narrower round the papilla than at the periphery; here and there was a sort of partial constriction, the papilla was very clear; the veins were the seat of remarkable pulsations a little later than the radial pulse." . . . "The central vein dilated and elongated itself so notably in the region of the papilla as to simulate a small aneurysm, but the pulsation was also visible in the smaller veins." In the right eye there were similar phenomena, but less well marked. The ophthalmoscopic examinations were verified by Galezowski. Under a course of electrical treatment, to which reference will subsequently be made, the patient recovered from the local asphyxia of the extremities, and also from his visual troubles; finally, the ophthalmoscopic examination revealed nothing abnormal.

The second case was in a young man, aged twenty-two, who was admitted into hospital with diabetes insipidus. He had local asphyxia of the upper extremities, and some blueness likewise of the face; his attacks, which were more common in the early morning, became well marked when he went out into the air, the blue regions of the skin becoming excessively cold. During the attacks the radial pulse was very small. "At the commencement of the cyanosis the patient complained of a notable obscuration of sight, which disappeared when the face and hands returned to their natural colour." Dr. Panas observed that at the beginning of the cyanotic attack the "arteries of the fundus oculi were definitely narrowed," and that "when reaction occurred they became widened." "The retinal veins were turgid, but presented no appreciable pulsation."

In the striking case of symmetrical gangrene of the fingers recorded by Weiss, there was considerable generalisation of these processes; for not only were there extensive transitory changes in the joints, to which reference will subsequently be made, but also remarkable eye phenomena, referred by him to the cervical sympathetic. As in Raynaud's first case of amblyopia, these phenomena occurred in attacks which alternated with some of the seizures of the extremities. For several days the patient had "retraction of one eyeball, narrowing of the palpebral fissure, contraction of the pupil with no reaction to light, and a slight degree of ptosis." . . . "At the same time there was reddening of the zygomatic region and of the external ear of the same side, some elevation of temperature, and hyperidrosis." . . . "As this attack subsided there was a little superficial gangrene of the skin of the zygomatic region in the shape of some small patches of first brown and then blackened epidermis, which ultimately separated." There were several attacks of this kind affecting the left side of the face and left ear, and some affecting the right side, and at times both simultaneously ; but only on the left side were the eye phenomena well marked. Weiss thought that the eye phenomena depended on ischæmia of the cilio-spinal region of the cord.

In a case of Mr. Hutchinson's, to be subsequently mentioned, there was iridoplegia on the left side : the pupils were large and unequal, the left being bigger than the right, and they were motionless, both to light and accommodation ; they contracted under the use of Calabar bean. The vision was good.

With regard to the generalisation of the malady, the next observation of importance is that of the occasional association of hæmoglobinuria with Raynaud's disease. It is strange, indeed, that Raynaud himself should never have noticed this connection. The first suggestion of it is found in the history of a case recorded by Mr. Hutchinson as far back as 1871. A woman, aged thirty, had suffered during the winter from frequent shivering fits after exposure to cold ; these attacks were accompanied or followed by general malaise, and the urine often became dark after them. One cold day, after returning home, her nose and left ear were found to be quite black, and small superficial sloughs gradually separated from these spots ; but during her stay in the hospital no blood was noticed in the urine. The patient also had iridoplegia.

Dr. Robert Druitt, in 1873, in recording his own case, maintained that he suffered from " obvious ague attacks, and also from distinct attacks of hæmatinuria related to cold, exposure, and worry." He describes these attacks as being associated with "numbness, tingling and blueness of the extremities, the blue patches being at times suggestive of imminent gangrene."

In 1879 Dr. (now Sir Samuel) Wilks recorded the case of a patient, aged sixteen, who had profuse suppuration from the bursa between the gluteus maximus and the great trochanter, which had followed some injury to the hip. When the boy was transferred to Dr. Wilks' care he was cyanotic in certain regions, and there was a systolic murmur at the third right space. The margins of the ears, the nose, and the toes became very blue ; and the tips of the thumbs and of several fingers became affected with gangrene, from which they slowly recovered. The urine was often dark in colour and gave the guaiacum test. Débris and granular casts were present, but blood corpuscles could not be found on several occasions when looked for ; at a later period, however, some blood corpuscles were present.

Dr. Southey, in 1880, described a case of symmetrical gangrene of the legs, and local asphyxia of the fingers, of Raynaud's type. Whilst under observation in hospital a trace of albumin was noted in the urine, but there is no record of the presence of hæmoglobin. Inquiry into the previous history of the patient elicited that she had passed black urine with some of the attacks in which the fingers became numb, black, and dead. In Dr. Southey's second case of local asphyxia and symmetrical gangrene (1883) intermittent hæmaturia occurred on several days after exposure to cold. It is recorded that the "blood was usually very apparent by its dark colour and the obvious sediment that it gave, but its presence was at times only detectable by the guaiacum reaction." Oxalates usually either preceded or accompanied the hæmaturia. There seems little doubt from the above account that the case was one of hæmoglobinuria.

The present writer, in 1883, recorded three cases of Raynaud's disease, in one of which there was typical hæmoglobinuria. The patient was a girl who, when three and a half years old, in the month of September, had her first attack of coldness and blueness, with pain affecting one foot, and lasting for several hours. Very soon after this attack began the child passed some very dark urine. She had repeated attacks during the following winter and spring; sometimes two or three during the week, with a duration generally of not more than three hours. The attacks occurred more commonly when the child went into the open air, but they also occurred indoors; they never appeared in the early morning, nor whilst the child was in bed. The usual time of the attack was about mid-day. There was complaint of pain before the coldness and blueness were noticed. The child did not pass dark urine with every attack, and never more than once with each attack. Along with the above symptoms she complained, on some occasions, of pain at the pit of the stomach; and in one attack the left hand became cold and blue up to the wrist. When she came under observation in February and March she was, for a time, having attacks daily; sometimes twice a day. The stomach symptoms usually preceded the pain, blueness and coldness of the feet, by an interval of two hours, though sometimes they succeeded these phenomena. The stomach ache was referred to the tip of the ensiform cartilage. There was no pain in the loins; the local asphyxia was quite typical, affecting sometimes one foot, sometimes both feet up to the ankles, sometimes both feet and one hand. The more widely-diffused attacks were less severe in duration and pain than the limited attacks. The dark urine was more common after limited than after diffuse attacks. Dark urine appeared within an hour or two of the local asphyxia; it was acid in reaction, and, on boiling, revealed but one-tenth of albumin, which came down in granular form, and was unaltered by the addition of nitric acid. There was a deep blue reaction with the guaiacum test. The deposit under the microscope showed no blood corpuscles, but brown granular pigment and crystals of oxalate of lime. The urine gave the characteristic spectrum of methæmoglobin. The urine, after some attacks, showed a copious deposit of lithates, but gave no reaction with the guaiacum test, and was free from albumin. There was no evidence of visceral disease; the spleen was never found enlarged, and there was no sign of disease of the blood-vessels. The child had never suffered from ague.

I then pointed out the marked parallelism between cases of intermittent hæmoglobinuria and characteristic cases of Raynaud's disease—
those, that is to say, in which the local asphyxia is paroxysmal, with
return to a normal state between the attacks. Neither are truly periodic,
but both are paroxysmal; and in both affections the attacks have a
remarkable relation to changes of temperature. By far the greater
number of cases of both affections occur in winter or cold weather, if
not exclusively at any rate primarily; and when the warmer weather
appears if the attacks do not vanish they notably diminish. In both
the attacks may be accompanied by some abdominal pain and slight
pyrexia; both may be followed next day by sleepiness, and by a
certain sallowness of complexion and of the conjunctivæ. It is rare for
intermittent hæmoglobinuria to occur when the patient is in bed, and
this exemption is also observed in many typical paroxysmal cases of
Raynaud's disease. I suggested that possibly other visceral paroxysmal
affections might be found, in these conjoined cases, comparable with the
temporary enlargement of the spleen sometimes found in cases of
hæmoglobinuria.

This suggestion I have verified in a recent, unpublished, case under my
own care. A young man was subject in cold weather to typical attacks
of local asphyxia of the four extremities and of the ears, with recurrent
gangrene of the margins of the helix on both sides. Some of these
attacks were associated with hæmoglobinuria, and with enlargement of the
spleen and slight pyrexia, followed on the next day by a little yellowness
of the conjunctivæ and sallowness of the skin. The question of malaria
was considered, as the man had lived for a time in a malarial district;
but the most careful examination of the blood during the paroxysms
showed no evidence of plasmodia.

Dr. Dickinson, in 1885, in his work on *Renal and Urinary Affections*,
Part III., is even more sweeping in his identification of these two diseases.
He holds that the two conditions "seem so to approach each other and
mingle as to make it impossible to make a distinct demarcation between
them." The most striking case narrated by Dr. Dickinson as bearing
on this point was that of a girl who was under observation in the
hospital for typical attacks of intermittent hæmoglobinuria. On one
occasion her usual attack was replaced by an attack of paroxysmal local
asphyxia affecting one hand, unattended by the usual alterations of
the urine.

Dr. John Abercrombie (1886) recorded a case of a boy who was
liable to attacks of local asphyxia affecting the hands, legs, cheeks, and
ears; and who in some of his attacks passed urine with sp. gr. 1023,
which contained one-tenth of albumin, gave the guaiacum reaction, and
showed amorphous material and oxalates, but no blood corpuscles. Dr.
Abercrombie suggested that paroxysmal hæmoglobinuria and Raynaud's
disease are of the same nature, and that the jaundice sometimes found
after the attacks of hæmoglobinuria is the result of arterial spasm of the
hepatic vessels. This is a debatable doctrine; but there is much to be

said in favour of the discoloration being due to the breaking up of hæmoglobin in the blood-current elsewhere.

Some reference must be made to the observations on the blood in cases of intermittent hæmoglobinuria. It is well known that, during an attack, blood drawn from a cold extremity shows marked changes in the corpuscles; they do not form rouleaux, they become extremely crenated, and granular masses appear in the serum. Murri maintains that corpuscular destruction occurs in the superficial vessels, and that arterial spasm is an essential factor. Boas found that corpuscular changes could be discovered in the blood from the finger of a certain patient, the subject of paroxysmal hæmoglobinuria, if the finger were put into iced water. Fleischer blistered one of his hæmoglobinuria patients during the inter-paroxysmal period, and found that after a paroxysm had occurred hæmoglobin could be discovered in the serum of the blister.

In the foregoing observations no special attention was directed to the question of local asphyxia of the extremities; but Dr. Myers recorded a case in 1885 which was singularly complete in this connection. A boy, aged seven years, when recovering from measles, suffered for the first time from paroxysmal hæmoglobinuria.[1] About the same time the ears became subject to attacks of coldness and blueness, and of aching as they became warm at the close of the paroxysms. Subsequently gangrene occurred on the margins of each ear; and there were several relapses, either of slight gangrene or of local asphyxia, during successive winters. The attacks of paroxysmal hæmoglobinuria continued, being more frequent in winter than in summer. Blood withdrawn during these attacks from the cyanosed ears, and from the hands, showed the following changes:—The coloured corpuscles showed an abnormal disinclination to form rouleaux; sometimes had crenated edges, and sometimes were fairly normal in outline. "Blood flakes" were found varying in colour from deep reddish black to a thin transparent red, and in size from about four to ten times as large as a normal coloured corpuscle.

Drs. Colman and Taylor, in 1890, recorded a case of Raynaud's disease not associated with hæmoglobinuria whilst under their observation, in which however there were local changes in the blood. A girl, aged ten, had attacks of local syncope of the fingers of the right hand, and sometimes of the left as well, preceded by pain behind the sternum. The blood carefully drawn from the fingers during the attack presented the following changes: "There was distinct coloration of the liquor sanguinis, the tint of the film being about half the depth of that of a healthy blood corpuscle, many of the red blood corpuscles were shrivelled

---

[1] The paroxysmal attacks in some cases, but by no means in all, were accompanied by a slight rise of temperature (to about 100° F.) for a few hours; after the attacks there was slight but distinct icterus, lasting as a rule about twenty-four hours. The spleen was very slightly enlarged, but no definite temporary enlargement during the paroxysms has been established.

and irregular, the projections being much blunter and less regular in size and form than the crenations seen in specimens of blood that have been allowed to evaporate." . . . "Some corpuscles were nearly normal in shape but quite colourless, whilst several were completely collapsed, and what appeared to be fissures could be seen in their walls." . . . "The individual white blood corpuscles were normal, but appeared to be relatively increased in number. There was no increase of hæmatoblasts, nor were there any blood plates." . . . "To check these observations blood was taken from an unaffected finger of the left hand, and also from the lobule of the ear." . . . "These specimens were completely normal."

Mr. W. G. Spencer, in 1892, recorded the case of a boy, aged thirteen, who, after sleeping two nights, in the month of February, in a van, with two other boys, was brought to hospital with dry gangrene of the ungual phalanges of all the toes of the left foot, and of those of the second and third toes of the right foot. No other boy suffered. Although it was stated that the circulation in the extremities had previously been good, yet inquiry elicited that, from the age of one year upwards, the boy had complained much of pain in the loins and between the shoulders whenever the weather was cold ; and that upon these occasions he passed urine as dark as port wine. When the boy was brought the day was cold, and he passed some urine which was dark coloured, gave the guaiacum reaction, but contained no red blood corpuscles. Although this case is described as one of frost-bite, it seems fair to regard it as a case of Raynaud's disease with hæmoglobinuria.

The skin.—Urticaria (brought on by a chill) is mentioned by Dr. Southey as occurring during some of the paroxysms in one of his cases ; and the same skin affection after exposure to cold has been recorded in paroxysmal hæmoglobinuria by Dr. Dickinson, Dr. Stephen Mackenzie, and Dr. Forrest. There are several cases on record showing the connection between Raynaud's disease and scleroderma. M. Ball, in 1871, reported the case of a woman who, for five years, during the winter, had suffered from hard yellowish patches on the extremities of the fingers, which subsided in the spring. She was liable to attacks, during which there was much pain, redness, ulceration, loss of substance, and tardy cicatrisation at the tips of the fingers ; the toes were affected also. M. Ball recorded this as a new variety of scleroderma ; but there was no trace of scleroderma in other parts of the body, and the case was claimed by M. Raynaud as a chronic form of local asphyxia and symmetrical gangrene. Dr. Colcott Fox has mentioned that in two of his cases of scleroderma, in which the hands were attacked, there had been for a long time a liability to dead fingers. "One of these cases continued to suffer from mild attacks of local asphyxia of the fingers after the onset of the scleroderma."

Dr. Finlayson records the case of a man, aged thirty-six, who had well-marked scleroderma of hands, feet, legs, front of chest and abdomen, neck and face. This patient was much influenced by exposure to cold ; he ultimately suffered from gangrene of the fingers and toes, for which no sufficient explanation was forthcoming at the necropsy. I had under my own care a lady in whom the succession of events was the reverse of that which occurred in Dr. Finlayson's case. The patient had typical attacks of local syncope of the finger ends, ending in symmetrical gangrene of the tip of each index finger; she recovered, but the fingers presented the atrophied, tapering, parchment-like character described by Raynaud, with very slight contractions of the last phalangeal joints; she was subsequently attacked by extensive scleroderma of the chest walls, and died marasmic.

The joints.—Raynaud referred to fibrous ankylosis of the terminal phalangeal articulations, and to thickening along the processes of the palmar fascia; and showed how remarkably such thickening may clear up on recovery from local asphyxia. Dr. Wardrop Griffith has recorded three cases of Raynaud's disease in which marked contractions occurred, with limitation of movements and some shortening of muscles. Mr. Hutchinson has described a group of cases which he calls "last joint arthritis"; these he believes to be related to Raynaud's disease.

Sometimes the larger joints are affected; in Dr. Southey's second case, during one of the attacks, effusion occurred in both knee joints. Dr. Weiss (1882) has given us a long series of observations on a case of symmetrical gangrene under his care. In the early attacks only the finger joints suffered; but in the later ones the left knee, the right elbow, the right shoulder, and the right wrist were affected. Weiss's summary is as follows :—"There was effusion in the joint cavities and infiltration of connective tissues above and below the joints; once there was synovitis of the metacarpo-phalangeal joint of the right middle finger followed by tendo-synovitis of the flexor tendons of this finger." . . . "On one occasion there was effusion into the knee joint associated with exudation into the cellular tissue of the thigh and knee. Sometimes the joint effusion was preceded by pain, in other cases it was painless." . . . "The swollen joints and the swelling of the soft parts were not specially tender to pressure. The skin was only reddened once, namely, in the case of effusion into the shoulder joint; the temperature was not raised at the outset, and the course was afebrile throughout." . . . "In most cases absorption was rapid, and the constituent parts of the joints returned to the normal state." Weiss, accepting frankly the view of the central origin of Raynaud's disease, was inclined to regard these joint affections as mild forms of an arthropathy dependent on some temporary change in the hypothetical joint centres of the cord.

Cerebral symptoms.—Many of Raynaud's cases were of neurotic proclivity. One of them was admitted to the Salpêtrière with "epileptiform attacks and notable alteration of intelligence and incoherence of ideas." In Dr. Southey's third case (1883), a boy aged nine, there were maniacal attacks in the early part of the illness, when gangrene of one finger tip was already present. Probably the severity and long continuance of the painful attacks, especially in poorly fed marasmic subjects, may be responsible for a certain amount of temporary mental instability. In a case under my own care, a middle-aged woman, during slight remission of her attacks of local asphyxia, became the subject of recurrent headaches, and of delusions which were always worse in the evenings, not unlike those associated with alcoholic neuritis. Removal, to an asylum was considered, but after a time she made a complete recovery. In another case of severe local asphyxia of the hands with threatened gangrene (in a young woman under my own care), marked chorea with maniacal delusions occurred. Dr. Southey has informed me that, since the publication of his papers, he has seen many asylum cases "which presented manifestations of local asphyxia." During one phase of the illness in Weiss's case, ataxic aphasia, without paralysis of limbs, appeared.

Spinal cord and Peripheral nerves.—The advance of histological research since Raynaud's time has led to more detailed investigation of the nervous structures in cases of gangrene; but it is open to question whether some of the cases in which extensive changes of these structures have been found would have been admitted by Raynaud, on clinical grounds, as belonging to the groups defined by himself.

Pitres and Vaillard (1885) narrate two cases with extensive changes. The first was that of a young woman, aged twenty-four, of feeble intelligence from childhood, who at eighteen began to suffer from tremors and stiffness of limbs with subsequent contracture and dementia. After a time the feet became cold, blue and insensitive, and then gangrenous; the left foot undergoing spontaneous amputation, and the right becoming almost separated. Many eschars appeared in various parts of the body, some of which suppurated; and the patient died from exhaustion. On necropsy the tibial arteries were seen to terminate in a cicatricial cul-de-sac, which was surrounded by fleshy granulations. In no part of the arteries of the lower limbs were adherent thrombi found, but soft clots only. The aorta and its branches and the veins of the limbs were healthy, and the viscera showed nothing special. There was chronic hydrocephalus of the lateral ventricles, some adhesion of pia mater to the cortex, and much thickening of the skull. There was a slight diffuse sclerosis affecting the whole of the antero-lateral columns and the greater part of the posterior columns in the dorso-lumbar region. The spinal ganglia and nerve roots, so far as they were examined, were normal. "The nerve trunks of the upper limbs and of the thighs were normal, the anterior and posterior tibials of both sides presented changes which were fairly symmetrical; these changes were extensive atrophy of nerve fibres with empty sheaths presenting numerous nuclei, and at intervals varicose dilatations which contained masses of granular protoplasm and drops of myelin." . . . "Between the fibres in many places there were leucocytes filled with small granules, and presenting the aspect of Gluge's corpuscles."

In the second case—that of a woman aged fifty-six, who for six months suffered from inability to feel the ground on which she trod—

bullæ had formed on the soles of the feet two months before admission. Subsequently the feet became swollen, painful, and covered with reddish patches on the dorsal surface; fresh bullæ formed, and there was complete anæsthesia over considerable areas of both feet. Gangrenous areas formed across the middle of the tarsus on both sides, and death followed from exhaustion. On necropsy, neuritis of the plantar and tibial nerves was found; but the vessels of the limbs were normal, as also were the brain, spinal cord, and other viscera. Pitres and Vaillard met the objection that the neuritis might have been consecutive to the gangrenous process, by giving the results of an examination of peripheral nerves in a case of embolic gangrene in which they found the nerves normal throughout. The only remark to be made about the above cases is that they did not conform or even approximate to the clinical type described by Raynaud; for example, in these cases there were extensive areas of persistent anæsthesia related to the neuritis, and possibly playing some part in the production of the gangrene.

Mountstein (quoted by Hochenegg, 1886) describes the case of a man, aged fifty-one, on whom amputation of the right leg in the upper third was performed, on account of gangrene of the foot, which had begun two months before. The necropsy showed many calcareous plates in the posterior tibial artery, but no adherent thrombi. The small vessels close to the gangrenous focus had only minute thrombi in them. The posterior tibial nerve showed interstitial neuritis, especially near the gangrenous area; and in the left (sound) lower limb similar changes were found in the posterior tibial nerve. Brain and cord were anæmic, and the examination of the viscera was negative. The clinical record is not adequate to show that this was a case of Raynaud's disease.

Hochenegg (1886) reports a case of a man, aged fifty-one, who had gangrene of the left hand with no obvious vascular disease. The necropsy showed chronic hydrocephalus and syringomyelia; there was but a slight degree of atrophy in the peripheral nerves, and this he regarded as secondary to the cord lesion. Hochenegg held that the gangrene was caused by the central lesion.

Dr. Wiglesworth (1887) has recorded a case of extensive peripheral neuritis in a woman, aged twenty-six, who was the subject of epileptic dementia and of chronic Bright's disease. She had suffered from repeated attacks of spontaneous gangrene of the fingers and toes, and presented extensive atrophy of the muscles of both hands. The sciatic, internal popliteal, external popliteal, posterior tibial, median and ulnar nerves on both sides, and the musculo-spiral on the right, were examined. Most of them showed overgrowth of connective tissue, with atrophy and degeneration of nerve elements. The spinal cord showed only a slight general thickening of the neuroglia, and some alteration of the posterior vesicular columns of Clarke. Dr. Wiglesworth held that the gangrenous areas were dependent on the nerve changes.

Dr. Affleck (1888) gives the results of the examination of the internal plantar nerve and the blood-vessels in a foot that was amputated for gangrene, which had followed attacks of pain and local asphyxia. The blood-vessels were normal, but the nerve showed extensive neuritis.

Rakhmaninoff (1892) describes a case of disseminated multiple neuritis, in a young man aged seventeen, following an attack of typhus fever two years before the patient came under observation. There were coldness and numbness in the hands and feet, twitching in the muscles of the hand and forearm, severe pains in the limbs, in the chest, and in the abdomen, much hyperidrosis of the body, redness and swelling of the dorsum of each foot, extending up to the ankles, and the lower parts of the feet became livid blue. A line of demarcation formed round the ankles, and amputation had to be performed below the knees. At the necropsy, besides pleurisy, pneumonia, and splenic enlargement, thickening of the vessels of the limbs, with narrowing of the lumen, was demonstrated. There was also neuritis in the nerves of the upper and lower limbs, rather in the small branches than in the trunks.

A case is recorded by Dr. Handford (1890) of disseminated myositis and neuritis, probably of alcoholic origin, in which at one time there was limited dry gangrene of the tips of the thumb and index finger. Although no autopsy was obtained, there could be no doubt about the neuritis; as there were extensive areas of persistent anæsthesia, and, besides remarkable thickenings of certain muscles, much atrophy also. But the limited areas of gangrene supervened on a process of sudden acute œdematous swelling, which was quite unlike Raynaud's disease in its course.

Dr. Samuel West (1889) obtained a necropsy in a case of Raynaud's disease in which there had been recurrent attacks of local syncope and local asphyxia of the hands and feet, and a purplish erythema of the face, which became blue and livid, especially at the tip of the nose and on the ears, when the attacks of blue fingers appeared. This purplish erythema was accompanied by a certain amount of branny desquamation. The patient died of an intercurrent pneumonia. On microscopic examination the radial artery at the wrist, the median and the radial nerves, were found normal. The spinal cord was normal.

For several years I had a man under observation who, in successive winters, presented typical Raynaud's disease in both feet. He had, first, attacks of local syncope in the left heel, subsequently in the toes, and then in corresponding parts of the other foot. He was able in part, and for a time, to ward off these attacks by sharp walking; and when the warmer weather came they diminished in frequency and severity. During the second winter the attacks assumed the character of local asphyxia of the toes, he presented blue patches (tachetées) on the thighs, and subsequently on the buttocks; and his finger ends became very cold, but not blue. He then had a little gangrene limited to the tips of the second and third toes of the left foot. In the succeeding winter, when his paroxysmal attacks returned, he was greatly benefited by the daily vigorous galvanic treatment to be described hereafter, and thus was enabled to resume his work. By the use of galvanism and shampooing during cold seasons he did well until the winter of 1886-7, four years after he had been first seen; then, he and his wife having become careless with regard to these measures, his malady gained upon him; the toes of both feet became very blue, and, in the spring of 1887, gangrene became imminent in the left foot and rapidly extended to the ankle. There was suppuration, the patient became extremely exhausted, and amputation in the middle third of the thigh was accordingly performed. The patient made a good recovery. The stump was carefully examined in respect of nerves, arteries, and veins: the nerves were quite healthy, the arteries were free from calcification or atheroma, but there was a definite thickening of all three coats, and a remarkable contortion and infolding of the elastic lamina. The walls of the veins were also thickened. For two years the patient had no serious recurrence of vascular trouble, though he still suffered from local asphyxia of the right foot; then, rather suddenly, gangrene supervened in the right foot, but less severely than in the former attack. The right leg was likewise amputated in the middle third; the patient made a good recovery, and has been in moderate health since.

Reviewing this case, there seems little doubt that it was primarily a case of Raynaud's disease. The attacks were paroxysmal; almost restricted to the cold weather; improved by going to bed; relieved by vigorous exercise, and almost cured by galvanism and shampooing: moreover, they were unaccompanied by clinical evidences of neuritis; that is to say, such atrophy as occurred was general, and did not pick out special groups of muscles. There was no reaction of degeneration, nor was there any persistent localised anæsthesia. As the attacks became very chronic the nutrition never really recovered itself between the paroxysms; and it would appear, in the light of the subsequent anatomical investigation, that the case approximated to one of Friedländer's obliterative arteritis. In this disease, as pointed out by Friedländer, the veins undergo thickening and narrowing as well as the arteries. It seems reasonable to suppose that ultimately recurrent spasmodic contractions of the vessels may at length bring about a permanent alteration in the walls and lumen.

Relation to diabetes.—Dr. Colcott Fox narrates a case of a man, aged fifty-one, who suffered from local syncope and local asphyxia of the fingers, and threatenings of gangrene of one great toe; besides some symmetrical gangrenous sores over the junction of each middle and lower third of the shins. The man proved to be the subject of diabetes; and Dr. Fox mentions that only in one of Raynaud's reported cases was this disease present, and that the local asphyxia in that case preceded the first definite diabetic signs by eight years. It seems probable, with regard to symmetrical gangrene following upon paroxysmal attacks of local asphyxia, that the association of diabetes is accidental; in the benign form, at all events, the progress is quite different from diabetic gangrene as commonly observed.

Relation to ague.—Raynaud does not appear, in his early memoir, or in his "new researches," to have considered the possibility of any connection between the disease which he described and malarial fever ; but in two of his earlier cases (VI. and VIII.) local asphyxia appeared a fortnight after an attack of tertian ague. The first patient described in his "new researches" had suffered from ague thirty years previously. In Raynaud's article on gangrene (40) he says, that "although, after repeated attacks of intermittent fever, œdema of the limbs, with or without thrombosis, may often be observed, no examples are known of gangrene special to the malarial cachexia." This is far too sweeping a statement. Several cases of local syncope, local asphyxia, and gangrene have been recorded as occurring in persons who either were suffering from ague at the time, or had suffered from it. Petit and Verneuil (1883) have given a complete review of the subject ; the forms of gangrene described by them are very varied. Some of them resemble the variety which has been found as a complication of different exanthems, and these are not strictly comparable with Raynaud's type. But there are others, indistinguishable from Raynaud's cases in that they occur in young subjects, are symmetrical, terminal, dry, and limited. It would seem, moreover, that in some cases, both of local asphyxia and of gangrene, there was some response to the use of quinine.

M. Mourson (1880) is inclined to place the local asphyxia of malarial subjects alongside some of the anomalous central and peripheral nerve affections which occur as sequels and "larval" forms of ague.

I have had four cases of Raynaud's disease under my own care, in which there was reason to believe, from the history, that previous malarial attacks had occurred. In one of these (*vide* p. 595), during the paroxysms of local asphyxia, symmetrical gangrene, and hæmoglobinuria, although the spleen was enlarged, no plasmodia could be found, and no benefit resulted from prolonged use of quinine and arsenic ; in the other cases there appeared to be no other indication of active malaria at the time of the attacks : the only determining factor was cold. It seems possible, nevertheless, that ague may bring about some change in the economy, in consequence of which the vaso-motor control or vaso-motor resistance may be lessened, and the influence of external cold become thereby a more powerful factor than under normal circumstances.

Relation to syphilis.—Two of the patients recorded by Raynaud (Nos. XVI. and XVII.), one a man aged thirty-four and the other a woman aged forty-six, had suffered from acquired syphilis in an aggravated form. A remarkable case of symmetrical gangrene was described to me by Dr. Henry Humphreys in a child who was the subject of congenital syphilis. Mr. F. Marsh has also described a case of the same kind in a syphilitic boy. From the character of the permanent upper median incisors, in one case of local asphyxia under my own care, the patient was suspected to be the subject of hereditary syphilis. It is conceivable that syphilis might be a co-operating factor in determining the occurrence of gangrene of the extremities, by causing disease of the inner and middle coats of the smaller and middle-sized arteries. But there are so many cases of Raynaud's disease in which syphilis can be excluded, that it is obvious we can at best reckon it as one only amongst other favouring conditions.

Relation to obliterative arteritis.—Friedländer's disease, in which there is proliferative overgrowth in the inner and middle coat of the arteries, with narrowing of their lumen and likewise thickening of the accompanying veins and narrowing of their lumen, and which is often though not always syphilitic, presents, when it affects the limbs, many features in common with Raynaud's disease. Local syncope and local asphyxia may certainly be induced; and there may be an entire absence of areas of anæsthesia or localised atrophy of muscles (thus separating it from peripheral neuritis); finally, gangrene of the dry mummified variety may supervene, and this may even be symmetrical, as in a case recorded by Mr. Pearce Gould. I am inclined to the opinion that some long-continued cases of Raynaud's disease, in which the paroxysmal phase has given place to persistent change, may, in their final stage, become examples of obliterative arteritis; a case under my own care, to which reference has already been made (p. 595), seems to support this view. But it is most important to recognise that, in Raynaud's disease, the pulsations of the principal arteries of the limbs can be felt distinctly at the outset, and in most cases throughout; during the paroxysm the pulsation often diminishes, but in the inter-paroxysmal periods it is obvious.

Summary.—It is possible that further pathological research may eliminate some of the chronic gangrenous cases from Raynaud's clinical groups. There can be no doubt about the occasional occurrence of multiple areas of gangrene in cases of peripheral neuritis, whether pure and simple, or associated with syringomyelia, Morvan's disease, or other central lesions. In these cases, when considering the causation of the gangrene, there is first the element of persistent and profound local anæsthesia to be reckoned with; and there is, also, the possibility of a concomitant obliterative disease of the arteries: for the experimental researches of Byvoets, Fraenkel, and others, would seem to show that damage to the main nerve trunks of a limb may induce some degree of obliterative disease in the arteries of the limb. In other groups of cases there is the possibility that the principal arteries of a limb may be normal so far as clinical investigation reveals, but that the smaller vessels may become affected with obliterative disease. There still remain, however, a large number of cases—(*a*) in which there are no areas of persistent anæsthesia; (*b*) in which there is no localised atrophy of groups of muscles; (*c*) in which the symptoms are paroxysmal with the return to the normal state in the inter-paroxysmal periods; (*d*) in which there is marked symmetry; (*e*) in which the arterial pulse, though narrowed during the attacks, becomes normal between the attacks; (*f*) in which the subjects are young and with no evidence of degenerative disease,—to which the title of Raynaud's disease is justly applied. Furthermore, when we consider the extension of some of these cases, the progress from one limb to another, and the occasional association of temporary amblyopia and hæmoglobinuria, we are led to ascribe the symptoms primarily to a pathological habit. The easiest explanation of this pathological habit appears to be Raynaud's hypothesis; namely, that vaso-motor centre or centres are unduly irritable, that the commonest irritant is from the periphery, for example, cold; and that the efferent impulses from the centre lead to the paroxysmal contraction of arterioles.

Treatment.—In Raynaud's last memoir he was led, by his view of the pathology of the disease, to try the effect of the continuous galvanic current. He employed the descending current down the spine, the positive pole being placed over the spinous process of the seventh cervical vertebra and the negative pole over the lumbar region. He used the sulphate of copper battery of Trouve and Onimus, beginning with twenty elements and progressively increasing up to sixty-four. The remarkable improvement which took place under daily applications of this treatment in the case of local asphyxia and alternating amblyopia before referred to, led him to apply it in other cases. Raynaud, however, was soon led to place the electrodes locally over the affected limbs as well as down the spine.

I submit the following method as one which has proved useful in the galvanic treatment of these cases :—Immerse the extremity of the limb, which is the subject of local asphyxia, in a large basin containing salt and tepid water; one pole of a constant current battery is placed in contact with the upper part of the limb, above the level of the water, and the other pole in the basin, thus converting the salt and water into an electrode. As many elements as the patient can comfortably bear should be employed; and the current should be made and broken at frequent intervals, so as to get repeated moderate contractions of the limb. The patient should also be instructed to make voluntary movements of the digits whilst the galvanism is applied. It will be found that in a typical paroxysmal case, if two limbs be similarly affected, the limb which is subjected to the above treatment will recover more rapidly than the one which is simply kept warm. In many cases during the acute phase of the attack shampooing is quite impossible; but if galvanism be first employed as above, it will then be found practicable to shampoo the limb; the painful spasm having been thus overcome.

In the chronic cases, although the relief is not so marked, galvanism unquestionably improves the nutrition of the limb, and aids in withstanding imminent gangrene. The cases which do best are those in which galvanism, shampooing, and Swedish movements are employed daily. In bad cases all these measures may be used twice daily; or indeed whenever a paroxysm occurs. The diffusible stimulants and vaso-dilators, such as nitrite of amyl, nitro-glycerine, and the like, have yielded little or no beneficial results, so far as my experience has gone. Alcohol relieves to a slight extent, but its employment is attended with the grave risk of inducing the inebriate habit. Opium is valuable when gangrene is threatened. Cannabis indica has been found helpful in a few cases. Hot applications are seldom useful. Dr. Southey found in one of his cases that an ice-bag applied over a painful extremity gave considerable relief. During convalescence Turkish baths and hot-air baths are very helpful; and a warm climate, with plenty of sunshine during the winter, is always to be sought for if feasible. Before exposure to cold, persons who are liable to Raynaud's disease should fortify themselves with nourishing food; and protect themselves by woollen clothing. Constipation and delayed digestion seem to play an accessory part in some of the attacks, and small doses of mercurials often appear to be helpful.

Gangrene is generally of a benign form, and then simple protection and rest are all that are needed; but severe cases should be treated on surgical principles, and, so far as experience goes, the outlook of amputation is more hopeful than in cases of extensive atheroma of the vessels; or in diabetes.

THOMAS BARLOW.

REFERENCES

1. ABERCROMBIE, J. "On some points in connection with Raynaud's Disease," *Archives of Pediatrics*, vol. iii. p. 567, Oct. 1886.—2. AFFLECK. "Observations on two Cases of Raynaud's Disease," *Brit. Med. Jour.* 1888, vol. ii. p. 1269.—3. BALL, B. "Une variété de sclérodermle," *Bulletins de la société médicale des hôpitaux de Paris*, vol. viii. 1871, p. 59.—4. BARLOW. "Three Cases of Raynaud's Disease," *Trans. Clin. Soc.* vol. xvi. pp. 179, 184 (1883); vol. xviii. pp. 300, 307.—5. *Idem.* "Some Cases of Raynaud's Disease," *Illustrated Medical News*, April 27, May 4, May 11, May 25, 1889. —6. BOAS. "Beitrag zur Lehre von der paroxysmalen Hämoglobinurie," *Deutsches Archiv für klinische Medicin*, 1883, p. 355.—7. BURY, JUDSON. *Treatise on Peripheral Neuritis*, p. 387; 1893.—8. CAVAFY. "Symmetrical congestive Mottling of the Skin," *Trans. Clin. Soc.* vol. xvi. p. 43; 1883.—9. COLMAN and TAYLOR. "Case of Raynaud's Disease not associated with Hæmoglobinuria, but in which there were local changes in the Blood," *Trans. Clin. Soc.* vol. xxiii. p. 195; 1890.—10. COUPLAND. "Case of Erythema Gangrenosum, or Raynaud's Disease," *Trans. Clin. Soc.* vol. xxi. p. 279; 1888. —11. *Idem.* "Second Case of Erythema Gangrenosum," *Trans. Clin. Soc.* vol. xxii. p. 280; 1888.—12. DICKINSON, W. H. "Renal and Urinary Affections, Part III.," *Miscellaneous Affections of the Kidney and Urine*, p. 1185; 1885.—13. DRUITT, R. "Two Cases of Intermittent Hæmatinuria," *Med. Times and Gazette*, April 19, 1873.—14. FLEISCHER. "Ueber eine neue Form von Hämoglobinurie beim Menschen," *Berl. klin. Wochenschrift*, 1881, No. 47, p. 691.—15. FINLAYSON. "Scleroderma and Gangrene," *Medical Chronicle*, vol. i. p. 316.—15a. FORREST. "Case of Hæmatinuria," *Glasg. Med. Jour.* 1879, p. 421.—16. FOX, COLCOTT. "Two Symmetrical Cases of Raynaud's Disease," *Trans. Clin. Soc.* vol. xviii. p. 300.—17. FRIEDLÄNDER. "Ueber Arteriitis obliterans," *Centralblatt für die medicinischen Wissenschaften*, Jan. 22, 1876, p. 66.—18. GOULD, A. PEARCE. "Spreading Obliterative Arteritis," *Trans. Clin. Soc.* vol. xviii. p. 95; sequel in vol. xx. p. 252.—19. *Idem.* "Symmetrical Gangrene of the Feet from obliterative Disease and Thrombosis of Arteries and Veins," *Trans. Clin. Soc.* vol. xxiv. p. 134.—20. GRIFFITH, WARDROP. "Three Cases illustrating Affinities of Raynaud's Disease, *Med. Chron.* vol. xv. p. 89; 1891.—21. HADDEN. "Obliterative Arteritis," *Trans. Clin. Soc.* vol. xviii. p. 105; 1884.—22. HANDFORD. "Disseminated Myositis and Neuritis probably of alcoholic origin, unilateral in distribution, accompanied by terminal Gangrene and by pigmentation of the skin, and followed by muscular Atrophy," *Trans. Clin. Soc.* vol. xxiii. p. 242; 1890.—23. HOCHENEGG. *Ueber symmetrische Gangrän und locale Asphyxie*. Vienna, 1886.—24. HUTCHINSON, J. "Gangrene of tip of Nose and part of Ear; Iridoplegia," *Med. Times and Gazette* for 1871, vol. ii. p 678.—25. *Idem.* "On certain local Disorders more or less cognate with Raynaud's Malady," *Archives of Surgery*, vol. i. p. 227.—26. MACKENZIE, STEPHEN. "On Hæmo

globinuria," *Lancet*, 1884, vol. i. pp. 156, 198, 243.—27. MAKINS, G. H. "Spontaneous Gangrene of Toes in a Child," *St. Thomas's Hosp. Rep.* vol. xii. p. 154 ; 1882.—28. MARSH, F. "Raynaud's Disease associated with Hereditary Syphilis," *Brit. Med. Jour.* 1892, vol. i. p. 1083.—29. MORGAN, J. H. "Progressive painful Obliteration of the Arteries," *Trans. Clin. Soc.* vol. xiv. p. 183 ; 1881.—30. MOURSON. "Observation d'asphyxie locale des extrémités survenue après un accès de fièvre intermittente," *Arch. de méd. nav.* vol. xix. p. 364 ; 1873.—31. *Idem. Arch. de méd. nav.* vol. xxxiii. p. 340 ; 1880.—32. MURRI. *Dell' emoglobinuria da freddo.* Bologna, 1880.—33. MYERS, A. T. "Case of Raynaud's Disease," *Trans. Clin. Soc.* vol. xviii. p. 336 ; 1885.—34. MYRTLE. "Anæmic sphacelus," *Lancet*, 1863, vol. i. p. 602.—35. PETIT and VERNEUIL. "Asphyxie locale et gangrène palustres," *Rev. de chirurgie*, 1883, pp. 1, 161, 432, 699. —36. PITRES and VAILLARD. "Contribution à l'étude des gangrènes massives des membres d'origine névritique," *Archives de physiologie normale et pathologique*, 1885, p. 106.—37. RAKHMANINOFF. "Contribution à la névrite périphérique : un cas de gangrène symétrique et deux cas de paralysie alcoolique," *Rev. de médecine*, vol. xii. p. 321 ; 1892.—38. RAYNAUD. *On Local Asphyxia and Symmetrical Gangrene of the Extremites.* Thesis, 1862.—39. *Idem.* "New researches on the Nature and Treatment of Local Asphyxia of the Extremites," *Archives générales de médecine*, Jan. 1874. Translation of (1) and (2) by Thomas Barlow, M.D. Selected monographs, with Appendix by the translator. New Sydenham Society, 1888.—40. *Idem.* Article on "Gangrene," *Nouv. dict. de méd. et de chir. prat.* pp. 592, 679.—41. SMITH, T. "Case of Spontaneous Gangrene of the Thumb and Fingers of the right Hand," *Trans. Clin. Soc.* vol. xiii. p. 196.—42. SOUTHEY. "Case of Symmetrical Gangrene, with some remarks on the Disease," *St. Bartholomew's Hospital Reports*, vol. xvi. p. 15 ; 1880.—43. *Idem.* "A Case of Local Asphyxia ; Symmetrical Gangrene," *Trans. Clin. Soc.* vol. xvi. pp. 167, 172 ; 1883. —44. *Idem.* "Case of Symmetrical Gangrene," *Trans. Path. Soc.* vol. xxiv. p. 286.— 45. SPENCER, W. G. "Frost-bite in a Boy, the subject of Hæmatinuria upon exposure to cold," *Trans. Clin. Soc.* vol. xxv. p. 287 ; 1892.—46. TREVES, F. "Case of pulsating Tumour of the Head with Raynaud's Disease," *Trans. Clin. Soc.* vol. xx. p. 12 ; 1887.—47. WALSHAM, W. J. "Acute Obliterative Arteritis," *Trans. Clin. Soc.* vol. xix. p. 304 ; 1885.—48. WEISS. "Ueber symmetrische Gangrän," *Wiener Klinik*, Oct. and Nov. 1882.—49. WEST, S. "Case of Raynaud's Disease with a peculiar Eruption on the Face, scaly at first, subsequently like erysipelas : Death from pneumonia : post-mortem negative," *Trans. Clin. Soc.* vol. xxii. p. 146 ; 1889.—50. WIGLESWORTH. "Peripheral Neuritis in Raynaud's Disease (Symmetrical Gangrene)," *Trans. Path. Soc.* vol. xxxviii. p. 61 ; 1887.—51. WILKS. "A Case of Hæmoglobinuria : Gangrene of the Fingers, etc. associated with prolonged suppuration," *Medical Times and Gazette*, vol. ii. p. 207 ; 1879.

T. B.

ERYTHROMELALGIA

SYN.—*The Red Neuralgia*

Der. : ἐρυθρὸς, red ; μέλος, a member ; ἄλγος, pain.

Definition.—"Erythromelalgia is a chronic disease in which a part or parts of the body—usually one or more extremities—suffer with pain, flushing, and local fever, made far worse if the parts hang down."

Historical note.—The above definition states in Dr. Weir Mitchell's own words his latest summary (1897) of the essential features of the malady which he first described in 1872, and to which he gave a descriptive title in 1878. So far back as 1843 Graves had cautiously stated his opinion that the nerves and arteries of a part of the body could influence local circulation, independently of the heart; and he recorded two cases which conform to Weir Mitchell's type, and are quoted by Mitchell. Graves describes another case, also quoted by Raynaud, which seems to lie half way between the group of cases designated as "Local Syncope" and that now under consideration. In 1871 Sir James Paget also had described what may be called an intermediate case between these two groups.

In Weir Mitchell's first paper exclusive attention was given to the lower limbs, and no better clinical picture of the disease can be given than as it occurs in a single foot. But, in 1878, other examples were recorded by Weir Mitchell in which the hands also were affected; and some in which the hands were affected exclusively. Moreover, in the more generalised cases a great variety of clinical phenomena were observed, which pointed to widespread organic or functional disease of the nervous system. With a wise reserve Weir Mitchell refused to attempt to declare the origin of the malady; though he inclined then to the view that it is due to spinal or cerebro-spinal disorder, and that some distinct lesions of definite regions might therein ultimately be found. Since 1872 several new examples have been described, and brief former records have been reconsidered in the light of recent cases.

Some of the most important cases are those of Vulpian, Sigerson and Lannois, Senator, Gerhardt, Bernhardt, Eulenberg, Allen Sturge, Morgan, Dreschfeld, and Stephen Mackenzie.

Since the appearance of Lannois' thesis in 1880, the best synopsis of the literature of the subject has been that of Lewin and Benda, who have analysed forty-one cases, and classified them under the three following groups: namely, (i.) those in which a true organic central nervous disease exists: (ii.) those in which the disease of the nervous centres is functional; (iii.) those in which the nervous disease, organic or functional, is only peripheral. For the most part the malady has been regarded as a vaso-motor neurosis, or as a vaso-motor paralysis; but a later conception, to which, indeed, Weir Mitchell now inclines, rather ascribes it to peripheral neuritis; of this, however, there is as yet no conclusive anatomical proof. Moreover, the claim for erythromelalgia to be distinctly classified has been contested; it has been maintained that it should rather be designated as an unstable symptom-complex which may be variably associated with many different diseases. However, the special symptoms described by Weir Mitchell occur, sufficiently often, apart from any others; and so uniformly grouped that, even in the absence of a satisfactory pathology, they deserve clinical definition and a name.

Symptoms.—*Typical case.*—A man of early middle age, who is engaged in heavy physical work, standing through a long day with exposure to varying temperatures, has had some illness, and returned to his work with lessened vigour. He begins to suffer in the evening with a burning pain in some part of the sole of one foot. The pain is made worse by the standing posture, and by voluntary movement; it is relieved by lying down, or by raising the leg to the horizontal position. If he is able to rest entirely in bed for some days, not only may the pain vanish during the rest, but he may get relief for a time; if, as is more commonly the case, he goes on with his work, the pain, though temporarily relieved by the rest, returns a little earlier each day, and lasts for a longer time. At this period physical examination gives no clue to the cause of the pain, and an attack of this kind may subside entirely. In the course of a few weeks the pain, after a walk or some other prolonged exertion, may recur with renewed violence; then there supervenes the second characteristic symptom, namely, redness of the foot. At first this is circumscribed; it may affect the ball of the great toe, one or other toes, the heel, the outer or inner side of the foot. Sometimes there are several small patches. The redness increases in depth and area as the vertical position is maintained, as the veins become distended, and the arterial pulsations excessive. After a time the vascular storm, as it is called by Weir Mitchell, partly subsides; the throbbing ceases, but the foot remains for a time of a purplish red colour. During the red phase the pain markedly increases in severity, and there may be excessive tenderness to the slightest touch over the red area. Sensibility to heat and cold is increased in the affected foot. Both superficial and deep pressure are resented, but sensation seems otherwise unaltered. The plantar reflex is either normal or exaggerated. During the attack there is unquestionably a local elevation of temperature; this is obvious to the hand of the observer: a surface thermometer may indeed show that the temperature of the affected foot does not rise as high as the mouth temperature, but it is sometimes two or three degrees higher than that of the unaffected foot, and it rises during the dependent posture; whereas in the normal state of health, as shown by Weir Mitchell, the surface temperature of the foot is a little lower in the dependent than in the horizontal position. There is a certain amount of swelling; occasionally the part pits on pressure, but more commonly this is not so: in many cases, however, the swelling has been such as to lead to the suspicion of a true inflammatory affection of the deeper structures or tissues of the periosteum, especially of the os calcis; and fruitless incisions have in many instances been made, even down to the bone.

As with the pain in the early stage, so with the redness and swelling, the vertical position and voluntary movement aggravate, whilst the horizontal position and rest relieve them. It is also found that cold days, cold applications and free exposure to air bring a certain amount of comfort; whilst hot weather or hot compresses, and any degree of pressure, increase the severity of the symptoms. Thus the sufferer refuses to walk; or, if he walks, he treads on the part of the foot which is unaffected: indeed, when the attack is very severe, he goes on his hands and knees. He prefers a bare slipper to a boot and stocking; and when he lies down he likes to have the weight of the bedclothes removed by a cradle, or to have his foot exposed to the air, and to bathe it with cold water. There are all degrees of severity. The mild cases may be cured by horizontal rest. Many cases relapse, and generally with increasing severity. The individual attacks, when the disease is established, may last for several hours, even in spite of recumbency ; during the intermissions the foot tends sometimes to become unduly pale. The disease may last for many years ; in one of Morgan's cases it continued for twenty-seven years, limited to one sole. In general, and in the chronic cases, after long periods the severity of the pain tends to diminish, as also do the changes of colour on alteration of position.

Taking the above case as one in accord with the type, there are many variations from it to be considered. The burning pain, though not so striking as the vaso-motor phenomena, is really the most important symptom, because almost invariably it is the initial one. It is important, however, to note that, in Sigerson's case, which was a multiple one, there were vaso-motor phenomena corresponding to the type, but in the history no record of pain.

Also some of the other multiple cases, which showed in certain extremities the triple symptoms—pain, redness, and swelling, nevertheless presented severe pains elsewhere also, which were unaccompanied by vaso-motor signs : namely, pains in the back of the head and neck, both before (Benda (18)) and subsequent to the erythromelalgia (Gerhardt) ; pains in one shoulder and elbow, along with and succeeding erythromelalgia in the feet (Strauss) ; slight burning in the feet with erythromelalgia in the hands (Weir Mitchell's case V.)

In Sir James Paget's case, which is probably one of the connecting links with Raynaud's disease, the pain appeared with occurrence of extreme pallor (local syncope) in the feet, which preceded the redness and swelling. During the red swollen stage the pain abated.

The characteristic pain is increased more by deep than by superficial pressure. In some of the cases pressure on the distant nerve trunk, or on the adjacent branch, increased the burning ; for example, on the sciatic in a case of Weir Mitchell's, and on the internal plantar in a case of Morgan's).

In many cases the adjacent nerves, when they could be reached by local pressure, were not tender ; and in other cases, when palpable nerves generally were found to be tender on pressure, this was not more marked in those which could be felt in the neighbourhood of the red areas than elsewhere.

Distribution of erythromelalgia.—Whether it be the foot or the hand, the disease at the outset most commonly attacks one extremity only ; and in the simple cases is limited to that extremity. Thus it is primarily asymmetrical. There are several cases recorded of hand affection, though it is not so common nor generally so severe as in the foot. When one or both hands suffer it is a characteristic attitude for the patient to keep them either crossed over the breast, or raised above the head ; thus bringing about the greatest possible physiological emptying of the vessels. The disease may attack portions of the other extremities at successive shorter or longer intervals. Further study has shown a still wider distribution. Thus in Woodnut's case, after successive invasion of some of the toes first of one foot then of the other, areas of erythromelalgia appeared on the lower part of one leg and over the middle of the back.

In Benda's case (18) there were rose-red areas on both sides between the mastoid regions and the neck, which were hot and painful, both spontaneously and on pressure, and accompanied by distinct erythromelalgia of the outer side of the right foot. In the case recorded by Auché and Lespinasse, along with erythromelalgic attacks in one upper and one lower extremity, there was much congestion of the face, eyes, and external ears; and one testicle became swollen and tender. Finally, Seeligmüller's case shows a still more remarkable distribution: a woman, aged fifty-six, had for two years burning pains in the left hand and right foot; then came redness and swelling of finger points as well as of the toes and ball of the foot. At the beginning of the periodical attacks she had the feeling as of a hot ray from the shoulder down to the fingers; and the head, neck, and mucous membrane of the mouth, throat, and gums became markedly hyperæmic.

Skin.—Weir Mitchell lays great stress on the colour in erythromelalgia, as distinguished from the livid colour of the local asphyxia of Raynaud; a rosy red at first, and ultimately, in the later stage of the vascular storm, purplish red. But in several of the chronic cases, in which the painful phases had lessened in severity, it is expressly recorded that the extremities became cold and either pale or livid.

With respect to other skin changes; vesication is sometimes found in the acute stage, and small nodules may appear on the red areas. Hardening of the cellular tissue, tense and shiny finger ends, or actual clubbing and thickening of the nails, occasionally result. Œdema has been recorded, in some of the chronic cases, as a late condition. The occasional simulation of a deep inflammatory effusion in erythromelalgia, especially in the sole, has been already mentioned. The surface temperature of the feet in the chronic cases is generally notably lower than that of the mouth.

The muscles of the affected limbs usually show slight general wasting. It is doubtful whether this is more than is to be explained by the pain and enforced disuse of the limb. It is certainly insignificant in amount as compared with that commonly seen in well-marked peripheral neuritis; and, as a rule, muscles are not picked out individually. The only important instance of extensive wasting was in Eulenberg's case—that of an anæmic woman, who, after her second attack of erythromelalgia, presented muscular dystrophy, of Erb's juvenile type, affecting the upper arm and shoulder of both sides. In no case are degenerative reactions to the constant current recorded. In Allen Sturge's case there was slight diminution of electric irritability; and in one of Weir Mitchell's cases slight quantitative increase to both currents, but no qualitative change.

Only in one case, under the care of Dreschfeld and Morgan (25), is the knee-jerk recorded as absent. In Weir Mitchell's last two cases it was increased.

We have now to enumerate briefly some of the various symptoms which have been found in the subjects of erythromelalgia, concerning which, in our present knowledge, it is impossible to say exactly how far the relation was an essential, and how far an accidental one; these relate almost entirely to the nervous system.

There are several examples of psychical changes, some of which are probably hysterical, or at all events temporary; others, however, are persistent or progressive, and associated with definite paralytic signs, such as hemiplegia, speech defects, or spinal cord degeneration. Thus Weir Mitchell's second patient, a man aged thirty-five, about six years after the onset of his erythromelalgia, became very morose, and would only answer questions in whispered monosyllables. He had some seizures, in which he became rigid and was drowsy. He complained of girdle pain, and showed for a time a fine tremor on muscular effort, ankle drop, and weakness of grasp. He ultimately presented excessive reflexes, spastic knee-jerks, and ankle clonus. Weir Mitchell's judgment was, that during the twenty-three years that this patient suffered, hysteria and some spinal cord lesion supervened on the erythromelalgia; which disorder, indeed, during the latter years of his life underwent marked diminution.

A woman, aged forty-four, who was under the care both of Gerhardt and Eulenberg, had well-marked erythromelalgia in all four extremities. In one of her attacks she got pains in the tongue, and some difficulties of speech. By degrees the painful element in her limb attacks diminished, and the extremities became cold and livid; but signs of central disturbance appeared. Besides suffering from pains in the head and neck, and giddiness, she became uncertain in her gait. Gradual failure of intelligence and memory with hallucinations supervened, and changes in the fundus oculi were discovered. In Benda's case a woman, aged fifty-seven years, was the subject of erythromelalgia of the back of the neck, shoulders, and one foot. On this there supervened some weakness of memory. The speech was described as slow and difficult; the pupils were immobile and the knee-jerks were exaggerated. Although in this case syphilis was denied, it was a possible factor, as double sixth nerve paralysis had preceded the erythromelalgia, and there was a history of three still-born children. There was also partial improvement after the use of iodide of potassium, and of baths and faradism. In several cases vertigo and pain in the head were induced by assuming the erect posture. A medical student, aged twenty-one, whose case is described by Lewin and Benda, was the subject of severe megrim with hemianopsia; and without any obvious cause got erythromelalgia of the left hand. Whilst suffering from this affection, a temporary paralysis of the left arm and leg followed upon three days' vomiting and giddiness. But the erythromelalgia remained unchanged, and he suffered pains in the right hand, though without redness or swelling. In Graves' case, a woman of eighty-two, there was a slight attack of left hemiplegia with headache, vertigo, and sight troubles. This was followed, in one month, by erythromelalgia of the right foot, which, after considerable suffering, subsided in about three months. In another month she suffered a second stroke and died. Henoch records the case of a gentleman, who, whilst undergoing a bath cure at Schlangenbad, was seized with paresis and anæsthesia of the left half of the body. From this after a few weeks he recovered, but a liability to frequent sweating on the left side persisted. Six months later erythromelalgia of the left foot appeared; after this came angina pectoris, and albuminuria with signs of arterio-sclerosis, and finally he died of cerebral hæmorrhage. In Machol's case erythromelalgia appeared in the last stage of a case of paralytic dementia; and there are two cases (Landgraf's and F. P. Henry's) in which it appeared in patients who were suffering from myxœdema.

There is at least one case (namely, that of Edinger) in which erythromelalgia occurred in the course of tabes; and another (Woodnut's) in which lightning pains in the arms and legs, and some lessening of sensation in one lower limb, apart altogether from the red areas, were suggestive of early tabes. Dr. James Collier has recently reported six cases of disseminated sclerosis, two cases of tabes dorsalis, and one case of chronic myelitis in which erythromelalgia occurred. Pospelow has recorded a case of syringomyelia in which erythromelalgia supervened in one hand and one foot.

Pathology.—*Age.*—Out of the forty-one cases analysed by Lewin and Benda the majority occurred in middle life. There are, however, a few examples amongst young people, namely, at the ages of sixteen, twenty, and twenty-one respectively. Baginsky records a case in a boy aged ten; and Henoch has referred to one case occurring in a child during teething.

Sex.—Of forty-one cases twenty-nine were male and twelve female. So far as they go these figures give a definite predominance to the male sex.

Occupation.—There seems some ground for the opinion that long hours of standing, associated with heavy work and stress, and also exposure to varying temperatures, may play some part as remoter causes.

The following is a list of the trades which were followed by some of the victims of erythromelalgia: iron-worker, copper-polisher, alkali-worker (who stood for hours in front of a furnace, his hands being held in cold water for long periods), locomotive driver, seaman, postman, baker, waiter, collier (who worked in a coal-mine with his feet in two feet of water ten hours at a stretch). It is important to note, however, that well-marked instances are also recorded of patients who were not subjected to any physical strain, and who were in easy circumstances of life.

Previous health.—The nervous constitution has been regarded as a predisposing factor ; but although there are a few instances in which hysteria became manifest during the progress of the case, there are a considerable number in which it could be confidently excluded. Of the female cases, there is one of Eulenberg's, an anæmic young woman in whom the symptoms of erythromelalgia began soon after her confinement ; there are two other patients, namely, Graves's, aged sixteen, and Stillé's, aged twenty-nine (reported by Weir Mitchell), in which the symptoms supervened upon cessation of the menses. In the first of these the cessation was associated with an exhausting diarrhœa ; but in the second it was sudden, after falling into a river.

In Weir Mitchell's first case the antecedents of prolonged erythromelalgia were insolation on the African coast followed by a severe attack of coast fever, which left behind it a weak heart with an apical systolic murmur. Another of his patients had had severe remittent fever ; and he lays stress on the fact that this patient had used a geological hammer with great persistence.

Eulenberg had one case in a patient who had suffered from severe malaria. Ross, quoting Elliotson, draws attention to gonorrhœa as being sometimes responsible for erythromelalgia, especially when radiating from the heel. Morgan gives one severe case which may support this view.

There are two cases in which it seems fair to believe that injury may have played a part in the production of the symptoms. The first was recorded by Lewin, and was that of a man who was shot in the right elbow and got ankylosis of the elbow joint ; some months afterwards erythromelalgia appeared in his right index, ring, and little fingers. The other case is recorded fully by Weir Mitchell in his last memoir ; the symptoms followed upon the fall of a heavy piece of stone on the patient's foot in front of the right ankle ; the wound was superficial, but there was considerable swelling of the foot and leg. Six weeks later a swelling on the sole was incised, but there was no evidence of suppuration and only slight bleeding. Signs of erythromelalgia gradually appeared with the addition of fine rhythmical tremor affecting the whole leg, an increase of the knee-jerk, and ankle clonus.

Weir Mitchell was of opinion that neuritis of the foot was set up by the injury. At his suggestion portions of the internal saphenous and musculo-cutaneous nerves were resected, and the two plantar nerves were stretched. Some anæsthesia was induced ; marked relief of the pain followed, and gradual subsidence of the flushing. In two months' time the patient could walk ; and six months later he was at his work and free from pain. It is important to note, however, that the microscopic examination of portions of the exsected nerves showed no morbid change.

Morgan attributes one of his cases of limited erythromelalgia of the hand to long-continued hammering.

Exposure to fatigue (as in long marches) seems to have played an important part in the causation of several cases. Whatever the primary cause, a long walk has sometimes precipitated a relapse.

Dreschfeld and Morgan's case, of a collier who worked for hours in the mine with his feet in cold water, has already been mentioned; and this may be paralleled by Sir James Paget's case of a gentleman who endeavoured to harden himself every morning by cold shower-baths, and by standing in cold water up to the knees. After eight days of such experiments the limbs became cold, numbed, and marble-like.

From the fact that this group of symptoms, striking as it is, has so many different antecedents, and exists in so many different combinations, it may well be asked is the pathology always the same? in other words, is one constant mechanism always present whatever the superadded conditions may be? To this question no answer can be given; chiefly because the results of anatomical and microscopic investigation are so meagre. There are at least three directions in which inquiry should extend: namely, first, to the peripheral nerves; secondly, to the brain and cord, especially with regard to the vaso-motor centres; and, thirdly, to the blood-vessels.

The doctrine now extensively held with regard to erythromelalgia, as well as with regard to Raynaud's disease, is that the symptoms are due to peripheral neuritis. That this change may play some ultimate part in them is possible; but there are many objections to its acceptance as the primary lesion. It is true that pain is the initial symptom, but in the typical cases the amount of wasting is not at all marked; moreover, such wasting as occurs is general, affecting all the muscles of the extremity instead of picking out special groups. There is no record hitherto of reaction of degeneration in any of these cases; moreover, of definite persistent damage to sensory function there is scarcely a trace. The temporary alteration of sensation in the paroxysms may fairly be referred to the vascular storm. In two cases recorded in Weir Mitchell's last memoir the portions of resected nerves were carefully examined microscopically and, as I have said, found normal. Also in a very important case, recorded by Dehio, in which part of the left foot and part of the left hand were affected with erythromelalgia, a portion of the left ulnar nerve removed above the wrist was found normal (*vide* p. 617). It is possible, of course, that the special form of neuritis in these cases may be entirely terminal; or it may be a neuritis of the vaso-motor fibres, but both of these views are mere speculation.

Lewin and Benda, in their final summary of the simple uncomplicated cases of erythromelalgia, divide them between neuritis and neuralgia; they lay great stress on the pain preceding the vaso-motor disturbance. They are inclined to regard erythromelalgia as comparable with one of those trigeminal neuralgias in which there is circumscribed temporal flushing. But when we consider the striking and pathognomonic symptom of erythromelalgia—namely, its precipitation by the vertical posture—the parallel soon breaks down.

Following the teaching of physiology, it would seem inevitable that some alteration of function in the vaso-motor centres must form at least one link in the chain of the morbid process of erythromelalgia. During what Weir Mitchell calls the vascular storm, there is either a paralysis of vaso-constrictors or a stimulation of vaso-dilators. In the generalised cases to which reference has been made, not the extremities only, but the neck, face, and even the mouth may undergo painful flushing ; the testicle may become temporarily swollen ; and painful erections may occur : here we must assume a widespread disturbance of the vaso-motor centres.

Does the change start centrally ? Probably so, in some instances, especially in the generalised cases in which the erythromelalgia supervenes on cerebral or spinal disease. But in the uncomplicated cases, limited to one or more limbs or to part of a limb, it would seem more reasonable to believe that the primary change starts at the periphery itself.

Unquestionably the peripheral irritation must be transmitted by afferent nerves, but the initial fault may be in tissues other than the nerve-endings themselves, or indeed in some altered blood state ; and if some limited form of neuritis ensue it is quite possible that this may be a late and secondary change.

With respect to the tissues it has been assumed rather too readily that, because no gross change can be found in the larger arteries, the blood-vessels can be excluded from any important part other than that of an alteration of calibre during a vascular storm. But we have to consider not only atheroma, with its accompanying calcareous deposits as it occurs in larger arteries, but likewise changes in the small and middle-sized arteries of the kind described by Friedländer, namely, the obliterative form ; and this may be difficult to detect during life.

Referring once more to the list of cases analysed by Lewin and Benda, it is of interest to observe that in Graves' second case, an old lady aged eighty-two, the affection of the right foot, which succeeded her attack of left hemiplegia, is stated (in a final note by Graves) to have been very like one of threatening senile gangrene. In Henoch's case the erythromelalgia supervened on a hemiplegia ; which in its turn was followed by angina pectoris, albuminuria, and general signs of arteriosclerosis, ending in fatal cerebral apoplexy. In at least four cases there was reason to believe that syphilis had occurred. Previous alcoholism was known in several of the cases.

Syphilis is one of the most potent factors of disease of the middle-sized arteries, and Friedländer claims the changes so minutely described by Heubner as one of the kinds of his obliterative form of arteritis. The blue extremities of alcoholic subjects are well recognised, and it is well known that alcoholism favours widespread vascular degeneration ; though its details have not been worked out so thoroughly as in alcoholic neuritis.

But the most important cases bearing on the question of disease of the middle-sized arteries in this malady are—(i.) the one recorded by

Dehio; and (ii.) the last case described by Weir Mitchell in his last memoir. Dehio's case was of a woman who presented erythromelalgia of the left hand and foot, with vertigo and other symptoms. Four centimetres of the ulnar nerve and a similar length of the ulnar artery were removed just above the wrist. The little finger became anæsthetic, and its colour became normal; though, so far as the rest of the hand was concerned, there was no improvement. The interest of the case is, however, pathological. As already stated, the piece of nerve was found to be absolutely normal; but the portion of the accompanying artery showed marked arteritis affecting the middle and inner coat, and some narrowing of the lumen.

Weir Mitchell's case LIX. (his last memoir) is in some respects still more important. It was a well-marked case of erythromelalgia of the right foot occurring in a medical man aged forty-eight. Having seen the marked benefit which, in his other case, followed excision of portions of the musculo-cutaneous and internal saphenous nerves, and stretching of the two plantars, Weir Mitchill recommended the same operation for this case; but the result was not satisfactory. Some signs of gangrene appeared along the margin of the incisions, and subsequently amputation was attempted by another surgeon, when the patient died upon the operating table. A complete autopsy was not obtained; but the amputated limb was examined, and all the vessels showed thickening of the middle coat. This was demonstrable even in the smallest arteries in the sole of the foot; while in the larger vessels, here and there in addition were calcareous deposits. It is also noteworthy that the pieces of excised nerve were carefully examined microscopically, and found quite normal. These two cases support the contention that in erythromelalgia arterial disease (especially of the small and middle-sized arteries) ought not to be excluded as a possible factor, even when clinical examination does not reveal its presence.

But, even if this be granted, the actual part played by the arterial disease, and the exact stage in which it comes into the chain of causation, are open to differences of interpretation, and may, indeed, vary in different cases. There is a certain amount of experimental evidence to show that abnormal dilatation of the artery leads to compensatory thickening of the intima (Thoma); and there is also some evidence that arterio-sclerosis can be brought about by section of nerve trunks (Fraenkel and others). In a case of severe left-sided supra-orbital neuralgia, Thoma found the left temporal artery in a far more advanced state of sclerosis than the corresponding artery on the other side; he ascribed this to alteration of the arterial walls brought about by the accompanying vaso-motor disturbance.

Thus, in the absence of obvious nerve disease to explain the arterio-sclerosis, we are led back to the hypothesis that the chief fault lies with the vaso-motor centres and their abnormal efferent vaso-motor impulses, leading to dilatation of the vessels with consecutive disease thereby induced.

But how is the fault in the vaso-motor centres brought about? In the limited cases there is often some long-standing local exhausting strain which, exerted at the periphery, may have been transmitted to the vaso-motor centre. If we suppose that, either by lowering of general nutrition or by some congenital weakness in the vaso-motor centre, there is diminished resistance, then abnormal efferent impulses may ensue, and the vascular changes at the extremities occur.

Allen Sturge's comparison with writers' cramp seems to be a very fruitful one :—"Just as over-exertion of the co-ordinating centres of the hand will, in certain cases, induce writers' cramp, so a prolonged over-excitation of the vaso-motor centres may be supposed to induce irregular action on their part."

In the generalised cases the affection of the vaso-motor centre may be brought about by extension from some central organic, or, indeed, functional brain or cord disease with which the vaso-motor centre is in active relation.

There remains one other question to consider, namely, the relation between erythromelalgia and Raynaud's disease. As between typical examples the clinical differences have been summarised, as follows, by Weir Mitchell :—

LOCAL ASPHYXIA (RAYNAUD).	ERYTHROMELALGIA (WEIR MITCHELL).
Sex, four-fifths females.	In twenty-seven cases two were women.
Begins with ischæmia.	Little or no difference of colour is seen until the foot hangs down in upright posture, when it becomes rose-red.
The affected parts become bloodless and white. In certain cases there is the deep dusky congestion of a cyanosed part, with or without gangrene.	The arteries throb, and the colour becomes dusky red or violaceous in tint.
Pain may be absent or acute, and comes and goes ; has no relation to position ; may precede local asphyxia.	Pain usually present ; worse when the part hangs down, or is pressed upon. In bad cases, more or less at all times.
Unaffected by seasons. In many cases all the symptoms can be brought on by cold.	Worse in summer, and from heat. Eased by cold.
Anæsthesia to touch.	Sensation of all kinds preserved.
Analgesia.	Hyperalgesia.
Temperature much lowered, and unaltered by posture.	Temperature greatly above normal. Dependency causes in some cases increase of heat, in others lowering of temperature.
Gangrene local and limited, likely to be symmetrical.	No gangrene ; asymmetrical.

There are a few criticisms to be made on this table.

The difference in respect to sex is not so striking with a larger number of cases as in Weir Mitchell's series; but this point is not a very important one.

In the reaction stage of many cases of local asphyxia there is distinct evidence of heat and of local throbbing of arteries, and there is likewise complaint of the burning pain. On the other hand, in some cases of erythromelalgia there is an early stage of marked ischæmia; this occurred in Paget's case. Moreover, in one of Weir Mitchell's examples—that of a man who had suffered from remittent fever, and who had used a geological hammer with great zeal—the attacks of erythromelalgia were followed by "notable pallor and coldness of the hands."

In Graves' first case (a girl aged sixteen) the lower limbs during the attacks presented an appearance like that of a half-ripe black cherry, but subsequently the parts were pale and corpse-like.

In the later stages of other recorded examples (for example, Gerhardt's, and Benda's) the extremities became cold and livid blue.

Intermediate cases, between erythromelalgia and Raynaud's disease, have been recorded by Morell, Lavallé, and Rolleston.

Although, in the typical example described of erythromelalgia, the disease began in one extremity, there are several cases of symmetrical affection of both limbs, which must be regarded as undoubted instances of the disease.

If in both maladies the hypothesis be accepted of an unstable condition of the vaso-motor centres, brought about in a variety of ways, it would seem possible to regard erythromelalgia, and the three clinical types of Raynaud's disease, as differing from one another in the extent of the vascular storm, and in the order in which spasm and paresis follow one another.

Treatment.—The slight cases of erythromelalgia, and probably the initial stage of all cases, can certainly be benefited by prolonged rest in the horizontal posture.

In the early stage, and also in the mild generalised cases, faradism to the extremities and to the neck has been in a few examples beneficial, but in the severe cases useless. Heat aggravates, but local application of cold during the paroxysms is often soothing.

Massage is of doubtful value, and during the paroxysms is unbearable.

Morgan, in a severe case affecting the feet, found that recovery followed the hypodermic injection of morphia and atropia, twice daily for three weeks.

Alcohol sometimes relieves the pain of the attacks temporarily; but Weir Mitchell learnt that one of his patients became a drunkard in consequence of too frequent recourse to this remedy, which he began on his own initiative.

Good food seems to lessen the severity of the attacks (Sturge). In case of any syphilitic history iodides and mercury should be given. Amputation of a toe or a finger has been performed in several cases, but the operation wounds have been slow in recovering, and no benefit has resulted. Incisions of the swollen red areas of the affected parts of the feet have been made in several instances, but without advantage.

Summing up his second series of cases, Weir Mitchell gave as his conclusion that "they were rarely amenable to treatment; they were aided for a time by cold and by rest, but either they remained unchanged for years, or, in rare instances, became gradually worse." To this conclusion, however, it ought to be added that, even after all therapeutic remedies have failed, some of the severe cases have manifested a tendency to slow spontaneous recovery.

Allen Sturge's case, which was a severe one, appears to have ended in recovery after several years; the cure was attributed to "faith healing."

In Weir Mitchell's last memoir he records the recovery of one case of traumatic origin; and immediate benefit seemed to have ensued upon exsection of certain portions of nerve and stretching of other nerves (*vide* pp. 614, 617). In a second case in which this was tried gangrene ensued.

Thomas Barlow.

REFERENCES

1. Auché and Lespinasse. "Sur un cas d'érythromélalgie ou névrose congestive des extrémités," *Rev. de méd.* p. 1049. Paris, 1889.—2. Baginsky. *Verhandl. der Berl. med. Gesellschaft*, 1892, p. 241.—3. Bernhardt. *Berl. klin. Wochenschr.* p. 1129. —4. Bury, Judson. "Erythromelalgia," *Treatise on Peripheral Neuritis*, 1893, p. 386. —5. Collier, James. "The occurrence of Erythromelalgia in Disease of the Spinal Cord: an account of ten cases," *Lancet*, Aug. 13, 1898.—6. Dehio. *Berl. klin. Wochenschr.* 1896, p. 817.—7. Edinger. *Neurolog. Centralblatt*, 1893, p. 657.—8. Eulenburg. *Verhandlung der Berl. med. Gesellschaft*, erster Theil, 1892, p. 239. —9. *Idem. Neurolog. Centralblatt*, 1893, p. 657.—10. Fraenkel. "Ueber neurotische Angiosklerose," *Wiener klin. Wochenschr.* 1896, pp. 147, 170.—11. Gerhardt. "Ueber Erythromelalgie," *Berl. klin. Wochenschr.* 1892, p. 1127.—12. Graves. "Painful Affections of the Feet," *Clin. Lect.* vol. ii. p. 586. Sydenham Society's edit. 1884.—13. Henoch. *Berl. klin. Wochenschr.* 1893, p. 1146.—14. Henry, F. P. "Myxoedematoid Dystrophy," *Journ. of Nerv. and Mental Diseases*, 1890.—15. Koch. *Berl. klin. Wochenschr.* 1892, p. 1146.—16. Landgrat. *Berl. klin. Wochenschr.* 1892, p. 1146.—17. Lannois. *Paralysie vaso-motrice des extrémités ou érythromélalgie*. Paris, 1880.—18. Lewin and Benda. "Erythromelalgie," *Berl. klin. Wochenschr.* 1894, p. 53. —19. Machol. "Erythromelalgie bei einem Paralytiker," *Berl. klin. Wochenschr.* 1892, p. 1319.—20. Mackenzie, Stephen. *Brit. Med. Journal*, 1879, i. p. 704.—21. Mitchell, Weir. "Painful Affection of the Feet," *Philadelphia Med. Times*, 1872, pp. 81, 113.—22. *Idem.* "On a rare Vaso-motor Neurosis of the Extremities and on the Maladies with which it may be confounded," *American Journal of the Medical Sciences*, July, 1878, p. 17. The title Erythromelalgia was given to the disease in this paper.—23. *Idem. Erythromelalgia: Clinical Lessons on Nervous Diseases*, 1897, p. 177.—24. Morel-Lavaliée, "Un cas d'érythromélalgie (maladie de M. Raynaud et maladie de Weir Mitchell)," *Bull. soc. franç. de dermat. et syph.* Paris, 1891, ii. 354.—25. Morgan. "Erythromelalgia," *Lancet*, Jan. 5, 1889.—26. Paget. "A Case illustrating certain Nervous Disorders," *St. Barth. Hosp. Rep.* 1871.—27. Pezzoli. *Wiener klin. Wochenschr.* 1896, p. 1263.—28. Prentiss. "Two Cases of Erythromelalgia," *Trans. of the Association of American Physicians*, Philadelphia, 1897, p. 303.—29. Rolleston. "Case showing some of the features of Erythromelalgia," *Lancet*, 1898, p. 783.—30. Ross. *Diseases of the Nervous System*, vol. i. p. 662; 1883.—31. Seeligmüller. Wreden's Sammlung. kurzer Med., *Lehrbuch der peripheren Nerven und des Sympathicus*, Bd. v. p. 37; 1882.— 32. Senator. *Berl. klin. Wochenschr.* 1892, p. 1127.—33. Sigerson. "Note sur la

paralysie vaso-motrice généralisée des membres supérieurs," *Progrès médical*, 1874, pp. 229, 246.—34. STRAUSS. "Paralysie Vaso-motrice des membres inférieurs," *Soc. méd des hôpitaux*, March 26, 1880.—35. STURGE, ALLEN. "Rare vaso-motor Disturbance in the Leg," *Trans. Clin. Soc.* 1879, vol. xii. p. 156; Sequel, vol. xxii. p. 381.—36. THOMA. "Ueber die Abhängigkeit der Bindgewebsneubildung in der Arterienintima von den mechanischen Bedingungen des Blutumlaufes," *Archiv für patholog. Anat.* 1883, Bd. xciii. p. 496.—37. *Idem.* "Ueber das Verhalten der Arterien bei supraorbital Neuralgie," *Deutsches Archiv für klin. Medicin*, 1888, p. 409.—38. VULPIAN. "Congestion symétrique des extrémités," *L'appareil vaso-moteur*, vol. ii. p. 623.—39. WOODNUT. *Journal of Nervous and Mental Diseases*, Oct. 1884, p. 627.

T. B.

POSTSCRIPT.—As these lines pass through the press an important paper on erythromelalgia appears by Weir Mitchell and Spiller.[1] The great toe was removed from a patient aged 62, who suffered from this disease. The nerves of the part were found "intensely degenerated;" but a few fibres, standing out in the background of connective tissue,—hardly more than three or four in a section,—were seen with axis-cylinder and medullary sheath perfect. The vessels were also much degenerated; and here we are reminded of the relation, discussed by Friedländer, between arterial disease and nerve degeneration. Whether in this case the arterial or the nervous degeneration were the antecedent is difficult to say; unless, at the age of 62, the arterial disease may be assumed to have taken the lead. Auerbach,[2] on the other hand, reports a case, with necropsy, in which the nerves of the lower limb were found perfectly normal, even in the feet; but the related posterior roots were degenerated. Yet we know that posterior roots may be degenerated often enough without erythromelalgia. For the present Weir Mitchell seems to think that interruption of sensory fibres anywhere between (or within) the spinal cord and the periphery may, under certain ill-understood circumstances, cause erythromelalgia.

DISEASES OF THE NERVOUS SYSTEM

DISEASES OF THE NERVES

PARTICULAR DISEASES OF THE SPINAL NERVES

INTRODUCTORY.—If we examine the medullated fibres of a mixed nerve, such as the sciatic, we find that the axis-cylinder—an integral part of the neuron—is its active constituent; the myelin sheath, or the white substance of Schwann, being but a protecting and isolating covering. The myelin is supported by the funnels of Golgi and Rezzonico, which are proportionately more numerous in the medullated fibres of the cord than in those of the peripheral nerves. The slits of Lantermann are probably dependent on the existence of these funnels, and the effect of various fixing solutions upon them. The neurilemma is an outer enveloping sheath divided into segments, each segment possessing a large nucleus, and each of them acting as a complete outer covering for the nerve fibre between the two nodes of Ranvier. The nucleus of the neurilemma, or the segmental nucleus as it has been not inappropriately called, is probably of far greater importance than is generally supposed. It has unquestionably a trophic influence over the portion of the myelin sheath belonging to its segment, and where the axis-cylinder of the segment has suffered it is rarely, if ever, found normal; conversely, when the segmental nucleus is healthy, the axis-cylinder is apparently healthy also. The segmental nucleus proliferates and acts as the agent for removal of myelin

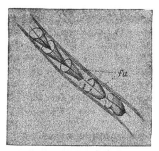

FIG. 31.—Funnels of Golgi and Rezzonico, from the posterior tibial nerve of a case of diabetic neuritis. *fu*, Funnels of Golgi.—R.A.F.

where a nerve fibre degenerates; and where regeneration of a nerve fibre occurs, an essential part of the process consists in the reappearance of the neurilemma envelope cells with their nuclei.

We are concerned just now with the process, not with the cell; and therefore to know how the process fares, when separated from its cell, becomes a very important matter. Does the law of Waller hold good, that a process, when separated from its trophic cell, necessarily under goes complete and speedy destruction? Nelaton, Wolberg, Ogston, and a number of other writers, recount cases of neuroma, and of section and other lesions of nerves, which had caused, for months or even for years, loss of sensory and motor power in the realm of the nerve affected, yet in which after reunion, by suture or other means, sensation had been restored in a few days, and motor power more slowly, but still more or less completely, in course of time. We have seen several of these cases.

What explanation can be given? Is it possible that, by means of collaterals, unaffected nerves may by anastomosis take the place of the nerve destroyed? This suggestion has been advanced by Vanlair, but it seems extremely improbable. If the distal end of the axis-cylinder process of a multipolar cell in the anterior cornu of the cord be completely separated from its trophic cell it will degenerate. Strœbe and many others have described the segmentation of the myelin; the removal of the debris either by proliferated nuclei of the neurilemma, or more probably by invading leucocytes; the gradual breaking-up of the axis-cylinder, often along with the segmentation of the myelin; and the gradual loss, moreover, of staining capacity, and therefore loss of recognition of the axis-cylinder altogether. We have repeatedly seen, in experimental sections and ligatures performed on rabbits, that a portion of the axis-cylinder, isolated in an oval-shaped ball of myelin, may persist for a long time, certainly for months, if the nucleus of the segmental neurilemma cell remain perfectly healthy—if, in other words, it has not proliferated. This is, however, only a temporary salvation, and time alone will effect its complete destruction. It is by no means necessary to take for granted that the motor end organs in muscle have no local trophic influence; and, so far as researches on this subject agree, they certainly tend to show that, notwithstanding great changes after nerve section, these end organs have a more persistent vitality than the nerve fibre running down to them.

Very different are the changes after section of sensory fibres. These fibres emanate, it is true, from trophic cells in the ganglia on the posterior nerve roots, or in the cord; but the sensory end organs are known to exert a powerful trophic influence over the fibres belonging to them, and accordingly we find in the peripheral end of a divided mixed nerve many fibres, more or less healthy in appearance; some of them apparently having given rise to a number of young fibres, probably by division of the axis-cylinder or in some other way. Here, then, we have an explanation of the rapid return of sensation after bringing divided ends of nerves together, amounting almost to union by first intention; and of the far more slow, and often far more imperfect, restoration of motor power.

The process is a part of the cell; but a process may have two trophic centres. A motor cell and its axis-cylinder process is a more easily explained entity than a sensory cell with its axis-cylinder process and its dual trophic centres. It is here that Waller's law comes into direct antagonism with surgical experience. It has been stated by Meyer, Neumann, and more recently by Kennedy, that the peripheral portion of a divided nerve is capable of such vitality that numerous young or proliferated axis-cylinders are found ready to be united by first intention whenever the surgeon's hand brings the two ends of the nerve together; but overwhelming evidence proves that, while such proliferation may take place in the sensory fibres in the peripheral end of a divided nerve, it cannot take place in the motor.

It will be convenient to refer to the vaso-motor fibres, using the term in the widest sense, in mixed nerves. These fibres are extremely fine, are medullated in most cases, and have, for their function, the supply of the vessels belonging both to the nerves and to the tissues which the nerves supply. These fibres play a very important part in the life-history of axis-cylinders, especially in disease; more particularly

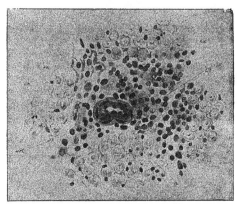

Fig. 32.—Right sciatic nerve from a case of alcoholic neuritis, showing recent leucocyte exudation around arteriole. *art*, Arteriole; *l*, leucocytes; *ex*, exudation; *n*, normal nerve fibres; *nx*, degenerated nerve fibre.—R.A.F.

in peripheral neuritis. In this affection the toxin, acting either on these fibres or directly on the capillaries in the nerve, causes not merely definite changes in the cells of the intima of the capillaries and smaller arterioles, but also small hæmorrhages, exudation of lymph, and lymphoid cells, all of which most probably interfere by pressure with neighbouring nerve fibres. But, further, it is these fine fibres, of which many must be vaso-motor, which are degenerated in an affected nerve in toxic neuritis; moreover, they are more degenerated than any other fibres. There is also strong presumptive evidence in favour of the degeneration of vaso-motor nerve fibres both in the central and peripheral ends of a divided nerve, whenever the fibres by such division have lost their function. Some evidence in favour of this will be given in treating of amputation-neuroma.

A nerve fibre is then much more complicated than Waller supposed, and it must be recognised as a specialised part of a very highly differentiated cell.

Nerve fibres generally conduct impulses in one direction only, some
to, and others from, the cells in the cord or brain; but although a fibre

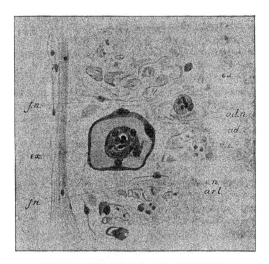

Fig. 33.—From the left sciatic nerve of a case of alcoholic neuritis showing exudation, with commencing
   organisation, and the changes in the coats of the arteriole. *arl,* Arteriole; *ex,* exudation; *f.n,* newly-
   formed connective tissue fibres; *e.n,* endothelial nuclei; *me,* media; *ad,* adventitia; *ad.n,* nuclei of
   adventitia.—R.A.F.

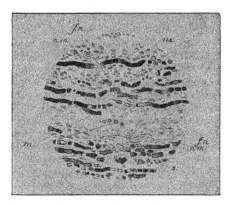

Fig. 34.—The right anterior tibial nerve from a case of alcoholic neuritis, showing greater segmentation
   of small sized than of average sized fibres. *n.m,* Small sized nerve fibres mostly degenerated; *n.x,*
   degenerated nerve fibres of larger size; *f.n,* connective tissue nuclei, proliferated in relation to fine
   fibres; *s,* segmental nuclei enlarged in size; *m,* myelin droplets.—R.A.F.

may thus conduct physiologically in one direction,—for example, centri-
fugally,—it does not follow that an injury or irritant applied to such a
fibre will not seriously affect the cell to which the process belongs, and

from which nerve stimuli pass. Whether nerve fibres conduct away from the cell, or towards it, the cell itself suffers; often only temporarily, but sometimes permanently. The changes found in the cell include alteration in the size of the cell itself; change in the position and the size of the nucleus; in the number and size of Nissl's granules, and other modifications: changes which may be temporary or permanent.

We know something of the conditions under which the telegraph wire carries on its function: now Gotch and Horsley prove by experiments that nerve fibres appear to conduct electrical currents in the direction in which they usually carry nerve stimuli; and that currents passed in an opposite direction meet with considerable resistance.

Dr. Althaus pleads in favour of the hypothesis that nerve stimuli are of an electrical nature. He considers the nerve cell to be a battery jar, as well as an accumulator of electrical or nerve energy, and that the myelin sheath of medullated fibres acts as an insulating medium to prevent escape of energy in transit. One neuron must communicate its electrical stimulus to another by induction, as there is no direct contact. Certainly, as Althaus points out, stimulation with the faradic current makes nerve cells take up more colouring matter than before; by means of these currents the cell may, he thinks, exercise a trophic influence on its processes.

CLASSIFICATION.—The consideration of the subject will be facilitated by its subdivision into two groups: one, of a more general character, will contain the pathological and clinical features common to the different forms of disease; the other, of a more special character, the several forms themselves.

GROUP I.—GENERAL FEATURES.

The subjects which fall under this head are neuritis, tumours, pressure, and wounds.

NEURITIS.—**Local neuritis.**—Inflammation may arise in various structures of a nerve: (i.) in the outer fibrous sheath surrounding the nerve bundles; this is generally called *perineuritis;* (ii.) in the delicate connective tissue strands between individual nerve fibres in the interior of a funiculus or nerve bundle, generally called *interstitial neuritis;* (iii.) in the nerve fibres themselves, generally called *parenchymatous neuritis.* The two latter forms are often associated together—for example, in peripheral or multiple neuritis of toxic origin; and it is generally considered that the second form is in these cases a sequel of the third.

Local inflammations, which originally attack from without, generally cause the first form; they may, however, if more pronounced, cause the second; but only by contiguity do they induce the third. Here we shall discuss local neuritis, usually limited to one nerve.

Causes.—Rheumatism, gout, and exposure to "cold" may induce a localised perineuritis, much in the same way as other connective tissues become inflamed in these conditions; but it is quite possible that. the active agents in rheumatism and gout may in some cases attack the nerve fibres themselves, causing a true parenchymatous neuritis. Cold probably always causes interstitial inflammation, by means perhaps of a paralytic hyperæmia.

A nerve may also be injured by wounds, bruises, muscular strains, fractures or dislocations of bones, tumours, abscesses, bedsores, or any contiguous focus of inflammation. Obviously in all these cases perineuritis is first produced; although in time the funiculi may be involved, and eventually the nerve fibres themselves.

There are many well-known instances of such local neuritis. Not infrequently a suppurating joint, or even an acute non-suppurating synovitis, may induce a local neuritis in neighbouring nerves; sometimes in syphilitic and other inflammations of the membranes of the brain and cord, a localised neuritis may be set up in the cranial or spinal nerves which arise at the site of the lesion. After a fracture neighbouring nerves may be damaged by the callus thrown out.

Lastly, there are certain states of the blood in which a limited neuritis may be determined by some local cause. It is probable, as above stated, that rheumatism and gout can act in this way; certainly in acute tuberculosis with much ptomaine absorption, in alcoholism, and as the result of any of the toxic causes which generally give rise to a multiple neuritis, the lesion may be limited to one nerve. Diphtheria is perhaps the most striking illustration of such limitation of a truly toxic agent in its sphere of attack; although in some cases a more general invasion of many peripheral nerves may ensue. Syphilis, cancer, and leucocythæmia may bring about a toxic neuritis; either through the blood or by direct infiltration of the nerve tissue with specific cells, causing local inflammatory changes.

Pathological anatomy.—In perineuritis and interstitial neuritis there is exudation into the connective tissue; and, dependent on the nature of the inflammatory process, there may be complete absorption, organisation of inflammatory lymph, or in infective cases even suppuration. The effect on the nerve fibres themselves depends on the ˙amount of pressure exercised and the nature of the exciting cause. The affected part of the nerve is reddened and swollen; the exudation infiltrating the sheath is sero-fibrinous or jelly-like, containing numerous lymphoid cells, especially around the vessels, often in well-marked groups; and not infrequently capillary hæmorrhages may be noted.

Microscopically these changes are best studied where the funiculi are affected. Here the exudation is very distinct, especially just within the sheath of the funiculus and along the lines of the septa; it is always most marked near the vessels, and the lymphoid cells òr leucocytes may be seen in the effused lymph, especially around the vessels. As the sheath of a funiculus is proportionally strong and inelastic, any great amount of effusion implies serious pressure directly on the nerve fibres, which must inevitably suffer.

Parenchymatous neuritis is described under multiple neuritis, there-fore no reference need be made to it here. The inflammatory process may be limited to one portion of a nerve.

Clinical features.—The symptoms of local neuritis vary with the extent and position of the inflammation and the particular nerve concerned. There may be high temperature, malaise, and considerable constitutional disturbances, which disappear in a few days; in milder cases there may be none of these phenomena. The chief sensory phenomenon is pain felt in the nerve, often radiating towards its radicles, or diffused over the whole limb. The pain is burning, gnawing, or boring, and is increased by digital pressure over the affected nerve, or by movement if thereby the contracting muscles put any strain on the nerve. The pain is often worse at night, and is increased by exercise, as well as by dependent posture, or anything causing passive congestion of the limb. The skin is often extremely hyperæsthetic, and there may be local redness, or œdema. When the inflammatory condition has interrupted the conduction of nerve impulses local anæsthesia not infrequently appears; sometimes there is perverted sensation; and in some rare and inexplicable cases there are similar, though slighter changes in the corresponding part of the opposite limb. Palpation where possible may demonstrate a distinct increase in size of the affected nerve.

Where there are many motor fibres in the nerve concerned there is paralysis with wasting of muscle, in degree depending largely on the amount of interference with functions. The muscles may simply be weakened, or they may become absolutely paralysed, and give a well-marked reaction of degeneration. The muscles are often tender, extremely painful on attempted movement, and not infrequently show fibrillary twitchings.

The *trophic changes* are very varied. Not infrequently the skin becomes thin and glossy; sometimes reddened and swollen, as recorded above. More rarely the skin becomes thickened, especially on parts of the affected limb subjected to intermittent pressure, where a callosity may result. The fingers become thin, from atrophy of sub-cutaneous tissues and muscles. The nails suffer remarkably, becoming grooved, brittle, and often falling off. The hair of the affected part often becomes scanty, or is altered in colour or texture. There is some-times profuse local sweating; occasionally herpetic and bullous eruptions appear in the line of the affected nerve, and sometimes ulcers, which are most resistant to treatment. In very chronic cases the bones not infrequently undergo atrophy. The joints of the affected limb are some-times swollen, especially in very complete, long-standing cases; and fibrous adhesions may ensue, with eventual fixation. In most cases these graver symptoms are absent, and pain of an intermittent type is the prominent feature. In chronic cases pain may be less pronounced, but trophic changes in skin, muscles, and joints are common (*vide* pp. 545 and 569).

Diagnosis.—In the majority of cases of local neuritis the diagnosis presents little difficulty. Definite sensory and motor phenomena referable to one nerve, localised pain elicited on pressure along the line of the nerve, and the recognition of an etiological factor in the case, simplify the diagnosis. It must be remembered that the pain of neuritis is of much longer standing and more continuous than neuralgia, although the pain of localised neuritis might with justice be called neuralgia. Many neuralgias leave local œdema and distinctly painful spots, which correspond to nerve trunks or their branches; but a marked alteration in sensation, especially anæsthesia, and paralysis with muscular wasting are absolute proofs of neuritis. Rheumatism and gout may cause neuritis, but pain produced by either of these agents is more likely to be due to inflammation about tendons or joints.

Prognosis.—The prognosis depends largely on the nature of the individual case. Acute neuritis may disappear in a few weeks if the cause can be successfully and promptly removed. Perineuritis and interstitial neuritis must of necessity be tedious, because inflammatory lymph has been effused, and absorption must occur before cure can be effected. Rapid improvement under treatment always renders complete recovery more probable; while persistent inflammation, however slight, will almost certainly be very protracted, and the cure may be incomplete. Rheumatism and gout often cause neuritis lasting months instead of weeks; partly because of the difficulty of eliminating the toxic agent, and partly because inflammatory lymph, if not removed, organises: connective tissue is thereafter extremely apt, by contraction, seriously or even permanently to compress the nerve fibres in the affected funiculi. In such cases the axis-cylinders may not be interrupted; but the myelin sheaths are thinner than normal, and certainly clinical experience teaches that conduction of impulses is greatly hindered by such a condition. The best prognosis must therefore be assigned to neuritis which is the result of an injury. A less favourable prognosis should be accorded to toxic cases, where the toxin cannot be removed at once; a still more grave prognosis will be assigned to all chronic cases with a duration of months or years, even although a long-standing case may at last be treated successfully.

Treatment.—The cause must be searched for and removed. Any injury must be suitably dealt with, the utmost care being taken to prevent a nerve, exposed in a wound, from becoming septic. Rheumatism, gout, and syphilis must be met by specific management; it is good routine practice to give salicylate of soda, or salol, where, with no certain rheumatic history, there is even a faint probability of its existence.

In acute cases it is always useful to act on the bowels by one or more doses of a saline hydragogue cathartic, or blue pill followed by a suitable purge; to aid elimination by the kidneys with diuretics; and lastly, to increase diaphoresis by baths, especially Turkish and vapour baths. Rest, removal of inflammatory products by absorption, and suitable means for keeping up nutrition of muscles, must be specially referred to. Rest can be most satisfactorily secured by confining the patient to bed, or at least keeping the affected limb absolutely quiet. A splint, well protected by wadding, will be found useful for this purpose, and every care should be taken to impress the patient with the necessity for this procedure. Sedative applications are of great value for the relief of pain. Continuous bathing of the affected part with hot water; hot fomentations, with or without the addition of tincture of opium; poulticing the limb; and the use of liniments, such as the British Pharmacopœial belladonna, aconite, and chloroform liniment, are most soothing. Leeching is likely to be of value where the local inflammation is recent and severe. Where the pain is harassing, or unbearable, local hypodermic injections of morphine or cocaine are often most beneficial; but they should only be employed along with absolute rest to the affected part, as any use of the limb rendered possible by a hypodermic injection of morphine is certain to be harmful. Obviously counter-irritation and sedative applications are of most use in the acute cases.

But in every form of neuritis at present under consideration there is effusion of inflammatory lymph, and the absorption of this is greatly facilitated by more vigorous counter-irritation. Small fly blisters, or blistering fluid painted along the line of nerve, or even the application of stimulating liniments, such as linimentum terebinthinæ aceticum, should be used, provided there be no trophic change in the skin where they are to be applied. Any change in sensation, especially anæsthesia, or any evidence of incipient "glossy skin," should absolutely contra-indicate all vigorous counter-irritation, and should prevent attendants from applying very hot fomentations or poultices. The constant current is recommended, both for the relief of pain and for the removal of exudation; a mild current and the positive pole applied locally should always be used, care being taken to avoid causing muscular contraction by interrupting the current. Potassium iodide is often given, sometimes with marked success; and small doses of mercury and antimony are frequently of great service.

The nutrition of muscles supplied by the affected nerve will require attention; but the faradic or interrupted galvanic currents should never be resorted to for exercising muscles, so long as any acute or subacute inflammatory condition remains. After subsidence of inflammation the interrupted current is of great benefit; but before this occurs it is better either to disregard the muscles, or to try the most gentle of passive movements.

In chronic cases of neuritis, where some organisation of inflammatory lymph has occurred, friction along the line of the nerve, and energetic and long-continued massage, are often followed by progressive improvement in both sensation and in motor power.

Neuritis migrans.—One of the most extraordinary results of an injury to a nerve has been called neuritis migrans, although perhaps it might be more correctly named neuritis ascendens. The ordinary form consists in an inflammatory process beginning at the seat of injury, and advancing more or less quickly up the nerve, causing intense pain, often so excruciating and so incurable as to necessitate nerve section, or even amputation.　Dr. Weir Mitchell describes several of these cases, which appear to be more frequent after gunshot wounds or sword cuts; although other cases are on record, such as the case of a girl whose median nerve was transfixed by the thin spout of a watering can, and on whom, after excision of bits of the nerve had only temporarily relieved the intolerable pain, amputation of the arm was performed.　It appears probable that the inflammation spreads upwards by the lymphatics, the rapidity of the process depending largely on the intensity of an infective organism or toxin.　This is a very different process from the changes which occur in the central end of any mixed nerve after section, and where there is no infective agent.　The condition we are considering is a true inflammatory process, the lymph stream carrying the organisms or their toxins upwards.

Again, an injury to a nerve may keep that nerve in a hyperæsthetic state.　This is sometimes due to a neuroma, or where the sensory nerve fibres are nipped by connective tissue.　These cases are generally completely relieved by opening the wound and removing the focus of irritation.

And there is yet a third group often closely allied to both the preceding.　A neuritis, not due to a local infective agent or toxin, extends up to the cord (or brain), and invades a tract of cord, setting up a chronic or subacute myelitis, which may or may not involve the membranes. .This group would include all the cases of so-called "reflex paralysis." Gowers mentions, by way of example, that, from a vesical inflammation, paralysis of both legs may result; and he attributes such cases to an ascending neuritis.　Such cases are rare, so rare that their very existence has been disputed; many authors asserting that the agent must be infective, as in the other cases, or else that the paralysis is functional, not organic.

Nothing can be stated as to the anatomical changes in those cases of so-called reflex paralysis, because it is alleged that there may be no changes in the nerve, although a spinal myelitis may be set up apparently by irritation of some kind actually passing up a nerve or nerves.　It must be remembered that grave doubts are expressed of the existence of cases of paralysis produced in the way indicated; and certainly they do not seem to be true cases of ascending neuritis at all.

Closely allied to these groups of cases of neuritis migrans are those in which sympathetic neuritis occurs, the corresponding nerve on the opposite side becoming affected, without, so it is said, the nerve cells being necessarily involved.　Gowers explains these curious phenomena by suggesting that the sympathetic neuritis may really be of vaso-motor origin.

The *treatment* of these curious cases of ascending neuritis consists in removing the focus of irritation from the old wound, separating any strong cicatricial adhesions, and removing a neuroma if present.　If this measure fails a portion of the nerve should be excised above, or at the seat of the pain. Failing this, amputation is probably the only remedy, and even this is by no means surely successful.

TUMOURS OF NERVES.—New formations are found in the spinal nerves, as follows :—

Neuroma.—Nerve tumours may be *true*, implying an actual increase of nerve tissue, or *false*, in which the tumour is not made up of nerve tissue at all.

True neuroma generally consists of medullated nerve fibres, though there are cases in which the tumour is made up of non-medullated fibres only. Ganglion cells have been described in one or two rare cases, but their occurrence is quite exceptional.

Many forms of neuroma occupy an intermediate position ; they undoubtedly consist in an increase of true nerve tissue, but the large amount of interstitial connective tissue also present allies them closely to fibroma.

The forms of neuroma requiring separate description are :—

1. *Multiple neuroma.* — These growths are often intermediate in anatomical structure between the true and the false. They are found on practically all the nerves of the body ; though far more generally on cranial and spinal nerves, and much less frequently on the sympathetic system. They vary in size from a pea to a large tumour, but in the latter the fibrous far exceed the nerve-tissue elements. Multiple neuromata sometimes specially affect the terminal cutaneous branches of sensory nerves, forming painful little nodules—the so-called " Tubercula dolorosa," and these are often associated with similar tumours in the nerve trunks. We have seen one case in which hundreds of tumours could be made out by palpation.

Neuroma may be hereditary; and men generally are more often affected than women : otherwise little is known concerning them.

Pain, dull, sharp, or lancinating, which is curiously erratic and constantly changing in degree, is the most frequent phenomenon.

There may be hyperæsthesia or anæsthesia, often with premonitory numbness, and formication, and spasm ; or paralysis with wasting of muscles may result, dependent on the nerves involved and on the amount of interference with their functions.

Diagnosis is easy in most cases, because some of the tumours are generally palpable. Where they are not palpable the diagnosis must depend on the evidence of interference with sensory or motor nerve fibres.

2. *Multiple neurofibroma.*—A special form of multiple neuroma has been described by Recklinghausen, whose name is associated with it. Since he first drew the attention of neurologists to the condition, many papers have been written about the disease ; that by Feindel and R. Oppenheim, in the *Archives générales de médecine* of last year, being perhaps one of the most interesting.

The essential features are as follows : (i.) Numberless small soft fibrous nodules, some sessile, others pedunculated, varying in size from a millet seed to a small nut, situated in the thickness of the skin. Sometimes larger cutaneous or subcutaneous tumours occur, and these may be plexiform neuromata or fibromata on small subcutaneous nerves.

(ii.) Tumours on the nerve trunks, the peripheral nerves, sometimes the spinal ganglia, and sometimes even on the nerve fibres, at or near the nuclear cells from which they take origin. The superficial tumours are palpable ; those on nerve trunks and in central positions generally give rise to marked phenomena such as pain, cramps, contracture and paralysis, and are thus easily recognised. These tumours may grow rapidly, may vary greatly in size ; and usually certain of those superficially and also of those deeply situated are of the nature of plexiform neuroma. Neurofibromata have even been recorded in connection with the visceral nerves.

(iii.) Pigmentation of the skin occurs in small spots, or larger patches. The former are found on the trunk and upper part of the limbs, and are not generally met with on the face, hands or feet. The patches are of a brownish white colour and vary greatly in size. The small pigmented spots may disappear, the larger patches generally persist.

Not infrequently ordinary nævi are found in patients suffering from this disease.

(iv.) There are many sensory and motor phenomena resulting from the presence of the nerve tumours such as pain, paralysis, contracture, cramps, and weakness of muscles ; but in addition there are peculiar mental changes, which are very characteristic, including gradual loss of intellectual power and difficulty in speaking.

Cases occur which depart more or less from the typical description given here. The disease is, as a rule, congenital, or at any rate a hereditary predisposition is traceable in most cases.

The prognosis depends on the success and possibility of operative treatment, which consists in the removal of such tumours as are causing most inconvenience to the patient.

3. *Plexiform neuroma*, as suggested by the name, is a nodular and tortuous bunch of nerve fibres matted together, often by myxomatous tissue ; each strand consists of a small group of nerve fibres, partly normal and partly degenerated, surrounded by an inner coat of open, delicate connective tissue with many nuclei, and an outer laminated coat of stronger fibrous tissue.

This condition begins in fœtal life, and is generally associated with a branch of the trifacial nerve in the orbit or upper eyelid ; but it occurs also in connection with the cervical, brachial, lumbar, and solar plexuses, and sometimes in the penis or the mamma. It may be superficial or deep-seated, and is of very slow growth. Only a very few isolated cases are on record.

The causation is unknown. In rare cases this neuroma may cause pressure on other structures, and sometimes interference with the functions of nerve fibres.

Diagnosis is only possible where the tumour is palpable.

4. *Amputation neuroma.* — After an amputation, larger or smaller bulbous swellings form on the central ends of the divided nerves. These swellings are the expression of the enormous vitality and rapidity of growth of divided axis-cylinders, in their efforts to reach the structures to which they were formerly distributed.

The funiculi grow beyond the point of section, are arrested in their efforts to grow straight onwards, and, partly by the thickened peri-neurium and interstitial tissue between the funiculi and partly by other causes, become twisted into a bulbous swelling. But though the funiculi are arrested in their growth, the individual axis-cylinders continue their efforts; and many of these can be seen isolated or in little groups of two or

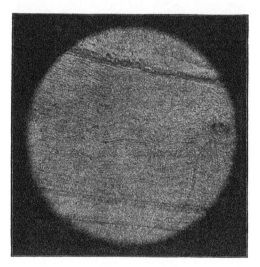

Fɪɢ. 35.—Funiculus of rabbit's sciatic nerve, healthy side, showing fine medullated fibres in groups or strands.—R.A.F.

three, making their way amongst the strong bands of connective tissue. Sections taken from the neuroma, and at short intervals above it, give an admirable picture of ascending degeneration in the nerve, especially if a number of nerves, obtained at varying dates after amputation, can be ex-amined. A few fibres have degenerated to some extent upwards; these are fibres whose chief trophic centre appears to be situated peripherally: they are few and far between, and some doubt has been expressed as to their existence. The majority of the larger fibres in the stump of a mixed nerve merely become thinner, less well covered with myelin; yet they persist as definite nerve fibres. But the most striking change is seen in the fine fibres, which are in all probability vaso-motor in function. Those which have lost their function—those, that is, passing downwards to vessels in the nerves or tissues below the level of division of the nerve —have degenerated, and their place is taken by connective tissue. This can be seen very clearly, because these fine fibres in a healthy mixed nerve are all, or nearly all, medullated; and, further, they are grouped together in the funiculi, and hence are readily recognised. Above a neuroma after amputation these fibres are replaced by connective tissue, and on microscopic examination these patches are very definitely seen. As the nerve is investigated farther upwards these fine fibres become less affected, because at a higher level there is an ever-increasing number of fibres whose function is still retained.

Further than this, one striking change in the vessels, which appears

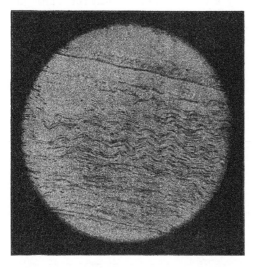

Fig. 36.—Funiculus of central end of rabbit's sciatic nerve, twenty-three days after application of a double ligature, showing thickened connective tissue, septa replacing fine medullated fibres.—R.A.F.

to be associated with the degeneration of the fine fibres, is well demonstrated. Where the fine fibres have degenerated the vessels show marked proliferation of the nuclei of the intima; to a less extent of the media; and to a still less extent of the adventitia. This proliferation of nuclei is well seen in the capillaries, arterioles, and venules; and it appears to decrease as the nerve is examined farther and farther upwards, away from the neuroma. It seems possible that the connective tissue replacing the degenerated fine medullated fibres, which have lost their function, may by compression have damaged neighbouring fine fibres, and so have produced, though to a gradual diminishing degree, this remarkable change in the vessels. The fact that in many cases of toxic neuritis three events are associated—namely, early degeneration of these fine medullated fibres, proliferation of nuclei in the vessels, and exudation of lymph with lymphoid cells and sometimes red blood corpuscles—seems to indicate that the fine fibres and the vessels are associated, and that they play an important part in many nerve conditions.

It only remains to be stated, that there are more nerve fibres in the neuroma itself than there are entering it; and this notwithstanding that the twisting of the fibres adds apparently to their number, and that many fibres are so compressed by fibrous tissue as in all probability to be arrested in their further growth. The cause of this is that the old nerve fibres, or as many of them as are able to do so, proliferate; and each old axis-cylinder may form several young ones, which rapidly acquire myelin sheaths.

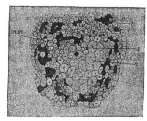

Fig. 37.—Funiculus from central end of sciatic nerve of rabbit, twenty-three days after double ligature, showing thickening of connective tissue strands between and partly replacing the fine fibres. *n*, Ordinarily sized nerve fibres; *n.m*, fine modulated nerve fibres; *t*, connective tissue strands; *s*, segmental nuclei.—R.A.F.

An amputation neuroma becomes pathological when it causes pain and discomfort. The pain is sharp, burning, or shooting; and is specially severe when any pressure is brought to bear on the neuroma. The pain may thus prevent the use of an artificial limb. In addition to sensory phenomena there is sometimes twitching or actual muscular spasm; and, as such phenomena are produced reflexly, they may be unilateral or bilateral. Even epileptic seizures have followed the irritation of such a neuroma; and, though rarely, profound mental depression may be caused by a painful neuroma.

The prognosis of such a case is not entirely satisfactory; operation will temporarily relieve the condition, but it may recur in course of time: much undoubtedly depends on the care taken by the surgeon.

The treatment is simply removal; and in so doing to make every effort to prevent inflammation in the stump, and to cause the formation of as small a bulbous end to the nerve as possible, and in a situation where it may escape most pressure.

Fibroma.—These fibrous tumours have been described already under false neuroma, and they are of fairly common occurrence. Multiple neuromata are generally largely fibrous in character.

Myxoma sometimes occurs on nerves, the interstitial tissues of the nerve forming mucoid material.

Glioma is rare on peripheral nerves; sometimes the auditory nerves are affected by these tumours.

Carcinoma and **sarcoma** also occur, the former more frequently; they are almost always secondary, but a number of primary sarcomata of the sciatic, musculo-spiral, and other nerves have been recently recorded.

Syphilis frequently affects the cranial nerves, but generally within the skull; and much more rarely affects spinal nerves. Where spinal nerves do suffer the inflammation is generally secondary to syphilitic inflammation of the spinal meninges, and it is the nerve roots which are the site of syphilitic exudation. In this way one or more nerves may become affected. It may be added that in some cases of locomotor ataxy the peripheral nerves are affected; although this is a secondary, and, according to some authors, mainly a degenerative change, and not a true primary inflammation. A gumma may by chance involve a peripheral nerve, and occasionally an interstitial inflammation in a nerve may be of syphilitic nature; but such cases are very rare. These forms of syphilitic affection of nerve are secondary or tertiary. No special anatomical description is requisite, and the symptoms and signs are in no way different from a local neuritis. The *diagnosis* will depend mainly upon the history of the case and coexistent evidences of syphilis. The *prognosis* is favourable in many cases, where early treatment is possible. The *treatment* consists in the administration of iodides and mercury, both together or alternately. These remedies act marvellously; and where there is any evidence of an acute, or what is more common, a subacute inflammatory process, mercury is invaluable.

There is no necessity to enlarge on the 'methods of using these remedies, but in the case of a local lesion mercurial inunction would certainly suggest itself.

PRESSURE ON NERVES.—Everyone is familiar with the "pins and needles" sensation, and most people with the inability to co-ordinate, or even in any way to put the affected muscles into motion, which follows prolonged pressure on a mixed nerve. Pressure, not in itself severe, will in time produce the well-known sleeping foot; or the more lasting paralysis of the upper extremity of the drunkard who falls asleep with his arm hanging over a chair; or the well-known crutch palsy of the cripple: the prickling begins with either a hot or cold sensation, and it passes away as soon as the pressure is removed. If a nerve is ligatured in an animal the distal part swells rapidly, often increasing to three times its former size; and, if the ligature is retained, this swelling persists and even increases for a long time. Is it not possible that pressure, in no degree approaching the severity of a ligature, may yet interfere with the circulation of blood or lymph in the peripheral part of a nerve? Pressure at least interrupts the conduction of nerve impulses, and moreover by its irritation causes very distinct paræsthesiæ or perverted sensations. Pressure must therefore break the nerve currents in some way, and it certainly generates currents of a remarkable kind, passing sometimes in the direction opposite to their ordinary route. This is difficult to explain, although there is some plausibility in the suggestion that as myelin is in a fluid state during life, any displacement of its molecules may interfere with its function as an insulating medium for the axis-cylinders; a suggestion which does not materially help us to understand the problem. In seeking for a workable hypothesis it certainly seems very much easier to take into account the disturbed circulation of blood or lymph.

In a case where there is prolonged pressure on a mixed nerve, in crutch palsy, for example, the motor is far more marked and more prolonged than the sensory paralysis. With almost complete paralysis, after the prickling feeling has passed away, there may be no lasting sensory change at all; or some formication may continue without actual loss of sensation, common or tactile. Perhaps this well-known symptom of pressure paralysis is one of the strongest arguments in favour of a dual trophic centre for most sensory fibres, if not for all. If there is a trophic centre in a touch corpuscle, and a greater trophic centre in a cell, either of a posterior nerve root ganglion or of the cord, surely these sensory fibres should recover with greater rapidity, and just in the same way be more capable of rapid union and early resumption of functions after suture of the two ends of a divided nerve.

Lastly, the result of pressure on a nerve depends greatly on the vitality and general state of health of the individual. The slightest pressure kept up for a short time on a nerve, which in health would not produce any effect, in a person debilitated by some illness may cause marked paralysis.

Etiology.—There are many causes of pressure; a complete list would necessitate a consideration of most of the nerves of the body separately. Besides pressure from without, instances of which have already been referred to, dislocations, fractures, and tumours of all kinds are among the common causes of pressure from within.

Anatomy.—Much which has been said under the general observations might be repeated here. Pressure kept up for a short time only, causes transient symptoms and signs, probably depending on changes interfering rather with functions of the nerve than with its anatomical structure. But prolonged pressure is apt to set up distinct local exudation, with subsequent organisation into connective tissue, constituting a form of interstitial neuritis; or it may, though much more rarely, cause the parenchymatous form.

But it is quite possible for pressure to interrupt all nerve impulses completely, to divide the nerve as by a ligature, without any real inflammatory process at all. This, however, is extremely rare.

Symptoms.—The symptoms vary greatly, as the pressure is slight and persistent, or sudden and severe.

Where the pressure is very gradual, as from the growth of a tumour, there is an extraordinary power of resistance in nerve fibres, and a capacity for adapting themselves to altered conditions; always provided that the pressure be exerted slowly enough. Everyone is familiar with instances of tumours apparently pressing on nerve fibres without causing any symptoms. Less gradual pressure, as by the finger on a nerve, and where there is no opportunity for the nerve fibres to adapt themselves to the compressing force, causes tingling in the area of skin supplied by the nerve, and a peculiar hot feeling; later anæsthesia or paræsthesia sets in, and then loss of motor power and of co-ordination in the affected muscles. When the pressure is removed motion and co-ordination in the affected muscles are regained, and sensation returns. The tingling may last for a longer time; but any protracted alteration in function implies either a definite nerve fibre lesion or inflammation resulting from the pressure. As already stated, the health of the individual determines the early appearance, the severity, and the duration of these sensory and motor phenomena; the slighter pressures causing more marked results in debilitated than in healthy subjects.

It must be remembered that in the palsied arm of the drunkard, who falls asleep with the arm hanging over the back of a chair, anæsthesia and motor paralysis may last for hours or days; implying a more severe interference with the conducting power and the molecular structure of the nerve at the site of pressure. There is most probably interference with the circulation of blood and lymph in the nerve, and thus is set up the condition which, in effect at least, is a local neuritis. Gradual recovery is the rule, even though a certain amount of atrophy of the affected muscles may have occurred.

Severe pressure causes a lesion closely resembling section or ligature of the nerve; and it produces the same changes as those described in full detail under nerve injuries.

The *diagnosis* should depend on the nerve affected, and whether it be one which is liable to compression. Generally a history of compression is obtainable, but each nerve requires separate consideration in this respect.

The *prognosis* is generally favourable; although in many cases days, or even weeks may elapse before sensory and motor power return.

The *treatment* is exactly the same as for nerve injuries, but suturing is unnecessary, unless the compressing force has caused complete division, or a fibrous nodule has formed at the site, preventing regeneration. Massage, electricity, and passive movements are indicated, care being taken to insure rest so long as there is any active inflammatory process in the affected nerve.

WOUNDS OF NERVES.—A nerve may be injured in many ways, especially by cuts, or stabs, and gun-shot wounds. The median, and sometimes branches of the ulnar nerve are injured by such accidents as occur in ærated water factories, or in work with sharp tools. The effect of such a lesion depends, firstly, upon the magnitude of the nerve or the nerve trunk damaged; secondly, and more especially, upon the amount of bruising and laceration; and, thirdly, and perhaps most important of all, upon the presence or absence of septic organisms. The larger the nerve which is injured the more likely are serious consequences to ensue. The most serious result is undoubtedly progressive ascending neuritis. It must, however, be remembered, that a nerve, after division, may unite by first intention, provided there be nothing to interfere with such union. Unfortunately, after many deep cuts or stabs, and certainly after gun-shot wounds, there is so much bruising and consequent exudation of inflammatory lymph, that union by first intention is absolutely impossible.

The division of a large nerve, such as the sciatic, is serious for three reasons : first, because it means a deeper wound, and therefore almost certainly more bruising and inflammatory lymph; secondly, because when a large nerve like the sciatic is injured, an extensive area of the body is cut off from the central nervous system; and lastly, the shock caused by the injury to a large nerve trunk is extremely great, and fainting is by no means uncommon; indeed, in a weak subject even fatal syncope may occur. The sciatic nerve is more frequently injured in warfare than in times of peace; but the scythe has been responsible for not a few accidental sections.

The *anatomical* changes resulting from a nerve injury depend much on the nature of the case. The severed fibres mostly undergo degeneration, as described in the general account of the neuron.

Beginning with Waller's account in 1862, many descriptions of the degenerative changes in the peripheral end of a divided nerve have been given; but it must be clearly remembered that some authors have begun to dispute the wholesale degeneration of the fibres in the peripheral end; indeed, as already stated, there are unquestionably not a few fibres, probably sensory, which do so escape destruction in the peripheral, although in the central end they may even degenerate. These fibres almost certainly possess a peripheral trophic centre in touch corpuscles or other sensory end organ; although their chief trophic centre is probably in the posterior nerve root ganglia or the cord.

The usual description of the changes in the peripheral end of a divided nerve is, briefly, as follows. About the third to the fifth day the myelin sheaths begin to break up, as described by von Büngner and others, forming ovoid balls, which sometimes break up into rows of globules; this division is undoubtedly modified to some extent by the spiral threads forming the funnels of Golgi and Rezzonico. The axis-cylinders sometimes divide at the ends of the ovoid balls of myelin, and the separated bits of axis-cylinder may be seen inside the balls. Certainly in two to three weeks the axis-cylinders either cease to take on any stain, or break up so that they disappear from observation. The debris of myelin —for the larger balls break up into smaller and still smaller globules—is removed by the segmental nuclei, which proliferate and, being set free, act as phagocytes; or leucocytes enter the neurilemma sheath, but this is unlikely. Now, unquestionably, certain factors determine the date when these changes begin, and their rate of progression. In experimental sections performed on dogs and rabbits by one of us, local inflammation, as, for instance, septic infection of the wound (a very common occurrence in a dog or cat), caused a marked acceleration of the degenerative changes.

It is not possible to make a similar statement with regard to human beings; we can only argue from analogy that similar conditions may reduce the powers of resistance of severed nerve fibres to the process of decay.

It is the rapid return of sensation, after surgical reunion of a divided nerve, which makes certain authors doubt this wholesale destruction, and assert that axis-cylinders in the peripheral end, probably formed by proliferation from pre-existing axis-cylinders, are awaiting the surgeon's help to effect a junction with central axis-cylinders, so as to conduct sensory impressions, at least, in a matter of twenty-four to forty-eight hours' time. One point is certain, that axis-cylinders do persist in the peripheral end of a divided nerve, not merely for three weeks, but for many months; although sufficient proof is still lacking for the statement that these axis-cylinders, staining so feebly as to be almost unrecognisable, do proliferate.

The changes occurring in the central end of a divided nerve have been referred to under the general description of the neuron, together with some general observations on the changes produced by such section on the trophic nerve cells.

A neuroma may form on the extremity of the central end, of the nature of the amputation neuroma already considered. The amount of inflammatory exudation, or hæmorrhage, in the neighbourhood of the divided fibres will greatly influence the future history of the case. A large amount of bruising, as in a gun-shot wound, means a great exudation of inflammatory lymph, probably hæmorrhage, and a proportionately more difficult task for the severed nerve fibres which are endeavouring to reunite. The presence of an infective organism implies the grave risk of ascending neuritis; and a large amount of organised lymph or blood clot will undoubtedly hinder reunion of the nerve fibres, and, by pressure on the central end, may keep up persistent irritative action which although certainly local, has been called a form of ascending neuritis. Indeed, it seems probable that in these cases a true ascending interstitial neuritis does occur, though it may be very limited and very slow in development.

The *symptoms* depend on the nature of the individual case. If a mixed nerve be completely divided there will be paralysis of motion and sensation in the affected part, with—unless union occur by first intention—well-marked reaction of degeneration. If the union be by first intention the reaction of degeneration may be partial or incomplete.

At the moment of the accident, if a large nerve be divided, there is frequently severe shock with faintness; and this may be increased by intensely agonising pain following on the injury, and only gradually abating.

With a gun-shot wound Weir Mitchell describes the sensations as very varied. Of ninety-one cases, investigated by him, in fully one-third there was no pain, although a nerve was known to be injured by the bullet: he describes the sensation in such cases as resembling a stroke with a stick, or as unperceived till the bleeding directs attention to the wound. In other cases there may be intense pain and faintness. Where a nerve is not completely divided there may be a spasm of muscles. After a complete division of a nerve there is anæsthesia; when it is partial there is often hyperæsthesia in the area of the skin involved, and the pain felt along the line of the affected nerve is of a burning and intensely agonising kind.

If the injury does not amount to division, very often there is more marked motor than sensory paralysis; and the sensory fibres appear to recover far more rapidly than the motor. This may indicate greater vitality, and consequently more rapid recovery of sensory fibres; or that sensory impulses require less perfectly insulated nerve fibres; or, lastly, that there may be anastomosis to some extent with sensory filaments of neighbouring nerves which are able to take the place of the damaged fibres. Certainly after a severe bruise of a nerve there may be motor paralysis, and extreme hyperæsthesia of the affected muscles when they are grasped, or stimulated to contract by electrical currents.

The electrical reaction of the affected muscles is that of degeneration. There is loss of reaction in both nerve and muscle to the faradic current (after complete division); and the irritability of the muscle to the galvanic current fails coincidently with the loss of irritability of the nerve. But in ten days to a fortnight the irritability of the muscle to the galvanic current becomes rapidly increased, till it far exceeds the normal; the well-known polar changes occur, and moreover, and perhaps of greater import, the character of the contraction alters: it begins more gradually, lasts much longer, and can be produced with a much weaker current. Where the nerve lesion is not recovered from, the increased galvanic irritability of muscle persists for a number of weeks, and gradually disappears with the increasing atrophy of the muscle fibres.

It must be remembered that in many cases, where a nerve is slightly injured, both nerve and muscles may be unduly irritable to both kinds of electricity, and especially to the faradic. As the reaction of degeneration proceeds, the muscles first become flabby and then waste; and their recovery depends on the restoration of continuity in the motor fibres conducting trophic impulses. With the abolition of sensation and of motor power the reflex arcs belonging to the affected area are abolished.

The vaso-motor and trophic changes in a severe case are very well marked. When the injury has set up local irritation, or inflammatory action, there may be extreme distension of vessels, with elevation of temperature and severe pain. In most cases there is simply œdema, with a temperature often below that on the opposite side. There may be excessive local sweating, rapid growth of hair or complete loss of hair, and, in addition to atrophy of muscles, diminution in amount of subcutaneous tissue, the skin becoming glossy, shining, and reddened. The fingers may be œdematous, and the long-standing œdema may tend to become more solid; but more commonly the finger-tips are shrivelled and tapering. The nails become brittle and thin, more rarely thickened; and in either case they are furrowed both transversely and longitudinally. Ulcers are not uncommon, and the skin is specially susceptible to irritation. The application of hot water, comfortably warm to the healthy hand, may cause vesication or the formation of blebs; and the superficial ulcers so produced heal with great difficulty. Where a large nerve with an extensive distribution is injured, so that recovery is much delayed, the joints of the affected limb are apt to suffer; effusion occurs into them, and fibrous adhesions and fixation may follow. This trophic inflammation is almost always chronic, and not infrequently in these cases marked wasting of bones occurs.

The *diagnosis* is not difficult, as the symptoms of either a slight or a severe nerve injury are distinctive, and the restricted area of the lesion defines such a nerve injury from multiple or toxic neuritis, should the history of the case permit of any doubt.

The *prognosis* is most important, because it is sometimes possible, by a careful examination of the affected limb, to predict the probable duration of the effects of the injury, and the ultimate result.

After the diminution in irritability of the nerve to the faradic current, which usually immediately follows a nerve lesion, accompanied as it is by a similar fall in excitability of the muscle to both currents, the continued preservation of faradic stimulation in the nerve and muscle is a good sign, indicating that the nerve fibres can still conduct. Incomplete quantitative and qualitative changes in the affected muscles to the galvanic current can be also construed into a more hopeful prospect of speedy recovery.

The reappearance of reaction to the faradic current, both in nerve and muscle, always indicates restoration of conduction of nerve fibres; although the galvanic changes, qualitative and quantitative, may still persist in the muscles for a long time after regeneration, and after the gradual return of conducting power has begun. Sensation generally returns long before motor power, as we have already stated; and therefore any return of common and tactile sensory phenomena in the affected area is hailed as an early sign of restoration of function.

When weeks pass by and there is a gradual loss even of the reaction of degeneration, no improvement in the condition of the muscles, no return of sensation, and perhaps trophic changes in the joints or bones, a grave prognosis should be given, unless operative interference be possible.

The *treatment* closely resembles that recommended for local neuritis. The first steps are rest to the affected part, reduction of inflammation, and the cleansing of any septic wound, should the injury have caused such a condition.

Where nerves have been severed by a wound, care should be taken to bring the divided ends into apposition by suture, if necessary. When time has been allowed to elapse without union of the divided nerves, an operation should be performed, the ends of the nerve being rawed, and brought together by suture. It is often difficult, after the lapse of months since the injury, to distinguish the peripheral end; but the removal of the bulbous extremity of the central end, and its union to the remains of the peripheral end, which may be mostly connective tissue, will often suffice to effect a complete regeneration of the peripheral part of the nerve.

Bowlby, Willard, and others have collected statistics of primary suturing of nerves, and, considering the number of septic wounds which had to be included in the tables, these are very satisfactory. Mr. Bowlby

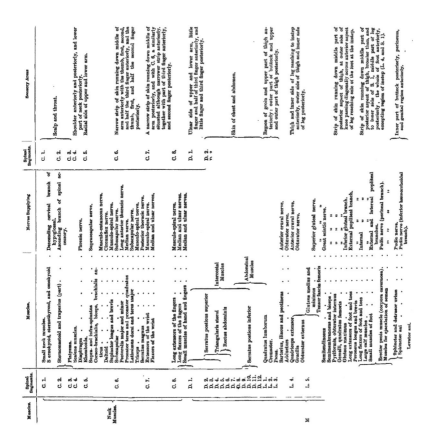

Muscles.	Spinal Segments.	Muscles.	Nerves Supplying.	Spinal Segments.	Sensory Areas.
	C. 1.	Small neck muscles.	Descending cervical branch of hypoglossal.	C. 1.	Scalp and throat.
	C. 2.	Sternohyoid, sternothyroid, and omohyoid	Ascending branch of spinal accessory.	C. 2.	
Neck Muscles.	C. 3.	Sternomastoid and trapezius (part).		C. 3.	Shoulder anteriorly and posteriorly, and lower part of neck posteriorly.
	C. 4.	Platysma. Scaleus muscles. Diaphragm. Rhomboids.	Phrenic nerve. Suprascapular nerve.	C. 4.	Radial side of upper and lower arm.
	C. 5.	Supra- and infra-spinatus Coraco-brachialis, biceps, brachialis anticus Deltoid	Musculo-cutaneous nerve. Circumflex nerve.	C. 5.	
	C. 6.	Subclavian Pectoralis major and minor Pronator teres and pronator quadratus Latissimus dorsi and teres major Triceps Serratus magnus Extensors of the wrist	Musculo-spiral nerve. Subscapular nerve. Long anterior thoracic nerve. Median nerve. Musculo-spiral nerve. Posterior thoracic nerve. Subscapular nerve.	C. 6.	Narrow strip of skin running down middle of arm anteriorly with the thumb, first, second, and half the third finger anteriorly, and the thumb, first, and half the second finger posteriorly.
	C. 7.	Flexors of the wrist	Musculo-spiral nerve. Median and ulnar nerves.	C. 7.	A narrow strip of skin running down middle of arm posteriorly, and with C. 8, a similarly situated although narrower strip anteriorly, together with part of third finger anteriorly, and second finger posteriorly.
	C. 8.	Long extensors of the fingers Long flexors of the fingers Small muscles of hand and fingers	Musculo-spiral nerve. Median and ulnar nerves. Median and ulnar nerves.	C. 8.	Ulnar side of upper and lower arm, little finger and half of third finger anteriorly, and little finger and third finger posteriorly.
	D. 1.			D. 1.	
	D. 2. D. 3. D. 4. D. 5. D. 6.	Serratus posticus superior Triangularis sterni } Intercostal Muscles Rectus abdominis		D. 2. " "	Skin of chest and abdomen.
	D. 7. D. 8. D. 9. D. 10. D. 11. D. 12.	Serratus posticus inferior } Abdominal Muscles			
	L. 1. L. 2. L. 3.	Quadratus lumborum Cremaster. Psoas. Sartorius, iliacus and pectineus Adductors.	Anterior crural nerve. Obturator nerve. Anterior crural nerve. Obturator nerve.		Region of groin and upper part of thigh anteriorly: outer part of buttock and upper and outer part of thigh posteriorly.
M	L. 4.	Quadriceps extensor Gracilis Obturator externus } Glutaeus medius and minimus Tensor fascia femoris	Superior gluteal nerve.		Thigh and inner side of leg reaching to instep anteriorly, outer side of thigh and inner side of leg posteriorly.
	L. 5.	Semimembranosus Semitendinosus and biceps Pyriformis, obturator internus Gemelli, quadratus femoris Glutaeus maximus Long extensors of foot and toes Peroneus longus and brevis Long flexors of foot and toes Small muscles of foot	Great sciatic nerve. " " " Inferior gluteal branch. External popliteal branch. Internal " " External and internal popliteal branches.		Strip of skin running down middle part of posterior aspect of thigh, at outer side of knee passing diagonally across anterior aspect of leg reaching side of the foot at the instep.
		Erector penis muscle (corpus cavernosum). Muscles for ejaculation, of semen	Pudic nerve (perineal branch). " " "		Strip of skin running down middle part of posterior aspect of thigh, broader than, and to inner side of S. 1, middle part of leg posteriorly, the whole of foot anteriorly, excepting region of instep (L. 4, and S. 1).
		Sphincter and detrusor urinae Sphincter ani Levator ani	Pudic nerve. Pudic nerve (inferior hemorrhoidal branch).		Inner part of buttock posteriorly, perineum, and genital region anteriorly.

records eighty-one cases; of these thirty-two were successful, twenty-two were partially successful, twelve doubtful, fourteen failed, and the issue of one was unknown. The sutures commonly recommended are sterilised silk or catgut.

In several cases of both primary and secondary suture, where there was a gap between the divided ends of the nerve, portions of rabbits' nerves, and sometimes a portion of a human nerve from an amputated part, have been used to form a link between the two ends, and in not a few cases with success. In a case of Tillmanns', in which 4½ cm. of a rabbit's sciatic nerve were inserted into the median and ulnar nerves, sensation returned in four weeks, and motor power in nine. Even years after division secondary sutures have been most successful (in one case of Marsh's, in which the ulnar nerve became reunited, twelve years had elapsed). Willard collected 130 cases, and found that 102 of these showed great improvement in motor power and sensation.

Unquestionably in young persons, and in persons in good health, the result of secondary suture is more favourable; whereas in old or debilitated subjects the prognosis after operation is less satisfactory. Massage, galvanism, and, later, faradism should be used with the utmost care after operation; for the greatest precautions must be taken to avoid setting up any inflammatory action in the nerve.

In a very few cases strychnine, administered hypodermically into the region of the affected muscles, is beneficial; but massage and electrical treatment are more generally useful. Passive movements should be begun early, and kept up until motor power returns; as it exercises the affected muscles and joints, and prevents adhesions and loss of free movement.

SPECIAL SECTION.—Under this head fall the individual affections of the different nerves. It will be convenient to review the diseases of the nerves of the trunk in the first place, and of the limbs afterwards.

The accompanying table of the spinal segments and their nerves and muscles has been compiled partly from original investigations, and partly from the results of previous observers, more especially Gowers and Kocher, to whom we desire to express our indebtedness. The table requires no explanation, and will be found of much use in elucidating the special phenomena now to be discussed.

Cervico-occipital neuralgia.—This form of neuralgia may affect any or all of the first four cervical nerves, most commonly perhaps the great occipital; less frequently the lesser occipital, the great auricular, the superficial cervical, and the supraclavicular nerves.

Causes. — A carious tooth, pressure of a heavy load on the neck, caries of the upper cervical vertebræ, cerebro-spinal meningitis, infective diseases such as influenza or malaria, cold, gout, and rheumatism are all included in the category of causes producing this form of neuralgia.

Clinical history.—There is generally a persistent dull pain, with acute lancinating paroxysms. It is generally bilateral; and there are the usual tender points, the more common being—(a) where the great occipital nerve emerges between the mastoid and the spine of the first cervical vertebra ; and (b) at the posterior border of the sterno-mastoid muscle, where the occipital nerves are grouped together. Movements of the head, such as are caused by walking rapidly, or sneezing, increase the pain ; and the head is generally held somewhat stiffly. In some cases the cervical glands swell and become painful ; and over the affected region of the scalp there may be hyperæsthesia of the skin, or even falling out of the hair.

Not infrequently trigeminal neuralgia accompanies this form, and the first and third branches are especially involved.

Diagnosis.—It is not difficult to distinguish this form of neuralgia from rheumatism because the pain in the latter is generally worst at night when the sufferer becomes warm in bed ; and in rheumatism the area over which pressure is painful is much more extensive than the tender points in neuralgia.

In hysteria there may be severe pain in this region, but the mental element in the case and the painful points differ distinctly.

The *prognosis* depends much on the patient. In older persons the condition may resist treatment for a long time, or may be intractable. In other cases the prognosis is much more favourable.

Treatment.—General treatment for neuralgia; but counter-irritation is of great value, and hence Paquelin's cautery, or the button cautery, applied on either side of the spinal column in the cervical region, is often most efficacious.

In one case, reported by Johnson, the superior cervical ganglion of the sympathetic and the cord below were fixed by adhesions. On freeing the sympathetic by operation the patient's symptoms, including the cervico-occipital neuralgia, disappeared.

Neuralgia of the phrenic nerve.—The phrenic nerves arise from the fourth, possibly also the third cervical roots.

Causes. — Neuralgia of the phrenic is rare. It is associated with diseases of the heart, pericardium, and larger vessels ; or it may be due to local irritation, as from a fractured clavicle (in one recorded case), a mediastinal tumour, and so forth.

Clinical features.—The pain shoots upwards from the region of the diaphragm to the throat or shoulder of the affected side, and generally it is the left phrenic in which the neuralgic pains occur. Breathing may be painful, especially if both sides are involved, which, however, is rare.

Diagnosis.—The pain closely corresponds to angina pectoris of organic origin ; indeed it may take the form of that complaint, and be brought about by the same causes, rendering a diagnosis extremely difficult.

Prognosis.—This is good, provided that there is no evidence of organic or vascular disease, and that the neuralgia is either purely functional or due to a removable or curable cause, such as fracture of the clavicle.

Paralysis of the phrenic nerve.—This may be unilateral or bilateral; if the former, there is often some difficulty in recognising the existence of the paralysis.

Causes.—Lesions of the spinal cord in the cervical region, of its membranes, or of the nerve roots (third or fourth cervical) may cause the condition. These include hæmorrhage, pachymeningitis, syphilitic meningitis, and, not uncommonly, fracture or disease of the spinal column. Wounds or tumours in the neck or thorax may injure or compress the nerve. In neuritis, perhaps most commonly of beri-beri and diphtheria, the phrenics may suffer; and in lead neuritis and multiple neuritis from alcohol these nerves are frequently included. In not a few cases of alcoholic neuritis, seen by ourselves, the implication of the phrenics along with the intercostals has been the immediate cause of death. Sir William Gowers is inclined to regard cold as a possible agent in the production of phrenic neuritis.

Clinical features.—A unilateral paralysis causes no special inconvenience to the patient. Bilateral paralysis implies loss of diaphragmatic breathing; and even on the deepest inspiration there is no protrusion of the abdomen. The breath-sounds at the base are feeble; and there is a great tendency to increasing congestion, especially of the lower lobes, and to bronchitis. Dyspnœa is not well marked except on exertion, unless advanced pulmonary congestion already exists. In neuritis there are often painful points over the scaleni muscles, or between the bellies of the sterno-mastoid muscle.

Diagnosis.—Diaphragmatic breathing is often in abeyance in hysteria, and in any case women do not use it much except on exertion. A useful test in such cases is more or less violent exercise, when, unless paralysis exist, diaphragmatic breathing must be evident. In pleurisy, especially diaphragmatic pleurisy, pain may prevent any movement of the diaphragm; and in those rare cases where the muscular fibres of the diaphragm undergo degeneration, some difficulty may be experienced in deciding whether one has to deal with a nerve or a muscle lesion.

Prognosis.—In diphtheritic neuritis and beri-beri, phrenic neuritis will probably terminate fatally; and in alcoholic cases of multiple neuritis the implication of the phrenics is very frequently of grave import. In rheumatism and hysteria a favourable opinion can be given. In other cases, due to aneurysm or tumour, the nature of the disease and the possibility of relieving the condition by operative or other interference, must govern our opinion.

Treatment.—Where treatment is possible, the essential point is to treat the cause by removing a tumour, if one exists; or by combating the toxic element in the case. Neuritic inflammation may be attacked by counter-irritation over the lower and inner parts of the anterior triangle of the neck, as advocated by Suckling. Hypodermic injections of strychnine have been used with advantage in diphtheritic cases. Lastly, it should be stated that all authors agree in considering electrical treatment, whether galvanic or faradic, absolutely useless.

Neuralgia of the intercostal nerves.—The anterior branches of the second down to the ninth or tenth dorsal nerves are most commonly affected, and more frequently on the left side.

Causes.—This affection is very common in women, both in adolescent and adult life; it is proportionately much less frequent in men, in old persons of both sexes it is found fairly equally.

Anæmia, cachexia, leucorrhœa, exhaustion following on lactation, severe illness especially fevers, sexual excess, and similar factors, not uncommonly cause the condition. Local injuries may also be responsible for not a few cases, such as a blow or injury over the thorax, fracture of one or more ribs (especially if reunion occurs with a large formation of callus directly interfering with intercostal nerves), scoliosis, or other spinal disease, and possibly pleurisy. But intercostal neuralgia may be reflex; and probably the frequency of its occurrence on the left side in cases of angina pectoris, actually constituting in some cases the alleged anginal attack, is a proof of this reflex irritative action. In aortic aneurysms, however, the sac may directly press on one or more intercostal nerves.

Clinical history.—The pain is dull and constant with sharp, lancinating paroxysms. Sometimes, though rarely, the pain is spasmodic, appearing to shoot through the chest; and the spasm is relieved only by a deep breath or other effort of the thoracic muscles.

The tender points are very noticeable, corresponding to the three branches—posterior, lateral, and anterior—of the intercostal nerves; although one or two of these are specially sensitive the nerve trunk is very rarely painful all along its course. The affected skin is not infrequently hyperæsthetic, and even the pressure of the clothes may be unbearable.

Herpes zoster is common, and the neuralgic pain may anticipate the herpetic eruption, and also continue long after it has disappeared. In a few cases, probably for the most part cases of angina pectoris, the pain spreads to the shoulder or arm of the affected side.

The diagnosis is generally easy; care should be taken to examine the condition of the heart, the lungs, the pleura, the breasts in women, and the spinal column.

The prognosis is generally favourable, although in some cases the pain persists for a long time. The heart, aorta, pleura, and spine should be examined before the probabilities of final and complete recovery can be estimated.

Treatment.—Counter-irritation, as by fly-blisters, mustard or the button cautery, is of great value. Where herpes zoster is associated, sedatives must be used. Tonics are generally indicated, and any irregularities of the alimentary tract should be rectified. Galvanism has been successful in one or two cases, but it is rarely of much benefit. Nerve section or section of the sensory roots should not be considered until all else has failed. Where callus presses on the nerve it should be removed.

Neuralgia of the breast; Mastodynia.—This curious form of neuralgia involves the branches of the intercostal nerves supplying the skin of the breast (2nd-6th), or the gland structure itself (4th-6th).

Causes.—The condition is met with in women almost exclusively, and generally about middle life. · It is· associated with excessive stimulation of the breast, as in over-lactation, or in pregnancy; but not infrequently it occurs in anæmic, neurasthenic, or hysterical women, without any functional activity of the affected gland at all; although in these cases it is generally more severe during menstruation. Tubercula dolorosa have been found on the nerves supplying the gland structure. Lastly, it may occur as the result of a neoplasm of the breast.

Clinical history.—The pain is sharp, and more often found on the left side; there may be circumscribed redness and swelling of the breast. Occasionally milky fluid exudes from the nipple (Erb), and herpes may be associated with the condition. The tender points are generally near the spinous processes of the vertebræ (2nd-6th dorsal).

Diagnosis.—The existence of a neoplasm can readily be recognised, especially if it be malignant, by the usual precautions, and so the swelling resulting from mastodynia alone can hardly be a source of error.

The *prognosis* depends almost entirely on removal of the cause, and the degree of benefit obtained from treatment. In many cases the condition is very intractable.

Treatment.—Attention must be paid to the general health, and any obvious cause such as excessive lactation must be dealt with. Supporting the breast by a bandage, the application of soothing liniments, painting the nipple with a strong solution of cocain, and the constant current are all useful.

Brachial neuralgia.—The brachial plexus is derived from the four lower cervical and the first dorsal nerves, with sometimes a branch from the fourth cervical. The neuralgic pain may affect the whole of the tributary nerves of the plexus, or may be limited to one or two alone; not infrequently other nerves, such as the intercostals, or the fifth cranial nerve, suffer in sympathy.

The *causes* consist frequently in a predisposition, such as may be produced by anæmia, debility, neurasthenia, rheumatism, or gout, with some exciting cause. Neuralgic pain not infrequently follows pressure, or bruising or injury of the brachial plexus, in whole or in part, and is of course one of the prominent symptoms in neuritis. Sometimes the cause is one acting reflexly, as for example a carious tooth, or an aortic or subclavian aneurysm. Diseases causing toxic neuritis, such as rheumatism, gout, diphtheria, typhoid, and influenza, may certainly cause brachial neuralgic pain; and peripheral injuries to nerves may produce ascending neuritis, accompanied by agonising pain. But in persons disposed to neuralgia the immediate causes may be of the same kind as those of the craft palsies. Pianists, violinists, telegraphists, and clerks, suffering from such palsy, generally complain also of neuralgic pain; and certainly in such cases the general health is often, if not always, below par.

The pain is of the usual neuralgic nature, dull and boring, with lancinating paroxysms more or less severe. The affected nerves are tender on pressure; and there are certain painful points in the axilla, over the circumflex nerve near the deltoid muscle, over the radial nerve where it turns round the humerus, over the ulnar nerve posteriorly and the median anteriorly at the elbow joint, and at other points in the lower arm. There may be anæsthesia or paræsthesia, herpetic eruptions, vaso-motor disturbances, and muscular atrophy, especially when neuritis is present. As a rule the pain is greatly increased on movement; and the limb is to be kept at rest as far as possible. If the pain be limited to a particular area the ulnar nerve suffers most frequently.

The *diagnosis* is easy; but it is more important to discover the cause of the condition with a view to successful treatment.

The *prognosis* in simple neuralgias is usually favourable; but here again the causation is of the utmost moment.

The *treatment* is that generally used for neuralgia; namely, rest, local sedatives or counter-irritants, together with active treatment of the etiological factors.

Brachial neuritis.—The nerve roots may be affected especially in spinal disease, or where growths affect the nerves at or near their exit from the spinal canal: and to this form the name of radicular brachial neuritis is given. When the nerve roots or the brachial plexus itself are affected the condition is generally a perineuritis.

Causes.—The radicular form, as indicated above, depends on injury from spinal or possibly meningeal disease. Brachial neuritis proper is rare, it is due to the ordinary causes of neuritis elsewhere, and is perhaps more especially associated with gout or rheumatism. It occurs more frequently in women, and generally in persons above middle life.

The *clinical history* is generally characteristic of a perineuritis. Pain is a constant phenomenon; slight at first and often referred to a distant part of the limb, such as the hand, back of the forearm, or near the axilla, or in the region of the scapula, it soon becomes more severe and more definitely associated with the plexus and the nerves arising from it. At first the pain may recur at considerable intervals; but later it becomes continuous, and generally there are paroxysms of an acute lancinating kind. It is increased on movement, and is frequently, during paroxysms at least, somewhat diffused; if on the left side it may closely suggest the pain of angina pectoris, the resemblance being rendered greater by irregular cardiac action or palpitation. There is often hyperæsthesia, hyperalgesia, or burning of the affected area, and there may be temporary anæsthesia. There may be loss of muscular power in hand or arm, with atrophy of the affected muscles; but this is generally a late phenomenon, and is usually slight in degree.

The trophic changes, in severe or long-standing cases, are frequently well marked; such as glossy skin, local subcutaneous œdema, wasting of muscles, and changes in the affected joints.

In radicular neuritis the pain felt near the spinal column, referable to the posterior cutaneous branches, and the presence, sometimes demonstrable by other phenomena, of bone disease or other cause of the condition, are generally sufficient, sooner or later, to clear up the nature of the case.

Diagnosis.—Neuralgia is simply nerve pain; but it is generally easy to decide whether there is or is not neuritis by attending to two points, namely, the presence or absence of marked or persistent tenderness along the line of the nerves, and whether movement of the affected arm is painful or not. Neuritis is always accompanied by these features, and the appearance of trophic changes in muscle and skin render the diagnosis more certain.

In angina pectoris the pain shooting down the arm is not accompanied by so much tenderness on pressure over the nerves, and cardio-arterial faults are usually present.

Rheumatoid arthritis, with its peculiar joint changes, has a distinctive history, and there is no nerve tenderness.

The *prognosis* depends almost entirely on the severity of the neuritis, and the consequent interference with the integrity of nerve fibres. Once the skin becomes glossy, the muscles atrophied, and joints more or less fixed, a complete cure is very problematical; and the patient finds that the affected limb is not merely almost useless, but the source of continual trouble. On excessive attempts at using the limb there is generally considerable pain, much like rheumatism, increased by cold weather; and formication, tingling, or burning, sometimes accompanied by muscular spasms, are frequently induced by the same causes.

Neuritis is always tedious, and more so if severe; and in all cases where vitality is much below par the prognosis must be guarded. In some cases relapses occur; but such relapses are frequently due to carelessness on the part of the patient, or too vigorous treatment on the part of the medical man.

The *treatment* differs in no way from the treatment of neuritis elsewhere. Rest is of greatest importance, and should be as complete as possible, with the arm not merely in a sling, but bandaged to the chest, so as absolutely to prevent all movement. For the acute stage, poultices, hot fomentations, and, if necessary, morphia or cocaine hypodermically should be used. After the inflammation has subsided massage and passive movements may be carried out, but with the greatest care. Hot water is also of great benefit in combating contracture; and sometimes galvanism is efficacious, although more as a sedative than a restorative.

Paralysis of the brachial plexus.—The plexus, or the nerve roots forming it, may be injured in many different ways.

Sometimes the whole of the plexus is affected, frequently, however, a part only. Tumours or spinal disease may affect the nerve roots; and injuries in the neighbourhood of the plexus, such as dislocation of the humerus, or fracture of the head of the humerus or scapula, may cause a more or less complete paralysis of nerves arising from it. Brachial neuritis may cause paralysis, a condition described separately ; and in ascending neuritis, an injury to one nerve may set up inflammation, which may spread to the whole of the brachial plexus.

I. *The whole plexus may be affected and all the nerves paralysed.*—These cases are almost always traumatic in origin ; and the commonest causes are subluxation of the humerus, fractures in the region of the axilla, and injury during parturition ; very frequently the paralysis becomes more and more limited, until only one or two nerves remain affected—often the circumflex and musculo-spiral.

The clinical history varies greatly, beginning with a general weakness and heaviness of the limb, and going on perhaps to paralysis of motion and sensation, with wasting of muscles and trophic changes in the skin or joints ; but very frequently the injury becomes limited to one or more nerves.

The diagnosis is generally comparatively easy, and the prognosis depends greatly on the extent and nature of the injury, the electrical reactions, and the more or less rapid recovery of the functions of the affected nerves.

II. *Erb's paralysis, or the upper arm type.*—This is due to a lesion of the fifth and sixth cervical roots. The muscles affected are the deltoid, biceps, brachialis anticus, supinator longus, sometimes the supinator brevis, supraspinatus and infraspinatus. The cutaneous supply from the two affected roots includes the area of skin controlled by the circumflex and musculo-cutaneous nerves, including the outer side of the upper and lower arm.

Generally injuries produce this form of paralysis. Not infrequently it is caused by pressure above the clavicle close to the side of the neck ; thus mason's labourers and porters supply many of the instances of this somewhat rare type of paralysis.

When the arm is raised above the shoulder and carried backwards, or when from the weight carried the head is twisted round backwards to the same, or to the opposite side, the fifth and sixth cervical nerves are more liable to be compressed. In infants, traction on the neck at birth may cause Erb's paralysis ; and, lastly, in a few isolated cases the lesion was apparently of toxic origin.

The arm cannot be abducted, and, as the anterior part of the deltoid sometimes obtains some supply from the anterior thoracic nerves, it can only in these cases be feebly carried forward. The arm cannot be flexed at the elbow joint, and supination is impossible, especially when the supinator brevis is affected. The arm is also turned somewhat inwards, and the humerus cannot be rotated outwards. Generally in cases occurring in adult life the affected muscles waste ; the reaction of degeneration is obtainable, often complete sometimes only partial ; and the paralysis is severe and of long standing. The sensory changes vary greatly. There is often pain, and there may be anæsthesia in the sensory realms of both circumflex and musculo-cutaneous nerves, or in one alone.

The *diagnosis* presents no difficulty, unless, as sometimes happens, the paralysis is not limited to the fifth and sixth cervical nerves.

The *prognosis* should be given with care ; the cases are usually tedious, and the paralysis may persist without improvement.

III. *The lower arm type.*—One form of this is *Klumpke's paralysis*, in which the eighth cervical and first dorsal roots are affected. The muscles chiefly affected are the small muscles of the hand and the flexors of the fingers in the forearm.

In other cases the seventh and the sixth cervical roots suffer also, and involve paralysis of the extensors of the fingers, the triceps, pronators, and flexors of the wrist.

Tumours pressing on the nerve roots, syphilitic meningitis, and primary neuritis of the nerve roots are among the assigned causes of this condition.

The affected muscles waste, and the paralysis depends on the extent of the lesion. Pain, hyperæsthesia, and anæsthesia are more marked in the ulnar region of the forearm and upper arm, and sometimes in the area controlled by the median nerve. Not infrequently there are marked ocular phenomena dependent, probably, on the injury of communicating root branches ; these include myosis on the side of the lesion, sluggish contraction of pupil, and diminution in size of the palpebral fissure.

The *prognosis* varies ; recovery may occur in two to three months, or, where the nerve roots are permanently damaged or torn, operative interference may offer the only chance of cure.

Paralysis of the long thoracic nerve, or nerve to the serratus magnus.—This nerve is formed in the scalenus medius muscle by branches from the fifth and sixth cervical nerves. It runs a long course passing behind the brachial plexus, entering the muscle at its lower border.

Causes.—The nerve may be injured by pressure or by a punctured wound. The carrying of heavy weights on the shoulders, especially if a sharp edge press heavily into the neck, or constant muscular contraction of the scalenus muscle may set up neuritis in the nerve.

The condition is, therefore, much commoner in men, and is more frequently met with on the right side. Muscular contraction of the scalenus is almost continuous in trades where the worker has his arm continually raised, as in plastering ceilings, and like occupations.

Isolated invasion of this nerve by toxic neuritis has been found after diphtheria, typhoid, and influenza, although very rarely ; cold air blowing on the neck is a possible cause.

Clinical history.—The serratus magnus muscle carries the scapula outwards, forwards, and slightly upwards. It fixes the scapula when the arm is raised above the horizontal. When the arm is raised vertically, and the scapula fixed by the rhomboids, etc., it can raise the ribs, and by expanding the chest in this way greatly helps forced inspiration.

When the serratus is paralysed the scapula is nearer to the spinal column, is higher in position, and is not kept in close apposition to the chest. When the arm is brought forwards the scapula rotates vertically, the posterior border projecting like a wing, and the lower angle being rotated backwards towards the spinal column, and also upwards. In most persons with this paralysis the arm cannot be extended beyond the horizontal, unless the scapula be fixed artificially ; although in some individuals—according to Jolly, Bruns, and others—the middle fibres of the trapezius can act in this way. Forced inspiration is interfered with, and when the arms are raised vertically the deficient expansion of the chest on the affected side becomes obvious. There is generally more or less pain before paralysis becomes marked ; and the electrical reactions help to clear up the condition. The *diagnosis* presents no difficulty. The *prognosis* is favourable in toxic cases ; but where the nerve has been injured by pressure recovery is generally tedious.

The *treatment.*—Rest for the affected limb, care being taken to prevent contractions of the scalenus medius. This is best carried out by keeping the arm in a sling, and forbidding any attempt at raising the shoulder. Electricity, when the neuritis has subsided, may be of use to keep up the condition of the muscle.

Paralysis of the suprascapular nerve.—This nerve arises from the trunk formed by the union of the fifth and sixth cervical nerves, and a branch of the fourth. It may be damaged alone, or with the circumflex nerve. Dislocation of the humerus, falls on the shoulder or on the hand causing contusion of the shoulder joint, and the carrying of heavy weights, are all causes of this somewhat rare paralysis.

The nerve supplies the supra- and infraspinatus muscles. The supraspinatus, according to Duchenne, not merely helps to raise and also to bring forward the arm at the shoulder joint, but it also keeps the head of the humerus in close apposition to the glenoid cavity. Hence in cases of paralysis of this muscle there is difficulty in raising the arm, and also a tendency to subluxation of the head of the bone when the deltoid lifts the arm. The infraspinatus rotates the humerus outwards, although it does not act unassisted, as the posterior part of the deltoid and the teres minor act in this way, and tend to become hypertrophied when the infraspinatus is unable to undertake its share of the work. Hence writing, sewing, and any movements of outward rotation of the arm become difficult. The affected muscles waste, and the absence of the infraspinatus is readily distinguishable.

There may be some anæsthesia over the scapula, and a certain amount of pain on movement is not uncommon.

Paralysis of the circumflex nerve.—This nerve is derived from the posterior cord of the brachial plexus, and supplies the entire deltoid muscle (with the exception of a small anterior part which occasionally receives a small branch from one of the anterior thoracic nerves), the teres minor, and the skin over the region of the deltoid.

Causes.—The course of the nerve is one especially exposed to damage, therefore, in injuries to the shoulder ; it may suffer as in falls and dislocations, and sometimes it is pressed upon by the head of a crutch. Rarely does a toxic neuritis occur in this nerve. In rheumatism, in infectious diseases, and in one recorded case of lead poisoning, this nerve suffered alone. Oppenheim attributes the latter case to a toxico-traumatic cause, as the neuritis began after the patient had carried heavy weights on the shoulder. In rheumatic cases there is some doubt whether the neuritis may not be associated with arthritis of the shoulder joint; or whether the two conditions may not be confused.

Clinical history.—The deltoid is paralysed, and the arm cannot be raised, except by the comparatively feeble supraspinatus and, occasionally, the anterior part of the deltoid. The deltoid wastes, and the shoulder joint often becomes stiff from adhesions, because the nerve appears to supply some trophic branches to the joint. The teres minor paralysis is not apparent. There is often pain and generally anæsthesia over the lower part of the deltoid, but this may be absent.

Diagnosis.—Care must be taken in diagnosing anchylosis of the shoulder joint, as in cases of osteo-arthritis, from paralysis of the circumflex. In anchylosis the scapula follows the head of the humerus when the arm is moved, and the deltoid can be made to contract, although it may be unable to produce any effect; the absence of anæsthesia also is of importance in aiding diagnosis.

Paralysis of the musculo-cutaneous nerve.—The musculo-cutaneous is derived from the fifth and sixth cervical nerves, and supplies the chief flexors of the elbow and the skin over the radial side of the forearm. The nerve is rarely affected alone, more commonly it suffers with the brachial plexus; and injuries of different kinds in the region of the shoulder have caused the cases recorded.

The biceps and brachialis can no longer flex the arm at the elbow joint; and, if the hand is supinated, the supinator longus is unable to act as a flexor. The muscles waste, and there is generally anæsthesia over the radial side of the forearm, both anteriorly and posteriorly.

The nerve to the coraco-brachialis muscle, which is closely related to the trunk of the musculo-cutaneous, may escape.

Paralysis of the musculo-spiral nerve.—The musculo-spiral nerve is derived from all the roots making up the brachial plexus, excepting the first dorsal. It supplies the following muscles :—The triceps, the extensor carpi radialis longior, the extensor carpi ulnaris, the extensor communis digitorum, the three extensors of the thumb, the special extensors of the index finger and little finger, and the two supinators. The cutaneous supply includes the radial side of the forearm and hand, and a part of the upper arm.

Causes.—The course of the nerve and its exposed position render it very liable to injury by pressure; and in 242 cases of paralysis of the arm, collected by Remak, 105 were due to a lesion of this nerve. It should also be remembered that in topers and cachectic persons, pressure which would be trivial in the robust may cause paralysis. A misfitting crutch may press on the musculo-spiral; and the "Saturday night paralysis," brought on by falling asleep with the arm over the back of a chair, is generally due to a lesion of this nerve. Sometimes sleeping on the arm when in bed causes it, especially if the bed be unusually hard. The continental device of tying prisoners' hands together behind their backs frequently produces this paralysis; and the Russian custom of tying infants' arms to their sides has occasionally caused it.

Toxic agents may produce an isolated lesion of this nerve, but generally the site of the lesion is determined by a local injury of some kind. Lead, arsenic, and silver may bring about this paralysis, but here again the cause is generally toxico-traumatic. Rarely, violent muscular contractions of the triceps, especially the outer head, have produced paralysis; and lastly, hypodermic injections of ether, chloroform, or other drug, in the vicinity of the nerve, not necessarily into its substance, are responsible for a small number of cases.

Clinical history.—Not infrequently the triceps or the supinator longus escapes, especially if the site of the lesion be near the middle of the humerus. In most cases there is paralysis of the extensors of the elbow, the wrist, and the long extensors of the fingers, giving very typical wrist drop; the fingers being bent at the metacarpo-phalangeal joints, and the thumb somewhat opposed and sunk. In long-standing cases the flexors, not being properly opposed, lose their power, and the pronators become shortened. Sir William Gowers draws attention to the fact that in some cases there is a gradation of extensor paralysis in the fingers, being most marked in the fourth finger and less marked towards the first.

Not infrequently there is some tingling or even anæsthesia; but in pressure cases sensory phenomena are usually slight.

The affected muscles may waste, and the sheaths of the tendons may swell, and sometimes the joints.

Diagnosis.—It is generally easy to distinguish this condition from lead paralysis, because, first, only one arm is affected; secondly, the supinator longus muscle is usually affected; and, thirdly, the onset is sudden.

Prognosis.—Pressure paralysis for the most part is rapidly recovered from; but for determining the probable duration of the condition no test is so satisfactory as the electrical reactions.

The *treatment* is on general principles; the utmost care being taken to prevent pressure on the nerve, and, where neuritis has been set up, to give rest to the affected limb.

Paralysis of the median nerve.—The nerve is derived from the lower three cervical and the first dorsal root.

It supplies the two pronators, the flexors of the wrist (excepting the flexor carpi ulnaris) and of the fingers (excepting the ulnar half of the deep flexor), the opponens, the two flexors, the short abductor of the thumb and the radial lumbricales. Its cutaneous supply includes the radial side of the palm, the front of the first, second, and half of the third fingers, and sometimes the back of the last phalanges of the thumb and first three fingers.

Causes.—The nerve is generally injured in the forearm by fractures of the radius or ulna, or by wounds. Esmarch's bandage is responsible for a few cases; and in some occupations, such as cigar-makering (Coester), and carpet-beating (Reinhardt), paralysis of the median nerve has been recorded. Powerful contraction of the pronator radii teres may also cause the condition.

Clinical history.—If the injury include all the muscular branches pronation is impossible, and the patient endeavours by rotating the upper arm inwards to compensate for the paralysed muscles. The wrist cannot be flexed except towards the ulnar side; the thumb is constantly extended and abducted, and cannot be opposed to the tips of the fingers The fingers cannot be properly bent at the first interphalangeal joint, and only the last three fingers can be bent at the second. The interossei can flex the first phalanx; and their unopposed extensor action on the second and terminal phalanges causes a tendency to subluxation. Where the lesion is sufficiently low down the smaller muscles of the hand may suffer alone.

Not infrequently the lesion is severe and the thenar muscles waste, while sensory changes are common. Pain and tingling may be present, or anæsthesia more marked, as a rule, on the palmar surface. The affected skin is often cold and cyanosed, and herpes or even bullæ resembling pemphigus may appear. In some cases the nails become brittle or furrowed, or may fall off.

Diagnosis is easy. In *prognosis* the electrical reactions are important. The *treatment* is on the usual lines.

Paralysis of the ulnar nerve.—The ulnar arises from the last cervical and first dorsal roots, and is associated with the lowest part of the cervical enlargement of the cord. It supplies the flexor carpi ulnaris, the ulnar half of the deep flexor of the fingers, the muscles of the little finger, the interossei, the inner two lumbricales, and the adductors of the thumb. The cutaneous supply is confined to the ulnar side of the hand, and, according to most authorities, to the back of two and a half fingers, and the front of one and a half.

Causes.—This nerve is more commonly affected than the median, and may suffer along with it. When the injury is in the upper arm, one of the commonest sites of lesion is at the elbow joint, where fracture of the internal condyle of the humerus, or a supracondylar fracture may readily implicate the nerve. In some instances, months after such a fracture, the nerve may be pressed upon by callus. Dislocation of the shoulder or elbow, wounds at the elbow joint or in the forearm may all cause it. The nerve is also apt to suffer from prolonged flexion of the arm at the elbow joint; especially in feeble or cachectic persons, or in those liable to neuritis from alcoholism, lead poisoning, or other cause; hence it is a common form of sleep paralysis; and in not a few cases where there is predisposition, even bending of the elbow causes numbness or tingling along the line of the nerve. A neuritis may readily be set up in these cases.

Clinical history.—On flexion the wrist is bent towards the radial side ; the fingers cannot be flexed at the first or extended at the second joints, and especially is this the case with the last two fingers. The interossei are paralysed, producing eventually the claw-like hand or "main en griffe"; although it should be stated that the first two fingers are not claw-like, because the two radial lumbricals are not paralysed. The fingers cannot be separated or adducted ; the thumb sticks out prominently, and may be slightly rotated forwards. The muscles affected may waste, and the hypothenar eminence disappears.

The sensory changes are often severe, pain and tingling being common ; but not infrequently the presence or absence of anæsthesia is out of all proportion to the gravity of the lesion.

The *diagnosis* rarely presents any difficulty, the claw-like hand differing, as mentioned above, from that found in progressive muscular atrophy.

The *prognosis* is generally favourable, though a period from a few weeks to months may elapse before complete recovery ; or an operation, such as removal of callus, or the like, may be requisite before the nerve can resume its normal functions.

Neuralgia of the lumbar plexus, or lumbo-abdominal neuralgia.— As in intercostal neuralgia, so the nerves of the lower part of the trunk may be affected, and we may get lumbo-abdominal neuralgia.

There are certain painful points, often tender on pressure, and among these the most important are :—an iliac point near the iliac crest ; a hypogastric, over the lower part of the rectus abdominis muscle ; a scrotal point in males, and a labial point in females. Sometimes pain shoots along the spermatic cord ; and it is quite probable that irritable testicle is, in many cases, of neuralgic origin.

The *causes* are those productive of neuralgia elsewhere. First, of a general kind, such as prolonged ill health, anæmia, or neurasthenia ; and, secondly, some proximate cause capable of producing neuralgia in those rendered susceptible, and generally accounting for the selection of a certain nerve or nerves.

The local causes are pelvic disease—constipation very frequently, uric acid causing pain in the penis, and analogous agents. There is not infrequently cutaneous hyperæsthesia, and sometimes herpetic eruptions appear along the line of the affected nerves. Occasionally, although rarely, it causes sexual excitement, seminal emissions, and increased frequency or pain in the act of micturition.

Crural neuralgia may follow a lesion of the lumbar plexus, or it may be secondary to sciatic neuritis. The cutaneous branches of the anterior crural nerve are perhaps more frequently affected. Herpes and hyperidrosis are not uncommon accompaniments.

There may be pain of neuralgic nature in the line of the obturator nerve, but it is rare.

The *diagnosis* of these neuralgias is not difficult, especially where the cause of the condition is apparent. Tumours, or other pathological conditions of the pelvic organs should be sought for ; and special care should be taken to investigate the condition of the generative organs, the bladder, and the rectum.

The *prognosis* depends on the cause; an idiopathic neuralgia is of no great importance; where anæsthesia or paræsthesia is marked, there is much more probability that an organic lesion is present, and therefore a more guarded prognosis should be given.

The *treatment* must be conducted on general principles.

Paralysis of the lumbar plexus.—The lumbar plexus arising from the first three lumbar roots and half of the fourth, with a connecting link from the twelfth dorsal root, is formed in the substance of the psoas muscle, and supplies the flexors and abductors of the thigh, the extensors of the knee, and the cremaster muscle. It supplies also the skin over the lower part of the abdomen, including the scrotum and root of the penis or labia, the anterior and both internal and external surfaces of the thigh, and the inner surface of the leg and foot.

The lumbar plexus may be damaged in whole or in part by—(i.) Disease of the spinal column, such as caries or tumour; (ii.) Tumours of the meninges, or inflammatory or other exudations; (iii.) Disease of the cord; (iv.) Invasion of the roots, loops, or cords forming the plexus, by tuberculous or other affection of the retroperitoneal glands, by psoas abscess, rarely by a primary neuritis, or a neuritis secondary to disease of the sacral plexus.

More commonly the following component nerves of the plexus suffer :—

Paralysis of the obturator nerve.—This nerve may be injured by pressure during parturition; more rarely by pelvic tumours or obturator hernia.

Paralysis of this nerve implies loss of power in the abductors of the thigh; inability to cross the legs; difficulty in both inward and outward rotation of the leg; and anæsthesia over the upper third of the inner surface of the thigh, sometimes extending nearly as low as the knee.

Paralysis of the anterior crural nerve. — This nerve may be injured in many ways by spinal caries or tumour; by psoas abscess; by dislocation of the hip joint; not infrequently by wounds in the groin or thigh; and, rarely, during parturition. In disease involving the roots this nerve may appear to be specially affected.

Bruns records a case of diabetes mellitus in which the anterior crural nerve alone was diseased; generally, where there is a toxic cause, other nerves suffer in the same way, this nerve is rarely specially selected. The nerve is most commonly injured in the groin or thigh; where damage is sustained within the pelvis, the branch to the iliacus may be involved, in which case flexion of the hip is difficult.

When the lesion is complete the motor paralysis is serious, as the extensors of the knee are supplied by this nerve, and the muscles waste. The knee-jerk is abolished. The area of anæsthesia includes the whole of the thigh excepting a part of the posterior surface, the inner side of the leg down to the toes, including the great toe, and the adjacent side of the second.

Pain in the line of distribution of the nerve is common, especially when the lesion is situated near the spinal column, and when the condition is in the irritative stage. The anterior crural nerve is very commonly affected only in part; the motor and sensory phenomena being correspondingly limited in extent.

Paralysis of the superior gluteal nerve. — This nerve belongs to both lumbar and sacral plexuses, and it supplies both the gluteus medius and minimus. It is rarely affected alone, and when it is there is inability to abduct and circumduct the thigh.

Paralysis of the external cutaneous nerve. — This nerve supplies the outer surface of the thigh from the hip joint nearly to the knee. Neuritis of this nerve has been described by Roth as neuralgia paræsthesia, but it is generally of alcoholic origin, and is not confined to this nerve alone. Besides pains along the lines of distribution there is sometimes difficulty in standing and walking, probably due to the loss of some controlling influence of this nerve over the fascia.

Sciatica.—This most indefinite name is applied to three conditions, all producing pain in the sciatic nerve.

First, there may be a true neuralgia of the nerve or its branches. Secondly, there may be pain produced in the nerve or its area of distribution, secondary to a tumour of the pelvis, inflammation of the hip joint, or other cause. Thirdly, there is sciatic neuritis, which is the ordinary form of sciatica.

It is difficult to assert that neuralgia of the sciatic nerve cannot or does not occur. Neuralgia may be the expression of nerve exhaustion, and therefore after excessive use of the legs there is no reason why a sciatic neuralgia should not occur. But it rarely does occur in such circumstances, because it is not common to have both sciatic nerves affected at once. Still, just as a carious tooth may set up a trifacial neuralgia, so the sciatic pain felt in cases of hip-joint disease may be truly enough a secondary sciatica, but yet in reality neuralgia, and not due to pressure or direct inflammatory implication. Neuralgia of the sciatic, where it does arise, is generally easily traced to some definite cause.

Secondary sciatica, if it is not neuralgic, as first stated, is due to pressure or direct contact with an inflammatory focus. The pain is not increased by pressure on the nerve.

While it is necessary in describing sciatica to keep in view all these three forms, it is sciatic neuritis which is most common, and therefore most important. The form of neuritis generally met with is either perineuritis or interstitial neuritis.

The *causation* is simple. It occurs in men much more frequently than in women; the proportion varying from two to four times as many, the latter figure being more nearly correct. The period of life at which sciatica is most common is forty to fifty; it is rather less frequent between fifty and sixty; much less frequent between thirty and forty, and rarely occurs in either the earlier or later decades of life.

Rheumatism and gout are the principal predisposing, cold and wet the chief exciting, causes. Heavy muscular exertion has been found to be a cause, especially in gouty or rheumatic subjects. Occasionally after a severe attack of lumbago the sciatic nerve has become involved in a rheumatic perineuritis. Certainly in persons so disposed, pressure on a hard seat, or, as Gowers remarks, exposure in a cold, draughty water-closet, may bring on an attack. Syphilis is not a common cause, and generally in specific cases, where there is sciatic pain, there is a primary spinal meningitis or a cord lesion.

It is possible that a severe muscular contraction may in a few rare cases set up sciatic neuritis, but some preceding cause should be sought for.

Secondary neuritis is due to a pelvic tumour, sometimes in the uterus; occasionally the fœtal head, a greatly-distended rectum, pelvic inflammation, or hip-joint disease may produce it.

Neuralgia, as stated already, is due to an irritant, acting reflexly; the remoter causes, if any, being anæmia or malnutrition of the nervous system generally.

The *pathological anatomy* of sciatic neuritis is derived from the appearance and microscopic examination of the nerve in cases where stretching or removal of portions of the nerve trunk has been resorted to. The nerve is seen to be reddened and swollen, and there is marked exudation into the sheath, and especially into the connective tissue between the funiculi. Hæmorrhages have often been found. These changes may extend along the greater part of the nerve trunk, but are known to be most marked in two positions,—at the sciatic notch, and in the middle of the thigh.

In secondary sciatica and in neuralgia no anatomical changes necessarily occur.

The great *symptom* is pain. It may come on gradually, tending to increase in violence, and to get worse on muscular effort; on pressure over the nerve trunk, and often towards night; or the pain may come on suddenly, and may or may not be paroxysmal in character. Where it comes on gradually, only certain movements which cause pressure on the nerve are painful; but eventually even the slightest movement may be accompanied by pain. Walking may only be possible with the knee bent. The pain is often burning or gnawing, and may be constant, or may increase at times in severity. Certain painful parts can be indicated by the sufferer, the two commonest ones being the sciatic notch and the middle of the thigh. Not infrequently the pain, limited at first to the upper part of the thigh, spreads downwards to the heel. Pain is also specially referred to the following regions: above the hip-joint; in the popliteal space; below the head of the fibula; just behind the external malleolus, and on the dorsum of the foot. In protracted cases groups of muscles may waste, and, if so, cramps and fibrillary twitchings often appear in them. Among the muscles so affected are the hamstrings, the calf muscles, the tibialis anticus and peroneal muscles, and the gluteus maximus. It is not very uncommon in severe cases to hear of numbness, tingling, and formication; and sometimes there are areas of complete anæsthesia, although it is more usual to find areas of partial anæsthesia and analgesia on the back of the leg or thigh. These sensory phenomena imply a marked interference with nerve conductions; in other words, a severe interstitial inflammation in the nerve. Where the skin on the back of the thigh is anæsthetic the small sciatic nerve is involved also.

Sometimes herpetic eruptions occur, and occasionally œdema of the affected leg may be present; as a rule, however, vaso-motor and trophic phenomena are not prominent features.

The *diagnosis* is generally made by digital examination over the nerve. In primary sciatica pressure on the nerve, or putting the nerve on the stretch, is sufficient to cause pain. It is easy to effect this either by exercising deep pressure on the nerve in the buttock or in the middle of the thigh, or else by flexing the leg at the hip-joint and exerting pressure in the popliteal space.

Secondary sciatica can generally be diagnosed by investigating the pelvic contents by rectal or vaginal examination, when the underlying cause may be revealed; or again by exerting pressure upon the nerve when little if any pain is experienced.

In disease of the sacro-iliac synchondrosis pain may radiate widely, but not usually so far even as the upper part of the thigh. Hip-joint disease may cause a secondary sciatica, probably neuralgic; if it does not, the pain is at any rate circumscribed, and the position of the limb, although to some extent resembling the semi-flexed limb of a sufferer from severe sciatica, is characteristic.

In lesions of the cauda equina or nerve roots, whether by tumour or inflammation, there is generally a double lesion; and not, as in sciatica, a condition limited to one side.

In locomotor ataxy the lightning pains are generally bilateral; and the ataxic and other characteristic phenomena are amply sufficient for diagnostic purposes.

Cases of sciatica are apt to be obstinate, and may last for months or even years, with a certain amount of remission as regards degree of pain. Sciatica may even keep the sufferer completely confined to bed, but in these cases the sciatic neuritis is extremely severe and protracted. As a general rule, the prognosis is favourable and the treatment successful.

Muscular atrophy, with cramps and fibrillary tremors and anæs-thesia over a wide area, are indications of a considerable degree of inter-stitial neuritis, and of a definite, if not necessarily permanent, lesion of the nerve fibres themselves. The *prognosis* of most cases of sciatica is, however, favourable; but the probable duration of the attack, even with active treatment, should be estimated in a guarded manner.

In *treatment*, attention should always be directed at once to the possibility, or rather probability of a constitutional element in the case; and rheumatism should be assailed with salol or salicylate of soda, gout with colchicum and salines. If there be a distinct history of rheumatism, however slight, salicylates and a saline purge should invariably be administered at once.

Locally, in mild cases, it may be sufficient to counter-irritate with iodine, the button cautery, or a fly-blister; but generally *rest* should be insisted on, and the most effectual means of enforcing this is by putting on a long splint. Many cases in which rest has not been tried, and which have resisted every other local or general method of treatment, yield to the long splint. An inflammatory exudation is unquestionably apt to be increased by movement, and is most likely to disappear by rest with counter irritation.

Poultices are of great service where the pain is severe, but blisters or the cautery produce a more powerful effect. Ice is recommended by some authors, but if not actually harmful is certainly unsatisfactory. A hypodermic injection of an eighth to a quarter of a grain of cocaine in the region of the nerve is most soothing, and is preferable to morphia; the latter is indeed only permissible when the pain is agonising, and should never be administered by the patient himself. It must be always remembered that the risk of a sufferer from sciatica acquiring the morphine habit is considerable. Not infrequently an injection of distilled water into the nerve relieves the pain, and should be tried before resorting to morphine. Chloroform has been recommended for injection into the neighbourhood of the nerve, but it is hardly so serviceable, and is not free from the risk of increasing the interstitial exudation.

Acupuncture is a much-abused, but a very admirable remedy. Not infrequently a patient, hardly able to walk on account of the pain, is almost instantaneously relieved by this method of treatment; but a very chronic case is unsuitable. In practising acupuncture about six needles are required; these should be at least two and a half inches in length. The line of the nerve should first be marked out with ink or a dermatographic pencil; then the needles, after being rendered thoroughly aseptic, should be dipped into carbolic oil (1 in 20), and rapidly inserted for about two inches (dependent, of course, on the amount of fat and muscle to be penetrated), along the line of the nerve. Generally the highest needle is about the level of the fold of the buttock, and the lowest several inches above the popliteal space. Most of the needles actually pierce the nerve. If the operation be skilfully performed, the patient only perceives the first needle, and possibly the second; he cannot tell how many times he has been pricked, and has no conception that six long needles have been pushed into his leg. The needles should be kept in position for an hour or thereabout, the limb being covered by a cage to keep off the pressure of the bed-clothes. Acupuncture is not employed nearly so frequently as it was years ago, but its usefulness in some cases should not be forgotten.

Baths are of great use in sciatica, and especially hot baths of all kinds; hot under-current douches, in which, by means of a hose, hot water under considerable pressure is directed against the affected limb while the patient is seated or recumbent in an ordinary hot bath, are of service; warm mud baths are also beneficial.

Electricity is not of great benefit. Galvanism has been recommended, the one pole being applied to the sciatic notch, and the other to various points along the nerve; but the results are not very satisfactory.

When all else fails, nerve stretching or even excision of a portion of the nerve must be tried The amount of tension brought to bear on the nerve should be sufficient at least to lift the limb off the table. One advantage is the breaking down of adhesions, which in a small percentage of cases may have something to do with the pain; but the main advantage is counter-irritation very directly applied.

Massage for the muscles of the limb is desirable where there is any tendency to muscular atrophy.

Tonics should be given in most cases; iron and arsenic being perhaps the best possible remedies for rheumatic subjects.

Plantar neuralgia.—Occasionally, in place of sciatic neuralgia, the pain may be limited to a branch or branches of the nerve; very possibly in flat-foot the pain may be partly of neuralgic nature.

Metatarsal neuralgia, or Morton's affection of the foot.—This peculiar affection is probably of neuralgic origin. It consists in spasmodic attacks of dull, throbbing pain felt at the base of the fourth toe, sometimes of the second, and extending up the leg. It is increased by pressure over the head of the metatarsal bone, and, unlike rheumatism, is not specially severe at night.

Causes.—Tight or badly fitting shoes exerting pressure on the head of the metatarsal, especially on the fifth, may cause the condition in those otherwise disposed to neuralgia; and possibly much standing, in persons with a tendency to flat-foot, may be responsible for the condition in some cases. Oppenheim and other authors are dissatisfied with this simple explanation, and believe it to be insufficient. The *treatment* of this curious condition is often very troublesome. Broad shoes to prevent pressure over the heads of the metatarsals, or a bandage to support the plantar ligament where there is any tendency to flat-foot, may be efficacious in some cases; in others excision of the head of the metatarsal is the only certain and permanent cure.

Paralysis of the nerves of the sacral plexus.—The sacral plexus supplies the extensors and rotators of the hip, the flexors of the knee, and all the foot muscles; and it supplies the skin over the buttock, back of the thigh, outer side and back of the leg below the knee, and the greater part of the foot.

Causes. — The sacral plexus may be injured by diseases of the vertebral column or meninges, or by swellings compressing the nerve roots, such as cellulitis, tumours in the pelvis, and, rarely, in parturition when forceps have been used in a narrow pelvis. Sometimes neuritis extends upwards from the sciatic nerve to involve the plexus; and possibly in a few rare cases it may arise primarily. When the cause of the paralysis is pelvic, the phenomena are generally more marked in the area of the external popliteal nerve. It is much more common to find particular nerves affected, or branches of these.

Paralysis of the sciatic nerve.—The same causes which paralyse the sacral plexus may paralyse the sciatic nerve alone.

Among these causes pelvic tumours, instrumental delivery in narrow pelves, or even the pressure of the fœtal head, are not uncommon; and, as mentioned above, the paralysis may be most marked in the area of the external popliteal branch. D. Gerhardt suggests that the fibres belonging to this nerve may be more susceptible to injury.

Below the pelvis, wounds in the thigh, fractures or dislocations of the femur, tumours, hypodermic injections of ether or corrosive sublimate, and sometimes primary neuritis, may cause sciatic paralysis.

Clinical features.—The extensors of the hip, the flexors of the knee, and the muscles below the knee, may all be affected; or, if the lesion is situated below the middle of the thigh, the paralysis may be confined to the muscles last referred to. Not infrequently in a lesion of the whole sciatic the external popliteal suffers more severely; and this is especially the case when the primary cause is situated in the pelvis.

The affected muscles may waste, and there may be a greater or less area of anæsthesia within the domain supplied by the nerve. Other trophic changes may occur, especially herpetic eruptions in the line of the nerve. If one sciatic is paralysed alone the patient can still walk, because the quadriceps extensor cruris is able to fix the leg.

Paralysis of the small sciatic nerve.—This nerve is rarely paralysed except from a lesion of the sacral plexus.

It is entirely sensory and supplies the lower part of the buttock, the back of the thigh, and the upper part of the back of the leg, and it supplies a branch to the perineum.

Paralysis of the external popliteal nerve. — This nerve supplies the long and short extensors of the toes, the peronei, and the tibialis anticus muscles. The sensory supply includes the outer half of the front of the leg and the dorsum of the foot.

Causes. — The nerve is very superficial where it passes over the head of the fibula, and hence may be injured by fractures of the head of the fibula, and by wounds and blows in that region. Powerful extension of the leg has set up neuritis; and in certain occupations where there is much stooping, such as potato picking, or asphalt laying, the nerve may suffer; possibly by pressure between the biceps tendon and the head of the fibula. Unquestionably alcoholism renders the nerve in such cases more susceptible to injury.

The clinical features are marked foot drop,—the ankle cannot be flexed, and the first phalanges of the toes cannot be extended; the gait is characteristically altered, the foot being raised in walking so that the toes may clear the ground. In old cases talipes equinus sets in; and generally, by contraction of unopposed muscles, the first phalanges of the toes become bent. There may be wasting of the affected muscles and anæsthesia of the area of skin supplied by the nerve.

Paralysis of the internal popliteal nerve.—The nerve and its continuation supply the posterior tibial, the muscles of the calf, the sole of the foot, the tibialis posticus, the popliteus, and the long flexors of the toes. The sensory supply includes the outer side of the lower part of the leg, the outer side of the foot, and the sole.

Causes.—The nerve may be injured by a wound or blow, sometimes by a strain; but it is much more commonly affected, along with other peripheral nerves, by toxic agents.

Clinical features.—Extension at the ankle joint, flexion of the toes, and the rotation inwards due to the popliteus are lost. The patient cannot rise on tip-toe, and, as time goes on, talipes calcaneus sets in, and the toes, from secondary contraction, become claw-like. There may be wasting of the affected muscle, and more or less definite anæsthesia in the area supplied by the affected nerve.

Paralysis of the plantar nerves.—These nerves rarely suffer alone, unless from direct injury. The internal plantar supplies the flexor brevis digitorum, the plantar muscles of the great toe (excepting the adductors), and the first lumbrical muscle; while the sensory supply includes the inner side of the sole and the inner three and a half toes.

The external plantar supplies the flexor accessorius, the adductor of the great toe, all the plantar muscles of the little toe, all the interossei, and the outer three lumbricals; while the sensory supply includes the outer half of the sole and the outer one and a half toes.

Paralysis of the external plantar very seriously interferes with walking, as pointed out by Gowers; the toes cannot aid propulsion of the body forwards, and the interossei, being paralysed the toes, become flexed at the two distal, and extended at the proximal phalangeal joints.

Neuralgia of the genitals and rectum.—Sometimes there is neuralgia in the testicle or spermatic cord, with hyperæsthesia of skin, and, not infrequently, spasm of the cremaster muscle; more rarely priapism, and even discharge of semen are observed during the attacks of pain, and the affected testicle may swell. Generally a suspensory bandage and ordinary anti-neuralgic remedies are sufficient to effect a cure. Neuralgia may be· of perineal or more commonly of rectal origin. Perineal neuralgia is generally associated, as testicular neuralgia may be, with masturbation. Rectal neuralgia may be caused by a loaded rectum, by fistula or fissure, or any rectal irritation; but often rectal, perineal, testicular, and urethral neuralgic pains are more or less mental in origin; and not a few of these sufferers find their way eventually to an asylum.

Coccygodynia; Coccygeal neuralgia.—This is generally found in women, and consists in a severe pain in the region of the coccyx, which is caused by any pressure on it, or by contraction of muscles connected with it, such as may be produced by sitting, going to stool, or even by the muscular effort of passing urine. It may come on after a severe labour, or an injury to the spine; and is especially common in the subjects of hysteria. The condition may be a simple neuralgia; or there may be an actual inflammatory condition of the coccyx and the muscles, and other structures attached to it, especially when the pain follows an injury.

Anti-neuralgic treatment, opium, or cocain suppositories, and sometimes electricity, may be sufficient to effect a cure; or it may be necessary to resort to operative interference, either removing the coccyx or separating the bone from its attachments to surrounding tissues.

G. A. GIBSON.

R. A. FLEMING.

REFERENCES

A very comprehensive bibliography on neuritis and neuroma is found in the *Real-Encyclopädie der gesammten Heilkunde*, 3rd edition, published in 1898; and the Index Catalogue of the Library of the Surgeon-General's Office, U.S. Army, contains copious references to most of the conditions contained in the preceding pages.

The following references are a selection from the more recent literature:—

Introductory: 1. ALTHAUS. *Edin. Med. Jour.* 1898, p. 570.—2. GOTCH and HORSLEY. *Phil. Trans. Royal Soc. Lond.* 1891, p. 267.—3. KENNEDY. *Phil. Trans. Royal Soc. London*, 1897, p. 257.—4. MEYER. *Jahresbericht Virchow-Hirsch*, 1882, vol. i. p. 297.—5. OGSTON. *Brit. Med. Jour.* 1881, i. p. 391.—6. WOLBERG. *Deutsche Zeitschr. f. Chirurg.* 1883, vols. xviii. and xix.

Neuritis: 7. DÉJÉRINE, J. "Interstitial Hypertrophic and Progressive N. in Infancy," *Rev. de méd.* 1896, p. 882.—8. DILLER, T. *Penn. Med. Jour.* Pittsburg, 1897-98, i. p. 537.—9. FEINDEL, E. "Case of Traumatic N.," *Rev. Neurolog.* vol. iv. No. 18.—10. MARINESCO, G. "Nodular mesoneuritis," *Sem. méd.* vol. xvi. p. 324.—11. MEUSER, W. *Ueber Neuritis nach Verletzungen.* Jena, 1896.—12. MOLLE. "Traumatic N. of left Leg, with resulting Changes in right Leg," *Loire méd.* November 1896.—13. REMAK, E. "Acute multiple localised N." *Neurolog. Centralbl.* vol. xv. No. 13.—14. VEEDER, M. A. "After Shoulder Dislocations," *Internat. Journ. of Surg.* vol. xi. No. 3, p. 64.

Ascending Neuritis: 15. ANGIOLELLA. "Study of," *Manicomio Mod.* 1896, Nos. 2 and 3.—16. CARRIÈRE and RAINGUET. "Following on Injury," *Gaz. hebdom.* vol. xliv. No. 42.—17. DELORME. *Bull. méd.* 1895, No. 43.—18. FLEMING, R. A. *Edin. Med. Jour.* 1897, Jan. and Feb.—19. KAUSCH. "Case of," *Neurol. Centralbl.* vol. xv. No. 19.—20. KREHL, L. *Mitth. aus d. Grenzgeb. d. Med. u. Chir.* vol. i. p. 391 —21. DE MAJEWSKA. *Thèse de Paris*, 1897.—22. MERTENS, G. Diss. Göttingen, 1895.—23. MITCHELL, J. K. *Remote Consequences of Injuries of Nerves and their Treatment*, 1895.—24. TOURETTE, DE LA GILLES, and CHIPAULT. "La phase radiculaire" of traumatic ascending N. *Presse méd.* 1896; No. 46.

Neuromata: 25. BUSSE. "A Neuroma containing Ganglia Cells situated on the Sympathetic," *Deutsche med. Wochenschr.* 1898, Ver. Beil. 93.—26. KNAUSS, K. "True Neuroma," *Arch. f. path. Anat.* Berlin, 1898, p. 29.

Neuromata-False: 27. MITCHELL, J. K. *Univ. Med. Mag. Phila.* 1897-98, p. 62.

Neuromata-Multiple: 28. BRUNS, LUDWIG. *Die Geschwulste des Nervensystems.* Berlin, 1897.—29. PETREN. *Nord. Med. Ark.* Stockholm, 1897.

Multiple Neuromofibromata (Recklinghausen): 30. VON BUNGNER. *Verhandl. d. deutsch. Gesellsch. f. Chir.* Berlin, 1897, p. 298.—31. DUPIN and DIEULAFE. "A Case of," *Gaz. des hôp. de Toulouse*, 1898, p. 249.—32. FEINDEL. "Sarcoma in a case of," *Arch. gén. de méd.* 1897, p. 102.—33. *Idem.* "Incomplete Forms of," *Gaz. hebdom. de méd.* Paris, 1898, N.S. iii. p. 877.—34. FEINDEL and OPPENHEIM, R. *Archives gén. de méd.* 1898, July.—35. JEHL. *Thèse de Paris*, 1898.—36. LANDOWSKI. *Thèse de Paris*, 1894.—37. *Idem. Gaz. des hôp.* 1896, No. 95.—38. PETREN. "Study of," *Nord. Med. Ark.* vol. xxx. No. 10.—39. SPILLMAN and ÉTIENNE. *Gaz. hebdom.* 1898, p. 673.—40. VESELY. *Rev. Neurol.* 1897, No. 23.

Plexiform: 41. Bégouin. *Gaz. hebdom.* vol. xliv. No. 42.—42. Bobrow, A. *Annales de russ. Chir.* 1896, pt. ii.—43. Boccasso. "A Case of," *Giorn. della R. accad. di med. di Torino*, 1896, Nos. 10 and 11.—44. Chipault. "Two Cases of," *Tribune méd.* June 1896.—45. Delore, X., and Bonne, C. "Study of," *Gaz. hebdom. méd.* Paris, 1898, n.s. iii. p. 289.

Amputation: 46. Fleming, R. A. *Edin. Med. Journ.* Jan. 1897.

Tumours—Sarcomata: 47. Berry, J. *Lancet*, 1897, i. p. 1554.—48. Hartmann. "Secondary Malignant Neuroma," *Beitr. z. klin. Chir. v. P. Bruns.* vol. xvii. p. 177.—49. Mory. "Of Median Nerve," *Echo méd. du Nord*, Lille, 1897, i. p. 229.—50. Murphy, J. B. *Chicago Clinic*, 1897, p. 195.—51. Scheven, O. *Beitr. z. klin. Chir. v. P. Bruns.* vol. xvii. p. 157.

Pressure on Nerves: 52. Pershing. "Caused during Surgical Operations," *Med. News*, New York, 1897, p. 329.

Wounds of Nerves: 53. Bowlby, A. *Injuries and Diseases of Nerves.* London, 1889.—54. von Büngner. Ziegler's *Beitrage z. path. Anat.* 1891.—55. Knox. *Texas Med. Ass. Trans.* 1897, p. 93.—56. Mitchell, Weir. *Injuries of Nerves*, 1872.—57. Molle. *Loire méd.* November 1896.—58. Tillmanns. "Nerve Injuries," *Archiv f. klin. Chir. v. Langenbeck*, 1882, p. 1.—59. Smissen, C. van der. *Injury by Fracture*, Diss. Kiel, 1896.—59a. Williams, L. L. *New York Med. Journ.* 1896, p. 81.

Regeneration after Wounds of Nerves: 60. Laubie. *Gaz. hebdom. de sc. méd. de Bordeaux*, 1898, p. 43.—61. Weiting. *Beitrag. z. path. Anat. u. z. allg. Path.* Jena, 1898, p. 42.

Neuralgia of Phrenic Nerve: 62. Jenner, W. *Allg. med. centr. Ztg.* April 1896.—63. Jousset, André. "A new Symptom of," *Méd. mod.* vol. viii. p. 494.

Brachial Neuralgia: 64. Heinlein. *Münch. med. Wochenschr.* 1896, No. 3.

Brachial Neuritis: 65. Bostwick, W. W. "Excision of Part of Plexus for," *Med. Record*, N.Y. 1898, p. 385.—66. Oppenheim, H. *Aerztl. Rundschau*, Munich, 1898, p. 421.—67. Schuster, Paul. "Pathology of," *Neurol. Centralbl.* 1896, No. 14.

Paralysis of the Brachial Plexus: 68. Apert, E. "Case of Radicular P." *Bull. et mém. soc. méd. des hôp. de Paris*, 1898, p. 613.—69. Ballet, G. *Bull. méd.* vol. x. 1896, pp. 903, 927.—70. Beevor, C. E. *Lancet*, 1895, Nov.—71. Cibert, Maurice. *Radicular Paralysis of Obstetrical Origin*, Thèse de Lyon, 1896-97.—72. Déjérine. "Radicular Paralysis," *Rev. prat. de trav. de méd.* Paris, 1898, p. 233.—73. Guillemot. Thèse de Paris, 1896.—74. Helfond. Thèse de Paris, 1896.—75. Legry. *Union méd.* 1896, Jan.—76. Raymond. *Presse méd.* 1895.—77. Weile, E. "Radicular Paralysis of Obstetrical Origin," *Rev. mens. des malad. de l'enfance*, 1896, p. 484.

Erb's Type of: 78. Levy-Dorn. *Neurol. Centralbl.* 1895, No. 17.—79. Osann. *Münch. med. Wochenschr.* 1896, No. 2.—80. Rissom, O. Diss. Berlin, 1897.—81. Stern, R. *Deutsche med. Wochenschr.* 1895, No. 13.—82. Weber. *Neurol. Centralbl.* 1895, No. 4.

Klumpke's Type of: 83. Heubner, O. *Charité-annalen*, 1896, No. 14.

Paralysis of Serratus Magnus: 84. Berdach. "A Case of," *Wien. klin. Rundschau*, 1896, No. 41.—85. Fraser, Donald. *Glasgow Med. Journ.* 1897, p. 41.—86. Ketli. "A Case of," *Wien. med. Presse*, 1896, No. 32.—87. Placzek, S. "Uncomplicated Case of," *Deutsche med. Wochenschr.* 1896, No. 43.—88. Zillessen. Diss. Bonn, 1895.

Paralysis of the Suprascapular Nerve: 89. Göbel. "A Case of," *Deutsche med. Wochenschr.* vol. xxiii. No. 19.

Paralysis of the Circumflex Nerve: 90. Brothers. *Ibid.* Nov. 1895.

Paralysis of the Musculo-spiral Nerve: 91. Barlow. "Fracture of Humerus causing," *Glasgow Med. Journ.* 1896, p. 131.—92. Bennet, W. "Lesions of the," *Clin. Journ.* 1897, No. 10.—93. Gerulanos. "Paralysis from Strong Contraction of Triceps," *Deutsche Zeitschr. f. Chirurgie*, vol. xlvii. p. 1.—94. Lehmann, R. "Fracture of Humerus causing," *Monatsschr. f. Unfallhlkd.* No. 9, p. 269.—95. Mies. "A Case of," *Deutsche med. Wochenschr.* 1898, Ver. Beil. 92.—96. Potain. "Etiology and Pathology of," *Sem. méd.* 1896, p. 365.—97. Remak. "Two Cases of," *Centralbl. f. Nervenhlkd.* vol. xix. p. 511.—98. Sarbó, Arthur. "Bilateral Paralysis in two Cases of," *Pester med.-chir. Presse*, 1896, No. 43.—99. Tixier. "Fracture of Humerus causing," *Province méd.* 1897, No. 24.

Paralysis of the Median Nerve: 100. Bernhardt, M. "Pathology of," *Neurol. Centralbl.* vol. xvi. No. 14.—101. Destot. *Méd. mod.* vol. viii. p. 487.—102. Dubar. "Contused Wound of," *Echo méd. du Nord*, 1897, vol. i. No. 16.

Paralysis of the Ulnar Nerve : 103. DESTOT. "Paralysis from Compression," *Wien. klin. Wochenschr.* 1897, No. 1.—104. JANZER, R. Diss. Berlin, 1895.
Paralysis of the Anterior Crural Nerve : 105. GUMPERTZ. *Neurol. Centralbl.* 1895, No. 13.
Paralysis of External Cutaneous Nerve : 106. WARDA. *Neurol. Centralbl.* 1897, p. 948.
Sciatica : 107. AVULLANI. "Artificial Compression as Treatment of," *Gaz. med. di Torino*, 1897, April.—108. BIRO, DE MAX. "Contribution to," *Deutsche Zeitschr. f. Nervenhlkd.* vol. xi. p. 207.—109. DONADIEU-LAVIT. *Nouv. Montpell. méd.* 1895, July and Sept.—110. GIBBES, J. M. "Treatment of," *Austral. Med. Gaz.* Sydney, 1898, p. 62.—111. LAGO. Thèse de Paris, 1897.—112. RENTON, J. C. "Four Cases of, relieved by removing Adhesions," *Scot. Med. and Surg. Journ.* 1897, Jan.
Metatarsal Neuralgia : 113. BOSC. *Nouv. Montpellier méd. : supp. dimensuel*, 1895. —114. DALCHÉ, P. *Tribune méd.* Paris, 1898, p. 708.—115. FÉRÉ, CH. "Contribution to," *Rev. de Chir.* 1897, March 10.—116. GALLOIS. *Bull. méd.* vol. x. p. 1216. —117. HALSTEADT, A. E. "Three Cases of," *Med. Record*, N.Y. vol. li. No. 1.— 118. JONES, R., and TUBBY, A. H. *Ann. Surg. Phila.* 1898, p. 297.—119 LAMACQ, L. "Study of," *Rev. de méd.* 1896, p. 476.—120. MORTON, T. "X Rays in Diagnosis of," *Internat. Med. Mag.* vol. v. p. 322.—121. DE PIERI, G. *Rif. Med.* 1896, vol. xi. p. 292.—122. TARUFFI. "Two Cases of," *Arch. di Ortopedia*, No. 1, 1897.—123. TUBBY, A. H. "Study of, with four Cases,"*Lancet*, ii. 1896, pp. 425 and 1217.—124. WHITMANN, R. "Study of," *Med. Record*, N.Y. 1898, p. 189.
Paralysis of Plantar Nerve : 125. GOWERS. *Diseases of the Spinal Cord and Nerves*, 1892, p. 96.
Neuralgia of Genitals and Rectum : 126. ARNOLD, W. F. "N. of Rectum," *Med. News*, 1895, August.—127. BOYD, R. "N. of Penis," *Med. Record*, N.Y. vol. l. No. 6.—128. PEYRAUBE. *N. of Testicles*. Thèse de Montpellier, 1895-96.
Coccygeal Neuralgia : 129. ROHLEDER, W. *Ueber Coccigodynie*, Berlin, 1896.

G. A. G.
R. A. F.

MULTIPLE SYMMETRICAL PERIPHERAL NEURITIS

Introduction. — The name neuritis is usually understood to mean inflammation of a nerve ; but, as pointed out by Dr. Buzzard, this is not its original interpretation. The adjective neuritis, the substantive νόσος being understood, signifies etymologically no more than disease affecting the nerve. It has indeed become customary, and even necessary, to include under the name neuritis not only what is ordinarily called inflammation, but also degeneration, atrophy, and other lesions affecting a nerve.

Some of the chief characteristics of the affection to be considered in the present article are indicated by qualifying epithets. Thus the adjective *peripheral* indicates that the extremities of the nerves are most markedly affected ; *multiple* that many nerves are usually affected ; and *symmetrical* that corresponding nerves on the two sides of the body are attacked, often almost simultaneously.

The commonest cause of the disease is a chemical poison ; and it is important at the very outset to recognise (i.) that the action of the poison is not necessarily limited to the peripheral nerves ; on the contrary, there are frequently indications that it has impaired the functions of other parts of the nervous system : (ii.) that the name Peripheral Neuritis does not imply that the abnormal condition of the nerves, upon which the characteristic symptoms appear to depend, is due to the direct action of the poison, and is entirely independent of changes produced by the poison on the central nervous system. In other words, lesions of the peripheral nerves do not necessarily constitute the whole anatomical substratum of the disease, but are its most conspicuous features.

History.—The clinical features of multiple neuritis are described by many of the older observers. Thus admirable descriptions of alcoholic paralysis were given by Lettsom in 1789, and by Jackson in 1822; but Graves was probably the first to suspect that certain forms of generalised paralysis depend on disease not of the brain or spinal cord, but of the nervous cords themselves. "One of the most remarkable examples of disease of the nervous system commencing in the extremities and having no connection with lesions of brain or spinal marrow," he says, "was the curious epidémie de Paris which occurred in the spring of 1828." After describing the chief symptoms and progress of this epidemic, the author says, "Now here is another remarkable instance of paralysis creeping from the extremities towards the centre. Here is a paralysis affecting all parts of the extremities as completely as if it had its origin in the central parts of the nervous system ; and can any one, with such palpable evidence before him, hesitate to believe that paralysis or even hemiplegia, without any lesion of the brain or spinal cord, may arise from disease commencing and originating in the nervous extremities alone ?" In another passage Graves asks the question : "May not the decay and withering of the nervous tree commence occasionally in its extreme branches ? And may not a blighting influence affect the latter, while the main trunk remains sound and unharmed ?" Dr. Todd, too, appears to have recognised that lead palsy depends on disease of the nerves. In one of his clinical lectures he says : "I believe that the muscles and nerves are early affected, and that at a later period the nerve centres become implicated. The nervous system is thus first affected at its periphery, in the nerves, and, the poisonous influence continuing, the contamination gradually advances towards the centre."

The first case, however, in which the presence of neuritis was proved after death was published by Duménil, of Rouen, in 1864. The patient was a tailor, aged sixty-one years, who presented the symptoms now recognised as characteristic of peripheral neuritis; and the autopsy revealed disease of the small nerves of the hands and feet, the brain and cord being quite healthy. In 1866 Duménil made a second communication on peripheric paralysis, and reported another case of this disease with autopsy.

These important pathological observations appear to have attracted little notice ; and it was not until further observations were reported by Lancereaux in 1871, Eichhorst in 1875, Joffroy in 1879, Leyden in 1880, and Grainger Stewart in 1881, that the doctrine of peripheral neuritis was placed upon a sure pathological basis. The degeneration of the nerves of the palate in a case of diphtheritic paralysis, discovered by Charcot and Vulpian in 1862, and the changes described in the muscles and nerves taken from a case of lead paralysis by Lancereaux in 1871 threw much light on this subject.

During the last sixteen years many observations and monographs relating to the subject of peripheral neuritis have been published; it would be impossible, within the limits of the present article, to enumerate even the more important of them; but I would draw special attention to the work of Moeli and Leyden in Germany, of Ballet, Déjerine, Pitres, and Vaillard in France, and of Dreschfeld, Buzzard, and Ross in this country. My colleague, Dr. Dreschfeld, was the first in England to adduce anatomical evidence in favour of the neuritic hypothesis of alcoholic paralysis. The very interesting and valuable series of cases which formed the basis of the Harveian lectures delivered by Dr. Buzzard in 1885, and subsequently published in book form, gave a great impetus to a careful study of the subject; while the masterly articles by the late Dr. Ross on Landry's paralysis, and his suggestive classification of peripheral neuritis, in which for the first time prominent places are given to an irritative and a vaso-motor type, helped greatly to enlarge our field of inquiry, and to give us a more definite view of the clinical features of the disease.

Classification.—A study of peripheral neuritis brings out very clearly that in most cases the cause of the disease is some kind of poison. Hence it has been found convenient to classify its different forms according to our knowledge of the causes producing them. Thus peripheral neuritis may be caused by lead, arsenic, mercury, phosphorus, or silver; by alcohol, ether, bisulphide of carbon, dinitro-benzine, aniline, or carbon monoxide. It may also be caused by the micro-organisms which produce specific diseases, or by their products: for example, those of diphtheria, influenza, typhoid, and other fevers; of pneumonia, erysipelas, gonorrhœa, syphilis; of the various forms of septicæmia (including puerperal fever), and malaria. Of beriberi and leprosy it is an essential part, and it occurs, too, in rheumatism, gout, and diabetes. It is not improbable that the cases of peripheral neuritis found in association with anæmia, pregnancy, the cancerous and other forms of cachexia, and gastro-intestinal disturbance, and after over-fatigue and exposure to cold and wet, also owe their origin to some toxic agent.

An etiological classification is useful in bringing into prominence the fact that variations in the symptoms of peripheral neuritis are partly due to variations in the selective action of different poisons. Thus lead picks out certain branches of the musculo-spiral nerves, while alcohol shows a preference for the nerves supplying the flexors of the ankle.

It is, however, to be noted that no particular set of symptoms is exclusively related to a particular poison. Moreover in practice the first question to be answered is not what poison has injured the nervous system, but what part of the nervous system is affected; have we to deal mainly with disease of the peripheral nerves, or with disease of the central nervous system? In other words, we have first to diagnose the presence of peripheral neuritis, and thence to seek its cause; indeed, it is not until we have acquired a mastery of the symptomatology of the disorder that we are able to make a satisfactory inquiry into its causation.

I have therefore determined to adopt in this article a classification which seems to me to be both more logical, and also, from a clinical point of view, more desirable. If we take the commonest example of multiple neuritis, namely the alcoholic variety, as our guide to classification, we shall find the characteristic clinical feature to be symmetrical localisation of motor, sensory, and vaso-motor symptoms in the peripheral parts of the limbs. As a rule all these symptoms are present, though varying much in relative intensity in different cases, and at different stages of the disease. Careful clinical observations also show that any one of the three groups of symptoms may predominate, and in exceptional cases be present alone. It is not, indeed, uncommon, to see cases of alcoholic paralysis in which sensation is quite normal to the most careful testing; and occasionally cases occur in which sensory or vaso-motor symptoms, if not present alone, are at any rate the most conspicuous features.

Furthermore, if we consider the symptoms of alcoholic neuritis at different stages of the disorder, we find that symptoms indicative of irritation of nerve tissue are present in the early stages of the disease, and that symptoms indicative of destruction of nerve tissue are present in the later. Thus in the early stages we have, on the motor side, muscular spasms and cramps; on the sensory side, shooting pains, paræsthesia, and cutaneous and muscular hyperæsthesia; in the later stages, paralysis and anæsthesia are predominant. Now in some cases irritative phenomena are present alone from first to last; the motor being prominent in one set of cases, the sensory in another set. If then we meet with cases, alcoholic or other, in which muscular spasms, or irritative sensory or vaso-motor phenomena are the dominant features, and are symmetrically localised in the extremities, can we adduce evidence to show that such cases are really examples of peripheral neuritis; using the name, in the wide sense already proposed, to denote any abnormal condition of the peripheral nerves? In the course of this article the question will be discussed. In the meantime, the above considerations—together with the fact that the relations of neuritis to many of its causes have already been described in various parts of this *System of Medicine* (see diphtheria, leprosy, lead poisoning, etc.)—suggest the following simple classification as a basis for practice :—

I. *The common or mixed type;* motor, sensory, and vaso-motor phenomena being present in various combinations. Examples: alcoholic paralysis, arsenical palsy, beriberi.

II. *The motor type;* motor phenomena are dominant or alone.

(A) The spasmodic variety, reaching its maximum in tetany.

(B) The paralytic variety; under which head are included chronic local forms of paralysis, as exemplified by lead neuritis; and acute universal forms of paralysis, as exemplified by Landry's disease.

(C) The atrophic variety, in which the degree of paralysis appears to depend on the amount of muscular atrophy present.

III. *The sensory type.*

(A) Sensory symptoms exist alone, or in association with a varying amount of muscular weakness.

(B) Sensory symptoms are associated with muscular inco-ordination; this variety is sometimes called Neurotabes peripherica.

IV. *The vaso-motor type.*—Erythromelalgia, Raynaud's disease.

I. THE COMMON OR MIXED.

ALCOHOLIC POLYNEURITIS. — Causes. — It is usually stated that spirit drinking is the commonest cause of alcoholic paralysis; but it is probable, judging from observations made at the Manchester Royal Infirmary, that the disorder is quite as often brought on by excesses in beer.

Sex.—The severer degrees of this neuritis are certainly commoner in women; but the milder are met with as frequently in men.

Age.—By far the majority of cases of alcoholic paralysis occur in persons between 30 and 50 years of age; the affection is seldom met with under 20 or over 60 years. Occasionally, however, it occurs at the extremes of life. Thus Herter records a remarkable case of acute alcoholic intoxication in a boy aged three years. The child, after a large drink of whisky, suffered from convulsions and paralysis of cerebral origin; and subsequently from typical symptoms of multiple neuritis. He made a complete recovery. As an instance of alcoholic neuritis occurring in advanced age, may be mentioned the case of a gentleman, aged 76, reported by Dr. Maude, who presented marked symptoms of the disorder, including œdema, local asphyxia, and trophic phenomena.

Symptoms.—The complaints of a patient in the early stage of chronic alcoholic poisoning may usually be referred to disorders, (a) of the digestive system, or (β) of the circulatory system, or (γ) of the nervous system.

The subjects of the first group complain of morning retching and vomiting, and of abdominal pain or disturbed action of the bowels; an examination reveals evidence of congestion and catarrh of the mouth, pharynx, and other parts of the alimentary tract. The subjects of the second group complain of shortness of breath on exertion, and sometimes of dropsy; on examination the heart is found dilated. The subjects of the third group complain of numb or cold extremities, and of cramps or muscular weakness; or of symptoms, such as impaired memory, which indicate disturbance of the cerebral functions. Each of these groups of symptoms are met with in practice, either separately or in combination with the other groups, as the results of chronic alcoholism.

Thus a patient may suffer for a long period from dyspnœa, dropsy, and congestion of the liver, and yet be entirely free from any symptoms of nerve disorder; on the other hand, paralysis and mental impairment may steadily set in without any decided symptoms of gastric or cardiac disturbance. These differences are to be explained by the varying susceptibilities of the tissues of different individuals to alcohol, rather than by the kind of alcoholic drink indulged in. On the other hand, signs of slight degrees of neuritis may frequently be found in what may be called the *gastric* and *cardiac* types of alcoholism, as well as in cases of ascites from alcoholic cirrhosis of the liver.

Mode of onset.—In a few cases the onset of paralysis is quite sudden, as in the case of a man who, when smoking, found himself unable to lift up his hand to take his pipe from his mouth; but, as a rule, paralysis not only sets in insidiously, but is preceded by certain premonitory symptoms which have existed in varying degrees of intensity for many weeks, months, or even years. These are not separated abruptly from the symptoms of the fully established disease; indeed, they are often present during its whole course. Nevertheless it is desirable to give them a prominent place at the outset, because they are very frequent, and often appear long before any signs of paralysis, and at a time when the knee-jerks, instead of being absent, are either normal or exaggerated.

The symptoms I refer to are disorders of the tactile sensibility of the extremities, vaso-motor irregularities, and muscular spasms. The *disorders of tactile sensibility* are usually described by the patient as numbness and tingling, or "pins and needles," in the fingers and toes. The hands feel as if covered with gloves, and the feet as if something soft, like fur or wool, intervened between the soles and the ground. Patients in this state have frequently to rub their hands together several times before they are able to use them for writing, sewing, or other work. The *vaso-motor disorders* consist of cold hands and feet, and sometimes of hot, burning sensations in the extremities. A patient may notice that on getting up in the morning his fingers go of a dark livid colour; or that, when his feet are hanging down, the soles and the toes turn dark red. *Muscular spasms* may be present, in the form of tremors and twitchings of the extremities; but more frequently they appear as active cramps, which are most severe and persistent in the calves of the legs. These cramps are usually very troublesome at night, just as the patient is about to fall asleep, or in the early morning; he feels that the calf is drawn up into a lump, and is often obliged to get out of bed and press his toes on the floor, rubbing first one calf and then the other for some time before the spasm relaxes. Sometimes the flesh is so sore that he prefers to bear the cramp rather than suffer the pain of the rubbing.

Sensory disorders.—In addition to "numbness and tingling," patients also suffer from pains of various kinds, which occur most commonly and severely in the early stages of the disease, but are by no means confined to that period. They may be aching, burning, twisting, or shooting in character. Paroxysms of excruciating lancinating pains in the limbs, especially in the lower limbs, frequently deprive the patient of rest and appetite, and thus become important contributory factors in the general weakness and emaciation which characterise severe cases of alcoholic paralysis. At one time the patient has darting pains in the instep or in the sole of the foot; at another in the fingers; at another along the course of the sciatic nerves : in other cases, again, the sensory branches of the cervical or brachial plexuses, or the nerves of the trunk are implicated. The plantar nerves are very liable to be affected, and then the soles of the feet become sensitive to pressure, and cause the patient much distress in walking. In such cases certain parts of the sole are particularly tender, as at the centre of the heel where the internal plantar nerve leaves the fascia to become superficial ; and over points between the ends of the metatarsal bones where the nerve divides into its digital branches.

Some of the visceral nerves are occasionally the seat of neuralgic attacks. Thus the patient may be subject to griping intestinal pains, like lead colic ; or to paroxysmal attacks of severe gastralgia which, when associated with vomiting, may closely resemble the gastric crises of loco-motor ataxy. Of objective sensory phenomena in alcoholic neuritis, the sensibility of the skin, muscles, and nerves requires careful investigation. Besides the tenderness of the soles of the feet, spots of cutaneous hyper-æsthesia may be found also on the forearms and legs. The superficially situated nerve trunks,—such as the musculo-spiral, the ulnar or the popliteal nerves,—may be unduly sensitive, and sometimes even enlarged. But the most frequent and prominent sensory phenomenon in alcoholic neuritis is muscular hyperæsthesia. This is usually most marked in the calves of the legs, but is present in other muscles of the limbs also ; in slight degrees of tenderness the patient shrinks when the muscles are gently squeezed, and in severe cases he is unable to bear the slightest movement or pressure, so that even the weight of the bed-clothes may be intolerable, and the feet and legs have to be protected by cradles. Cutaneous anæs-thesia, although a less prominent symptom than muscular hyperæsthesia, is usually present in some degree. It is more common to meet with loss of sensibility to painful impressions than to tactile ; sometimes the sense of temperature is impaired also, all objects feeling cold ; or cold and hot bodies are not readily distinguished. As a rule, anæsthesia is partial, but it may be complete : it is found in the lower limbs as high as the knees, in the upper limbs as high as the elbows ; and occasionally in the arms and thighs.

Cutaneous anæsthesia and muscular hyperæsthesia often co-exist in advanced stages of the disease ; in the early stages either may exist alone. In fact, any disorder of sensation may be present at any period of the disease, and the chief points to bear in mind are—(i.) That numb-ness and tingling and aching and shooting pains are early symptoms ; (ii.) that muscular hyperæsthesia and cutaneous anæsthesia characterise the fully-established disease ; (iii.) that anæsthesia is very variable both in intensity and extent ; in some cases the most careful examination being required to detect it, whereas in others it is completely absent.

Motor disorders.—The tremor, twitching, and cramps which constitute the premonitory and early symptoms of alcoholic neuritis are also present, in varying degree, during its whole course. In addition to these symptoms of morbid over-action of muscular tissue, the further progress of the disease is indicated by muscular weakness which, beginning usually in the periphery, gradually spreads to the proximal segments of the limbs and, in some cases, to the muscles of the trunk. At first the patient finds that he is losing his spring in walking, or that he has a difficulty in ascending a stair; and he may also have noticed that he cannot execute certain special actions with the fingers, such as buttoning the clothes, as well as formerly. Subsequently the extensors of the toes, the flexors of the ankles, and the extensors of the wrist become paralysed, giving rise, when the limbs are not supported, to a double wrist and double ankle drop. The affected muscles are soft and flaccid, and undergo a progressive atrophy. This muscular atrophy, together with the unbalanced action of healthy muscles, gives rise to various abnormalities in the position and in the power of the limbs which will be now described.

The upper limbs.—The finer movements of the fingers and thumb require careful study, inasmuch as their weakness may occur before that of the extensor muscles, and constitute the first indication of the presence of neuritis. Thus abduction and adduction of the fingers may be feebly performed, and, when the small muscles of the thumb are weak, the patient is unable to touch the tip of the little finger with the point of the thumb, except by flexing its distal phalanx; and, when the opponens minimi digiti is also feeble, the point of the thumb touches the side instead of the end of the little finger. Weakness of the opponens pollicis allows the metacarpal bone of the thumb to be drawn backwards by the action of the long extensors, so that it lies nearly on the same plane as the other metacarpal bones. Then as the extensor secundi internodii pollicis becomes weak the distal phalanx of the thumb bends towards the palm; and when the extensor primi internodii pollicis is affected the basal phalanx is also bent, while weakness of the extensor ossis metacarpi is betrayed by approximation of the metacarpal bone of the thumb to that of the index finger. When the extensors of the wrist become weak the patient cannot perform certain movements, such as grasping an object, without the wrist becoming flexed; owing to the preponderating action of the flexor muscles. Similarly, in buttoning or unbuttoning the clothes the prominence of the curve of the flexed wrist and the fumbling of the feeble fingers are very conspicuous features. Before the extensor muscles of the fingers are completely paralysed their stretching by the flexion of the hand on the forearm causes extension of the first phalanges; the distal, however, are flexed by the long flexor. When the extensor muscles of the wrists and fingers are completely paralysed, and the patient is asked to raise his hands, the wrists are strongly flexed; while owing to the action of the interossei and lumbricales the fingers are slightly flexed at their metacarpo-phalangeal, but extended at the phalangeal joints. The attitude then frequently resembles that produced by active muscular spasm, as in tetany. As regards the upper arm the triceps is usually more paralysed than the biceps or supinator longus; hence the elbows are bent, and, owing to the necessary stretching of the shortened flexors, cannot be fully extended by passive movements without causing pain.

The progressive atrophy also contributes to the deformity of the limbs. The thenar and hypothenar eminences are flattened, and deep grooves appear on the back of the hand between the metacarpal bones; the space between the metacarpal bones of the thumb and index finger being especially hollow. The back of the forearm becomes flattened and the ulnar border loses its roundness; but the radial border usually retains its natural curve, because the supinator longus is comparatively spared. The biceps and deltoid are also often but little affected; the triceps, however, is usually much wasted. In other cases the deltoid, biceps, and supinator longus become weak and wasted.

The lower limbs.—Restriction of movement is not always due to paralysis, it may depend on great tenderness of the soles and of the leg muscles. But sooner or later paralysis sets in, and is usually first declared by the patient's inability to raise the toes from the ground in walking. When the foot is unsupported its anterior part falls down, forming an obtuse angle with the axis of the leg, instead of a right angle, as in health. In the first degree of paralysis, in addition to dropping of the feet, the toes are hyper-extended at the metatarso-phalangeal and flexed at the phalangeal joints, with the exception of the big toes which are hyper-extended at both joints. This hyper-extension of the big toes is a characteristic feature of the early stages of neuritis; and when, as some-times happens, it is associated with exaggeration of the knee-jerk and of the plantar reflex, the case might easily be mistaken for one of spastic paralysis, the result of disease of the lateral columns of the cord. In the second degree of paralysis the terminal phalanx of the big toe becomes flexed. In the third degree the whole of the big toe is bent down towards the sole, but the other toes still remain over-extended at the metacarpo-phalangeal joints. But in the fourth degree of paralysis these also become bent, and the whole fore part of the foot hangs loose and curved towards the sole; this tends to increase the concavity of the foot, although when it is placed on the ground it appears to be flatter than normal. In old-standing cases, in which the flexors of the toes and the muscles of the sole have undergone adaptive shortening, the concavity of the foot is persistently maintained; and during the stage of recovery from paralysis the patient may be unable to bring his heels to the ground.

In addition to the muscles on the anterior aspect of the legs the calf muscles also frequently become affected; and in advanced cases all the muscles below the knee are so wasted that anteriorly the skin appears to lie almost on the bones, while posteriorly the calves are represented by loose bags of skin. Frequently the thigh and pelvic muscles become affected, the extensors more than the flexors; and when this occurs to any serious degree the patient becomes bedridden. Then the anterior aspect of the thigh is much wasted, and the gluteal regions are flattened, soft, and pendulous; the gluteal folds feeling as if composed of little more than layers of skin. In such a case the hips and knees are flexed to about a right angle, while the ankles are hyper-extended, the anterior parts of the feet being strongly curved towards the soles; the outer lateral surface of one limb rests on the bed with the other limb lying upon it.

The peculiar gait, seen in all marked cases of alcoholic paralysis, depends chiefly upon the flatness of the feet and the weakness of the anterior muscles of the legs. Thus, when the heel of the foot to be advanced is raised, the toes drop, and are only prevented from trailing along the ground by an unusual degree of flexion of the knee and hip. The undue elevation of the knee at each step makes the gait resemble that of a high-stepping horse; and the drop of the fore part of the foot unduly exposes the sole to the view of an observer standing behind the patient.

Muscles of the trunk.—In some cases the muscles of the back and abdomen are affected, and in rare cases those of the neck also. When the lumbar muscles are feeble the hollowing of the back is deepened; and if the glutei are also paralysed the patient has a difficulty in rising from a chair or from the ground; in attempting to do so his attitudes closely resemble those seen in pseudo-hypertrophic paralysis. Feebleness of the abdominal muscles impairs the power of expelling the contents of the rectum or bladder, weakens the force of sudden expiratory acts like coughing and sneezing, and takes away the patient's power of raising himself from the recumbent position. When the muscles of the neck become paralysed the patient is unable to raise his head, or even to move it on the pillow.

The further advance of the disease is indicated by implication of the muscles of respiration. The diaphragm is first attacked, its paralysis being indicated mainly by the drawing in of the epigastrium during inspiration, and by over-action of the lower intercostal muscles. When the intercostals become feeble the patient complains of a tightness across the chest, and expansion of the chest is feeble or lost; whereas its elevation is carried on by the violent action of the extraneous muscles of respiration.

Muscles of the face.—Decided paralysis of the facial muscles rarely occurs in alcoholic paralysis, but slight feebleness is not uncommon. This feebleness is shown—(i.) by a loss of expression, the lines which give character to the face being little marked or even obliterated; (ii.) by a widening of the palpebral fissures, owing to weakening of the orbiculares palpebrarum and to retraction of the upper eyelids; and (iii.) by tremor of the lips in speaking, or on protrusion of the tongue.

Tremor and weakness of the tongue and lip muscles render articulation thick and indistinct; and in some cases this defective articulation, together with the want of tension about the lower facial muscles, presents a close resemblance to the facial and articulatory characteristics of general paralysis of the insane. Phonation, too, is frequently feeble and husky, and occasionally there is complete aphonia, these changes being due partly to laryngeal congestion and partly to weakness of the vocal cords.

Muscles of the eye.—As a rule the muscles of the eyeball are spared ; but in a few cases nystagmus, ptosis, convergent strabismus from weakness of the external recti, and even ophthalmoplegia externa have been observed. Ptosis and paralysis of the external rectus have been proved to depend on degenerative changes in the third and sixth nerves, but in cases of ophthalmoplegia there is usually a lesion of their nuclei. The pupils, if altered in size, are usually somewhat dilated. It is probable that they always contract to light and accommodation. Epéron, however, has brought forward some inconclusive evidence in favour of the occasional presence of the Argyll-Robertson phenomenon in alcoholic neuritis.

Inco-ordination of movement—Ataxy.—True ataxy occurs very rarely in multiple neuritis. In the large majority of cases the disorders of gait and other motor defects are due to muscular weakness, and not merely to errors in the balance or equilibrium of the contractions of muscles by which a particular movement is performed. Thus, if the lower limbs are partially paralysed, the patient (his eyes being closed) can usually give accurate answers with regard to the position of his legs in bed ; he can cross one knee over the other without any exaggeration of the necessary movement, and is often able to describe a circle in the air with his foot, and to stand with his feet together and his eyes shut, without any material increase of the unsteadiness due to his muscular weakness.

It is true that occasionally the gait of a patient suffering from multiple neuritis may present a superficial resemblance to that of ataxy ; as, for example, when there is considerable anæsthesia of the soles of the feet. Then when the patient's eyes are closed he may walk in an uncertain oscillating fashion. In other cases, too, it may be noticed that extension of the knees in walking is performed with abnormal vigour, and presents the sudden jerky exaggerated action of ataxy ; but a careful examination will show that weakness of the flexors of the knee determines the undue action of the extensors. In neither instance is the resemblance to ataxy a close one. It must be admitted, however, that a genuine inco-ordination of movement does very rarely occur in cases where the lesions are limited to the peripheral nerves, the posterior roots and root zones being free from disease. A well-marked instance of this condition is recorded in the section on neuro-tabes peripherica.

The bladder.—The sphincters, as a rule, are unaffected. When psychical disorders are prominent, patients who are able to empty their bladders in a normal manner may pass their urine into the bed ; or they may suffer from retention of urine and overflow-incontinence. When the patient's intelligence is unaffected, disorders of micturition have been occasionally observed ; of these dysuria and retention are the commonest : paralytic incontinence, apart from the presence of spinal cord disease, is excessively rare.

Disorders of reflex action.—Loss of the knee-jerks is one of the most valuable signs of peripheral neuritis ; but it is important to remember that the knee-jerks in the early stage, and in the milder varieties of the disease are frequently exaggerated. Thus it is not uncommon in out-patient and in private practice to find increased knee-jerks in association with slight motor defects, slight anæsthesia, and a moderate degree of muscular hyperæsthesia; on the other hand, I have never seen a well-marked case of alcoholic paralysis in which the knee-jerks were present.

The cutaneous reflexes are usually enfeebled or abolished; but they may be present, and even increased, as when cutaneous hyperæsthesia is prominent. Sometimes the plantar reflex is lost when the cremasteric and abdominal reflexes are active. The latter indeed, as a rule, are not lost until paralysis is both profound and widely distributed.

The *electrical reactions* of the nerves and muscles in cases of multiple neuritis are variable in character. When there is obvious paralysis and muscular atrophy, some form of the reaction of degeneration is usually present; but in the minor degrees of paralysis, when it is of great importance to recognise the nature of the disease, the faradic and galvanic irritability of the nerves and muscles are either normal, or present such slight variations, that an electrical examination can scarcely be regarded as of much diagnostic value.

Changes in the colour, moisture, and temperature of the extremities.—As already mentioned, subjective feelings of cold or heat in the extremities are common premonitory symptoms of peripheral neuritis, and they may persist during the course of the disease. Sometimes they are associated with perceptible changes; thus the fingers and toes may be white and cold, hot, red and dry, or warm, livid and moist. The hands and feet when hanging down, are often of a dark purple tint; but pale and bloodless when held above the horizontal position. In rare cases the three stages characterising Raynaud's disease have been observed in succession : namely, the stage of local syncope, in which the extremities are pale ; the stage of local asphyxia, in which they are blue, and the stage of local gangrene. Dr. Ross recorded a case of this kind : the patient was suffering from numbness and tingling of the extremities, nocturnal cramps, loss of the knee-jerks, tottering gait, and other symptoms of alcoholism; he had suffered for some time from alternating attacks of severe burning sensations in his hands and fingers, and coldness and deadness of them. When Dr. Ross saw him the palmar surfaces of the two distal phalanges of the index and middle fingers of the right hand and the dorsal surfaces of the last phalanges were of a dark livid colour ; the tip of the thumb was also affected. Dark-coloured bullæ had already appeared on the palmar surfaces of the affected digits, and the matrix of the nails had begun to ulcerate.

Profuse sweating is not uncommon ; this may be general, or restricted to certain localities, such as the forehead, the back of the hands and feet. The moisture, in which the feet are often bathed, is apt to be particularly offensive. At an advanced period of the disease the skin, especially that of the lower limbs, becomes excessively dry and covered by scales of dried epidermis.

Other local changes.—In many cases the skin of the palms of the hands and backs of the fingers loses its wrinkles, and becomes thin, smooth, and glossy; sometimes the soles of the feet are similarly affected. The nails and hairs tend to become dry and brittle; the former may be furrowed longitudinally, and jagged and cracked at their edges. Bedsores and perforating ulcers occur in cases of multiple neuritis, but with extreme rarity.

Changes in the joints.—Pain in the neighbourhood of the joints is not uncommon, and, in the absence of any evidence of the presence of gout or rheumatism, redness and swelling of the joints are occasionally seen; presumably as a direct result of the disease of the nerves. In chronic cases thickening of the affected joints may occur, and end in restriction of their movements. In one remarkable case, under my own care, pain over the right elbow with effusion into the joint appeared during the course of a most pronounced and characteristic case of multiple neuritis of alcoholic origin, and was followed by almost complete ankylosis. The joint affection was associated with much tenderness over the lower end of the humerus and the upper ends of the radius and ulna [*vide* also art. "Neurotrophic Diseases of Bones and Joints," p. 545].

Œdema is sometimes a noticeable feature of alcoholic cases. It is usually dependent on cardiac dilatation from muscle failure; but it may occur apart from heart disease, and when no feasible explanation, other than disease of vaso-motor nerves, can be given. In the latter case the œdema is usually limited to the lower extremities and to the backs of the hands; but in cases of alcoholic heart failure the dropsy is often widespread, and erratically distributed. Caprice of localisation is indeed a peculiar feature; the walls of the chest or the lower part of the back may pit on pressure, and the scrotum be greatly swollen, when the lower limbs are comparatively free from œdema. The arms and upper part of the trunk may be involved when there is no obvious dropsy elsewhere. The face and eyelids usually escape; but in a few cases œdema of the eyelids does occur, although it is difficult to be certain whether it depends on the heart or on associated Bright's disease.

The *course* of alcoholic neuritis presents many variations. As a rule the symptoms succeed each other gradually, and several weeks elapse before they attain their maximum intensity. Then, if the poison have been removed, there is a stationary period of one or two months, after which signs of improvement begin to show themselves; the pain and hyperæsthesia diminish in intensity, cutaneous sensibility becomes normal, and, finally, muscular power is completely restored. Sometimes the march of the affection is very slow, and its duration much prolonged; fibrotendinous contractions and even actual articular changes may cripple the patient for a long time; and occasionally muscular atrophy is a distinctive feature, and may persist for many years. In other cases the onset of the disease is sudden, paralysis spreads with great rapidity, and by invasion of the respiratory muscles quickly leads to a fatal issue. The description of such cases is given under "Landry's disease" (p. 694).

Complications.—For an account of the visceral disorders and other complications of chronic alcoholism, the reader is referred to the article by Dr. Rolleston (vol. ii. p. 852). I would here merely lay stress on the frequency of psychical disorders, and of the symptoms and physical signs of cardiac failure; and on the liability of subjects of alcoholic paralysis to suffer from pulmonary tuberculosis.

The psychical disorders were divided by the late Dr. Ross into four stages :—

(i.) The stage of exaltation, in which there are active hallucinations of sight and hearing associated with a gradual lowering of the intellectual powers. (ii.) The stage of depression, or melancholia, which is characterised by great restlessness, moroseness, mental irritability, insomnia, and horrid dreams; and frequently, too, by much morbid timidity, when the patient becomes suspicious and distrustful of his best friends. (iii.) The stage of delirium, mania, or melancholia with excitement, or of epileptiform convulsions, passing on to (iv.) The final stage, of dementia. Failure of memory is one of the earliest and also one of the commonest symptoms met with in cases of alcoholic neuritis, and is usually associated with a peculiar disorder in the appreciation of time and locality. Thus a patient may be unable to tell the day of the week, or to say whether he is in a hospital or at his own home. He cannot retain any fresh impressions in the memory; thus, if an object be shown to him or a word be repeated to him, he is unable a few minutes later to recall the word, or to remember the object. Ultimately the memory becomes almost a complete blank; and a patient who has been lying helpless in bed for weeks may give a circumstantial account of a walk in the morning, of the public-houses he visited, and of the boon companions he met by the way.

Pathological anatomy.—The results of necropsies in cases of alcoholic paralysis show that, while morbid changes are frequently found in the brain and spinal cord, the most frequent changes are in the peripheral nerves; and there is now abundant evidence in favour of a direct causal relationship between peripheral nerve changes and the peripheral paralytic phenomena.

The changes in the *nerves* may involve both the connective tissue and the nerve fibres, but the latter always suffer more severely. The condition then is mainly one of parenchymatous neuritis; perineuritis and interstitial neuritis being absent, or present to a slight degree only. Hence, to the naked eye the nerves and their branches appear quite healthy. In acute cases, however, when there has been acute inflammation of the sheath and connective tissue, the nerve may appear reddened and swollen; or, at a later stage, soft and pulpy. The microscopical changes have already been described in the previous article. As regards the distribution of the changes in the nerve fibres the rule is that they are most intense in the terminal branches to the muscles and skin, and become progressively less marked towards the larger branches; the trunk and anterior roots of the nerve are usually quite healthy.

In the diseased portions of the nerve the fibres are not affected equally; some may be quite normal, some may be slightly affected, others may have undergone complete atrophy. These differences, as shown by Fleming, are largely related to the presence or absence of local exudations in consequence of changes in the vessels.

The nerves of the limbs are principally affected, and, while all the terminal nerves of the limbs may be involved in some degree, the branches of the musculo-spiral and the anterior tibial usually suffer the most severely. Degenerated fibres have also often been found in the phrenic and vagus nerves.

The *muscles* in connection with diseased nerve present changes similar to those of experimental neuritis: they are pale and wasted, and their fibres are reduced in size. All the fibres are not affected to the same extent, and the variations are greater than in cases of experimental neuritis. There are changes, too, which appear to depend on some process other than simple atrophy. Thus the connective tissue of the muscles may be profoundly altered; its overgrowth in some cases is so great that it looks as if there had been a primary fibrosis of muscle with a secondary atrophy of its fibres. This interstitial myositis is chiefly found in cases of chronic neuritis, but it may appear in acute cases. Two causes may be suggested: that it is secondary to the irritating effects of the poison on the nerve branches; or is primary, and due to the action of the poison on the muscle itself.

The spinal cord has been found healthy in many cases, even when carefully examined by the most recent methods of investigation. For example, Déjerine reported the following case:—A man, aged 41, a spirit drinker, suffered from symptoms of severe multiple neuritis of arms and legs; marked hyperæsthesia, muscular atrophy, and contractures were present. Slow improvement went on for three years and the patient recovered the use of his arms completely; but his legs remained paralysed. He died the following year from cirrhosis of the liver. Pronounced changes were found in the nerves to the skin and muscles, but the cord and its anterior and posterior roots were quite normal. The microscopical examination of the nerve cells was made on sections treated by the method of Nissl, and that of Marchi and Weigert-Pal.

In other cases of alcoholic neuritis, changes have been found in the cord. As Dr. Tooth has pointed out, the cells of the anterior horns, although generally unaltered in form, may show heavy pigmentation. He says that the pigment in the cells of normal cords increases in quantity and depth of colour as the age increases; and he regards the heavy pigmentation referred to as a hint that premature old age of the cord may follow chronic alcoholism. But, in addition to increased pigmentation, the cells may present a vitreous appearance, or distinct vacuolation. More considerable changes have also been found: namely, chronic inflammation of the membranes, especially of the pia mater; an irregularly disseminated chronic myelitis; and in some cases an over-growth of connective tissue throughout the cord, often especially marked in the posterior columns. Slight degeneration of the columns of Goll is frequently mentioned in reports of cases of alcoholic neuritis.

Many other poisons, enumerated above as causes of peripheral neuritis, may produce what we have called the common or mixed type. Two, namely arsenic and the poison of beriberi, may be specially mentioned as giving rise to symptoms which closely resemble those of alcoholic paralysis.

ARSENICAL PARALYSIS.—The causes of arsenical poisoning have been considered by Dr. Oliver in the second volume of this work, and I will only here lay stress on the importance of remembering that peripheral paralysis has occasionally followed the medicinal administration of arsenic ; when for instance Fowler's solution has been given in large doses, or in small doses for a long time. As regards the *symptoms*, the lower extremities are attacked, as a rule in arsenical paralysis, before the upper ; in both cases the extensor muscles of the hands and feet are principally implicated, so that the patient cannot properly extend his fingers, toes, wrists, or ankles ; and in some cases there is complete wrist and ankle drop. Atrophy of the muscles occurs very quickly, probably more quickly than in the peripheral palsies of lead or alcohol. The muscles respond badly to the faradic current, and often show the qualitative alterations to galvanism which characterise the reaction of degeneration. The paralysis may spread to the small muscles of the hands and feet, or to the arms and thighs, and occasionally may become almost universal in distribution.

Tremors, general or localised, may be present, and spasmodic movements have also been described. Thus Pick observed spasmodic flexion of the great toes ; while in a remarkable case of arsenical paralysis, recorded by Kovacs, the fingers of both hands were the seat of movements like those of athetosis. The movements only occurred when the limbs were in a position of rest, and ceased directly during the performance of voluntary movements.

Arsenical paralysis is ushered in and accompanied by marked sensory disturbance. The patient complains of severe darting, smarting, burning, or rheumatic-like pains in the limbs, and of numbness and tingling in the fingers and toes. The spontaneous pains are often severe enough to prevent sleep. Painful cramps are also present, and there may be much cutaneous and muscular hyperæsthesia. These irritative phenomena are quickly followed, or accompanied, by diminution or loss of the cutaneous sensibility. The muscular sense is also frequently affected, so much so as sometimes to constitute a true ataxia. As a rule any incoordination of movement can be explained, or is overshadowed by muscular weakness ; but occasionally it is the dominant feature of the case which then closely resembles one of locomotor ataxy.

The tendon reflexes are almost invariably lost, while the superficial are usually present. In the only case of arsenical paralysis that has come under my own observation, the knee-jerks and plantar reflexes were both increased ; the other symptoms of the case were pricking sensations in the hands and feet, weakness of the muscles on the front of the legs, relative anæsthesia of the hands, feet, and outer side of the legs, and hyperæsthesia of the calves. The patient, a man aged 41, had worked in arsenic three months; he was only seen once, so that the subsequent history of the case cannot be given. It seems probable that the deep reflexes are often exaggerated in the early stages of arsenical as in alcoholic and other toxic palsies; but Kovacs holds the contrary opinion, namely, that their loss is much more frequent when the paralysis is due to arsenic than to other poisons.

Pathology.—The clinical history of arsenical paralysis justifies the assumption that the peripheral nerves rather than the spinal cord are implicated but the anatomical proof of this is not yet fully established. Jarschka, in 1882, was the first to suggest that the paralytic symptoms depend upon a multiple neuritis; and, according to Putnam, this view has been confirmed by the autopsy of a case reported in the *Canada Medical and Surgical Journal*, 1886, page 716. Quite recently Erlicki and Rybalken examined the nervous system in two cases of arsenical paralysis, and found disease of both the anterior horns and peripheral nerves. They believe that the degeneration of the spinal ganglion cells, which is sometimes found in toxic cases, is due to physiological and chemical peculiarities of the blood; not to the direct effect of the poison on nerve elements. It has also been shown that arsenic injected subcutaneously is capable of destroying adjacent nerves, apart from any changes in the nerve centres. The careful experiments of Vrigens, in 1881, make it probable that no part of the nervous system is exempt from the influence of the poison. Hæmorrhages widely distributed in the brain and cord are sometimes found; and are supposed to be due partly to paralysis of the vaso-motor nerves, and partly to changes in the constitution of the blood and vessels.

The distinction of arsenical from alcoholic paralysis is based on the absence of a history of intemperance, and on the discovery of a cause of arsenical poisoning; as well as on the presence of associated symptoms which are known to be the result of poisoning by arsenic. These are—(i.) certain skin lesions: (*a*) a peculiar pigmentation, sometimes closely resembling that of Addison's disease; (*b*) herpes zoster, which is present in a small percentage of cases; (*c*) bullous or erythematous eruptions: (ii.) loss of hair; falling off of the nails: (iii.) intermittent dysuria, or glycosuria: (iv.) œdema of the eyelids: (v.) ulceration of the gums and fauces: (vi.) the presence or history of acute unaccountable attacks of indigestion associated with nausea, salivation, and epigastric pain.

BERIBERI.—The peculiar features of this disease are the association of dropsy and signs of cardiac failure with symptoms of a multiple neuritis. Dropsy and dilatation of the heart are not uncommon in alcoholic paralysis, but they are constant in beriberi. For a full description of. the disease, including its pathology and bacteriology, the reader is referred to the article by Dr. P. Manson in the second volume.

DIPHTHERITIC PARALYSIS has been adequately described by Dr. Gee, and its morbid anatomy by Dr. Kanthack, in the first volume. It is mentioned here in order to emphasise the fact that, as a rule, it conforms, in the association of sensory with motor symptoms and in their distribution, to the common type of peripheral neuritis. Purely motor forms occur ; but, as might be inferred from the statements of some writers on the subject, they are not the rule.

Some of the distinctive features of diphtheritic paralysis are :— (i.) The early symptoms ; namely, paralysis of the palate followed by paralysis of accommodation of the eye from weakness of the ciliary muscle. (ii.) The slow spread of paralysis, which is rarely absolute, from one part to another; and the frequent implication of a large number of muscles, including those of the trunk, and sometimes those of the neck. (iii.) A slight or moderate degree of muscular wasting rather than marked atrophy. (iv.) A greater tendency to inco-ordination of movement than in cases of neuritis from other causes. (v.) The condition of the knee-jerks. I have already said that absence of knee-jerks in alcoholic paralysis may be preceded by their exaggeration. This is often the case in diphtheritic neuritis ; and, further, Dr. Bristowe has recorded a case in which increased knee-jerks were maintained throughout the whole period of paralysis, and did not disappear absolutely until the patient had completely recovered from paralysis. In diphtheria, as in diabetes, the knee-jerks may be lost in the absence of paralysis. (vi.) The occurrence of bulbar crises. In patients who are seen during the second or third week of diphtheritic paralysis, and who present slight weakness of the legs, nasal voice, paresis of the palate, and sometimes squint, the voice may suddenly become weak and hoarse, and the cough loose, ineffectual and noiseless. Then the respiration may give warning of approaching danger ; it is not necessarily swift, but inspiration is sudden, deep and forcible, and expiration short and weak ; and mucus accumulates in the air passages. The crises which occur, and which are very fatal, are marked by sudden and complete paralysis of deglutition, by complete aphonia, by alarming dyspnœa, and sometimes by repeated and uncontrollable vomiting. The pulse-rate rises to 140 or 150, and the temperature to 102° or 103°. It is probable that these attacks are attributable to a disorder of the vagi or their centres. Sudden heart failure, which is apt to occur in cases of diphtheria also, may be due to peripheral degeneration of cardiac nerves, or to changes in the myocardium.

II. THE MOTOR TYPE.

Under this heading I include cases of peripheral neuritis in which motor symptoms are dominant ; sensory phenomena being either absent, or present but in slight degree. Three groups may be distinguished ; namely, the spasmodic, the paralytic, and the atrophic group.

A. The spasmodic or irritative form of neuritis, in which spasm

predominates over paralysis.—In considering motor phenomena it is convenient to regard the motor tract as composed of two parts, an upper and a lower segment; or, as they are now designated, central and peripheral neurons. The upper segment comprises the motor cells in the cerebral cortex and the pyramidal fibres which extend between these cortical centres and the anterior horns of the spinal cord, or the corresponding nuclei in the medulla and pons. The lower segment includes the bulbar nuclei and the anterior horns, together with the motor fibres which extend from them to the muscles. A lesion situated in any portion of the upper segment of the motor tract gives rise to a spastic paralysis —that is, to a paralysis associated with rigidity or spasm of muscular tissue. A lesion situated in any part of the lower segment gives rise to an atrophic paralysis, in which weakness is combined with relaxation and wasting of muscular tissue.

Increased muscular tonus, then, is one of the distinguishing features of affections of the upper segment; diminished muscular tonus of affections of the lower segment of the motor tract. We may now ask, Does muscular spasm ever occur in cases where a lesion is limited to some portion of the lower segment? First, with regard to the *spinal nuclei,* will irritation of the motor cells in the anterior horns, and restricted to them, produce muscular spasm? Physiologists do not appear to be agreed as to the excitability of any part of the cord to direct electrical and mechanical stimuli; it is stated that the motor centres can be excited by blood heated above 40° C.; or by asphyxiated blood; or by certain poisons, such as strychnine (Landois and Stirling). The knowledge derived from a study of cord diseases does not lend any support to the opinion that spasm may be caused by a lesion limited to the anterior horns. How rare, for example, is it to meet with any signs of local muscular rigidity in infantile paralysis, even at the onset of the affection! And when it is present in this disease it is probably due to an associated lesion, such as meningitis; or possibly to peripheral neuritis.

In a few cases of infantile paralysis I have seen exaggeration of the knee-jerk and slight muscular rigidity of the non-paralysed leg. What is the explanation of this? Are these symptoms due to an associated peripheral neuritis, or to implication of the terminal fibres of the pyramidal tract?

Secondly, as regards the *peripheral nerves.* Irritation of motor nerves, by the electric current or other stimulus, tends to produce muscular spasm. Has disease a similar effect? The answer is that spasm of the ocular muscles may result from basal meningitis, in consequence of irritation of the motor nerve trunk; and that facial spasm may be caused by a tumour pressing on the facial nerve. With regard to the evidence afforded by the clinical history of multiple neuritis, I would draw attention to the frequency of tremor and local spasms, and to the occasional presence of exaggerated knee-jerk in the early stages of the disease.

Without entering into a discussion on the pathology of tremor, we may note how often a fine variety is met with in cases of multiple

neuritis.   Thus it occurs in alcoholic, in lead, and in arsenical paralysis.
It is a distinguishing feature of mercurial poisoning; and in cases of
poisoning, both acute and chronic, it may be followed or accompanied by
symptoms of neuritis.   The presence of tremor in exophthalmic goitre,
and during the course of severe typhoid or other specific fever—all
diseases which owe their origin to some toxin in the blood—and the
occasional association of evidence of peripheral neuritis with the tremor,
are also suggestive facts worthy of consideration in the pathology of
tremor.

The possibility that the tremor, spastic attitudes, and other symptoms
of paralysis agitans might depend on a chronic irritative form of neuritis
has often occurred to me, but it would be profitless to pursue the speculation further.   Turning now to muscular cramps and spasms, we have
seen that they are common phenomena in cases of alcoholic neuritis, and
are most persistent and troublesome in the muscles of the calves of the
legs.   The forearms, hands, and fingers also are liable to be attacked;
and the spasms are particularly apt to come on while the patient is
engaged in some kind of manipulation such as writing, sewing, or playing
the piano.   They are often complained of by patients suffering from the
slightest varieties of peripheral neuritis : thus a patient, who suffers from
numbness and tingling and impairment of the special movements of the
thumb and fingers, may state that his fingers feel drawn when he awakes
in the morning; sometimes they are so stiff and painful that vigorous
rubbing for a few minutes is necessary before they can be used.   Although
most prominent during the early stage of neuritis, active spasms are
often present throughout its course, and may be associated with considerable paralysis.

In a well-marked case of alcoholic paralysis, under my own care, the
position of the hands was much like that seen in tetany.   The dropped
wrists were the result of paralysis of the extensor muscles; but the
flexion of the first phalanges of the fingers and the extension of the
terminal ones were mainly caused by spasm of the interossei : this was
proved by the firmness with which the fingers were pressed together, and
by the resistance experienced on trying to separate them, or to extend
them at the metacarpo-phalangeal joints.   The fingers, too, were never
completely at rest, and their quivering movements appeared to be due to
intermittent contractions of the interossei.

Finally, exaggeration of the knee-jerk, suggestive of increased muscular tonus, has been met with in the early stages of diphtheritic and
alcoholic paralysis,—an increase which, during or even before the onset of
paralysis, had given way to diminution and loss of the reflex.

Is it possible to admit the existence of an irritative form of peripheral
neuritis clinically expressed by muscular spasm and by no other prominent symptom ?   We know that paralysis of the extremities may result
from disease of the peripheral nerves.   Are there cases in which a
spasmodic condition of the extremities can be attributed to morbid
irritation of a number of motor nerve fibres ?   This question naturally

suggests tetany, a disease the clinical features of which present certain affinities with those of multiple peripheral neuritis.

Tetany will be fully described in the following volume. Suffice it that the morbid anatomy demands reinvestigation; and that it is especially important that a careful histological examination should be made of all parts of the nervous system in cases where tetany has existed for many years. At present, evidence as to (*a*) the probable seat, and (*b*) the nature of the lesion, can only be obtained from a consideration of the causes and clinical aspect of the disease.

(*a*) As to seat.—We have seen that muscular spasm is chiefly met with in affections of the upper segment of the motor tract. In favour of the cerebral origin of tetany the following facts may be mentioned :—(i.) That interosseous spasms occur in some forms of brain disease; as, for example, in the spastic hemiplegia of infancy. (ii.) That tetany in infants is frequently associated with laryngismus stridulus, and is occasionally followed by general convulsions. (iii.) That headache, vertigo, and even psychical disorders have been observed; while bulbar disturbance has sometimes been suggested by the presence of polyuria and glycosuria.

Against the cerebral origin of tetany, according to Abercrombie, is the persistence of the tonic spasm during sleep, and chloroform anæsthesia. If, too, the spasms depended on cortical disturbance we should have to admit the limitation of this disturbance, in many cases at least, to certain portions of the hand and foot centres. It may also be noticed incidentally that the position of the hand in tetany differs from that seen in the eclamptic attacks of infancy. In both there is rigid flexion, but in eclampsia all the joints of the fingers are flexed, and the thumbs, instead of being pressed against the forefingers, are flexed and drawn inwards under cover of the firmly-bent fingers. Moreover, the convulsions which sometimes occur during an attack of tetany do not appear to have any influence over it. The features of tetany persist through the convulsive attack, and, although both are probably started by the same irritant, their independence suggests that different parts of the nervous system are being excited.

As to the upper segment of the motor tract in the cord, it may be observed that a spastic weakness of arms and legs sometimes occurs in consequence of degeneration of the pyramidal tracts, and, when unattended by muscular atrophy or sensory disturbance, is considered by some authors to point to a primary lateral sclerosis. But in these cases a careful examination will usually reveal impairment of the superficial abdominal reflexes, or other indications that the gray matter of the cord is also implicated. Moreover, ankle clonus is present, and the knee-jerks and tendon reactions in the arms are exaggerated; phenomena which, if they occur in tetany, must be very rare.

Coming now to the lower segment of the motor tract, we are ignorant, as I have said, of spasmodic conditions in lesions of the anterior horns : even physiological experiments do not give us much assistance. The spasms produced by strychnine are said to be due to the action of the poison on the spinal gray matter, but I am not aware that there is any direct proof of this.   Houghton and Muirhead believe that in strychnine tetanus some resistance is removed to the passage of impulses between the posterior horn and the terminal fibres of the sensory nerve roots which surround the motor cells.   They think it probable that the poison acts neither on the terminal fibres nor on the motor cells, nor yet on the cells of the posterior root ganglion.

The occasional occurrence of muscular atrophy in cases of tetany may be due to a lesion of the ganglion cells of the anterior horns, but it may also be accounted for by disease of the peripheral nerves.   Other arguments, too, bear testimony to the possibility of the peripheral origin of tetany. They are :—(a) The distribution of the disorder—in ordinary cases the hands and feet are the only parts of the body affected—which presents a resemblance to that of alcoholic neuritis.   The extremities are flexed by spasm in tetany, they are flexed in consequence of weakness in alcoholic paralysis.   (β) Evidence of disturbance of sensory fibres, namely, paræsthesia and, rarely, anæsthesia; also Hoffmann's phenomenon, namely, exaggerated excitability of the sensory nerves to mechanical and electrical stimulation.   (γ) The increased mechanical and electrical excitability of the motor nerves, as well as the occasional presence of fibrillary muscular contractions, of muscular paresis, and atrophy.

(b) The nature of the irritant.—Without entering into a discussion of the causes of tetany, two pathological facts of great significance may be briefly noticed: (i.) That tetany is frequently associated with some disturbance of the alimentary canal.   (ii.) That it often follows excision of the thyroid gland.

When present in infancy tetany is nearly always found in cases of rickets, but as a rule only in those cases where there are offensive stools or other evidence of bad digestion.   In adults tetany has been observed in cases of dilatation of the stomach.   Bouveret and Devic have written a valuable paper on this subject, in which they have collected twenty-three cases.   From a number of exhaustive experiments and analyses, they conclude: (a) that the tetany which occurs in patients affected with gastric dilatation is almost exclusively limited to cases where there is permanent hypersecretion of the gastric juice ; (β) that tetany is not produced reflexly by irritation of the stomach, but by the direct action of a chemical poison on the nervous system ; (γ) that the toxic substance is produced by the action of free hydrochloric acid on syntonin, and by the action of alcohol on that ; (δ) that the introduction into the blood of any animal of a solution of an alcoholic extract of the digestive fluids produces violent tetanic convulsions ; but the latter do not occur when the injection is made subcutaneously.

The occurrence of tetany after extirpation of the thyroid gland is difficult to explain.   It has been proved that tetany does not follow other operations in the neck, and that it follows total rather than partial removal of the thyroid.   The association of tetany with the myxœdema following the operation suggests that possibly the tonic spasms are excited by the poisonous effects of mucin; and it is significant that the injection of mucin into cats has sometimes been followed by tetany (Wagner and Hammerschlag). The probability that tetany, in a large number of cases, is due to the irritating effects of some poison in the blood is not only indicated by the facts of its relation to alimentary disturbance and to excision of the thyroid gland, but also by its occurrence after some of the acute specific fevers, after lead poisoning, and by the phenomena of ergot poisoning, which are almost identical with those of tetany.

It appears, then, reasonable to assume that the condition called tetany is due to irritation of some portion of the nervous system by the presence of a poison in the blood or lymph; and that the facts connected with the ordinary features of the disease are perhaps best explained on the supposition that motor nerve fibres and not nerve cells are selected by the poison. At the same time the action of the poison is not limited to the peripheral nerves; for symptoms indicating central disturbance are sometimes combined with those which, as just suggested, appear to be related to a morbid condition of the peripheral nerves.

B. The paralytic variety, in which paralysis is the dominant feature, the muscles being flaccid or wasted, while sensory and other symptoms are absent or inconspicuous. Can such a variety of peripheral neuritis be admitted? Is there adequate evidence that a purely motor paralysis may depend on disease limited to peripheral nerves? To answer these questions we must consider two groups of cases—(a) cases where paralysis is limited to certain groups of muscles, as in lead paralysis; (b) cases where paralysis is widespread, affecting a large number of the limb and often many of the trunk muscles.

Group (a).—Lead palsy has been described in the second volume of this work, and it is therefore only necessary to refer briefly to the two commonest varieties—the wrist-drop type and the upper arm type—as good examples of the present group. In the former type the extensor muscles of the fingers and wrists are successively attacked by paralysis and progressive atrophy. In the latter type there is paralysis of the deltoid, biceps, brachialis anticus, and supinator longus. Now in both cases there is adequate proof that the atrophic paralysis is dependent on what appears to be a primary degenerative neuritis. Examples of localised forms of motor neuritis also occur as a result of other poisons; as of alcohol, of influenza, of typhoid, and so forth.

With regard to Group (b) the matter is not so simple. Many cases of generalised paralysis are met with in practice in which the diagnosis, especially in the early stages, is very difficult. The peripheral portions of the limbs are mainly involved; the affected muscles are flaccid, the knee-jerks are lost, and sensory phenomena are absent or inconspicuous. Have we here to deal with disease of the nerves or with disease of the anterior horns? Some of these cases are quickly fatal owing to invasion of the respiratory muscles; others survive, and the affected muscles undergo a progressive atrophy. In the former case a microscopical examination of the nervous system may be inconclusive; and even in the latter the diagnosis has sometimes to be held in reserve until the ultimate result can be foreseen; a gradual improvement and ultimate recovery pointing to multiple neuritis, a steadily increasing weakness and muscular atrophy pointing to disease of the anterior horns.

That this distinction, however, does not always hold is shown by the history of a case published by Blocq and Marinesco. In this case the illness had extended over a period of twenty years. The attack was ushered in by fever and digestive derangement; there was generalised atrophic paralysis, which was succeeded by local recovery. Sensory symptoms were entirely absent, and the case was diagnosed as one of acute spinal paralysis. The autopsy revealed grave degeneration of the muscles and of the intra-muscular nerve branches; other parts of the nerves were healthy, and senile changes only were found in the spinal cord. Blocq and Marinesco point out that multiple neuritis was indicated in the above case by the presence of psychical phenomena, diarrhœa, vomiting, œdema, and vaso-motor derangements.

Examples of widespread motor paralysis have also been observed in connection with lead poisoning, diphtheria, influenza, and some other toxic causes. Dr. Buzzard has recorded a well-marked example of generalised motor paralysis after influenza, and I have recently seen two cases of this class.

A remarkable *case of generalised motor paralysis* in a young man was observed by myself in which, after an exhaustive inquiry, no possible cause could be ascertained. He lay in bed, completely helpless, for several weeks; then he slowly recovered. As already mentioned, a favourable course indicates a peripheral rather than a central origin; and suggests that the motor fibres of a large number of peripheral nerves may be attacked by certain poisons while the sensory fibres are wholly or comparatively spared.

The *acute cases of generalised motor paralysis* offer the greatest difficulties in diagnosis. For the most part they are included under the names of "Landry's" or "Acute ascending paralysis"; and this subject, owing to its importance, must now be considered in some detail.

LANDRY'S PARALYSIS.—Before entering upon a description of this disease, it is necessary to note: (i.) That authorities appear to differ as regards the limitations of the name. Some would restrict it to certain rapidly fatal cases of ascending paralysis, in which sensation is either unaffected, or affected to a slight degree only; others would give it a wider range, in order to include cases where sensation is decidedly affected or completely lost, and also cases in which recovery, whether partial or complete, occurs after a longer or shorter interval. (ii.) That an analysis of cases reported under the heading of Acute ascending or Landry's paralysis shows very clearly that they differ widely as regards their pathological phenomena; well-marked lesions being found in one group of cases in the spinal cord; in another group in the peripheral nerves; in a third group in both cord and nerves; while in a fourth group of cases careful microscopical examination failed to reveal any morbid changes either in the central or in the peripheral parts of the nervous system. In fact, Landry's paralysis has served as a convenient clinical name for a number of cases of rapidly progressive generalised paralysis in which the pathological diagnosis during life was uncertain ; in consequence, it may be, either of incompleteness of clinical examination, or of the similarity of symptoms produced by minute changes in the peripheral nerves to those produced by lesions in certain parts of the central nervous system.

The subject is a difficult one ; and it must be frankly admitted that, in the present state of our knowledge, the pathology and the classification of cases presenting the features of Landry's paralysis cannot be accurately given.   In the meantime there appear to me to be sufficient reasons for placing well-marked examples of the disease provisionally under the heading of acute multiple neuritis ; and I believe that the clearest conception of the subject will be obtained by basing the description of the symptomatology on the historical case described by Landry in 1859 ; for surely if the name Landry's paralysis is to retain a place in the classification of nervous disease, it must be used to designate cases presenting the features described by the discoverer, and not in other senses adopted by some writers on the subject.

The following is an abstract of the case referred to :—

A pavior, aged 43 years, entered the Hospital Beaujou, under M. Gubler, on 1st June 1859. He had suffered from some kind of intermittent fever in childhood, and had an attack of articular rheumatism at the age of 15 years ; but subsequently he enjoyed fair health up to about twelve months before his admission.   In July 1858 he was laid up for some weeks in bed by fever, which was ushered in by a rigor ; but he made an excellent recovery, and returned to his work. Three months later he had another rigor, followed by fever and vague pains in the extremities, which lasted three weeks ; and again he made a good recovery and returned to his work.   At the beginning of 1859 he suffered from slight difficulty of deglutition and a teasing cough ; but there was no fever or pain, and in the following March he was attacked afresh by rigors and fever, which was this time accompanied by pain in the side and free expectoration.   The medical man who attended him said he had a "fluxion of the chest," and bled him three times, administered emetics, blistered his side, and put him on a low diet.   From this illness he made a very imperfect recovery ; but at the end of two months he returned to his work.   A few days afterwards he felt tingling sensations in the tips of his fingers and toes ; and at the end of a week he was compelled to leave off work altogether, owing to the great general weakness from which he suffered.   A fortnight later he entered the hospital.   He walked a considerable distance to get to the hospital, and until nearly a fortnight after his admission he did not complain of any definite symptoms beyond general weakness. On 13th June the patient complained that in walking his knees gave way under him ; on the following day sudden flexion at the knees whilst walking became more frequent ; his feet felt heavy, and seemed as if "they were glued to the ground."   For some days the tingling sensations, which he had formerly experienced, began to extend ; and they gradually invaded the feet, the legs, and ultimately the thighs. In the superior extremities these sensations ascended as high as the arm ; and during this ascent the forearm felt as if it were surrounded by a tight bracelet, whilst the part below this line seemed if if it were benumbed by cold. On the fourteenth and subsequent days walking became more and more difficult, and on the seventeenth the patient was unable to raise his feet ; on making a few steps they trailed on the ground, but were never projected forwards in a disorderly manner. When lying on his back in bed he was unable to raise either lower extremity from the mattress, and experienced great difficulty in flexing the thigh slightly on the pelvis. In the effort to turn on his side he could move the trunk, but he could not draw the legs after it. With the upper extremities he could still grasp a little, but could neither raise his arms to the horizontal position, nor maintain them in that position when raised by the observer. He complained of a feeling of stiffness in his fingers, and when he tried to move them they felt as if surrounded by a bandage. There was no fever, no pain either in the limbs or along the vertebral column, no headache, and no contractures or convulsions. There was some degree of blunting of sensibility in the soles of the feet. The intelligence was clear. The reflex reactions were lost. The visceral functions were normally performed, although the appetite was not very good.

20th June.—The lower extremities were almost completely paralysed ; and, although the movements of the upper extremities were not entirely lost, the patient was unable to make use of his hands for any purpose. The tingling, which was formerly localised in the distal segments of the extremities, was now felt around the thorax and at the base of the neck. The patient also complained of a painful constriction round the chest ; and, on examining the chest, it was found that breathing was carried on by an elevation movement, whilst the movement of lateral expansion was lost. The epigastrium fell in slightly during inspiration, and was protruded during expiration. The patient's speech was somewhat broken, and his cough was wanting in energy.

25th June.—The muscles of both lower and upper extremities were almost completely paralysed, and the patient was unable to maintain a sitting posture without support. The abdominal muscles still contracted feebly, the intercostal muscles were paralysed, and the diaphragm was now manifestly implicated ; respiration being carried on chiefly by the action of the cervical muscles. Respiration was frequent, and there was marked dyspnœa ; the voice was broken and feeble, and the cough had so little energy that expectoration was almost impossible. The masticatory muscles were feeble, the tongue could hardly be protruded, and articulation was thick ; but the muscles of the face and eyeballs were not appreciably affected, although the patient complained of tingling and stiffness of the cheek. The paralysed muscles and nerves still reacted readily to the electrical (faradic) current. The reflex reactions were completely lost, but there was no retraction of the tendons, no contracture, and no convulsions. The sense of pain and of temperature, and the electrical sensibility were not affected ; but the muscular sense was lost in the feet and toes, and tactile sensibility was diminished in the distal segments of the limbs, and completely lost over the tips of the fingers. The patient complained of a feeling of torpidity and numbness in the limbs, which he compared to the effect of severe cold ; and he also stated that his limbs were always very cold. The limbs felt likewise cold to objective examination, and the feet felt to the observer's hand at a cadaveric temperature. The patient died suddenly in the afternoon as he was being propped up, by his own desire, to have some food.

Autopsy.—The results were chiefly negative. Strong adhesions were found between the visceral and costal pleuræ on both sides, and portions of the lungs were abnormally airless and friable ; but there were no tubercules. The most careful microscopic examination of the spinal cord by Bourguignon, Gubler, Robin, and Landry failed to detect any evidence of morbid change, either in the gray or white substance of the spinal cord. The nerve trunks were not examined.

In this case, then, the cutaneous sensibility of the extremities was considerably affected ; and Landry, in his description of the disease based on an analysis of ten cases, while admitting that generally "les troubles fonctionnels portent surtout sur le mouvement et sont alors caractérisés par la diminution graduelle de la force musculaire," also states that "la sensibilité et la mobilité peuvent être également compromises."

Now, as already pointed out, many recent writers, in their discussions of the nature of this disease, exclude cases in which sensory symptoms are conspicuous features ; for example, Bailey and Ewing, in an important paper, criticise the views of Nauwerck and Barth and Ross, who include such cases. But surely the latter authors are more correct than the former ; for if Landry's paralysis means anything, it means the disease originally described by Landry ; and although many cases of purely motor paralysis, presenting in other respects a clinical history similar to that described by Landry, may prove to have the same pathology, it is impossible to exclude from a description of the disease cases which fulfil the requirements of Landry himself.

With these considerations in mind I submit the following definition of the disease : Landry's paralysis is a disease which, ushered in usually by sensory symptoms, is characterised by a rapid advance of motor paralysis. This, as a rule, begins in the lower limbs, spreads rapidly to the muscles of the upper limbs and trunk, often invades the muscles of the face, tongue, palate, larynx, or eyeballs, and frequently proves fatal in a short time by respiratory paralysis. Sometimes, however, improvement begins and progresses gradually to partial or complete recovery. The cutaneous sensibility is nearly always affected, but not often in a profound degree. The bladder and rectum are but rarely implicated. After death no constant changes are found in the nervous system.

Causes.—The disease affects men about three times oftener than women. It occurs chiefly between the ages of twenty and forty years ; but it has been observed in children, and in elderly people. Severe exposure to cold has sometimes been the most noteworthy antecedent, but in about two-thirds of the reported cases the poisons known to lead to peripheral neuritis appear to have been the probable causes. Thus it has followed excesses in alcohol ; it has come on during convalescence from some general disease, as small-pox, typhoid, influenza, measles, diphtheria ; or has occurred in connection with the puerperal state, syphilis, septicæmia, or phthisis. In a few cases no distinct cause could be ascertained.

Symptoms.—*The period of invasion.*—The course of evolution in Landry's disease varies in different cases. In some cases the onset of paralysis is quite abrupt; in others it is preceded and ushered in by certain premonitory symptoms which have existed for periods of time varying from a few hours to several weeks. The most frequent premonitory or initial symptoms are sensory in character, and consist of numbness, tingling, formications, and other paræsthesiæ which mainly affect the fingers and toes and the peripheral parts of the limbs. Pains of various kinds may also be present; thus there may be diffuse aching of a limb, or of the back; or acute pains shooting along the course of some of the chief nerves, or localised to one nerve, as the sciatic. Attacks of gastralgia or diarrhœa have also been noticed. The muscular masses of the limbs, especially the calves, may be painful and tender; and pain may be readily produced by any active or passive movement of the body. Occasionally anæsthesia of the extremities precedes the paralysis. In other cases feelings associated with muscular weakness have been present; such as langour, heaviness of the limbs, and fatigue after slight exertion. Fidgets, restlessness, stiffness of the muscles of the limbs, back, or neck, general malaise and loss of appetite have also been observed in different cases. Occasionally the premonitory symptoms have been motor in character; weakness of the legs being present for a few weeks before the rapid advance of ascending paralysis. Vaso-motor and secretory disorders have also been observed during the initial stage; such as dead, cold, or livid extremities, or clammy sweating of the palms and soles. It is probable that the premonitory stage tends to be longer when the disease is set up by the action of a definite poison like alcohol, or that producing diphtheria or septicæmia, than when it occurs in persons who have not been exposed to the action of any well-known toxic agent.

The period of paralysis.—The sensory symptoms of the premonitory stage may persist. Sometimes the cutaneous sensibility is distinctly blunted; and, although a firm touch is recognised, a slight stroke with the finger is not perceived, nor can distinction be made between the head and point of a pin. In some cases marked anæsthesia has been observed, painful impressions being as a rule more impaired than tactile.

In the majority of cases of Landry's paralysis sensory symptoms are not conspicuous features; but, judging from an analysis of reported cases, and from one case seen in consultation in which I found the cutaneous sensibility—thought to be normal—distinctly impaired, and from my experience of cases of multiple neuritis from alcohol and other causes, I believe that slight impairment of cutaneous sensibility is frequently overlooked. The investigator must not be content with pricking and touching the skin, but he must test its sensibility to hot and cold objects, and to the faradic current. Still more is it necessary to insist on the importance of comparing corresponding parts of the limbs with one another; for it is a common experience to find that sensation has been pronounced normal when a pin prick, for example, although recognised on both sides, is much less perceptible on one limb than on its fellow.

Cutaneous and muscular hyperæsthesia and tenderness on pressing over the nerve trunks have also been observed in several cases. In a typical case of Landry's paralysis, described by Albu, in which a microscopical examination of the nerves and cord gave negative results, there was intense tenderness of the whole body. In a case recorded by Curschman, and in one recorded by Giuzetti, there were pain and tenderness over the vertebral spines. These symptoms, in the last case, were apparently explained after death by the presence of degeneration in the spinal roots.

Disorders of sensation, however, although usually present in some degree, are completely overshadowed in intensity by the motor paralysis which dominates the disease. Generally indeed, the first striking symptom is weakness of the lower limbs, one limb being often affected before the other. The weakness increases, and the power of walking or standing without support is quickly lost. When lying down the patient may still be able to move the toes or feebly to flex the ankle and knee; but in a few days, or even a few hours, every trace of motor power in the lower extremities may be abolished; they then lie flaccid and powerless, and the feet and toes assume the dropped position imposed upon them by the action of gravity and by the pressure of the bed-clothes.

Soon after the onset of weakness in the legs, or even simultaneously with this, the arms become attacked. At first the finer movements of the fingers and thumb are enfeebled; then the grosser movements of the wrist, elbow, and shoulder, until in a short time the upper limbs may become as completely paralysed as the lower. The muscles of the pelvis, loins, and abdomen are now invaded. The power of sitting up is soon lost; while, owing to the weakness of the abdominal muscles, the acts of coughing, sneezing, and defæcation become weak and ineffective. In many cases, too, the muscles which move the head are attacked; thus the power of rotating the head or of raising it from the pillow may be lost.

Probably in about half the cases of Landry's paralysis the muscles supplied by the cranial motor nerves are implicated; the muscles which preside over the movements of swallowing and speech are those most commonly affected. Difficulties in swallowing may depend on paralysis of the soft palate, or on paralysis of the epiglottis; in the former case fluids regurgitate through the nose, in the latter case food is apt to enter the larynx. When there is a great or a complete inability to swallow, which sometimes occurs, it may be assumed that the pharynx and upper part of the œsophagus are paralysed; then the patient has to be fed through a tube.

Indistinct, or nasal, speech and other disorders of articulation have been described, and depend in different cases on paresis of the tongue, lips, and soft palate. Sometimes phonation is affected, the voice being hoarse, feeble, falsetto, or completely lost. A feeble voice may depend on commencing paralysis of the muscles of respiration; but qualitative

changes in phonation or complete aphonia have been found in a few cases
to depend on paralysis of some of the laryngeal muscles.

In several cases facial paralysis, unilateral or bilateral, has been
observed; more rarely paralysis of the masseters. Occasionally evidence
of paralysis of the ocular muscles has been present; for example, ptosis,
external strabismus, inequality of the pupils, and impaired reaction of the
pupils to light and accommodation.

Further progress of the disease is usually indicated by implication
of the muscles of respiration. As a rule, the diaphragm is attacked before
the intercostal muscles; when the latter are paralysed, breathing is carried
on partially or entirely by the extraordinary muscles of respiration.
Soon those, too, fail and the patient after a short struggle dies from
asphyxia. During the progress of respiratory paralysis there is not, as a
rule, much obvious dyspnœa; the rate of breathing may be moderately
accelerated, but violent respiratory struggles are usually absent.

The nutrition, tone, and electrical reactions of the paralysed muscles.—It
is persistently stated in books that the muscles neither undergo active
atrophy nor present changes in their electrical irritability. This is doubtless true as regards acute cases which end fatally in a few days; then
the characteristic feature is early flaccidity of the limb muscles, and there
is no recognisable atrophy. But the statement is untrue when applied
to cases which end in recovery, or in which life is prolonged for a few
weeks or months. The evidence bearing on this inquiry was ably
analysed by the late Dr. Ross, and need not be further discussed here;
for he clearly showed that many cases have been reported, which, in the
early stages, were clinically indistinguishable from cases of rapidly fatal
ascending paralysis, in which, when convalescence was protracted, some
of the muscles became atrophied and gave the partial or complete reactions
of degeneration to electrical tests. In these cases the limbs, owing to
the wasting of some of their muscles, presented distortions, such as the
"main en griffe" and double ankle drop; as in other cases of chronic
muscular atrophy.

Reflexes.—The knee-jerks are quickly lost, and in the fatal cases are
lost till death. When recovery takes place the knee-jerks may slowly
return; but not, as a rule, until all traces of paralysis have disappeared.
The same remarks apply to the wrist and elbow jerks. Probably the
plantar and the other superficial reflexes are also lost, but information on
this point is incomplete.[1]

The bladder and rectum.—Retention of urine and obstinate constipation
occasionally occur, and are probably due mainly to weakness of expulsive
efforts, owing to paralysis of the abdominal muscles and the diaphragm.

---

[1] In two patients at least under my own care such was the case. In the later of the
two, a typical case in a young lady aged 20, seen in 1898 with Dr. Holden of Sudbury,
although trunk and limbs were completely paralysed, there was no trace of sensory disturbance, subjective or objective; touch, pain, and temperature were quickly and truly perceived;
for instance, on tickling the soles of the feet, although there was no reflex, she laughed and
exclaimed at once. The respiratory muscles were threatened in the first week, but on my
visit, ten weeks later, the functions of organic life were normally performed.—ED.

In a few cases paralysis of the sphincters has occurred, giving rise to incontinence of fæces and urine; but generally the latter is the incontinence of an over-distended bladder.

Other symptoms.—It is quite exceptional for the disease to be ushered in or accompanied by fever. Towards the end of life, however, the temperature is often raised and the pulse quickened. Profuse sweating, albuminuria, and enlarged spleen are phenomena that have been observed occasionally. Psychical disorders are rarely present, and the patient who cannot move a limb, and can scarcely express himself by speech, may give evidence that his mental functions are unimpaired. In this respect Landry's paralysis presents a marked contrast to alcoholic multiple neuritis.

Course, duration and termination.—The usual course followed by Landry's disease cannot be better summarised than in the words of the discoverer. He says the first phenomena always manifest themselves at the extremities of the limbs, and most frequently at the extremities of the lower limbs. The paralysis pursues an ascending course, and attacks the muscles in an almost constant order; namely, in the first place, the muscles which move the toes and feet, then the posterior muscles of the thigh and pelvis, and, lastly, the anterior and internal muscles of the thigh; in the second place, the muscles moving the fingers, the hand, the arm upon the scapula, and, lastly, the forearm upon the arm; thirdly, the muscles of the trunk; fourthly, the muscles of respiration, and finally, those of the tongue, pharynx, and œsophagus.

As pointed out by Dr. Ross, the term "ascending" was used by Landry, in the sense of "centripetal," to indicate that the paralysis first attacked the distal segments of the limbs, then gradually ascended to the proximal segments, and finally invaded the muscles of the trunk. Sometimes the arms are attacked before the legs; sometimes they are attacked simultaneously; and a few cases have been recorded in which the muscles supplied by the bulbar nerves were paralysed as soon as those of the upper extremities, or even before them—the muscles of the lower limbs being the last to be implicated. But in whatsoever order the muscles become paralysed there appears to be no justification for the use of "ascending" in the anatomical sense implied by some writers, who state that the order in which the muscles are attacked corresponds to the order in which they are innervated by the spinal cord; or, in other words, that the disease begins in the lumbar portion of the cord, and pursues an upward or ascending course till it reaches the bulbar nuclei.

The rate of progress and the duration of the disorder vary greatly in different cases. An analysis of the records of a large number of fatal cases shows that in about 60 per cent death occurred before the tenth day, and in about 40 per cent either at the end of the second or during the third or fourth week. Occasionally the disease pursues a very rapid course and ends fatally in forty-eight hours; but the most common time for death to occur is at the end of the first week.

The mode of death is nearly always by asphyxia in consequence of respiratory paralysis—the diaphragm being usually attacked before the intercostal muscles; sometimes, however, the latter become paralysed as soon as the former.

There can be no doubt that cases presenting symptoms identical with those of the fatal cases do occasionally end in recovery. Thus paralysis may rapidly invade the muscles of the limbs until they become absolutely powerless, and then cease to spread; and after a varying interval power is slowly regained, the muscles last attacked being the first to recover. A patient may indeed lie completely powerless, with marked symptoms of respiratory paralysis, and yet make a complete recovery. The paralysis may cease to advance at any stage of its progress.

The length of the stage of convalescence varies from a few weeks to several months; and must obviously depend upon the degree of morbid change which has taken place in the nervous system and muscles.

Pathology.—It has already been pointed out that the condition of the nervous system, in cases reported under the heading Acute ascending or Landry's paralysis, is very inconstant even when the symptoms during life have been almost identical. In one set of cases no changes were found, even when the cord and nerves had been submitted to a thorough microscopical examination. The case already referred to, reported by Albu, is a good example: the nerves and cord were quite normal, and a bacteriological examination gave negative results. In another set of cases distinct changes have been found in the spinal cord: sometimes these are widespread, in the sense that they are not limited to any one histological element of the cord, and are often similar to those met with in acute myelitis.

Thus Oetlinger and Marinesco report the following case:—

A man, aged 20, during an attack of variola had retention of urine, marked flaccid paresis of the lower limbs, absent knee-jerks, and diminution of the cutaneous sensibility. Two days later the upper limbs and the respiratory muscles became paralysed, and death ensued on the fourth day. Necropsy:—The dorso-lumbar cord was soft and there were capillary hæmorrhages. The changes in the cord followed the distribution of the vessels; the vessel walls were thickened, and were filled with leucocytes containing basophilic granules; in some vessels thrombi were found. Cocci were found in a few of the ganglion cells, and in many of the circumvascular spaces and in the leucocytes; they were also present in the central canal.

The nerve cells showed degenerative changes. The lesion was most marked in the gray matter, and was most severe in the dorso-lumbar region of the cord; though it was also present in the cervical region and in the medulla and pons. The nerves to the lower limbs were quite normal. The kidneys were congested and the spleen presented recent infarcts.

The authors attribute Landry's paralysis to the action of microbes or their soluble products in the nervous system, that the microbes are several, and, thus, the forms of the disease several; the cord being affected in one case, the nerves in another, and both in a third case.

Sometimes the changes are limited to the anterior horns, and are similar to those found in the early stage of acute anterior poliomyelitis; as in a case recorded by Bailey and Ewing. The authors found acute poliomyelitis of the cord and medulla; vascular and exudative changes in the motor cortex, basal ganglia, and cerebellum; degeneration of ganglion cells and slight vascular changes in the nerve roots. The cells of the anterior horns, when stained by Nissl's method, showed partial or complete absence of the chromophilic masses which, in a healthy ganglion cell, are grouped concentrically about the nucleus, are arranged in rows along the cell borders, and are prolonged as slender rods into the dendrites. The peripheral nerves were not examined.

In a third series of cases changes have been found in the peripheral nerves only. Eisenlohr reports such a case; he found degenerated fibres in the right hypoglossal and right phrenic nerves, in the anterior roots of the cervical nerves, and in other peripheral nerves. The spinal cord was normal. The spleen was much enlarged. A thorough bacteriological examination of the cord, nerves, blood and spleen was completely negative. Finally, in a fourth series of cases morbid changes were found both in the central and peripheral parts of the nervous system; examples of which are recorded by Giuzetti and Ballet. Kruger believes Landry's disease to be the terminal phase of a chronic multiple neuritis, which has spread by direct continuity to the cord—the disease in the cord spreading very quickly to the bulbar nuclei.

C. The Atrophic variety.—The proportion between muscular atrophy and paralysis presents considerable variations in different cases of multiple neuritis. As a rule paralysis occurs first, and is succeeded by muscular atrophy, which then progresses side by side with the paralysis. In some cases paralysis is predominant, in others muscular atrophy; and the latter may progress to an extreme degree. There are indeed certain groups of cases in which wasting of muscular tissue is a primary feature, and appears sufficient to account for the degree of weakness present; and in many of them there is good evidence that the disease is a chronic form of peripheral neuritis.

Two groups may be briefly considered :—

(i.) *Localised forms of muscular atrophy as illustrated by the Aran-Duchenne type.*—This form is characterised by paralysis and atrophy of the small muscles of the hands; namely, the interosseous muscles and the thenar and hypothenar eminences. Atrophy is the conspicuous feature, and accompanies rather than succeeds the loss of power. The type is named from the close resemblance the condition and attitude of the hands bear to the type of progressive muscular atrophy described by Aran and Duchenne, which is known to depend on degeneration of the ganglion cells of the anterior horns. One of its commonest causes is lead poisoning, of which it may be the sole manifestation ; but as a rule it complicates the common or wrist-drop type of paralysis. In one case of this kind, reported by Madame Déjerine-Klumpke, the spinal cord was found quite healthy, but extensive changes were found in the nerves of the brachial plexus and their terminal branches.

Another cause is over-fatigue of the hand muscles from some occupation, such as sewing. A patient, now under my own care, besides marked atrophy of the intrinsic muscles of the hands, has weakness and wasting of the flexors of the left wrist and fingers. The condition began a few years ago with "prickling pains" and a feeling of numbness in the fingers, ball of the thumb, and palm of the left hand. A year later she began to suffer from the same sensations in the right hand; and she soon became unable to follow her occupation of tailoring. There is tenderness to pressure over some of the affected muscles, and a slight impairment of the cutaneous sensibility of the fingers and thumb.

I have seen other cases of this kind in which no cause could be discovered. The occupation did not involve fatigue of the hands, and there was no evidence that the muscular atrophy was due to lead, alcohol, or other poison.

(ii.) *Generalised forms of muscular atrophy* occasionally come under observation, in which the association of pains and other sensory disorders with paralysis in the early stages of the disease suggests that they have been caused by disease in the course of the nerve trunks and their peripheral branches. Rheumatism has sometimes been the most noticeable antecedent. One variety of extensive muscular atrophy must be especially noticed; namely, the peroneal type of family amyotrophy, as described by Dr. Tooth: or, as it is sometimes called, the Charcot-Marie form of amyotrophy. This form usually begins in the second half of childhood, and may affect several members of the same family. It has sometimes followed an acute specific disease, especially measles. The muscles of the feet and legs are first attacked; then, after an interval of some years, those of the hands and forearms. The muscles of the thighs and arms may be affected at a later period; but the atrophy is always most extreme at the periphery, and progressively diminishes towards the proximal portions of the limbs. It is symmetrically distributed. Slight fibrillation of the affected muscles may be observed. The tendon reactions are feeble or abolished. The reaction of degeneration is often present. The patient sometimes suffers from pains and cramps in the limbs; and the cutaneous sensibility, though often normal, may be impaired or lost over the distal portions of the limbs.

The nature of the disease cannot yet be fully explained; but the most constant lesions found are those of the peripheral nerves and the posterior columns of the cord. The lesion of the nerves consists in a marked change of the nerve fibres with proliferation of the intra- and peri-fascicular connective tissue. The lesion of the posterior columns is very similar to that of tabes. Between this peroneal type of muscular atrophy and the idiopathic or myopathic type, as it is called, there are many transitional forms; and it is impossible to separate those of neuritic from those of purely muscular origin, or to say how far the muscular atrophy and the nerve disease are caused by a virus in the blood, or are dependent on a congenital tendency to early slow degeneration. Myopathic atrophy is described elsewhere, and is only mentioned here because there can scarcely be a doubt that some of its forms are associated with disease of the peripheral branches of motor nerves, if not directly dependent on it. Before leaving the subject, however, it is desirable to mention a condition described by Déjerine and Sottas, which they call Progressive hypertrophic interstitial neuritis of infancy. The disease runs a slow and progressive course, and is characterised by the following symptoms :—Ataxy of the four limbs with muscular atrophy ; lightning pains and very marked disturbances of sensation with delay in its transmission ; nystagmus ; myosis and the Argyll-Robertson phenomenon ; kypho-scoliosis ; marked hypertrophy and hardness of all the nerve trunks of the limbs accessible to palpation. A necropsy in one case revealed very pronounced hypertrophic sclerosis of the limb nerves, and of the anterior and posterior roots of the spinal cord ; as well as a sclerosis of the posterior columns presenting the same distribution as in locomotor ataxy.

III. THE SENSORY TYPE

Under this heading I refer to cases in which sensory symptoms, symmetrically distributed to the extremities of the limbs, are the conspicuous features. The symmetry, the association with motor defects, and frequently also with impairment of the knee-jerks, together with the fact that complete recovery is the usual result, strongly suggest that the symptoms depend on an abnormal condition of the peripheral nerves. Such cases may be broadly divided into two classes, according to the association of weakness or of inco-ordination of movement with the sensory phenomena.

Class A.—*Sensory symptoms are prominent, motor weakness is inconstant or inconspicuous.*—The slighter degrees of multiple neuritis are represented sometimes by motor defects, such as spasm or weakness of some of the special movements of the fingers and thumb, but far more commonly by various sensory disturbances. Patients often consult a physician for numbness and tingling in the fingers and toes ; very often these sensations are worse at night, and may be severe enough to keep the patient awake. Sometimes they are associated with severe cramps in the extremities. On examination the cutaneous sensibility may be normal; but, when carefully investigated, it is often found impaired or lost over the tips of the fingers, or at the sides of the hands. Frequently, too, the first dorsal interosseous muscle is tender ; and in many cases, especially those of alcoholic origin, there is much hyperæsthesia of a considerable number of muscles. The knee-jerks are increased, diminished, or lost. The above symptoms may be the only ones present ; or they may be accompanied by slight weakness of the movements of the digits, or even of those of the hands and feet.

When cases of slight neuritis can be traced to an obvious poison, as that of alcohol or rheumatism, and this is removed or destroyed, then a complete recovery is the rule; but often no cause can be discovered, and then the symptoms, although they do not increase in severity, tend to persist; or they improve for a time and then relapse.

Dyspepsia is a common antecedent. One patient told me that, after her meals she suffered from numbness and tingling in the fingers and elbows, and from pain down the middle of the forearm; the finger-ends also became quite cold, and the left arm red in colour.

Diabetes, which rarely produces obvious multiple neuritis, often leads to symptoms of slight neuritis; such as neuralgic pains in the legs, cramps, numbness and tingling, hyperæsthesia, and absence of knee-jerks. Paralysis, however, is of rare occurrence.

I have already given a full description of the marked sensory phenomena of alcoholic neuritis which characterise the early stages of the disease, and have now to add that sometimes they are the only symptoms, even when alcohol has been taken in large quantities for a long time. The patient suffers from severe darting pains in the limbs, or aching pains in the joints; and the case may be mistaken for one of rheumatism. The soles of the feet are so tender that to walk is agonising: their cutaneous sensibility, nevertheless, may be much diminished, the condition *anæsthesia dolorosa* being present. Muscular hyperæsthesia is extreme. There is no paralysis and no ataxy of movement. The cutaneous reflexes, and often too the knee-jerks, are much increased. Great emaciation is common, partly as a result of prolonged gastric disturbance and insomnia, but partly also as a direct result of pain. The patient's weakness, pallor, and emaciation render him particularly liable to pulmonary tuberculosis.

Gouty subjects often suffer from numbness and "tingling pains" in the finger tips; and in persons who inherit a strong tendency to gout these symptoms appear to be easily excited by small quantities of alcohol. Thus Dr. Ross knew a gentleman, of gouty parentage, who experienced numbness in the finger tips after taking a single glass of beer; and if he persisted in taking beer to dinner for a few days, his finger nails became dry, and cracked longitudinally. This susceptibility to certain alcoholic drinks makes it difficult to decide how far symptoms indicative of a peripheral neuritis, occurring in a gouty subject, are to be attributed to alcohol or to gout. The difficulty is illustrated by an interesting series of cases described by Dr. Buzzard, in which symptoms suggestive of slight neuritis were present, and appeared to depend on gout; but, as many of the patients partook pretty freely of alcohol, its direct influence could not be absolutely excluded.

The symptoms presented by Dr. Buzzard's cases were: numbness and tingling in the fingers; acute pains radiating along a limb, often especially severe in the thumb or in one finger; cutaneous hyperæsthesia. Dr. Buzzard mentions one place in particular where exquisite pain was felt on pressure. "It lies just inside the inner and upper angle of the scapula, and the pain caused by the pressure there seems to travel down to the hand. Apparently there is neuritis of the posterior branch of a spinal nerve, the anterior branch of which enters into the formation of the brachial plexus." These sensory phenomena are soon followed by muscular weakness and atrophy, sometimes affecting the greater portion of a limb, but as a rule limited to certain parts—such as the intrinsic muscles of the thumb, or some of the forearm muscles.

Mr. Hutchinson has drawn attention to the occurrence of attacks of neuro-retinitis in gouty subjects : in one of his cases the third cranial nerve was implicated ; in another case, the left facial nerve ; while another member of a gouty family suffered from neuritis of the brachial plexus.

A patient, under the care of Drs. Ross and Mules, an old gentleman who was the subject of chronic gout in both feet, had almost lost the power of walking. All the muscles of the lower extremities were the subjects of fibrillary contractions ; these being found more especially in the extremities of the thighs and legs. These muscles showed also manifest signs of wasting, and the patellar tendon reactions were lost. Under massage the patient gained an inch in the circumference of the calves, and an inch and a half in that of the thighs ; and the fibrillary contractions disappeared. The joints of the feet were anchylosed, but the patient regained his power of walking in great degree, although the gait remained awkward.

The neuritis of leprosy is also largely sensory (vol. ii. p. 58). Cases have been published, by Chauffard and others, in which the alterations of cutaneous sensibility, so characteristic of syringomyelia, have been observed, namely, loss of sensation to pain and temperature associated with preservation of the tactile sensibility. The connection between leprosy and syringomyelia and Morvan's disease appears in some respects to be a close one ; indeed some authorities, as Zambaco, believe syringomyelia to be a variety of leprosy.

Class B.—Sensory symptoms are associated with muscular inco-ordination.

Neuro-tabes peripherica.—Under this heading two groups of cases require discussion :—

(*a*) Cases of ataxy in which the main lesion is disease of the posterior columns of the spinal cord—that is, ordinary tabes dorsalis—but in which changes are found in the peripheral nerves also.

(*b*) Cases of ataxy in which the main or only lesion is disease of the peripheral nerves.

It is now well established, from the researches of Westphal, Pierret, Pitres and Vaillard, Oppenheim and Siemerling, Déjerine, and others, that disease of the peripheral nerves, both cranial and spinal, is very frequently found in association with disease of the posterior columns in ordinary cases of locomotor ataxy. Déjerine has shown that in many cases there is a close correspondence between the distribution of anæsthesia and that of changes in the peripheral nerves ; and it is highly probable also that the trophic lesions of the skin, bones, and joints depend on the process of degeneration in the peripheral nerves (*vide* p. 563). How far then is the incoordination in any given case due to central or to peripheral lesions?

The independence of these lesions is shown by the combination of symmetrical cord lesions with unilateral neuritis; and by the absence of any relation between the gravity of nerve lesions and the duration, extent, or gravity of cord lesions. Thus, as Oppenheim demonstrated, considerable changes may be met with in the peripheral nerves at the onset of tabes when cord lesions are limited; and, conversely, the peripheral nerves may be intact when sclerosis of the posterior columns, of considerable extent, has existed for a long time. The latter point is substantiated by abundant evidence; and there cannot be a reasonable doubt that, in many cases, ataxy occurs as a direct consequence of disease of the posterior root zones.

We may now consider group (*b*), and ask whether genuine ataxy ever occurs from lesions of the peripheral nerves alone; other parts of the nervous system being healthy. At first sight such a question appears to be superfluous, because numbers of cases of ataxy in connection with peripheral neuritis have been reported; but it is to be noted that in many of them the evidence of ataxy is not conclusive; and it is beyond question that the high stepping gait of multiple neuritis has often been ascribed to ataxy when it was really due to paralysis of certain muscles of the legs.

A little consideration of the subject suggests either that many of the published observations are inaccurate, or that there is sometimes a real difficulty in discriminating between abnormal movements which are the result of incoordination and those which depend on muscular weakness. To assign definite limits to the use of the term ataxy is not indeed so easy a matter as might at first sight appear. Accurate adjustment of muscular action is necessarily impaired by weakness or by spasm of any muscle employed in a particular movement; but such imperfections of movement are not all to be included under the term "ataxy." Ataxy, or incoordination, implies errors in the balance of the contractions and relaxations of the groups of muscles required for a given movement, apart from alterations in their strength; and although paralysis or spasm may be found in association with ataxy, the latter, as in tabes dorsalis, frequently exists without the former. Nevertheless, there is sometimes a difficulty in deciding whether a defective movement be due to an alteration in the strength of certain muscles, or merely to a want of proportion between their respective actions. In some cases of "writer's cramp," for example, where there is no obvious weakness or spasm of any of the muscles used in writing, it may be difficult to give a mechanical explanation of the muscular irregularities displayed in the attempt to write; and the same remark applies to the motor defects sometimes met with in cases of multiple neuritis. The difficulty referred to, however, is found mainly in the minor defects of muscular action; for, as a rule, a careful examination will enable us to decide whether certain defects in the movement of a part be due to incoordination, or to paralysis. Also when the two conditions are combined—as, for example, in ataxic paraplegia—the incoordination of movement is still recognisable, unless paralysis be profound. Hence in the earlier stages of multiple neuritis, when the muscular weakness is moderate in degree, incoordination of movement should, if present, be detected readily.

In the following case of alcoholic multiple neuritis signs of ataxy were unmistakable :—

The patient was a woman, aged 37, with a strong history of drunkenness. The mental condition was characteristic, and the heart was dilated. Muscular hyperæsthesia was severe in both arms and legs. There was marked anæsthesia in the lower limbs, and partial anæsthesia in the hands and forearms. The sense of movement and position was very defective : thus when the toes or feet were moved she felt nothing ; she could tell, however, when the legs were raised from the bed, but was unable to say whether they were crossed or not. A weight of several pounds suspended from the foot or ankle was not felt ; and when weights were placed on the feet the patient was not aware of their presence. She could tell when a finger was moved, but could not say which finger ; she said she felt that something about her hand was moving, but could not tell anything more, nor did she feel anything when her wrist or elbow was moved ; but she could distinguish movements at the shoulder, and movements at the elbow were referred to the shoulder. The weight sense was lost in the hands as well as in the feet. The knee-jerks, the plantar reflexes, and in all probability the abdominal reflexes were quite absent. As regards motor power, the patient was able to move any part of the lower limbs ; but the movements were feeble, and the flexors of the ankles were especially weak ; she could partially extend the wrists and fingers, but only by the exercise of great effort, and the power of grasp was almost completely lost. While there was considerable muscular weakness there was not complete paralysis of any movement. The patient was unable to stand or walk without assistance ; when supported, her gait presented the most striking resemblance to that of tabes dorsalis ; the legs were jerked forcibly forwards, and the feet brought down with a stamp ; sometimes they became entangled, and were thrown hither and thither in the greatest disorder. It was particularly noticed that the anterior part of the advancing foot was raised ; the gait, in fact, was totally unlike the ordinary high-stepping one of alcoholic paralysis.

The patient was treated at first with salicylate of soda and iodide of potassium, subsequently with strychnine and massage ; in two months' time she was much better, and when I saw her again, eight months after the appearance of the first symptoms of neuritis, the movements of the limbs were almost quite natural, but the knee-jerks were still absent.

Similar cases have been reported by Déjerine, Leyden, Dreschfeld, and others, in which multiple neuritis was found on necropsy. Ataxic conditions have also been described in connection with diabetes in cases of lead and arsenic poisoning; and as following diphtheria, measles, and other acute diseases.

In most of the reported cases of ataxy occurring in connection with peripheral neuritis, other motor and sensory symptoms were present; and this is to be expected from the constitution of the mixed peripheral nerves. Does ataxy ever occur as the only symptom in cases of multiple neuritis? That this may happen when disease is limited to certain tracts in the spinal cord we know; are there fibres in the peripheral nerves which, when picked out by disease, give rise to incoordination of movement, and to this alone? It is impossible to give a complete answer to such a question at present, but we may remember that cases occur in which, while ataxy is pronounced, muscular weakness and sensory disorders are quite insignificant; and where complete recovery strongly suggests peripheral rather than central lesions. These conditions obtained in the following case of acute ataxy recorded by Leyden :—

A man, aged 55, after working in a cold room when his feet were sweating, felt creeping sensations in the legs and numbness in the feet. Five days later, after a hard day's work, these sensations returned, and for the first time his legs felt weak ; on the next day he could only walk with the help of a stick. He was then compelled to take to his bed. When lying down he was free from pain, and the abnormal sensations in the legs became less troublesome.

His condition on the eighth day from the onset of symptoms, when he came under Professor Leyden's care, was as follows :—

All the symptoms were limited to the lower extremities ; an examination of the cranial nerves, the upper extremities, and the thoracic and abdominal organs revealed nothing abnormal. The motor power of the lower limbs was not impaired ; the patient could perform all the movements at the different joints perfectly well, and he offered strong resistance to passive movements. All the movements of the lower limbs presented marked ataxy ; with closed eyes he was unable to touch the knee of one limb with the heel of the other. He was unable to stand, and when supported his gait was distinctly ataxic ; Romberg's phenomenon was also present. Tactile sensibility was but slightly impaired, yet painful sensations were severely felt ; and he complained of numbness and creeping sensations in the extremities. The knee-jerks were abolished ; the cremasteric reflex could not be obtained on the left side, and was diminished on the right side. He was unable to pass urine ; when withdrawn by a catheter it was found to be alkaline, but did not contain albumin or sugar.

A week later urine was passed spontaneously, but only in small quantities at a time ; the patient could walk better, but ataxia was still conspicuous, and he complained of darting pains in the feet. Subsequently improvement went on rapidly ; in a month from the onset of the first symptom the knee-jerks had returned, the functions of the bladder were normally performed, and, with the exception of slight unsteadiness in walking, the patient was almost quite well. The most important antecedent was syphilis, from which the patient had suffered in early life ; but Leyden is inclined to attribute the symptoms to a peripheral neuritis, which had been started by exposure to damp and cold.

Obviously there is a difficulty in locating the lesion in some cases of ataxy. Rapid loss of the knee-jerks and of the muscular sense, in association with sensory disturbance and motor weakness, speak for a peripheral rather than a central lesion ; but duration appears to be the only certain test, and speedy recovery may be regarded as strongly in favour of peripheral neuritis. It is highly probable, then, from the clinical and pathological evidence adduced, that cases of ataxy, presenting no striking difference from ordinary tabes dorsalis, may result from disease of the distal parts of the spinal nerves, especially of the nerve fibres which occur so abundantly in the "muscle spindles"; while the well-known case, reported by Hughes Bennett, in which the posterior spinal roots were involved in a series of isolated sarcomatous tumours, suggests that disease limited to the proximal ends of sensory nerves may also produce ataxy. In this case it is unfortunate that the cutaneous and muscular nerve endings escaped examination :.but it is clear, as Dr. Bennett points out, that the primary disease did not originate there ; and it seems fair to regard the case as an important pathological link between the classical lesion in the posterior root zones and the cases of "nervo-tabes périphérique,' described by Déjerine.

A study of the relation of ataxy to peripheral neuritis brings out two points: —

1. That ataxy is a rare symptom in cases of multiple peripheral neuritis, even when cutaneous and muscular sensibility are profoundly affected.

2. That it occurs occasionally when signs of muscular weakness and of diminished cutaneous sensibility are slight or absent.

It is probable that the presence of ataxy in cases of multiple neuritis points to disease of sensory muscle nerves and their end organs, the "muscle spindles" (which, as shown by Batten, are diseased in cases of tabes). But it is very remarkable that extreme degeneration of terminal nerve fibres to both skin and muscle has been found in cases which presented no signs of incoordination during life. It is highly important in all cases of multiple neuritis which come to post-mortem examination, that the results of histological investigation of the condition of the "muscle spindles," and of nerve fibres to both muscle and skin, should be carefully studied in relation to any indications of ataxy exhibited during life.

IV. THE VASO-MOTOR TYPE

In the study of symptomatology we are constantly impressed with the absence of boundary lines between different diseases ; we notice that, while cases which closely approximate to the type stand out clearly from one another, there are numerous transitional or aberrant forms, the diagnosis of some of which is difficult, or may be impossible. These observations are well illustrated by the various groups of symptoms met with in peripheral neuritis. Thus, in the preceding sections, we have noticed cases in which muscular spasm, or motor paralysis, or ataxy was the chief or only evidence of neuritis. Cases grouped under the heading "Landry's paralysis" are particularly striking in this respect, and teach us how closely the symptoms of disease of nerve cells may simulate those of disease of their fibres.

If now we pass to the subject of vaso-motor symptoms in the limbs, we find that here also a gradual transition may be traced between the group of symptoms which belong to typical cases of multiple neuritis and the group of vaso-motor phenomena which belong to Raynaud's disease (p. 577). This condition is characterised by the presence of skin lesions, which are either temporary or permanent.

Three stages or forms of the disease may be distinguished : (i.) The stage of local syncope, in which there is a paroxysmal condition of pallor of the extremities; (ii.) the stage of local asphyxia, in which there is a paroxysmal condition of blueness of the extremities; (iii.) the stage of local gangrene.

The pallor, the lividity, and the gangrene are usually symmetrical in distribution ; but by no means invariably so. They may affect the fingers, the toes, the tips of the ears, or nose. In the simplest cases there is a series of attacks of local syncope or local cyanosis, in which the affected parts become cold, and present either a dead white or a livid appearance; their sensibility is blunted and their motive power diminished, and they are frequently the seat of severe pains resembling those of frost-bite. These colour changes are excited by very slight variations in the surrounding temperature, and tend to become "marked and prolonged out of all proportion to the stimulus" which starts them.

In severe cases the condition of local syncope, or more commonly that of local cyanosis, is succeeded by spontaneous gangrene. This is generally of the dry variety; and in a large number of cases is remarkable for its limited and superficial distribution.

Now in alcoholic paralysis, as we have seen, the fingers and toes may become cold, dead, and white or livid ; while in severe cases the extremities may become gangrenous : indeed, in a few rare cases, as in Dr. Ross's case (see p. 682), the three stages of Raynaud's disease have been observed.

The following is a brief abstract of a remarkable instance of gangrene occurring in a case of peripheral neuritis which was recently under my own care in the Manchester Royal Infirmary :—

A man, æt. 34, began, in February 1897, to suffer from dragging pains in the calf of the right leg, and subsequently from pains in the left leg. These pains continued for four or five months, and were followed by weakness of the leg. The patient, however, was able to walk until June, although he became soon tired. He took to his bed on 22nd June. At this time his knee-jerks were said to be exaggerated, and his speech, power of swallowing, and eyesight were affected to a slight degree. No satisfactory evidence of the cause of the disease could be obtained. He was admitted to the infirmary at the end of

September, and in spite of careful treatment he gradually got worse, and died at the end of January 1898.

The following is a summary of his symptoms up to December : Complete paralysis and atrophy of the muscles of the lower limbs ; partial paralysis of the upper limbs. The neck and shoulder muscles not implicated, but all the muscles of the arms, forearm, and hands weak and wasted—the extensors of the wrists and fingers, and the right supinator longus, being the most affected. Cutaneous sensibility of the hands slightly impaired, that of the lower limbs not at all. Moderate cutaneous and muscular hyperæsthesia in the lower limbs ; the small muscles of the hands tender when squeezed. Knee and wrist jerks abolished ; plantar reflexes not obtainable, but cremasteric and abdominal reflexes normal.

There was considerable œdema of the lower extremities, but none elsewhere. The œdema diminished when the limbs were raised, and the feet, livid when dependent, became white on lifting them up from the bed. The skin of the face, trunk, and limbs had a purplish appearance ; and the white streak of a scratch with the finger nail was slowly replaced by a dusky erythema, accompanied by slight swelling.

The bladder and rectum were unaffected, and the heart and other viscera showed no signs of disease. The memory and other mental functions appeared to be unimpaired. From the first there was some stomatitis of an ulcerative character, and the pharynx and epiglottis were congested. The left vocal cord was less curved, and moved much less freely than the right one. The voice became high pitched and falsetto. There was occasionally a difficulty in expectorating, but never any real difficulty in swallowing. Early in December the lividity of the feet began to increase, and at the end of the month the toes and distal portion of the left foot were gangrenous ; the three inner toes being quite black, cold, and shrivelled. On 19th January the right toes became slate coloured, and gangrene was well marked during the last week of life.

Dr. Williamson, who kindly undertook the histological examination, reports as follows :—"The spinal cord and the peripheral nerves were examined microscopically, and the case proved to be one of peripheral neuritis of the parenchymatous form. Degenerative changes were found in the anterior tibial nerve, in the musculo-spinal, and in the posterior interosseous nerves. The anterior tibial and the dorsalis pedis arteries were atheromatous, and a thrombus was found in the latter artery."

As a contrast to the above case may be mentioned one described by Rakhmaninoff :—

A youth, aged 17, was admitted to hospital suffering from gangrene of both feet and the lower parts of the legs. His illness dated from an attack of typhus two years previously. He became anæmic, and suffered from a feeling of coldness and numbness in the hands and feet. Lancinating pains in the limbs and trunk ensued ; he became liable to profuse sweats, and ultimately gangrene of the feet set in. A line of demarcation formed around the ankles, and it was deemed advisable to amputate the legs a little below the knees. The wounds healed quickly, but the patient became worse, and died of pleuropneumonia about sixteen days after the operation. Rakhmaninoff found signs of degenerative neuritis in the nerves of the upper, as well as in those of the lower limbs, and he regarded the neuritis as the main cause of the symmetrical gangrene. In the hypertrophic tissue around the nerve fasciculi he found vessels with thickened walls and narrowed or obliterated channels; but he was unable to decide whether these thickened vessels were to be regarded as secondary to the neuritis, or as primary and the direct cause of it.

In this case it is to be noted that, with the exception of pains, the ordinary symptoms of multiple neuritis were absent; and this has also been observed in other cases of symmetrical gangrene wherein degenerative neuritis was discovered after death. Peripheral neuritis has not, however, been found in all cases of Raynaud's disease, even after a careful histological examination; hence neuritis cannot be regarded as a constant or even an essential feature. Nevertheless the connection between the two conditions is a very close one; and in forming an opinion regarding the pathology of Raynaud's disease the following facts should be kept in mind :—

1. Degenerative neuritis has been histologically demonstrated (i.) in cases presenting well-marked motor and sensory symptoms of multiple neuritis in association with vaso-motor phenomena, succeeded or not by gangrene; (ii.) in cases presenting typical symptoms of Raynaud's disease either (a) when the ordinary symptoms of multiple neuritis were present, or (b) when these were absent, as in Rakhmaninoff's case.

2. Careful histological examinations have failed to reveal changes in the peripheral nerves taken from some cases of Raynaud's disease (vide vol. vii. p. 602).

These facts tend to indicate (a) that occasionally vaso-motor nerves may be picked out by disease, the symptoms resulting therefrom being identical with those of Raynaud's disease; (b) that the symptoms of Raynaud's disease do not always depend on lesions of the vaso-motor nerves, but in some cases may be related to a morbid condition of vaso-motor centres. In my treatise on "Peripheral Neuritis," after a full discussion of the subject now under consideration, I have stated my belief as follows : "At present it appears to me impossible to suggest a better hypothesis than that brought forward by Raynaud." His views will be set forth at length in a later article; briefly, however, he attributed the spasm of the capillary vessels to the morbid activity of vaso-motor centres in the brain and cord. I argued "that the peripheral neuritis, sometimes present, must be regarded as an epiphenomenon, either as the direct result of arterial disease, as suggested by Rakhmaninoff's case, or as a nerve degeneration due either to the imperfect supply of blood, or to changes in those central cells which preside over the nutrition of the peripheral nerve endings."

I am now inclined to regard these views as incomplete; I believe that they are applicable to many but not to all cases. In all probability the name Raynaud's disease, like Landry's paralysis, includes different groups of cases which, although presenting similar or even identical clinical features, are dissimilar in the site of the morbid action.

To put the matter in another way, I think it not unlikely that future investigations may distinguish two or three pathological varieties of Raynaud's disease: the chief lesion in one series of cases implicating vaso-motor centres ; the chief lesion in another series implicating vaso-motor nerves ; while, possibly, in a third series of cases morbid changes will be found along the whole vaso-motor tract, nerve cells as well as nerve fibres being affected.

General pathology of Multiple peripheral neuritis.—The limits of this article do not permit a complete discussion of the pathological anatomy of peripheral neuritis. The morbid changes found in cases of alcoholic paralysis and of Landry's disease have already been briefly sum- marised, and I need now only consider some of the leading features of the general pathology of the subject.

At the outset it may be stated that the work of the last sixteen years has demonstrated, in the clearest possible way, the existence of a group of cases characterised by the presence of certain well-defined symptoms, and by the limitation of pathological changes, wholly or chiefly, to the peripheral parts of the spinal nerves—the spinal cord, roots, and proximal portions of the nerves being often quite healthy. In applying the name Multiple peripheral neuritis to this group it must be clearly understood that it is used in the wide sense indicated at the beginning ; namely, to signify that the peripheral portions of the nerves are the chief seat of the morbid action ; they are in an abnormal state, not necessarily inflam- matory, while other parts of the nervous system are inconstantly or are less specially affected.

The abnormal condition may be demonstrable on necropsy, or may conceivably be so temporary or slight as to leave no changes that can be detected by the highest powers of the microscope. The inclusion, therefore, of many conditions under the heading Peripheral neuritis can only be justified by a consideration of their clinical analogies with other conditions where the peripheral nerves show definite organic change.

Perhaps the most characteristic clinical feature of multiple neuritis is symmetrical localisation of motor and sensory symptoms in the peripheral parts of the limbs. The chief motor symptom is weakness of the dorsal flexors of the feet and of the extensor muscles of the hands ; while the sensory symptoms comprise diminution and perversion of cutaneous sensibility, together with tenderness of the nerve trunks and muscles. Such being the case, it appears not unreasonable to suppose that symp- toms other than the classical, if they present a similar distribution, may be dependent on an abnormal state of the peripheral nerves. In other words, if, in place of paralysis, muscular spasms or vascular disturbances form the dominant features, but have the same symmetrical localisation in the extremities, is it not probable that they too may be due to peri- pheral neuritis ? These questions have been partially discussed in con- nection with tetany and with Raynaud's disease. But, while admitting the importance in diagnosis of symmetrical localisation in peripheral parts, we must remember how widely the symptoms of multiple neuritis vary, both in character and distribution; and how difficult it is in some cases to decide whether the lesion be situated in the cord or in the nerves. In peripheral neuritis, instead of a symmetrical, we may have a random distribution of symptoms; instead of evidence that many nerves are affected (as we should expect from the presence of a poison in the blood) the symptoms may be confined to the territory of a plexus, or to that of a particular nerve. Buzzard and Brissaud have each drawn attention to partial forms of alcoholic neuritis; Leudet to a case in which the muscular branches of one ulnar nerve only were affected. Furthermore, isolated neuritis has been observed also in connection with diabetes, influenza, and other diseases.

The difficulty in diagnosis is further illustrated by cases of widespread atrophic paralysis—such as those which occur in connection with influenza and lead poisoning, and as in the case described by Blocq and Marinesco, which has been already mentioned.

How are we then to explain the variations in the distribution and character of the symptoms met with in multiple neuritis? The commonest cause of the disease is admitted to be a chemical poison, which may be assumed to circulate freely in the blood, and to be conveyed to all parts of the nervous system. Its frequent action on the brain is shown by the prevalence of psychical phenomena; the extent of its action on the spinal cord is not easy to define; and, with regard to changes found in the nerves, pathologists are not yet agreed how far such changes are primary, or how far they are secondary to minute lesions in the cord. In other words, does the central nervous system exercise any influence on the distribution and character of the symptoms presented by peripheral neuritis; and are variations in the motor and sensory phenomena to be explained by differences in the selective action of the poison on nerve fibres, or on the ganglionic cells which preside over their nutrition?

There are three possible ways in which a limitation of changes to the peripheral nerves may be explained:—(i.) The poison selects and attacks those parts solely or predominantly: (ii.) it primarily attacks nerve cells; and, as a consequence, those portions of the nerve fibres which are farthest removed from their influence undergo degeneration, namely, the peripheral: (iii.) the poison acts with equal intensity on nerve cells and nerve fibres; the former recover, but the latter, having been robbed of vitality for a time, have lost resisting power, and degeneration, already started, steadily progresses.

At first sight it appears reasonable to conclude that if the peripheral branches of nerves are diseased alone, the poison has singled them out for attack, and has had no affinity for nerve trunks, cord, or brain. But we are faced by the difficulty that occasionally a trophic change, such as muscular atrophy, is met with, apart indeed from demonstrable lesions in any part of the nervous system, but where there are reasons for attributing it to central disturbance. Two instances of this are particularly suggestive—

arthritic muscular atrophy, and the atrophy which in some few cases affects hemiplegic limbs.

The occurrence of muscular atrophy in hemiplegia, and sometimes (as in a case recorded by Babinski) when no spinal or neuritic changes can be discovered, suggests that the cerebral cortex may play a part in the dispensation of trophic lesions.   This is also indicated by the occurrence of trophic lesions in limbs affected by hysterical paralysis; and, further, by such cases as those related by Dr. Bristowe under the heading of Hysterical peripheral neuritis; and again by cases (which I have seen) in which symptoms of peripheral neuritis were manifested shortly after severe blows on the head.

With regard to arthritic muscular atrophy the evidence is against neuritis, and is in favour of the hypothesis of Charcot, namely, that the nutrition of the motor cells of the cord is deranged in a reflex manner, morbid impulses being conveyed to them from the joint nerves; and that their derangement or torpor determines the alterations in the muscles. That the process is reflex has indeed been demonstrated by Raymond, who found that a previous division of the posterior spinal roots prevented the wasting of the muscles.

Again, in all probability, slight changes in the anterior horns will be discovered when the histology is reinvestigated by modern methods; for it has been shown that an experimental lesion of the posterior roots will occasionally lead to wasting of some of the cells in the anterior horns. This is an indication that the vitality of motor cells depends to some extent on the integrity of sensory fibres, and is one of the links in a further conception of the pathology of the nervous system which new histological methods are daily bringing to light.   The method of Nissl, especially, has added to our knowledge of the anatomy of the nerve cell, and has demonstrated slight pathological changes hitherto undetected. Hence it is necessary to wait for the further information to be expected from the use of these methods before we can clearly understand the relations between central and peripheral disease.   It is true that before Nissl's method came into use changes in nerve cells were found in many cases of peripheral neuritis.   Dumenil, thirty-five years ago, in one of the cases already mentioned, found disseminated lesions in the spinal gray matter and a rarefaction of the cells of the anterior horns. Degenerative changes in these cells have also been described by Monakow, Œller, Oppenheim, and other observers, as occurring in cases of peripheral neuritis from lead, alcohol, or arsenic; but they were very inconstant, and the partisans of a central hypothesis for polyneuritis were obliged to fall back on supposed dynamic changes in nerve cells.   Nissl's method of staining the cells, introduced in 1885, opened up a new field of inquiry; and we may now take a brief glance at some of its results, as regards the motor neuron, derived from the researches of Marinesco and other observers.

Two distinct substances are said to enter into the constitution of a motor cell, namely, a chromophile or chromatic substance which takes up

basic colouring matter, and an amorphous fundamental substance which
presents no affinity for colouring matters.   The chromatic substance,
called also kinetoplasma, is represented by a number of granules
arranged for the most part around the central nucleus, and also
in rows along the cell border; they are prolonged as slender rods
into the protoplasmic processes or dendrites of the cell, but do not occur
in its axis cylinder.   The latter is a prolongation of the achromatic
amorphous substance, called also trophoplasma, which in the cell body
binds the chromatic granules together.   Now the researches of Marinesco,
Ballet, and Deutil have proved conclusively that when the axis cylinder is
cut, injured, or diseased, as in peripheral neuritis, certain changes take
place in the kinetoplasma.   The chromophile granules disappear partially
or wholly, and the nucleus, instead of being in the centre, approaches the
periphery of the cell.   If the lesion of the nerve fibres be slight and
curable, the chromatic substance may regain its normal characters ; but if
the lesion be severe other changes set in.   The fundamental achromatic
substance disintegrates both in the axis cylinder and in the cell body, and
the whole neuron becomes atrophic.   These changes then are secondary to
lesions of the nerves.   Do they differ from primary changes in the nerve
cell due to the action of some poison directly upon it ?   Marinesco believes
that a difference may be distinguished.   He says that when anæmia of
the cord is produced by a temporary ligature of the aorta there is a dissolution of the chromophile elements in the form of a band at the
periphery of the cell ; but, in addition to this, the trophoplasma quickly
disintegrates, vacuoles are produced, and ruptures occur in the protoplasmic processes.   It is this precocious disintegration of the trophoplasma which Marinesco regards as particularly characteristic of primary
lesions of the nerve cells.

Leaving out of consideration this suggestive structural distinction
between primary and secondary lesions of nerve cells, the chief value of
the above researches is the proof they afford that minute changes in nerve
cells are very common in cases of neuritis, and that many of them are
secondary to it.   They show that while nerve fibres depend for their
vitality on nerve cells the condition of the cells is influenced by that of
the fibres ; not only may central changes lead to peripheral lesions, but the
latter also in turn may initiate lesions in nerve centres.   But although it is
anatomically correct to regard the neuron and its axis cylinder as one
body rather than as two distinct bodies artificially linked together, and
although it is difficult to exclude central influences from the explanation of
the phenomena of peripheral neuritis, it will be granted that a predominance of pathological changes in peripheral nerves is evidence that
they have been specially selected by a particular poison ; now, if this be
admitted, it is logical to infer that cases exist in which these parts are
attacked alone, the neurons themselves presenting no affinity for the
particular poison.   This inference is proved to be correct by such a case
as that reported by Déjerine, to which I have already referred (p. 685).

The view that nerves alone may be picked out by certain poisons receives further support from the frequent implication of sensory fibres in peripheral neuritis ; for it seems more reasonable to believe that a poison will attack two adjacent structures, like the motor and sensory fibres in a peripheral nerve, than two widely-separated organs, like the anterior horns and the ganglia on the posterior roots which preside over the functions of the sensory and motor fibres. From a clinical standpoint the differences between affections of the nerve fibres and nerve cells are usually well marked ; but this is not always the case, as has already been indicated in connection with acute affections of the neuron, as exemplified by cases grouped under the title Landry's disease. When sensory phenomena are well marked, as in Landry's own case, there can be little doubt that the disease is acute multiple neuritis ; but when motor phenomena are solely or predominantly present it is very difficult to say which part of the peripheral neuron is affected. In some cases motor fibres are picked out, in others motor cells ; in others, again, both may be affected by a toxin in the blood. The pathological selection is probably due mainly to the kind of poison, and to its dose ; but partly also to antecedent weakness of the part of the neuron which is attacked.

Further, it is to be noted that toxins act not only on nerve cells and nerve fibres, but also, in many cases, on the vessels supplying them. The careful investigations of Dr. Fleming show that degenerative changes in weakened nerve fibres are greatly expedited by local effusions depending on vascular conditions. In two cases of alcoholic neuritis he found effusions particularly well marked "around the arterioles and capillaries in the endoneurial septa, and often between the nerve fibres and the perineurium, and separating the inner lamellæ of the perineurium." The exudation is greater in one part of the nerve than in another, and acts injuriously by compressing the nerve fibres in its neighbourhood, thus causing degenerative changes in them, not merely at the level where it occurs, but also to a greater or lesser extent peripherally. The effusion was always accompanied by changes in the walls of the vessels, and these vascular changes became better marked as the nerves were traced peripherally. Dr. Fleming believes that the greater the interstitial effusion the less the chance of subsequent recovery.

In conclusion, some of the main pathological features of peripheral neuritis may be summarised as follows :—(i.) The chief cause is a chemical poison. (ii.) The poison affects all parts of the nervous system, though to a very unequal degree in different cases; partly because the nature of the poison varies, and partly because individual portions of the nervous system present varying susceptibilities in different persons. It may, indeed, be safely assumed that sometimes the peripheral nerves are solely implicated ; while it is probable that particular fibres—motor, sensory, or vaso-motor—may be picked out by special poisons. In many cases, however, there is evidence that the brain, or cord, or both, may be attacked together with the nerves.

The treatment of peripheral neuritis. — The first essential in dealing with any case of peripheral neuritis is to find out the cause, and to remove it, or to stop its action, as soon as possible. The cause, as we have seen, is nearly always some poison; and, if the patient be withdrawn from its influence and placed under favourable conditions, complete recovery is the rule. There is abundant proof that muscles extremely atrophied as a result of neuritis may completely regain their normal bulk, strength, and electrical reactions. Hence it is clear that nerve fibres profoundly degenerated may be entirely reformed; new axis cylinders may develop, and become covered with myelin; and ultimately a new set of nerve fibres may convey healthy impulses to healthy muscles.

In cases due to alcohol the patient should be deprived at once of alcoholic drink in any form; even in old, broken-down topers the deprivation is rarely attended with danger, if suitable nourishment be administered and careful attention be given to the digestive organs. To provide against deception on the part of the patient, and to insure the complete withdrawal of alcohol, it is often necessary to remove the patient from the care of his friends, and to place him in the charge of trained and trustworthy nurses.

In all except the slightest cases rest in bed is advisable. The patient is thus protected from exposure to cold, the pernicious effects of movement are reduced to a minimum, and local treatment can be carried out more readily and satisfactorily.

In the acute stage the suffering of some patients is extreme; and it is of the utmost importance to relieve this as promptly and effectively as possible. The severest cases require a water-bed; this not only relieves pain better than an ordinary bed, but also gives more support to a weak patient, and thus lessens the danger to life arising from a feeble, dilated heart or paralysed respiratory muscles.

In feeding the patient, or in attending to his evacuations, the nurse should exercise the greatest care and gentleness; so that all unnecessary movements on the part of the patient may be avoided. For the relief of tender nerves and muscles there is nothing better than warm fomentations. It is best to apply them intermittingly; a warm fomentation may be put on the painful part for half an hour, and the application repeated every four hours; a layer of hot cotton-wool taking its place in the intervals. Mills recommends rapidly alternating applications of very hot and very cold water; "a large sponge or soft towel is dipped in very hot and another in very cold water, and one is made to follow the other rapidly up and down the limb." Occasional vapour baths often afford the patient great comfort; but they should not be used when the action of the heart is much impaired. As regards drugs; in the early stages of multiple neuritis, salicylate of soda and iodide of potassium, either alone or in combination, appear to be of service; Mills speaks highly, too, of oil of gaultheria. Neuralgic pains may also be relieved by the administration of antipyrin, phenacetin, or exalgin; but when the suffering is very great the hypodermic injection of morphia becomes necessary.

The drugs mentioned are of value in all forms of peripheral neuritis, but special treatment is called for in particular cases. Thus quinine must be given when paralysis is due to malarial poisoning; mercury and iodide of potassium in syphilitic cases; when the neuritis depends on anæmia or on septicæmia, perchloride of iron in large doses deserves a trial. The weak, dilated heart of alcoholism requires digitalis and strychnine, to which small doses of cocaine may often be added to lessen the craving for stimulants.

But of far greater importance than drugs is the regular and careful administration of nourishment, in the form of boiled milk, beef tea, beef extracts, soups and broths. Benger's food or peptonised gruel may be required; and when vomiting is a prominent symptom nutrient enemas should be administered.

Complete rest in bed in a well-ventilated room, careful feeding, and exposure to sunlight are the essential points in the treatment of the early stages of multiple neuritis.

When the acute symptoms have subsided, recourse may be had to massage, electricity, and tonic treatment. In the acute stage massage would be unendurable, and no doubt hurtful; but its application should not be delayed too long. It may be employed as soon as extreme pain and tenderness have disappeared. At first massage should be employed in the gentlest manner, and only for short periods of time; but as soon as the patient stands it well, it ought to be regularly and vigorously applied. The patient should also be encouraged to make voluntary movement against resistance; and other modes of Swedish exercises can be employed with advantage. By these means the nutrition and strength of the muscles are improved, while any tendency to contractures is overcome. Moreover, the patient's capacity for assimilation of food is thus steadily increased.

The restoration of the degenerated nerves and muscles may also be aided by the daily application of electricity. The constant current is the most useful in stimulating the nutrition of the affected muscles. Large electrodes are desirable in order that as much muscular tissue as possible may be reached by the current. As soon as the muscles respond to a weak faradic current this form of electricity may also be employed with advantage. A daily warm bath, followed by vigorous friction to the skin, is of value, whilst tonics and cod-liver oil often prove of great service.

When should the patient be allowed to get up? Not until pain and tenderness have subsided, and there is evidence that the process of repair has become established.

From first to last abundant fresh air and sunlight are of the greatest importance; and as soon as the patient is able to take outdoor exercise a change of air is often advisable: in many cases, however, it will be some time before local massage can be entirely dispensed with.

As to the efficacy of drugs in the elimination of poisons from the system fresh investigations are needed. The experiments made by Professor Dixon Mann show that iodide of potassium has no appreciable influence on the elimination of lead. He made a systematic examination, extending over several months, of the urine and fæces taken from cases of lead poisoning, and found that no medicinal treatment had any effect on the rate of elimination of this poison. A certain proportion of lead forms definite combinations with organic matter, and may remain in the system for an indefinite time; but a small proportion undergoes progressive elimination independently of any treatment. Professor Mann believes, however, that warm baths and general massage do contribute to a slight extent to increase the rate of normal elimination.

JUDSON S. BURY.

REFERENCES

A full bibliography of multiple neuritis up to the year 1890 is given in the *Treatise on Peripheral Neuritis* by Drs. Ross and Bury. The following references comprise the more important contributions to the subject since the year 1890; when, as in some of the articles, references are given to other published work on peripheral neuritis, these are not repeated.

Neuritis generally: 1. ANDERSON, W. "Acute Peripheral Neuritis, followed by Multiple Ankylosis," etc., *Lancet*, 1894, i.—2. ANDERSON, T. M·C. "Multiple Neuritis," *Glas. Med. Jour.* 1895—3. BABINSKI, J. (Article with bibliography,) *Traité de méd.* Charcot et B., 1894.—4. BALLET, G. *Le prog. méd.* 1896.—5. BREVOR. *Quart. Med. Journ.* Sheffield, 1894-95.—6. BERNHARDT, M. *Nothnagel Sp. Path.* Bd. xi. 1 Theil, Wien, 1896.—7. BONNET. *Acute infectious P. N.* Lyon, 1892.—8. BUZZARD. *Lancet,* 1893, ii.—9. CAGNEY. *Lancet,* 1895, ii.—10. CRAIGMILE. *Lancet,* 1894, ii.—11. DÉJERINE. "Hypertrophic Progr. Neuritis of Infancy," *Rev. de méd.* 1896.—12. ESKRIDGE. *Med. News,* 1895.—13. ETTLINGER. *Gaz. des hôp.* 1895.—14. FINOTTI. *Arch. path. anat.* 1896.—15. FLEMING. *Brain,* 1897.—16. FRANKEL. *Deutsche med. Woch.* 1892, 1896, 1897.—17. FUCHS. *Deutsche Zeitschr. f. Nerv.* 1893-94.—18. GOLDSHEIDER and MOXTER. *Fortschr. d. Med.* 1895.—19. GIBSON and FLEMING. "Fatal Terminations," etc., *Edinb. Hosp. Rep.* 1895.—20. GIESE and PAGENSTECKER. *Arch. f. Psych.* 1893.—21. GOWERS. *Clin. Journal,* 1896-97.—22. HAMMOND. "Cases in Infants," *Journ. Nerv. and Ment. Dis.* 1895.—23. JOLLY. *Charité-Ann.* 1897.—24. KRAUSS. "Peroneal Atrophy," *Journ. Nerv. and Ment. Dis.* 1895.—25. KORNELOW. "Acute Primary Polymyositis," *Deutsche Zeitschr. f. Nerv.* 1896.—26. MARTIN. *Journ. Path. and Bact.* 1892-93. —27. MARINESCO. *Compt. rend. soc. de biol.* 1895, 1897.—28. OPPENHEIM. "The Senile Form," *Berl. klin. Woch.* 1893.—29. PUTNAM. *Amer. Journ. Med. Sc.* 1895.—30. RAYMOND. *Clin. des mal. de syst. nerreux,* 1897.—31. REMAK. *Neur. Cent.* 1896.—32. ROHDE. *Z'schr. f. klin. Med.* 1894.—33. SCHLESINGER. *Neur. Cent.* 1895.—34. STEPHENSON. "Acute Ataxia," *Med. Chron.* 1894.—35. SHARKEY. *Brit. Med. Jour.* 1896, i.—36. SIEMERLING. *Neur. Cent.* 1897.—37. SORGO. *Ztschr. f. klin. Med.* 1897.— 38. SOUKHANOFF. *Arch. de Neurol.* 1896; also *N. icon. de la Salpêt.* 1897.—39. STEIN. "Senile Neuritis," *Münch. med. Woch.* 1897. **Landry's Paralysis:** 39a. ALBU. *Zeit. f. klin. Med.* 1893.—40. BAILEY and EWING. "Analysis of Forty-Three Post-mortems," *New York Medical Journal,* 1896. 41. BEHMER. "Septicæmia," *Neur. Cent.* 1890.—42. BERNHARDT. "Puerperal," *Deutsche med. Woch.* 1894. —43. BEHREND. "Alcohol," *Deutsche med. Woch.* 1895.—44. BURGHART. *Charité-Ann.* 1897.—45. CARTER. "Diphtheria," *Brit. Med. Journal,* 1890, i.—46. CHURTON. *Trans. Clin. Soc.* 1895.—47. CANE. *Brit. Med. Journal,* 1892, ii.—48. DILLER and MEYER. *Amer. Journ. Med. Science,* 1896.—49. ELLISON. "Measles," *Lancet,* 1896, ii.—50. EICHHORST. "Malaria," *Virch. Arch.* Bd. lxix.—51. HUN. *New York Med. Journal,* 1891.—52. JAMES. *Edin. Med. Journal,* 1896-97.—53. JOLLY. "Alcohol," *Berl. klin. Woch.* 1894.—54. KLEBS. "Tubercle," *Deutsche med. Woch.* 1891.— 55. KRUGER. *Ztschr. f. kl. Med.* 1897.—56. LEYDEN. "Influenza," *Ztschr. f. kl. Med.* 1894.—57. LOVENSTEIN. *Neur. Cent.* 1889.—58. LUNZ. "Alcohol," *Neur. Cent.* 1890. —59. ORMROD. *St. Barth. Hosp. Rep.* 1892.—60. PAILHAS. "Influenza," *Arch de neur.* 1895.—61. REMLINGER. *Compt. rend. soc. de biol.* 1896.—62. REYNOLDS. *Med. Chron.* 1895-96.—63. RICOCHON. "Rabies," *Gaz. hebdom. méd.* 1892.—64. STEVEN. *Glasgow*

Med. Journal, 1896.—65. TOTHERICK. *Brit. Med. Journal*, 1892, ii.—66. WATSON. *Brit. Med. Journal*, 1892, ii.—67. WALTON. *Boston M. and S. J.* 1895. **Alcoholic Neuritis:** 68. CAMPBELL. "Morbid Anatomy," *Liverpool Journal*, 1893.—69. COLE-BAKER. *Brit. Med. Journal*, 1893, i.—70. DÉJERINE. *Compt. rend. soc. de biol.* 1897.—71. EICHHORST. "Apoplectiform variety," *Virch. Arch.* Bd. cxxix.—72. GUDDEN. "Analysis of Forty-three Post-mortems,"*Arch. f. Psych.* 1896.—73. HERTER. *New York Med. Journal*, 1896.—74. JAMES. *Edinburgh Med. Journal*, 1896-97.—75. LESZYNSKY. *Journ. Nerv. and Ment. Dis.* 1892.—76. LÉPINE. *Rev. de méd.* 1898.—76a. MAUDE. *Brain*, 1895.—77. NOTHNAGEL. *Allg. Wien. med. Ztg.* 1895.—78. RENNERT. *Deut. Arch. f. klin. Med.* 1892.—79. TOOTH. *Path. Trans.* 1894, vol. xlv.—80. WHITE. *Intern. Clinic*, 1895. References to paralysis from carbonic oxide, bisulphide of carbon, aniline, roburite, lead, arsenic, mercury, phosphorus, and other poisons, will be found in vol. ii. of this *System of Medicine*. Other references are : 81. ANKER. "Lead," *Berl. klin. Woch.* 1894.—82. ADAMS. "Arsenic," *Lancet*, 1894, i.—83. BARRS. "Arsenic," *Brit. Med. Journal*, 1895, vol. i.—84. BRAUER. "Mercury," *Berl. klin. Woch.* 1897.—85. BROU-ARDEL. "Arsenic, tabular analysis of sixty-eight cases," *Arch. de méd. expér.* 1896.—86. CARLO CENI. "Lead," *Arch. f. Psych.* 1897.—87. COMLEY. *Neur. Cent.* 1897.—88. VON ENGEL. "Mercury," *Prag. med. Woch.* 1894.—89. HELLER. "Mercury," *Deutsche med. Woch.* 1896.—90. JOLLY. "Arsenic," *Deutsche med. Woch.* 1893.—91. LANCEREAUX. "Arsenic," *Neur. Cent.* 1897.—92. LEYDEN. "Mercury," *Deutsche med. Woch.* 1893.—93. MEIROWITZ. *Journ. Nerv. and Ment. Dis.* 1895.—94. MÜLLER. "Arsenic," *Wien. med. Presse*, 1894.—95. SPILLMAN and ETIENNE. "Mercury," *Rev. de méd.* 1895.—96. SINKLER. "Lead," *Med. News*, 1894.—97. THOMSON. "Arsenic," *Med. Rec. New York*, 1898.—98. WHITE. "$C.S_2$," *Prov. Med. Journal*, 1892. **Pregnancy and the Puerperium:** 99. DANZIGN. *Neur. Cent.* 1897.—99a. ELDER, *Brit. Med. Journal*, 1896, i. —100. EULENBERG. "Analysis of Thirty-eight Cases," *Deutsche med. Woch.* 1895.—101. HIGIER. *Neur. Cent.* 1897.—102. JOHANSEN. *Münch. med. Woch.* 1896.—103. KOSTER. *Münch. med. Woch.* 1896.—104. LAMY. *Arch. de toxol. et de gynéc.* 1893.—105. LUNZ. *Deutsche med. Woch.* 1894.—106. MADER. *Wien. klin. Woch.* 1895.—107. MÖBIUS. *Münch. med. Woch.* 1892.—108. REYNOLDS. *Brit. Med. Journal*, 1897, ii. —109. SANGER. *Neur. Cent.* 1898, ii.—110. STEMBO. *Deutsche med. Woch.* 1895.—111. STIEFEL. *Abstr. neur. Cent.* 1893.—112. TURNEY. *St. Thomas's Hosp. Rep.* vol. xxv. p. 1. **Septicæmia:** 113. KRAUS. (Reference to other cases,) *Wien. klin. Woch.* 1897. **Tubercle:** 114. CARRIÈRE. *Neur. Cent.* 1897. **Influenza:** 115. ALLYN. *Journ. Amer. Med. Assoc.* 1897.—116. DRESCHFELD. *Med. Chron.* 1898.—117. PUTNAM. *Boston M. and S. J.* 1892.—118. STEVENSON. *Lancet*, 1893. **Diphtheria:** 119. GOODALL. *Brain*, 1895.—120. GUTHRIE. *Lancet*, 1894.—121. HASCHE. *Münch. med. Woch.* 1895.—122. HAWTHORNE. *Glasg. Med. Journ.* 1893.—123. MELSON. *Birm. Med. Rev.* 1892.—124. MACKENZIE. *St. Thomas's Hosp. Rep.* 1893.—125. PASTEUR. *Brit. Med. Journal*, 1895, i.—126. TOOTH. "Deafness," *Brit. Med. Journal*, 1893, i.—127. TOWNSEND. *New York Med. Journal*, 1894. **Rheumatism:** 128. HANDFORD. *Brit. Med. Journal*, 1892, ii.—129. KAHNE. *Cent. f. klin. Med.* 1892.—130. ORD. *Clin. Journ.* 1892-93.—131. RISSE. *Deutsche med. Woch.* 1897.—132. STEINER. *Deut. Arch. f. klin. Med.* Bd. lviii. **Whooping Cough:** 133. MACKAY. *Brit. Med. Journal*, 1894, ii. **Diabetes:** 134. WILLIAMSON, R. T. *Diab. Mellitus and its Treatment.* (This book contains a full list of references.) **Varicella:** 135. GAY. *Brit. Med. Journal*, 1894 i. **Measles:** 136. MONRO. *Lancet*, 1894.

J. S. B.

TRIGEMINAL NEURALGIA

Introduction. — The word neuralgia, strictly used, signifies a pain which follows the course of some peripheral nerve or nerve root, but is caused by no gross organic lesion of any part of the nervous system. However, such a use of the word is impossible in practice, for it involves the introduction of pathological qualifications.

Vulgarly, neuralgia is used to signify any pain which appears to shoot along the course of a nerve. But since a large number of such pains are caused by definite well-known organic diseases of the nervous system, the name neuralgia has been clinically used to denote any pain of this character which cannot be attributed to some one of these. For, if the character of the pain only were relied upon, it would be impossible to separate the lightning pains of tabes, or the pain which follows herpes ophthalmicus, from true neuralgia; yet both are now known to be due to organic disease. Again, the discovery of neuritis at once removed brachial and sciatic neuralgia to a position amongst the symptoms of this newly-formed disease group. Thus the more our knowledge of organic and functional disease of the nervous system advances, the smaller becomes the group of pure neuralgias.

Again, the group of pure neuralgias has been much diminished of late by observations in another direction. It was well known before Valleix's time that a pain clinically resembling neuralgia might be produced not only by disease of the nervous system, but also by disease of some internal organ. Valleix is careful to explain that in none of his cases of neuralgia was visceral disease present; a statement that an examination of his records, in the light of our present knowledge, by no means bears out. Thus an increased knowledge of the referred pains of visceral disease has further reduced the group of idiopathic neuralgias, by referring such pain to the position of a symptom of visceral disease.

Progress in both directions has been so great of late years, that we are almost justified in believing that all neuralgias will ultimately be classified as symptoms of disease in some part of the nervous system (either peripheral or central), or as the expression of the reaction of the nervous system to visceral irritation. Thus neuralgia is in most cases not a disease, but a symptom; and the greater part of the contents of this section are and should be broken up and distributed about this *System of Medicine.* As, however, the word is in popular use, and the determination of the true focus or cause of the neuralgic pain is often extremely difficult, an attempt will be made to treat of the various affections still known as neuralgia, and to show how far we are able to assign them to their proper places.

As many different conditions are included under the name neuralgia, they will be considered in the following order :—

1*st.* Neuralgia quinti major (tic douloureux, epileptiform neuralgia).

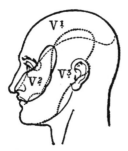
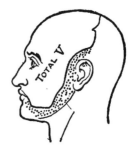

FIG. 38.—To show the supply of the three branches of the 5th nerve obtained by dissection.

FIG. 39.—To show the analgesia produced by total extirpation of the Gasserian ganglion in man.

I propose to show that this is a definite disease of the nervous system, with a distinct course and character.

2*nd.* Neuralgia secondary to disease of the nerves of the head ; for example, tumours involving the fifth nerve, post-herpetic neuralgia, and the like. These conditions are often extremely difficult to discriminate

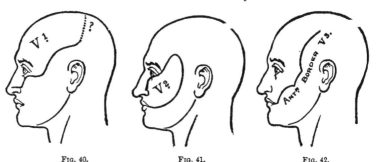

FIG. 40.   FIG. 41.   FIG. 42.

To show the full supply of the three branches of the 5th nerve in man.
In Fig. 40 the 2nd and 3rd branches were divided and removed ; in Fig. 41, the 1st and 3rd ; and in Fig. 42, the 1st and 2nd for the relief of neuralgia quinti major. In each case the area outlined represents the parts of the skin over which sensation to pain stimuli remained intact.

during life from neuralgia major or minor. Such pains as are part of multiple neuritis will be considered elsewhere.

3*rd.* Neuralgia minor. This group contains—

(*a*) True visceral referred pains due to disease of the intimate structure of some organ of the head.

(*b*) Pains due to disease of the membranes or tissues surrounding some organ, or to actual implication of the finer nerve twigs by the morbid process.

(*c*) Neuralgias of the head and face arising as direct consequences of disease in organs other than those of the head.

4*th*. Neuralgias arising from general bodily states, such as neurasthenia, hysteria, and the like.

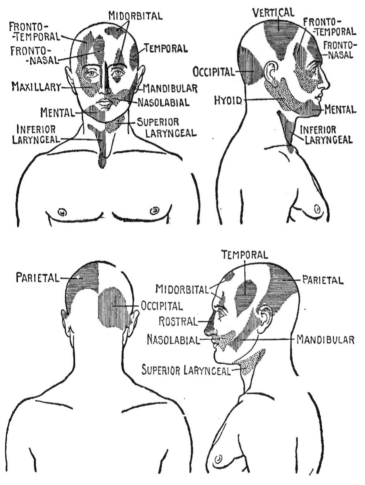

Fig. 43.—The "segmental" area of the head and face.

Central and peripheral nervous supply to the head and neck.— (1) *Distribution of the trigeminal.*—The peripheral distribution of the branches of the fifth nerve can be mapped out by three methods—

(*a*) By dissecting each branch to its finest termination. This is extremely laborious, and must always fail to show the complete supply of the nerve, owing to the difficulty in determining the limits of supply for the finest branches. Fig. 43 shows the supply given in *Quain's Anatomy.*

(β) By observing the anæsthesia produced when one or more branches have been divided. This method shows only the area on the skin supplied solely by the nerve divided, and the result will therefore fall short of its full supply. In cases, however, where the third method is inapplicable, we are forced to fall back upon the distribution of anæsthesia. This is particularly the case with the delimitation of the posterior border of the fifth, where it is overlapped by the supply of the cervical nerves. I therefore give Fig. 39 to show the extreme limits of the loss of sensation produced by extirpation of the Gasserian ganglion.

(γ) On the other hand, we can avail ourselves of an ingenious method, invented by Prof. Sherrington, for mapping out the posterior roots upon the body. This method, which may be called that of "residual

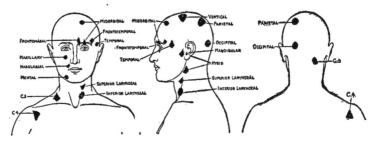

Fig. 44.—The "maxima" of the segmental areas shown on Fig. 43.

æsthesia," can best be elucidated by an example. Supposing the first and second divisions of the fifth nerve to have been divided, the border of the anæsthesia so produced will represent the extreme anterior limit of the supply of the third division of the fifth, excepting where it meets the cervical nerves of the vertex. In the same way, if all three branches of the fifth have been divided, the limit of the anæsthesia will represent the anterior border of the posterior root of the second cervical. I have taken advantage of those cases where the different branches have been divided for the relief of neuralgia quinti major to consider the sensory results so produced from this aspect, and give three figures to represent the results so obtained on man. They very closely correspond to those obtained by Sherrington from experiments on monkeys.

The posterior border of the fifth nerve cannot be mapped out by this method; for this purpose division of the posterior root of the second cervical nerve would be required. To show the extreme limits of the supply of the third division of the fifth, we are therefore forced to fall back upon the second method, and to note the anæsthesia produced by extirpation of the Gasserian ganglion (Fig. 39).

(2) "*Segmental*" *areas of the head and neck.*—When an organ, such as the eye or one of the teeth, is affected, pain is not situated only in the organ itself, but is referred to parts at a distance on the scalp or face. Such visceral referred pains, when of sufficient severity and duration, are accompanied by areas of superficial tenderness. These areas are supposed to represent the segmental origin of the nerves for pain, heat, and cold to the head ; and, at any rate, to whatsoever level of the central nervous system they may belong, they do not represent the distribution of the peripheral branches of the cranial nerves. Fig. 43 is given to show their character and distribution, in order to facilitate reference in later parts of this article. When the tenderness is not very severe these areas may be present only in part. Certain spots in each area are then found to become tender sooner, and to remain tender longer than any other parts of the area. These maxima are of practical importance, because they are the spots to which the patient refers his pain, whether the pain be accompanied by superficial tenderness or not (Fig. 44).

Neuralgia quinti major.—*Tic douloureux, epileptiform neuralgia.*— This form of neuralgia has been placed in a group apart, owing to the marked similarity that one case bears to another, both in course and symptoms. In the earliest stages each case appears to be one of simple neuralgia, and under this impression relief has been sought in removal of teeth or other operative procedures. At last the full clinical picture of this hideous disease unrolls, varying only in unessential details from the classical type.

The story of most of these cases is somewhat as follows—a man or woman, between thirty-five and sixty years of age, apparently in fair health, is suddenly attacked with pain within the peripheral course of one of the branches of the trigeminal. The pain is continuous for some hours or days. The teeth are attended to without relief ; or perhaps the removal of a tooth, apparently sound, is coincident with the cessation of pain, and the patient imagines he is cured. But after a varying interval the pain recurs, and at last no day passes without an attack of greater or less duration. Throughout this time the patient is able to continue his work without much interruption ; but gradually the attacks increase in severity and frequency till all consecutive work becomes impossible. The onset of the first attack is usually, as far as the patient can tell, without obvious cause. Later attacks may seem to be due to some change in the weather ; and for this ill-defined influence of weather there is an analogue in the lightning pains of tabes. Abnormal physical states of the body, such as constipation, and more particularly such mental conditions as a sudden shock, anxiety, business worry, and the like, are peculiarly apt to induce an attack in this stage of the disease. At first the attacks of pain may be limited to the territory of one branch of the nerve, to that of the inferior dental branch of the third division, for instance. But, sooner or later, the pain spreads to other branches on the same side of the face, until at last all three divisions may be more or less implicated. The attacks also alter in frequency. Throughout the space of many hours daily the patient is racked by paroxysms of pain at regular intervals enduring from a few seconds to many minutes. Sleep, except under anodynes, becomes impossible; the patient dare not eat, talk, or smile, for fear of precipitating a paroxysm. Life thus becomes utterly unbearable, and is not uncommonly ended by suicide.

In the simplest cases the pain affects one spot in the jaw or face; but generally more than one spot is affected, and from these spots the pain radiates along the course of some nerve branch. In a case where the pain was situated at a single spot in the upper jaw, it was said to resemble "the sudden thrust of a red-hot gimlet into the flesh." More commonly the pain starts at one spot, and rapidly radiates along the course of the nerve. It cannot be said to shoot from one point to another, but, starting at one focus, the pain radiates along the course of the nerve "as if a red-hot electric wire was plunged into the face and the current affected the whole nerve." If two spots form radiating foci the pain in any paroxysm may start from them simultaneously or successively, but does not definitely dart from one to another. Uncommonly, radiation may take place into the occipital region or into the neck; although, since the pain in this region is removed by ablation of the Gasserian ganglion, there is no reason to suppose the territory of these nerves to be primarily affected.

The pain never starts at a spot outside the territory of the fifth nerve, though radiation may take place beyond its boundaries. It is rarely bilateral; Krause describes one such case, and I have seen this bilateral distribution in an old woman of seventy-five, in whom the disease had lasted twenty-five years.

The spots from which the pain radiates are always described as situated below the skin. Thus a not uncommon distribution is for the pain to start from a spot exactly above the highest point of the curve of the ala nasi, and thence to dart around the eye on the inner and the outer side, until a patch is affected on the forehead about the size of the palm of the hand, extending from the upper lid to the root of the hair. Here the pain is throughout "just under the skin." Another common starting-point is just posterior to the canine of the lower jaw. Here the stab of pain begins, and rapidly radiates along the whole lower jaw. It may then stop, but sooner or later it will pass from a deep course in the lower jaw to radiate over the posterior part of the temporal fossa. Not uncommonly a second painful focus is perceived over the posterior part of the zygoma. Another extremely common spot is exactly over the infra-orbital foramen, and from this point the pain radiates over the cheek and anterior part of the temporal fossa. Sometimes the lateral border of the tongue is the seat of a focus of pain, from which radiation takes place over the same half of the tongue, excepting only the posterior part of the dorsum. Thus the pain tends to start at certain points which mostly correspond to the exit of nerve bundles from the deep structures of the face, or to their terminations upon the surface. From such foci radiation takes place mainly along the distribution of the nerve branch implicated. But the matter is not quite so simple as it seems at first sight. For although the pain may start at the angle of the nose, and affect the eye and forehead, complete extirpation of the first division of the fifth may still leave the nasal point unaffected. Moreover, after such an operation the anæsthesia of the scalp extends back to the parietal eminence, and is of wider extent than the previous pain.

I have already alluded to Valleix's "points douloureux." Krause states, and in this respect my experience absolutely bears out his statement, that pressure with the finger may start a paroxysm, or may simply increase that dull sense of pain which exists over the area of radiation between the paroxysms. Moreover, in such cases tender points can frequently be found over the exit of nerves other than those directly implicated in the paroxysm. When the paroxysm occurs at stated intervals pressure or even the lightest touch in such a point will not uncommonly precipitate a paroxysm; whilst immediately after it has passed pressure, whether heavy or light, is without obvious effect. Moreover, in the paroxysm itself most patients firmly press the hand or some hard object to the face, and apparently gain some ease by this action. Lastly, there are a certain number of cases of undoubted severity in which no tender point can be detected.

As I have said, the first attack starts without any obvious cause and when the patient is not conscious of any deviation from his general health. I have seen one case, however, in which the first attack began two weeks after a blow on the side of the head from the main boom of a yacht.

After the disease is once established the season of the year may determine an attack. In a case of Krause's the attacks came on in the spring, and only for a period of six weeks; for the rest of the year she remained free. One of my patients suffered from February to October for many years; but the period shifted, and he then suffered in the winter months only.

Any marked deterioration of physical health, such as may be due to a common nasal catarrh or constipation, will tend to bring on an attack.

Mental shock is a potent factor in inducing these attacks. One of my patients remained free from attacks for sixteen months after the inferior dental nerve had been stretched. But within an hour after seeing a fellow-workman killed by a fall the pain came on worse than ever it had been before. Business worry or family anxiety acts in a similar way, or even an access of anger may induce an attack.

During the period of an attack the actual paroxysms are affected by the most diverse conditions. A breath of wind, a slight touch on the beard or hair, talking, drinking, deglutition, or even swallowing the saliva, will precipitate a paroxysm or increase its severity. Thus the patient lets his hair and beard grow, the saliva may dribble from his mouth upon the pillow, the tongue and cheeks may become foul from decomposing food; yet he dare not utter his wants. The act of defæcation is commonly attended by an increase in the severity of pain, and the patients therefore shun going to stool, and thus aid in the production of the constipation so commonly present. As a general rule during the attacks a cold blast of air from an open window is unpleasant, and is said to increase the severity of the paroxysm. But atmospheric heat and cold cannot be said to have any definite effect in determining the attacks in a patient already suffering from the disease. The effects of hot and cold water in the mouth are extremely variable. In some cases, especially those which do not affect the lower jaw and tongue, neither hot nor cold water have any effect on the paroxysms. Sometimes hot water seems to relieve the pain, sometimes it is unpleasant; in other cases cold water may be without effect, or sometimes it may increase the paroxysms. Thus each patient will regulate the temperature of his food according to his particular experience.

In the earlier stages of the disease the attacks last a shorter time; but each attack tends to be continuous, and is not made up of a chain of paroxysms separated from one another by longer or shorter periods of freedom from pain. In one of my cases the first sign of disease was an attack, of sudden onset, lasting continuously for over a week. Later he suffered from one short attack daily of about half an hour's duration; ultimately a paroxysm appeared every five minutes throughout the three days I had him under close observation. When periodicity is well established the paroxysms may return at almost any interval. The most frequent I have seen recurred with almost precise regularity every forty seconds for several days in succession; on the other hand, some patients have only one short daily paroxysm at exactly the same hour.

In the earlier stages the pain ceases if the patient can get to sleep, and does not return during the time he is asleep; but during the later stages the paroxysms continue with the same regularity day and night, for sleep becomes impossible.

The pain is accompanied by marked vascular trophic and secretory changes. A more or less permanent red flush suffuses the affected side, which may deepen with each paroxysm. The conjunctiva is reddened. The hair and beard change colour, or may fall out. Or again, either or both may be rubbed away by the pressure exerted by the patient on his face during the paroxysm. The affected cheek not uncommouly appears peculiarly greasy. The patient may complain that some part of his face, such as the lip, feels swollen, and he is convinced that it is larger than normal. A similar feeling of swelling also exists over those parts of the jaw which are tender. In one of my cases the two painful spots were marked out by trophic changes over an area of the skin about the size of a sixpence; the skin here appeared raised, thickened, and very dark in colour. These spots disappeared entirely when after treatment the pain left her, and she stated that they always came and went coincidently with the pain.

During an attack, especially within the territory of the first and second divisions of the nerve, tears flow copiously, and intense photophobia may exist. With an attack over the third division saliva may be secreted. Occasionally a discharge of thin fluid takes place from one nostril, apart from lachrymation.

. A metallic taste may also be complained of over the affected side of the tongue. Apart from the foulness of the mouth, the appetite is, as a rule, unimpaired, and the patients do not waste. Constipation is commonly present during the period of attack, owing in part to the dread of defæcation.

The mental condition is at first merely that of a person suffering pain—irritable and depressed, but fairly cheerful in the inter-paroxysmal periods. Later, partly owing, no doubt, to the enormous doses of hypnotics and anodynes necessary to still the pain, the patient may become insane. The form assumed is that of an acutely suicidal melancholia. Krause states that even when of considerable duration this insanity is curable after the pain has been relieved by operation. But, apart from insanity, suicide is extremely common, and every patient in the later stages of the disease should be looked upon as a possible suicide. Neither hallucinations nor delusions are common, but the memory becomes extremely bad for all recent events.

During each paroxysm the agony causes the patient's face to be drawn up. But, apart from this expression of emotion, the facial muscles seem in some cases to participate reflexly in the paroxysm. Each slight attack is then accompanied by a fibrillary tremor that can have nothing to do with expression.

Causation.—In spite of all that has been written on the subject of the heredity of this neurosis, nothing can be clearer than that the subjects of neuralgia major are in no sense of the word neurotic; nor have they a neurotic heredity. To say that some ancestor suffered from "paralysis" no more constitutes a neurotic inheritance than a similar history of "dropsy" would necessarily indicate a tendency to renal disease. In the clinical records of cases of neuralgia major it is striking how few cases are hereditary neuropaths. Krause is particularly emphatic in the statement that the cases that came under his observation were in no way inheritors of nervous disease. Horsley in his large experience has only found one case in which there was a history even of "paralysis." In ten consecutive cases I could find none in which there was a history of any nervous disease or insanity in the family. Again, the subjects of neuralgia quinti major, unlike so many of those who suffer from neuralgia minor, are not themselves neuropaths. With the exception of their one ailment, they are healthy persons. To say that a man, who has suffered from agonising pain every four seconds day and night for a fortnight, is neurotic because he is disposed to be irritable or to cry, betrays a lack of imagination in the observer. Once relieve the pain by operation, and these patients will prove to be quiet, intelligent, and normal human beings. They may perhaps show a tendency to early arterial degeneration; although, as most of them have already reached the age at which slight arterial degeneration might be expected, such observations are of but little value. The great age to which many of these patients live is in itself a testimony to their inherent soundness.

With regard to sex Krause found three men and nine women; Rose, five women and no men; Horsley, eleven men and eight women. My cases comprise seven men and four women. These numbers are too few to form any conclusion, but they go to show that the cases which come to operation yield a preponderance of women.

Horsley's youngest patient was twenty-six at the time of onset; his oldest fifty-eight; the ordinary age of onset lies between forty and fifty.

Pathology.—If we look back from the history of each case we find that the disease has invariably been mistaken for neuralgia minor at first, but has rapidly shown that it belonged to the graver type. Very commonly it begins in the upper or lower jaw, in the region of one of the teeth, but never, as far as my experience goes, in the tooth itself. It may start at one point in an edentulous jaw, or in the whole of one side of the jaw as far forwards as the point of insertion of the canine. The subsequent history is always the same. A dentist is applied to, who rightly clears the jaw from decayed stumps, and then proceeds to remove sound teeth. This gives the patient transitory relief, or no relief at all; the pain then rages as before in an edentulous jaw. The pain may also start about an eye that is absolutely healthy. Thus, unlike neuralgia minor, and especially unlike referred visceral pain, no obvious cause or connection can be found between the onset of the pain and disease of any peripheral organ to which the nerve terminals are distributed.

Many observations have been made on portions of nerves extracted by surgical operation, but up to the present time without satisfactory results. Dana found no change in the nerve elements, but an endarteritis of the vessels of the nerve sheath. Putnam found the same endarteritis, but also changes in the nerve elements and the endoneurium. Horsley and Rose found no change in the vessels, but change in the nerve elements. Krause found here and there thickening of the nerve sheath, accompanied in one case by thickening of the nerve fibres; in all cases the arteries were normal. Thus, considering that the material for examination was obtained by twisting the nerve from the canal, the microscopical changes were surprisingly small, and of little pathological importance.

Several observers have examined the Gasserian ganglion, and described changes in the ganglion cells. But slight changes, such as pigmentation and the like, are common after middle life, and in no case have observations with newer methods of nerve-cell staining been published. I examined a ganglion (removed by Mr. Jonathan Hutchinson) by Nissl's method; it showed nerve cells so perfect that they could be used as standard specimens of normal staining of the cells of the ganglion by this method. There was, perhaps, some thickening of the periganglionic tissue, but this was doubtful. Thus as yet the pathological lesion at the bottom of this disease has to be discovered.

Treatment.—(a) *Drugs.*—The drugs which have been recommended

for this malady are innumerable; but the favourable effects attributed
to many of them are probably due to a confusion between the major
and minor forms of the disease.   Large doses of quinine once a day
have been recommended, and in the earlier stages certainly seem to
have some effect.   The antipyrin group have a palliative effect, even in
comparatively late stages of the disease.   Salicylates have a similar
effect in some cases.   Two drugs, gelsemium and butyl chloral, definitely
ease the pain in the earlier stages, and Mr. Horsley states that if
gelsemium is pushed to produce its toxic effects (one drachm every two
hours), the patient is relieved, even in the later stages.   He states that
no relief is obtained until a feeling of sickness with numbness in the
extremities of the fingers comes on; relief so obtained is, however, but
temporary.   In lighter cases opium often gives marked relief, but it
tends to increase the constipation from which these patients so commonly
suffer.   Morphine is only a palliative, and so great is the danger of
establishing a morphine habit that Krause forbids its use altogether;
cocaine is in this respect even worse than morphine.   There is, however,
one method of administering morphine which I have seen to succeed after
every operation short of removing the Gasserian ganglion had failed.
The patient was placed in a room apart, away from all noise or disturb-
ance.   An injection of $\frac{1}{4}$ to $\frac{1}{3}$ grain of morphine was given every four
hours for ten days, and he was carefully fed with fluid diet at the time
the injection was given.   The frequency of the dose was gradually
diminished, and in three weeks was discontinued.   The paroxysms of
pain, which had ceased, remained absent for some months; but ultimately they recurred.   The aim of this treatment is to keep the patient
at absolute rest for a long period; not simply to keep him free from
pain.   In the earlier stages above all things the general health must
be regulated, constipation corrected, and all sources of worry or mental
anxiety avoided.

(b) *Local applications.*—Counter-irritation over the painful spots, or
the application of the actual cautery, may afford temporary relief.   In
the same way a paint of equal parts of camphor and chloral rubbed up
together, menthol in oil, or aconite ointment, may give relief in the earlier
stages; but later in the disease they are absolutely without effect.

The application of ethyl chloride spray, such as is commonly used in
minor surgical operations, will also give marked relief for a time, even
in severe cases, and is worth a more extended trial in those cases
where the paroxysms occur once or twice a day only.   The skin of the
face should be first protected with a thin coat of grease, and the eye
carefully guarded.

(c) *Galvanism.*—At one time the constant current, with the anode
resting on the painful point and the kathode on the neck, was considered
a valuable cure in trigeminal neuralgia.   This error undoubtedly arose
from a want of discrimination between neuralgia major and the minor
forms.   This method of treatment should always be tried, but it rarely
affords more than a temporary alleviation, if any.   Mr. Horsley mentions

a striking case (which I had an opportunity of seeing), where a sufferer from a tolerably severe major neuralgia, who had come into the hospital for operation, was cured, at any rate for a considerable time, by a three weeks' application of the constant current.

(*d*) *Climate.*—A quiet life in a warm, sunny climate seems to benefit many of these patients, but does not cure the cases which have already become severe. Many patients are undoubtedly worse by the sea; and, as in some cases of brachial neuritis, sea-bathing often increases the paroxysms.

(*e*) *Operative.* —The minor operations, such as resection or nerve stretching, are to be looked upon as no more than a profound kind of counter-irritation. For the details of these operations Krause's work or some text-book of surgery must be consulted. They afford relief for a considerable time in suitable cases, especially where the pain lies completely within the territory of one branch of the nerve; but ultimately the pain returns in nearly every case.

Rose attempted to reach the Gasserian ganglion at the base of the skull, and performed several operations by his method. But it was not until Krause and Hartley independently performed what is now known as the Krause-Hartley operation that excision of the ganglion became so far practicable as to need mention in a text-book of medicine. The operation is shortly as follows:—

A flap is turned down over the temporal fossa with its base at the zygoma. Krause forms an osteoplastic flap, but Horsley removes the bone with forceps after trephining; he then enlarges the opening until the lower and anterior third of the temporo-sphenoidal lobe has been laid bare, when, if the opening is of sufficient size, the temporo-sphenoidal lobe is seen covered by dura mater. The dura mater is next detached from the floor of the middle fossa of the skull, and the temporo-sphenoidal lobe, covered by dura mater, is held up with a retractor. Krause ligatures the middle meningeal and then divides it; but Horsley cuts it and finds it gives no trouble. The foramen rotundum and ovale now come into view. The cavum Meckelii, in which the ganglion lies, is now opened, and the ganglion is freed as far as possible. Then the second and third divisions are divided at the foramen rotundum and ovale, and the ophthalmic division is divided close to the ganglion (some of the ganglion is left attached to the stump) in order not to injure the fourth and sixth nerves which lie close to it. Lastly, the ganglion is steadily twisted and drawn upon, when the greater part of the root of the fifth nerve comes away attached to it. Those who have never seen this operation cannot realise how clearly the parts can be seen and individually dealt with.

The wound should heal by first intention, and no unsightly scar be left. The movements of the jaw are of course impaired, but not to such an extent as materially to interfere with the patient's comfort. Krause has performed thirty such operations, Hartley four, and Horsley eight, without a death. The first was performed five years ago, and in no case as yet has the disease recurred on the operated side. Thus we seem at last to have found a means of cure for the most terrible of all diseases.

Neuralgia due to organic lesions of the trigeminal nerve, or of its roots.—Certain neuralgic pains which accompany organic lesions of the nerves or nerve roots must be briefly mentioned here; not because they come within the true scope of this article, but because the diagnosis between them and neuralgia major is often extremely difficult during life.

Tumours of the cranial nerves not infrequently cause intense neuralgic pain radiating over the territory supplied by the fifth nerve. At other times the pain, though paroxysmal and aching in character, is local, and not referred along the course of the nerve. In both cases, however, there is usually marked loss of sensation over the area to which the affected branch is distributed. The root of the fifth nerve is not uncommouly involved in tumours growing from the meninges. Krause mentions a case of one of these tumours, around the root of the fifth nerve in a woman, which caused pain so exactly resembling neuralgia quinti major that he operated and successfully removed the ganglion. Fifteen days after the operation she complained of headache, the wound reopened, and finally, after a second exploratory operation, she died. A cholesteatoma of the arachnoid the size of a walnut was found lying in the middle fossa of the skull. Krause makes no mention of the presence or absence of anæsthesia; but in the cases I have seen of a similar pathological condition the loss of sensation was very well marked. In one of them, where the mass was malignant, the pain was characteristically neuralgic, but it occupied the whole of one-half of the face. In the second case a growth of small size on the root of the fifth nerve caused the headache, vomiting, and optic neuritis of a cerebral tumour, together with the progressive anæsthesia of the face so characteristic of a lesion of the trigeminal root. Without testing the sensation of the face the former of these closely simulated neuralgia major, the latter an ordinary cerebral tumour. Thus before operation in every case of neuralgia it is well, if possible, to take the opportunity of a period of freedom from pain to test the face carefully for anæsthesia, and to consider whether the symptoms might be due to an undiscovered neoplasm.

The outburst of herpes ophthalmicus, like herpes zoster, is frequently preceded by severe neuralgic pains which usually subside somewhat after the rash has come out, giving place to intense soreness due to the condition of the skin. Sometimes, especially in elderly people, or in those broken down in health, pain follows the rash, pain of agonising intensity and typical neuralgic character. This pain is confined to the area occupied by the eruptions, and is most marked in those portions of the skin where the scarring is deepest (*vide* article on "Herpes," in a later volume).

Tumours of the skull, especially gummata (nodes), cause intense neuralgic pain apart from implication of meninges. The anterior part of the temporal fossa is a not uncommon situation for a syphilitic gumma.

In this position it causes neuralgia over the whole of the temporal fossa, accompanied by marked tenderness of the superficial structures, not only over the actual gumma itself, but over a wide area in front of it, spreading out above and in front somewhat like a fan. This area corresponds to the distribution of the ascending branches passing from the deep parts of the fossa forwards and upwards to the scalp. It does not correspond to any area or combination of areas of referred pain such as are shown on Figure 44.

Some time after a fracture or injury to the skull neuralgic pains may arise, apart from neurasthenic or hysterical states. In a case where there had been a compound fracture of the centre of the frontal bone intense neuralgia came on, in attacks of considerable frequency, lasting for a week or more at a time. This pain, though unrelieved by trephining, was probably due to adhesions between the meninges, the scar, and the skin. In another case an intense neuralgic headache, limited to a spot two inches in diameter over the temporal fossa, followed a direct blow received in hunting. There was no pain elsewhere, and the patient was in no sense of the word neurasthenic. The pain was accompanied by intense tenderness, both superficial and deep, limited to this small area only ; and, although it throbbed and darted, it did not radiate elsewhere. Gunshot injuries of the skull are said occasionally to produce somewhat similar results ; I have, however, no experience of such injuries.

Neuralgia minor.—Within this group are included all those pains which, whether associated with localised pain in some organ or not, have certain characteristics which cause the patient to speak of them as "neuralgia." It may be that he suffers from an aching tooth accompanied by a shooting or boring pain over some part of the face ; or pain in the face may be present without any local manifestation pointing to affection of a tooth or other organ of the head.

In this section are grouped two forms of neura gia of different origin, but so closely resembling one another, if the pain only be considered, that they have been habitually confused : (i.) Visceral referred pain ; (ii.) True neuralgia minor.

(i.) *The characteristics of a visceral referred pain.*—Many of the pains to be dealt with in this group have not the neuralgic character, they do not give the impression to the patient of shooting along a nerve. Thus the majority of patients speak of the supraorbital pain produced by some error of refraction as a headache ; some, however, speak of it as a neuralgia. Again, iritis will cause intense neuralgia in the temple and cheek ; but if less acute the pain is described simply as aching. Thus it becomes necessary to include in this article on neuralgia all referred pains in the head, for it is a mere matter of severity and of the idiosyncrasy of the patient whether they are called neuralgia or not.

When the pulp of the tooth is exposed to irritation the patient frequently complains of pain in the face. This pain is of greater or less intensity and extent, and comes and goes in paroxysms of varying duration. Each paroxysm is either the single response of the inflamed pulp to stimulation, or is associated with some general state, such as hunger or fatigue. Pain is accompanied by tenderness of the skin and subcutaneous tissue of the face over an area of greater or less extent, according to the tooth affected. Whenever it accompanies visceral referred pain this soreness lies within areas (*vide* Fig. 43), which do not correspond to the distribution of peripheral nerves. During the actual paroxysm of pain tenderness of the skin is not usually perceived ; but it remains as a constant and troublesome consequence when the actual sharpness of the pain is passed. Thus the neuralgia itself is intermittent ; but so long as the attacks are not too far removed from one another tenderness is persistent. To demonstrate this tenderness, pick up the skin and subcutaneous tissues lightly between the finger and thumb ; as soon as the tender spot on the face is reached, the patient will complain that there he feels sore, tender, or bruised. Even a better way, in some cases, is to make light pressure with the spherical top of a common pin : when this is done, provided the hyperalgesia be considerable, the patient may complain that he is being pricked ; or, if less intense, that the head of the pin touches a sore, bruised place. In this way one or more areas can be marked out following the lines of those on Fig. 43.

The more prominent the pain the greater will be the tendency of the patient and of his medical attendant to call it neuralgia ; the greater the tenderness as opposed to pain, the more likely are they to call it headache or faceache.

Thus the characteristics of a visceral referred pain are—(*a*) The presence of pain over areas other than those peripheral nerves ; (*b*) the association of this pain with tenderness of the superficial structures of the head.

(ii.) *True neuralgia minor.*—There is, however, a second form of neuralgia minor which differs fundamentally from that just described, although in many cases it stands in relation to discoverable disease about some organ in the head. If, for instance, the periodontal membrane, lining the socket of one of the teeth of the upper jaw, be inflamed, it is not uncommon for the patient to complain of darting pain up the jaw and below the eye. Now such pain is typically " neuralgic " in character, but does not follow the lines laid down for a visceral referred pain. It is, as a rule, unaccompanied by superficial tenderness ; but when tenderness is present, the tender area represents the peripheral distribution of the affected nerve trunk. An exactly analogous phenomenon appears when the socket of the eyeball is invaded by a growth which does not invade the eye itself. It also appears in innumerable diseased conditions of the jaws and skull.

Such neuralgic pains follow the course seen in neuralgia quinti major ; and in the early stages of the latter disease it is often quite impossible to say whether the case will turn out to be of the major or the minor form. We can, however, say definitely at once that, by its distribution and the absence of true superficial tenderness, it is not a true referred visceral pain.

Thus we can formulate the differences between the two groups of pain included in neuralgia minor as follows :—

Referred Visceral Pain.	*Neuralgia Minor Proper.*
1. Pain usually accompanied by superficial tenderness.	1. Pain not usually accompanied by superficial tenderness.
2. Pain and superficial tenderness follow lines in the nervous system central to the peripheral nerves.	2. Pain (and when present tenderness) follows a distribution representing that of the main branches of the trigeminal.

Thus it is evident that the tender points described by Valleix can be of little importance in the diagnosis of "neuralgia." He states that in neuralgia certain tender points are to be found corresponding to the positions where nerves rise to the surface. He described four such "points douloureux" for the first division of the fifth, five for the second division, four for the third division, and twelve for the neck and arm. He stated that in every case upon which his observations were founded no visceral cause existed for the pain, which was therefore a pure neuralgia. An examination of his records at once proves this to have been erroneous. The majority were just those to which we should look for the appearance of more or less widespread visceral referred pain. Trousseau always held that Valleix had been misled by anatomy, and that in reality these tender points were areas of cutaneous hyperæsthesia representing the expansion of a nerve ; moreover, he showed that these tender areas may appear as the accompaniments of visceral disease. At this point he stopped, misled by an attachment to the word neuralgia ; and he did not draw the obvious deduction that such pains might arise from the disease of any organ.

A most characteristic feature of all these minor neuralgias is their tendency to cause pain in remote and unaffected organs. This is more particularly the case with visceral referred pain ; but it is also a marked feature of some neuralgias following a peripheral distribution. Thus glaucoma may cause the teeth of the upper jaw to ache and be tender to percussion, exactly as if they were affected with periodontitis. Exposure of the pulp of a molar tooth in the lower jaw may cause such intense pain as to mislead both patient and physician into thinking that the ear is diseased. I have once seen a perfectly healthy membrana tympani incised under such conditions for the relief of pain that entirely ceased with the destruction of an exposed nerve in the second molar of the lower jaw. In a second case where exploration of the mastoid was suggested, all pain and tenderness disappeared with removal of a carious lower molar tooth. Malignant disease of the lateral border of the tongue causes pain in the ear ; and I have seen a case in which much valuable time was lost owing to the patient's conviction that he was suffering from earache only. Again, pain produced by one tooth is particularly apt to be referred to another in the same or the opposing jaw. This reference, in my experience, is very rarely made to a tooth of the opposite half of the jaw.

Associated with both the referred visceral and the peripheral nerve form of neuralgia are certain interesting reflex effects. Referred pain from an exposed pulp in the upper jaw will sometimes cause marked conjunctival injection, or a reflex flow of tears. Salivation is also a well known accompaniment, especially of pain of dental origin. Tomes mentions a case in which by touching the exposed nerve of a first upper molar tooth he could at will produce injection of the conjunctiva, a profuse flow of tears, and an outpouring of saliva. I have seen pin-point pupils dilate to their normal size on the removal of a tooth that had caused persistent neuralgia from periodontitis.

All these minor neuralgias are remarkably affected by general states of the body. They are usually at their worst during hunger or fatigue, and improve or disappear to a remarkable degree after a meal or a night's rest—except, of course, in cases where the mastication of food stimulates an exposed pulp. Alcohol in most cases causes a marked improvement ; unless, again, the pain be due to a collection of pus at the root of a tooth, under which circumstances the throbbing pain, so characteristic of this condition, may be increased by the alcoholic stimulation of the cardio-vascular system. Of the effect of heat and cold within the mouth, when the neuralgia is due to affections of the teeth, I shall speak later. When the neuralgia is a true visceral referred pain—for example, from a tooth with an exposed pulp—sudden alterations in the temperature of the surrounding air are in all cases unpleasant. Thus, if a patient go from a warm room to the cold winter air the pain is increased, or a fresh attack induced ; but in most cases a continuous sojourn in the cold outer air is followed by marked diminution of the pain, or even by its disappearance. A return to the warm atmosphere of a room starts a fresh attack at once, which does not, as a rule, disappear, as was the case in the cold air. An attack nearly always comes on as the patient becomes warm in bed, and such patients are often at their worst when sitting by a fire. A clergyman who, until his teeth were removed, suffered for years from neuralgic pains of the visceral type, told me that for this reason he could never visit his parishioners during the winter. On the other hand, that form of neuralgic pain which is due to periostitis, or periodontitis, is decidedly increased by exposure to cold air, and is usually lessened by sitting over the fire, " or baking the face."

Of all general states of the body that have a profound influence on these minor neuralgias, anæmia is perhaps the most distinct. A patient may be anæmic, and yet suffer from no pain or tenderness. But as soon as some cause for referred pain is present, widespread and diffuse neuralgias make their appearance out of all proportion to the original focus of disease. In an anæmic person menstruation, hypermetropia, or caries of a tooth, may cause widespread pain and tenderness of the head and neck. A similar effect is produced by that cachexia which in some cases precedes, by a considerable period, the specific manifestations or signs of pulmonary phthisis. Pregnancy, again, is frequently accompanied by facial neuralgia, possibly owing to the readiness of the teeth to decay during gestation. A sudden rise of temperature will frequently produce an increase in a pre-existing neuralgia, especially if it be of the referred visceral type. But in some cases a sudden rise of temperature will produce widespread pain and tenderness of the scalp without our being able to recognise any area of primary disturbance. This condition is produced most easily by epidemic influenza; in this disease the patient complains of pains all over, and especially in the head. Careful examination shows that in many cases these pains, like referred pains, are associated with tenderness of the superficial structures of the forehead and scalp. Sometimes an attack of influenza will leave behind it persistent neuralgic pains which may belong to both the visceral and peripheral nerve types.

Abnormal mental states, neurasthenia and hysteria, also intensify these minor neuralgias. These will, however, be dealt with later, as more frequently they generate the neuralgia.

One thing that has tended to keep up the belief in the substantial existence of neuralgia as a disease has been the effect of treatment directed not to the cause, but to the pain itself. A leech or blister may relieve the pain for a considerable time, even though it be definitely referred from some visceral lesion. Thus a leech applied over the temples has a profound effect on the referred pain and tenderness of acute glaucoma. Violent counter-irritation seems to produce some effect upon the nervous system which prevents the generation of these pains, even though the focus of disease be untouched. Thus I have seen an operation on the skull, in which nothing was done to the nerve, abolish the most profound neuralgia major for nearly a week. A purge, or a full dose (5 to 8 grains) of quinine taken at night will often abolish a neuralgia definitely due to the exposure of an inflamed dental pulp. But the results of such treatment are extremely misleading, and in spite of the apparent cure the focus of disease should always be looked for carefully.

In neuralgia quinti major we saw that heredity played but a small part. With these lesser neuralgias, on the other hand, it is extremely common to find a tendency to nervous or mental disease. That in some cases even a direct tendency to neuralgic pains seems to be inherited cannot be a matter for wonder when we consider that errors of refraction and other painful eye affections tend to run in families, and that a tendency to early caries of the teeth is frequently hereditary. But since we no longer look upon neuralgia as a uniform disease the question of its heredity is of but little interest.

Neuralgia minor secondary to diseases of the teeth.—The first stage of caries of a tooth consists in the removal of the enamel and excavation of the underlying dentine. During this process pain may or may not be present, but can generally be elicited by stimulation of the affected tooth. The most effective stimuli in this condition are heat and cold; for in many cases, even where the carious part of a tooth can be cut away without pain, a jet of hot or cold water upon the exposed dentine will produce a twinge of pain. As long as the pulp cavity is not exposed the pain remains local, and the patient suffers simply from toothache, pointing to the peccant tooth as the source of his woe. The pain may dart and shoot, but the darting and shooting are practically confined to the aching tooth. Local stimulation produces local pain and neuralgia is absent. As soon as the pulp cavity is exposed the pain alters in character and distribution. It may start in the affected tooth and dart into the face, forehead, neck, or ear. Each stab of pain lasts a few moments, only to be followed more or less rapidly by a second twinge. Eating or any other such act stimulates the exposed pulp, increases the pain, or starts a paroxysm. Heat and cold taken into the mouth usually much increase the pain.

On testing the face or neck within the areas affected by this neuralgia more or less tenderness of the skin and superficial structures will be found over areas more or less corresponding to those shown in Fig. 43. On the face the tenderness is superficial; but parts of the jaw, mouth, and tongue may be tender at a distance from the affected tooth, owing to their participation in the area affected. Thus teeth at a distance from that affected may ache, and be tender to the touch.

Many patients are aware of the presence of this tenderness, and state that they first feel the darting and shooting pain, which seems to leave a soreness behind it. When such a tender area on the face is tested for tenderness it is not uncommon for the patient to complain that a touch within its limits seems to make the pain in the tooth worse. This tenderness does not arise until the neuralgia has lasted several hours, and it usually disappears, without further treatment, within twenty-four hours of the removal of the tooth. But in a few cases the pain and tenderness spread widely, extending even to the arm; such cases are best treated by cleaning out the wound produced by the extraction, and applying some preparation of cocaine. Such cases usually last about a week or ten days in the acute form, and then subside gradually. It may happen when the patient comes under observation that the pain has ceased for many hours; in such cases tenderness will probably be absent, and yet, from the account he gives of the nature and cause of his pain, it is certain that it was a visceral referred pain from some tooth. For instance, pain in the ear represents the maximum point of the hyoid area (vide Fig. 44); this area is peculiarly associated with the teeth of the lower jaw from the second bicuspid backwards. Thus we can argue that the patient who complains of referred pain in the ear is probably suffering from irritation of one of these teeth, although the pain may be unaccompanied by tenderness at the time of his visit.

Where the pulp becomes fibrous or calcareous it is not uncommon for the nerve, or part of the nerve, to retain some vitality in one root, although the pulp and nerve of the other root be dead. Irregular calcification, with the formation of pulp-stones, frequently leaves some living pulp, and is a potent cause of neuralgia. In all such cases attacks of neuralgia of the visceral referred type accompanied by superficial tenderness are apt to appear from time to time; and it is under these conditions more particularly that the dental origin of the neuralgia is most likely to be overlooked. There is no toothache, but the dying contents of a root tend to light up into activity from some indefinite cause; or the patient's general health deteriorates, and he suffers from a sharp attack of neuralgia which is put down purely to his lowered vitality. The pain passes off under general treatment, and its origin in a tooth remains unsuspected. The presence of superficial tenderness over one or more of the segmental areas of the face should have made the case clear, and directed attention to certain of the teeth amongst which the affected tooth would have been found.

So long as the pulp or contents of the root are living, inflammation of the cavity of the tooth will produce neuralgic pain of the referred visceral type. After caries has reached the pulp cavity many different changes can occur. The pulp and nerve become inflamed and reddened, and may die rapidly and steadily. Sometimes this inflammation and death of the pulp takes place with extreme rapidity, and four or five hours of agonising pain are followed by perfect peace. Sometimes, however, death takes place much more slowly; one part, or the whole of the pulp in the chamber of the tooth may die, and with it the nerve in one or more roots, yet the nerve in one root may remain alive and potent for harm for a long while. Again, the inflammation and death of the pulp may go on slowly under a cap of sodden dentine. Under all these conditions referred pain, accompanied by more or less superficial tenderness over the segmental areas of the face, is almost certain to make its appearance at some time or another.

The exact innervation of each tooth from the segmental areas seems to vary somewhat, but the following table gives the approximate supply, as it has been worked out at present :—

Upper Jaw.			*Lower Jaw.*	
Incisors . . .	Fronto-nasal.		Incisors . .	Mental.
Canine . . .	Naso-labial.		Canine . .	,,
1st Bicuspid .	,,		1st Bicuspid	,,
2nd Bicuspid .	Temporal or maxillary.		2nd Bicuspid	Doubtful.
			1st Molar .	Hyoid.
1st Molar . .	Maxillary.		2nd Molar .	,,
2nd Molar . .	Mandibular.		3rd Molar .	Superior laryngeal or hyoid.
3rd Molar . .	,,			

When the pulp and nerve are dead a tooth may still be a source of pain of neuralgic character, owing to inflammation of the periodontal membrane or abscess about the root; but this pain is usually local and situated in the tooth itself. If, however, the pain shoot from the tooth into the jaw and neuralgia appears, the distribution and the accompaniments of the pain in the vast majority of instances differ fundamentally from that produced by inflammation of the pulp: it closely follows that already described in neuralgia quinti major, and superficial tenderness over the visceral segmental areas of the face is extremely rare. A tooth in this condition frequently seems as if it were "too long" or "longer than the teeth around." Intermittent pressure on such a tooth, as in chewing, causes pain, but steady pressure relieves the pain for a while. The patient frequently pulls at such a tooth, moving it backwards and forwards for the sake of the subsequent ease produced by this momentarily painful manipulation. Cold water taken into the mouth usually eases the pain, but hot water nearly always increases it. Pressure sometimes causes a twinge of pain which travels beyond the limits of the tooth; thus when the periodontal membrane is inflamed pressure on a canine may cause a neuralgic pain which darts into the upper jaw and below the eye. Pressure on a lower bicuspid causes a pain to run along the jaw and affect all the teeth behind; this pain, however, does not come out upon the face, as with the upper canine. Thus in neither case does the pain follow the lines of segmental areas, but we see at once how closely it follows the distribution with which we are familiar in cases of neuralgia quinti major.

This neuralgic pain may arise without any conscious stimulation of the tooth, and the differential diagnosis then becomes of great importance. It can only be made by noting the direction of the pain and the absence of superficial tenderness.

Periodontitis or alveolar abscess may produce a pain away from the tooth affected in two ways. In the instances just given branches of the nerve (not the nerve endings to the pulp) are probably involved in the inflamed tissue; pain then radiates up the nerve exactly as pain radiates up the ulnar when the divided peripheral end has been caught in scar tissue. But periodontitis can cause radiating pain in another manner. Suppose a non-erupted dead wisdom tooth to lie below the gum, and to set up inflammation around it which involves the trunk of the nerves to the teeth in front: under such conditions the pain radiates along the branch of the nerve, and is felt in all the teeth of the lower jaw. This phenomenon corresponds to the radiation of pain to the little finger produced by implication of the trunk of the ulnar nerve in inflammation about the elbow joint.

Thus in tracing the dissolution of a tooth we first find local pain and tenderness due to early caries and exposure of the dentine with a healthy pulp; then referred pain of the visceral type, accompanied by more or less superficial tenderness, the consequence of chronic inflammation and destruction of the pulp tissue; and, lastly, after the death of the pulp, local pain and tenderness, with or without neuralgia, appear in consequence of periodontitis or abscess formation at the root; such pain follows the distribution of peripheral branches of the trigeminal and not segmental areas.

Before concluding this section I must allude to a curious form of neuralgia often accompanied by all the signs of widespread visceral referred pain, due apparently to what is known as "cross-bite."

Neuralgia minor secondary to changes in the eye.—Errors of refraction do not commonly give rise to neuralgic pain of any severity. Though an extremely fruitful source of headache the pain so produced is rarely paroxysmal, and its steady aching character leads patients to speak of it more often as a headache. Yet if the patient become anæmic, or the general health fail, this headache may present characters which lead the patient to complain of frontal neuralgia. It is necessary therefore to consider shortly the position and peculiar features of the headache due to errors of refraction. If asked to point out the situation of the pain the patient's right hand is usually placed over the forehead, with the hypothenar eminence over the centre of the right eyebrow and the second phalanges of the fingers over the centre of the left eyebrow. This position of the hand has led to the common statement that the headache is situated over the centre of the forehead; but the patient himself states that the headache is "over the eyes;" and if asked to point with two hands to its position he will place the tips of the fingers of each hand over the centre of each eyebrow.

This headache, as usual with referred pains of visceral origin, is associated with more or less superficial tenderness, which, in errors of refraction, lies over the mid-orbital area (*vide* Fig. 43). As a rule only the maximum of this area is present; but occasionally, especially if the patient be seen immediately after reading or sewing, the whole area may be tender.

This headache comes on in the morning as soon as the eyes are opened; and, unless the patient engage in near work, it gradually wears off during the day. It is intensified by reading or sewing; it disappears if the eye is put under atropine, and is worse over the eye with the more marked error of refraction, provided that this eye be not amblyopic.

Astigmatism of all kinds is a fruitful source of headache, and of the errors of refraction hypermetropic astigmatism is the most likely to cause headache. For whilst a simple error of $+1_D$ or $+2_D$ can frequently be neglected, an astigmatic error of $+1_D$ will not uncommonly produce the most definite pain and tenderness.

Simple myopia, however high the error, causes no such headache and tenderness. The myope sometimes complains of a tired, aching feeling over the forehead, which is never, either in intensity or character, the least like neuralgia. It is not accompanied by tenderness, and is always absent on awaking from a night's rest. In those uncommon cases, however, where myopia is associated with spasm of accommodation, referred visceral pain of considerable intensity and wide distribution may be present. It entirely disappears if the eye be put under atropine.

The gradual breakdown of accommodation which accompanies the establishment of presbyopia in a hypermetropic person of about forty, is not infrequently associated with very considerable discomfort. This entirely ceases when presbyopia is fully established, and headache ceases as vision fails for near objects. If, moreover, the patient is a woman, the association of the climacteric with the presbyopic failure may be responsible for much troublesome pain of the referred visceral type.

In all these conditions pain and tenderness originally lie over the mid-orbital region of the forehead; but if severe they tend to spread both forwards to the middle line of the forehead and backwards into the temporal fossa, and upon the vertex.

Usually the presence or absence of a headache, due to errors of refraction, depends directly upon the extent to which the eyes have been used. But in some cases the headache assumes a curious paroxysmal character. The patient may use his eyes continuously for near work, yet suffer from one or more attacks of headache only during the week. Such headaches are, however, extremely severe, are sometimes accompanied by vomiting, and not uncommonly interrupt the patient's work. They are then called megrim; but they differ from true megrim in the presence of marked superficial tenderness of the referred visceral type, in their bilateral distribution, and in the absence of any of the higher visual phenomena such as fortification figures.

When the deeper layers of the cornea are affected, as for instance, by a deep or ragged ulcer, or if the depth of the anterior chamber of the eye be increased by disease, very marked pain of a definitely neuralgic character may come on. The pain and tenderness are situated primarily over the fronto-nasal area, and the pain down the inner side of the nose is sometimes very decided. Later, if the lesion be very severe or the patient in ill-health, both pain and tenderness may spread backwards to the temple and scalp.

Of all the diseases of the eye iritis and glaucoma produce the most definite neuralgic pain. In both diseases the pain is primarily situated over the temporal and maxillary regions, but may spread forwards up to the middle line, or backwards and upwards to include the vertex. In iritis this neuralgic pain may be severe; but in glaucoma it may become agonising, and is frequently accompanied by vomiting and considerable prostration. In acute glaucoma the pain in the eye itself is so acute that, except from gross carelessness, there is no chance of an error in diagnosis; but in chronic glaucoma the neuralgia (referred visceral pain) may become so prominent a feature that its dependence on disease of the eye remains unrecognised. I once saw a patient who had been treated for intractable attacks of neuralgia for a month before it was recognised that she was suffering from glaucoma; by this time the sight of the affected eye was irretrievably lost. During an attack of glaucoma it is not uncommon for the teeth of the upper jaw to ache on the side affected; this is due to the frequency with which the maxillary segmental area becomes tender in consequence of rise of tension within the eyeball. If the pain and tenderness spread forwards to affect the frontal area, the teeth of the upper jaw ache up to the middle line; if they spread back, as is not uncommon in an attack of glaucoma, the teeth of the lower jaw may ache also. Occasionally the teeth affected are tender to percussion, as if affected with periodontitis. That this tenderness is reflex, and not due to any actual change in the sockets of the teeth, is shown by the daily variation in the position and number of the tender teeth, coincident with changes in the condition of the eye, and by its occurrence in an edentulous jaw.

Changes in the retina and optic nerve are, as a rule, unaccompanied by any marked pain. But there is a peculiar primary optic atrophy, due to some unknown cause, in which the progressive loss of vision is marked by severe pains in the head which are invariably called neuralgia. These pains are accompanied by soreness of the scalp. There are no associated signs of disease in any other part of the body or of the central nervous system. The three cases I have seen were all in women, and vision was completely lost. Beyond this point the disease, whatever its nature, does not seem to progress. Thus neuralgia of the forehead or scalp, with progressive loss of vision, should always lead us to look to the tension of the globe and the condition of the optic nerve.

Orbital growths, on the other hand, cause pain which is either local or follows the nerve, and is unaccompanied by tenderness of the forehead or scalp.

Neuralgia minor produced by disease of the ear.—Pain produced by lesions of the auditory meatus, from its opening to the membrana tympani, is local, though frequently severe. If, however, the membrana tympani or middle ear be affected, the pain will be referred to some point at a distance from the source of irritation, and may be accompanied by superficial tenderness. It is particularly prone to all those characters which lead the patient to speak of it as neuralgia. During suppuration in the middle ear, before perforation of the membrana tympani, the pain is intense; it is situated over the side and top of the head (vertical and temporal areas), and in and behind the ear (hyoid area). The former ceases when the discharge appears, but the pain and tenderness over the hyoid area usually remain. This persistence of tenderness over the hyoid area is probably due to inflammation of the membrana tympani, which continues to cause referred pain after the tension in the middle ear has been relieved.

A similar set of symptoms may be caused by the blocking of an already established opening in the membrana tympani.

Thus for practical purposes the hyoid area is that which most commonly appears in ear disease. The vertical and temporal areas of the scalp, which might lead to errors in diagnosis, are only present when tension in the middle ear rises to such an extent that the aural origin of the pain can scarcely be overlooked.

Neuralgia minor secondary to diseases of the tongue.—It is a well-known fact in surgery that malignant disease of the tongue may cause pain in the ear, or over the back of the head; in addition to the pain in the tongue itself. Gumma of the tongue may also cause pronounced neuralgic pains of the visceral type.

If the disease involve the anterior part of the tongue, pain is felt over the spot where the mental nerve rises through the deeper structures of the jaw to supply the skin. (The maximum of the mental area.) If the lateral part of the tongue only is implicated the patient complains of pain in the ear and behind the ramus of the lower jaw on the side affected. In such cases the hyoid area is tender. But as the disease is rarely confined to one part of the tongue, tenderness is generally found in some other area besides the hyoid. If the dorsum of the tongue is affected, the pain may be situated in the occipital region, and take the form of occipital neuralgia. But the presence of superficial tenderness at once reveals its true nature as a visceral referred pain.

Thus lesions of the tongue are associated with tenderness over three main areas: (a) mental area in disease of the anterior portion; (b) the hyoid area in disease of the lateral portion, and (c) the occipital area, when the disease is situated over the dorsum.

Diseases of the tonsil frequently cause pain behind the jaw, associated with superficial tenderness over the hyoid area. Though severe, this pain cannot possibly lead to any confusion.

Neuralgia minor due to diseases of the nose.—Few nasal affections are painful, and even in those that cause pain it is rarely acute enough to be spoken of as neuralgia. In inflammatory conditions of the olfactory portions of the nose and frontal sinuses, pain may appear over the fronto-nasal and mid-orbital areas of the forehead; but pain from this cause rarely reaches the intensity of a neuralgia, unless the patient be highly neurotic, or in a low state of health. Under such conditions operations directed to the removal of the primary cause do not always cure the pain.

With syphilitic disease of the bones of the nose much pain may be present. I have seen but few cases of this pain in its acuter form, and cannot say therefore whether it follows the lines of a referred visceral pain or not. It is situated over the forehead and over the eyes.

In many affections of the brain intense pain is felt which, till the nature of the disease is discovered, is not infrequently called neuralgia. Such pains, though in some cases neuralgic in character, do not come within the scope of the present chapter (*vide* article " Cerebral Tumour ").

Neuralgia and headache secondary to disease of the organs within the thorax and abdomen.—It has long been known that disease of the abdominal and thoracic viscera can cause pain in various parts of the head. But it was not until the discovery of the importance of superficial tenderness that the headache due to general diseased states, and those due to direct reference of visceral pain from the thorax and abdomen to the head, could be distinguished. In this section I shall only treat of the latter kind, reserving those pains in the head which are due to general diseased states for the succeeding section.

Any organ of the chest and abdomen may, under favourable con-ditions, cause referred visceral pain to the head. These pains in the head, like all other visceral pains, are associated with scalp tenderness. The head is not mapped out into areas, each of which represents some organ of the thorax and abdomen, as some would have it, but the areas on the head are segmentally coupled with those on the body, and thus stand only indirectly in relation with any particular organ in the body. For instance, the temporal area of the scalp is usually associated with the seventh dorsal area, which runs round from the back, below the angle of the scapula, to the epigastrium. Now, speaking broadly, it is quite immaterial, for the production of temporal headache with tenderness over the temporal area of the scalp, whether the disease be phthisis destroying the base of the lung, gastritis, certain forms of mitral disease, or anæmic gastralgia. The only necessary condition is that one of these diseases should produce a certain segmental area of cutaneous tenderness on the surface of the body (seventh dorsal), when the temporal area will appear irrespective of the nature of the disease.

I give a table showing the areas on the scalp which are coupled up with the areas on the trunk; upon it are marked the organs which, when diseased, are apt to cause the appearance of these segmental areas of the trunk with their accompanying areas on the head :—

Associated Area on Scalp.	Area on Body.	Organs in particular Relation with these Areas.
Fronto-nasal (? rostral) .	Cerv. 3	Apices of lungs, stomach, liver.
Fronto-nasal . . .	Cerv. 4	Aortic orifice (?)
Mid-orbital . . .	Dorsal 2	Lung, heart (ventricles), ascending arch of aorta.
,, . . .	Dorsal 3	Lung, heart (ventricles), arch of aorta.
	Dorsal 4	Lung, heart (ventricles).
Fronto-temporal . .	Dorsal 5	Lung, heart (occasionally).
,, . . .	Dorsal 6	Lower lobe of the lungs, heart (auricles).
Temporal	Dorsal 7	Bases of lungs, heart (auricles), stomach (cardiac end).
Vertical . . .	Dorsal 8	Stomach, liver, upper part of small intestine.
Parietal . . .	Dorsal 9	Stomach (pyloric end), upper part of small intestine.
Occipital	Dorsal 10	Liver, intestine, ovaries, testes (? stomach).
None . . .	Dorsal 11	Intestine, Fallopian tubes, uterus.
,, . . .	Dorsal 12	Intestine (colon), uterus, etc.

The degree to which these pains in the head intrude on the patient's consciousness varies greatly. Thus sometimes he is quite unaware that the scalp is tender, and the associated tenderness is only discovered by examination. Again, he may be aware of the soreness of the scalp, but he complains not of pain, but simply of tenderness over certain areas of the skin when he brushes his hair. He may, however, complain of headache, or finally of shooting neuralgic pains which, when they pass off, leave behind them a feeling of intense soreness. Thus the patient's indications give a clue solely to the intensity of this associated phenomenon. The acuter the pain in the body the more intense and "neuralgic" is the pain in the head likely to be. Thus in some cases of aortic disease, especially those with paroxysmal attacks of referred pain (secondary angina pectoris), patients complain bitterly of shooting and darting pains in the forehead and side of the head.

Neuralgia secondary to general disease.—(*a*) *Anæmia.*—Simple anæmia, as such, is not a cause of neuralgia ; for in cases of pernicious anæmia and of profuse hæmorrhage we observe no tendency to these pains. However, a referred visceral pain once started in such patient will spread widely. The majority of young girls suffering from anæmia (chlorosis) suffer from widespread neuralgi s of the referred visceral type associated with widespread areas of superficial tenderness. As, however, in a certain proportion of quite definite cases of this disease neuralgia is absent throughout, it seems rational to suppose that when neuralgia is a promi- nent feature it arises from some visceral disturbance, however slight, which, owing to the diminution of resistance within the nervous system, spreads widely and reaches an intensity out of all proportion to the original cause.

(*b*) *Diabetes.*—Neuralgias are common in diabetes, especially about the jaws and the face. These may possibly be due to the frequency with which the teeth decay, especially in the severer cases of diabetes. The presence of these pains has been said to vary with the quantity of sugar in the urine, but of this I have no experience. Whatever the cause of these neuralgic pains about the face there is no doubt that diabetics are prone to painful affections of the neuralgic kind, possibly due to neuritis, as is shown by the frequency of sciatica in this disease.

(*c*) *Malaria* is apt to produce the well-known "brow ague" now so little seen in this country. In the few cases I have seen this pain pre- ceded the paroxysm, and in one case seemed to alternate with the attacks or to replace them. It closely resembled the frontal pain of influenza.

(*d*) *Rheumatism* is frequently cited as a cause of neuralgia ; but amongst the many manifestations of acute and subacute rheumatism (of the kind associated with cardiac disease) there is no especial tendency to neuralgias of the head. Even "muscular rheumatism" (of the lumbago type) is not associated with neuralgia of the scalp or face. That these pains are relieved by salicylic acid and its derivatives is no proof that rheumatism is a factor in their production, for this drug relieves other pains which are obviously not of rheumatic origin. Thus to say that rheumatism is the cause of any particular neuralgia is but a cloak for our ignorance, and is particularly pernicious in that it tends to relieve the observer of further search for a cause. I have even heard the referred pain of an acute iritis called "rheumatic neuralgia." Now, whatever the cause of the iritis may have been, the pains it produced were exactly what we should expect from acute inflammation of the iris, and these, as such, should have attracted attention to the eye at once.

(*e*) *Hysteria and other mental states.*—Neurasthenia and hysteria are fruitful sources of neuralgia. The pain so commonly present in the back is associated with shooting pains in the occipital and vertical regions. Such local pains in the head may precede a hysteroid attack, or a true hystero-epileptic convulsion, by some hours or days. After such an attack such patients exhibit intense and widespread superficial tenderness of the whole body, including the head and neck; probably due to the diffusion of visceral pain consequent on the decreased resistance in the nervous system. An exactly similar condition may follow a true epileptic attack in which consciousness is lost, urine passed, and the tongue bitten.

Hypochondriacs and sufferers from visceral delusional insanity may suffer from extremely local and permanent pains of the head. These pains will be discussed in other articles; but I want to draw attention to certain cases where an outburst of insanity is heralded by a minor neuralgia exactly similar to that produced by disease of the teeth. In one such patient every possible care had been taken to see that there was no focus of disease in the teeth, yet for a few weeks preceding each relapse he was troubled with marked neuralgic pains exactly resembling those produced by caries of the lower molar teeth. In a second case an outburst of neuralgia was always the signal for a relapse into a condition of violent delusional insanity. All pain ceased immediately when the relapse fully declared itself.

Treatment.—The first and foremost rule in the treatment of these minor neuralgias is to find out the organ from which they arise, and to treat the conditions found there. To aid the discovery of this primary focus of disease has been the aim of the previous pages; yet after all we must confess that too often in cases of minor neuralgias the cause eludes us.

It is also of great importance to treat the general condition of the patient, even though the local cause of the neuralgia be already known. For, whatever the cause of the pain, it is always intensified by inanition, cachexia, anæmia, or any general diseased state of the body. Thus in the case of widespread headache due to hypermetropia in an anæmic person, the anæmia must be treated, as well as the error of refraction.

Wherever the neuralgia is supposed to bear any relation to syphilis or malaria the specific remedies will, of course, be tried before any other treatment is adopted.

The antipyrin group has an extremely good palliative effect on the minor neuralgias, and even when they depend on a definite visceral lesion will often completely remove them for a time. Phenacetin, the mildest of the group, in doses of from ten to fifteen grains, will completely relieve a referred visceral pain in the head whatever its origin. The primary minor neuralgias are less amenable to this group of drugs, but generally yield for a time to antipyrin or antifebrin.

Gelsemium and butyl chloral are invaluable in all minor neuralgias within the territory of the trigeminal, whether they be referred or not. These two drugs, and especially gelsemium, seem to act readily in those cases of primary minor neuralgia in which the antipyrin group is not so effective.

Nitroglycerine ($\frac{1}{100}$ to $\frac{1}{50}$ gr. three times daily) in some cases relieves these pains.

Bromides are extremely unsatisfactory, except where the pain has spread widely. Strychnia and nux vomica are often far more efficacious, probably by their tonic effect on the nervous system.

Of local treatment nothing is so good as a small blister, or a couple of leeches, applied to the spot of maximum pain. We do not know how either of these remedies acts, but in most cases of minor neuralgia they give ease with surprising rapidity and certainty, especially where the pain is referred.

Galvanism is often very useful, the anode being applied steadily over the painful spot and the kathode over the spine.

In all forms of minor neuralgia hypnotic suggestion has been used in many cases with considerable success, even in persons by no means hysterical.

HENRY HEAD.

REFERENCES

1. BENEDIKT. "Ueber Neuralgien und neuralgische Affectionen," *Klinische Zeit. und Streitfragen*, 1892.—2. BERNHARDT. Article in Northnagel's *Textbook*, Bd. xi. 2.—3. BOEUNEKEN. "Beitrag zur Aetiologie der Trigeminusneuralgie," *Berlin. klin. Wochenschrift*, 1893, No. 44.—4. DANA. *Journal of Nervous and Mental Disease*, 1891, No. 1.—5. HARTLEY. *New York Med. Journal*, vol. lv. 1892.—6. HORSLEY. *Brit. Med. Journal*, 1891; *Clinical Journal*, 1897.—7. KRAUSE. *Neuralgie des Trigeminus.* Leipzig, 1896.—8. MITCHELL, WEIR. *Injuries of Nerves.* Philadelphia, 1872.—9. NOTHNAGEL. "Schmerz und cutane Sensibilitätstörungen," *Virchow's Archiv*, liv. S. 121.—10. PUTNAM. *Boston Med. and Surgical Journal*, 1891.—11. ROSE. *Surgical Treatment of Neuralgia of the Fifth Nerve.* London, 1892.—12. TOURETTE, G. DE LA. "Note sur quelques paroxysmes hystériques peu conuUs," *Progrès médicale*, 1891, No. 31.—13. TROUSSEAU. *Clinique méd. de l'Hôtel-Dieu*, Lecture liv.—14. VALLEIX. *Traité des névralgies.* Paris, 1841.

H. H.

THE DISEASES OF THE CRANIAL NERVES

Prefatory note.—In the following chapter the cranial nerves have been studied chiefly from the side of the paralytic conditions which affect them ; a short anatomical account has been added, based largely on the recent work of Kölliker, and the pathological observations of many workers, to which I have added my personal experiences.

In the space allotted to me I can do no more than describe cursorily the clinical phenomena of the cranial nerve diseases. The subject of spasm as it affects these nerves is dealt with elsewhere ; and the important condition known as labyrinthine vertigo will find a place in a later article.

Treatment has been dealt with on general principles only, as its methods are in harmony with the therapeutics of other affections of the nervous system. For special forms of treatment the reader is referred to the articles upon diseases of the nose, eyes, ears, and throat.

THE OLFACTORY APPARATUS.—Situated in the Schneiderian mucous membrane is a large number of bipolar cells, whose protoplasmic processes ramify towards the surface, and whose axis-cylinder processes pass as olfactory nerves through the cribriform plate of the ethmoid bone. Entering the ventral surface of the olfactory bulb these fibres break up into end-tufts in the glomeruli of that body. In this situation they are in contact with the end-tufts of the protoplasmic processes of the so-called "mitral" cells of the olfactory bulb, whose axis-cylinder processes are continued along the olfactory tract towards the cerebral hemisphere. Some of the axis-cylinders of the "mitral" cells end in the cortex of the olfactory tract, the cells of which also send fibres to the hippocampal region and to the anterior commissure.

At the anterior perforated spot the olfactory tract divides into two roots, the external of which, passing towards the apex of the temporal lobe, contains fibres which end in the cortex of the hippocampal lobule; the mesial or smaller root is composed of the fibres which cross by the anterior commissure. According to Obersteiner another root passes directly to the optic thalamus, the existence of which is indicated chiefly by the presence there of "amyloid bodies."

For a complete comprehension of the olfactory centres a study of this apparatus, as it occurs throughout the mammalian series, is essential. But as it is impossible in a work of this nature to deal exhaustively with this subject a few principal facts only are given.

(a) All that remains in man of the great rhinencephalon of macrosmatic mammals is the olfactory bulb and tract, the anterior perforated spot, the two olfactory roots, and the uncinate gyrus,—a structure only seen on the mesial surface, and hidden by the temporo-sphenoidal lobe.

(b) In the anosmatics, such as the narwhal, the lobus hippocampi is a moderately well-formed structure. As this mammal does not possess an olfactory apparatus some other function must be fulfilled by it—a fact which indicates that this lobe is not concerned entirely with the sense of smell.

(c) The only structure which wholly disappears in the anosmatic mammal is, according to Hill, the *fascia dentata*, and this part varies with the relative development of the olfactory apparatus. According to the same observer, the anterior commissure and fornix vary in thickness with the relative development of the rhinencephalon; although neither is absent from anosmatic brains.

If we are asked therefore what is the present knowledge of the intracerebral course of the olfactory fibres, the following statements might be made : (a) That a certain number of fibres cross in the anterior commissure, forming the "pars olfactoria" of that structure ; (β) that a considerable number of fibres pass to the uncinate gyrus on the same side ; (γ) that some olfactory fibres are to be found in the neighbourhood of the internal capsule and optic thalamus ; and (δ) that a part of the anterior commissure forms a connecting strand between the hippocampal lobules on opposite sides.

Symptoms.—Anosmia, or loss of the sense of smell, is a rare symptom of nervous disease. Much more commonly it is due to local conditions within the nose; hence the value of a careful rhinoscopic examination in all cases in which this sense is either blunted, lost, or perverted. In testing the sense of smell, substances should be used which stimulate only the olfactory nerve and do not irritate the trigeminal branches; such are oil of cloves, camphor, musk, and assafœtida. Anosmia may arise from—

(1) Local inflammatory and other changes within the nasal chambers.

(2) From arrest of secretion and "trophic" changes in the mucous membrane in cases of paralysis of the trigeminal nerve.

(3) In fracture of the base of the skull involving the ethmoid bone and the branches of the olfactory nerve which perforate it.

(4) From diseases involving the olfactory bulb and tract in the anterior fossa. Besides local meningitis, syphilitic necrosis, and bony tumours in this situation, unilateral anosmia is of value for the topical diagnosis of tumours of the frontal lobe (see also p. 823).

(5) From disease involving the cortical centres of smell. In the recorded cases of this condition the most prominent symptom has been a perverted sensation of smell rather than a deprivation. Thus in the cases of Jackson and Beevor, Sander and M'Lane Hamilton, in which a new growth involved the tip of the temporo-sphenoidal lobe and the adjacent uncinate gyrus, an olfactory aura preceded an attack of unconsciousness. But for further facts upon this subject the reader is referred to the article on "Cerebral Localisation" in the next volume.

Anosmia occurs in hysterical patients in association with hemi-anæsthesia and other sensory disturbances characteristic of this condition, and its existence in several cases of tabes dorsalis has also been recorded.

Concerning the **treatment** of anosmia little need be said. In the majority of cases it is the treatment of the local nasal condition: if, on the other hand, intracranial disease is present, treatment will be carried out on the appropriate principles.

THE VISUAL SYSTEM.—**Course of the fibres.**—Recent investigation has shown that the optic nerves, chiasma, and tracts are composed of several bundles of fibres occupying more or less definite positions. The observations of Gudden, v. Monakow, Henschen, and others have demonstrated the existence of, first, a *direct bundle* of fibres passing between the central ganglia and the eye of the same side, and occupying the external part of the nerve. Upon the internal (mesial) aspect of the nerve is found a second bundle, which is continued into the opposite optic tract, to this the name *crossed bundle* has been applied; while, in a position relatively between the two, and occupying the more central parts of the nerve, is the *foveal* or *papillo-macular bundle*. The existence of this bundle, originally pointed out by Leber, has since been amply confirmed. In certain forms of retrobulbar neuritis, characterised clinically by central colour scotoma and blanching of the temporal side of the optic disc, a localised area of degeneration has been described in the optic nerve (Samelsohn, Nettleship, Uhthoff). In a case of this nature which I examined (21), the area of degeneration occupied, just behind the globe, a wedge-shaped zone on the temporal side, with the apex pointing towards the central artery ; but in front of the optic foramen the bundle extended across the middle zone of the nerve—facts which are in harmony with the observations of Samelsohn, Nettleship, Vossius, and Bunge.[1]

At the chiasma the direct bundle occupies an external and also slightly superior situation, and maintains, in the more anterior parts of the optic tract, a relatively similar position ; though Williamson's observation places it in a central position. The crossed bundle lies superior (Henschen) and inferior (Monakow) in the chiasma, internal and inferior in the optic tract ; while the macular bundle, occupying the central part of each symmetrical half of the chiasma, lies in the middle of the optic tract. As these tracts approach the central ganglia the fibres of the several bundles intermingle, so that it has been found as yet impossible, by the degenerative or other processes, to distinguish the one from the other.

It is apparent from these observations that the fibres from the temporal halves of the retina (nasal field) occupy a corresponding (external) position in the optic nerve and tract ; those from the nasal halves (temporal field) occupy a corresponding (internal) site in the optic nerve of the same and in the tract of the opposite side ; the macular bundle occupying a relatively central position in both the nerve and the tract.

Having in this way ascertained the presence of these bundles let us now inquire how they arise and where they terminate.

According to the recent investigations of Ramon y Cajal and others upon young mammals, there exists in the retina a layer of large ganglion cells, each of which has protoplasmic expansions, spreading in a horizontal direction in the internal plexiform stratum, and an axis-cylinder process which becomes an optic nerve-fibre. These axis-cylinders, passing by one or other of the bundles in the optic nerve and tract already described, reach the basal ganglia, where they terminate in the now well-known end-tufts of Golgi.

Optic tract fibres may be traced into three basal ganglionic structures : the anterior corpus quadrigeminum, the pulvinar thalami, and the external geniculate body. In the anterior quadrigeminal bodies the nerve-fibres do not appear to pass beyond the superficial stratum ; but in the pulvinar and external geniculate body there is a more general disappearance of tract fibres throughout the entire structure of these ganglia. In the external geniculate body the fibres of the crossed bundle of the nerve and tract form chiefly the ventral part of the capsular lining, while those of the direct bundle occupy the mesial and lateral aspects (Henschen).

---

[1] The recent experimental observations of Usher and Dean (22), following upon similar researches by Pick (10), show that secondary degeneration may be obtained in the optic nerve in the position of the macular bundle after destruction of the retina between the macula lutea and the optic disc.

The anatomical description of these structures is corroborated by experimental and pathological results. Von Monakow found, after unilateral ocular ablation in animals, atrophy of the optic nerve and of the opposite tract, along with atrophy of the external geniculate body and pulvinar thalami, the ganglion cells in these structures being preserved; but there was a disappearance of the cells of the superficial layer of the anterior quadrigeminal bodies: and Henschen, in several cases of complete unilateral optic atrophy in man, found degeneration in both external geniculate bodies—an observation confirmed by the researches of Leonowa in anophthalmic fœtuses.

Henschen has investigated a case of great interest bearing upon the whole visual pathway. In an old-standing case of complete blindness, due to destruction of the eyeballs from small-pox in early life, there was observed atrophy of both optic nerves, the chiasma, and the tracts; atrophy of the cells of the external geniculate body and ventral part of the pulvinar thalami; atrophy of the optic radiations, chiefly the middle portion, which is continued as part of the centrum ovale of the occipital lobes, and atrophy of the cortex of these lobes, more especially that of the calcarine fissure, and of Vicq d'Azyr's line.

As already stated, the observations of von Monakow have shown that enucleation of the eyeball in young animals is followed by atrophy of the cells in the superficial stratum of the anterior quadrigeminal bodies, while the cells of the pulvinar and external geniculate body remain intact.

Key and Retzius have pointed out that the fibres of the optic nerve and tract are of two kinds, the thick and the thin fibres; and Gudden showed that after lesion of the anterior quadrigeminal bodies in some animals (rabbit) the thin fibres suffered atrophy. In a case of complete unilateral optic atrophy, examined by Henschen, a certain number of fibres remained unaltered in the atrophied nerve; these were of fine calibre and occupied a dorsal position in the optic tract; and in another of Henschen's cases (Pt. 3, No. 20), in which the hemiopic pupillary reaction was obtained, a small softening of one optic tract was found on post-mortem examination, from which a degenerated strand on the dorso-mesial surface of the tract was traced. From these and other observations, it would seem that in the peripheral optic apparatus there are two sets of fibres having different functions: one associated with the transmission of visual impressions as such, while the other subserves the reflex contraction of the pupil.

It seems probable that the optico-pupillary fibres differ in appearance from the visual fibres, that they are of fine calibre, and arise in the cells of the anterior quadrigeminal bodies; and that, although they occupy a definite position in the optic tract, they are in all likelihood distributed equally over the whole retinal surface, ending, according to Ramon y Cajal, in relation with the expansions of the bipolar cells of the internal granular layer: the visual fibres, on the other hand, of large size, take origin in the multipolar cells, and terminate in end-tufts in the pulvinar thalami and external geniculate body.

Let us now consider the degenerations of the posterior visual segment, those which occur after removal or destruction of the occipito-angular region.

A. There are the experimental investigations on young mammals of Tartuferi, Gudden, Ganzer, and chiefly of von Monakow. Extirpation of the occipital lobe was found by the last observer to be followed by atrophy of the cells in the substance of the external geniculate body and the pulvinar thalami, and of the white matter of the anterior quadrigeminal body. On the other hand, division of the optic radiations was attended by a descending degeneration into the anterior corpora quadrigemina, and an ascending degeneration towards the cortex cerebri; from which he concluded that centrifugal fibres passed from the cortex to the anterior quadrigeminal bodies, and centripetal fibres from the basal ganglia to the cortex.[1]

B. There are the results of disease of the hind part of the brain in man, and chiefly of the occipital region. Here we are brought face to face with a large number of conflicting statements. After eliminating a vast array of partial or ill-recorded observations, we have chiefly to consider the facts detailed within the past few years by von Monakow, Vialet, and Henschen. A critical study of the observations of the two former show (*a*) that lesions of the hind brain involving the optic radiations are followed by degeneration of these tracts, the external geniculate bodies, the pulvinar thalami, and the anterior quadrigeminal bodies; (*b*) the observations of Vialet, more particularly, have shown that the fibres in relation with the calcarine fissure and the adjacent parts of the cuneus and lingual lobe occupy the middle and inferior portions of the optic radiations, and are distributed to the posterior and external parts of the pulvinar and external geniculate body—the most inferior of the strata in the radiations being localised in the lingual and fusiform gyri, the middle strata more especially in the cortex of the calcarine fissure; (*c*) that lesions involving the angular gyrus and convexity of the occipital lobe are followed by degeneration in the superior strata of the optic radiations, the anterior and superior parts of the optic thalamus and pulvinar thalami.

The observations of Henschen, on the other hand, and of Flechsig, working by the myelination method, indicate that the external geniculate body and the radiation from it to the calcarine fissure should alone be considered as visual in function.

It appears, therefore, that the optic radiations of Gratiolet may be divided into three distinct strata, having definite relations with the basal ganglia on the one hand and the cerebral cortex on the other; and if Henschen be correct in his view that the cortical centre of vision is localised in the lips of the calcarine fissure, the middle stratum of these radiations alone deserves this designation.

It is still a question how far the optic tracts and nerves undergo

---

[1] The recent experimental work on this subject by Dr. Ferrier and myself is published in *Phil. Trans.* vol. cxc. p. 1.

secondary degeneration after lesion of the occipito-angular region. Von Monakow found degeneration in these structures and atrophy of them after cortical and subcortical lesions, and in three out of five cases traced degeneration into the optic tracts and nerves; and this was observed also in the cases of Moeli and Zinn: but it is necessary to point out that the equally well-recorded cases of Vialet failed to show any change in these structures. And in a number of experiments upon excision of the occipital lobe and angular gyri, performed in association with Dr. Ferrier, no degeneration was observed in the optic nerves or tracts. The probability is that the basal ganglia—external geniculate body and pulvinar thalami — form, so to speak, a half-way house, where the fibres proceeding from the cerebral cortex on one side and from the retina on the other are broken by the intervention of end-tufts and cells, so that degeneration is effectually arrested; although in old-standing cases an atrophy of the secondary neurons, as is now known to happen, probably occurs. It would, therefore, be a point of great importance to investigate the degenerations following lesion of the basal ganglia alone; and this we are able to do by means of a case recorded by Henschen. As a result of complete destruction of the external geniculate body, accompanied by slight secondary implication of the pulvinar and posterior part of the internal capsule, this observer traced degeneration, on the one hand, through the middle and inferior parts of the optic radiations to the cortex of the occipital lobe; and, on the other hand, he found atrophy of the optic tract on the side of the lesion and a degenerated strand in both optic nerves occupying the position of the direct and crossed bundles already described. It is possible, however, that a direct tract may exist between the retina and the cortical centre for sight, although its existence is so far chiefly hypothetical.

By these means I have attempted to show that the visual path is composed of two distinct segments, an anterior (inferior) and a posterior (superior). It is essential to bear this arrangement in mind when discussing the symptoms due to interference with the optic apparatus. It is demonstrated that of the fibres composing the optic nerve some come from the temporal side of the retina, others from the nasal side, and a third from the papillo-macular region; that at the optic chiasma some of the fibres pass directly into the optic tract of the corresponding side, while others decussate into the opposite optic tract; that, of the fibres which form the optic tract, some come from the superficial layers of the anterior quadrigeminal bodies, others pass into the external geniculate bodies, and a third set into the pulvinar thalami, while, according to some observers, a fourth set is continued directly into the optic radiations; that fibres pass out of the external geniculate body and pulvinar thalami to be continued towards the posterior part of the cerebrum as the optic radiations of Gratiolet; that the fibres occupying the superior layer of this radiation pass towards the cortex of the angular gyrus, those occupying the middle stratum towards the cortex of the calcarine fissure, and those of the inferior layer towards the cortex of the lingual and fusiform gyri.

Henschen has located the cortical centre for vision in the cortex of the calcarine fissure. It is highly improbable, in view of many physiological and clinical phenomena, that the cortical centre is thus narrowly circumscribed. It would appear indeed, from the degenerations already mentioned, that the cortical visual centre in man is situated in the region of the angular gyrus, the cuneus, the calcarine fissure, and probably also the lingual and fusiform gyri.

But, in addition to the great system of visual projection fibres just described, certain other tracts have important connections with the cortical centre for sight. The observations of Monakow, Déjérine, and Vialet have shown that after ablation or destruction of the occipital lobe degeneration may be traced through the forceps corporis callosi and the splenium into the occipital lobe of the opposite side. These are, no doubt, commissural fibres connecting similar portions of the occipital lobes on opposite sides; just as the experimental observations of Muratoff have shown that analogous portions of the Rolandic area are commissurally related through the corpus callosum.

Déjérine and Vialet have also observed a band of degeneration passing forwards into the temporal lobe in cases of softening of the occipital lobe, and more especially of the gyrus lingualis. In their opinion this bundle —fasciculus longitudinalis inferior—connects the cortical centre for sight with the auditory speech-centre in the first temporal gyrus.

The optico-pupillary fibres.—The course of the fibres subserving the pupillary light-reflex is not yet definitely known. There is sufficient evidence at hand, however, to show that in the optic nerve lie two kinds of nerve fibres, large and small; and it has been suggested that those of small calibre are more especially related to the action of the pupil (*ante*, p. 756). Several statements have been made regarding the position of the pupillary fibres posterior to the optic chiasma, chiefly from experiments upon animals. Bechterew has stated that the pupillary fibres pass from the posterior border of the optic chiasma into the gray matter surrounding the third ventricle, and thence directly to the nucleus of the third nerve—a view which has received some confirmation from the clinico-pathological observations of Moeli and Henschen. But it is impossible to believe, in view of the hemiopic pupillary reaction which accompanies lesion of the optic tract, that all the pupillary fibres take this course. Whether the results of experiments obtained by Darkschewitsch and Mendel reveal the actual course of the fibres as happens in man is also open to doubt. According to these investigators, the pupillary fibres leave the optic tract in the region of the external geniculate body and pass to the ganglion habenulæ, from which they proceed by the posterior commissure to the nucleus of the opposite third nerve. The most recent histological investigations of Ramon y Cajal and Kölliker indicate that fibres leave the optic tract and terminate in cells in the superficial layers of the anterior corpora quadrigemina, which cells send their protoplasmic processes and collaterals to the nucleus of the third nerve. These fibres are seen in sections of this region passing from the anterior quadrigeminal bodies to the third nerve nucleus in the Sylvian gray matter. Should they be shown eventually to be the optico-pupillary fibres, as there is reason to believe they are, the view originally expressed by Meynert again comes to the front. In this connection an observation of Ross is of importance, for he showed (12), in a case of tabes dorsalis, that the abolition of the pupillary light reflex was associated with the degeneration of Meynert's fibres.

But these are not the only fibres of the visual system which come to the anterior quadrigeminal bodies. It has been shown already that atrophy of these structures has been found, by von Monakow and others, to follow ablation of the occipital lobe; and in my experiments with Dr. Ferrier fibres were traced along the optic radiations and through the pulvinar thalami to the middle zone of the anterior quadrigeminal bodies after excision of the occipital lobe, but not after destruction of the angular gyrus.

When the hemiopic pupillary reaction is considered later from a clinical point of view, further facts will be adduced to show that the pupillary fibres probably do not pass either into the external geniculate body or pulvinar thalami, but pass directly into the superficial layers of the anterior corpora quadrigemina; and that a partial decussation of pupillary fibres must occur at the optic chiasma, along with the partial decussation of visual fibres, and in relation to them.

Symptoms of disease of the visual apparatus. — Disease may affect the several parts of the visual apparatus just described. It is unnecessary in this article to describe the ophthalmoscopic appearances of the general conditions affecting the optic nerve—optic neuritis and optic atrophy (primary and secondary)—concerning which the reader is referred to the chapter on medical ophthalmoscopy (p. 826), and to special works on the subject.

Optic nerve. — Besides optic neuritis and optic atrophy, as significant of inflammatory and degenerative changes in the central nervous system, the functions of the optic nerve may be arrested under local conditions, such as inflammation and hæmorrhage within the nerve sheath, traumatism, and embolism of the central artery. As a result of such lesions vision may be suddenly lost; but this is not necessarily associated at the outset with any obvious ophthalmoscopic change. Atrophy of the nerve usually ensues, preceded in some instances by slight inflammation of the optic papilla.

Neuritis of the optic nerve, apart from that associated with intracranial tumours, is seen in the acute retrobulbar form attributed to certain toxic agents, such as lead; or to general diathetic conditions, such as rheumatism, anæmia, influenza, and the exanthems; while a more chronic and specialised variety is seen in the common tobacco or toxic amblyopia.

As regards vision in lesions of the optic nerve, it may be stated that in optic neuritis vision may be entirely unaffected, even in an advanced stage of the disease. On the other hand it may be lost suddenly. Various forms of hemianopsia may coexist with optic neuritis depending upon interference with the visual fibres in higher portions of the brain.

Loss of vision again may be gradual, as occurs in tabetic or primary atrophy from other causes, such as disseminated sclerosis. Such loss of vision does not necessarily take place throughout the whole extent of the visual field; on the one hand peripheral contraction may be found, or on the other hand loss of central vision only. In illustration of the former may be mentioned a case of primary tabetic optic atrophy with marked contraction of the whole visual field, while a small area of central vision remained acute, so that the patient saw $\frac{6}{12}$ with the right eye, and $\frac{6}{9}$ with the left. A perimetric chart in such cases shows merely a small central spot of clear vision around the point of fixation.[1] Examples of the latter are seen in the cases of "toxic amblyopia," where central vision, at first for colours and later for light in severe cases, may be abolished, but with good peripheral vision. The explanation of this would seem to be due to the implication of the papillo-macular bundle in the latter forms, as pathological examination of the nerve has shown; in the former variety this bundle escapes, or is implicated in the late stages.

In disease of the optic nerve the reaction of the pupil to light becomes impaired, and with the abolition of the light perception the reflex pupillary contraction is arrested. If the optic nerve is completely divided both light perception and the pupillary light reaction are abolished. There are instances, however, in which the pupillary light-reflex is recorded with complete blindness and optic atrophy. A possible explanation of such cases is, that the pupillary fibres remain free from the sclerotic degeneration—an argument, however, for which there is little pathological evidence.

In addition to abolition of pupillary reflex, arrest of the functions of the optic nerve is accompanied by dilatation of the pupil. Should the nerve be but partially destroyed a characteristic feature is the dilatation which occurs after the contraction on exposure to light.

Chiasma.—The arrangement of the fibres in this structure explains the features brought out by disease. The characteristic symptom of lesion of the optic chiasma is *bitemporal hemianopsia*, due to interference with the fibres from the nasal halves of the retina.

The chief causes of this condition are tumours (syphilitic or other) in the pituitary fossa, or of the third ventricle (chiefly dilatation). Acromegaly, a condition accompanied by, if not actually due to hypertrophy of the pituitary body, with secondary enlargement of the pituitary fossa, is not uncommonly associated with bitemporal hemianopsia; from pressure upon the nasal fibres of the optic tracts. A curious case in which an aneurysm divided the chiasma in the middle line has been recorded by Weir Mitchell. Although in simple cases lesion of the chiasma would be accompanied by this form of hemianopsia, yet in practice various forms of scotoma

[1] Some instructive charts illustrating this are to be found in Dr. Byrom Bramwell's *Atlas*, vol. xi. p. 50.

are seen, due to unequal pressure upon its fibres, or unequal destruction of them. In one of Henschen's cases a gummatous tumour of this region caused blindness in one eye and temporal hemianopsia in the other; in the later stages vision may be entirely abolished in both eyes.

. If a lesion involve the non-decussating fibres of the chiasma on one side nasal hemianopsia results. A very rare condition is *binasal hemianopsia ;* a case of this kind has been recorded by Knapp as a result of bilateral pressure from calcified carotid arteries.

It may be supposed that a lesion may be so situated in the chiasma as to cause lateral hemianopsia (homonymous). This symptom, however, is characteristic of lesions of the visual path above the chiasma, and will therefore be considered next.

It is well also to bear in mind that a growth in the pituitary fossa may reach a considerable size without causing any such localising symptoms as have been described.

Homonymous hemianopsia, or blindness of the corresponding halves of both retinæ, is due to interruption of the visual fibres in the optic tract, basal ganglia, and optic radiations, and destruction of the centres in the cerebral cortex. As this subject, in relation to cerebral localisation, will be considered in detail in another article, it will be treated here from a general standpoint rather than in respect of lesions of any particular part of the visual tract.

The line of demarcation between the seeing and the blind halves of the retina may or may not pass through the fixation point; which point corresponds to the macular region, and is supplied by the papillo-macular bundle of fibres of the nerve. According to Sir William Gowers, it is doubtful whether the fixation point ever proves to be completely divided when carefully tested. If this be so, it is always included in the seeing, never in the blind half. This fact presupposes a special immunity on the part of the central bundle, its origin from both cerebral hemispheres, or its separate representation in the cerebral cortex, distinct from the retinal halves. The first supposition does not hold, because we have seen that the macular bundle is peculiarly liable to the influence of certain toxic agents; the second is probable, although there are not yet any definite anatomical facts bearing on the subject, the statement having been made by some, however, that at the chiasma, macular fibres pass from one optic nerve into both tracts; but both experimental and clinical evidence support the third (3).

It is not to be supposed, however, that there is a hard and fast line of demarcation between the portion of the retina supplied by the macular fibres and the general retinal area. In homonymous hemianopsia the blind halves, although not including the fixation point, pass over and involve a portion of the area supplied by the macular fibres; and, conversely, destruction of the angular gyrus, which is by some regarded as the cortical centre of the macular region, produces, temporarily at least, defect of vision over more than the papillo-macular area of the opposite eye (crossed amblyopia). It is therefore seen that an admixture of general retinal and macular fibres obtains, owing to which recovery may take place to some extent, blindness remaining permanently in that portion which is chiefly represented in the fibres or centres destroyed. Thus homonymous hemianopsia may clear up from the centre towards the periphery, so as to leave a symmetrical peripheral loss (Gowers); amblyopia from lesion of the central (foveal) fibres lessens from the periphery towards the centre.

In studying perimetrically a case of homonymous hemianopsia, in addition to the loss of vision in the correlated half-fields, more or less peripheral restriction of the seeing halves is not uncommonly found. This does not characterise lesion of any particular part of the visual path, for it may be met with from lesions situated anywhere between the optic chiasma and the cerebral cortex. That this is not necessarily due to implication of the angular gyrus, in addition to the occipital lobes or optic radiations, is shown in a case recorded by Dr. Bramwell, where a limited softening of the posterior part of the cuneus caused homonymous hemianopsia with peripheral restriction of the seeing halves. According to Wilbrand this is due to a superadded functional element.

There are various individual differences in the position and course of the dividing line. In some cases it is vertical, in others oblique ; or it may be straight, or irregular. It is probable that these variations are due to peculiarities in the decussation of the optic fibres at the chiasma, rather than suggestive of lesions in particular localities.

Although complete homonymous hemianopsia is the rule, several irregular and incomplete forms have been observed. Thus a sector or *quadrant hemianopsia* has been described, in which correlated retinal quadrants have been rendered blind ; it has been supposed that this form is due to lesion of corresponding portions of the cortical visual centre, as in the cases recorded by Hun and Doyne.

But the clinico-pathological evidence on this point is meagre and unsatisfactory, especially when it is borne in mind that *complete* homonymous hemianopsia results, not only from lesion limited to the calcarine fissure (Henschen, Nordensen), but also from lesions involving the anterior or posterior parts only of the cuneus, or the lingual gyrus. So far as observation has yet gone, there is not sufficient evidence to affirm that the several retinal segments are related to distinct areas in the cortical centre for sight.

There are also various forms of *irregular hemianopsia*, giving peculiar perimetric tracings, which cannot be put down to any definite lesion, but which are probably due to local inflammatory or other destructive change in the retina, optic nerve, or tract. A *monocular hemianopsia*, due to partial lesion of the optic nerve from fracture through the optic foramen, has been described by Wilbrand.

In the vast majority of cases hemianopsia is absolute ; that is to say, there is loss of colour, form, and light senses : there are, however, several cases on record in which the loss of colour sense only was observed ; but, as Mackay has pointed out, it is very improbable that on careful testing this ever proves to be the case. Mackay has shown, both from recorded and from original cases, that in these examples there is defect of form-sense as well as a peripheral defect of the light-sense. The view most in accordance with the facts, so far as yet ascertained, is that loss of colour vision in the half-fields, be it partial or complete, and hemianopsy, partial or complete, are merely manifestations of varying degrees of visual disturbance in the cerebral centres of sight. This is well illustrated in a case recorded by Vialet where, with complete hemi-achromatopsia, there was associated partial hemianopsia,—a condition, however, which passed into absolute hemianopsia before death. On this hypothesis the loss of colour-sense is regarded as the earliest manifestation of implication of the visual centres; and, depending upon the extent and intensity of the destruction, more or less defect of form and light-senses is associated with it. In central colour scotoma from toxic causes, loss of the senses of red and green may be looked upon merely as antecedents to complete loss of form and light, which latter are met with in severe and advanced cases. No support can, therefore, be given to the opinion that separate centres exist for colour vision of the correlated retinal halves, or separate tracts of fibres for the conduction of colour impressions.[1]

Let us now briefly consider how far we may discriminate between lesions of the several parts of the visual path. Homonymous hemianopsia, occurring without any other associated localising symptom, is due to destructive lesions of the half-vision centres in the cerebral cortex, or of the subjacent optic radiations in the occipital lobe. Right-sided hemianopsia may or may not be associated with one or other, or with both forms of sensory aphasia (word-blindness or word-deafness). If such symptoms coexist the combination shows not only an implication of the optic radiations, but also of the cortical gray matter of the angular gyrus, the first temporal convolution, or both. Word-blindness existing by itself points conclusively to the fact that the subjacent optic radiations are not involved, but the angular gyrus alone.

When hemianopsia is associated with hemiplegia and hemianæsthesia, or with the latter alone, the lesion may with confidence be placed in the retro-lenticular part of the internal capsule and in the posterior limb of the same. Destructive lesions of the basal ganglia are usually accompanied by hemianopsia; but it is still doubtful how far this is due to direct interference with the functions of the ganglia, or to indirect implication of the optic radiations at the posterior part of the interior capsule. Henschen believes that destruction of the external geniculate body alone is productive of hemianopsia; but the case from which he deduces this statement is by no means conclusive, as the pulvinar thalami was

---

[1] The view expressed here is in accordance with the general principle that the more fundamental the form of sensation the more widespread is the provision for its representation and conduction. Hence we find that specialised forms of sensation, such as the appreciation of colour, are lost earlier than the more fundamental one of light, whether the lesion involve the conducting tracts or the cortical centres.

partially involved : and Dr. Ferrier and I have recorded an experiment in which destruction of the pulvinar thalami was followed by homonymous hemianopsia, the external geniculate body being intact. Lesion of the optic tract causing hemianopsia may or may not be associated with localising symptoms, such as hemiplegia or paralysis of the oculo-motor or other cranial nerves. There is one sign, however, which is supposed to be diagnostic of a lesion of the optic tract, and that is the hemiopic pupillary reaction.

The hemiopic pupillary reaction. — This symptom, originally described by Wernicke, has been regarded as diagnostic of lesion of the optic tract. It has recently been considered critically by Henschen, who has collected all the cases in which the observation of this symptom was followed by a necropsy.

When a narrow pencil of light is thrown upon the blind halves of the retina no pupillary contraction is observed, or merely a sluggish one ; when, on the other hand, the light is turned on to the seeing halves the pupil contracts normally. This symptom, therefore, presupposes the existence in the optic tract of pupillary fibres corresponding to the visual fibres from correlated retinal halves. Fifteen cases have thus far been recorded in which this symptom was noted during life, and a necropsy obtained. The lesions consisted of softenings, hæmorrhage, and tumours involving the optic radiations, the basal ganglia, and the optic tract. The general conclusions which may be drawn from them are—

(*a*) That softenings or tumours involving the optic radiations do not give rise to the hemiopic pupillary reaction, unless indirectly by pressure upon the optic tracts.

(*b*) That lesions of the optic tracts, whether these parts are involved directly or by pressure from a distance, are accompanied by this form of pupillary reaction.

(*c*) That lesions of the basal ganglia—external geniculate body and pulvinar thalami—do not of necessity give rise to the hemiopic pupillary reaction. They are not uncommonly associated with it, but merely by secondary implication of the tract fibres.

The hemiopic pupillary reaction has also been observed in the bitemporal hemianopsia occurring in acromegaly (Asmus) and other affections of the optic chiasma (Peretti, Seguin). In a case of left-sided monocular temporal hemianopsia, mentioned by Wilbrand, due to fracture through the optic foramen, the hemiopic pupillary reaction was present in the left eye.

As pointed out when the course of the pupillary fibres was being discussed, and as the observations on the hemiopic pupillary reaction clearly show, it is impossible to support the view of Bechterew as to the passage of all the optico-pupillary fibres by the floor of the third ventricle in man. It is as yet, however, impossible to say whether the views of Darkschewitsch and Mendel, or those originally proposed by Meynert, state truly the course of these fibres.

THE OCULO-MOTOR NERVES.—Under this head are included the third, fourth, and sixth pairs of cranial nerves. These nerves may be affected by disease together or individually; while the symptoms thus produced may be unilateral or bilateral, according to the position of the lesion. In associated actions they work harmoniously, showing that an intimate connection exists between the several nuclei. It is my intention to describe first their anatomical relations and connections; then to give in detail the symptoms of paralysis of individual muscles and nerves; and, finally, to consider associated paralyses and ophthalmoplegia.

The third nerve nucleus.—The groups of cells forming the nucleus of the third cranial nerve lie in the anterior part of the Sylvian gray matter, corresponding to the position of the anterior quadrigeminal bodies and the posterior part of the third ventricle. The nucleus is segmented, and in this respect is analogous to what is seen both in the facial and hypoglossal nuclei. The several cell-groups lie laterally as well as anteroposteriorly to each other. Various observers have described the character and arrangement of the cells (Gudden, Perlia, and others), but that given by Bruce is the one adopted here.

According to Bruce, whose terminology is consistent with the erect posture, the arrangement of the cell-groups is as follows: inferior, superior, anterior, and external groups; postero-internal and postero-external, and an unpaired median nucleus. The anterior group is composed of large cells, and extends from the lower end of the nucleus to immediately below the superior group; and commissural fibres unite the nuclei of opposite sides. Composed also of large cells is the postero-external group, having a distinct outline external to the posterior longitudinal bundles, and forming the external group. The postero-internal group is characterised by its pale colour, and the superior nucleus is formed of small cells, and lies well in advance of the other cell-groups, and external to them. This is the antero-lateral nucleus of Darkschewitsch, which lies amongst the fibres of the posterior longitudinal bundles, and is in direct relation with many of the fibres of the posterior commissure. Kölliker denies the relation of this group to the third nerve nucleus, from the facts that many of the fibres of the longitudinal bundles end in it, and that a large number of posterior commissural fibres spring therefrom.

As Bruce's terminology and description of this nucleus has not as yet been adopted by text-books, I append a table showing the connection between the groups here described and those met with in the current literature on the subject:—

Anterior nucleus { inferior group—postero-ventral.
                 { main group—antero-ventral of Siemerling.
Posterior-external—Dorsal nucleus of Edinger and Siemerling.
Median nucleus—Nucleus impar.
Posterior-internal—Edinger-Westphal nucleus.
Superior group { Antero-lateral nucleus of Darkschewitsch.
               { Deep nucleus of the posterior commissure (Kölliker).

It appears from Bruce's observations, that between the lower end of the true third nucleus and the fourth or trochlear, there is a small group of cells which he has named the inferior group. It is possible that this may correspond with that which Siemerling has described as the nucleus of the levator palpebræ muscle, and with that which Kausch regards as the true trochlear nucleus; but on neither of these points is the evidence yet sufficiently definite.

The several cell-groups supply root-fibres according to their position; thus the innermost root-fibres of the nerve spring from the median and postero-internal groups, the outermost from the postero-external and external groups; while the superior group gives rise to the uppermost fibres.

Notwithstanding the experimental researches of Hensen and Volckers, and the clinico-anatomical observations of Kahler and Pick, Starr, Siemerling, and others, the relations of the various groups of cells to individual ocular muscles are as yet quite undefined. One fact, however, is ascertained, that the cells which subserve the internal muscular mechanisms of the globe and the light-reflex of the iris lie in the superior part of the nucleus, and give fibres to the uppermost roots; those supplying the external ocular muscles situated in the posterior part send their processes by the mesial and the lower root-fibres. In spite of the views of Kölliker the superior cell-group appears to be the centre for some at least of the internal ocular movements, probably for the pupillary light-reflex, and not the postero-internal group as Westphal suggested.

It is reasonable to suppose that the cell-groups already described, instead of supplying individual muscles, are centres of innervation for muscular movements. For example, the superior rectus, inferior oblique, and levator palpebræ superioris, being influential in raising the eyeball and upper lid, are probably supplied from the same or adjacent nuclei; and the contraction of the pupil which occurs with the associated action of the internal recti muscles in convergence suggests one centre, or closely related centres, for this action.

Kahler and Pick have given the following relations as those probably existing in the third nerve nucleus in man. Belonging to the median groups of cells are—from above downwards—the ciliary muscle, the sphincter iridis, the rectus internus, and the rectus inferior; served by the lateral groups are the levator palpebræ superioris, the rectus superior, and the obliquus inferior. In Starr's arrangement the ciliary muscle is placed in the lateral group; while, according to Siemerling's observations, the levator palpebræ superioris occupies the most inferior position of the group.

The *connections of the third nerve nucleus* are—

(i.) With the cerebral cortex through the pyramidal tracts. The exact position of these fibres is not yet definitely determined, but they probably lie in the anterior limb of the internal capsule, in close relation to the "knee." In the crus they lie mesially, but just external, and mingling with the fibres of the fronto-pontine tract.

(ii.) With the posterior longitudinal bundles, which connect the third nucleus with those of the fourth and sixth nerves, and with the other motor cranial nuclei and probably also with the anterior horns of the spinal cords, through their continuations—the antero-lateral ground bundles.

(iii.) With the optic tracts. This again is not yet definitely determined; but fibres pass from the superficial layers of the anterior quadrigeminal bodies, in which certain of the optic tract fibres terminate, to the Sylvian gray matter (*vide* p. 756), and we have already seen the very close relation which exists between the superior nucleus and the fibres of the posterior commissure, by which route, according to Darkschewitsch and Mendel, the pupillary fibres of the optic tract are supposed to reach the third nucleus.

(iv.) A connection probably exists, although not yet definitely determined anatomically, between the third nerve nucleus and the trunk of the facial nerve (*vide* under "Seventh nerve").

A point of some practical importance, namely, the connections between the two third nuclei and the third nerves, is still under discussion. There is undoubtedly in some animals (for example, in the rabbit) a half-crossed origin of third nerve root-fibres. The most recent observations of Perlia and Kölliker show that a similar decussation of root-fibres occurs in man; but it is doubtful whether the mesial root-fibres decussate (Perlia), or those which lie laterally (Kölliker). Throughout the greater part of the nucleus commissural fibres exist.

Lying in the peripheral part of the Sylvian gray matter, external and dorsal to the third nerve nucleus, is a crescentic layer of large cells, giving origin to the so-called "descending" trigeminal root. These cells have normally no connection with the fibres of the third nerve; but in some rare cases, to be described later (p. 783), it would appear as if such a connection were possible and might exist abnormally.

The structures through which the root-fibres pass from the nucleus to the base of the brain should be remembered in their topographical relations. Leaving the anterior part of the Sylvian gray matter, the rootlets of the third nerve pass archwise through the tegmentum cruris, the red nucleus and superior cerebellar peduncle, the substantia nigra, and the mesial portion of the pes cruris (later p. 780).

The nucleus of the **fourth** or **trochlear** nerve lies in the dorsal part of the posterior longitudinal bundles, opposite the cerebral end of the posterior quadrigeminal bodies. There is no sharp line of demarcation between the superior end of this and the lower end of the third nucleus; though, according to Siemerling, a distinction may be traced between them, chiefly by an alteration in the size of the nerve-cells. At the level of the trochlear nucleus and in the longitudinal bundle there is a cell-group, composed of smaller cells, which may be traced upwards and seen to merge into the third nucleus. The special value of this nucleus seems to lie in the fact that it gives origin to the nerve-fibres supplying the levator palpebræ superioris muscle (Siemerling).

Kausch (8) has recently endeavoured to show that the classical *trochlearis* nucleus does not give origin to the fibres of the fourth cranial nerve, but that these fibres have origin in the posterior ventral cell-group of Westphal, the inferior group of the anterior nucleus as described by Bruce. This statement is based chiefly on the fact that in a case of *ophthalmoplegia nuclearis* both the third and fourth nerves were degenerated and their muscles paralysed, but the so-called trochlearis nucleus was normal.

The trochlear root-fibres leave their nucleus and pass down in the central gray matter as far as the superior medullary velum. Here the nerves of opposite sides decussate and, passing over the superior cerebellar peduncle, course ventrally forwards towards the cavernous sinus. The position and relations of the trochlear decussation is of importance, as the superior oblique muscle may be paralysed from the pressure of a tumour involving the anterior end of the vermis cerebelli, the posterior quadrigeminal bodies, or the superior medullary velum (Gowers). The trochlear nucleus, from its position on the posterior longitudinal bundles, is thus closely associated with the third nucleus above and the sixth nucleus below.

Sixth nerve.—The nucleus of this nerve occupies a prominent position in the hind part of the tegmentum pontis. It is formed of large first-type cells, whose axis-cylinder processes pass as root-fibres vertically through the tegment and pyramids, and emerge on the ventral aspect of the pons Varolii at its lower margin. The nucleus lies in a bend.(genu) of the issuing root of the facial nerve, the fibres of which have no connection with the cells of the nucleus.

The connections of this nucleus are numerous and important.

(i.) With the cerebral cortex—posterior end of the second frontal gyrus—by means of the pyramidal fibres; although, as is the case with the oculo-motor nerves as a whole, the position of these fibres in the internal capsule and pes cruris is closely allied with those of the fronto-pontine tract.

(ii.) By means of the posterior longitudinal bundle with the opposite third nucleus, which relation subserves the conjugate movements of the eyes (*vide* under "Conjugate Movement").

(iii.) With the superior olivary body through its peduncle, whereby an extensive indirect connection is established between the sixth nucleus and the auditory nerve, the corpus trapezoides, the lateral fillet, and the posterior quadrigeminal bodies.

(iv.) With the flocculus cerebelli (Bruce).

Paralysis of individual ocular muscles.—The muscles which move the eyeball are the four recti and the two obliques; but more than a single muscle is required to produce most individual ocular movements; for example, elevation of the globe is caused by the associated action of the superior rectus and the inferior oblique; depression by the combined action of the inferior rectus and superior oblique. The cause of this is not far to seek: the insertion of the superior rectus being lateral to its origin, its contraction produces rotation inwards as well as elevation, which is counteracted by the outward rotatory action of the inferior oblique; and the outward rotatory action of the inferior rectus is negatived by the inward rotation caused by contraction of the superior oblique. Movement of the globe outwards and inwards is performed solely by the external and internal recti respectively; while conjugate movement of both globes is carried out by the associated action of the external rectus of one side and the internal rectus of the opposite side (see "Conjugate Movement"). The two internal recti acting together produce the movement of convergence of the globes. Applying the same principles to more complicated movements we find that *rotation upwards and outwards* is affected by three muscles acting in harmony, the superior and external recti with the inferior oblique, the last-named counteracting the wheel-rotation of the superior rectus. *Rotation downwards and outwards* is carried out by the inferior and external recti, with the superior oblique to counteract the wheel-rotation of the inferior rectus. In like manner *rotation upwards and inwards* and *downwards and inwards* is brought about by the superior and internal recti and inferior and internal recti respectively, being associated in the upward movement with inferior oblique, and in the downward movement with the superior oblique.

Paralyses of individual ocular muscles are productive of two series of phenomena—those of which the patient complains, and those observed by the physician. To the first belong erroneous projection of the visual field and double vision; to the second, strabismus and limitation of ocular movement.

(*a*) Erroneous projection and diplopia. By the degree of effort necessary to contract the ocular muscles we are informed of the relative position of objects to our bodies. For example, when we turn our eyes to an object towards the right we are aware, from the amount of innervation necessary to contract the muscles, how far towards this side the object lies, and the hand is correctly guided to lay hold of it; but (to continue the example) should the right external rectus muscle be paretic a greater amount of nerve energy is required, so that the impression conveyed to the mind is that the object lies really farther to the right than is actually the case, so that on attempting to lay hold of it the hand goes beyond. From this it appears that there are two ways by which the impression of erroneous position may be produced: either by the excess of energy given to the paralysed muscle, or by the increased action of the healthy muscle, either of which would convey to the sensorium a sense of false position.

If in a case of paresis of the right external rectus muscle an effort be made to turn the eyes to the right, the patient, in addition to the erroneous projection, sees two objects—one blurred, the other distinct. If a coloured glass disc be placed before the paralysed eye he will notice that the image seen by this eye lies to the right of that of the sound eye; the diplopia is, in fact, homonymous, and the following is the explanation. When the eyes are at rest in the mid-position no muscular action is taking place, and the image of an object falls directly on the macula lutea of each eye; and on deviation of both eyes—to the right, for example—the parallelism of the optic axes is maintained, while the object is seen as single, the image still falling directly on the maculæ. Should, however, the external rectus be paralysed the macula of the affected eye is not rotated inwards to the same extent as it is outwards in the sound eye, and the image of the object is thrown upon the right retina at a place where, in the healthy state, the macula should have been. Thus, as in the instance given, this is inside the macular region, and the image appears to the patient to be to the right of that of the sound eye. If, however, instead of the right external rectus being paralysed, the right internal rectus be weakened—that is, a divergent strabismus—the false image, for a like reason, would be to the left of the true image formed in the left eye, that is, crossed diplopia. Hence the rule is stated, that *in convergent strabismus the diplopia is homonymous, in divergent strabismus it is crossed.*

(*b*) Strabismus and limitation of movement. When an ocular muscle is paralysed the globes lose their natural parallelism. The unopposed action of the normal internal rectus muscle, in the event of paralysis of the right external rectus, produces convergent strabismus of the affected eye. If, in this condition, the left eye being covered, a person is asked to fix an object to the right side with the right eye, owing to the excess of effort necessary to move the paretic eye outwards, the associated internal rectus muscle of the sound eye is thrown into over-action, and the sound eye is turned inwards more than normally—*secondary deviation.* Paralysis of the internal rectus muscle gives rise to divergent strabismus from the unopposed action of the corresponding external rectus. In the event of the right internal rectus being paretic, and the person being asked to fix an object to the left with the right eye (the left being covered), the secondary deviation is seen in an excessive outward rotation of the left globe.

In concomitant squint, commonly met with in cases of hypermetropia, and arising to a large extent from the association between accommodation and convergence, the primary and secondary squints are the same in degree. In paralytic squint, for the reasons above mentioned, the secondary squint (secondary deviation) is always larger than the primary.

Paralysis of individual ocular nerves.—The nerves supplying the eyeball and its appendages are the third, fourth, and sixth cranial, and the sympathetic nerves. The fifth nerve is the sensory nerve of the eyeball, but its relations and symptoms are described later.

A. *The third nerve.*—Lesion of this nerve causes paralysis of all the external ocular muscles, except the external rectus and the superior oblique; also paralysis of the levator palpebræ superioris, the sphincter iridis, and the ciliary muscle. The symptoms, therefore, are—ptosis, inability to move the eyeball upwards, downwards, or inwards, external strabismus from over-action of the unimpaired external rectus, a wheel-rotation of the globe on asking the patient to follow the examiner's fingers downwards and outwards (from the unimpaired action of the superior oblique), dilatation and immobility of the pupil, and paralysis of accommodation. A slight protrusion of the eyeball may also be noticed.

As paralysis may be due either to a nuclear or a peripheral lesion, the symptoms vary both in degree and in extent. Ptosis is usually a common and an early symptom in both varieties. In the nuclear lesion the internal muscles may escape, while the external are paralysed.

If the paralysis of the nerve be only partial an examination of the double images may be made. The strabismus being divergent the diplopia is crossed when the patient looks to the side opposite the palsy; on looking up the false image will be higher than the true; on looking down the false image will be lower than the true and inclined towards it, from the wheel-rotation of the superior oblique.[1]

B. *The fourth nerve.*—Paralysis of this nerve affects only the superior oblique muscle. As this muscle is concerned in the downward and inward movement of the globe, the diplopia is only seen in this direction; actual defect of movement is difficult to determine without the aid of the double images. The diplopia is homonymous, and the false image is lower than the true, and is inclined towards it.

Although the extra-cerebral course of the nerve is long, yet isolated trochlear palsy is infrequent (twice out of 116 cases of ocular palsy, Collins and Wilde). Double trochlear palsy would indicate a lesion in the neighbourhood of the anterior medullary velum, the posterior corpora quadrigemina, and anterior end of the vermis cerebelli.

C. *The sixth nerve.*—Paralysis of this nerve retards the outward movement of the globe, as the action of the external rectus muscle is impaired. The strabismus is convergent; and the diplopia therefore homonymous. A slight and otherwise imperceptible weakness of this muscle may be brought out by a study of the double images; the false image lies to the side of the weakened muscle when the eyes are turned in that direction. On looking upwards and outwards, or downwards and outwards, the false image is inclined away from the true.

Unilateral abducens paralysis is not uncommon, and when co-existing with other symptoms of intracranial disease is a valuable localising sign. Owing to the long intracranial course of the nerve it is implicated in disease of the basal meninges, of the pons, of the cerebellum, and of the middle cranial fossa. Abducens palsy with opposite hemiplegia indicates a lesion of the ventral part of the pons Varolii; but it is more common to find paralysis of the combined action of the internal and external recti muscles of opposite eyes (paralysis of conjugate movement), a symptom which points to lesion of the sixth nucleus and tegmentum pontis (*vide* p. 782). According to Wood, simple non-

---

[1] A good "artificial memory" for the position and relations of the double images in ocular palsies is that of L. Werner given by Swanzy, *Handbook*, 5th ed. 1895, p. 491.

rheumatic abducens palsy indicates in adults syphilis, but tuberculous disease in children.

D. *The sympathetic nerve.*—The symptoms of an affection of this nerve from lesion in the neck are :—contraction of the pupil from palsy of the dilating fibres of the iris contained therein ; narrowing of the palpebral fissure, which may give the appearance of a false ptosis, and a sunken condition of the eyeball in the orbit (enophthalmos).

OPHTHALMOPLEGIA.—I propose to include under this name chiefly those forms of ocular palsies which are due to lesions in or about the nuclei in the gray matter of the Sylvian aqueduct ; namely, palsy of the external ocular muscles—chiefly of nuclear origin, and palsy of the internal ocular muscles—cycloplegia and iridoplegia.

(i.) *Cycloplegia*, or paralysis of accommodation, is a feature in paralysis of the trunk of the third nerve ; but it is also met with alone, chiefly as a result of diphtheria and syphilis, in which latter condition it may indicate an early degenerative change in the central nervous system (tabes, for example).

As a post-diphtheritic phenomenon it is bilateral, and usually occurs unassociated with any other intra-ocular palsy ; as a syphilitic lesion, however, it is often unilateral, and is usually accompanied by loss of the iris light-reflex. Recent investigation on the post-diphtheritic paralysis has shown that the toxic agent affects chiefly the intra-muscular terminations of peripheral nerves ; and in several cases of such palsy I have been unable to detect any microscopical change in the nerve centres or extra-muscular portions of the nerves. Hence we incline to the view that post-diphtheritic cycloplegia may not improbably arise from the lesion of the nerve filaments within the ciliary muscle itself, although no direct evidence on this point is yet forthcoming. Its association with reflex iridoplegia, as met with in syphilitic affections on the other hand, points in some cases to a central nuclear affection ; in others, to a lesion of the uppermost of the rootlets of the third nerve.

(ii.) *Iridoplegia.*—The commonest form of iridoplegia is met with in the loss of the pupillary light-reflex ; if at the same time contraction on convergence is present, the condition known as the Argyll-Robertson pupil is obtained.

In testing the reaction of the pupil to light, which should not be more intense than that to which the eye is usually accustomed, two actions are to be noted—the direct and the consensual pupil contraction. It is direct when light falling on one eye, the other being closed, a pupillary contraction is noted ; it is consensual when, on light being thrown on one eye, the pupil of the opposite eye contracts.

The observation of the consensual pupillary reaction is of much value, for by it we are enabled to gauge the condition of the commissural connections and intercommunications between the centres and the afferent and efferent limbs of the reflex arc. For instance, direct reflex pupillary immobility in one eye may be associated with a consensual contraction of that pupil when light is thrown into the other eye ; this reaction necessitates an intact state both of the pupil-contracting centres and of the commissural fibres between them. If, on the other hand, both the direct and consensual reactions are abolished in one eye, the lesion is limited to the centre of the sphincter iridis, or to the fibres arising therefrom on one side, which is the only site where blocking both of direct and crossed pupillary fibres is possible, supposing the lesion to be single. If, in homonymous hemianopsia from lesion of the optic tract, light be thrown on the seeing half of one retina, both pupils contract, the reaction suggests both a semi-decussation of pupillary fibres at the optic chiasma, and a free communication between opposite pupil-contracting centres.

The Argyll-Robertson reaction—that is, loss of the pupillary light-reflex with pupil-contraction on convergence—may be associated either with a large or a small sized pupil. If the pupil be large the condition is called paralytic mydriasis or simple iridoplegia ; if small it is known as paralytic myosis. A small pupil, arising from paralysis of the cilio-spinal fibres alone, may, however, contract further on the stimulus of light, and this condition is known as spinal myosis. The cause of myosis in such cases is usually ascribed to interference with the cilio-spinal fibres in the cervical region of the spinal cord ; the loss of the light-reflex being due to the blocking of impressions along the fibres from the anterior quadrigeminal bodies to the third nerve nucleus (Meynert's fibres). This view presupposes either a double lesion or an extensive area of degeneration implicating structures so far apart as Meynert's fibres and the cilio-spinal region. In a considerable number of cases reflex pupillary immobility is met with as an isolated symptom ; there being no evidence of interference with the ascending trigeminal root, or gelatinous substance of the medulla, in which the cilio-spinal fibres probably lie (see under " Fifth nerve "). Hence we are led to assume in many cases that a single lesion is the cause both of the myosis and of the reflex iridoplegia ; and that the situation of this lesion can only be where the pupil-contracting and pupil-dilating centres are situated : now these centres lie in the fore part of the third nerve nucleus, probably the superior nucleus of Bruce (antero-lateral of Darkschewitsch).

Myosis, or a contracted state of the pupil, is regarded as irritative or paralytic. The former variety is seen in the early stages of cerebral tumour, in meningitis, in cerebral abscess, and in apoplexy, especially of the pons Varolii ; the latter is most commonly observed in tabes, general paralysis, and some forms of cerebral syphilis.

Mydriasis, or dilatation of the pupil, has also been ascribed to irritative and to paralytic lesions. The former is seen in cases where there is reason to suppose the existence of an irritative lesion in the upper part of the spinal cord, or of irritation of the sympathetic dilating fibres in the neck ; the latter in disease affecting part of the third nerve nucleus, and in states of great intracranial pressure.

It has long been a matter of dispute whether dilatation of the pupil

is due to inhibition of the pupillary contracting fibres or to stimulation of a dilator muscle. The recent observations of Langley and
Anderson seem to indicate the existence of such dilator fibres—a fact
which may explain the clinical observation that in paralytic myosis a
partial dilatation of the pupil may be obtained by the instillation of
mydriatics. But, notwithstanding this, there are many facts in favour
of the view that dilatation of the pupil is due to inhibition of the
sphincter iridis, an action comparable to others in the body.

A condition is sometimes met with, the converse of the Argyll-
Robertson phenomenon, namely, the presence of the pupillary light-reflex,
associated with loss of contraction on attempts at convergence. The
lesion which causes this condition is situated in a different part of the
third nerve nucleus from that which occasions reflex pupillary immobility.
From these and other observations it would seem that the centre subserving pupillary movements is subdivided into—

(*a*) A sphincter-contracting centre closely associated with a sphincter-
inhibitory centre, which two subserve the pupillary light-reflex.

(*b*) A centre for contraction of the pupil with convergence, in close
relation with the centre for the associated action of the internal recti
muscles.

Lesion of the sphincter inhibitory centre, or of the fibres coming from
it, gives rise to the condition known as "spinal myosis." If the fibres
passing to the centre only be involved, reflex pupillary immobility alone
results; but if both the afferent fibres and the centre be diseased, the
contracted Argyll-Robertson pupil is obtained. Interference with the
functions of the sphincter-contracting centre occasions the dilated Argyll-
Robertson pupil; the pupil contraction on convergence being retained in
both instances by means of a special centre (*b*) for this action (see under
"Paralysis of convergence ").

In some cases of reflex pupillary immobility, with or without other
symptoms of tabes dorsalis, anæsthesia over the distribution of the trigeminal nerve has been found. This is indicative of a sclerotic lesion,
either in the trunk of the fifth nerve, or more probably in the so-called
ascending trigeminal root in the medulla oblongata.

The peripheral course of the pupil-contracting fibres is through the
uppermost of the rootlets of the third nerve, the trunk of the nerve, the
ciliary ganglion, and the short ciliary nerves. It is associated in its
course with the nerve filaments for the ciliary muscle. The course of
the pupil-dilating fibres is more circuitous: they pass from the centre
in the Sylvian gray matter through the pons Varolii, medulla oblongata,
·and cervical region of the spinal cord, to issue by the anterior root of the
second dorsal nerve, and to be conveyed in the cervical sympathetic, the
ophthalmic branch of the fifth, the ciliary ganglion, and the long ciliary
nerves to the iris.

From experiments upon the fifth nerve and its intra-medullary roots
referred to elsewhere (*vide* under " Fifth nerve "), it is evident that the
pupil-dilating fibres pass chiefly in the gelatinous substance of Rolando or

adjacent tissue ; for section of the so-called ascending trigeminal root and destruction of the tubercle of Rolando were invariably followed by contraction of the pupil on the side of lesion. That the sensory root of the trigeminus between the side of the pons and the Gasserian ganglion also contains pupil-dilating fibres, is clear from the fact that on cutting the nerve contraction of the pupil is observed.

(iii.) *Ophthalmoplegia interna.*—This name is given to a condition in which all the internal ocular muscular mechanisms are paralysed. It presents the clinical features of paralysis of accommodation, mydriasis, and pupillary immobility. The condition may be unilateral or bilateral ; or it may be complete on one side and partial on the opposite side. It may or may not be associated with paralysis of the external ocular muscles. When these symptoms occur alone, the lesion is situated almost invariably in the nucleus of the third nerve ; but in several cases of this nature I have observed a slight degree of ptosis, which would indicate that a partial lesion of the nerve trunk itself may be the causal agent.

(iv.) *Ophthalmoplegia externa.*—Under this name are included those forms of ocular paralysis in which more than one external ocular muscle is paralysed. Hence there exists a large number of ocular palsies due to lesions in various situations, of different nature, and arising from many causes, both acute and chronic. The form, however, which may be taken as the standard or type is that arising from chronic degeneration of the cells of the oculo-motor nuclei ;—*chronic nuclear ophthalmoplegia.* This condition presents many clinical varieties ; it may exist alone as a pure ophthalmoplegia for a number of years, as in the cases of Strümpell (20 years), Hutchinson (17 years), and others ; or it may become associated with a like degeneration of the bulbar nuclei ; or again, it may be concomitant with the symptoms of tabes dorsalis. In a complete case all movements by means of the external ocular muscles are paralysed, with or without drooping of the upper eyelid. In partial cases diplopia is a constant and troublesome symptom. A common symptom also, and probably characteristic of nuclear affection, is an alternating ptosis, sometimes more marked in one eye, sometimes in the other ; there is also a tendency to remission and exacerbation, which is seen likewise in the other defective ocular movements.

Both eyes are usually affected, but not always to the same extent ; and, in the pure cases, the internal ocular muscles and the reflex action of the iris to light are unaffected, or not involved till the later stages. The movement of convergence of the globes may be impaired along with the other defective ocular movements ; in this case the contraction of the pupil on attempted convergence is lost or diminished. Weakness of the orbicularis palpebrarum has been observed in cases of nuclear ophthalmoplegia, and would probably be more frequent if looked for. If this is present a nuclear degeneration may with confidence be diagnosed. Although in these cases the lagophthalmos met with in facial paralysis is not seen, yet by the examiner's finger the upper lid may be raised against resistance more readily than is possible in a healthy condition. In one of Dr. Hughlings Jackson's cases the patient stated that, although he was able to close the lids, he had not sufficient power to prevent water getting into the eyes when washing his face.

I have seen weakness of the orbicularis palpebrarum in three cases of nuclear ophthalmoplegia ; in one of them the frontalis was also so largely paralysed that the patient was unable to frown.

Although, as already mentioned, paralysis of the external ocular muscles from chronic nuclear disease may be met with alone, yet it is not uncommonly associated with paralysis of the motor division of the fifth cranial nerve, with weakness of the facial muscles, and also with paralysis of the bulbar nerves (hypoglossus and vagus). In these cases the ocular palsy is usually in advance of the bulbar form ; whereas in cases beginning as a bulbar paralysis, ophthalmoplegia rarely reaches a marked degree of intensity.

This affection is due to a very clear pathological condition. Since Sir William Gowers originally found a degenerative atrophy of the cells of the oculo-motor nuclei in a case of this nature, a vast number of observations have been brought forward in confirmation. But a point which does not seem to have received sufficient attention, yet one which is apparent in some cases and in the closely-related chronic progressive bulbar palsy, is the evidence of vascular degeneration. Small hæmorrhagic extravasations in the neighbourhood of the nerve nuclei, fatty infiltration of the walls and dilatation of the arterioles, thickening of the vessel walls and of the ependyma ventriculi have been frequently observed ; and this not in one situation only. In a case of amyotrophic lateral sclerosis with bulbar symptoms, I found marked dilatation of the arterioles in the spinal cord and medulla oblongata, with enlargement of the periarterial lymph spaces ; and changes of the nature of fatty infiltration of the walls of the small vessels have been found in the cortex cerebri (Joffroy and Achard). Should it be proved eventually that the chronic atrophy of the cells is due to a change in the vessels of the central nervous apparatus, support will be given to Gowers' view that a toxæmic influence is the directly causal agent ; thus the chronic progressive degenerative forms will be brought into close etiological relation with the acute form to be described immediately, and which is undoubtedly of a toxic nature.

A form of ophthalmoplegia, differing from the above in its method of onset but probably allied in its etiological features, is the so-called *polio-encephalitis superior* (Wernicke). In this we meet with an ophthalmoplegia of sudden origin, not uncommonly associated with general symptoms, such as delirium, somnolence, and sometimes optic neuritis. In some recorded cases the symptoms pointed to an implication of the gray matter of the floor of the fourth ventricle and of the anterior horns of the spinal cord, giving rise to acute bulbar symptoms and paralysis of the limbs. These cases, whether the symptoms be limited to the oculo-motor nerves, or be indicative of a simultaneous affection of the bulbar and spinal gray matter, are often fatal; and post-mortem examination has shown hæmorrhagic extravasations in the gray matter around the Sylvian aqueduct, and in the walls of the third ventricle with vascular distension and thrombosis; while a similar pathological condition has been observed in the bulbar and spinal gray matter. This form of paralysis occurs usually in chronic alcoholism, but there is reason to suppose that it may be due to the effects of other toxic agents, such as influenza, diphtheria, and, in rare cases, lead.

It is more common for the alcoholic poison to produce ocular paralysis in this way than by a neuritis of the oculo-motor nerves; for in a case of alcoholic paralysis with ophthalmoplegia Jacobæus found evidence of a polyneuritis of the nerves of the limbs, and hæmorrhagic extravasations into the Sylvian gray matter; and in Boediker's case of acute alcoholic ophthalmoplegia, the ocular nerves presented normal microscopic appearances; several cases of acute hæmorrhagic ophthalmoplegia have been recorded, and its pathology is now well known (Kojewnikoff, Thomsen, Eisenlohr).

But there are cases of acute nuclear ophthalmoplegia, occurring without such well-marked general symptoms, which do not present any evidence of implication of the central gray matter elsewhere. Such cases are not rapidly fatal, and in many recovery takes place. For this reason the underlying pathological condition is unknown; but it is not unlikely that thrombosis of small vessels, minute hemorrhagic extravasations, and small arterial dilatations give rise to the clinical phenomena. It is also probable that in these cases the causal agent is to be found in some blood poison—syphilis, diphtheria, influenza, and others still undetermined. It should also be borne in mind that temporary oculomotor palsies occur as an early feature in some cases of tabes dorsalis; and that, in rare instances, complete or partial ophthalmoplegia has been described as a sequence of migraine, a condition which usually undergoes spontaneous resolution.

In studying the two forms of ophthalmoplegia now described from a comparative point of view, the one due to chronic progressive atrophy of the nerve-cells, the other to acute thrombotic or hæmorrhagic destruction of the gray matter, we note localised manifestations of two conditions occurring throughout the bulbo-spinal centres. From the same causes there may arise acute and chronic bulbar palsy, if the disease is limited to the gray matter of the medulla oblongata; or acute and chronic anterior poliomyelitis, if the pathological processes are at work in the spinal cord. In the cord the symptoms usually point to a limited affection either in the cervical or lumbar enlargement. On the other hand, such acute or chronic conditions may implicate the whole extent of the bulbo-spinal nuclei, more or less simultaneously. As an example of the chronic form may be mentioned amyotrophic lateral sclerosis with bulbar palsy and ophthalmoplegia; while the acute form is seen in the cases of Guinon and Parmentier.

As a connecting link between these two extremes mention is specially made of a subacute variety of polio-encephalomyelitis, a well-marked case of which has been described by Kalischer. Here a patient presented paralysis of all the muscles, from the eyes to the lower limbs inclusive, which had arisen during the course of six months. The necropsy revealed hemorrhagic extravasations of various sizes and of different dates in the central gray matter, from the Sylvian aqueduct to the sacral region of the spinal cord. The blood-vessel walls were thickened and showed aneurysmal dilatations and patches of fatty degeneration; while here and there the cells of the anterior horns were atrophied. In this form is to be found the link between the acute and the chronic varieties already described; the pathological process being essentially of a vascular origin, through which the nutrition of the nervous elements is impaired.

Brief reference may here be made to a form of ophthalmoplegia, which is rarely acute in onset or complete in range. It is associated with such general symptoms as staggering, optic-neuritis, and sometimes impairment of hearing. In these cases the lesion is not limited to the Sylvian gray matter, but encroaches upon it from above, as in tumour of the corpora quadrigemina; or from behind, as in tumour of the vermis cerebelli. The oculo-motor disturbances consist chiefly of palsy in the region of the third and fourth nerves, rather than in that of the sixth; while palsy of convergence, ptosis, and loss of the upward movement of the globes have been the chief ocular phenomena noted in such cases [*vide* "Lesions of the corpora quadrigemina," in art. on "Cerebral Localisation"].

Varieties of ophthalmoplegia. — 1. *Cortical ophthalmoplegia (so-called)*.—Ophthalmoplegia, defined in its proper sense as impairment of the movements of the eyeballs in all directions, does not occur in purely cortical lesions. As an experimental result of destructive lesion of the area in which stimulation causes deviation of both eyeballs to the opposite side, or of extirpation of the frontal lobe in monkeys, and in some cases of disease of this region in man, temporary paralysis of conjugate movement of the eyes to the side opposite the lesion has been observed; but both frontal lobes, containing the excitable areas for such ocular movements, may be completely extirpated without any evidence, other than temporary, of defective conjugate movements. That the area in the frontal lobe presiding over the conjugate movements also contains centres for other (upward and downward) movements of the globe has been shown experimentally by Dr. Risien Russell (13); but yet within a short time of the bilateral extirpation of this centre a monkey is able to move the eyes in any direction.

Nor is there any clear proof, either experimental or from disease in man, that lesions of the inferior parietal lobe or angular gyrus occasion ophthalmoplegia; as described by Grasset, Landouzy, Wernicke, Henschen, and others. Experimental destruction of the angular gyrus was not followed by any oculo-motor paralysis, either alone or when destroyed conjointly with the extirpation of the frontal lobe.[1] As regards the evidence from man, it may be stated that lesions of the inferior parietal

---

[1] From experiments made in association with Dr. Ferrier, *Phil. Trans.* vol. cxc. p. 1. See also chapter on "Cerebral Localisation," in the next volume.

lobe and angular gyrus are not always accompanied by conjugate deviation of the eyes; nor is there any evidence that bilateral lesions determine ophthalmoplegia.

Nor has the existence of a cortical centre for the elevator of the upper lid in the angular gyrus been established ; although cases pointing to this have been described by Chauffard, Lemoine and Surmont, Herter, and others. Experimental evidence is certainly not in agreement with these observations, nor is the evidence from disease in man sufficiently conclusive ; for, of fifty cases of lesion in the region of the angular gyrus collected by Surmont (*Thèse de Lille*, 1886), eleven only showed more or less complete blepharoptosis, while in many the oculo-motor nerves do not appear to have been examined microscopically. (For further evidence on this subject see hereafter " Localisation of Cerebral Disease.")

2. *Subcortical ophthalmoplegia*, or paralysis of the ocular movements from disease affecting the fibres between the cortex and the oculo-motor nuclei, as in the so-called cortical form, is unknown, except a temporary paralysis of conjugate movement which occurs as an early and fleeting effect of hæmorrhage within, or in the neighbourhood of, the internal capsule and the basal ganglia. As previously shown (p. 767), the tract by which the oculo-motor fibres pass from the cortex to their nuclei in the pons Varolii and Sylvian gray matter is probably to be found at the "knee" of the internal capsule, and occupying the mesial third of the pes cruris ; the most internal of such fibres coming directly from the prefrontal or non-excitable portion of the frontal lobe.

A lesion situated so as to involve the oculo-motor fibres in the pes cruris would at the same time implicate the issuing roots of the third nerve, so that the ophthalmoplegia thus produced would arise from peripheral or infra-nuclear causes.

3. *Nuclear ophthalmoplegia* has already been described.

4. *Infra-nuclear (or basal) ophthalmoplegia.* — Under this name are included those ocular palsies due to a lesion situated between the oculo-motor nuclei and the sphenoidal fissure.

A lesion which involves both the third nerve and the crus cerebri produces one form of alternate paralysis—paralysis of the third nerve on one side and of the limbs on the opposite side (Weber's symptom). But this paralysis may arise from lesion (tumour usually) within the substance of the crus (intra-peduncular) ; or from basal meningitis (sub- or extra-peduncular). Are there any points by which these two forms may be distinguished ? In the intra-peduncular form the third nerve is not usually paralysed completely, the internal ocular muscles often escaping ; ptosis being the most frequent and most marked effect. Owing to the linear expansion of the nerve rootlets the paralysis, from the progressive picking out of the several branches which occurs, may resemble a nuclear one. If in association with these features there are tremors, hemichorea or hemiathetosis, cerebellar titubation and ataxy, an intra-peduncular lesion may be confidently diagnosed. Brissaud has pointed out that if the lesion involve the third nerve and only the mesial portion of the crus cerebri, a facial palsy of the cerebral type without palsy of the limbs may coexist.

The causes of such palsies are to be found in tuberculous or syphilitic inflammations or new growths, affecting the basal membranes, or situated within the cerebral substance. Syphilitic obliterative arteritis of the basilar artery or its branches, leading to softening in its area of distribution, is no uncommon lesion in this situation. Indeed, an oculo-motor palsy with hemiplegia of the opposite side coming on simultaneously is suggestive of a specific lesion.

Basal meningitis in the neighbourhood of the sphenoidal fissure, or thrombosis of the cavernous sinus occasions complete oculo-motor paralysis (third, fourth, and sixth nerves), with affection of the fifth nerve causing anæsthesia of the face, and cornea, and keratitis; many cases present an associated optic neuritis.

5. *Orbital ophthalmoplegia.*—Various conditions within the orbit may give rise to oculo-motor palsies (gunshot or other wounds, new growths, cellulitis, etc.), the oculo-motor nerves being in whole or in part involved; but in this situation the ophthalmic branch of the fifth rarely escapes, and the optic nerve itself is not uncommonly implicated, especially when the lesion is in the neighbourhood of the sphenoidal fissure and optic foramen. The association of such paralytic phenomena with proptosis is suggestive of an orbital affection, as distinguished from one in the neighbourhood of the cavernous sinus or sphenoidal fissure.

6. That a truly peripheral ocular palsy may occur from lesion of the intra-muscular terminations of the nerve is probable from what is known of the action of certain toxic agents in other situations. Thus it is not unlikely, as already pointed out, that the post-diphtheritic cycloplegia is due to an intra-muscular affection of the ciliary nerves, while the palsy of the external rectus met with in post-diphtheritic palsies may be due to a similar affection of the sixth nerve. Direct pathological observations are still wanted in this respect.

Associated paralyses.—*Paralysis of convergence.*—There are several facts indicating the existence of a centre for the convergent action of the internal recti muscles, apart from that presiding over their associated action with the external recti in lateral deviation. For example, there are cases on record, and I have seen one such, in which the internal recti were paralysed for convergence, but acted normally in lateral deviation of the globes. With the palsy of convergence there was loss of the associated pupil contraction, but the pupillary light-reflex was retained;—facts which strongly support the view, already stated (p. 775), that there are two centres for the contraction of the pupil, one subservient entirely to the light-reflex, the other associated with convergent movement. With the paralysis of convergence is paralysis of accommodation; for although we may accommodate without converging, convergence cannot occur without accommodation. Thus paralysis of accommodation may exist alone (*vide* "Cycloplegia"), but I have never seen paralysis of convergence without paralysis of accommodation. In palsy of convergence the unopposed action of the external recti muscles may occasion a slight bilateral divergent strabismus.

Paralysis of convergence, without loss of the other muscular movements supplied by the third nerve, is invariably due to disease of the centres; but it is not yet known what group of cells in the third nerve nucleus presides over this function.

Paralysis of conjugate movement.—The eyeballs are normally moved to either side by the associated action of the internal and external recti muscles. In certain forms of disease of the central nervous system this normal action may be impaired; on the one hand, the eyes may be forcibly deviated to one or other side from tonic spasm of the associated muscles; or, on the other hand, the patient may be unable to turn the eyes to one or other side owing to paralysis of the associated mechanisms. The former is due to an irritative lesion above the centre, in the pons Varolii, for the associated action of the internal and external recti muscles; and will be more fitly described when the cortical and subcortical relations of the ocular muscles are considered (p. 779); the latter, as already stated, is caused by destructive lesion of the centre in the pons. The following is the probable course of the fibres for conjugate movement of the globes:—Arising from cortical centres in the frontal lobe the fibres pass in the anterior limb of the internal capsule, and occupy a mesial position in the pes cruris. They cannot be traced farther than the upper part of the pons Varolii, but the probability is that they find their way through the tegment to the nucleus of the sixth cranial nerve.[1]

The sixth nucleus appears to be the pontine centre for conjugate movement; for it is impossible to turn one eyeball outwards without at the same time causing the other to turn inwards. This nucleus also has an extensive connection with adjacent structures which appear to be associated with the movements of the eyes. Thus it is directly connected with the superior olivary body, a structure which undergoes degeneration after destruction of the accessory auditory ganglion; by this means the sixth nucleus is indirectly brought into relation with the posterior corpora quadrigemina, the lateral fillet and the lateral column of the spinal cord. It appears also to be directly connected with the flocculus cerebelli (Bruce); while through the nucleus of Deiters it has indirect relations with the middle lobe of the cerebellum. From the sixth nucleus, probably by way of the posterior longitudinal bundle, fibres pass to a group of cells in the third nucleus which supply the internal rectus muscle of the opposite side. That this group of cells is distinct from that which innervates the internal rectus muscle for movements of convergence is clear from the fact that palsy of convergence may exist without palsy of conjugate movement.

A lesion, therefore, in order to cause palsy of conjugate movements must be either in the course of the fibres above the sixth nucleus, or must involve the nucleus itself. The latter is the commonest situation. Several cases have been recorded of this lesion (Bennett and Savill, Blocq and Guinon).

---

[1] *Trans. Ophthal. Soc.* vol. xviii. p. 395.

Commonly but not invariably associated with this paralysis is facial palsy on the same side ; that is to say, there exists paralysis of the face of the peripheral kind on the side to which the patient cannot turn his eyes. The cause of this association is apparent when it is borne in mind that the sixth nucleus lies in the "genu" of the facial nerve-root. Loss of conjugate movement is therefore a pontine lesion, and is never due to an affection of the third nucleus. It is commonly caused by gross disease, such as tumour or thrombotic softening ; there is no recorded instance of its origin in chronic degeneration of the sixth nucleus, probably because this nucleus is not affected alone.

It is still doubtful how far a lesion limited to the posterior longitudinal bundle may cause palsy of conjugate movement. No such limited case has been recorded in human pathology.

Of *other associated ocular movements* may be mentioned a pupillary contraction which is stated to occur on forced closure of the palpebral portions of the orbicularis palpebrarum (6). Gifford noted in some cases, more especially in these associated with blindness, that on forced contraction of the lids,—as, for instance, when an attempt is made to close them against resistance,—a contraction of the pupil takes place with the normal upward movement of the globe. It appears that this reaction occurs independently of convergence or accommodation, and points to a close relation between the centres of pupillary contraction and closure of the lids. Some fibres of the third nerve may pass directly to the palpebral portion of the orbicularis palpebrarum muscle by way of the supraorbital branch of the fifth nerve.

Another curious associated action has been described between certain movements of the lower jaw and the upward movement of the upper eyelid. Numerous cases have now been recorded, and according to Sinclair (14) may be divided into three groups : first, cases of one-sided congenital ptosis, in which the drooping eyelid is raised when the mouth is opened, and when the jaw is directed to the opposite side ; secondly, cases of one-sided congenital ptosis, in which the lid is raised when the jaw is depressed only ; and, thirdly, those cases in which elevation occurs only with lateral movement of the jaw : other cases again have been noted in which no ptosis was observed, but in which the upper lid jerked when the jaw was moved. The probable explanation of such cases lies in a connection between the nuclei of the third and fifth nerves. It is elsewhere shown that the so-called "descending" trigeminal root, which arises in the Sylvian gray matter in close relation to the third nerve nucleus, contains motor fibres for certain depressor muscles of the lower jaw (mylohyoid and anterior belly of the digastric). In the recorded cases the abnormal congenital condition leading to ptosis may be associated with an abnormal connection between the third nerve nucleus and the descending trigeminal root.

A rare association is that between the internal rectus and the levator palpebræ muscles on the same side, which contract and relax together (18). But a still more curious associated movement has been recently described in some cases of paralysis of one external muscle where movement inwards of the affected eye is associated with contraction of the orbicularis palpebrarum and retraction of the globe (Sinclair, *op. cit.*).[1]

Causes of ocular palsies.—Various conditions both of the nerve centres and nerve trunks lead to paralysis of the ocular muscles.

Of these the commonest is *syphilis*. In this condition the nerve trunks are involved either by the pressure of a gummatous basal meningitis, or by a gummatous growth in the nerve itself. On the other hand, peripheral ocular palsy is not common in simple meningitis, although a perineuritis of the cranial nerves may be associated with and directly due to it. Syphilis also leads to a chronic progressive degeneration of the cells of the oculo-motor nuclei, analogous to what is seen in the bulbar nuclei and in the anterior horns of the spinal cord. This form of degeneration is, however, by no means characteristic of the disease. Another, but rarer form of ocular paralysis, arises from vascular thrombosis in the basilar artery and its branches, with consequent softening in the region of the nerve nuclei.

There is nothing pathognomonic in the clinical phenomena of syphilis, but certain associations make them highly suggestive. For example, such partial affections as reflex pupillary immobility on one or both sides; unilateral cycloplegia and iridoplegia with or without ptosis; and such ocular affections as are not necessarily late manifestations of this disease. (For further evidence on this point see later, in article on "Intracranial Syphilis.")

Common also is the peripheral ocular palsy due to cold—the so-called *rheumatic form*. Actual pathological evidence of this is still wanting; but reasoning from what has recently been described by Minkowski in the so-called rheumatic facial paralysis (see under "Seventh nerve"), the lesion may be of the nature of a parenchymatous neuritis.

Ocular paralysis is also a sequel of *diphtheritic infection*. This usually involves the ciliary muscle; but either the third or the sixth, or both nerves may be bilaterally affected. The action of the diphtheritic virus is probably upon the intramuscular termination of the nerves, although no direct evidence of this, as regards the ocular muscles, is yet forthcoming. Hæmorrhagic extravasations into the trunk of the third nerve and its sheath have also been described and are a rare cause of oculo-motor palsy, as in a case described by Dr. Gibson and myself (20).

Various ocular palsies, sometimes of a temporary, sometimes of a permanent nature, chiefly of the external muscles (third and sixth nerves), are observed in association with *chronic degenerative lesions*, such as tabes dorsalis and general paralysis of the insane. Such palsies occur early in the course of the disease, and may indeed be the first symptom to attract attention; hence the importance of a guarded prognosis in all cases of oculo-motor palsy in which a specific history has been obtained. One cause is, undoubtedly, the toxic agent causing the primary lesion, and giving rise either to a nuclear degeneration or a peripheral neuritis; but

---

[1] Cases observed by Nettleship, Parker, and MacLehose.

no definite pathological facts have as yet thrown light on the palsies of temporary nature met with in these diseases.

Trauma also plays a part in the causation of these paralyses ; all the oculo-motor nerves as well as the optic nerve may be paralysed from fracture in the region of the optic foramen and sphenoidal fissure. The abducens may be implicated alone, and the commonest site for implication of this nerve in fracture of the base is the apex of the petrous temporal bone (Purtscher). In addition to direct implication of the nerve-trunks in such fractures, palsy may result secondarily from pressure of hemorrhage, or inflammatory exudation, or suppuration ; and it is possible that an injury may cause hæmorrhage directly into a nerve nucleus.

Ocular palsies may be due to several other causes, such, for example, are pressure on the oculo-motor nuclei by a tuberculous or other tumour, or by periostitis of the orbit ; and in rare cases they have been due to lead and alcoholic poisoning.

The *treatment* of ocular palsies is conducted according to the general principles laid down for the treatment of the cause. As peripheral ocular palsies are almost invariably due to specific causes (syphilis, rheumatism, diphtheria, and other toxic agents), the respective antispecific remedies in common use should be administered. Local remedies, such as leeching or blistering the temples or forehead, are often of the greatest service, more especially in the early stages, and when the palsy is accompanied by headache, which is not uncommonly the case.

In the acute ophthalmoplegias arising from nuclear causes the same antispecific remedies may be applied as in the peripheral cases. In the chronic degenerative forms not much benefit is likely to be obtained by drugs. In these cases the local application of electricity, chiefly in the form of weak galvanic currents, has been recommended, and in some cases has seemed to be of value ; but it should be borne in mind that a tendency to remission is one of the features of the disease, and that the degenerative process may be spontaneously arrested for a longer or a shorter time.

THE TRIGEMINAL NERVE.—**Anatomy.**—When seen at the base of the brain this nerve consists of two distinct parts ; but its central connections have to be studied in three divisions :—the so-called "ascending" or sensory root, the motor root, and the "descending" root, which is regarded by some investigators as also motor in function.

(i.) The *sensory division* of the nerve may be readily traced amongst the fibres of the middle cerebellar peduncle into the lateral part of the tegmentum pontis. Here some fibres pass directly into the so-called sensory nucleus (convolutio quinti), which is nothing else than the expanded proximal termination of the substantia gelatinosa Rolandi (Kölliker and Bruce). The remainder of the division may be followed through the pons Varolii and medulla oblongata, in the distal part of which it forms the layer of white matter covering the gelatinous expansion or tubercle of Rolando. The recent observations of Kölliker and Held, working by Golgi's method, show that the fibres composing this root are the axis-cylinder processes and collaterals of the cells of the Gasserian ganglion. Throughout its extent such fibres are being given off into the gelatinous substance, to terminate in end-tufts which embrace cells lying in this region. These cells in turn give off axis-cylinder processes, which pass as arcuate fibres across the raphé and, entering the tegmentum of the opposite side, pass towards the cerebrum as longitudinal fibres. In this manner the *substantia gelatinosa Rolandi* is regarded by these authors as the end-nucleus of the sensory trigeminal fibres; just as the caput cornu posterioris is the end-nucleus of the direct fibres of the posterior spinal roots, and the posterior vago-glossopharyngeal nucleus, as will be shown later, is the end-nucleus of some of the afferent vago-glossopharyngeal root-fibres.

This view is corroborated by the facts of experiment; for section of the sensory division between the Gasserian ganglion and the brain, or its implication in disease, is followed in man by degeneration and atrophy of the fibres entering the so-called "sensory nucleus," by sclerosis of the "ascending" root, as far as the second cervical nerve, and of the fibres which pass from this root through the gelatinous substance into the posterior horn of gray matter. The probability is that such degeneration is here arrested in the cells of the substantia spongiosa which forms the end-nucleus of the nerve; so that it has not yet been found possible to trace degeneration beyond this in the tegmentum.

It is evident therefore that the central course of the sensory trigeminal fibres is still doubtful; that they pass towards the cerebrum in close relation with the sensory fibres from other parts of the body is clear from various experimental and clinico-pathological observations. The mesial or chief fillet is regarded by some observers as the central sensory pathway; but as this may be completely sclerosed, and the nuclei from which it arises destroyed, without any impairment of common sensation, we must look for some other route by which such impressions are conducted towards the brain. Bechterew places the sensory fibres of the cranial nerves mesial to the fillet in the pons Varolii and in the substantia nigra of the cerebral peduncle; but it is still a matter of conjecture by what route these fibres pass brainwards.

(ii.) *The motor roots.*—These consist of fibres coming, on the one hand, directly from the cells of the motor nucleus; on the other from the "descending" trigeminal root.

The cells of the motor nucleus consist of large, multipolar first-type cells, which send their axis-cylinder process directly into the motor root, and form the *efferent* fibres of the nucleus. A crossed connection has been described by many observers, and Kölliker confirms its presence in new-born animals. A well-marked strand of fibres may sometimes be observed in the situation of the crossed root. These are, without doubt, the most proximal fibres of the *genu facialis*, and the issuing limb of that nerve; and have probably been mistaken in some cases for a crossed trigeminal root. The *afferent* fibres of the nucleus are the pyramidal fibres from the cerebral cortex, but their situation has not as yet been definitely determined. Arguing, however, from what occurs in the hypoglossal nucleus, these fibres probably reach the nucleus by way of the raphé and the reticular formation. In the internal capsule they lie at the "knee" in close approximation with the fibres of the other motor cranial nerves.

The *descending trigeminal root* or "trophic root" of Merkel is still the subject of discussion. It was long disputed whether the root joined the motor or the sensory division of the nerve. The most recent work on this subject shows conclusively that it joins the motor division, and, as will be shortly shown, probably contains motor fibres.

From personal observations upon the functions and connections of this root the following may be stated :—

(*a*) In an experiment, in which the motor root of the fifth nerve was destroyed in its course through the pons Varolii, atrophy of the fibres of the descending trigeminal root, and of the cells from which they spring, was detected.

(*b*) In an experiment upon the superior cerebellar peduncle, in which the descending root was divided where it lies under cover of this structure, degeneration of some of the fibres of the issuing motor root was observed, the motor nucleus itself being intact.

(*c*) In an eight-months' human fœtus the passage of the medullated fibres of the descending root could be clearly traced directly into the motor division of the nerve.

It is more difficult to determine what is really the function of the root. The original view of Merkel (1874), that it is the trophic root of the fifth nerve was based on insufficient grounds, and was distinctly negatived by experiments carried out by Eckhard two years later. Merkel's view has, however, recently received support at the hands of Mendel, who observed atrophy of the descending trigeminal root in an old-standing case of facial hemiatrophy (see "Facial Hemiatrophy, p. 485"). More recent observations, however, would seem to show that this root, in part at least, has motor functions. Kölliker states that it probably supplies motor fibres for the tensor palati and tensor tympani muscles, and probably also the mylohyoid and anterior belly of the digastric; and this view receives corroboration from the experiments of Réthi on stimulation of the motor root of the fifth within the cranial cavity.

In a case in which the muscles of mastication were paralysed, the motor nucleus of the fifth was found after death to be almost completely degenerated; on the other hand the fibres of the descending root, and the cells from which they spring, were quite normal: this observation eliminates the possibility of a motor supply by this root to the muscles of mastication—at any rate, in man.

In opposition to the view of Merkel, and in harmony with Eckhard's experiment, division of this descending trigeminal root was not followed by any detectable trophic alteration in the eyeball.[1]

---

[1] This statement is based upon several experiments performed in association with Dr. Ferrier. *Phil. Trans.* vol. cxxxv. p. 763.

The existence of a cerebellar trigeminal root has been described by Meynert and others, but its presence has not been corroborated by recent investigators. According to Edinger this is the trigeminal portion of a "direct sensory cerebellar tract," connecting the auditory and vago-glosso-pharyngeal nerve-roots with the cerebellum. After section of the sensory division of the fifth nerve no tract of degeneration was observed passing up into the cerebellum ; but, on the other hand, *after extirpation of the vermis cerebelli* an area of degeneration in the position of this cerebellar root was observed, and its termination was found in the nucleus of Deiters, or large-celled external auditory nucleus. The cerebellar root of the trigeminus, therefore, appears to be a portion of an efferent tract from the middle lobe of the cerebellum.

The view here taken of the central connections of the fifth cranial nerve differs materially from that of the older writers, and is based upon the most recent researches, chiefly of Kölliker. The fibres of the sensory division arise as axis-cylinder processes of the cells in the Gasserian ganglion, and terminate in the long end-nucleus known as the *substantia gelatinosa medullæ*. This root and nucleus are sensory, but appear to contain, as shown by experiment as well as by disease, some pupil-dilating fibres. The motor root has two separate nuclei of origin : first, in the classical motor nucleus situated in the pons Varolii internal to the expanded upper end of the sensory end-nucleus ; and, secondly, from the layer of cells situated in the peripheral part of the Sylvian gray matter, as far up as the anterior quadrigeminal bodies.

Some points in the physiology of the trigeminus.—It has long been held, chiefly as a result of the experiments of Majendie and others, that progressive destructive changes in the eyeball occur after intracranial section of the fifth nerve, and more especially of its ophthalmic branch : but the reason of this destruction has long been a moot question. The corneal and conjunctival anæsthesia accompanying division of the nerve was regarded by many as aiding the retention of irritating extraneous matter ; for it was observed that if the eye were protected from the effects of such irritants no inflammation followed. But this view did not receive corroboration at the hands of other observers ; and disorganisation of the eye was also seen even though the anæsthesia were not complete. There are on record numerous cases of anæsthesia of the cornea in which no "trophic" corneal alteration was detected ; nor was the view altogether acceptable that the ocular changes differ according as the lesion is in front of the Gasserian ganglion or behind it.

The general conclusion at which Gaule arrived, as a result of his experiments upon rabbits, was that the "trophic" alterations in the cornea which he described were due to lesion of the ophthalmic branch or of the Gasserian ganglion, while they were not observed to follow lesion of the nerve behind the ganglion. But when it is stated that the changes, which consisted in atrophy and hypertrophy of Descemet's membrane in patches, and necrosis and atrophy of the corneal ground substance, occurred within a short time after the actual division of the nerve, it is difficult to believe that they were due entirely to the lesion thus practised.

In a series of experiments on monkeys, performed by Dr. Ferrier and myself, the fifth nerve trunk, its ophthalmic branch, and the intra-medullary roots were divided. Of seventeen experiments, in which anæsthesia of the cornea was the prominent symptom, two only showed evidence of destructive changes and panophthalmitis; and in both of these there was evidence of septic irritation. In the remaining fifteen, with the exception of slight drying of the corneal surface, no opacity or ulceration was detected, although the duration of life varied from forty-eight hours to four months after the section of the nerve.

Looking more especially at the cases in which the ophthalmic branch was divided, it was found that of the series of seven such, one only showed destructive corneal change, and in that also there was post-mortem evidence of septic meningitis. But of more interest in these cases is the fact that in one of them the cornea of both eyes was touched with a point of lunar caustic. As a result, a small central corneal ulcer formed, but no progressive change ensued, and the process of repair proceeded as well in the cornea on the side on which the ophthalmic branch was divided as on the sound side.

The general conclusion to be drawn from a study of these experiments is that no strictly trophic influence is exerted by the Gasserian ganglion upon the cornea; and that, provided septic organisms are excluded, the ophthalmic branch may be safely divided, or the Gasserian ganglion removed, without. fear of disorganisation of the eye. The destructive changes which occur with inflammatory conditions of the basal meninges, without the existence of an external wound, would seem, on this hypothesis, to be due to the presence of pathogenetic organisms causing local irritation (*Brit. Med. Journal*, 1895, vol. ii.) And these facts are corroborated by the cases of extirpation of the Gasserian ganglion in the human subject. Of the series of five such cases recorded by Rose only one showed disorganisation of the eye, and this was clearly due to accidental causes; while in Richardson's, Krause's, and Doyen's cases the cornea one week, two months, and one year respectively after the removal of the Gasserian ganglion, showed no alteration.

It may therefore be stated' that the so-called neuro-paralytic phenomena associated with lesion of the trigeminal nerve are evidence of irritation of the nerve, and not of paralysis. This statement holds good whether the lesion be situated so as to implicate the ophthalmic branch, the nerve trunk, or the intra-medullary root.

Paralysis of the fifth nerve.—The symptoms of paralysis of the trigeminal nerve resolve themselves into two sets, according as the motor or sensory branches of the nerve are implicated.

Paralysis of the *motor branch* is indicated by weakness of the muscles of mastication. The feebleness or inability to contract may be detected manually in the case of the temporal and masseter muscles; while unilateral loss of power in the pterygoid muscles is shown by the deviation of the lower jaw to the paralysed side when the mouth is opened, and by inability to move the jaw to the non-paralysed side.

As Gowers states, there is no sign of the paralysis of the tensor tympani and tensor palati muscles in affections of this nerve ; nor, likewise, is there any evidence of paralysis of the mylohyoid and anterior belly of the digastric, although, as already shown, these muscles are probably innervated through the motor fifth.

The *causes* of this paralysis are similar to those affecting the other motor cranial nerves. Thus, the motor nuclei of the nerves may be affected in the chronic form of progressive bulbar palsy. Usually this is a late phenomenon, but it has been observed in the early stages, more especially in association with primary affection of the oculo-motor nuclei. A possible and occasional connection between the third nerve nucleus and the descending trigeminal root has been described already (p. 783).

The roots of the nerve are involved in the pathological conditions affecting the dura mater of the base, alone or in association with adjacent nerves, chiefly the oculo-motor nerves. Unilateral motor trigeminal palsy, with or without implication of the auditory nerve on the same side, and associated with symptoms of cerebellar disease, is characteristic of lesion of the middle fossa, and is usually diagnostic of tumour or pressure upon the middle cerebellar peduncle.

It is still a point of doubt how far cortical and sub-cortical lesions may produce masticatory paralysis. There is as yet no really crucial case of palsy of these muscles from a purely cortical lesion, although cases in which this condition formed one of the symptoms have been described by Barlow, Dalmont and Kirchhoff. Cases of trismus have indeed been recorded (Hirt and others), but there is reason to suspect that these cases were complicated by other lesions ; in Hirt's cases, for example, there were clear signs of tabes dorsalis.

Oppenheim and Siemerling, in their recent work on pseudo-bulbar or subcortical bulbar palsy, have described weakness of this muscular group ; but they have also shown clearly that in the majority of these cases careful microscopic examination reveals hæmorrhages, thrombosis, etc., in the medulla and pons Varolii.

Palsy of the masticatory muscles, on the other hand, may be due to coarse lesions in the pons Varolii ; for example, tumours, hæmorrhages, etc. involving the nucleus or roots of the nerve.

It has been already pointed out, when describing the physiology of the fifth nerve, that trophic alterations do not necessarily follow lesion, either of the nerve trunk or of the ophthalmic branch ; and that when they occur they are evidence of irritation, and not of paralysis. *A constant feature*, however, *of palsy of the sensory division* is anæsthesia (of the peripheral type) over the distribution of the branches of the nerve. This anæsthesia extends from the vertex over the face to the margin of the lower jaw, and affects also the mucous membranes of the nose, mouth, the tongue, the soft palate and its anterior pillars, the cornea and the conjunctiva. According to the branch or branches involved and to the intensity of the destruction, depends the extent and completeness of the anæsthesia. A usual symptom of disease of the roots of the fifth nerve is the loss of taste on the same side as the lesion (*vide* "Sense of Taste").

There are several points of importance to be considered in estimating the value of trigeminal anæsthesia as a localising symptom.

Anæsthesia over the area of the first division of the nerve suggests implication of the ophthalmic branch; but this being associated with oculo-motor paralysis, and indicating meningeal affection in the region of the sphenoidal fissure, rarely occurs as a solitary feature.

Anæsthesia over the distribution of the whole trigeminal nerve on one side, with or without coexistent affection of the motor root, indicates as a rule lesion of the root of the nerve between the Gasserian ganglion and the surface of the pons Varolii; but it is not unlikely that the same symptom may arise from a localised lesion in the pons, without any impairment of the motor or sensory function of the limbs. Not uncommonly, however, along with such an anæsthetic area, symptoms of cerebellar disease are present, pointing conclusively to an affection of the middle cerebellar peduncle, involving the trigeminal root.

Anæsthesia over the area of trigeminal distribution on one side may be found associated with some impairment of the common sensibility of the body and limbs. In a series of experiments upon destruction of the tubercle of Rolando in monkeys (1), it was found that this lesion produced certain sensory alterations in the body and limbs on both sides in association with complete tactile and painful anæsthesia over the distribution of the fifth nerve upon the same side. The sensory disturbances varied according as the examinations were made immediately after the operation, or after a short interval. In the first instance tactile anæsthesia and loss of the sense of localisation on the side of lesion were associated with analgesia on the opposite side; but later a restitution of tactile sensation was established, while painful sensibility remained defective. Closely analogous phenomena were noted by Herzen and Lœwenthal in their experiments upon cats; and Bechterew records a case in which somewhat similar phenomena were observed after a wound in the region of the occipito-atloid joint. Hence we are justified in stating that should complete trigeminal anæsthesia on one side be associated with loss or defect of tactile sensibility in the body and limbs on the same side, and analgesia on the opposite side, the lesion may with confidence be referred to the level of the spinal-medullary junction, involving more especially the tubercle of Rolando and the origin of the ascending trigeminal root.

It is doubtful, however, whether the same dissociation of sensory phenomena obtains with lesions higher up in the medulla or pons Varolii. Should the "ascending" trigeminal root be involved, complete trigeminal anæsthesia will result on the side of lesion; and if this lesion be sufficiently extensive a coexistent impairment of sensibility of the body and limbs will arise on the side opposite to the facial anæsthesia (16).

The presence of trigeminal anæsthesia on the same side as that of the body and limbs points to a lesion above the entrance into the pons of the sensory root of the fifth nerve ; and, according to the associated phenomena, it may be placed either in the upper part of the pons, the crura cerebri, or the posterior part of the internal capsule.

Such are the general indications by which trigeminal anæsthesia may be used as a localising sign. It is less easy to state definitely what structure in the central nervous apparatus conveys the sensory impressions from the face to the cortex cerebri. According to Hösel, this is to be found in the mesial fillet or lemniscus ; but evidence may be brought forward against this view, the chief of which is that this strand of fibres may be entirely sclerosed, and the structures from which it arises destroyed, without any impairment of sensation.

It has been shown already that impressions are conveyed by the fibres of the ascending trigeminal root as far down as the tubercle of Rolando at the spinal-medullary junction : the assumption is that they then cross the raphé and ascend in the tegment of the medulla and pons of the opposite side, although no direct evidence from degeneration is yet forthcoming.

The sense of taste.—In addition to the tongue, the mucous membrane of the soft palate and palatine arches subserves the sense of taste. Two nerves are stated to preside over this function, the chorda tympani, a branch of the facial nerve for the anterior two-thirds of the tongue, and the glossopharyngeal nerve for the posterior third ; the soft palate and palatine arches receiving branches from the spheno-palatine or Meckel's ganglion. There is, however, reason to suppose that the fibres for taste do not pass into the brain by the roots of the same nerves as those by which they are peripherally distributed. Hence their position has to be studied in connection with their peripheral distribution, as well as with the channels by which they pass into the brain.

Most observers are agreed that the taste fibres for the anterior part of the tongue are distributed with the branches of the lingual nerve, for section of this nerve was found by Lussana and others to be followed by loss of taste on the anterior two-thirds on the same side. But whether all the fibres pass into the chorda tympani, or whether some pass directly along the lingual, is less certain, as some observations by Schiff and Ferrier indicated that section of the lingual nerve above its union with the chorda tympani produced in some cases a partial loss of taste.

It is a well-known fact that implication of the facial nerve, either in disease of the middle ear, or in inflammatory conditions implicating the nerve in the *aqueductus Fallopii*, is associated with loss of taste on the anterior two-thirds of the tongue ; and the experimental observations of Urbantschitsch showed that electrical excitation of the facial trunk, when exposed after suppurative disease of the middle ear, gave subjective sensations of taste. Sir William Gowers, moreover, points out that in this condition taste may be lost over the posterior third of the tongue as well as on the anterior parts.

It seems now to be proved that disease of the root of the facial nerve within the skull is not associated with any loss of taste; while there are numerous recorded cases (Erb, Gowers, and others) in which disease affecting the sensory division of the trigeminus between the Gasserian ganglion and the brain was associated with such loss. In some of the cases this loss was detected over the whole tongue on the side of lesion (Erb, Gowers), in others it was limited to the anterior two-thirds (Ferrier and others), while in a unique case recorded by Bruns no such loss was made out either on the front or back of the tongue. Undoubtedly many cases of peripheral trigeminal palsy are met with in which no loss of taste is detected; but in these it is found either that the implication of the nerve is not complete, or that the lesion is in the medulla, the anæsthesia being due to implication of the so-called ascending root.

There is much contradictory evidence as to the branch or branches of the fifth nerve which transmit the fibres of taste. The first or ophthalmic branch may with certainty be excluded. There are, on the one hand, numerous cases of abolition of taste (Salomonsohn, Heusner, Zenner) in which the distribution of anæsthesia indicated a lesion of the first and second divisions and an intact state of the third. On the other hand, cases exist in which the anæsthetic area pointed to a lesion of the third division only, yet in which taste also was lost (Romberg, Ziehl). Or again, a case of Erb's shows paralysis of the third trigeminal branch with an intact state of the first and second, and retention of taste; while cases by Jaffé, Stamm, and Schmidt show retention of taste where the third branch was free, and the first and second nerves, either in whole or in part, paralysed. The evidence on this part, therefore, is conflicting, and on the whole is divided as to whether the taste fibres pass by the second or the third divisions of the nerve.

Two points are, however, established: first, that the facial nerve within the Fallopian aqueduct contains fibres of taste; and, secondly, that they are also present in the root, and in the second and third divisions of the trigeminus. How then and by what route are these two nerves connected? The answer appears to be given by a case recorded by Ferguson (4), in which a small exostosis was found after death to press upon and to divide the left Vidian nerve. Now, during life complete loss of taste had existed upon the anterior two-thirds of the tongue upon the left side, while the posterior part of the tongue, the fauces, and the soft palate were normal. Subsequent microscopic examination showed degeneration of the great superficial petrosal nerve, which was found to enter the ganglion geniculum faciale, and to pass through the facial trunk as far as the chorda-tympani, from which it was traced to the lingual nerve.

This case, which stands alone, affords conclusive proof of the passage of the taste fibres for the anterior two-thirds of the tongue through the Vidian and great superficial petrosal nerves to the facial trunk, from which they pass by the chorda-tympani to the lingual branch of the third division of the trigeminus. Owing to the connection between the Vidian nerve and the spheno-palatine, or Meckel's ganglion, it would have been expected that excision of this structure should occasion loss of taste on the anterior two-thirds ; such, however, according to the observations of Prevost and Bastian, is not the case.   But, on the other hand, Schiff has stated that section of the superior maxillary division above the spheno-palatine ganglion was followed by loss of taste on the anterior two-thirds.

In the rare cases of disease of the roots of the bulbar nerves in the subdural space, without coexistent implications of the roots of the fifth, taste has usually been retained ; although Ziehl mentions a partially recorded case in which taste was lost on the posterior third, all the nerves from the sixth to the twelfth being involved ; but there was no necropsy.

Lesions of the glossopharyngeal trunk are accompanied by loss of taste on the posterior third of the tongue ; and the experiments of Vintschgau and Honigschmied showed that division of the nerve was followed by atrophy of the circumvallate papillæ and taste bulbs.   But the more recent experiments of Baginsky failed to confirm this observation.

In a case recorded by Lehmann a basal fracture caused paralysis of the facial, auditory, hypoglossal, and vagus nerves on the right side, on which side, throughout the length of the tongue, taste was abolished.[1]

A unique case is recorded by Pope (11), in which aneurysm of the left vertebral artery pressed upon the roots of the glossopharyngeal nerve. Here taste was abolished on the left side of the tongue, but only partially in the anterior portion.

There are also cases on record of complete uncomplicated paralysis of the sensory root of the trigeminus in which taste was retained on the posterior third of the tongue (Ferrier).

The evidence, therefore, regarding the ultimate destination of the taste fibres contained in the glossopharyngeal nerve is conflicting, for the test case—complete isolated unilateral glossopharyngeal root palsy—is not yet recorded, although Pope's case comes near to it.

There is some evidence to show that implication of the tympanic plexus and the nerve of Jacobson may be associated with loss of taste on the posterior third of the tongue.

The general conclusion to be drawn from these observations is, that the taste fibres contained in the trunk of the glossopharyngeal nerve may on the one hand pass into the roots of the nerve, or on the other escape through the nerve of Jacobson and enter the small superficial petrosal nerve, from which they pass through the otic ganglion to the inferior maxillary division of the trigeminus.

The taste fibres having then reached the brain through the root of the fifth nerve, what is their further course ? on this point there is no clear evidence, except one observation recorded by Gowers.   In this case

---

[1] There is no post-mortem record, but it is suggested that the loss of taste on the anterior part is due to involvement of the facial nerve, as it passes through the petrous temporal bone, which was evidently invaded by the fracture.

paralysis of taste was associated with loss of the conjugate movement of the eyeballs to the same side, but without anæsthesia over the area of the fifth nerve—indicating the separation of the taste fibres from those of common sensation after entering the pons Varolii; and a case recorded by Dana proves the converse. Here the symptoms were paralysis of the limbs on one side, with palsy and anæsthesia of the face on the opposite, but without loss of taste—a combination clearly pointing to a lesion within the medulla involving the so-called ascending trigeminal root.

What the further course of the taste fibres may be is doubtful. They probably pass brainwards in relation with the fibres of tactile and painful sensibility. That they have decussated at the internal capsule is clear from the fact that lesions of the posterior limb have been associated with defect of taste on the opposite side; while a cortical centre for taste has been located in the tip of the temporo-sphenoidal lobe.

Treatment.—Little need be said about the treatment of paralysis of the fifth nerve. In the majority of cases the internal administration of specific remedies with local counter-irritation is all that can be done medicinally.

In paralysis of the muscles of the jaw from lesions of a degenerative nature, the hypodermic injections of strychnine are to be recommended, in conjunction with local electrical treatment (faradism or galvanism as the case may require), according to the reaction of the muscles.

For an account of trigeminal neuralgia the reader is referred to the article on "Neuralgia," p. 724.

THE FACIAL NERVE.—The *nucleus of origin* of the facial nerve is situated in the ventral portion of the tegmentum pontis, immediately dorsal to and outside the superior olivary body. As in the case of both the third and hypoglossal nuclei it is segmented. Kölliker follows Huguenin in describing two such segments, a dorsal and a ventral; but it is, so far, quite uncertain whether they correspond to special divisions of the facial nerve trunk.

The nerve-roots pass dorsally, in a series of fasciculi, towards the floor of the fourth ventricle; on reaching which position they are collected into a compact bundle, to be seen mesial and somewhat dorsal to the sixth nucleus. The root-fibres, which hitherto have held a vertical course, now pass horizontally under the floor of the ventricle, as far as the upper (proximal) end of the sixth nerve nucleus. Here they turn obliquely outwards, and passing through the tegmentum and transverse fibres of the pons, reach the surface in a position between the trigeminal and abducens nerves, and ventral to the auditory nerve. The following important connections of the nucleus and nerve may be said to be established either directly by anatomical, or indirectly by clinical evidence.

(i.) That it is associated with the cortex cerebri, and that the cortico-peduncular fibres pass in close relation with the like fibres of the other cranial nerves, is undoubted. Bechterew places them immediately posterior to the "knee" of the internal capsule; in the crus cerebri they form the innermost of the bundles of the pyramidal system, and lie immediately external to the fronto-pontine tract, which is the most mesial of the bundles in this region. Spitzka observed degeneration of this bundle after a destructive lesion of the cerebral cortex involving the facial and hypoglossal areas.

(ii.) A direct connection is believed to exist between the hind-part of the third nerve nucleus and the issuing root of the facial nerve. I have observed in two cases in which the facial nucleus was degenerated and the oculo-motor nuclei were healthy, a large number of normal nerve-fibres passing into the otherwise atrophied facial nerve-root from the opposite posterior longitudinal bundle—an observation which has been confirmed by Oppenheim and Muratoff in similar cases. The experiments of Mendel, so far as they go, tend to corroborate this connection; and there is some recent clinical evidence also in support of it, to which reference will later on be made.

(iii.) A similar connection is stated to exist between the hypoglossal nucleus and the facial nerve—a relation originally pointed out by Lockhart Clarke. Direct anatomical evidence of this is so far wanting, but some clinical facts lend support to the view.

(iv.) Minor connections are stated to exist between the facial nucleus and the corpus trapezoides and the sensory trigeminal root.

Reference has still to be made to the *portio intermedia*, or nerve of Wrisberg. It was supposed by Huguenin that this nerve arises in the accessory auditory nucleus, and forms the sensory root of the facial trunk; but the observations of Martin and His showed that the fibres arose in the ganglion geniculi facialis, and, according to Duval, belonged entirely to the facial nerve, and formed the fibres of the chorda tympani. The cerebral termination of this nerve remains obscure: His traced it into the "solitary bundle" or ascending vago-glossopharyngeal root; but the recent observations of Kölliker do not confirm this relation. Kölliker is rather of opinion that some of the fibres enter by the facial nerve and others by the auditory.

Facial paralysis.—This is one of the commonest forms of cranial nerve palsy, and arises both from central and peripheral causes. Facial palsy of central origin will be considered later, as it shows certain features by which it may be distinguished from the more common peripheral type. By far the commonest variety of this is the so-called "rheumatic" facial paralysis, caused in the majority of cases by cold. According to the statistics of Philip and Hubschmann, from 72 to 73 per cent are due to this agent; from 6 to 9 per cent are due to otitis media, 5 to 6 per cent are of traumatic nature, and about 3 per cent are syphilitic.

The pathological anatomy of the common form of facial palsy has recently been described. In a case of rheumatic facial palsy, accompanied by loss of taste on the anterior two-thirds of the tongue, hyperacusis, and the reaction of degeneration in the facial muscles, in which death occurred from an intercurrent affection, Minkowski found a true degenerative neuritis, with disintegration of the medullary sheaths, but without evidence of interstitial inflammation. The important feature detected in this case was the intensity of the inflammation at the outer end of the Fallopian canal and in the peripheral distribution of the nerve, with lessening intensity when traced along the nerve towards the geniculate ganglion. In a case of facial paralysis arising from disease of the middle ear Darkschewitsch and Tichonow also found a parenchymatous neuritis extending peripherally from the site of the lesion, but without any interstitial change. There is not yet, therefore, sufficient pathological evidence on which to base the statement that in the rheumatic form of facial palsy the nerve is compressed by inflammatory material, either in the Fallopian canal or at its issue from it. The meagre pathological evidence at our disposal locates the change chiefly in the nerve branches distributed over the face, and in the outer part of the Fallopian canal; while the pathological state of the nerve is a parenchymatous and not an interstitial inflammation.

This may explain some of the features observed in the purely peripheral facial palsy, such as greater implication of some groups of muscles; simultaneous affection of one or more branches of the trigeminal nerve, which is occasionally observed; the curious relation which has been noted between herpes zoster facialis and herpes zoster of the cervical plexus with facial palsy; and the rare instances in which the palsy has extended from one side of the face to the other, as in the case recorded by Hubschmann.

Regarding other aspects in the pathology of facial paralysis, there are to be noted the forms associated—(*a*) with chronic degenerative atrophy of the cells of the facial nucleus; (*b*) with implication of the nerve-roots by lesions situated in the tegmentum pontis; (*c*) with destruction of the nerve-roots by gummatous or other new growths involving the dura mater of the base of the skull; (*d*) with the form associated with other peripheral palsies as sequels of diphtheria, in which no pathological change at all has been detected; and, lastly, the form which is observed in the true myopathies, such as have been described by Landouzy and Déjérine.

The *symptoms* of a complete facial palsy are so characteristic that a detailed description of the condition is unnecessary. There is loss of movement over the whole of the affected side of the face, and when the patient is requested to close the eyes, the eyeball on the paralysed side is seen to roll upwards, owing to the absence of descent of the upper lid. Whistling is impossible, and the tongue, when protruded, may give a false impression of deviation to the paralysed side. Food collects between the jaw and the cheek; and in drinking, the fluid may run out at the angle of the mouth.

Taste may or may not be abolished on the anterior two-thirds of the tongue. In mild cases, characterised by slight facial palsy and quantitative diminution of the faradic excitability, taste may not be affected at all, indicating a limitation of the affection to the peripheral distribution of the nerve; while in more severe cases, as shown in that recorded by Minkowski, taste is lost by an extension of the neuritis into the Fallopian canal towards the geniculate ganglion. Ageusia, therefore, implies either an extension of the neuritis into the Fallopian canal, or, according to some investigators, a concomitant lesion of the fifth nerve, which sometimes shows itself in diminished sensation over the paralysed side of the face.

In facial palsy from lesion of the nerve-trunk paralysis of the soft palate does not occur. The association of these symptoms, which is commonly described, is due to simultaneous affection of the facial and vago-glossopharyngeal nerves (*vide* "Paralysis of the Palate," p. 820).

Hearing is often implicated. Should the lesion causing the facial palsy be middle ear disease, air conduction of sound may be abolished ; but in cases where the nerve to the stapedius muscle is involved, without otitis media, an increased sense of hearing may exist, especially to musical sounds.

Many cases are met with in which no such complete invasion of the facial muscles is detected, especially when submitted to electrical stimulation. In illustration of this I have observed cases in which faradic excitability had been lost in all the facial muscles, excepting the frontalis and orbicularis palpebrarum, which, however, have shown quantitative diminution ; while the palpebral portion of the orbicularis palpebrarum is especially retentive of faradic excitability—a fact which may indeed suggest the possibility of its further innervation directly from the third nerve nucleus, through the connection which exists between the third and fifth nerves at the sphenoidal fissure : it is a common observation that the oculo-facial group recovers its electrical irritability earlier than the other facial muscles.' I have also notes of a case of apparently peripheral nature, in which the levator anguli oris on one side appeared to be the muscle mainly affected. Cases are also on record of escape of the orbicularis oris, and of the triangularis and quadratus menti ; but it would appear that these are probably of congenital origin, and as such are due to nuclear degeneration.

The escape of the orbicularis oris in the cases of congenital facial palsy recorded by Schultze and Bernhardt, tell in favour of the innervation of this muscle from the hypoglossal rather than from the facial nucleus— a fact which is also emphasised by the unique case described by Gowers, in which the orbicularis oris escaped when the facial nucleus was affected by acute polio-myelitis.

Another and minor symptom met with in facial paralysis, due indirectly to the nerve lesion as such, may be mentioned; namely, an apparent increase in the secretion of tears (epiphora), a condition which is caused by the defective movement of the lower lid and the associated palsy of Horner's muscle.

Varieties of facial paralysis.—(i.) *Cortical and subcortical facial palsy.* —Paralysis of the face, having features to be described presently, follows destructive lesions of the cerebral cortex at the lower end of the ascending frontal gyrus and of the fibres which pass from this centre to the facial nucleus in the pons Varolii. These fibres lie at the knee of the internal capsule, and in the pes cruris they lie innermost of the pyramidal fibres. They are distinct from the oculo-motor fibres and may be paralysed alone. The lesion may be either on one or on both sides of the brain.

The characteristic feature of cerebral facial paralysis lies in the greater implication of the lower facial muscles, the upper being relatively intact. It is a mistake, however, to suppose that the oculo-facial group is not weakened in this form; although the eyelids may be closed voluntarily, yet on the side of the paralysis the patient is usually unable to resist attempts to open them. Should there be weakness on both sides, as is seen in the so-called *pseudo-bulbar paralysis*, the weakness of the oculo-facial group is bilateral, but it is not complete. As stated by Oppenheim, the patient may be able to close the lid momentarily, but the lagophthalmos, so characteristic of peripheral facial diplegia, is never seen in this condition. It has also been stated, as characteristic, that although the patient is unable to keep the lids closed, yet he can wink reflexly (Tilling and Wernicke).

In the cerebral form, also, although the voluntary movements of the mouth are paralysed on one side, the emotional are as a rule retained; in the peripheral type both forms are abolished. Facial weakness, as described from cortical and subcortical causes, rarely, if ever, occurs alone, being associated with paresis of the tongue movements and defective articulation, and paralysis of the limbs on one or both sides. The electrical irritability of the muscles is unchanged, or at the most presents a slight general quantitative diminution.

(ii.) Should the lesion, however, be situated in the lower part of the pons Varolii, one of the forms of alternate hemiplegia is met with; there is paralysis of the face, of the peripheral type, on one side, and of the limbs on the opposite side. This condition is rarely found alone, being in the majority of recorded cases, in which the lesion is situated within the pons, associated with paralysis of conjugate movements of the eyes to the side of the facial palsy. This association of symptoms—unilateral facial palsy, and loss of conjugate movements to the same side, with or without hemiplegia of the opposite limbs—is diagnostic of a lesion of the tegmentum pontis, involving the nucleus of the sixth, the "knee," and the issuing root of the seventh nerve.

(iii.) The diagnostic signs of a *nuclear lesion* are not yet sufficiently explicit, for chronic degeneration of the facial nucleus rarely occurs alone, being associated with degeneration of the hypoglossal, motor fifth, and sometimes the oculo-motor nuclei. A case of acute isolated infantile palsy of the face is mentioned by Sir William Gowers; in this the orbicularis oris escaped. An example will be brought forward to show that the nerve-fibres supplying the sphincter oris may arise from another nucleus, probably the hypoglossal. Other facts lending support to this view are the well-known association which exists between the movement of the lips and tongue, and their simultaneous implication as an early symptom in bulbar palsy, and the escape of the orbicularis oris in the cases of congenital facial palsy already mentioned.

There is reason also to suppose that some of the fibres for the frontalis and orbicularis palpebrarum muscles may arise in the posterior part of the third nerve nucleus. Reference has been already made to the course which these fibres probably take.

I have seen weakness of the orbicularis palpebrarum in three cases of nuclear ophthalmoplegia, in one of which the frontalis was so much paralysed that the patient was unable to frown. Hughlings Jackson has also recorded two cases of this association; others again have been referred to more recently by Hanke and Goldflam.[1]

(iv.) The facial nerve is not uncommonly involved in disease (gumma, tubercle, etc.) of the dura mater of the base of the skull, with or without associated paralysis of the auditory nerve; in such cases the symptoms are those of a complete palsy of the peripheral type, with the important difference that taste is unaffected. The condition is not uncommonly bilateral, and gives rise to *diplegia facialis* to be presently described. Other cranial nerves may be affected simultaneously; more especially the auditory, which in the subdural space lies immediately superior and dorsal to the facial.

Several cases of diplegia facialis with bilateral deafness are on record. The cause in such cases is usually a gummatous meningitis of the posterior fossa, but fracture of the base of the cranium produced the combination in one instance (Bristowe).

(v.) Unilateral facial palsy of the peripheral type has been described already. Several cases have been recorded in which the condition was bilateral, simulating, in symptoms, that met with in double lesions of the dura mater of the base. In these cases one side is usually affected before the other, the cause, according to Hubschmann, being the passage of the inflammatory condition from the nerves of one side across to the other.

The most common agent, however, in the production of peripheral facial diplegia is the diphtheritic poison. This is usually a grave symptom, being associated with paralysis of other important muscles. In the cases which I have seen, the ocular muscles, the diaphragm, the soft palate, and the muscles of the limbs have also been involved, and death has occurred from cardio-pulmonary paralysis. As already mentioned, when dealing with ocular palsies, a lesion in these cases may be found in the intra-muscular portions of the motor nerves. So far as ascertained this has not been definitely proved for man. In those personally examined no change was detected either in the nerve centres or in the trunks of the peripheral nerves, so that the evidence on this point is chiefly negative.

Simultaneous bilateral otitis media has been known to cause peripheral diplegia facialis (Wright); as also the application of the forceps at the time of birth (Edgeworth); an association between dental periostitis, teeth extraction, and facial paralysis has also been observed (Hochwart).

The *prognosis* of facial paralysis is based upon—first, the seat of the lesion ; and, secondly, in peripheral cases upon the electrical reactions.

---

[1] It is possible that the frontalis receives a direct nerve-supply from the third nerve, through the anastomosis which exists between this and the ophthalmic branch of the fifth at the sphenoidal fissure.

In the nuclear variety the prognosis is grave, because the facial weakness is merely an element in a degenerative process occurring throughout the bulbo-spinal centres. In this form there is generally a quantitative diminution to both faradic and galvanic stimulation.

If the palsy be of the type associated with disease in the subdural space, the prognosis also is bad, as it is seldom that the affection remains limited; although, if it be of a syphilitic nature, a certain amount of recovery may take place under suitable treatment.

Of the purely peripheral forms, that due to disease of the middle ear is the least satisfactory; only in rare instances do these forms show any marked improvement, although the aural disease may be carefully treated and cured. Secondary contracture and over-action of the muscles on the paralysed side is, in this form, not uncommon.

In the peripheral forms of rheumatic nature, already shown to be by far the commonest variety of facial palsy, an *electrical examination* is essential in order to form a satisfactory prognosis. If from a week to ten days after the onset of the paralysis there is no quantitative diminution, but rather an increase to faradic stimulation, recovery will take place in three or four weeks. If at about the same time after the onset the faradic irritability be distinctly lessened quantitatively, recovery is likely to take place in from six weeks to two months. Should the faradic excitability be entirely lost in seven to ten days after the onset, recovery is likely to be delayed for three months. In this case, in addition to the loss of faradic reaction, there is likely to be qualitative galvanic alterations, seen in the reaction of degeneration. If the faradic excitability remain in abeyance three, four, or more months after the onset, the prognosis as to recovery should be guardedly given. In such cases the onset of secondary contracture and over-action is highly probable.

Treatment.—This is, for all practical purposes, limited to the purely peripheral type of palsy. In the mildest forms, characterised by a slight diminution of the faradic excitability of the muscles on the weakened side of the face, little or no active treatment is required; the application of a mustard leaf or small fly blister behind the ear and the prevention of fresh exposure to cold are all that is needed, as recovery will take place in from three weeks to one month.

In the more severe forms of facial palsy, especially in those associated at the outset with considerable pain, care ought to be taken in the use of counter-irritants. I have seen a case in which the injudicious use of croton oil, as a counter-irritant, provoked most intense cellulitis over the parotid region; in such cases the careful use of small mustard leaves, repeated several times, may be of greater service than the application of a cantharides blister.

In cases arising from disease of the middle ear the treatment of this latter condition is absolutely essential before any measures may be taken for the relief of the paralysed side of the face. On the whole such cases are distinctly unsatisfactory, especially if the ear disease be of long duration; for the nerve becomes so irretrievably disorganised as to obliterate all means of reorganisation.

As regards the use of electricity in facial palsy, the variety to be adopted is that to which the muscles respond. As long as faradic excitability is absent the galvanic current may be used with advantage.

Care should be exercised in the use of faradism as a remedial agent. In the mild cases, as I have already said, it is better not to use it at all; in cases of severer nature and of longer standing, in which a diminished faradic reaction is obtained, it may be used with advantage twice or thrice weekly for a short time. The too frequent or too prolonged use of the faradic current undoubtedly tends in some cases to the production of secondary contracture.

THE EIGHTH NERVE.—Anatomy. — The eighth nerve-trunk, having arrived at the side of the pons Varolii, divides into two nerve-roots, one of which passes mesial to the restiform body, the other dorsal and external to it; the former is the anterior, mesial, or *vestibular* root, the latter being the posterior, lateral, or *cochlear* root. Upon the cochlear root is situated the anterior or accessory auditory ganglion; while in the dorso-lateral part of the pons there lie two other auditory nuclei, the dorsal or chief auditory nucleus, and the external or Deiters' nucleus. It should be stated at the outset, in order to prevent inevitable confusion, that we have here to deal with two distinct nerves, having separate origins, separate terminations, and different functions.

1. *The vestibular nerve.*—The fibres of this nerve, arising in the lining membrane of the semicircular canals, pass in the trunk of the eighth nerve, and enter the pons Varolii between the restiform body and the ascending trigeminal root. Some of the fibres terminate in end-tufts around cells in Deiters' nucleus, while others pass into the dorsal nucleus. It is not clear whether any pass directly into the so-called descending auditory bundle, although Kölliker makes a statement to this effect. According to Bruce, the descending auditory bundle arises from the cells of the *nucleus cuneatus medullæ;* but degeneration in this bundle was not observed either after destruction of the cuneate nucleus or after section of the eighth nerve. According to Bechterew the chief part of the vestibular root passes on to the nucleus vestibularis, which lies at the outer angle of the fourth ventricle; but upon this point also there is considerable diversity of opinion. Baginsky, after destruction of the labyrinth in rabbits, found atrophy of the anterior root, and of the gray matter at the outer angle of the fourth ventricle, in which Bechterew places the vestibular nucleus, but which is regarded by Bruce as merely a dorsal extension of Deiters' nucleus. There was also noticed atrophy of the inner portion of the restiform body of Meynert, which corresponds to what is now known as the descending auditory bundle.

Given, therefore, as end-nuclei of the vestibular nerve, Deiters' nucleus and the dorsal auditory nucleus, how is this nerve brought into association with the other parts of the central nervous system ? This is effected, first, through the indirect connections which these nuclei have with the middle lobe of the cerebellum. It has been shown elsewhere that Deiters' nucleus stands in close relation with the *vermis cerebelli*—extirpatiou of which structure was followed by degeneration of the "direct sensory cerebellar tract" of Edinger and of the nucleus of Deiters. Hence these fibres arise as axis-cylinder processes of the cells of the roof nuclei, and terminate in end-tufts around the cells of the nucleus of Deiters, as implied by the degeneration just described. Kölliker states that axis-cylinder processes of the cells of Deiters' nucleus, the dorsal auditory nucleus, and of Bechterew's vestibular nucleus, pass towards the cerebellum ; but many of these processes appear to pass also into the formatio reticularis. And this leads to the consideration of the second connection which the vestibular end-nuclei have with other parts, namely, as the *fibræ arcuatæ internæ*. These fibres pass from the several vestibular end-nuclei into the tegmentum pontis ; others pass into the posterior longitudinal bundles, while others cross the raphé and appear to enter the lateral fillet.

A third connection of Deiters' nucleus, and one of much importance, is with the antero-lateral tract of the spinal cord. Von Monakow found atrophy of the cells of Deiters' nucleus after hemisection of the cervical portion of the spinal cord ; and Held has shown, by the myelination method, that this nucleus has both crossed and uncrossed connections with the antero-lateral ground bundles, and the lateral limiting layer of the spinal cord. In two experiments, performed in association with Dr. Ferrier, there was found, after destruction of Deiters' nucleus, a tract of degeneration in the antero-lateral periphery of the spinal cord on the side of the lesion.

Two other connections of Deiters' nucleus have also been described : one by Bruce with the inferior olivary body, and the other with the nucleus of the sixth nerve.

It is therefore clear that Deiters' nucleus has manifold connections with other parts of the hind-brain and spinal cord. This explains the observations of Onufrowitz and Baginsky, that the nucleus of Deiters does not atrophy after section of the auditory nerve ; for we have shown that a large part of Deiters' nucleus has no direct connection with the vestibular root. Its chief function, indeed, seems to be what Deiters originally stated, namely, an internode in a great cerebellar spinal system.

2. *The cochlear nerve.* — The fibres of this, the second division of the auditory nerve, arise as axis-cylinder processes of the cells of the cochlea, and pass in the trunk of the nerve to the anterior or accessory nucleus (auditory ganglion) situated outside the medulla oblongata on the trunk of the nerve. Here many of the fibres terminate in end-tufts around the ganglion cells, while others pass dorso-externally over the restiform body to terminate in a similar fashion in the so-called *tuberculum acusticum*, which lies on the dorso-lateral aspect of the medulla.

The cochlear fibres differ from the vestibular in two respects : first, they are of smaller size; and, secondly, they receive their medullary sheaths at a later date, so that on a section of the nerve the two sets of fibres may be distinguished.

There is reason to believe that the auditory tubercle and the accessory ganglion are parts of the same structure; and as the fibres of the cochlear nerve end therein, the term *cochlear end-nucleus* may be appropriately given (Kölliker). And in this relation also lies the explanation of the fact that section of the auditory nerve-trunk, as it enters the internal auditory meatus, is not followed by degeneration beyond the cochlear nuclei just described, or the vestibular end-nucleus to which reference has already been made.

Contained in these end-nuclei are large multipolar nerve-cells, whose axis-cylinder processes pass into the tegmentum medullæ, as the central connections of the cochlear nerve. Of these, let us first examine the fibres from the tuberculum acusticum, namely, the *striæ acousticæ*. It is probable that some of these fibres have a direct connection with the cochlear nerve; for after destruction of the auditory ganglion degenerated fibres were seen in the dorsal part of the tegmentum; the majority, however, do not thus degenerate after section of the nerve-trunk. Leaving the acoustic tubercle they pass more or less deeply into the reticular formation and cross the raphé. It is not certain where they end, but some are supposed to enter the posterior quadrigeminal bodies by the lateral fillet.

The central connections of the auditory ganglion are of great importance, as there is reason to believe that they form the *central auditory tract*. What these connections are will be described from cases in which the auditory ganglion was experimentally destroyed. The observations recorded here were made by Dr. Ferrier and myself from an experimental study of the central auditory tract in monkeys. As a result of this lesion, degeneration was traced through the fibres of the corpus trapezoïdes, across the raphé, into the lateral fillet of the opposite side. In connection with the degeneration of the trapezoid body, the mesial of the two portions into which the superior olivary bodies are divided showed extensive degenerative changes on both sides. Degeneration was followed through both lateral fillets, which was more extensive on the side opposite the lesion, of the tegmentum cruris and the internal geniculate body. The posterior corpora quadrigemina appeared to be ganglia accessory to the central auditory tract, rather than to be situated in it. There is reason to suppose that the internal geniculate body stands in a relation to the auditory tract similar to that of the external geniculate body and pulvinar thalami to the visual fibres.

Held has recently shown that the axis-cylinder processes of the cells of the auditory ganglion pass directly into and become fibres of the trapezoid body, some of which end in the superior olives, others merely giving off collaterals to them; the remainder passing on through the lateral fillet to the posterior quadrigeminal tubercles and internal geniculate body.

Von Monakow found that lesion of the lateral fillet was followed, among other changes, by atrophy of the superior olivary body, the posterior quadrigeminal body and its brachium, and the ventral tegmental radiation.

Situated on the external surface of the crus cerebri is a bundle of fibres known as the "bundle of Turck," or "lateral pontine system." Bechterew, Zacher, Winkler, and others have shown that this tract degenerated downwards into the upper portion of the pons Varolii; and it has been more recently pointed out by Déjerine that after a lesion of the second and third temporal gyri it degenerates downwards. On the other hand, destructive lesion of the first temporal gyrus, performed experimentally by Dr. Ferrier and myself, was followed by degeneration of this bundle, which could be clearly traced as far as the upper part of the pons Varolii. From this it is apparent that the temporal lobe has a double connection with the hind-brain : one, a projection system, from the temporal gyri to the pons Varolii; the other, an afferent system, passing from the accessory auditory ganglion by way of the trapezoid body, the lateral fillet, and internal geniculate body. As already said, there is reason to believe that this constitutes the central auditory tract.

Symptoms of nerve deafness.—When a person complains of deafness, it is essential to ascertain, in the first instance, whether this symptom be due to obstruction in the external auditory meatus, to disease of the middle ear, or to causes impairing the reception of sound by the internal apparatus and its conduction by the auditory nerve and central nervous mechanisms.

In many cases the history of the onset of deafness is of value in directing the physician's attention to the apparatus affected ; and if no objective sign is obtained of the existence of external or middle ear disease, the following symptoms and signs may be taken as indicative of disease of the auditory nervous mechanism.

1. Impairment or loss of the bone conduction of sound; the aerial being retained as tested by the tuning-fork of Gardiner-Brown, Weber, and Rinne. For example, when the note of a tuning-fork is no longer heard when held against the mastoid process, if it be placed off the concha and its sound again perceived, we suspect labyrinthine deafness (Rinne). If in a case of unilateral deafness the base of a vibrating tuning-fork be applied to the vertex in the middle line, the sound will be heard better towards the deaf ear, if this is due to the conducting apparatus, and better, or altogether in the sound ear if due to labyrinthine affection (Weber) ; or again, if a vibrating tuning-fork be held upon the root of the nose or on the vertex, and the patient told to indicate when he ceases to *hear* the sound, the examiner is able to compare the length of time before he ceases to *feel* the vibrations. In labyrinthine disease the patient ceases to hear the sound from half a second to several seconds before the examiner ceases to feel them (Gardiner-Brown). At or after sixty years of age senile changes occur which render bone conduction defective.

2. Impairment or loss of perception of notes of a high pitch ; the

voice, for example, being heard better than a watch. Galton's whistle is of value in testing such impairment.

3. The existence of vertigo and vomiting.

4. The presence of associated symptoms indicating disease of adjoining nervous structures. There is, as yet, no objective method by which deafness arising from disease of the auditory nerve may be distinguished from that due to lesion of the cerebral conducting tracts or centres, except by the presence of the associated symptoms referred to later.

Of certain phenomena, which may be taken as suggestive of labyrinthine disease, but which are in no wise conclusive, the following may be stated: audition is worse in a noise, whereas in middle-ear disease hearing is usually better under such circumstances (paracusis Willisii). There may be also a perversion of pitch, and a sensation of jarring produced by certain sounds. In such cases, also, inflation of the middle ear by a Politzer's bag not only fails to improve the hearing power, but frequently makes it temporarily worse.

Varieties of auditory anæsthesia.—(i.) Cortical and subcortical deafness. Cases of this nature due to tumour or softening involving the temporal lobe, and more especially the first temporal gyrus, are rare; but a sufficient number of clinico-pathological facts are on record to confirm the existence and the site of a cortical centre for hearing which experiment has indicated. As in a large number of such cases there has been no local examination of the ear, either clinically or pathologically, it has been deemed advisable not to refer to them here; but the subject is considered in greater detail in the subsequent chapter on "Cerebral Localisation."

A crucial case has, however, been recorded by Wernicke and Friedländer, in which complete deafness resulted from bilateral softening of the first temporal gyrus, while the examination of the ears both before and after death showed an entire absence of any local changes; and a case presenting somewhat similar features has more recently been reported by Mills.

Unilateral deafness has been observed from destructive lesion of the first temporal gyrus of the opposite side (Kaufmann, Ferguson), but this lesion is not commonly associated with impairment of hearing other than temporary.

The symptom more commonly met with as a result of unilateral destruction of the first temporal gyrus, and chiefly that on the left side in right-handed persons, is *word-deafness*, which may or may not be accompanied by some degree of deafness to ordinary auditory impressions.

(ii.) Deafness of varying degree has been met with as a result of lesion, chiefly tumour, of the corpora quadrigemina. It has been shown that the lateral fillet which degenerates after destruction of the external auditory ganglion stands in close relation to the posterior quadrigeminal bodies; and section of the lateral fillet itself was followed by degeneration in the nucleus of the posterior body on the same side. But it is still uncertain whether the posterior quadrigeminal bodies are in the central auditory tract, or merely lie in close relation to it. Hence it is doubtful whether the deafness observed in many cases of quadrigeminal tumour be due to direct lesion of these bodies, or merely to pressure upon the adjacent lateral fillet. In the records of nineteen cases of quadrigeminal tumour, Weinland found deafness in nine; and of these five showed impairment of hearing on both sides. In three hearing was defective on the side opposite the tubercles mainly destroyed. It appears therefore that hearing is chiefly impaired on the side opposite the lesion in such cases; but, owing to the mental dulness and apathy which frequently accompany tumours in this locality, it is difficult to obtain definite facts in this regard.

(iii.) In local lesion of the pons Varolii hearing is rarely impaired; this may be explained by the fact that morbid states in this region chiefly affect the tegmentum. It has been shown that the auditory tract is to be found in the corpus trapezoides and lateral fillet, structures which respectively lie ventral and lateral. In the pons, although the superior olivary bodies stand in close relation to the cochlear fibres of the trapezoid body, and degenerate after destruction of the external auditory ganglion, it is doubtful whether they play any direct part in the act of hearing, being more probably associated with the reflex movements of the eyeballs; their connection with the nucleus of the sixth nerve, through the so-called peduncle of the superior olive, being very intimate. Of thirty cases of pons tumour, collected by Bernhardt, in five only was there defect of hearing. In some of them this sense was not mentioned. In the three in which details are given, the impairment of hearing was upon the same side as the lesion, which was of considerable extent, and appeared to involve the auditory nerve at the surface of the pons.

(iv.) Deafness, unilateral or bilateral, is not uncommonly due to morbid processes affecting the auditory nerve in the posterior fossa. The nerve may be involved, either alone or in association with the facial nerve or other nerves, by gummatous or other morbid states of the dura mater of the base, by inflammatory conditions extending from the bones of the skull, by meningitis, or by aneurysm. Unilateral deafness associated with cerebellar symptoms is indicative of a tumour involving the middle cerebellar peduncle. (Such conditions have been referred to already, and further mention is made of them under "Multiple cranial nerve paralyses," p. 823.)

(v.) The commonest causes of "nerve deafness" are to be found in affections of the nerve terminations within the labyrinth. These conditions come properly into the sphere of the aural surgeon, but reference is more particularly made here to such affections in tabes dorsalis and other degenerative processes in the central nervous apparatus. Recent observations have shown that in tabes, not only is primary atrophy of the auditory nerve and its branches possible (Strumpell, Oppenheim, and Siemerling), but that actual degenerative changes occur in the structure of the labyrinth, giving rise to deafness, usually of a bilateral character;

the middle ear in such cases presenting a healthy appearance (Morpargo, Hochwart).

On the other hand, Lucae has found the labyrinth and auditory nerve normal in tabetics with defective hearing, a fact suggesting invasion of the central auditory apparatus by the sclerotic process characteristic of this disease. It should also be borne in mind that the lining membrane of the labyrinth undergoes atrophic degeneration in the old. Little is known regarding auditory phenomena in multiple sclerosis.

Less can be said regarding the *treatment* of nerve deafness than of any other form of cranial nerve palsy. For the various methods of treatment which have been from time to time recommended and adopted the reader is referred to special works on the subject. In other respects general principles should be applied in the treatment of deafness arising from intracranial disease.

THE HYPOGLOSSAL NERVE.—**The hypoglossal nucleus.**—The *hypoglossal chief nucleus* consists of a column of cells lying ventral to the central canal as long as this remains closed ; but when it has opened out into the fourth ventricle the nucleus forms the mesial part of the mass of gray matter forming its floor. The cells of the nucleus are roughly divided into three groups—internal, external, and posterior (Bruce). In sections prepared by the osmium-silver method the cells are seen to be large multipolar structures conforming to Golgi's first type. The axis-cylinder processes become chiefly the issuing roots of the nerve (Held). A few processes are seen to cross the middle plane, so as to form a commissure between the two nuclei.

Within and around the nucleus are many medullated nerve-fibres. Some of these are the terminations of the pyramidal fibres around the cells of the nucleus, the *fibræ propriæ* of Koch ; others belong to the " dorsal " and " posterior " longitudinal bundles.

Two accessory nuclei have been described in connection with the hypoglossal nerve—Roller's small-celled nucleus and the nucleus of Duval. The former lies ventral to the chief nucleus, and, according to the observations of Roller and Koch, it gives origin to some root fibres of the hypoglossal nerve, but it is doubtful whether this be so. The latter consists of large multipolar first-type cells, lying in close relation to the roots of the hypoglossal nerve. An analysis of the records of published cases of bulbar paralysis, in which the state of these nuclei was specially noted, as well as my personal observation, in two cases, indicate that they are not implicated in this disease. That they do not give origin to hypoglossal root fibres is also shown by the experiments of Mingazzini.

Duval's nucleus appears to be one of the many groups of large multipolar cells, which lie in the reticular formation and tegmentum, and whose physiological value is yet unknown. It is not improbable that many of these nuclei are stations in long commissural fibre systems uniting the cranial nerve nuclei with each other and with the spinal nerve nuclei. The nucleus of Deiters, as already described, is in part at least, a station in the cerebello-spinal system ; and the observations of Held and others have shown the presence of long internuncial fibres descending between the corpora quadrigemina and the antero-lateral columns of the spinal cord.

The *efferent* hypoglossal fibres are the root fibres or axis-cylinder processes of the cells of the nerve nucleus. Atrophy of the cells of the nucleus, which occurs in bulbar paralysis, is associated with atrophy of the root fibres in direct proportion to the amount of cell degeneration. The root fibres spring from the nucleus of the corresponding side.

The connections of the hypoglossal nucleus through afferent fibres are numerous. First, there are pyramidal fibres connecting this nucleus with the cells of the cortical centre for the movements of the tongue. These fibres pass in close relation with those of the other motor cranial nerves, already described. That they decussate in the raphé is probable, although there is, as yet, no anatomical evidence on this point. Secondly, fibres are said by Kölliker to pass from the fillet to the hypoglossal nucleus. Thirdly, afferent fibres reach the nucleus from the reticular formation ; they are of fine calibre, and are clearly seen in cases of bulbar paralysis, where the large issuing root fibres have disappeared ; but it is as yet impossible to say whether they are collaterals of long commissural systems in transit through the medulla, or whether they arise in cells scattered throughout that formation. It seems most probable that they are associated with the reflex mechanisms of the tongue.

A direct connection between the cells of the hypoglossal nucleus and the issuing vagus roots has been described by several observers (Lockhart Clark, Bruce, and others), and it has been suggested that this may be a source of innervation for the muscles of the soft palate and of the vocal cords. It seems more probable, however, that these fibres are really efferent vago-glossopharyngeal fibres passing from the cells of the posterior nucleus into the hypoglossal nucleus where they terminate in end-tufts (Kölliker).

Paralysis of the tongue—Glossoplegia.—The hypoglossal, like the motor fifth, is purely motor, hence the effects of its paralysis are found entirely in motor disturbances ; sensation in the cavity of the mouth, whether common or special, being normal when this nerve is affected alone. Palsy of the tongue may occur upon one or both sides ; in unilateral palsy defect is rarely apparent as long as the tongue lies still on the floor of the mouth ; but on protrusion it is seen that the tip deviates towards the paralysed side, from the unopposed action of the unaffected genio-hyglossus muscle : a patient with this affection may also have difficulty in moving the tongue within the mouth towards the paralysed side. A false appearance of paralysis of the tongue is commouly seen in facial paralysis ; here it appears as if the tongue deviates to the side of palsy owing to the asymmetrical movement of the mouth.

In complete bilateral palsy the tongue cannot be protruded at all, it lies motionless on the floor of the mouth. Owing entirely to the mechanical difficulty thus produced both articulation and swallowing are impaired. Should wasting of the muscular tissue of the tongue be present, in addition to paralysis, as occurs in nuclear and infra-nuclear affections, the mucous membrane is thrown into a number of prominent folds.

Paralysis of the tongue rarely occurs alone, being usually associated with a like affection of the lips, if from nuclear disease ; with the soft palate and the vocal cords, if from disease of the nerve-roots. If met with as an isolated symptom it is unilateral, and accompanied by wasting, from lesion of the nerve itself in the neck or floor of the mouth.

It will be found convenient to study hypoglossal paralysis, from the point of view of the localisation of the seat of disease, by the same methods as adopted for the other motor cranial nerves. Thus there may be—

(i.) *Supra-nuclear paralysis* (including the cortical and subcortical varieties). It is rare for a cortical or subcortical lesion to be so limited in extent as to involve the centre at the most posterior end of the third frontal gyrus, or the fibres proceeding from this in the centrum ovale, internal capsule, or pyramid, without injuring the adjacent centres or tracts. Edinger, however, has recorded a case in which a small focus of softening beneath the cortical centre produced paralysis of the tongue alone on the opposite side. In epilepsy the onset of a fit is sometimes heralded by a feeling of, or actual twitching on one side of the tongue.

Much more commonly does a lesion in this region give rise to palsy of the opposite side of the tongue with implication of the lower facial region ; or the palsy of the tongue may merely form an item of a hemiplegia.

In the so-called pseudo-bulbar paralysis bilateral hypoglossal palsy is observed, but not alone, being invariably associated with weakness of the facial muscles, and sometimes with weakness of the limbs. This condition is distinguished from the bilateral lingual palsy of nuclear disease by the absence of wasting and by the retention of the faradic excitability of the lingual muscles.

(ii.) *Nuclear paralysis.*—Atrophic degeneration of the cells of the hypoglossal nucleus is the earliest, and usually the chief pathological condition found in bulbar palsy. It is also met with as a concomitant lesion in tabes dorsalis, just as we have already observed atrophy of the oculomotor nuclei to give rise in this disease to ophthalmoplegia externa, or of the cells of the anterior horns of the spinal cord to localised atrophy of the muscles of the limbs. Other pathological conditions giving rise to nuclear palsy are met with in bulbar syphilis, in general paralysis of the insane, in localised hemorrhage and softening, involving the hypoglossal nucleus and the adjacent parts of the medulla oblongata ; and more recently the nucleus has been found implicated in the changes underlying the symptoms found in syringomyelia.

In addition to the paralysis of the lingual muscles observed in the chronic form of bulbar palsy, those other structures which stand in close physiological relation in the act of articulation—the lips, the soft palate, and the vocal cords—are also largely involved. This close physiological and degenerative association suggested an innervation of these structures from similar or closely related nerve nuclei; but more recent pathological investigation in cases of chronic bulbar palsy has shown that the muscles of the tongue are supplied exclusively from the hypoglossal nucleus, while those of the soft palate and vocal cords receive their nerve-supply from the nucleus ambiguus (p. 813). Although, as yet, there are no definite pathological facts to go by, it is not improbable that the orbicularis oris and lingual muscles are innervated from the same nucleus.

Nuclear palsy is characterised by bilateral and usually symmetrical atrophy of the tongue, with inability to protrude it. Fibrillary tremors are not uncommonly observed, and the faradic excitability is sometimes diminished, though rarely lost. The reflex action of the soft palate, fauces and larynx is also considerably lessened (see also "Bulbar Paralysis" in a later article).

(iii.) *Infra-nuclear paralysis.*—There are three situations where the hypoglossal nerve, in common with the other cranial nerves, may be implicated between the nucleus and the periphery.

First, where the roots pass from the nucleus in the floor of the fourth ventricle to the surface of the medulla. A lesion in this situation, involving the hypoglossal nerve-roots and the pyramid on one side, is productive of a rare form of alternate hemiplegia; the tongue being paralysed on one side and the limbs on the opposite side, as in the case recorded by Goukovsky.

Secondly, where the roots lie in the subdural space prior to their exit through the anterior condyloid foramen. In this situation the hypoglossal root fibres lie in close proximity to those of the vago-glossopharyngeal nerve, so that the one set is rarely involved without the other; and the symptoms of a lesion in this situation are highly characteristic; namely, unilateral paralysis of the tongue and of the soft palate and of the vocal cord on the same side. Disease in this situation is either of tuberculous, cario-necrotic, carcinomatous, or syphilitic nature, involving the meninges of the posterior fossa.

Thirdly, in the course of the nerve during or after its exit from the skull. The nerve trunk is not uncommonly thus engaged in disease of the occipito-atloid articulation; merely, however, from its close proximity to this joint and its ready invasion by inflammatory exudations connected therewith. Hemiatrophy of the tongue may indeed be the only localising symptom of suboccipital caries.

Idiopathic inflammation of the trunk of the hypoglossal nerve, such as is seen more especially in the facial nerve, is rare; a fact which is probably explained by the depth at which this nerve lies amongst the sublingual tissues.

The so-called "rheumatic" inflammation of this nerve rarely occurs, but its existence seems probable in the cases recorded by Montesano and Marina. There are cases on record in which it has been injured by wounds inflicted high up in the neck ; and its implication (along with the sympathetic, the spinal accessory, the vagus, and sometimes the glosso-pharyngeal nerves) in tumours or glandular enlargements behind the angle of the lower jaw, has been recorded from time to time.

Isolated hemiatrophy of the tongue from extra-cranial causes is so infrequent that it is necessary to exclude meningeal affections of the posterior fossa, which are not uncommon, before such a diagnosis is permissible.

Hemiatrophy of the tongue has also been observed occasionally in association with facial hemiatrophy (*vide* " Facial Hemiatrophy ").

The treatment of hypoglossal paralysis is to be conducted according to the same general principles, and upon the same lines as described for the other cranial nerves. Electricity may be applied to this organ with advantage in cases of hemiatrophy, as well as in complete paralysis. The occasional association between lingual hemiatrophy and suboccipital caries should not be forgotten.

THE VAGO-GLOSSOPHARYNGEAL NERVE.—Considerable confusion has existed both in the nomenclature and in the descriptions of mutual relations of the bulbar nerves—glossopharyngeus, vagus, and accessorius. Except outside the skull, where their distribution is clear, no means exist of distinguishing, anatomically, one from the other, either as regards their root fibres or nuclei of origin, except inferentially by their position ; the glossopharyngeal nerve being regarded as the uppermost, the accessory as the lowest of the series

It is commonly stated in text-books that the group of cells lying posterior to the hypoglossal nucleus so far as the central canal remains closed, is the nucleus of origin of the accessory nerve ; while after the canal has expanded into the fourth ventricle, the cell-column external to the hypoglossal nucleus gives origin, from its upper end, to the glosso-pharyngeal, and, from its lower end, to the vagus fibres.

But before considering the results of recent investigation into this complicated subject, let us inquire whether the nomenclature, as used in the text-books, is quite correct. As Spencer has pointed out, the descrip-tion of the roots of the bulbar nerves, as given by Willis, has not been universally followed. The term " accessory " was applied by this anatomist to the special nerve which is accessory to the vagi or " wandering pair," and which passes to the sterno-mastoid and trapezius muscles. Owing to a misuse of the term "accessory," it came to be applied to the lowest fibres arising from the bulb, which fibres do not belong to the accessory nerve, but to the vagus, as Willis indeed had shown. Hence the nerves of bulbar origin are, in addition to the hypoglossal, the glossopharyngeal and vagus ; while the accessory nerve, or nerve of Willis, is of purely spinal origin. In the accompanying detailed account of the nuclei of origin of the bulbar nerves, it is shown that the glosso-pharyngeal and vagus are really parts of one great mixed nerve ; that they have a common nucleus of origin of their efferent (motor) fibres ; and that their afferent fibres terminate in the so-called posterior end-nucleus on the one hand, and on the other in the so-called "ascending" glossopharyngeal root and its related end-nucleus.

The vago-glossopharyngeal nuclei.—These nuclei are considered as two segments of one structure, an anterior and a posterior : the former is the origin of the motor (efferent) root fibres of the vago-glossopharyngeal nerve, and forms the so-called *nucleus ambiguus ;* the latter is a portion of the end-nucleus of the afferent fibres of the vago-glossopharyngeal nerve-roots.

(a) *Nucleus ambiguus.*—According to Kölliker, to whom we are indebted for a very full and clear account, this nucleus extends from the level of the fillet decussation, proximally, as far as the exit of the upper glossopharyngeal root fibres. It is, therefore, coextensive with the posterior division of the nucleus, but occupies an antero-lateral position in the medulla. It is recognised by the position of its cells, which lie *upon* and *mesial* to the vago-glossopharyngeal root fibres. By the osmium-silver method it is found to be composed of large multipolar cells of Golgi's first type, the long axis of the cell lying parallel to the root fibres. From the fact that the nucleus alters its position in higher and lower portions of the medulla it has to be carefully defined from the *nucleus antero-lateralis medullæ* and the *nucleus centralis inferior* respectively. The former, which in the upper parts of the medulla lies immediately on its outer side, is characterised by the large amount of neuroglia in which its cells are buried ; the latter, in the lower parts of the medulla, lies *mesial* to the *nucleus ambiguus.* The *efferent* fibres of the nucleus are the axis-cylinder processes of its cells. In the lower portion of the medulla these fibres pass directly outwards from the nucleus as the lowest roots of the vagus nerve ; while in the upper portion they assume a dorso-internal direction before bending outwards as the upper fibres of the vagus and glossopharyngeal nerves (Kölliker).

In many cases of bulbar paralysis the cells of this nucleus have been found atrophied. But whether atrophy occurs at all, or is only slight, depends upon the amount of nuclear implication and the stage of the disease at the time of death. A comparison of the clinical symptoms with the pathological facts in this disease indicates that the *nucleus ambiguus* is the nucleus of origin of the motor fibres for some of the muscles which move the vocal cords, and probably also for the levator palati muscle.

The pathological evidence in favour of this view has been obtained from cases of bulbar paralysis, wherein during life paralysis of the soft palate and of the internal thyro-arytenoid muscles was observed ; and on post-mortem examination atrophy of the cells of the *nucleus ambiguus* was detected. When this observation is considered in connection with the clinical combination of paralysis of the soft palate and of the vocal cords (Hughlings Jackson), and with the physiological experiments upon the vagus roots (J. Reid, Bernard, and others), all evidence points to the *nucleus ambiguus* being the motor nucleus for the elevators of the soft palate and the tensors of the vocal cords.

(*b*) The *posterior vago-glossopharyngeal nucleus* is the end-nucleus of some of the afferent fibres of the combined vago-glossopharyngeal nerve (Kölliker and Held). The roots of this nerve are composed of two kinds of fibres : first, those efferent fibres which have been already shown to arise in the *nucleus ambiguus ;* and, secondly, afferent fibres which are the axis-cylinder processes of the cells situated in the jugular and petrosal ganglia and the ganglia of the vagus (Kölliker). This observer has further shown that some of these afferent fibres break into end-tufts in the posterior vago-glossopharyngeal nucleus. In osmium-silver preparations many cells of this nucleus are multipolar, and conform to the first type of Golgi ; but they are distinctly smaller than those of the hypoglossal nucleus and nucleus ambiguus, and are usually spindle-shaped.

The *afferent* fibres of the nucleus have been already shown to be the axis-cylinder processes of the cells in the ganglia upon the glosso-pharyngeal and vagus nerves.

The *efferent* fibres are the axis-cylinder processes of the cells composing the nucleus. The connections of these fibres are as yet uncertain. Kölliker both in Golgi and Weigert preparations has found fibres passing into the fillet layers. It seems probable that some fibres may also pass into the hypoglossal nucleus, while others, crossing the raphé, enter the posterior longitudinal bundle of the opposite side ; other fibres, as were seen in osmium-silver preparations of the kitten's brain, passed into the reticular formation, where they were lost to view.

(*c*) *The fasciculus solitarius, or "ascending" glossopharyngeal root.*—A third factor is to be studied in connection with the vago-glossopharyngeal root fibres. According to His and Kölliker, the *fasciculus solitarius* derives its fibres from both the ninth and tenth nerves (vago-glossopharyngeal). This bundle is traced from the level of the uppermost glossopharyngeal roots as far as the lower end of the medulla oblongata. Bruce localises its lower end in a group of cells situated dorso-externally to the posterior vago-glossopharyngeal nucleus in front of the funiculus gracilis. Surrounding this bundle, which is composed of axis-cylinder processes and their collaterals, is a considerable amount of gelatinous substance, into which the fibres pass and terminate (Kölliker). In the gelatinous substance cells are found which send their processes into the reticular formation, and in this way they associate the fasciculus solitarius with other parts of the brain.

Division of the glossopharyngeal nerve-roots in the monkey was followed by degeneration of many of the intra-medullary root fibres ; these could be traced both into the *fasciculus solitarius* and, to a less extent, into the posterior glossopharyngeal nucleus. The whole of the fibres of this so-called ascending root were not degenerated, supporting the view of His and Kölliker that some fibres are derived from the vagus roots. At the level of the fillet decussation the degenerated bundle was found lying in the reticular formation external and ventral to the internal arcuate fibres.

A full corroboration of Kölliker's statements followed the examination of the osmium-silver preparations. The *fasciculus solitarius* is by this method seen to be surrounded, chiefly on its mesial aspect, by gelatinous substance very rich in end-tufts, into which the fibres of the bundle have broken up. Amongst the end-tufts are seen cells, chiefly of the second type, whose axis-cylinder processes branch and pass into the reticular formation.

From these observations it is seen that the so-called ascending glossopharyngeal root is analogous with the so-called ascending trigeminal root, both of which are composed of afferent fibres, passing to their end-nuclei, and springing from the cells of ganglia which are situated on the nerves outside the brain. It is clear therefore that in this nucleus we have to deal with a complex structure, which, both in the extent of its peripheral distribution and in the complexity of its central connections, may be compared with the trigeminal nerve.

The condition of these structures in bulbar paralysis has been variously stated. By some observers both the solitary bundle and the dorsal end-nucleus have been found atrophied, but in those I have personally examined neither structure was pathologically altered.

I have endeavoured to show that the great bulbar nerve, described under the term vago-glossopharyngeus, has a double function, being in motor part, in part afferent. The peripheral distribution of the nerve, which is scarcely necessary to follow in detail here, as it may be studied in any anatomical text-book, is most extensive; structures so far differing in position and in function as the soft palate, the vocal cords, the pharynx and œsophagus, the lungs, the heart, the stomach, and to some extent the intestines, receive a portion of their nerve-supply through this nerve.

Ever since the time of Bischoff (1832), John Reid (1838), and Claude Bernard, the functions of the vagus roots have been studied experimentally; and they are still the subject of careful anatomical, physiological, and pathological inquiry. It is impossible in an article of this nature to give even a brief summary of the valuable communications upon this nerve, or even to refer to the functions of its several parts in detail. I therefore reproduce, with slight modifications, the table of the functions of the vagus roots given by Spencer in the article already referred to; a table which shows at a glance what may be taken as the latest views regarding its functions and distribution :—

[TABLE.

TABLE showing Functions of the Vago-glossopharyngeal Roots, modified from W. G. Spencer (*op. cit.*)

	Afferent.	Efferent.
Upper roots: 9th or glossopharyngeal nerve	Respiratory regulating fibres Respiratory exciting fibres (Inspiration) Superior laryngeal	Cricothyroid (?) Stylopharyngeus Œsophagus Pharyngeal constrictors
Middle roots—10th or vagus nerve	Respiratory inhibitory fibres (expiration) Bronchial	Gastric branches Bronchial muscles
Lower roots of vagus nerve	no afferent fibres	Inferior laryngeal Cardio-inhibitory; levator palati
Spinal accessory nerve (of Willis)	no afferent fibres	Sterno-mastoid Trapezius (upper part)

It is not to be supposed that there is a hard and fast line between the upper and middle roots, or between the middle and lower, as might be implied by this table; the general statement may be made that experiment has shown that the upper vagal roots are more concerned in inspiration than the middle, which chiefly subserve expiration. The fibres more especially related to inhibition of the heart lie in the lower root bundles.

Vago - glossopharyngeal paralysis. — A. *Paralysis of the glossopharyngeus.*—There is no case of localised unilateral paralysis of the glossopharyngeal root fibres on record; so that the derangement of function produced by such a lesion has to be inferred by a process of exclusion from the connections it forms with other adjacent nerves, and from the facts of experiment. It is stated that the trunk of the nerve contains the fibres subserving taste for the posterior third of the tongue, but it is doubtful whether such fibres reach the brain by the glossopharyngeal roots. There is evidence on record of taste being retained in this locality when the roots of the nerve have undoubtedly been involved in disease; while taste has been lost on the hind-part of the tongue and the soft palate in disease of the root of the trigeminal nerve. But this subject has been fully discussed on a previous page ("Sense of Taste," p. 792).

In a series of experiments upon rabbits performed by Kreidl it was shown that the nerve fibres for the muscular apparatus of the œsophagus pass outwards in the uppermost of the vago-glossopharyngeal roots. Outside the skull these fibres enter the vagus, nerve-trunk through which they are distributed by its recurrent laryngeal branch. But the pharyngeal plexus may play a part in this connection, for it is probable that it receives its motor fibres directly from the vagus, through the pharyngeal branch; it was found that the section of the glossopharyngeal nerve-trunk had no effect upon the innervation of the œsophagus (Kreidl). As the stylo-pharyngeus muscle receives a branch from the glossopharyngeal nerve it is inferred that it receives its motor supply from this source.

But whether these fibres are contained in the glossopharyngeal root, or are derived from the facial, is unknown. It is still a moot point how far the glossopharyngeus is the nerve of common sensation for the posterior part of the tongue, the palatal pillars, and the soft palate. These parts have been found anæsthetic in cases in which coexistent symptoms pointed to disease of the root of the fifth nerve.

B. *Laryngeal paralysis.*—This is the most important factor in vago-glossopharyngeal palsy. As is well known the larynx is supplied by two branches of the vagus; the superior laryngeal, which is the sensory nerve of the mucous membrane in the upper portions of the larynx, and is motor for the cricothyroid muscle and the epiglottideus; and the recurrent laryngeal supplying the remaining muscles and the mucous membrane of the part below the vocal cords and the trachea. The vagus roots which transmit the laryngeal motor fibres are, according to the observations of Grabower (cats and dogs), the middle bundle; as stated in the preceding table. Whether these results may be applied directly to man has yet to be decided; but it has been shown, when describing the nuclei of origin of the nerves, that the motor fibres of the vagus arise in the nucleus ambiguus, and that the spinal accessory nerve, which by many is said to transmit to the vagus its motor fibres, has in reality no medullary origin, but is a spinal motor nerve.

The kinds of laryngeal palsy, partial or complete, have been described (vol. iv. p. 851 *et seq.*), but I may indicate their bearing on our present subject.

(α) Total bilateral palsy. Aphonia, no cough, and stridor only in deep inspiration. Both vocal cords motionless and in the cadaveric position. Due to organic causes only.

(β) Total unilateral palsy. Voice hoarse, no cough, stridor usually absent, but may be present on deep inspiration. The paralysed cord is motionless in the cadaveric position. Due to organic causes.

(γ) Bilateral abductor palsy. Voice normal, cough normal, inspiration difficult and accompanied by a loud stridor. Cords approach on phonation, but do not separate on inspiration. Usually organic, but appears to be occasionally of functional nature.

(δ) Unilateral abductor palsy. Voice and cough scarcely affected. Paralysed cord immobile during inspiration. Both cords approach on phonation. Usually organic.

(ε) Adductor palsy (always bilateral). Aphonia, no cough or stridor. Cords normal during inspiration; no movement on attempt at phonation. Usually functional.

(ζ) Internal thyro-arytenoid palsy. On phonation an oval space is seen between the margin of the cords. Met with in the early stage of bulbar palsy.

Varieties of laryngeal paralysis.—(i.) *Cortical and subcortical laryngeal palsy (so-called).*—Experimental research has shown that, in the case of certain of the lower animals, the stimulation of a certain cortical area causes adduction of the vocal cords. This centre was found to be bilaterally situated, for if it were excised on one side stimulation of the corresponding area on the opposite side evoked the adductor movement of both cords. The more recent observations of Dr. Risien Russell have shown that, in addition to adduction of the vocal cords, abduction of the same may also be produced by cortical stimulation. It would appear that from this cortical area a tract of fibres passes through the internal capsule, in close relation with the fibres for the tongue, to the centre for the laryngeal muscles in the medulla oblongata.

It is still doubtful how far the results of such experimental observation may be applied to man. A number of cases have been recorded in which palsy of the vocal cords is said to have resulted from cortical and subcortical lesions. Among the number of recorded cases, which, however, do not stand a critical examination, one recorded by Déjérine (2) is specially recalled. He ascribes the paralysis of the right vocal cord found in this case to a subcortical lesion below Broca's convolution on the left side, which was also associated with motor aphasia and hemiplegia. But it is hardly logical to argue a principle from one case, especially when such an association is confronted by a large number of negative observations at the hands of experienced observers. In order to establish the relation of cause and effect, it is essential that there should have been, first, a laryngoscopic examination during life; secondly, a single cortical or subcortical lesion in the positions experiment has indicated, and, thirdly, a microscopic examination of the nucleus ambiguus in the medulla oblongata and of the nerve-roots issuing therefrom. Now, in none of these recorded instances, so far as I am aware, have all these conditions been fulfilled. It is, therefore, scarcely desirable, in an article of this kind, to do more than refer to the cases of so-called cortical laryngeal palsy.

The general statement may be made that, so far as clinico-pathological observation has yet shown, there is no clear evidence that a unilateral cortical lesion is followed by palsy of the vocal cords on one or both sides.

(ii.) *Nuclear paralysis.*—In chronic nuclear degeneration the muscles of the larynx are rarely paralysed alone; there is an associated paralysis of the muscles of the soft palate and usually also of the pharynx. When in association with such symptoms there exists palsy of the lips and tongue, the condition known as chronic progressive bulbar paralysis is obtained. Nuclear paralysis of the degenerative type is usually bilateral; but limitation of the symptoms to one side has been found in such conditions as tabes dorsalis and syringomyelia.

In the cases of chronic bulbar palsy, personally observed, the laryngeal muscles chiefly involved have been the internal thyro-arytenoids, or internal tensors of the vocal cords; but in nuclear disease usually, as well as generally in paralysis from lesion of the vagus trunk or its recurrent laryngeal branch, the crico-arytenoideus posticus or abductor of the vocal cord is that primarily involved, as originally pointed out by Semon and Rosenbach. In general paralysis of the insane, Permewan observed abductor paralysis not unfrequently, which was probably caused by degenerative changes in the bulbar nuclei.

The extent of the laryngeal palsy in all such cases is due to the amount of degeneration of the nucleus ambiguus, for it is rare even in advanced cases of bulbar palsy to find this nucleus completely atrophied. The great longitudinal extent of the nucleus and its close connection with the functions both of phonation and deglutition, as suggested by Gowers, probably account for much of the variation which has been observed.

Associated with the palsy of nuclear degeneration is usually to be found a diminution or loss of reflex action from the soft palate, pharynx, and larynx; but common sensibility is retained. Should the reflex irritability be increased, the lesion is situated above the level of the nucleus, and implicates the cortico-medullary fibres (pseudo-bulbar paralysis).

But nuclear degeneration is rarely limited to this situation. In bulbar paralysis there is an associated degeneration of the cells of the anterior horns of the spinal cord, with wasting of the limb muscles; and we have seen that the laryngeal palsy may be a phenomenon in tabes dorsalis, general paralysis of the insane, and syringomyelia.

(iii.) *Peripheral laryngeal paralysis.*—The course of the trunk of the vagus and its recurrent laryngeal branch is so extensive that it may be involved by disease, usually from compression, both in the neck and the upper part of the chest. Experimental section of the vagus trunk is followed by complete palsy of the vocal cord upon the side of lesion; but should the section be performed above the point of emergence of the superior laryngeal branch, anæsthesia above the level of the paralysed cord is also obtained.

It is, however, rare for a tumour or other growth, at all events in the early stages, to destroy the continuity of all the nerve-fibres so effectually as to produce this result. The symptom most commonly obtained is paralysis of the abductor mechanism only. It is scarcely necessary to enter here into this much debated question, for it is now a well-recognised clinical phenomenon; but the following facts may be stated in this relation :—

(*a*) In some forms of nuclear disease, as already mentioned, the abductor fibres are implicated before the adductors (Semon).

(*b*) In disease of the trunk of the nerve, or of its recurrent laryngeal branch, the abductor fibres are invariably affected before the adductor (Semon, Rosenbach); and, conversely, during healing the adductor recover before the abductor.

(*c*) In the process of death the abductor fibres lose their electrical excitability before the adductors (Onodi).

(*d*) In slow cooling of the nerve the abductor die before the adductor fibres (Semon).

(*e*) The abductor and adductor fibres occupy distinct and separate bundles in the nerve trunk and its branches (Risien Russell).

Why in every case the abductors should be implicated earlier than the adductors is more difficult to explain ; but it is not unreasonable to compare them to the extensors of the limb, which are invariably affected by disease before the flexors.

A curious point, and one not altogether easy of explanation, is the fact that with complete palsy of one vocal cord, as, for instance, from the pressure of an aneurysmal tumour in the thorax, partial (abductor) palsy of the opposite cord may be detected.

C. *Paralysis of the soft palate.*—Although it is a commonplace in neurology to say that the elevator of the soft palate is innervated by one of the bulbar nerves, yet it is stated in many anatomical text-books, and in some on clinical medicine of recent publication, that this muscle receives its nerve-supply from the facial nerve, and is paralysed in some forms of peripheral facial palsy. It was probably from the writings of Bell that this statement found its way into the English anatomical text-books ; and cases over which no doubt can be thrown have from time to time been recorded of an associated palsy of the soft palate and of the face on the same side. Amongst the earlier recorded cases of this association the state of the uvula only was taken as a diagnostic sign, but this is now known to be of no practical value. In the cases in which paralysis of the velum palati was observed it is not unreasonable to suppose, from the facts now at our disposal, that a double lesion was the cause of the palatal and facial palsies.

Experimental evidence can scarcely be said to support the view that the nerve-supply of the levator palati muscle is through the portio dura and its branches. Indeed almost all recent experimental and clinical evidence is in favour of the bulbar innervation of this muscle. But whether this occurs through the vagus or its accessory nerve has been long disputed.

The older observers held, and this is still the view expressed in many of the text-books, that the accessory nerve contains the palatal motor fibres ; but this view is based on a wrong impression of the origin of the accessory nerve. It has been recently shown that atrophy of the nucleus ambiguus, from which all the motor fibres of the vagus arise, and which does not give origin to any spinal accessory fibres, is associated with, among other phenomena, paralysis of elevation of the soft palate. Given therefore, the nucleus ambiguus as the origin of those fibres, it follows that they pass through the roots of the vago-glossopharyngeal nerves as some of its efferent fibres, and find their way into the trunk of the nerve. From these reasons, therefore, there comes a simple explanation of the associated palsy of the soft palate and the vocal cords which obtains invariably in disease of the bulbar nucleus and of the nerve-roots in the subdural space.

From the trunk of the nerve the palatal fibres in all likelihood find their way into the pharyngeal plexus, and thence to the elevator muscles, while the laryngeal nerve fibres continue in the vagus trunk.

It is still doubtful how far the tensor palati muscle is innervated through the vagus nerve. The old view that fibres passed through it from the motor division of the trigeminus by way of the optic ganglion, although not entirely proven, has had some confirmatory observations made upon it recently by Kölliker and Réthi.

Paralysis of the soft palate, whether uni- or bilateral, is only recognised when the patient is made to phonate. In complete bilateral palsy there is no palatal movement on saying the vowel "ah," and the pronunciation of those words requiring closure of the naso-pharynx is rendered imperfect; hence "rub" is pronounced "rum," and "egg" as "eng." Bilateral palsy may exist in all degrees, from the complete form best seen as an earlier post-diphtheritic phenomenon to the incomplete variety of early bulbar palsy. In unilateral paralysis there is said to be, when at rest, a lowered and less arched condition of the velum pendulum palati, but this sign, if it exists, is not to be relied upon. The only true evidence of palsy of one side of the palate is the absence of movement of that side on phonation, the opposite side being freely elevated. The position of the uvula is of no clinical value in this relation.

In the *treatment* of vago-glossopharyngeal palsy the same principles should be borne in mind as in like affections of the other cranial nerves. Owing to the extensive distribution of the nerve and the long course of its trunk in the neck and chest, it is much more liable to implication by disease of an extra-cranial nature than any of the other cerebral nerves.

The degenerative diseases do not permit of any satisfactory form of treatment, but the most favourable methods are given under bulbar paralysis. For the treatment of local laryngeal affections the reader is referred to special text-books.

THE SPINAL ACCESSORY NERVE.—It has been held that the accessory nerve consisted of two parts,· the spinal and the vagal accessory, and such is the description given in most text-books. But it has been shown (p. 812) that the vago-accessory roots (so-called) are none other than the most distal of the root-fibres of the vago-glossopharyngeal nerve, and arise from the lower end of the motor nucleus of this nerve—the nucleus ambiguus.

The eleventh nerve of Willis, or spinal accessory nerve as it should be called, arises from a group of cells situated on the dorso-lateral aspect of the anterior horn of the spinal cord, over an area corresponding to the origin of the first five cervical nerve-roots. The cells of both these sets of nerve-roots lie in the anterior horn; but the root-fibres of the spinal accessory pass dorso-laterally through the lateral column of the spinal cord to make exit ventral to the posterior horn, while those of the cervical nerves pass antero-laterally to form the anterior nerve-roots.

The spinal accessory roots may be traced as high up as the lower end of the inferior olivary body; that is to say, to the place where the most distal of the hypoglossal root-fibres make their appearance.

Formed by the union of nerve-roots, arising in the manner just described, the spinal accessory nerve takes an upward course, and passes into the cranium through the foramen magnum. Here it approaches the vago-glossopharyngeal nerve, and issues with it through the jugular foramen. In this situation also it lies in close proximity to the root of the hypoglossal nerve.

It supplies two muscles, the sterno-mastoid and the upper part of the trapezius.

Paralysis of the spinal accessory nerve.—As just shown this nerve has a spinal origin, and a cranio-spinal course; while it passes out of the cranial cavity in company with and in close relation to purely cranial nerves. Hence we find that it may be implicated in disease of the spinal cord and in disease of the subdural space, either of the upper part of the vertebral canal or of the posterior fossa of the skull. The sterno-mastoid and trapezius muscles may therefore be paralysed as a result of chronic degenerative atrophy of the cells of the anterior horns, as occurs in progressive muscular atrophy, or in that form in which the bulbo-spinal centres are affected throughout their extent; palsy of them has also been found in tabes dorsalis and syringomyelia. On the other hand, they may be paralysed in company with the soft palate, pharynx, vocal cords, and tongue, as a result of disease implicating the nerve-roots of the posterior fossa. Or again, they have been found paralysed from disease of the membranes or bones in the occipito-atloid region, or from injuries inflicted in this neighbourhood. The nerve may be paralysed alone outside the skull either from injury or from the pressure of new growths, or by implication in inflammatory conditions situated deeply in the upper part of the neck.

The *symptoms* of paralysis of this nerve are to be found in the altered conditions of the sterno-mastoid and trapezius muscles. Paralysis of the former muscle occasions impairment in the rotary movement of the head to the opposite side. This movement is not entirely lost, owing to the unimpaired action of the deeper neck muscles, which are also rotators of the head at the atlo-axioid joint. The paralysis is associated with wasting and consequent loss of the prominence which the normal muscle occasions at the side of the neck.

Of the three divisions into which Duchenne divided the trapezius, the upper two, and chiefly the uppermost, are affected. As this portion is largely a muscle of extraordinary respiration, its absence is conspicuous in forced inspiration; and the rounded contour of the neck and upper part of the shoulder is lost from the atrophy which accompanies the paralysis. In bilateral paralysis the movement of shrugging the shoulders in which this muscle takes a part is impaired, and the chin tends to fall forwards on to the sternum. The second and third parts of the trapezius are completely involved in progressive degenerative atrophy of the anterior horns only, as the second part is largely, and the third part entirely supplied by branches of the spinal nerves.

The *treatment* of paralysis of the spinal accessory nerve is that of the morbid condition, general or local, causing the paralysis; while the nutrition of the muscles is to be maintained by the application of electricity, faradism, or galvanism, according to the muscular reaction.

MULTIPLE PARALYSES OF THE CRANIAL NERVES.—Under this heading it is intended to give a short description of paralysis of the cranial nerves which occur commonly in groups of two or more ; especially with reference to disease of the nerve-roots as they pass through the subdural space and basal membranes to find exit by the foramina at the base of the skull. The term "multiple" has been used to distinguish them from the "associated" paralyses, which have already been described under paralysis of convergence and of conjugate movement.

A superficial examination of the base of the skull shows that it is readily subdivided into three divisions : the anterior, middle, and posterior fossæ respectively ; while an inspection of the mode of exit of the cranial nerve-roots indicates that each fossa has a group or groups of nerve-roots passing from it.

Thus the anterior fossa, formed by the orbital plate of the frontal and the cribriform plate of the ethmoid bones, contains the olfactory bulbs and tracts, and, quite at its posterior extremity, the optic nerves and chiasma ; the fossa itself containing the frontal lobe.

In the middle fossa, which contains the temporo-sphenoidal lobe, lie two groups of nerves : in the anterior part the oculo-motor nerves (3rd, 4th, and 6th), with the ophthalmic branch of the fifth ; and, posteriorly, the Gasserian ganglion with its three divisions ; while the optic chiasma occupies an important mesial position.

In the posterior fossa are situated the cerebellum, the crura cerebri, pons, and medulla oblongata ; and from the side of the latter structures issue several groups of nerves. Quite at the anterior margin of this fossa, mesially, is the origin of the third cranial pair. Immediately behind, but lying laterally, are the motor and sensory roots of the trigeminus. The motor root arising higher up and somewhat dorsally to the sensory, turns round the latter so to lie in the middle fossa ventral to the Gasserian ganglion. Passing posteriorly and mesially, the sixth pair are seen to pierce the dura mater to enter the middle fossa. Lying immediately outside this pair are the facial and auditory nerves, hidden from view when exposed from above by the flocculus cerebelli and its peduncle. Of these two nerves the auditory is the more dorsal, and they both leave the fossa by the internal auditory meatus. Immediately behind them, and in the same line, lies the vago-glossopharyngeal and accessory group ; and parallel with this set, but more mesial, is the series of hypoglossal root bundles.

The cranial nerves may be paralysed in groups by disease in the several fossæ ; and a study of the combinations thus induced may lead to an exact diagnosis of the site of the lesion.

Unilateral loss of the sense of *smell* from disease of the anterior fossa is rarely met with ; but if it occurs with other symptoms pointing to a tumour of the frontal lobes, its presence is of great localising value.

The symptoms of lesion of the *optic chiasma* and tracts have been already referred to in detail (p. 761), so that it is only necessary here to accentuate the fact that lesion of the optic chiasma, the common cause of which is tumour or enlargement of the pituitary body, is characterised by the phenomena of bitemporal hemianopsia.

But the *middle fossa* is not uncommonly the seat of inflammatory or other conditions of the dura mater involving the cranial nerves. Paralysis of the oculo-motor nerves together with the ophthalmic branch of the trigeminus is the combination of nerve palsies characteristic of disease of the anterior part of the middle fossa, chiefly about the cavernous sinus; and in inflammatory states and new growths protrusion of the eyeball has been observed.

A unilateral lesion of the sensory trigeminal nerve, complete or partial, without affection of its motor root, is highly characteristic of a meningeal affection of the posterior part of the middle fossa, in the neighbourhood of the Gasserian ganglion. These conditions are usually associated with the so-called neuro-paralytic keratitis, for the reason already given—that it is due to an irritative (inflammatory) condition in addition to the paralysis.

Coming now to the *posterior fossa*, the auditory and facial nerves are usually paralysed together, either on one or both sides; the latter combination causing the peculiar condition of diplegia facialis, with bilateral deafness.

In basal affections of the anterior part of this fossa, involving the roots of the fifth nerve, motor and sensory trigeminal palsy are associated.

The vago-glossopharyngeal, accessory, and hypoglossal group are usually paralysed together; seeing that they arise, pass through the subdural space, and eventually issue from the skull, in close proximity to each other.

It is not to be supposed, however, that these are the only combinations of cranial nerve palsies. Thus there are cases on record in which a meningeal affection of the middle fossa paralysed all the nerves from the third to the sixth inclusive; and, again, a similar condition in the posterior fossa led to palsy of the nerves from the fifth to the twelfth inclusive; while the curious combination of a bilateral palsy of the motor fifth and seventh nerves has also been observed (Ferrier).

In respect of the causation of this condition, the several processes of disease which occur at the base of the skull have to be considered. Of these by far the commonest is syphilis. From this cause a gummy basal meningitis arises which grips, and eventually compresses, the nerve-roots as they pass through the subdural space; or, according to Kahler, a true neuritis of the roots may be set up.

Next in frequency come new formations, either carcinoma or sarcoma of the bones of the base of the skull.

Tuberculosis of the basal dura mater appears to be distinctly rarer than the forms already described. Tuberculous caries of the bones of the basis cranii has also been described.

A not uncommon cause, but one usually fatal, is fracture of the base of the skull, whereby the nerve-roots are either torn, or involved in hæmorrhagic or inflammatory effusions.

WILLIAM ALDREN TURNER.

REFERENCES

For reference to the subject as a whole the reader should consult standard text-books in Neurology, both in the English and German languages. Such are:—
1. GOWERS. *Diseases of the Nervous System*, vol. ii. 2nd edit. 1893.—2. STRUMPELL. *Lehrbuch d. spec. Path. ü. Therap. der Inneren-Krankh.* vol. iii. 1896.—3. DERCUM. *A Text-book of Nervous Diseases*, 1895.—4. PEPPER. *A System of Medicine*, vol. v.—5. BERNHARDT. *Nothnagel Spec. Path. ü. Therap.* vol. xi. pts. 1 and 2, 1895.—6. BRUCE. *Tracts of the Mid and Hind Brain*, 1892.—7. HILTON FAGGE. *Text-book*, vol. i.—8. BRISTOWE. *Theory and Practice of Medicine.*—9. BASTIAN. *Paralyses: Cerebral, Bulbar, and Spinal*, 1886.—10. MILLS. *The Nervous System*, 1898.

Special references.—A few references in the text are given below. For those desirous of a fuller knowledge on special points the following are given:—
A. **Olfactory:** 1. RAMON Y CAJAL. *Nuevo Concepto, etc.* Barcelona, 1893.—2. HILL. *Phil. Trans.* vol. i. 184 (B.) 1893.—3. Sir WILLIAM TURNER. *Journ. of Anat. and Phys.* 1890.—4. ALTHAUS. *The Lancet*, 1881.—5. JACKSON and BEEVOR. *Brain*, vol. xii. B. **Optic:** 1. HENSCHEN. *Pathologie des Gehirns.* Upsala, 1890 *et seq.*—2. VIALET. *Centres cérébraux de la vision.* Paris, 1893.—3. VON MONAKOW. *Archiv f. Pysch.* vols. xxii. xxvi. *et seq.*—4. FERRIER. *Anat. des centres nerveux*, 1895.—5. ALLEN STARR. *Amer. Journ. Med. Sci.* 1884.—6. FERRIER. *Croonian Lectures*, 1892.—7. WILBRAND. *Hemianopsie*, 1881.—8. DÉLÉPINE. *Trans. Path. Soc.* 1890. C. **Oculo-motor nerves:** 1. BRUCE. *Proc. Roy. Soc. Edin.* 1889-90.—2. OPPENHEIM. *Archiv f. Psych.* 1892.—3. SIEMERLING. *Achiv f. Psych.* (supplement), vol. xxii.—4. COLLINS and WILDE. *Inter. Journ. Med. Sci.* 1891.—5. SWANZY. *Diseases of the Eye*, 1895.—6. BLEULER. *Deut. Arch. f. klin. Med.* 1886.—7. BOETTIGER. *Diss.* 1889.—8. WESTPHAL. *Arch. f. Psych.* vol. xviii.—9. KALISCHER. *Deut. Zeitsch. f. Nervenheilk.* 1894.—10. MAUTHNER. *Vorträge*, 1885. D. **Trigeminal nerve:** 1. FERRIER. *Trans. Odontol. Soc.* 1889.—2. TURNER, ALDREN. *Brit. Med. Journ.* 1895; and *Journ. of Anat. and Phys.* vol. xxix.—3. KÖLLIKER. *Handb. d. Gewebelehre*, 1894.—4. HEAD. *Brain*, 1893 *et seq.*—5. SCHMIDT. *Deut. Zeitsch. f. Nervenheilk.* 1895.—6. KRAUSE. *Neuralgie des Trigeminus*, 1896. E. **Facial nerve:** 1. PHILIP and HUBSCHMAN. *Neur. Centralb.* 1894.—2. TOOTH and TURNER. *Brain*, 1891.—3. HUGHLINGS JACKSON. *Lancet*, 1893.—4. MENDEL. *Neur. Centralb.* 1887. —5. MINKOWSKI. *Archiv f. Pysch.* vol. xxiii. F. **Eighth nerve:** 1. KÖLLIKER. *Handb. d. Gewebelehre*, 1894.—2. GRUBER. *Text-book, Diseases of the Ear* (trans. by Law and Jewell), 1890.—3. POLITZER. *Text-book, Diseases of the Ear* (ed. by Dalby), 1894.—4. HOCHWART. *Nothnagel Spec. Path. und Therap.* 1895.—5. GOWERS. Bradshaw Lecture, *Lancet*, 1896. G. **Vago-glossopharyngeal nerve:** 1. TURNER and BULLOCH. *Brain*, 1894.—2. SPENCER. *Lancet*, 1895.—3. SEMON, *Brain*. —4. GRABOWER. *Archiv f Laryng.* 1894. H. **Hypoglossal nerve:** 1. ERB. *Deut. Arch. f. klin. Med.* vol. xxxvii.—2. *Idem.* *Archiv f. Psych.* vol. ix. K. **Multiple cranial nerve palsies:** 1. MÖBIUS. *Centralbl. f. Nervenh.* etc. 1887.—2. BERNHARDT. *Neurol. Centralb.* 1890.—3. JOLLY. *Berl. klin. Wochenschr.* 1892.—4. PYE SMITH. *Guy's Hosp. Reports*, 1894.

The following authors are referred to in the text:—1. TURNER. *Brain*, 1895, p. 231.— 2. DÉJÉRINE. *Compt. rend. de soc. de biol.* 1891.—3. EWANS. *Brain*, 1893, p. 475.—4. FERGUSON. *Medical News*, 1890, p. 395.—5. FERRIER and TURNER. *Phil. Trans.* 1898, p. 1.—6. GIFFORD. *Archiv f. Ophthal.* 1895, p. 402.—7. GOUKOVSKY. *Nouv. Iconog.* 1895.—8. KAUSCH. *Neur. Centralb.* 1894, p. 518.—9. KREIDL. *Pflüger's Archiv*, 1894, p. 9.—10. PICK. *Deut. Akad. der Naturforscher.* 1895, No. 1.—11. POPE. *Brit. Med. Journ.* Lond. 1889.—12. ROSS. *Brain*, 1885.—13. RUSSELL, J. R. *Journal of Physiology*, 1890.—14. SINCLAIR. *Ophthal. Review*, 1895, p. 307.—15. SPENCER. *Lancet*, 1895, i. p. 476.—16. STARR, ALLEN. *Journ. of Nervous and Mental Disease*, 1884.—17. TAMBOURER. *Neur. Centralb.* 1892, p. 494.—18. *Trans.*

Ophthal. Society, 1887 and 1890.—19. TURNER and BULLOCH. Brain, 1894.—20. TURNER and GIBSON. Edin. Med. Journ. 1897.—21. TURNER, W. A. Journ. of Anat. and Phys. 1889. — 22. USHER and DEAN. Trans. Ophthal. Soc. 1896, vol. xvi. p. 248.—23. WEINSTRAND. Deutsch. Zeits. f. Nervenheilk. 1894-5, p. 393.—24. WILLIAMSON. Brain, 1892, p. 230.

W. A. T.

MEDICAL OPHTHALMOLOGY

THE work of the physician comes into contact with that of the ophthalmologist at many points and in frequently occurring circumstances. Sir Thomas Watson, in his classical lectures on the *Principles and Practice of Physic*, laid stress upon the fact that the transparency of the cornea and of the aqueous humour, coupled with the accessible position of the eye, rendered it possible to watch, in this organ, the progress of morbid changes identical with or analogous to those which are concealed from view in other parts ; and he used the phenomena of inflammation of the iris to illustrate the course of pleurisy, and the phenomena of inflammation of the conjunctiva to illustrate the course of bronchitis. Since his day, living nerve and blood-vessel, with the alterations wrought in them by disease, have been rendered visible by the ophthalmoscope ; and accurate investigation of visual function has thrown some light upon morbid conditions of the nerves or centres by which that function is exercised or controlled. Briefly, it may be said that impairment of vision, although it be the first symptom com-. plained of by the patient, may point to the existence of extensive disease elsewhere ; and that the diagnosis of disease primarily affecting other organs may be assisted and rendered more precise by the investigation of departures from the normal conditions of the eyes.

The whole subject of the relations between *ocular and general diseases*, or between diseases of the eyes and those of other organs, was first comprehensively dealt with by Professor Förster in 1877, and has recently been made the subject of a more extended work by Knies. The association of eye disease with diathetic conditions has been dwelt upon in many text-books ; but, with a few exceptions, the evidence appears to me to be inconclusive. There can be no doubt that iritis is a common manifestation of syphilis, or that other affections of the eye are met with in the later or even in the inherited forms of that disease ; nor can there, I think, be any doubt with regard to the occasional dependence of iritis upon a rheumatic tendency. Farther than this I am seldom inclined to go ; although frequently urged by patients to admit that their ocular maladies are consequences of "gout," the pre-existence of which there is nothing else to indicate. Acute glaucoma, before its nature was understood, was commonly described as "acute internal arthritic ophthalmia," and Mr. Hutchinson has endeavoured to show that certain cases of retinal hæmorrhage are often associated with a gouty family history; while Wagenmann (12), more recently, has framed against the *Morbus Dominorum* of our ancestors a still more comprehensive indictment. For my own part, I am disposed to agree with Förster in regarding a belief in the alleged connection between gout and eye disease, or between rheumatism and eye disease (other than certain forms of iritis), mainly as a survival from an earlier period of pathology. It must be remembered that any widely-diffused diathetic condition must either afford immunity from diseases of the eye, or must sometimes be found coexisting with them; and the opportunities for coexistence are so frequent as to call for weighty evidence before we can assume a relation of cause and effect. Physicians who are largely concerned in the treatment of declared gout do not recognise any special liability to ocular troubles among their patients, although both Sir Alfred Garrod and Sir Dyce Duckworth mention a form of conjunctivitis as thus occurring; and, conversely, there seems reason to believe that purulent ophthalmia in infants or children may give rise to an articular affection, due to the migration of cocci or to the absorption of their products, and strictly analogous to the form of masked pyaemia once known as gonorrheal rheumatism. It is essential, in any consideration of diathetic eye disease, to define precisely what is meant by the term denoting the diathesis; and the word "gout," even without the prefix of a qualifying adjective, is exceptionally elusive in this respect. Moreover, in declared gout I do not recognise any hæmorrhagic tendency in parts which are unquestionably affected by it—no such tendency, for example, as is produced by degeneration of arterioles in some of the forms of renal mischief in which retinal hæmorrhage is not infrequent. A necessity for caution in accepting a diathetic origin for eye disease arises from the fact that the diathesis, if believed in, may predominate over the local affection in the mind of the practitioner, who may content himself with the treatment of assumed rheumatism, or assumed gout, when he ought to be treating acute iritis or acute glaucoma. There are few ophthalmic surgeons who could not compile a dismal record of disasters hence arising, in which patients have lost their sight from conditions which would have been cured if their nature had been recognised, but which were regarded as diathetic rather than as ophthalmic, and in which the eyes were suffered to perish while the assumed diathesis was being treated by remedies which possibly did no harm, but which were powerless to control the local affection for which they were prescribed. It has been my custom to urge upon students that, in the presence of glaucoma or of iritis, the importance of the local condition overshadows that of any suspected diathesis; and that constitutional treatment, although never to be neglected, can only be regarded as subsidiary in its character. I am quite sure that the opposite manner of regarding the question is fraught with danger to all concerned, with danger of loss of sight to the patient, and with danger of loss of reputation to the doctor.

The symptomatology of the eyes with reference to more general conditions is chiefly valuable in relation to diabetes, to diseases of the

kidney, and to diseases of the · nervous system.   The first-mentioned
malady is sometimes attended by *cataract*, less frequently by degenerative
changes in the retina, and occasionally by turbidity of the vitreous body ;
and any of these may be present in a marked degree, prior to the appearance of other symptoms of glycosuria.   In diabetics of advanced age we
may sometimes see senile cataract pursuing its ordinary course, apparently
uninfluenced by the disease ; but the form peculiar to diabetes may be
met with in comparatively young subjects, and differs widely from senile
cataract both in its appearance and in the manner of its development.
Diabetic cataract begins in the superficial cortex of the lens ; at first often
resembling exaggerated fluorescence under focal illumination ; and it
increases as a general cloudiness rather than by opaque striation, the
lens at the same time becoming somewhat swollen, so that the iris is
pushed forward and the tension of the eyeball is raised.   In its completed
stage the opacity is commonly uniform over the whole surface of the
lens, and presents a bluish white semitranslucent aspect, like that of
opalescent glass.   In any case in which a recent impairment of vision is
traced to cloudiness of the vitreous body, or to changes in the lens,
especially if these changes are not of the ordinary senile character, or if
they appear prior to the period of life at which senile cataract becomes
common, there should be a careful examination of the urine.   The
control of diabetes by dietary and treatment may sometimes retard the
progress of the cataract, but fails to do so as a rule.   Seegen (10)
professes to have seen two cases in which the cloudy lenses were restored
to transparency ; but his statements have not been confirmed by other
observers, and nothing of the kind has ever occurred in my own
experience.   In the absence of other ocular changes a diabetic cataract
may generally be removed by operation with fair prospects of success,
provided, of course, that the case be not one in which a fatal termination
of the disease may be regarded as imminent.   The senile cataracts of
elderly diabetics are to be dealt with on general principles, and will seldom
present any remarkable difficulty.

The *retinal degenerations* of diabetes, constituting the "diabetic
retinitis" of some authors, are practically undistinguishable from the
similar degenerations of albuminuria, and indeed may sometimes indicate
that the two conditions coexist.   Degenerations of an analogous character
occur also in leukæmia and in pernicious anæmia ; and they cannot be
regarded as essential complications of these conditions, but merely as
consequences of impaired local nutrition produced by arterial disease or
by depravation of blood.   Endeavours have been made to describe or to
depict differences between these several forms of "retinitis," but such
differences appear to have been due to the personal peculiarities of the
individuals in whom they were displayed, rather than to the form of malady
with which they were associated.

The eye symptoms in renal disease have already been dealt with in
Dr. Dickinson's article on the main subject, and need not here be further
considered.   [Vol. iv. p. 390.]

In diseases of the nervous system the eyes may afford information by their tolerance or intolerance of application to visual work, by their positions and movements, by the positions and movements of the lids, by the varying states of diameter and of contractility of the pupils, by the appearances presented by the optic discs, the retinal vessels, and the interior of the posterior hemispheres generally, and by alterations in or within the boundaries of the fields of vision.

Intolerance of application to visual work, incapacity, that is, to continue the use of the eyes upon near objects of any kind, is frequently due simply to *errors of refraction*, and may easily, if these errors be not corrected, lead on to symptoms which may appear to be of serious import, such as disabling headache, vertigo, palpitations, or sickness. Such consequences may be produced, in uncorrected hypermetropia, by the strain thrown upon the nervo-muscular apparatus of accommodation; and, in uncorrected myopia, by the strain thrown upon the nervo-muscular apparatus of convergence. Whenever such symptoms, or, indeed, distressing symptoms of any kind are produced by employing the eyes, and are relieved by resting them, the state of refraction should be the first subject of inquiry, and any departure from the normal conditions should be corrected by the aid of spectacles.

When no error of refraction is discovered, or when, in the presence of such error, carefully selected spectacles fail to give more than partial or temporary relief, it will often be found, especially in patients presenting a variety of vague neurotic symptoms, that the eyes, when passive, do not occupy correct relative positions, or, in other words, that *they are not directed to the same point in space*. The visual axes of passive eyes should be either parallel or equally convergent, but this ideal is frequently unfulfilled. A simple test is afforded by using as an object a spot of light, furnished by a lamp placed behind a screen having a small perforation. The patient should be seated several feet from the spot, the left eye covered by an opaque disc, and the right by a cylindrical lens, or a disc of fluted glass, of sufficient refractive power to convert the spot into a line, the direction of which should at first be vertical. The attention being directed to the line, the left eye should be uncovered, so that it may see the spot; and then, if both eyes are directed to the same point, the line will necessarily appear to bisect the spot. If the right eye be more convergent than the left, the line will be to the right of the spot; and, if it be less convergent, the line will be to the left of the spot. The cylinder may then be turned so as to render the line horizontal, in which position it may appear either to bisect the spot, or to be above or below it; the apparent position above showing that the right eye is directed to a lower point than its fellow, and the apparent position below showing that it is directed to a higher point. The test turns upon the fact that, although both eyes are looking at the same object, its appearance is different to the two, so that there is no mental stimulus to the combination of the retinal images, and the eyes remain in their static or resting position, which may often be described as one of "latent squint."

As soon as both eyes are uncovered, and the spot presents the same appearance to them both, the consciousness that there is only one object comes into play, the eyes are called from their static position into correct convergence, and the object is seen singly. The general result is that when the eyes are unoccupied, when their external muscles may be said to be "standing at ease," there is more or less deviation from correct relative position; and this deviation, which would produce double vision if it were maintained during the attentive examination of near objects, as in reading, must be corrected before any such examination can be carried on. In other words, the eyes have to be called from "ease" to "attention," and to be held, during the continuance of occupation, in a relative position which is more or less unnatural to them, and which can only be preserved at the cost of a muscular effort commensurate with the degree of the deviating tendency. This effort may not only become a source of difficulty and pain in using the eyes, but it may produce, especially in neurotic subjects, a variety of indefinite symptoms, some of which have little or no apparent connection with the eyes, and which have been attributed by American physicians, by whom they have been chiefly studied, to a continued and unnatural expenditure of nerve force in counteracting the deviating tendency. The condition described may be palliated by the use of prismatic spectacles, in which the refracting angles of the prisms are so placed as to neutralise the effect of the deviation and to render the muscular effort unnecessary; or it may be cured by carefully planned operations on the muscles themselves. Such operations, in the great cities of America, have been performed upon hundreds, perhaps upon thousands, of patients; but my own experience leads me to believe that they are called for only in a comparatively small number of well-marked or severe examples of the state which they are employed to relieve. In such I have performed them with satisfactory results; but the great majority of the cases would probably be curable by a combination of prismatic spectacles with exercises intended to strengthen the weak muscles. In some, the difficulty of maintaining correct convergence may be avoided by reading with one eye only, the trick of maintaining closure of the other being easily acquired by most people. But, whatever may be the most appropriate remedy in any individual case, it is necessary to remember that incorrect equilibrium of the external ocular muscles may undoubtedly be a cause of neurotic symptoms, and that the possible existence of such a condition should be borne in mind whenever such symptoms prove rebellious to ordinary treatment. The question is partly one of degree, partly of the demand made upon nervous energy in overcoming a faulty position; for I believe that a state of absolutely correct equilibrium of the external eye muscles is comparatively rare, and that minor deviations are habitually and unconsciously corrected by the great majority of people. It is said, and with high probability, that upward or downward deviations occasion more distress, and are less amenable to palliative treatment, than deviations towards convergence or divergence.

In the cases last described, although a trained observer may often detect some slight fault of position when the eyes are passive, this fault will not be remarkable, and there will be no manifest limitation of the power of movement in any direction. When deviation is conspicuous, mobility will be diminished in the opposite direction to the deviation; and such a condition may arise either from ordinary squint, or from paralysis or weakness of one or more of the external muscles of the eyeball. The scope and limits of this article do not embrace the consideration of cases of ordinary squint arising from error of refraction, or from the external deviation of an eye which has become blind—neither of which conditions possesses any symptomatic value as far as, regards general medicine ; but the case is otherwise with *squints of recent origin*, produced by paralysis or paresis of one or more of the external muscles. Such conditions may be due to interference with conduction by hæmorrhage or effusion within the sheath of the implicated nerve, or by pressure exercised by some growth or morbid formation without. In the affections of the sixth nerve, producing paralysis of the corresponding external rectus, or in those of the fourth, producing paralysis of the corresponding superior oblique, only one muscle can be concerned, and hence the fact of paralysis does not indicate the seat of the lesion, which may be peripheral, nuclear, or intermediate. According to Sir W. Gowers, the sixth nerves, by reason of their longer intracranial course, are more likely than others to be compressed during the growth of an intracranial tumour. When the third nerve is concerned, which supplies the remaining external muscles of the globe, the levator palpebræ, the muscle of accommodation, and the sphincter pupillæ, the number of these which suffer may afford a clue to the precise position of the mischief ; but, even then, it must often be doubtful whether this be nuclear, affecting only one or more centres, or whether it be in the nerve trunk, at a spot anterior to that at which the unaffected branches are given off. If all the parts supplied by the third nerve suffer, and still more if the fourth and sixth, or either of them, participate in the defect, it almost follows that the cause of pressure must be seated at a spot where the third trunk is entire and complete, and where the others are in close proximity to it, as immediately within or beyond the apex of the orbital cavity. Such a position may often be held to exclude brain lesion, and to afford reasonable hope of recovery under treatment.

I was once consulted by a gentleman who had been shot by a very small conical revolver bullet. The muzzle of the pistol had been almost in contact with the skin of his right temple, opposite the position of the apex of the orbit, and the bullet had elevated the temporal bone at a corresponding point on the other side. It had cut through or destroyed all the nerves entering both orbits, except the left sixth. Both eyes were absolutely blind, and both were immovable—the right in a central position, the left in a position of outward deviation. The pupils neither contracted to light nor expanded under cutaneous irritation, and the optic nerves were completely atrophied. There had been no brain symptoms, and the intelligence was perfect.

A man supposed to have an orbital tumour was sent to St. George's Hospital. I found his right eye moderately prominent, and immovable in a central position. The condition was of recent origin, was not attended by headache, and the sight was beginning to suffer. Nothing could be felt in the orbit, the only displacement of the eyeball was directly forwards, and could be rectified by gentle pressure, but soon returned when the pressure was removed. The optic disc was slightly swollen, and there was a distinct syphilitic history. My diagnosis was complete paralysis of all the external muscles, from compression of their nerves, as well as compression of the optic nerve, by the growth of a gumma at the apex of the orbit. Full doses of potassium iodide were given, and the patient quickly recovered.

When a seeing eye assumes a position of deviation on account of recent muscular paralysis, the chief complaint made by the patient, and that which usually impels him to seek relief, is the inconvenience occasioned by the suddenly occurring double vision, which of itself may be enough to produce vertigo. The less the deviation the greater will be the inconvenience, because, the less the deviation, the nearer to the macula lutea will be the image received by the deviating eye, and the less easily will it be distinguished from the image received by the other. If the deviation be considerable, the false image will be remote from the true one, and, falling upon a peripheral portion of the retina, it may, like the false image of ordinary squint, be easily neglected by the consciousness.

Endeavours have been made, by many ingenious persons, to draw pictures illustrative of the relative positions of the true and the false images in every possible form and combination of paralysis of the external muscles of the eye. The drawings have usually been founded upon simple subtraction of the effect of the paralysed muscle or muscles, and they are seldom trustworthy. The position of the eye will not be governed solely by such subtraction, but by a rearrangement, so to speak, of the aggregate of the remaining forces. This aggregate will differ in different people, according to varying conditions of original equilibrium, and it may be modified, in any particular case, as one or more of the remaining muscles may be strengthened by exercise or weakened by inactivity. In a general way, the loss of power to move the eye in some given direction is too evident to permit any doubt concerning the seat of the paralysis to remain after a single careful examination. The direction of the false image, of course, will always be exactly opposite to that of the deviation.

While the causes of paralytically disturbed ocular motility are, in the majority of instances, orbital in their position, and also, it may be said, syphilitic in their character, a very different account must be given of the disturbance of motility next to be considered, namely, the state of nystagmus or oscillation.

Nystagmus.—The customary steadiness of the ocular muscles, and the power of sustained fixation which this steadiness confers, appear to depend entirely upon early education of the centres of visual perception. In an infant with defective vision, however occasioned, whether by congenital cataract, high degrees of hypermetropia or astigmatism, albinism, turbidity of the corneæ from purulent ophthalmia, or disease of the optic nerves, unless good vision can be speedily afforded, the eyes will remain permanently in an oscillatory condition. It would seem that imperfect visual impressions during the first few weeks or months of life, especially when due to conditions which reduce the sensibility of the macula lutea to the same level as that of the surrounding parts of the retina, are insufficient to afford the necessary stimulus to the establishment of correct relations between the centres of visual perception and the efferent nerves proceeding from these centres to the muscles of the eyes; and no subsequent improvement or restoration of sight appears to be capable of making good the early deficiency. *Congenital nystagmus* is distinguished from that which is acquired in after life by the history, by the presence of evidences of the condition to which the original defect of sight was due, such as corneal nebulæ, congenital cataract, albinism, etc., etc., and by the fact that objects of vision do not appear to the subject to be unsteady.

Acquired nystagmus is seen under two principal forms, in miners, as a result of the conditions of their occupation, and in the sufferers from various forms of cerebral or spinal disease. Miners work in a dim light and in a constrained position, which frequently involves considerable and sustained upward rotation of the eyes, so that they are exposed to a combination of defective sight and of irregular innervation of the eye muscles. The occupation, and the absence of other symptoms, will usually be sufficient to establish the nature of the case.

As a consequence of disease of the central nervous system, nystagmus is most frequently seen in disseminated sclerosis of the brain and spinal cord, and it is usually first evident when both eyes are strongly directed to the right or left. In contradistinction to the congenital or infantile form, it produces apparent movement of the objects of vision, sometimes attended by vertigo. According to Robin (9) it generally indicates a lesion at the base of the brain, or on the convexity behind the fissure of Sylvius, but does not furnish sufficient ground for precise localisation; while other writers attribute it to changes which obstruct, but do not altogether destroy, the channels for the conduction of motor impulses from the cortical centres to the muscles of the eyes, so that the movements of the latter become irregular and indeterminate. In some instances nystagmus is attended by oscillatory movements of the head, which may be partly compensatory in their character. Acquired nystagmus is seen in some cases of subdural or cerebral hæmorrhage, in meningitis, and in tumours, as well as in disseminated sclerosis, and must usually be regarded as an evidence of advanced structural disease.

The **positions and movements of the eyelids** are liable to be modified in weakness or paralysis of the levator palpebræ, in paralysis of the orbicularis, and in the earlier stages of that group of symptoms, now commonly referred to the cervical sympathetic, which is collectively described as exophthalmic goitre, or as Graves's or Basedow's disease. Paralysis of the levator palpebræ may be either partial or complete, and may be either part of general loss of power of the third nerve, or limited to the branch by which the levator is supplied. When it is complete the upper lid falls absolutely, remains unwrinkled, and cannot be raised by any effort of the will. When it is partial the lid droops more or less below the level of its fellow, and can be raised in some degree by strong effort, in which the occipito-frontal muscle is often obviously made to participate. When complete paralysis is part of an affection involving the whole nerve trunk, it will be seen, when the lid is raised by the fingers, that the pupil is dilated and the eye immovable in an everted position; while, if any branch of the trunk has escaped, the muscle supplied by it will retain its functions. Paralysis of the orbicularis muscle can only be produced by disease or compression of the facial nerve, and manifests itself by imperfect power of closing the eye, coupled with a sinking downward of the lower lid, which is no longer closely applied to the surface of the globe, and no longer keeps the lachrymal punctum in such a position as to receive the tear secretion, which therefore tends to overflow upon the cheek. As with the third nerve, the affection of the facial is mostly due to compression of its trunk at some portion of its course, either by swelling due to periostitis, by gumma, by some tumour, or by hæmorrhage. The cause must generally be discovered by the aid of other symptoms.

In the normal condition, when the eyes are cast down, the upper lids follow the movement of the globes, not by any effort of the orbicular muscles, but almost as if the mucous surfaces clung together by a sort of adhesion. It was first pointed out by von Graefe that, in an early stage of exophthalmic goitre, this attendant movement of the upper lids is frequently absent, the form and position of the lid opening remaining unaltered when the eyes are directed downwards. Such absence of the upper-lid movement is often called "von Graefe's symptom," and it is usually one of considerable significance. Another symptom which is sometimes precursory of exophthalmic goitre, and which was first described by Stellwag von Carion, is a tucking-up of one or both of the upper lids, often to a sufficient extent to expose the white of the eye above the cornea. This elevation does not seem to be produced by the levator, but by the assemblage of unstriped fibres known to anatomists as "Müller's muscle," which is probably thrown into action by the sympathetic. I have, however, more than once seen Stellwag's symptom affecting one eye, and was once called upon to remedy by a plastic operation the unsightliness of appearance which it occasioned, although there was no other manifest departure from health, and although no other symptoms of exophthalmic goitre ever displayed themselves. The patient operated upon was a young lady, shortly about to be presented, and I united the external quarter of an inch of her lid margins in order to render her fit to appear at the drawing-room. Possibly nervousness at the prospect of presentation had something to do with her condition, but she has ever since remained quite well. I have seen one instance, in a healthy young man, in which Stellwag's symptom on one side followed an operation for the removal of polypi from the corresponding nostril.

The measurements and movements of the pupils are often of great symptomatic value, and cannot be understood without constant reference to the origins and distribution of the nerves by which these conditions are controlled. There are some points, with regard to this distribution, which remain unsettled or obscure; but the general facts are fairly well established, and have recently been very clearly set forth by Dr. Alexander Hill. The retinæ may be regarded as functionally divided into halves by lines which are generally vertical, but which curve in the centre so as to enclose the regions of the maculæ. The fibres from the right halves of the two retinæ meet at the chiasma, and pass into the right optic tract, and the fibres from the left halves pass into the left optic tract; while those from each macula are divided at the chiasma, and pass some into the right optic tract, and some into the left. It follows that visual impressions coming from the left-hand side of the subject, and impinging upon the right-hand sides of the two retinæ, will be conveyed to the right side of the brain; while visual impressions coming from the right-hand side of the subject are conveyed to the left side of the brain. Impressions derived from objects in front, on which the eyes are fixed, are received upon the two maculæ, and are conveyed from each macula along both optic tracts, and so to both sides of the brain. The optic tracts themselves enter the quadrigeminal bodies, in the anterior pair of which are seated the centres of visual sensation, from which efferent fibres proceed to the motor oculi nerve; the centres of the two sides being so connected by commissural filaments that impulses received by either may react simultaneously through both. Behind the quadrigeminal bodies the afferent fibres of visual conduction pass backwards to the centres of visual perception as distinguished from sensation—centres which are situate in the occipital regions of the cerebral hemispheres, and from which also efferent fibres proceed to the motor nerves of the eyes. Through the intermediation of the ciliary ganglion the iris receives motor filaments not only from the third nerve, but also from the sympathetic, in addition to sensory filaments from the fifth.

The contraction of the pupils under the influence of light is a reflex act, which only requires for its performance the integrity of the nervous apparatus between the eyes and the quadrigeminal bodies. There may be complete arrest of conduction between these bodies and the occipital lobes, and consequent absence of perception of light, although the contractility of the pupils may remain unimpaired. On the other hand, if the arrest of conduction be in the optic tracts, perception of light and contractility will both be destroyed.

It will be manifest, from what has already been said of the arrangement of the ocular nervous apparatus, that a complete arrest of conduction on either side, whether in one of the optic tracts or between the quadrigeminal bodies and the occipital lobes, would be productive of blindness of the corresponding halves of the two retinæ, while central vision, as provided for by the macular region, and vision with the other halves of the retinæ, might be unimpaired. In such a condition the reflex action of the pupils to diffuse daylight would be retained; and reflex action to a pencil of light made to fall on the blind half of either retina would also be retained, if the lesion were posterior to the quadrigeminal bodies, but would be lost, or at least greatly enfeebled, if the lesion were anterior to them. In the latter case, any reflex action would be due to light dispersed in the refracting media, and thus enabled to reach the portions of the retinæ which still ministered to sight.

A yet more complicated condition, first investigated by Wernicke (13), and often called by his name, may arise when total blindness is occasioned by an arrest of conduction which is anterior to the quadrigeminal bodies on one side, say on the right, but posterior to them on the other. In such a state there would be no perception of light, but both pupils would react to diffuse daylight. More exact observation would show that the reaction was produced by the light which fell upon the left half of either retina, and that, if focal illumination were so arranged as to fall only on the right half of either retina, no effect would follow. In such a case the total blindness might be described as double hemianopsia; and the loss and the retention of light reflex on the respective sides would afford evidence which might assist in localising the disease on either. In Wernicke's original case a tumour was found in the occipital lobe on one side, while on the other side the optic tract was compressed by an enlarged and distended vein.

The normal diameter of the pupils in health is a result of the antagonistic forces exerted by the third nerve in exciting contraction of the sphincter pupillæ, and by the sympathetic in exciting contraction of the dilatator, in inhibiting the action of the sphincter, in regulating the amount of blood contained in the vessels of the iris, or in all of these methods at different times or in combination. Some observers have denied the existence of a dilator muscle; but the opposite view commands what appears to me to be a preponderance of assent. Under ordinary conditions, and apart from cases in which the eyes differ greatly from each other in acuteness of vision or in refraction, the two pupils are of equal diameter; and contract equally under the stimulus of light applied to either, or in convergence and active accommodation. In repose of accommodation the pupillary diameter is subject to considerable range of variation, which Woinow estimated at from 2·5 to 5·8 millimetres, and differences between individuals are very marked. The largest pupils are found, as a rule, in young people, especially in young myopes; and the diameter usually diminishes through middle life to advanced age, probably as a result of an instinctive effort to supplement failing power of accommodation by cutting off the lateral portions of pencils of light. A difference of diameter between the two pupils, under equal stimulation and equal effort, is usually a local symptom, although it may be the forerunner of other signs of intracranial disease. When the difference does not amount to extreme contraction or dilatation of either, it is not always easy to decide which of the two should be regarded as abnormal, unless a clue should be afforded by impairment of vision on one side, or by diminished mobility under ordinary stimuli.

Dilatation of the pupil may occur in one or in both eyes, the former being usually dependent upon some local cause, such as paralysis of the sphincter muscle or its nerve from a contusion, or the application of some drug (atropine, daturine, cocain, duboisin, scopolamine, hyoscyamin, etc.) Among other possible causes must be reckoned increased tension of the affected eye, or excitation of motor fibres on one side only, as by irritation of the cilio-spinal region by some morbid growth or injury, or of the sympathetic by rickets, tumours in the neck, or other morbid conditions. Or there may be paralysis of the motor oculi on one side, behind the point at which the branch to the ciliary ganglion is given off, from syphilis, ataxy, or other causes ; or there may be inhibition of the third nerve by irritation of the fifth, as from carious teeth. When both eyes are affected there may have been the application of one of the above-mentioned drugs to both, or belladonna may have been taken internally, or there may be grave intracranial disease, such as tumour or hæmorrhage, which would usually be recognisable by other symptoms, or there may be some local affection of the nerves or muscle of the iris, as in paralysis following diphtheria. Dilatation occasioned by the local action of a drug is usually complete, and is attended by complete paralysis of accommodation, producing a disturbance of vision which may be corrected by a lens; while paralytic dilatation is usually incomplete, and admits of being increased by atropine and its congeners, or of being diminished by eserine or pilocarpine. 1 have lately seen a young lady, apparently in perfect health, to whose eyes a solution of atropine was applied, nearly a year ago, in order to test their refraction. In the left eye the effect was, as is usual, only temporary ; but in the right it has so far been permanent. The pupil remains fully dilated, and the accommodation is paralysed. The pupil contracts to eserine, but becomes dilated again as soon as the effect of this agent passes away.

Contraction of one or both pupils may be occasioned by drugs locally applied (eserine, pilocarpine, etc.), or by irritation of the third nerve. Contraction of both is seen as an effect of poisons (morphia and other preparations of opium, tobacco, aconite, etc.), in profound sleep, in general paralysis, meningitis, encephalitis, hysterical convulsions, in certain stages of chloroform narcosis, and, as a result of defective action of the sympathetic, in locomotor ataxy, in which it is commonly associated with loss of contractility to light, while further contraction still occurs during accommodation. This combination constitutes what is often called the "Argyll Robertson" pupil, in consequence of its having been first described by Dr. Argyll Robertson in 1869. I have once met with a typical Argyll Robertson pupil, on one side only, as a consequence of an attack of frontal herpes, attended by keratitis, which had occurred several months previously. The iris had not been implicated, and the cornea, when I saw it, had regained its transparency.

In order rightly to estimate the contractility of the pupils the necessary examination must be conducted with some care, and with due reference to the fact that the commissural connection between the quadrigeminal bodies will produce contraction of both pupils from the incidence of light upon either. The eyes must therefore be examined separately. The patient should be seated facing a window, but not in direct sunshine, and one eye should be completely closed by a covering of opaque material, such as several folds of a handkerchief. The hand of the examiner should then be so held as to screen the open eye from the light, when the pupil should undergo moderate dilatation, expanding rather slowly. The screening hand being then suddenly removed, the pupil should contract quickly; and the same results should be obtained from the other eye. In any case of hemianopsia, or if the pupils contract to light, although the patient does not perceive it, the examination should be repeated by artificial illumination in an otherwise darkened place, and a pencil of rays should be so directed by a lens as to fall first upon one side, and then upon the other, of each retina. If the pupils are very small, so that their movements are not conspicuous, it will in any case be best to use artificial light, as in focal illumination, and to magnify the pupil under observation as the light falls upon or is withdrawn from it. This may often be most conveniently done by a strong convex lens, or from 16 to 20 dioptres, placed behind a small ophthalmoscopic mirror, a very slight movement of the mirror sufficing to apply or to remove the light, while the pupil remains in the focus of the lens. The same combination is convenient for testing contraction during accommodation, the patient being directed to look past the edge of the mirror towards the other side of the room, and then, at a given word, to look at the central perforation of the mirror. In this way the presence or absence of movement to light, or during accommodation, may be rendered clearly manifest even when the pupils, as often happens in cases of spinal disease, are of extremely small diameter.

The contractility of the pupils having been determined, it is usually necessary to proceed to **examination with the ophthalmoscope**; and it is often most convenient to employ the indirect method first, in order to obtain a general survey of the background of the eye, and the direct method subsequently, for the more precise examination of individual portions. Whether the pupil should be artificially dilated or not must depend partly upon its diameter, partly upon the position and nature of the changes to be investigated, and partly upon the skill of the observer; but it may be said, generally, that a great deal may be seen through a very small pupil after sufficient experience in the use of the instrument has been gained. If dilatation is necessary, a drop of a one per cent solution of homatropia hydrobromate is one of the best applications for the purpose, on account of the temporary character of its effect; or, in some cases, a solution of cocaine may be employed for the same reason.

When the ophthalmoscope is used on account of complete loss of vision in one or both eyes, it may sometimes be found that the light from the mirror will not penetrate *the media*, or is absorbed in them, so that no return of it can be obtained, except perhaps a reddish glow when the eye is directed laterally. In such cases the view is obscured by blood, sometimes effused into the substance of the vitreous body, sometimes retained between the hyaloid membrane and the retina. Such large hæmorrhages, in both eyes, may arise from hæmophilia or from purpura, and the nature of the case would be rendered plain by the history. They may occur also in one eye only, or in the two at different periods, in persons apparently in perfect health, usually young adults; and, in my experience, more frequently in males than in females. Mr. Hutchinson is of opinion that the subjects of these hæmorrhages usually suffer from habitual constipation; and it may doubtless happen that straining at stool may be the immediate cause of the rupture of a retinal vessel. Under gentle regular purgation, with a limited supply of fluid, the blood is usually absorbed in the course of a few weeks or months, vision gradually improving as absorption continues, and being often to a great extent restored in time. As soon as the eye-ground becomes visible, it may usually be seen that the veins of the retina are winding and distended, showing that the blood must have been furnished by the venous system; but I have never been able to detect the place of rupture, which is probably anterior to the field of view of the ophthalmoscope. In some cases I have seen nothing but gradual clearing, as if the effusion had remained between the retina and the hyaloid; while in others the last remains of the blood have appeared as clots floating in the vitreous, which must then have been broken into and disorganised.

Hæmorrhages smaller in quantity, and more circumscribed in area, may frequently be seen scattered over the eyeground, or even covering a considerable portion of its surface. It is often possible to discover, by their contour, colour, and general appearance, whether they are arterial or venous, and in what portion of the retina they are situate. The larger vessels, of both kinds, lie immediately beneath the limiting membrane, and any blood which may escape from them is usually spread out in an uniform layer beneath this membrane, is bounded by a sharp line, and entirely conceals the subjacent structures. As the vessels divide they sink more and more deeply into the retina, and hæmorrhages from them will not only be smaller in amount, but will also be seated in the retinal tissue, and will derive a fibrillated appearance, and an irregular, brush-like, pointed, or flame-shaped outline, in consequence of the blood passing between, and more or less separating and disturbing, the retinal fibres. Frequently the vessel which has given way may be discovered, either by its close proximity to one of the patches, or by its ceasing to convey blood, and showing only as a white line beyond the point of rupture. Sometimes the other vessels of the eyeground will not appear to depart from their normal condition; at other times they will be more or less winding and distended. The optic disc may be of normal aspect, or it may be swollen and with blurred edges, and the general surface of the retina may be studded with white spots, which are sometimes conspicuous as a stellate figure in the region of the macula.

Venous hæmorrhages between the retina and the limiting membrane are most frequently met with in women of middle age, in connection with irregularity or with cessation of the menses; and they are sometimes absorbed without injury to vision. When "flame-shaped," that is, situate in the fibre layer of the retina, they are apt to do permanent mischief to sight, probably because the nervous tissue is more or less torn and injured as the blood forces a way among its meshes, or because the blood, when there, may excite irritation and effusion. Mr. Hutchinson, as already mentioned, has striven to connect these flame-shaped hæmorrhages with a gouty family history, but I do not think we are materially assisted by the hypothesis. The last patient in whom I saw them was a gentleman who had been rendered thin by chronic diarrhœa in China, but from this he had completely recovered long before the occurrence of the bleeding, and two eminent physicians, who examined him at my request, both reported that they could not find any other departure from health, or any indication for treatment. I have met with many instances in which the sight of one eye has been practically destroyed by flame-shaped hæmorrhages, and in which the patient has continued in good health for many years, insomuch that I have come to regard the condition as the result of some local changes in the vessels themselves. When hæmorrhages are associated with nerve-swelling, or with patches of degeneration, they are usually indications of diabetes, of albuminuria, or of leukæmia; and these conditions cannot be certainly distinguished from each other by the changes in the eyes. Slight differences have, indeed, been described by authors; but, as I have said with reference to "retinitis," they appear to have been differences due to the individuals affected rather than to the maladies under which they were suffering. It is superfluous to say that every case of intraocular bleeding calls for the most complete inquiry into all the conditions by which it may have been promoted or produced; and that arterial retinal hæmorrhage, in persons in the decline of life, points to probable atheroma and to great danger of apoplexy.

The occurrence of changes in the appearance of the *optic disc* is a matter which always requires serious consideration, and such changes may be at least of two kinds, either of which may be the precursor of atrophy and blindness. There may be *simple swelling, œdema, or "choking" of the disc*, with or without consecutive inflammation of the connective tissue elements, or there may be "optic neuritis" properly so called. These conditions, in the descriptions of cases, are not always sufficiently distinguished from each other.

When swelling of the optic disc, with distension and tortuosity of the retinal veins, was first recognised as a frequently occurring condition, especially in connection with intracranial growths, it was explained as a consequence of increased intracranial pressure, by which subarachnoid fluid was forced down the space between the dural and pial sheaths of the optic nerve, and was arrested at the termination of this inter-vaginal space in such a way as to distend the dural sheath and to compress the ocular extremity of the nerve, thus retarding the return of venous blood from the retina, and producing mechanically a dropsical swelling of the disc. It is certain that in some cases the described distension of the ocular end of the dural sheath has been found in post-mortem examinations. Opportunities for such examinations have not, however, been as frequent as could be desired, and, when afforded, the original condition has often been obscured by subsequently occurring changes. A certain school of pathologists began to assert that evidences of inflammation of the disc tissues were always to be found in these cases when sought for, and to describe swelling as "optic neuritis." It is common to read, in reports of brain tumours, that "optic neuritis" was among the symptoms.

We are now, I think, fairly well acquainted with "neuritis" as a pathological condition liable to occur in many regions of the body ; and I also think we should be fully justified in the assertion that, whenever "neuritis" is present, the function of the affected nerve will be disturbed, suspended, or destroyed. It is a matter of familiar knowledge that the optic disc, the intraocular termination of the nerve, may be swollen to a very considerable extent, and for a very considerable time, without the slightest alteration of the visual function. It is equally a matter of familiar knowledge that, in undoubted optic neuritis, great impairment or total loss of vision will be an early and prominent symptom.

The records of the National Hospital for Paralysis and Epilepsy would furnish a very large number of cases in which symptoms indicative of intracranial gumma or other tumour were attended by swelling of the optic discs without diminution of vision ; but perhaps the most remarkable example of the kind is one which occurred in New York. At the International Ophthalmological Congress, held there in 1876, a patient apparently in perfect health, but with two swollen discs, was exhibited to the members. He had applied at a dispensary three years previously on account of some trivial ailment ; and the dispensary doctor, who was in the habit of using the ophthalmoscope systematically, discovered the condition of his discs. There was not the smallest impairment of vision, either centrally or laterally ; and the disc swelling remained unchanged during the three years. I myself saw this patient at the Congress, where he was examined by a large number of skilled observers, all of whom recognised the condition, and the majority of whom were of opinion that the man must be the subject of an intracranial tumour. Towards the end of the same year great loss of life was occasioned by the burning of a theatre in New York, and post-mortem examinations were made of some of the charred bodies found among the ruins. In the cerebellum of one of these there was discovered a passive tumour, the size of a small cherry; and the discovery led to the identification of the body, by the remains of clothing and other indications, as that of the man whose optic discs had been exhibited at the Congress. For more than three years, therefore, this man had had swollen discs, arising from the most common cause of the condition; but, considering his perfect vision, we cannot say that he had had optic neuritis without reducing the use of the word "neuritis" to an absurdity.

As said above, it seldom happens that a post-mortem examination of a case of swollen discs can be obtained at the time when it would be most valuable, or prior to the occurrence of secondary changes; but the abundant clinical evidence seems to me to point to the conclusion that such swelling may in its origin be purely dropsical, produced either by distension of the intervaginal space or by some other impediment to the free return of venous blood. As long as the dropsy is not excessive in amount, there is no reason why it should either arrest or impede conduction through the nerve fibres, or should excite irritation in the connective tissue. If the effused fluid should possess an irritating character, or if it should increase beyond certain limits, which would probably differ greatly in different individuals, it may do both these things. Arrest of conduction would produce impairment of vision, either general, or limited to portions of the field corresponding to the parts of the nerve on which the greatest pressure was exerted; while irritation and inflammation of the connective tissue, analogous to the erythema of a dropsical leg, would be liable to produce plastic effusion between the nerve fibres, which effusion, by undergoing gradual shrinkage, might ultimately produce complete strangulation, and blindness from consecutive atrophy.

A young woman came under my care in the National Hospital, in whom there was enormous swelling of the left optic nerve, coupled with loss of a large sector of the temporal portion of the field from the fixing point outwards. The swelling continued to increase and the blind area to extend, and patches of hæmorrhage appeared on and about the disc from obstruction to the veins. I detached the external rectus muscle, exposed the optic nerve, and slit up the dural sheath from near the eye as far as possible towards the apex of the orbit. The result was an immediate diminution of the swelling, and restoration of vision over a portion of the previously blind area. Shortly afterwards, in the middle of the night, the patient was roused from sleep by the bursting of an abscess into her nares, her mouth being filled with stinking pus by which she was half choked, and which excited free vomiting. Except for a small remaining blind spot she recovered completely, the nerve regaining its natural level and aspect, and the central vision being unimpaired. The locality of the abscess could not be determined, and she had left the hospital before its spontaneous evacuation occurred.

As a contrast to these cases, we may take one of general "*optic neuritis*," and we shall find it afford us some such picture as the following:
—A complaint is made of dimness of vision in the affected eye, dimness

which may cover the whole field, but which is apt to be more remarkable, perhaps because contrasting more strongly with the normal condition, over the central area and the vicinity of the fixing point. If the other eye be sound, the affection may have made some progress before it is discovered by the patient, and it is therefore seldom possible to fix the date at which it commenced; but, when once attention has been called to it, increase is usually somewhat rapid, and, even in the course of two or three days, sight may be wholly lost. The inflammation is usually seated behind the eye, somewhere in the orbital portion of the nerve, and most frequently near the optic foramen, and from thence it creeps downwards to the eye. In its course, sometimes before vision is lost, sometimes not until afterwards, it reaches the optic disc, which then usually displays, not the swelling and œdema already described, but changes of a much less conspicuous character, requiring some practice with the ophthalmoscope for their recognition; such as a little increase of the normal capillary vascularity, a little fulness of the larger vessels, a little veiling or uncertainty of the outlines of the disc. These changes, unless recovery should be brought about, will before long be followed by manifest atrophy, usually commencing in the outer and lower quadrant of the disc, and ultimately extending over its entire area.

Apart from "neuritis" Dr. Buzzard has called attention to the probability that the localised morbid process which, in its final stage, is known as "*sclerosis*" of nerve tissue, may commence in some portion of the track leading from the eye to the occipital lobe, may interfere with conduction of visual impressions, and may be recovered from, without at any time producing any intraocular manifestation of its presence. The diagnosis, in such a case, would rest upon the association of temporary impairment of vision with the signs of sclerosis affecting other portions of the nervous system.

Impairment of vision, occurring in a person who to all appearance is otherwise healthy, will be obviously more likely to direct the patient to an ophthalmic specialist than to a general physician; and the manifold causes of such impairment could not be discussed, could hardly even be enumerated, in the space here at my disposal. But such impairment, occurring in the case of a malady for which the patient is already under treatment, will be most likely to exhibit as its immediate cause, under examination by the ophthalmoscope, either turbidity of the vitreous body, or hæmorrhage (with or without patches of retinal degeneration, such as may arise in connection with albuminuria, with diabetes, with leukæmia, with mere arterial degeneration, or with syphilis), or swelling of, or vascular or atrophic changes in, the optic disc.

In cases which do not present impairment of vision, but in which the symptoms, such as headache or vertigo, point to the possibility of intracranial mischief, the diagnosis may be confirmed by the presence of swelling of the discs, a symptom which will be found in nearly every case of intracranial tumour, probably in every case at some stage of its progress, and probably in every case of cerebral abscess. A perfectly normal aspect of the discs would, I think, be almost sufficient to dispel a belief in the existence of either condition; but the swelling, when it occurs, does not materially assist us to localise the disease. In suspected sclerosis of any portion of the visual tract, nothing more than very slight appearances in the discs must be expected, such as a trace of blurring of the margins, a trace of capillary congestion, or a just perceptible dimming of the outlines of the larger vessels; but these slight appearances may usually be interpreted as possessing very grave significance.

The results obtained by ophthalmoscopic examination may be either confirmed or modified by examination of the visual function; and this examination should be threefold, including first, acuteness, secondly, colour-vision, and thirdly, the integrity of the field.

Acuteness, or the **integrity of form vision,** may be roughly tested by covering each eye alternately, and directing the patient to survey the objects in the room; but it is better to use Snellen's types and measured distances whenever possible, because by this method an exact numerical statement of the existing acuteness can be obtained, and improvement or deterioration can be exactly measured from time to time.

In estimating **colour-sense,** it is necessary to ascertain whether the patient was originally of normal vision in this respect; and it must be remembered that, among the male population of this country, about 3 per cent are more or less colour-blind, and are not necessarily acquainted with the fact. *Congenital colour-blindness* may be readily discovered by the use of Holmgren's wools. Acquired colour defect, as a rule, commences in the centre of the field. The retinal image of a large object, such as a skein of wool, may easily be of sufficient magnitude to pass beyond the limits of the affected area, so that the colour may still be correctly perceived by the surrounding parts. It is therefore necessary to test with very small objects, many of which have been suggested by different persons. Discs of coloured paper, a millimetre in diameter, fixed upon a black ground, or pins, the heads of which have been coated by red or green sealing wax, are among the things commonly employed. In use, the object selected should be held in front of the patient, a little to one side of his direct line of vision, but so that he can recognise the colour. It should then be brought exactly into his line of vision, and, if there be central defect, the colour will either disappear, or will appear less bright than, or in some way different from, what it was before. A very ingenious test has been devised by Captain Abney, and consists of a number of pellets, like small pills, brightly coloured in different tints. These are thrown into a white plate, and the patient, looking at the centre of the plate, will at once declare that some of the pellets, the images of which fall upon portions of the retina outside the macula, are red. When asked to pick up a red pellet he will be unable to do so. As soon as the eyes are directed to any particular red pellet, its image will fall upon the macula, and its red colour will no longer be recognised.

This central impairment of colour vision is an almost pathognomonic sign of what is commonly called "*toxic amblyopia*," that is to say, of a neuritis which is limited (at the beginning) to the macular fasciculus of retinal fibres, and is caused by the excessive use (excess either absolute or relatively to the idiosyncrasy of the patient) of tobacco, of alcohol, and possibly of other agents, either singly or in combination. Endeavours have been made to connect particular poisons with the size and outline of the affected area, but these have not been successful. In every case inflammation would at first be limited to the macular fasciculus, and the defect to the region supplied by it; while, if the disease continues, adjacent nerve fibres are likely to become implicated, and additional tracts of retina to be affected. It is said that central defect for colour may exist without impairment of form sense; but, in my own experience, I have never met with such an instance. The subjects are not usually very observant, and it is common for the disease to make considerable progress before advice is obtained. It is even common to see marked evidences of degeneration of the lower and outer quadrant of the disc, the region in which the macular fibres are collected together at their exit from the eye; although, as this portion of the nerve surface often differs somewhat from the nasal side in either colour or brightness, it is necessary to be careful in arriving at any positive conclusion as to its state. A certain blending of opacity with pallor may be regarded as a positive indication of the presence of morbid changes. The whole question has been investigated in an exhaustive manner by Uhthoff, and his papers contain some interesting statistics. Among 1000 patients detained in hospital for alcoholic excess, he found amblyopia in 6 per cent, the peculiar nerve lesion without amblyopia (which presumably was on its road) in 6·5 per cent more, and other pathological conditions of optic nerve or retina in 5·3 per cent. Among 238 cases of retro-bulbar neuritis he attributed 64 to alcohol, 23 to tobacco, 45 to these agents in combination, 3 to diabetes, 1 to poisoning by lead, 2 to poisoning by sulphuret of carbon, 14 to syphilis, 5 to multiple sclerosis, and the rest to various unknown or accidental causes. It is probable that such figures would present great variations in different communities. In this country we are more familiar with impaired vision from tobacco than from alcohol, and are most familiar with tobacco disease among seafaring men; while Mr. Priestley Smith has pointed out, I think with much reason, that, as a rule, the disease is not produced by tobacco alone, but by some cause of depression acting upon a large consumer, such as shipwreck and its attendant hardships upon a sailor, or financial anxieties upon a great smoker who is engaged in trade. From the point of view of general medicine, it is sufficient to say that the central defect of colour vision, and the changes in the appearance of the outer and lower quadrant of the nerve disc, which commonly, sooner or later, become manifest, tend to show that the mischief is situate in the orbital portion of the nerve, and to exclude the probability of any intracranial affection.

The **field of vision**, which next calls for attention, is the area in front of the eye from which light can enter the pupil, and this area is necessarily limited by the conformation of the anterior opening of the orbit. As a consequence of this conformation, it is more limited upwards and towards the median line than in other directions, and it presents an irregular oval outline. According to numerous measurements made by Landolt, the minimal limit in health is 55 degrees in a direction upwards, upwards and inwards, inwards, and inwards and downwards; 60 degrees directly downwards; 70 degrees upwards and outwards; 85 downwards and outwards; and 90 degrees directly outwards. Anything falling short of these measurements should be regarded as abnormal.

Vision may be impaired or lost over certain portions of the field of one or both eyes from various causes, which may be roughly arranged under the three heads of interception of light, retinal insensibility, and arrested or impeded conduction of visual impressions.

An opacity in the vitreous body posterior to the lens, or even in the anterior layer of the retina itself, will cut off light from a corresponding area, and will, according to its density, either exclude or obscure objects of vision which occupy points in the field corresponding to its position. If the affected eye were directed towards a white surface, the position and magnitude of the object would be indicated by a dark cloud or spot, corresponding to the depth and extent of the shadow which is cast upon the retina. Such a cloud or spot is described as a *positive defect* in the field. When, on the other hand, a defect is due to want of nerve perception, or of nerve conduction, the defect is *negative*, the patient seeing nothing which occupies a corresponding position, and not being conscious of his loss otherwise than negatively. The state is precisely analogous to that produced by the blind spot in the normal eye. The objects of which the images fall upon the affected area are not seen, just as they would not be seen if they were behind the spectator, or beyond ordinary visual limits on his right hand or on his left. It follows that a patient may be unaware of the existence of a considerable defect, unless its position be such as to prevent him from performing some customary action. Thus, a defect immediately to the right of the fixing point, in both eyes, would render it impossible to look forward in reading; but a defect on the left of the fixing point might scarcely attract attention, unless it were of considerable extent, in which case, of course, the subject of it could hardly remain unconscious of his inability to see objects in positions in which it would be usual for them to be visible.

Defects in the field of vision may be roughly determined by any convenient object, moved into various positions while the eye under examination (the other one being covered) is fixed upon that of the observer; but their precise determination and localisation require the assistance of the perimeter, which is essentially a quadrant or arc capable of being placed in any desired meridian, and on which an object of vision may be made to move either towards or away from the fixing point.

In estimating the value of the perimeter as as instrument of diagnosis, it is necessary to remember that it furnishes results which depend for their value upon the accuracy, the capacity, the attention, and the trustworthiness of the patient. If these qualities, or any of them, be subnormal in degree, the correctness of the perimetric chart may be diminished in corresponding proportion. Were it not for this consideration, the instrument might with propriety be furnished with scales calculated to be read by a vernier. As a matter of fact, it is seldom possible to obtain more than an approximation to identity in two charts taken from the same eye, with a short interval of rest between them; and it is often difficult even for a careful observer to state precisely at what point he first becomes aware of the presence of a peripheral white spot, or of the colour of a coloured one. With regard to either the eye will recognise the presence of a moving object, while this is still too far from the centre to be seen when stationary. The slightest change in the position of the eye may also appear to give a more or a less extended field than actually exists; and, as the patient must sit with his back to the light, very small movements may easily escape the notice of the examiner. In a protracted examination, moreover, the peripheral and less active portions of the retina are found to undergo diminution of sensitiveness from exhaustion. On all these accounts charts of the field must generally be regarded only as approximations to the truth; and hence there is but little advantage to be gained from the use of costly and elaborate perimeters. The various "self-registering" forms are, I think, specially to be avoided, on account of the fatal facility which they offer for making an indelible mark upon the chart, in response to a possibly misleading statement from the patient. A very good and light instrument, made to pack into a portable box, can be obtained from Fritsch of Vienna, or, in a somewhat improved form, from Mr. Hawksley of 357 Oxford Street. I need hardly add that it is unnecessary to follow the example of some Continental authorities, and to convert perimetry into a solemn function, to be accomplished by means of a black instrument supported upon a black table, and to be presided over by a person wearing black clothes and black gloves. The patient should be comfortably seated, with his back turned towards an interval between two windows, and the slide of the perimeter should be moved by means of a hook of blackened wire, twelve or fifteen inches in length, and set in a convenient handle. In this way, even without black gloves, the hand of the operator will not guide the eye of the patient to the moving spot.

Quite recently, a cheap and still more simple perimeter for frequent use has been introduced by Dr. Ascher, of Frankfort on the Maine (1). It consists of a very light and nearly hemispherical bowl of transparent celluloid, so mounted on a handle that it can be held before either eye by the patient. A central aperture permits the observer to watch the position of the eye that is under examination; and the moving object, which consists of a square of any desired colour and magnitude, carried upon a black stem, is kept in contact with the external surface of the bowl. By means of a pencil of water colour the outline of the field can be traced upon the celluloid itself, and the examination can be made with great ease and rapidity. The instrument is calculated to render perimetric observation practicable in every consulting-room, and therefore to extend the applications of what is often a valuable aid to diagnosis. It can be supplied by Mr. Hawksley.

It is the custom of many foreign observers to take a chart of the field not only for white, but also for green, for red, and for blue, and much importance has been attached to the maintenance of the usual proportion between the zones of vision for these colours. Captain Abney has shown, however, in experimenting with white light and with the pure colours of the spectrum, that the area over which a spot can be seen does not depend upon its colour, but upon its luminosity ; and that a coloured spot is visible over a smaller area than a white one, not because it is different from the white in colour, but because it is less luminous. By using spots of different colour, but of equal luminosity, that is, by subduing the more luminous to the level of the less luminous, he found the field to be the same for all. It is obvious that a white spot, which reflects all the elements of the spectrum, must be more luminous than a spot of equal area which reflects only red, or only green ; and, at least in healthy eyes, the colour fields mark the retinal areas which are responsive to comparatively feeble stimulation. I have no reason to doubt that the same thing is true in disease, and that impaired nutrition of the retina, or impaired conduction through fibres proceeding from its periphery, will narrow the field of colour vision by narrowing the area over which a feeble stimulus will excite sensation. Again, while the area over which a coloured spot is visible as an object depends upon its luminosity, the area over which its colour can be recognised depends greatly on the degree of saturation of that colour, and it follows that colour names must often be misleading. In my own Fritsch's perimeter the green object is a square of rather bright green paper with a reflecting surface, and the green itself is pale, or diluted with white. If I replace this object by a disc of Marx's green cloth, which is highly saturated, and less luminous, I obtain a diminished field for the object, and an enlarged field for the colour. I think it would be better if the colours were laid aside, and if objects of graduated shades of gray were used instead of them, so that the test might be put upon its true basis, as one of sensitiveness to comparatively feeble luminosity alone. For the present, however, observers who are unacquainted with Abney's work (Wilbrand, Baas, etc.,) continue to make frequent reference to the *zones of colour-vision,* and to the changes of contour and of extension which they may undergo.

The alterations in the field which may be discovered by the perimeter, or sometimes by rougher methods of testing, are of many varieties, some of them depending upon changes in the retina itself, others upon conditions impeding the conduction of impressions along the fibres of the optic nerve, others possibly upon changes in the receptive ganglia. We may find general narrowing, frequently most declared with regard to objects on the nasal side ; deficiency in a sector or sectors, sometimes increasing until it produces blindness over one or other of the vertical halves of the field; and deficiency over an islet or islets, either central or scattered. In ordinary chronic glaucoma we find a narrowing which begins, and long continues most marked, on the nasal side, but which ultimately contracts the boundaries in every direction. The cause of this form appears to be that the anatomical conditions of glaucoma interfere with the normal activity of the retinal circulation, first on the temporal side, and ultimately at the whole of its periphery, and that the perceptive elements are reduced, by the diminution of their customary blood-supply, to a condition of partial or complete inefficiency. It is possible that the more or less concentric contraction observed in certain cases of hysteria may sometimes be a phenomenon analogous to ·the contraction in glaucoma, the interference with the circulation being brought about through the agency of vaso-motor nerves, instead of by the mechanical operation of direct pressure. Contraction is also seen as an early symptom of the participation of the visual apparatus in the changes productive of tabes dorsalis, and is then usually attended by a contraction of the colour fields as well as of the field for white. In a case of doubtful tabes, with slight central impairment of the vision of one eye, and with a tendency to pallor of the optic disc, it will often be found that the field is narrowed, not only in the eye obviously affected, but also in its fellow, and such a combination will afford adequate foundation for a very grave prognosis. It would seem, from the ordinary history of such cases, that the hardening or overgrowth of the connective tissue of the affected portions of the nervous system pursues such a course as to extend its influence from the peripheral to the axial fibres of the optic tracts or nerves.

A loss of vision over the right or left half of the combined field is a state which may be brought about by very various causes, and is conditioned by the distribution of the conducting fibres. As already mentioned in relation to the contractility of the pupils, the fibres of the right optic tract proceed to the right hemisphere of each retina, and those of the left optic tract to the left hemisphere of each retina, while the region of the macula on either side has been usually supposed to receive fibres from both tracts. It follows that arrest of conduction through the right optic tract would render the patient blind to all objects on the left of the fixing point; and that arrest of conduction through the left optic tract would render him blind to all objects on the right of the fixing point—the blind portion of each field being usually defined by a vertical line with a slight central curvature, which leaves the macula within the seeing portion. On the other hand, morbid changes may be so localised in the chiasma, or in one or both of the optic nerves in front of it, as to produce loss of the temporal half of the field in one or both eyes, or of the nasal half of one or both, or of the upper or lower portions of one or both; and the resulting phenomena may be of assistance in determining the position of some aneurysm, gumma, or other tumour, by which the visual apparatus is compressed or interfered with. Such conditions are, nevertheless, little more than curiosities of pathology.

Dr. Harris has recently called attention to a class of cases, chiefly of transient hemianopia, in which the dividing line between the blind and the seeing portions bisects the macula, instead of curving round and including it in the seeing half. Willbrand has described the same condition, and states that in 77 cases of lateral hemianopia the dividing line was central in 29, but only in 9 out of 32 of bi-temporal hemianopia. Dr. Harris is of opinion that these cases of transient hemianopia afford complete proof that the macula is innervated on the same plan as the rest of the retina, and that there is no special decussation of the macular fibres. He has examined the position of the dividing line with especial care, not trusting to the perimeter alone, but using a method suggested by Sir William Gowers. The patient is made to sit facing the observer with one eye shut, at a distance of about two feet. The observer then closes his own eye opposite to that shut by the patient, who is directed to gaze steadily into the open eye of the observer, who, in turn, watches the patient's pupil. The line of fixation is therefore the same for both eyes, and the slightest wavering of the patient's eye is seen and allowed for by the observer. A very small spot of white, carried upon a black stem, being used as an object, may be slowly brought from the periphery of the field towards the centre; and it can be exactly determined by the observer, after repeated trials, whether or not the object is seen by the patient before it reaches the line of fixation. It is so seen in most cases of persistent hemianopia, but not in transient cases, and Dr. Harris thinks that the apparent discrepancy may be accounted for in one of two ways. The cortical centre of the macula may either have escaped destruction or may have regained some of its functions; or the patient may have developed by education a new fixation point in his retina close to the original fovea centralis.

Speaking generally, it may be said that a vertical division of the two retinæ into blind and seeing halves is an indication of intra-cranial disease on the same side as the blindness; that is, on the side opposite to that of the objects which are not seen. It means, of course, complete arrest of conduction at some point between the chiasma and the occipital lobe on the side concerned; and, as already mentioned, if the place of arrest be anterior to the quadrigeminal bodies, the reflex contractility of the pupils to light falling upon the blind parts of the retinæ will be lost; while, if the arrest be posterior to the quadrigeminal bodies, the contractility may be retained. The only other symptom likely to assist in localising intra-cranial disease would be some interference with the power of speaking or of writing, which, according to its precise nature, might indicate the probable seat of a blood-clot or of a tumour.

The existence of complete right or left blindness is usually unmistakable, and may be ascertained by very simple methods; while the limits of the defect are determined by the anatomy of the parts concerned, and hardly require to be pointed out by the patient. In the case of regular or irregular contraction of one or both fields, or in the case of isolated or scattered defect in either, the conditions are somewhat different, and, before placing too much reliance upon the outlines of the perimetric chart, it is necessary to ascertain the trustworthiness of the patient. An easy means of doing so is afforded by the blind spot in each eye; and it is my custom to begin the examination by an endeavour to map out the spot on the chart. If this can be done with fair accuracy the patient may be depended upon and the examination proceeded with; but, if the limits of the blind spot are irregular or uncertain, and still more if it cannot be found at all, it may be assumed that the eye wanders from the fixation point, and that an elaborate drawing will represent nothing more than a period of wasted time. The defect caused by the blind spot is roughly elliptical in outline, with its major axis vertical. It extends from just above the horizontal meridian to just below the meridian of 60°; and covers horizontally, at its widest part, a space extending from about 14° to about 17° from the fixing point. Eccentric isolated or scattered defects in the field of either eye are usually dependent upon disease within the organ itself, as of the retina or choroid, just as central defect is usually dependent upon retro-bulbar neuritis, whether toxic or of some other origin; but contraction, whether general or in a sector or sectors, is usually due to an arrest of conduction consequent upon the morbid change which, in its completed form, is described as "sclerosis," and which is liable to occur in small patches, irregularly and apparently capriciously distributed over many parts of the nervous system, and producing symptoms and results varying with its position and extent, but always involving, when the morbid process is carried to completion, absolute loss of function in each patch of nerve tissue which is affected. Contraction is also seen in a class of cases first described by von Graefe (5), and styled by him "retinal anæsthesia." Von Graefe described the condition as one which occurred chiefly in children at or near the age of puberty, or in hysterical women, and he gave as its characteristic symptoms a slight lowering of central vision, a marked contraction of the field, and a morbid sensitiveness of the eyes to light or occupation; while phosphenes could be produced, as in healthy eyes, by pressure even over those eccentric portions of the retinæ which had lost their visual sensibility. Other writers, following von Graefe, have described as "hysterical," apparently only because they terminated in recovery, cases in which, along with the contraction of the fields, there was considerable diminution of central vision; and, taking the general literature of the subject, I think it may be said that the described symptoms of "hysterical" amblyopia are quite as worthy of the epithet "Protean" as those of hysterical affections of any other kind. I have seen cases in which the patient, examined by the perimeter, acknowledged only to fields about ten degrees in diameter, and in which I convinced myself, by a simple test, that there was, in reality, little if any real contraction.

I once operated for strabismus upon a young lady, a native of Australia, who suffered from some form of intracranial disease in early childhood, and in whom this disease was followed by complete arrest of conduction through the fibres proceeding from the peripheral portions of both retinæ, while the fibres of the macular bundles remained intact. Each eye has normal central vision, and she reads brilliant type with perfect facility, but she cannot see the whole of the face of a person sitting opposite to her at a distance of four feet. If she looks at the eyes she cannot see the mouth, and conversely. She gives a graphic description of the difficulties which her small fields entail. In childhood she was always falling over foot-stools and other things which she could not see, and it was a long time before her falls were attributed to anything but "awkwardness," or before she realised the difference between her own vision and that of the persons around her. On entering a room it takes her some time to search it in every direction to see what things or people it may contain; and on meeting an acquaintance at whom she is so looking as to recognise the features, she cannot see whether or not a hand is held out to her. Her difficulty in this matter suggested to me a test which I have found useful in determining the reality of alleged extreme contraction. Engage the attention of the patient in such a way as to make him or her look you straight in the eyes, and then suddenly hold out a hand as if to shake hands, but at a somewhat low level. If the contraction is simulated, the hand will be taken instinctively; and in this way I have been able to detect not only hysterical girls, but, in one instance, a plaintiff who had been in a railway accident, and who had become a great proficient in the art of sitting to the perimeter.

Even with all the aid which can be afforded by general symptoms, the physician will sometimes be perplexed to distinguish undoubted contraction of the field, such as, in the great majority of cases, must be taken to indicate serious lesion in some part of the nervous system, from real or apparent contraction which leads to nothing, which is recovered from, and which therefore, after recovery, is often described as "hysterical." I think the clue to some of the difficulties hence arising has been furnished by Dr. Buzzard's valuable suggestion, already mentioned, that the morbid process which usually terminates in sclerosis may also terminate in restoration of the affected patch to health, even after changes which may have sufficed materially to impede, or even wholly to arrest, nerve conduction through the diseased portion. The acceptance of this conclusion will not diminish the difficulties of diagnosis, but it will afford a reasonable explanation of events for which the easy hypothesis of "hysteria" does not always seem sufficient to account.

R. BRUDENELL CARTER.

REFERENCES

1. ASCHER. La clinique ophtalmologique, 25 Mars, 1898.—2. BAAS, KARL. Das Gesichtsfeld. Stuttgart, 1896.—3. BUZZARD. Transactions of the Ophthalmological Society of the United Kingdom, vol. xvii.—4. FÖRSTER, Prof., of Breslau. "Beziehungen

der Allgemein-Leiden und Organ-Erkrankungen zu Veränderungen und Krankheiten des Sehorgans," *Handbuch der gesammten Augenheilkunde* (Gräfe und Sämisch), Bd. vii. —5. VON GRÄFE. "Anaesthesia retinae mit concentr. Verengerung d. Gesichtsfeldes," Zehender, *Monatsblätter*, 1865.—6. HARRIS. "On Hemianopia," *Brain*, vol. xx. p. 307. —7. HILL, ALEX. Norris and Oliver's *System of Diseases of the Eye.*—8. KNIES, MAX. *Die Beziehungen des Sehorgans und seiner Erkrankungen zu den übrigen Krankheiten des Korpers und seiner Organe.* Wiesbaden, 1893. (Translated in America.)—9. ROBIN. *Des troubles oculaires dans les maladies de l'encéphale,* 1880.—10. SEEGEN. *Diabetes Mellitus.* Berlin, 1875.—11. UHTHOFF. Grafe's *Archiv,* Bd. xxxii. Abth. 4, 1886 ; Bd. xxxiii. Abth. 1, 1887.—12. WAGENMANN, Prof. (of Jena). "Einiges uber Augenerkrankungen bei Gicht," *Arch. f. O.,* Bd. xliii.—13. WERNICKE, CARL. "Hemianopische Pupillar - Reaction," *Fortschritte der Medicin,* 1883, Bd. i. S. 49. —14. WILBRAND, HERMANN. *Die Erholungsausdehnung des Gesichtsfeldes unter normalen und pathologischen Bedingungen.* Wiesbaden, 1896.

R. B. C.

DISEASES OF SPINE

DISEASES OF VERTEBRAL COLUMN, TUMOURS, AND COMPRESSION PALSIES

COMPRESSION of the spinal cord gives rise to a very definite group of symptoms, the differential diagnosis of which is often difficult, but now admits of a considerable approach to accuracy.

A certain degree of compression of the cord is caused by pachymeningitis; but for the treatment of this subject reference must be made to the next article.

The subject divides itself under the following headings :—

I. Seat of origin, and nature of the causes of compression; II. Symptomatology and diagnosis; III. Site of the mischief; IV. Treatment.

I. Causes of compression of the spinal cord.—The spinal cord may be compressed by disease or injury of the vertebræ, of the intervertebral discs, of the membranes and tissues in the neighbourhood of the spine by growths springing from the meninges of the cord, or by intrathecal hæmorrhage. Of these, invasion of the neural canal, as a result of tuberculous caries, is the commonest. Next to caries must be placed fracture of the spine; then new growths; and lastly, parasites.

From what has just been said it follows that the causes and their nature are best considered under the heads of—(A) the extrinsic; (B) intrinsic : the plane of separation being the dura mater sheath, or theca, of the cord.

The first class, therefore, will consist of extra-thecal causes, and the second class of intra-thecal.

A. Extra-thecal sources of compression.—The vertebræ are liable to become the seat of the following destructive processes :—(a) *Tuberculous disease or caries of the spine.*

This disease has three chief seats of origin :—The first occurs just beneath the vertebral bodies at their articular surfaces; the second seat is the cancellous tissue of the laminæ, and, subsequently, the periosteum; the third is the perithecal tissue. Probably, however, the occurrence of tuberculous disease here is secondary to mischief arising primarily in the bone.

Tuberculous disease of the bodies of the vertebræ produces, as a rule, an abscess as well as the marked deformity which is referred to on p. 856. When an abscess is present it forces its way down the bodies of the spine, under the anterior common ligament, and then along the fibres of the psoas muscle, provided it takes origin from a point not higher than the middle of the posterior mediastinum. It also extends, however, horizontally backwards, and then, meeting in the middle line the opposition of the posterior common ligament, it projects into the neural canal as two lateral swellings, usually of unequal size ; these swellings press the spinal cord back against the laminal arches, and compress it laterally also. When the operation of laminectomy is performed these swellings are found as elastic, reddish, rounded eminences at the side of the theca. They are readily opened, their contents scraped and removed, and the cavity disinfected and drained. The proximity of the abscess causes a certain degree of perithecal pachymeningitis.

(*b*) *Caries sicca* is the next disease of the bone to be considered ; by it is to be understood a progressive rarefactive osteitis in which the enlarged spaces in the bone are filled with a deep red granulation tissue, the microscopical appearances of which resemble those of a small spindle-celled sarcoma. This is a form of tuberculous caries, and may bring about a severe compression of the cord without producing much deformity, or occasionally indeed without producing any; as its name denotes, it is not attended with abscess formation.

Unquestionably syringomyelia, whether accompanied by gliosis surrounding the cystic space or not, may be confounded in diagnosis with the other conditions which are now under discussion. At the same time, it is so different in character that it should be easily distinguished from genuine compression of the spinal cord; the cardinal points of difference are undoubtedly the early and patchy occurrence of analgesia in syringomyelia, and the early atrophy of muscles under the rapid and injurious invasion of the anterior cornual centres. Of gliosis accompanying the formation of the central cystic spaces the extension upwards of the symptoms is perhaps the best indication. In such cases no amelioration can be obtained by operation; but in simple syringomyelia some temporary improvement can unquestionably be gained by tapping the dilated cavity in the cord.

(*c*) The next commonest cause is *new growth* arising from the periosteum, or from the substance of the bone, and gradually involving the spinal cord by penetrating the intervertebral foramina, and thus encroaching on the space of the neural canal.

. The bodies of the vertebræ frequently become the seat of new growth, either of sarcoma or secondary carcinoma. So, too, sarcomata arising in the tissues, that is, in the muscles or tendons, whether primarily or as part of a general sarcomatosis, may likewise produce paraplegia.

(*d*) *Trauma* may lead to compression in one or other of the following ways :—

(a) Separation of contiguous bodies of the vertebræ combined with fracture or subluxation—where such subluxation is possible—of the articular processes of the vertebræ, with the effect of allowing the relative positions of the vertebræ to be distorted, and so to cause a narrowing of the neural canal.

(β) Crushing of the body of one vertebra, combined with fracture of the laminæ and articular processes, so that the cord is compressed by the sharp edge of the body of the lower vertebra projecting into the neural canal, the upper part of the spine being displaced forwards.

(γ) Displacement of an intervertebral disc, which may be squeezed backwards from its normal position between the damaged bodies.

(δ) Hæmorrhage.

Though it might be expected that, in view of the rich vascular supply of the perithecal tissue, free hæmorrhage in the neural canal, as a direct result of trauma, would be common, such is not the case ; and though intra-thecal traumatic hæmorrhage is sometimes severe in its effects, and intramedullary hæmorrhage always so, perithecal bleeding is not, practically speaking, a source of compression.

Of other but much rarer sources of compression must be mentioned (e) aneurysm and (f) hydatid.

(e) Aneurysm.—A very dangerous cause of paraplegia from compression is aneurysm of the descending aorta. This, when situated in the posterior mediastinum, causes erosion of the bodies of the vertebræ, and consequent collapse of the same, if the progress of the mischief be considerable ; the disease is not very common, is very difficult to treat, and must always be carefully borne in mind in forming a differential diagnosis. It is to be detected, of course, by the ordinary physical signs of aneurysm, and by the peculiar boring character of the pain. It most commonly occurs in the lower half of the dorsal region.

(f) Parasitic disease.—Echinococcus cysts, if they develop retro-peritoneally or in the thoracic region, may invade the neural canal in the same way as new growths, that is, through the intervertebral foramina ; they may also produce a certain amount of erosion in the bodies of the vertebræ, but do not produce collapse or the same angular deformity as in the case of neoplasms. Deformity may be present, however, as in Cruveilhier's classical case. The pressure effected by hydatid cysts is always very severe, and the consequent destruction produced in the cord, by the ischæmic disturbance of the circulation therein, is but slowly recovered from after laminectomy has removed the cause ;—slowly, that is, as compared with the relatively rapid recovery in cases of caries. The treatment, of course, is early laminectomy with, as far as possible, thorough extirpation of the cysts.

II. Symptoms and diagnosis.—**Local conditions of the spine in cases of disease causing compression of the spinal cord.**—*Deformity of the spinal cord.*—The various diseases which produce compression-paraplegia affect the spinal column very diversely. It will be best, therefore, to group the cases according to whether the disease actually causes a certain amount of physical destruction of the bone, and hence a yielding of the same, so that either the natural curves of the different regions of the spine are exaggerated—for example, the dorsal region becomes kyphotic, —or an aberrant curvature makes its appearance at some one point in the column, when the curvature is definitely angular, or sometimes, in a combination of these causes, it is both angular and lateral.

There is another condition often to be taken into account, namely, that the spine is not infrequently held by the patient in an unusual attitude on account of pain; or, by reason of pain, the natural tone of certain supporting muscles is interfered with, so that the spine automatically assumes a curve resulting from the functional paresis of the muscles in question. It may be stated that under such circumstances the spine usually presents a large kyphotic curve.

The conditions under which deformity of the spine is especially to be looked for and expected are (i.) tuberculous caries; (ii.) fracture dislocation; (iii.) new growths, attacking the bodies of the vertebræ.

The details of these conditions must be sought for in surgical works; but for the purposes of diagnosis attention must here be directed to the fact that, in certain regions of the spine, it is very difficult to detect a deformity which, if harmony with other symptoms is expected, ought inferentially to be present. Thus in the cervical region it is perfectly possible for a complete fracture dislocation of the body of the fifth or sixth cervical vertebra to exist without any disturbance of the lines of the cervical spine; and this may occur, and any deformity still be invisible, even when the spines and laminæ are denuded of the muscles and ligaments, as in a laminectomy. So too in the lumbar region, extensive tuberculous (non-suppurative) caries, producing the severest paraplegia, may be present without the slightest deformity of the spine.

This is the suitable place to estimate the influence of deformity of the spine in producing compression-paraplegia of the spinal cord. It is well known that, in the case of tuberculous caries, it is possible to have serious curvature without any apparent pressure effects on the spinal cord. On the other hand, a limited fracture of the body of a vertebra may lead to complete division of the spinal cord. The whole problem resolves itself into the question whether the dural canal is or is not diminished in diameter. In a caries case, such as that first mentioned, the change in the curvature of the spine is exceedingly gradual; and, unless there be also an abscess sac pressing backwards, or tuberculous granulation tissue invading the loose perithecal tissue and fat, practically no mechanical diminution of the neural canal, of any importance, is produced.

On the other hand, in fracture of the spine the neural canal is narrowed very suddenly and severely. It is true no serious degree of narrowing may be found during an operation, or at death, because the bones may spring back; and no doubt they commonly do so as soon as the compressing force, which produced the fracture, is taken off. The sharp angular edge of a fractured body of the vertebra cuts like a sharp-edged instrument under such circumstances, and may hopelessly injure the soft cord by the brief but powerful compression which is exerted. So too when the vertebræ are the seat of new growths the bones thus attacked undergo rapid rarefactive change, they readily break or are crushed, and consequently the deformity caused and the compression - paraplegia resulting therefrom are often very sudden in onset.

Other local conditions of the spine.—The spinal region at or about the seat of compression, when the source of mischief is extra-dural, is very commonly tender on pressure, whether applied directly, or indirectly, in the axis of the body, by pressing on the neck and shoulders. Furthermore it is often hypersensitive, as shown by the application of a hot sponge ; and sometimes the skin is locally reddened from the paralysis of vaso-motor fibres running in the nerve roots which themselves are opposite the seat of disease or injury, and are implicated in the mischief. In diagnosis by physical examination great care must be exercised to distinguish between true local pain and the pains of mere neur-asthenia (especially traumatic neurasthenia), which are spoken of as the hysterogenetic points or zones of Charcot, and occupy the well-known situations ; the chief of these are the sixth and twelfth dorsal spines, the posterior iliac spines, and the coccygeo-sacral articulation.

In addition to the local signs just mentioned there is frequently the limitation of movement and fixation of the spine, due to pain causing the patient, voluntarily or involuntarily, to hold the spine in one position. This also must be carefully discriminated from the somewhat stiff attitude in which a traumatic neurasthenic patient often holds the dorso-lumbar region of his spine.

Finally, as regards local examination of the spinal column, it must be remembered that congenital absence or shortening of a spinous process is not infrequently met with, and has often been mistaken for a result of injury.

Pain.—The occurrence of pain in cases of pressure upon the cord by new growths has been recognised from classical times ; hence the name Paraplegia dolorosa, given to the cases of malignant disease of the vertebræ leading to paraplegia by force of compression of the cord. Though a striking and almost invariable accompaniment of tumour cases, pain is practically absent in other kinds of spinal com-pression. We will begin, therefore, with the pain of new growths. It is necessary to consider this pain from two points of view : namely, first, its character ; secondly, its precise situation.

Character and mode of production.—The character of the pain in such cases is almost always burning and stabbing ; this paroxysmal condition is not infrequently preceded, or accompanied, by steady aching which is only relieved at times by change of posture. This aching should be compared to that often observed in traumatism. A very important

TABLE

Nerve Root	Motor	Sensory	Visceral	Reflex	Vaso-motor	Superficial origins of spinal nerve roots	Apices of spinous processes	Nerve Root
C. 1.	1. Small flexors of head. Depressors of hyoid bone.	C. 1.	...	C. 1.	...	Cervical 1		C. 1.
2.	2. Small rotators of head. Complexus. Splenius.	2. Occipito-parietal region of scalp.	...	2.	...	2	1 Cervical	2.
3.	3. Sterno-mastoid.	3. Posterior triangle of neck.	...	3.	...	3		3.
4.	4. Levator anguli scapulæ. Scaleni. Trapezoid. Diaphragm.	4. Trapezoidal region of neck and shoulder and subclavicular region.	...	4.	...	4	2	4.
5.	5. Levator anguli scapulæ, Scaleni, Supra-spinatus, Rhomboids, Subclavius, Infra-spinatus, Teres minor, Biceps, Brachialis anticus, Deltoid, Supinator longus, Supinator brevis (?), Pectoralis major (clavicular part), Serratus magnus.	5. Delto-bicipital region of arm.	...	5.	...	5	3	5.
6.	Subscapularis (? C. 5), Pronators, Teres major, Latissimus dorsi (? C. 5), Serratus magnus (? C. 7), Pectoralis major (spinal part ? C. 8).	6. } Pre-axial border of forearm and hand.	...	6 Radius tap. Scapular.	...	6	4	6.
7.	7. Triceps. Extensors of the wrist and digits.	7.	...	7.	...	7	5	7.
8.	8. Flexors of the wrist and digits. Interossei and small muscles of the hand.	8. Mid line of forearm and hand.	...	8 Triceps tap.	...	8	6	8.
D. 1.		D. 1. Post-axial border of forearm and hand, i.e., little finger.	D. 1.	D. 1.	D. 1.	Dorsal 1	7	D. 1.
2.	2. } Dilator fibres of Pupil.	2.	2. } Secretion submaxillary gland.	2. } Pupil dilatation to shade.	2. } Blood vessels, head.	2	1 Dorsal	2.
3.	3.	3.	3.	3.	3.	3		3.
4.	4. } Intercostales.	4. Nipple level.	4.	4.	4. } Blood vessels, lung. Acceleration of heart.	4	2	4.
5.	5.	5.	5. } Sweat glands of hand (probable).	5. } Epigastric	5.	5	3	5.
6.	6.	6. Ensiform level.	6.	6.	6. } Vaso-constrictor to upper limb.	6	4	6.
7.	7.	7.	7.	7. } Subdivide according to sensory areas. (See Diagrams.?)	7.	7	5	7.
8.	8.	8.	8.	8.	8.	8		8.
9.	9.	9. Umbilical level.	9.	9.	9. } Fibres to renal vessels, chiefly vaso-motor.	9	6	9.
10.	10. Rectus abdominis. Obliquus internus.	10. }		10 Abdominal	10.	10	7	10.
11.	11. Obliquus externus. Transversalis.	11.		11.	11.	11	8	11.
12.	12.	12. Upper gluteal border.		12.	12.	12	9	12.
L. 1.	L. 1. Quadratus lumborum.	L. 1. Mid buttock.	L. 1.	L. 1. } Cremasteric.	L. 1. } Vaso-constrictor to lower limb.	Lumbar 1	10	L. 1.
2.	2. Cremaster.	2. Outer side and front of middle of thigh.		2.	2.	2		2.

feature is that the stabbing and burning pains are frequently called forth by movement, that is, by bending or rotatory twisting of the spine.

Pain of the kind just described is probably due to pressure on the sensitive dura mater and cord within it; but there is also a concurrent manifestation of pain produced by implication of the nerve root. Under these circumstances the pain begins in the pricking and stabbing manner, and then has a special character shooting along the distribution of the nerve whose root is directly pressed upon. However, such localised pain soon becomes merged in the diffuse pain due to pressure on the cord as a whole.

Site of the pain.—Considering that every aid is required to establish a correct topographical diagnosis of the lesion, the importance of the fact that the pain is never referred to any part above the seat of the lesion is self-evident. This fact is doubly significant when the bifurcating character of the posterior root-fibres entering the cord is remembered, as also their association, each respectively, with reflex centres situated lower down the cord. If, of course, the lesion involve a nerve root, the pain along which is a very definite feature, then this pain becomes of the utmost value in topographical diagnosis; but, unfortunately, as a rule, the pain is derived from the cord fibres, and then is referred to parts some distance below the lesion. Thus in a case of compression of the lower part of the dorsal region the severe pains complained of were referred below the knees. Here I need only mention, as a warning, that in view of this fact that the localisation always tends to be too low, the occurrence of any apparently trivial pain must be carefully noted, and its distribution along the course of any given root accurately observed.

The general effect on spinal centres.—The effect upon the spinal centres, generally of compression of the spinal cord at some point above them, is so to exaggerate their functional excitability as to produce over-action with resulting spasticity and exaggeration of reflex movements; but in very severe cases (for example, in traumatic severance of the cord) a loss of functional activity ensues (Bastian), the knee-jerks disappear, and in extreme cases remain absent, but in moderate ones they return. The permanency of the loss of function suggests the existence of a diffuse traumatic myelitis.

The accompanying table shows the special representation of the various functions of the cord at the level of each segment; that is, at the level of each nerve root.

Ocular symptoms.—The nerve fibres, the excitation of which causes dilatation of the pupil, start from a centre in the floor of the posterior part of the iter, as yet not accurately localised. Such fibres run down in the lateral columns of the cord, and leave the latter by the second dorsal nerve root to reach the inferior cervical ganglion of the sympathetic, and so pass up to the eye. This bundle of fibres is so well localised that, if at a focus in the cervical region compression be exerted with a little more strength on one side than on the other, the pupil of that side will be smaller. The very rare phenomenon of congestion of the disc in the same eye may occasionally be observed; it resembles an early stage of optic neuritis.

Cardiac symptoms.—Fibres which accelerate the heart run from a centre in the upper part of the floor of the fourth ventricle down the lateral columns of the cord, leave the cord by the dorsal nerve roots from the fourth to the ninth, and reach the cardiac plexus by the sympathetic. These fibres, on careful examination, may be found functionally affected in compression of the spinal cord in the cervical region; and thus in one of two ways they may be excited, this being the commoner: or they may be paralysed, as in acute compression of the cord. If the pressure be not very severe, and excitation occur, the pulse-rate will be found very high, that is, up to 140 per minute, without any corresponding constitutional condition to account for it. Very frequently this over-action on the part of these fibres is parox-ysmal; the pulse-rate may rise rapidly, and after remaining up for a certain time fall again; and then, after an interval of some hours, may rise again, and so forth. In the paralytic state the heart-rate is slow, below the normal, the vagus being, apparently, no longer antagonised. It must also be noted whether the compression of the spinal cord affect the vaso-motor channel, in which case it causes, as a rule, hyperæmia and œdema of the paralysed parts, or the so-called heat fibres, that is, the ther-motactic, in which case the temperature may rise to 104° independently of any inflammatory mischief with which such pyrexia is usually associated.

Respiratory symptoms. — The fibres conveying the innervation of respiratory movements must be divided into those supplied to the diaphragm and to the intercostal muscles respectively. Of these two groups the diaphragmatic are by far the most important, because the intercostal muscles are more distant from the respiratory centre, as is evidenced by the fact that, when the compression of the cord is opposite some point above the fourth cervical nerve, the intercostal muscles may be completely paralysed while the diaphragm continues in full action. From this it is clear that the phrenic fibres in the cord are, practically speaking, more resistant (because possibly more numerous) than those for the intercostal muscles. "Deficiency" of the action of the inter-costals is very commonly observed to result from compression of the cord as low as the second dorsal root, and is relatively quickly recovered from as soon as the source of the compression is removed.

The failure of respiration is not, of course, wholly one of affection of conducting channels alone; but this point cannot be further discussed here. The relative share taken by the bulbar and spinal portions of the central respiratory nerve mechanism, even in the case of the lower mammals, is itself an undecided matter.

Vaso-motor symptoms.—(a) *Constriction.*—The vaso-constrictor fibres probably leave the spinal cord, in man, at the following levels, indicated on the table at p. 859.

The conditions under which vaso-constrictor spasms appear to be maintained, or at any rate in which the calibre of the vessels is reduced, and in which vaso-dilatation does not occur, are seen in those cases in which there is long-standing compression of the cord, and where atrophic changes have been set up in consequence of subacute degenerative changes. In these cases it will be observed that, besides the pallor and coldness of the paralysed parts, there are also evidences of narrowing of the vessels in the dry, harsh condition of the skin; coupled with which is often an accumulation of epithelium, producing a kind of exfoliative state of the epidermis, in patches and spots.

(b) *Vaso-dilatation.*—Whereas vaso-constriction is marked in a case running a slow course, vaso-dilatation is a sign of acute and severe compression of the cord. It shows itself in the paralysed limbs, causing swelling; and very commonly also in a pink flush. Sometimes the tumefaction of the tissues is practically limited to the synovial membrane of the chief joints of the limb; the knees or ankles, for example, constituting the so-called arthritis observed in some cases of acute myelitis. It must not, of course, be confused with the acute synovitis of a pyæmic nature, which occasionally arises in connection with the bedsores of acute myelitis, and which goes on to suppuration —a stage which the congestive synovitis of vaso-dilator origin never reaches.

Visceral symptoms.—The abdominal viscera, whose innervation is disturbed by compression lesions of the spinal cord, are chiefly the alimentary canal and bladder.

Alimentary canal.—In extensive crushing lesion of the cord, with probable intra-medullary hæmorrhage, causing compression if not destruction of the centres from which the fibres passing into the splanchnics take origin, the small intestine is sometimes paralysed.

(a) *Intestine.*—Under these circumstances meteorism is produced, the abdomen is notably distended, and, though there is no acute pain connected therewith, the patient very often has severe discomfort nevertheless, or curious sensations of oppression connected with the dilated condition of the paretic gut; especially a sense of peristaltic movements involving successive segments down to a certain point where they stop, suggesting a block. In the large intestine the expulsive force is very greatly diminished; but the bowel can be caused to contract by suitable local stimulation, as by the faradic current, or by injection of castor oil or turpentine. In extensive lesions of the sacral root portion of the lumbar enlargement the sphincter may be completely paralysed.

(b) *Bladder.*—The chief site of the representation of this important viscus in the lumbar enlargement is opposite to the second sacral root. And in all conditions of compression of the cord every possible variety of interference with the action of the organ may be observed as follows :— (α) In an early spastic stage there may be retention due to tonic spasm of the sphincter vesicæ. (β) In all forms of gradual compression there is diminished holding power of the sphincter ; as the paresis increases this becomes a complete loss of control, and then the flow is incessant or occurs at brief intervals.   As an intermediate grade what is called the overflow condition is sometimes observed.

(c) *Secretory glands.*—A clinical condition, comparatively speaking overlooked, and yet one of considerable value for the purposes of diagnosis, is the condition of the secretory glands and notably of the sweat glands in the skin of the paralysed parts, which are found, in an early stage, to exhibit paralytic hypersecretion ; in the later stage there is failure of the normal function.

(a) Sweat glands.—Strauss employed pilocarpine in facial paralysis to test the loss of function of the secretory fibres of the seventh nerve.   It occurred to me that this method could be employed to map out in like manner the area of skin below a compression lesion of the cord by comparing its condition with that of the skin above the lesion, and thus obtaining a line of demarcation.   In the majority of cases the injection of a quarter of a grain of pilocarpine will produce a sharp contrast between the two areas, the line of junction being marked by a line of drops of sweat.   With such a test, of course, care must be taken that there is no tendency to bronchorrhœa, a matter of special importance in cases of fracture in the cervical and cervico-dorsal regions when the intercostal muscles may be thrown out of gear.

(β) Other glands (kidneys, mucous glands, etc.)—The secretory activity of the kidneys may be diminished by lesion in the lumbo-sacral region (see topographical table, p. 859), and this diminution aids in estimating the degree of loss of function and injury due to the lesion. Similarly the mucous glands of the bowel sometimes exhibit hypersecretory activity.

Trophic changes.—This is not the place to enter into a discussion of the mechanism by which trophoneuroses are set up (p. 574), but it is necessary to recite shortly what alterations are produced by compression of the cord.   In the first place, there is the great difference between the trophoneuroses produced by an extra-medullary or intra-medullary lesion, or by a very circumscribed, or by a general lesion, respectively. For example, a restricted extra-medullary lesion will hardly cause bedsore, and will lead but very gradually to inflammatory conditions in the skin where it is pressed upon, and most likely in proportion as the lesion invades the functional activity of the cord.   It is quite otherwise in an intra-medullary lesion, or in a very extensive extra-medullary compression of a large portion of the cord; in such instances, unless the nurse be vigilant, bedsores are rapidly formed ; the skin, after being reddened for perhaps two or three days, becomes œdematous, and soon the centre of the red œdematous area is found to be necrotic, and an eschar is formed, the depth of which may reach to the nearest bony surface.   Such trophic changes are not confined to the parts pressed upon as the patient lies on the bed—for instance to the sacral region, or the heels, but may occur wherever the skin surfaces are in contact.

Relief of the pressure on the cord by laminectomy always stops this kind of mischief, and brings about the healing of it. Unless the mechanical pressure be re-established there is no relapse. It is plain, therefore, that wherever these trophic lesions are pronounced active and serious pressure may be inferred. In long-standing cases of severe compression-para-plegia the skin of the paralysed parts becomes harder, the epithelium tends to desquamate, and, as there is little or no normal secretion from the sweat or sebaceous glands, the surface is harsh and dry. There . is seldom any glossy skin such as is seen in disease or injury of the peripheral nerves.

Site of the lesion.—The very important problem of the precise seat of the mischief in the cord must be considered under the following headings: (i.) Determination of the level of the lesion in the cord. (ii.) Determination of the corresponding point on the exterior of the body. (iii.) Determination of the nature of the lesion. Of these headings the last rests entirely on the facts of pathology, to works on which subject reference is made; there remain, therefore, for notice Nos. (i.) and (ii.)

(i.) *Determination of the level of the lesion in the cord.*—The site of a lesion in the cord must be determined by observing the disturbance it effects in the functions of the following parts: (*a*) of the conducting channels from encephalon to nerve roots; and reversely (*b*) of the nerve centres.

(*a* 1) Conducting motor channels.—The exact seat of a complete transverse lesion of the cord can be estimated by observation of the highest of the muscles, innervated from points below the lesion, that are visibly thrown into action by voluntary effort. Unfortunately, whereas this is easy of analysis when the muscles in question are those of the limbs, it is difficult to be sure when an intercostal muscle or a single segment of the rectus abdominis or erector spinæ is concerned; here in a great measure the whole mass seems to move, although only certain portions are really in action.

The seat of an incomplete lesion must be ascertained by reference to the table, wherein the local innervation of the respective muscles and groups of muscles which are paralysed can be ascertained.

(*a* 2) The conducting sensory channels.—As in the case of interference with the outgoing channels of conduction from the encephalon, so the lowest possible border of æsthesia that can be marked is taken as the chief means of determining the segment involved; but here we have to discriminate carefully between the precise edge of the area of absolute loss of sensation, from pressure on the conducting channels, from the zone of paræsthesia, or often of hyperæsthesia, due to the local implication of nerve roots immediately above the anæsthetic area (*vide infra*). The topographical outline of the various nerve root-zone areas are shown in the accompanying diagrams taken from Dr. Head's work *On the Disturbances of Sensation of the Skin*, 1898 (German edition), a scheme which certainly seems to be more in accordance with clinical facts than

the other well-known schemes that have been published. They are to
be similarly applied in determining the position of incomplete lesions.

The foregoing applies to the tactile sense and to the temperature
sense, which channels run partly in the posterior and lateral columns of
the cord, and in the gray matter, the two latter including the internuncial and collateral fibres.

To the channels mentioned above must be added the direct cerebellar
tract and the antero-lateral tract, which probably subserve equilibrial
and "muscular sense" functions.

(a 3) The channels for conduction of pain.—The existence of analgesia produced by compression of the channels of conduction of painful
impressions is a most important symptom; because, since the original
experimental discoveries of Schiff and the subsequent clinical researches
into the pathology of syringomyelia, there seems to be little doubt but
that the channels for the transmission of painful impressions lie
in the gray matter of the cord near the central canal. Consequently
the presence of analgesia signifies, as a rule, the existence of a lesion
(that is, myelitic or hæmorrhagic), greatly affecting the viability and
recuperability of the central mass of the spinal cord. As regards exact
localisation, since these channels are internuncial in character, it follows
that, excepting where a complete transverse lesion of the cord occurs,
the determination of the border of analgesia will always be less definite
than that of the areas of other affections of the senses.

(b) Nerve centres.—Of course discrimination must be made in every
case between the amount of failure due to the disorganisation of a centre
and that caused by interruption of a channel of connection with the
encephalon. Systematic localisation of a lesion causing disorder of the
various central mechanisms of the cord may be arranged advantageously
by exploring the following functions in the order given:—Systemic
muscles; motion. Systemic surfaces; sensation. Sensation. Reflexes;
superficial, deep. Orbital, that is, intraocular, movements. Cardiac
movements. Respiratory movements. Vaso-motor movements; constriction, dilatation. Innervation of the alimentary and renal viscera.
Innervation of the secretory glands.

Trophic changes.—The details must be worked out by the table.

(ii.) *The determination of the corresponding point on the exterior of the body.*—
The correspondence between definite points in the cord and the bony
prominences of the spine and surface markings is stated on the table;
but there are a few points worthy of mention.

Thus the fixing of the vertebral prominences is sometimes difficult;
but the spot can be made out in a stout subject as the first spine felt on
drawing the finger firmly down the ligamentum nuchæ.

In a thin person, where confusion may arise from the number of
palpable spines, the 7th cervical can be distinguished, as a single knob,
from the bifid 6th cervical.

The 3rd cervical arch is commonly quite concealed under the
laminæ of the 2nd vertebra.

EXPLANATION OF PLATES III., IV.

Plates III., IV. show the division of the segmental areas from the 3rd cervical to the 4th sacral zone. The form and dimensions of each area (which is drawn here) are derived from :—

1. The relative appearance of the tender skin in visceral disease.
2. The division of the eruptions in sixty-two cases of herpes zoster.
3. The limits of the analgesia (or loss of pain) in organic diseases of the spinal marrow and spinal roots.

C 3 = Sterno-mastoid or 3rd cervical area.
C 4 = Sterno-nuchal or 4th cervical area.

Here follows a blank which is not generally represented in visceral diseases. The same corresponds with 5th, 6th, 7th, and 8th cervical segment.

D 1 = Dorso-ulnar or 1st dorsal area.
D 2 = Dorso-brachial or 2nd dorsal area.
D 3 = Scapulo-brachial or 3rd dorsal area.
D 4 = Dorso-axillary or 4th dorsal area.
D 5 = Scapulo-axillary or 5th dorsal area.
D 6 = Sub-scapulo inframammary or 6th dorsal area.
D 7 = Sub-scapulo ensiform or 7th dorsal area.
D 8 = Middle epigastric or 8th dorsal area.
D 9 = Supra-umbilical or 9th dorsal area.
D 10 = Sub-umbilical or 10th dorsal area.
D 11 = Sacro-iliac or 11th dorsal area.
D 12 = Sacro-inguinal or 12th dorsal area.
L 1 = Sacro-femoral or 1st lumbar area.
L 2 = Gluteo-crural or 2nd lumbar area.

Then follows a second blank, which is not primarily represented in visceral diseases. It corresponds to the 3rd and 4th lumbar segment area.

L 5 = Fibulo-dorsal or 5th lumbar area.
S 1 = Sole or 1st sacral area.
S 2 = Sciatic or 2nd sacral area.
S 3 = Gluteo-pudendal or 3rd sacral area.
S 4 = Coccygeal or 4th sacral area.

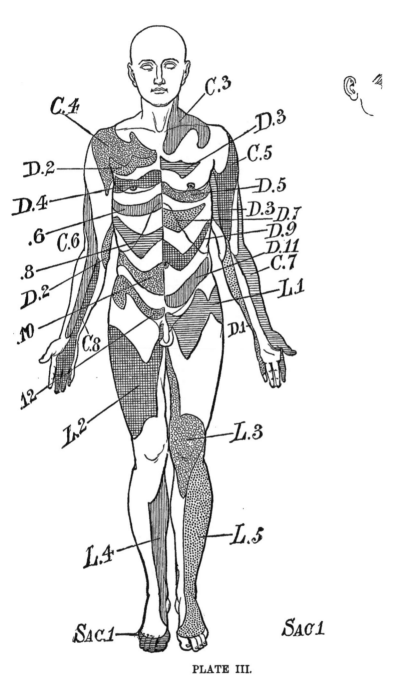

C.3

C.4

D.3

C.5

D.2

D.5

D.4

D.3 D.7

.6   C.6

D.9

D.11

.8

C.7

D.2

L.1

.10

D.1

C.8

.12

L.2

L.3

L.4

L.5

SAC.1

SAC1

PLATE III.

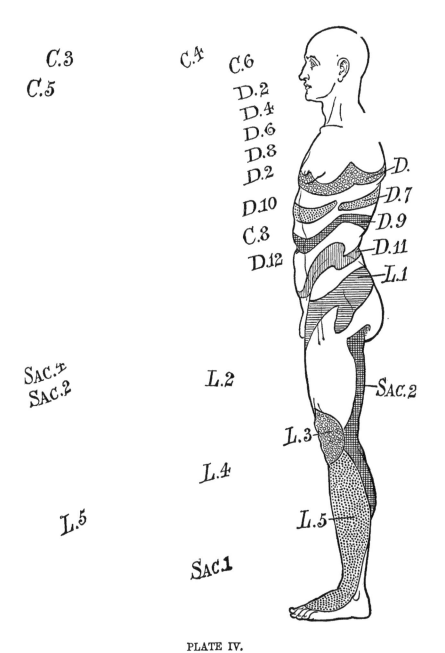

C.3 C.4 C.6

C.5   D.2

    D.4

    D.6

    D.8

    D.2   D.

        D.7

    D.10   D.9

    C.8   D.11

    D.12   L.1

SAC.4

SAC.2   L.2   SAC.2

       L.3

      L.4

L.5   L.5

    SAC.1

PLATE IV.

The 12th dorsal can often be made out more correctly by tracing up the last rib to the spine than by counting down from the 1st dorsal.

The 3rd 'lumbar can be estimated correctly by drawing a horizontal line at the level of the iliac crests.

Treatment.—*Treatment of caries of the spine.*—Caries of the spine is a very different disease in the young child, in persons of early adult age, and in those of advanced age, respectively. It may safely be said that in the first case adequate rest and extension will, in the majority of instances, cure the disease; that in the last class the condition is an exceedingly intractable one whatever is done; and in the middle group that the most active steps are necessary to obtain a satisfactory result. The next point to be determined in any given case is the presence or absence of an abscess,—to determine, in short, whether the compression of the spinal cord be due to the bony deformity, or to the pressure of an abscess sac. In the latter condition operation becomes an immediate necessity, whereas in the former it should be resorted to after other measures have failed.

The diagnosis of the presence of an abscess, simple enough when the seat of mischief is the lamina of a vertebra, is by no means easy when the disease is in its common position, that is, in the bodies of the vertebræ. We shall note that, as stated above, the coexistence of pyrexia (often very slight), with increased spasticity and contracture of the paralysed limbs, forms the best foundation for the suspicion of an abscess. When the abscess has been exposed by laminectomy it must be opened by the side of the theca, thoroughly scraped out with a sharp spoon, disinfected with strong 1 in 500 perchloride solution, and the cavity drained and dressed assiduously, so as to obtain obliteration of the sac. In this connection the difficulty of determining when the compression in the spinal cord is thoroughly relieved must again be called to mind; for in some instances it is necessary to repeat the scraping out and disinfection several times before the tuberculous mischief is arrested and restoration of the cord established.

To adopt a rough general rule for the influence of age the following is justifiable:—Any case seen at its very beginning should be treated by extension of the spine, with a modification of the apparatus in which the head and arm-pits are fixed by suitable straps and bands to elastic accumulators, the other ends of which are attached to the wall; and then counter-extension, of a similar kind, is to be provided by laced-up anklets to which rubber accumulators, fastened to the end of the bed, can be attached. The duration of such extension varies, of course, according to the signs of improvement, which ought to begin to show itself within two months. If in the young adult a favourable change is not noted at the end of this period a laminectomy should be performed. In persons of advanced age operation affords the only possible assistance. It is rare that in the young adult any treatment is very serviceable, unless it be laminectomy in an early stage of the disease. A certain proportion of cases, however, which bear extension well, can be cured by such treatment.

In strong contrast with such cases are those of persons suffering from senile tuberculosis, in whom the disease tends to progress rapidly, and to attack, not the bones only, but also the theca ; leading to a very definite myelitic softening of the cord. If, then, the patient's condition renders it possible a complete laminectomy ought to be performed.

In connection with this general subject of treatment of caries producing compression of the spinal cord, attention must be paid to other points than those which have been referred to under the heading of motor and sensory paralysis ; these are body weight, and condition of the paretic parts (for example, swollen or red suggesting vaso-motor paralysis). If there be any such symptoms the inference follows that the spinal cord is already beyond the possibility of amelioration, and in a condition of diffuse myelitis.

Treatment of deformity of the spine due to caries.—Recently the old and somewhat barbarous treatment of the kyphosis due to caries by immediate reduction has been revived, and often improperly regarded as treatment of caries. It is very questionable whether any mechanical advantage accrues to the patient from straightening out the curve.

On the treatment of new growths compressing the spinal cord.—Intra-dural and extra-medullary.—As soon as a local lesion is diagnosed, and the assumption that it is a neoplasm sufficiently justified, then laminectomy should be performed, care being taken that the part of the cord exposed corresponds with the highest nerve root whose function can be found in any degree altered, even in the slightest. When the tumour is shelled out the bleeding is to be stopped ; this can be easily done with a little gentle pressure, or by taking up any obstinately oozing vessel with a very fine needle and horse-hair ligature.

Intra-medullary.—These are sometimes met with in cases where an exploratory operation has been performed, cases in which it was not possible to diagnose the seat of the growth correctly ; but, as a rule, it is very difficult to detect their presence in the intact cord. Further, it is impossible in the present state of surgery to remove them without injury to the remainder of the cord.

Extra-dural.—In cases of extra-dural sarcoma of the spine operative interference to preserve life is, of course, useless ; but it may be undertaken, if necessary, to relieve extreme pain, which can easily be done as the latter is produced purely mechanically. Cases of primary sarcoma considered inoperable may with advantage be treated with injection of Coley's fluid, and local necrosis thus induced, with consequent relief of the pressure.

Treatment of traumatism.—(*a*) Immediate reduction.—A moderate degree of fracture dislocation of the spine, with consequent compression of the cord, has in some cases been treated fairly successfully by immediate reduction under an anæsthetic, and fixation of the spine with suitable plaster of Paris or other apparatus.

(*b*) Operative treatment.—In the majority of cases fracture dislocation of the spine produces such severe compression of the cord as to make the symptoms during the first few days very urgent, and the condition of the patient a perilous one. In this condition of affairs it is better to postpone any active interference for a few days until the immediate effect of the shock has passed off, and then to do a laminectomy. The object of the operation is not so much to deal with blood extravasated into the neural canal, which, as stated before, is rarely present in such quantity as to cause compression symptoms, but to remove fractured laminæ, or projecting portions of the vertebral bodies, or, not infrequently, invertebral discs, which are the most frequent means of compression. Contusion of the cord, with resulting hæmatomyelia, cannot be satisfactorily dealt with, as the extravasation is diffused through the substance of the cord (art. "Hæmatomyelia," in the next volume).

V. A. H. HORSLEY.

AFFECTIONS OF THE SPINAL MENINGES

THE most important morbid conditions of the spinal meninges are the following :—

I. Vascular disturbances :—1. Hyperæmia. 2. Hæmorrhage.

II. Inflammations :—1. External pachymeningitis. 2. Internal (hæmorrhagic) pachymeningitis. 3. Cervical hypertrophic pachymeningitis. 4. Syphilitic meningo-myelitis. 5. Leptomeningitis : (*a*) Acute simple ; (*b*) Cerebro-spinal ; (*c*) Tuberculous ; (*d*) Chronic leptomeningitis.

III. Tumours of the meninges.

Besides these conditions there are certain morbid states which are only of interest from the pathologist's point of view, and concern us but little, as they give rise to no clinical manifestations by which they can be recognised, or which call for treatment.

IV. Calcification of the dura and arachnoid.

V. Pigmentation of the arachnoid.

VI. Hydrorrhachis.

VII. Varicosity of the veins of the pia mater.

I. VASCULAR DISTURBANCES.—1. **Hyperæmia of the spinal meninges.** —It is common on necropsy to find hyperæmia of the spinal meninges, the vessels being so engorged as to suggest a pathological process. This, however, is not the true explanation in the majority of instances in which there had been no symptoms during the patient's lifetime to suggest such a process. As a rule, the cadaver is placed on its back, so that gravity determines the flow of blood into the dependent vessels of the spinal meninges, a state of things no doubt accentuated by the long time that many of these patients have been lying on their backs during a protracted illness which has ultimately proved fatal. In addition to the engorgement of the vessels there may be a diffuse redness consequent on decomposition of the blood, with diffusion of its colouring matter. It may be very difficult, therefore, to determine whether the hyperæmia has any other significance, even where the clinical manifestations had led us to expect changes of the kind; and to detect anæmia of the meninges, even if this had existed during life, may be impossible. Much error has resulted from attempts to formulate a group of symptoms by which hyperæmia manifests itself clinically, and by the supposition that the diagnosis has been borne out by the morbid changes met with after death; whereas in reality the changes to which so much importance has been attached have been none other than those occasioned by gravity and by decomposition.

Diseases attended by convulsions during life show distinct hyperæmia of the spinal meninges after death, as a consequence of disturbance of the respiration and circulation. Notably is this the case in tetanus, eclampsia, dentition convulsions, and chorea. Similarly, poisons which give rise to convulsions or asphyxia, such as strychnia, prussic acid, and carbonic oxide, are attended with a like result.

In the early stage of a meningitis, if death have resulted before the stage of exudation, we may find no more than an intense congestion of the meninges, which are of a rosy hue, the vessels being dilated and engorged; and, what is of great importance in establishing the pathological significance of the changes, the presence of minute hæmorrhages, which may often be detected, if carefully looked for.

Whether hyperæmia of the meninges may exist apart from the above conditions is a difficult question to decide. Those who hold that such is the case assign as its causes, accidents and other conditions attended with pain in the back and lower extremities, tremors, and weakness, amounting, it may be, to actual paralysis; to these spasm may be added. So, too, suppression of the menses or of a hæmorrhoidal flux, chronic uterine and abdominal diseases, and pregnancy have been held responsible for the condition.

Prominent among those who have upheld the view that congestion of the spinal meninges is a definite process are Frank and Ollivier. The clinical picture of the condition, as represented by the latter observer, resembles the course of a Landry's paralysis; for the onset is attended with weakness of the lower extremities, the loss of power spreads upward until the upper part of the trunk is reached, and it is accompanied by painful subjective sensations of pins and needles, and the like. There is then a stationary period during which the pulse and respirations remain slowed, and the paralysis incomplete; and this may be followed by complete disappearance of all symptoms in the reverse order to that of their advance. He includes cases of suppression of the menses, chills, abdominal affections, and so forth—in which there is pain in the spine radiating to other parts and accompanied by incomplete paralysis. The variations and irregularity of the course, together with the rapid recovery in some of the cases, are explained by the variations in the amount of blood contained by the meninges. Ollivier further adduces, in support of his contention, that on necropsy in these cases hyperæmia of the spinal meninges is found, while the spinal cord itself is intact.

Plausible and even justifiable as these arguments may seem, we shall hesitate to attribute cases in which the symptoms are at all severe to a mere congestion of the spinal meninges ; and cases in which such symptoms exist during life, and in which, nevertheless, congestion of the meninges alone is found after death, without any evidence of implication of the spinal cord itself, appear to belong rather to the category of spinal cord affections in which toxic influences disturb nerve function, and perhaps arrest it, without producing lesions capable of detection by methods hitherto in use. We know of no group of symptoms indicative of congestion of the spinal meninges to the exclusion of any other affection. Nevertheless, when we meet with pain in the back, radiating it may be to the lower extremities, which are weak, in association with suppression of the menses or of a hæmorrhoidal flux, it is not unreasonable to assume that the symptoms may be due to congestion of the spinal meninges. Similarly, when we know that backward pressure in the circulation exists, and we meet with pain in the back, and subjective sensations and weakness in the lower extremities, a like assumption seems warranted. So too in the course of fevers, when pain in the back and weakness of the lower extremities are present, as is especially apt to occur in variola and enteric fever, congestion of the spinal meninges serves as a reasonable explanation ; whether alone, or in conjunction with the effects of the action of a toxin on the nerve elements, must remain for future research to determine.

When variations in the intensity of the symptoms are rapid and transitory, it is reasonable to assume that they may be due to hyperæmia ; and, according to Brown-Séquard, the most certain sign of congestion of the spinal meninges is a greater paresis in the morning than in the evening in patients who are up during the day, an increase due to increase of the congestion consequent on the recumbent position during the night.

2. **Hæmorrhage into the spinal meninges.** — (Hæmatorrhachis ; Meningeal apoplexy.)—In this condition blood is found extravasated either between the dura mater and bone of the walls of the neural canal (extrameningeal hæmorrhage), or within the dura mater (intra-meningeal hæmorrhage). In the latter case the blood either exists in the arachnoid cavity between the dura and arachnoid (subdural hæmorrhage), or between the arachnoid and pia mater (subarachnoid hæmorrhage).

Causation. — (i.) *Extra-meningeal hæmorrhage.*—This is the most common form, and is usually the result of some trauma in which the spinal column is injured, and in which the dura mater participates ; or in which there is simply shock. The blood is derived from the rich plexus of veins which surrounds the dura. Another cause of extravasation of blood in this situation is the rupture of an aneurysm into the spinal canal; and in operations on the spinal column blood-clot may, of course, be found lying on the dura. So too, in diseases like tetanus, when the patient dies during the spasms, blood may be found outside the dura mater. Indeed any of the conditions under provocative spinal congestion may be attended by such hæmorrhages; among these may be mentioned more especially various intoxications, eclampsia, trismus neonatorum, dentition spasms, and the like. In diseases of the heart or lungs, in which there is backward pressure in the portal system, hæmorrhages may also occur. In many of these conditions it is probable that the blood was only extravasated during the last hours of life, or actually in the agony.

I have recently met with an instance in which a considerable amount of fresh clot existed outside the dura, in the lower cervical and upper thoracic regions, in connection with a purulent external meningitis, evidently of septic origin.

(ii.) *Intra-meningeal hæmorrhage* is almost as common as the extra-dural variety. In these cases the blood may be either derived locally from rupture of veins in this situation, or it may find its way into the arachnoid sac from elsewhere, usually from the intracranial cavity. When of local origin, the cause may be an injury which has resulted in fracture of the spinal column, with tearing of the dura, or rupture of the vessels of the pia, with or without laceration of the spinal cord. It is well to remember, however, that, without fracture of the spine, blows on the back or falls on the buttock or feet may give rise to meningeal hæmorrhage. Spontaneous non-traumatic hæmorrhage is very rare and its mode of origin uncertain; probably some of the cases are due to strain: but whether any are to be accounted for by arrested menstrual or hæmorrhoidal flux is doubtful. This accident may happen to children at the time of birth, either when forceps are used to aid delivery, or, more commonly, in cases of extraction by the feet, when there is separation of a vertebra at the epiphysial line with rupture of the anterior vertebral ligament. Ruge met with this condition in eight out of sixty-four cases of the latter mode of delivery. But spinal meningeal hæmorrhage may occur apart from luxation of the spinal column; Litzmann found such hæmorrhage in thirty-three cases out of eighty-one in which the spinal canal was opened in autopsies on new-born children; but, as has already been said, in twenty-three of these cases the blood was wholly extra-dural.

In operations on the spinal cord, or on the nerve roots, necessitating opening of the dura mater, blood may be found extravasated in this situation.

As in the case of extra-meningeal hæmorrhage, so here the hæmorrhage may be met with in cases of death from convulsive affections, such as tetanus, puerperal eclampsia, epilepsy, or strychnia poisoning.

In the infective fevers small hæmorrhages are not uncommonly met with : this is notably the case in hæmorrhagic small-pox ; so again in diseases where there is a general tendency to hæmorrhages,—such as scurvy, or morbus maculosus, such small hæmorrhages occur ; they may be plentiful in meningitis when death results before the stage of pus formation is reached ; or a large collection of blood may be met with in association with purulent meningitis.

But, as aforesaid, instead of originating locally, the blood may find its way into the neural canal from elsewhere ; the largest of such hæmorrhages result from rupture of an aneurysm of the basilar or vertebral artery at the base of the brain.   In operations on the posterior fossa of the skull, necessitating opening of the dura mater, blood may escape into the spinal meninges, as I have seen both in man and experimentally ; but the amount is never sufficient to be of any serious moment.   So too a cerebral hæmorrhage which bursts into the lateral ventricles may find its way to the spinal meninges, instances of which I have also met with ; or the hæmorrhage may be derived from the base of the brain as the result of an injury.   In cerebral apoplexy of the new-born, the result of difficult labour, the blood may find its way into the spinal canal ; in the cases in which Litzmann found hæmorrhage in the spinal arachnoid cavity he found also hæmorrhage in the intracranial cavity, mostly meningeal blood extravasations.

Morbid anatomy.—It must be remembered that, owing to the usual position of the cadaver on the back, the veins outside the dura mater become greatly distended ; and when they are divided, as the neural canal is opened, a good deal of blood may escape.   A hæmorrhage of ante-mortem origin may thus be looked upon as merely of this accidental character ; but more commonly the error consists in regarding the post-mortem condition as of ante-mortem origin.

In the extra-dural variety of hæmorrhage the blood is usually clotted and not large in amount ; it is derived from the plexus of veins between the dura and bone, and the blood escapes into the loose cellular tissue in this situation.   Partly because the space between the dura and bone is larger dorsally than ventrally, and partly because of gravitation, the blood tends to remain more or less confined to the dorsal aspect ; but where the hæmorrhage is more extensive the blood-clot may be found extending along the nerves through the intervertebral foramina.   It is rare, however, to meet with an extravasation sufficiently large to give the dura a compressed or flattened appearance ; though the soaking of the membrane in blood may give rise to staining which is obvious on looking at its inner surface.

When the hæmorrhage is intra-meningeal it may be small in amount, or it may fill the greater part of the subdural sac ; when beneath the arachnoid it may, similarly, be limited to a few segments of the spinal cord, or it may extend throughout the greater part of the length of this structure.   In the subarachnoid variety the blood is usually derived from vessels of the pia mater ; and when thus local in origin the hæmorrhages are rarely large, but they may be so when the blood gravitates to the spinal from the cerebral meninges. The reverse of this may obtain, as in a case recorded by Leprestre, in which a spinal hæmorrhage into the arachnoid cavity not only reached the pons but also burst through the valve of Vieussens and reached the lateral ventricles of the brain. On the other hand, independent hæmorrhages may arise in the intracranial cavity and neural canal as the result of a common cause. The spinal fluid is frequently blood-stained, as Coluguo also observed in new-born children dead of asphyxia. When the hæmorrhage is subarachnoid in situation the spinal cord is especially liable to damage; and, apart from this, the various levels of the cord may be compressed in variable degrees.

Symptoms.—It is impossible to formulate any distinctive symptomatology for extra-dural hæmorrhages. Where they result from an injury it is not possible to distinguish the symptoms consequent on the hæmorrhage from those directly due to the injury; and it is exceedingly rare to meet with an extra-dural hæmorrhage large enough to produce symptoms of compression of the spinal cord. Such a result may, however, come about through rupture of an aortic aneurysm into the neural canal.

The smaller multiple hæmorrhages, whether extra- or intra-meningeal, as a rule give rise to no symptoms; and symptoms may be absent or ill-defined even where the intra-meningeal hæmorrhages are larger; or symptoms, if present, may be masked by those of the disease in the course of which the hæmorrhages had occurred. So also when intracranial hæmorrhage coexists with that into the spinal meninges the symptoms due to the former condition may completely overshadow those of the spinal affection; or death may approach so rapidly that the spinal symptoms have not time to appear.

When symptoms of meningeal hæmorrhage do exist they are almost the same in extra-meningeal and intra-meningeal cases; and, in the absence of any serious concomitant lesion of the spinal cord, irritative phenomena preponderate over the paralytic.

Pain.—Sudden and severe pain in the back is usually the first, and is certainly one of the most frequent signs of the condition; its position corresponds to that of the hæmorrhage, and, as the cervical region of the cord is most commonly the seat of such extravasations, it is frequently felt between the shoulders and in the neck; but it may also be spread out over the greater part of the length of the spinal column, and is often severe in the loins. This pain is not increased by pressure on the spinous processes of the vertebræ, although it is made worse by movement of the patient, such as turning round and sitting up.

In addition to the pain in the back there are usually paroxysmal attacks of lancinating pain along the course of the nerve roots which pass through the meninges at the seat of extravasation, and are irritated by the clotted blood. These pains are generally very severe, and may be burning or darting in character, and accompanied by various paræsthesiæ, such as feelings like pins and needles, tingling and the like, referred to the parts affected by the pain, and felt in the intervals between the paroxysms. The distribution of these sensory phenomena depends on the seat of the hæmorrhage : when in the cervical region they are referred to the neck and upper extremities ; when in the thoracic region girdle pain appears ; and when the meninges of the lower part of the cord are affected the lower limbs are the seat of these abnormal sensations.

Hyperæsthesia and Hyperalgesia.—Pressure on the skin, or muscles, causes a varying degree of discomfort, which may amount to actual pain ; this is most common in the lower extremities. Erections may be attended with pain ; as may the passage of urine and fæces.

Anæsthesia may exist over a wide area in association with hyperæsthesia, but it subsequently becomes much more restricted. Such residual anæsthesia is especially prone to involve the perineum, the genital organs, the bladder, and the rectum.

Muscular spasms.—This may give rise to stiffness of the back ; a condition which may be due also to voluntary contraction of the back muscles to prevent the pain of movement. The spasms are probably reflex in origin, and may be so severe in the back as to cause opisthotonos. Rigidity and active jerkings are more frequently met with in the lower than in the upper limbs. Sometimes, however, the convulsive movements are general, while in other cases certain muscles are in persistent contraction.

Motor paralysis.—True loss of motor power, which is commonly met with in the lower limbs, must be distinguished carefully from abstention from movement on account of pain. It is not common for the loss of power to be complete, though it occurs in some cases. When power is lost at the onset it means either that the cord is compressed by a large extravasation of blood, such as may result from the rupture of an aneurysm, or that there has been hæmorrhage into the cord as well as into the meninges. When the cervical meninges are the seat of the hæmorrhage a diplegia brachialis may result.

Tendon jerks.—These are absent in the lower limbs at the onset, and remain so when the lesion is in the lumbar region ; but when the meninges of the thoracic cord are involved the tendon jerks may be preserved.

Sphincters.—Retention of urine is frequent ; incontinence also occurs, though more rarely.

Priapism is especially frequent at the outset, and is, of course, more common when the hæmorrhage is in the cervical region.

Such are the symptoms which indicate an affection of the spinal meninges which is interfering with the functions of the spinal cord, and of its afferent and efferent nerve roots. The precise grouping of the symptoms in a given case will, of course, depend on the seat of the lesion. Thus, when the meninges of the cervical region of the cord are affected, the pain and rigidity are in the neck and arms ; paretic symptoms may be present in the latter as well as in the legs ; respiration may be interfered with ; there may be difficulty of swallowing, and one or both

pupils may become dilated. Girdle pain, with a varying degree of paraplegia and, usually, with preservation of the reflexes, characterises a lesion
of the thoracic cord; while when the lumbar region is concerned the
pain is referred to the legs, in which signs of loss of motor power come
on early, with absence of the tendon jerks, and paralysis of the sphincters
allowing incontinence of urine and fæces. Cerebral symptoms are absent
as a rule; when present they are usually due to a simultaneous intracranial lesion, either independent of the spinal hæmorrhage, or giving
rise to escape of blood from the intracranial cavity into the neural canal.
Or again, a hæmorrhage, primarily spinal, may find its way into the
intracranial cavity, and thus give rise to cerebral symptoms. Apart
from this, however, consciousness may be lost for a short time, owing
probably to shock; and delirium and even coma have been observed.

In turning to consider the signs of hæmorrhage as opposed to any
other lesion of the spinal meninges, the sudden apoplectic mode of onset
is of primary importance. Not only is the onset sudden, but the
maximum effect of the lesion is rapidly reached—in two or three hours
as a rule; though sometimes a day or two may intervene. It must be
remembered, however, that in very exceptional cases this sudden onset
with rapidly increasing intensity of symptoms up to the maximum is
replaced by a gradual mode of onset in which there is no pain, and in
which paralytic phenomena are developed slowly.

When moreover there is a history of an injury capable of inducing
a meningeal apoplexy, the probability of hæmorrhage is of course
strengthened.

The course of these cases varies according to the amount of hæmorrhage, its seat, the degree of concomitant damage to the spinal cord, and
the presence or absence of complications, due on the one hand to a
simultaneous cerebral lesion, and on the other to secondary effects of the
spinal lesion, such as bedsores and cystitis.

The usual course, in favourable cases, after the maximum primary
effect of the lesion is reached, is a diminution of the symptoms for the
next few days, to be followed by an increase during the period of
inflammatory reaction. This exacerbation usually takes place between
the second and the fourth day. The amount of increase of symptoms at
this time and their duration vary; there may be some pyrexia, and death
may ensue; but more commonly, after lasting not more than a fortnight,
permanent improvement sets in, absorption of the blood-clot takes place,
and in the course of four to six weeks the symptoms may yield or
even disappear, provided that proper rest and therapeutic measures have
been enforced.

Yet such a favourable course may be interrupted by severe meningitis, by the occurrence of acute bedsores, or by cystitis. So too, where
there has been concomitant injury to the cord, the meningeal symptoms disappear only to leave the phenomena due to a lesion of the cord
more prominently in relief; whether that lesion be purely traumatic,
or aggravated by secondary myelitis. The most common indications of

the implication of the spinal cord itself are marked paralysis, especially of the sphincters, during the time that the meningeal symptoms are prominent, and the persistence of paralytic phenomena, accompanied it may be by muscular atrophy, after the more characteristically meningeal symptoms have passed off. But it is always a matter of great difficulty to ascertain how much of the clinical picture may be accounted for by the meningeal hæmorrhage alone, and how much ought rather to be attributed to concomitant injury of the cord; this question will be considered more in detail when we discuss the diagnosis of meningeal hæmorrhage.

Death occurs most commonly a few hours after the onset of the symptoms, and may be due to shock or exhaustion from the intense pain; on the other hand it may be due to respiratory difficulties consequent on the combined effects of paralysis and spasm; or blood may find its way into the intracranial cavity and thus cause death; or this result may be brought about by a simultaneous hæmorrhage in the intracranial cavity. Indeed, in the last contingency, the intracranial lesion may be so severe as to cause death before symptoms of the spinal lesion have had time to make themselves manifest.

Diagnosis.—The most important indications on which a diagnosis may be based are the sudden onset of symptoms; foremost among them being pain in the back, which may be so violent as to cause the patient to cry out, and the signs of meningeal or nerve root irritation predominating over any paralytic symptoms present. In the very exceptional cases in which onset of symptoms is gradual and without pain it is impossible to arrive at a certain diagnosis. When an injury precedes the sudden appearance of the above symptoms, diagnosis is made considerably easier in so far as the question of hæmorrhage is concerned; but not necessarily so as regards a discrimination between extravasation limited to the meninges and concomitant hæmatomyelia. Severe paralysis of motion and of the sphincters always indicates a simultaneous lesion of the spinal cord; moreover, such paralytic symptoms are present from the outset, and, even if not pronounced at first, rapidly become so. In uncomplicated meningeal hæmorrhage, on the other hand, irritative phenomena precede paresis. In attempting to distinguish an uncomplicated case of hæmatomyelia from one of hæmatorrhachis, we have to rely on the fact that in the former condition paralytic phenomena predominate over those due to irritation of the meninges and nerve roots. Pain in the spine is more commonly absent in hæmatomyelia than in meningeal hæmorrhage, and when present is more localised and does not tend to radiate. In patients who recover a residuum of paralysis is usually left; together with, it may be, some muscular atrophy, some affection of the sphincters, or other indication of structural damage to the spinal cord itself.

We have seen that meningitis may result as a secondary effect of a meningeal hæmorrhage; but, apart from this, the inflammatory affection may be distinguished from a spinal apoplexy by the gradual onset of the symptoms and the presence of pyrexia from the beginning. The absence of pain, and of signs of irritation of the meninges and nerve roots, together with the presence of well-marked paralytic phenomena, serve to distinguish a myelitis.

Prognosis.—In attempting to formulate a prognosis much depends on the exact time when the patient is seen and the probable seat of the hæmorrhage; extravasation in the cervical region being especially grave, owing to interference with respiration. Death may result at the onset, or soon after; but the prognosis improves when the maximum effects of the hæmorrhage seem to have been reached. But, the initial danger past, there are still grounds for fear until the inflammatory stage is over; after four to six days, however, without evidence of meningitis, the prognosis, so far as life is. concerned, becomes very good.

As regards recovery otherwise, meningeal apoplexy, in common with hæmorrhages in general, is relatively curable; but the degree of recovery to be expected largely depends on the effect upon the spinal cord. In the absence of much damage complete cure may result, and this with a degree of rapidity depending on the severity of the initial lesion, and on the contingency of bedsores or cystitis; or there may be some residuum in the form of paræsthesia, slight paralysis, weakness of the sphincters, or, perhaps, muscular atrophy; yet under proper treatment even these may be recovered from in the end. It is needless to say that the presence of a simultaneous lesion of the spinal cord very greatly reduces the chances of complete recovery.

Treatment.—Absolute rest and careful nursing are all-important in the treatment of meningeal hæmorrhage; and it is equally important to attend to the posture of the patient. Even passive movements are best avoided in these cases as much as possible; and the patient ought not to lie on his back, but should be carefully propped in position on one or other side by means of cushions or bolsters; moreover, a few hours should be spent in the prone position every day. Indeed, many such patients are unable to lie on their backs for the increase of pain which this posture occasions, and there can be little question that a supine . position may aggravate the damage. Furthermore, the head and upper part of the trunk ought not to be allowed to lie too high.

Some observers recommend venesection in robust subjects, with a view to lower blood-pressure, and thus to facilitate the arrest of hæmorrhage. When this procedure is not thought advisable, local blood-letting may be tried, by means of wet cupping or leeches applied over the supposed seat of hæmorrhage; or the leeches may be applied to the anus. In feeble persons, where even these measures are best avoided, dry cupping over the supposed seat of the hæmorrhage is sometimes tried. In any case ice should be applied to this part of the spine, and ergotine may be administered, by the mouth or subcutaneously. In order to relieve the violent pain, and to keep the patient as quiet as possible, morphine should be administered subcutaneously, or some other anodyne substituted. In the next place free action of the bowels must be secured.

Where there is reason to suppose that the spinal cord is being compressed by blood-clot, removal of the neural arches, to relieve the pressure, may be advisable. Such surgical treatment could be adopted with least risk of ill effects in cases in which the hæmorrhage is extra-dural; but, unfortunately, these are the very cases in which the operation is least likely to be called for, for it is rare to meet with compression symptoms from hæmorrhage in this situation. Yet even where there is reason to suppose that the hæmorrhage is intra-meningeal, surgical intervention is undoubtedly justified where life appears to be threatened by the effects of the compression; and even when this is not the case, but there is reason to suppose that irreparable damage is being done to the nerve elements, the operation deserves our careful consideration.

For the treatment of meningitis, bedsores, and cystitis the reader is referred to other portions of this work which deal specially with these subjects.

Any residual paralysis and sensory disturbances must be treated on the recognised lines by massage, electricity, baths, gymnastics, and so forth. Of drugs, the iodides are most serviceable in the earlier stages, while iron and strychnine are called for later.

II. INFLAMMATIONS.—1. **External spinal pachymeningitis.**—This condition is also designated "peripachymeningitis," or simply "peri-meningitis," either name agreeing well with the state of things present in these cases; for the inflammatory process takes place in the loose cellular tissue which surrounds the dura, and occupies the space between this membrane and the bony wall of the neural canal. As in the cervical region the cellular tissue is more scanty and closer, this form of perimeningitis rarely gives rise to any symptoms in connection with the meninges of this part of the cord; moreover, there is no tendency for the process to spread to the intracranial cavity. In the neural canal the process may be diffuse, affecting a considerable extent of the long axis of the canal; or it may be more circumscribed, and limited to a small part of it. The process goes on to pus formation, and occasionally is found associated with a purulent leptomeningitis.

Causation.—In the vast majority of instances in which this state of things is met with there is clear evidence that it is secondary in origin; indeed, it is very doubtful if the process is ever primary.

(*a*) Spinal caries is responsible for no mean proportion of the cases; abscesses originating in the bodies of the vertebræ make their way into the neural canal, or secondary inflammatory processes without pus occurring in the peridural cellular tissue find their way into this space directly from the bone. As a rule, this variety of perimeningitis is tuber-culous in character; and a caseous condition may be met with, a thick layer of this material occupying the space between the bone and the dura, to the outer surface of which membrane it is intimately adherent. Sometimes fibrous tissue proliferation is well marked, originating in granu-

lation tissue, and leading to the formation of thick masses. The leptomeninges may become affected secondarily.

(*b*) Inflammatory processes in the neighbourhood of the spinal canal,
such as psoas abscesses, angina Ludovici, and the like. Pus may make
its way into the neural canal by way of the intervertebral spaces, and
thus set up a meningitis.

(*c*) Bedsore.—Closely allied to the last mode of causation is the way
in which this external meningitis may arise as a consequence of deep bedsores which, extending down to the sacrum, may perforate into the lower
part of the neural canal; and, under rarer circumstances, may even lead
to a necrosis sufficiently extensive to lay bare the spinal cord.

(*d*) Trauma.—Contusion of the muscles of the lumbar region or loins,
hæmatoma of the back muscles, and, the like, have all been known to lead
to purulent perimeningitis.

(*e*) Metastatic.—I recently examined a case in which perimeningitis,
with pus formation and hæmorrhagic extravasation, existed in the lower
cervical and upper thoracic regions of the neural canal; it was associated
with other evidences of septic conditions in other parts of the body:
there was no bone disease or other local process to account for the
occurrence of the meningeal disease.

Symptoms.—As in all meningeal affections, pain in the back is a prominent symptom; but it varies a good deal in degree. It may be referred
to the greater part of the length of the spine, or it may be felt chiefly in
the loins, or between the shoulders. So too lancinating pains may occur,
and may be referred to the trunk or limbs, commonly giving rise to the
girdle sensation.

Stiffness of the back is another common complaint; but it may not
be so obvious as in many of the other affections of the meninges, as
the part in which it can be most readily recognised, namely, the cervical
region, is the very part of the neural canal which, as we have seen, is least
commonly affected. It is not common to meet with spasms in the
muscles of the limbs; they do occur, however, in some cases; yet
usually even then they are only brought out, in any notable degree,
on movement.

Motor paralysis may, of course, result from pressure on the spinal
cord, and, as it is so rare for the cervical region to be affected, paraplegia of the legs is the most common form of paralysis. We are, of
course, speaking of pressure on the spinal cord as a result of the perimeningitis, not resulting directly from a common cause of the perimeningitis, namely, spinal caries, which not infrequently affects the
cervical region, and may give rise to paralysis of all four limbs. It
is worthy of note that the paralytic phenomena dependent on a perimeningitis may precede the symptoms already described as so characteristic of meningeal affections.

In association with the other phenomena of irritation, hyperæsthesia
of the skin may be present, especially in the legs; but there may be
anæsthesia, corresponding in distribution with the paraplegia.

The sphincters may be affected ; the usual sequence of events being that retention of urine occurs first, and is followed by incontinence.

Diagnosis.—From what has been said with regard to the symptoms to which this condition gives rise, we can see how impossible it may be to distinguish this from any other form of meningitis ; even if we bear in mind that paralysis is common, and occurs early in this variety, and that spasm of the neck is usually absent. There are certain signs, however, which may lead to a correct diagnosis in such cases ; notably the discovery of any collection of pus in the neighbourhood of the spinal column, and again of any condition to which the affection is known to be secondary, such as spinal caries, angina Ludovici, a deep bedsore with, perhaps, necrosis of the sacrum, and so forth.

Prognosis.—As in many cases the diagnosis must of necessity be doubtful, it is difficult to estimate the proportion of them which terminate favourably ; for where recoveries occur there is no means of ascertaining whether the diagnosis had been correct or not ; and, even of cases ending fatally, the number of autopsies published are not sufficient to support any very definite conclusions.

Where the condition arises in association with spinal caries, the whole process may certainly become arrested, and even cured.

2. Internal hæmorrhagic pachymeningitis.—This condition, also known as hæmatoma of the spinal dura mater, is a rare one ; it is of the same nature as the hæmatoma which occurs in connection with the cranial dura, with which condition, indeed, it is commonly associated.

Causation.—If we except trauma, all the conditions which give rise to this form of pachymeningitis do so in conjunction with a similar affection of the cranial dura. This is the case in general paralysis of the insane, and chronic alcoholism. A third condition with which internal hæmorrhagic pachymeningitis may be associated is tuberculous meningitis, which, as we shall see, rarely exists apart from the same affection of the cerebral meninges.

Morbid anatomy.—The inner surface of the spinal dura is covered by a fibrinous-looking membrane, which is comparatively easily separated from it, and in which hæmorrhages of various sizes are seen. Parts of this membrane may be quite free from any extravasated blood, especially if the condition happen to be seen in its earliest stages. The extravasations are usually small, though large hæmatomata may occur. The blood may be encysted or undergoing transformation, when the false membrane with the contained blood presents various shades of brown, from red to yellow. In some cases the whole length of the spinal dura is affected in this way ; in others, the process is partial, and may be limited even to a small part of the caudal end of the cord. This form of pachymeningitis may be associated with the external variety.

Occasionally adhesions form between the dura and pia-arachnoid ; but, on the other hand, the pia may be hæmorrhagic in appearance only, from absorbed blood, or it may even be perfectly natural. The cerebro-spinal fluid is blood-stained to a variable extent.

Pathology.—For the different views that have been advanced concerning the primary nature of the morbid process, the particular membrane in which it originates, and the source from which the hæmorrhage is derived, the reader is referred to a later section on hæmatoma of the cerebral dura mater. I will only say that my opportunities of studying the condition lead me to conclude that Virchow's view— that the process is primarily inflammatory with secondary hæmorrhages into the newly-formed membrane—accords best with my experience. These observations also lead me to conclude that the primary seat of the affection is the dura mater, not the pia-arachnoid, as contended by Bondurant; and, moreover, that the source of the hæmorrhage, in the earlier stages at any rate, is the vessels of the dura mater.

Symptoms.—The symptoms are those of a subacute cerebro-spinal meningitis, as there is concomitant affection of the cerebral meninges; or the spinal symptoms may be quite overshadowed by the cerebral. When spinal symptoms can be detected they consist in pain in the back, pain radiating along the course of the nerve roots, stiffness of the vertebral column, spasms of the muscles of the trunk and limbs, and perhaps hyperæsthesia and other signs of irritation.

Diagnosis.—Where symptoms, such as those that have just been narrated, come on in the course of general paralysis of the insane, or of chronic alcoholism, especially if accompanied by others referable to a similar condition of the cerebral membrane, the diagnosis may be made with comparative confidence.

Treatment.—Measures such as have been recommended in the treatment of hæmorrhage into the spinal meninges are of service in these cases also.

3. Hypertrophic cervical meningitis.—It is very doubtful whether this affection deserves to be described separately, or whether it would not be more correct to regard the clinical picture as the result of a more or less accidental limitation of a morbid process to the meninges of the cervical region of the spinal cord, which process, if affecting any other region, would of course give rise to a different picture. Further, it becomes a question whether any morbid condition of the meninges of the cervical region of the cord, resulting in its compression and in interference with the nerve roots at this level, is not capable of producing a clinical picture indistinguishable from that which we have hitherto regarded as distinctive of hypertrophic cervical pachymeningitis, as represented to us chiefly in the writings of Charcot and of Joffroy. Nevertheless, as it has been customary to describe this condition separately, I propose thus to deal with it for the present; clearly recognising, however, that other morbid processes of the spinal meninges, similarly limited, are likewise capable of reproducing the clinical phenomena which are supposed to be characteristic of hypertrophic cervical pachymeningitis.

Causation.—There is considerable uncertainty as to the causes of this form of pachymeningitis; though it has usually been attributed to exposure to cold, to injury, or to over-exertion. There can be little question, however, that some of the cases owe their origin to syphilis; and to my mind this is one of the most potent arguments for regarding the condition as but a sub-group, for that syphilis may and does give rise to pachymeningitis of other regions of the spinal cord cannot be gainsaid.

Morbid anatomy.—The hypertrophic thickening of the dura mater, which may be as much as 0·5 cm., is consequent on the deposition of concentric layers of fibrous tissue, the result of inflammatory proliferation of the membrane. The greatest thickening usually occurs on the posterior aspect; and here the dura becomes adherent to the periosteum of the neural arches, and to the posterior vertebral ligament. The dura is also intimately united with the pia-arachnoid; so that it is quite impossible to separate the different membranes from each other. The thickened dura is sometimes very tough; and the appearance may suggest the formation of an outer and an inner layer. The walls of the vessels are thickened.

By the pressure the spinal cord is flattened dorso-ventrally; moreover, inflammatory and other changes are met with in its substance, especially at the periphery. Here there is a marginal sclerosis in which several factors are probably operative; foremost among them probably being the spread of inflammation from the meninges to the cord along the septa of the pia mater, and along the vessels; but direct pressure on the periphery of the cord—with consequent destruction of the marginal nerve elements, interference with the vascular supply by compression of the pial vessels, and hindrance to lymph flow by similar compression of the lymph channels, must be concomitant factors. A diffuse myelitis, thus initiated, extends for a varying distance into the substance of the cord, especially affecting the posterior and lateral columns, and leading to secondary ascending and descending degenerations. The process may, however, become more extensive, affecting the cord throughout its whole thickness, and giving rise to considerable sclerosis with consecutive atrophy. There is much to be said for Koppen's view that only the marginal changes in the spinal cord are to be attributed to the thickened membranes; and that the inflammatory changes in the cord may owe their origin to the action on the interstitial tissue of the same cause which induced the meningeal affection. This view appears to me to be specially applicable to those cases where syphilis seems surely responsible for the vascular and sclerotic changes in the meninges and in the cord itself. Other changes in the cord substance, met with in some instances, consist in softening, even to excavation. The nerve roots are compressed, and show degeneration of the nerve fibres, with proliferation of the interstitial tissue.

Symptoms.—The clinical course of the affection, in conformity with the teaching of Charcot, may be described in three stages.

Pain is the leading feature of the first period; it is exceedingly severe and is referred to the neck, spreading up even over the occipital region to the vertex, and also radiating downwards into the arms, in the larger joints of which it is often seated. Though present, as a rule, in some degree, it is prone to paroxysmal exacerbations, when the suffering may be intense. There may be a feeling of constriction in the upper part of the thorax, and various paræsthesiæ are common in the arms. Moreover herpes may appear in the distribution of some of the irritated nerve roots. Movements of the head and upper limbs increase the pain, while tenderness is provoked by any pressure or percussion on the cervical spines. There is rigidity of the cervical muscles, with stiffness of the neck, as in cervical caries; this condition being reflex in part, and in part the result of voluntary effort to prevent the increase of pain on movement. This period of the affection is thus marked by the phenomena of nerve root irritation; it usually lasts for two to three months. Apart from the rigidity of the muscles of the neck, and more or less perhaps of the arms, the motor functions are little interfered with during this stage; though a slight degree of weakness and some twitching of the muscles of the upper extremities may be noted.

The second stage is characterised by paralysis and atrophy of certain muscles of the upper limbs consequent on extension of the morbid process to the anterior nerve roots. The muscles supplied by the median and ulnar nerves are thus affected; those supplied by the radial either escape altogether, or are affected in slight degree only, or not until late in the course of the affection. The atrophy of the muscles becomes pronounced, and on electrical examination they show the reaction of degeneration. As the flexors are considerably affected, while the extensors escape, unopposed action of the latter results in hyperextension of the hand at the wrist, with extension of the first phalanges, and flexion of the second and third; this gives rise to a peculiar position of the hand which has been named the "preacher's hand": however, this position of the hand is neither constant in cases of hypertrophic cervical pachymeningitis, nor peculiar to it, as Charcot was himself aware. In addition to the loss of certain movements consequent on the affection of the groups of muscles already referred to, there is a varying degree of general enfeeblement of the arms from the shoulders downwards; sometimes it is no more than a general stiffness and clumsiness of execution, but at other times it amounts to complete paralysis of one or both limbs.

The severe pain of the first stage of the affection is much mitigated during the second period, though the paræsthesiæ usually persist and even increase. Anæsthesia, consequent on destruction of the sensory nerve roots, now appears, in a manner comparable to the muscular atrophy which results from destruction of the motor roots; and, as in the latter case, this does not pervade the skin of the whole arm, but only that corresponding to the distribution of certain roots. This sensory defect is a further factor which interferes with movement, more especially with the finer movements of the fingers; so that the picking up of small objects, for instance, is clumsy.

The third stage is characterised by phenomena consequent on compression of the spinal cord; by spastic paraplegia without muscular atrophy, but later by contracture; anæsthesia may become manifest on the legs and trunk, the functions of the bladder and rectum may be interfered with, and bedsore, if not prevented, may soon follow.

Pain, so prominent a feature of the first stage, usually disappears before the third stage is reached, when paralytic phenomena, as a rule, completely replace those due to irritation of the sensory nerve roots.

It remains to be said that while the above description forms the type of the affection many variations in its course are met with. I have said that the characteristic position of the hand may not be present; the patient may be spared the intense suffering caused by pain in the earlier stages; and affection of the lower limbs, bladder, and rectum may be met with quite early in the course of the malady.

The course of the disease always extends over several years, death usually resulting from the secondary consequences of cystitis, or from bedsore.

Diagnosis.—As the same symptom-complex may be anticipated in any chronic meningo-myelitic process of this part of the cervical cord, however induced, it follows that considerable difficulty may attend the diagnosis. The several affections with which the condition may be confounded depend on the stage at which the case is seen.

However much we may suspect that the pain of the earliest stage is consequent on irritation of the posterior roots by some organic process in the meninges, it may be impossible to exclude with certainty its dependence on an idiopathic neuralgia; or, again, where girdle sensation is well marked, it may be difficult to exclude tabes, and even more so to decide that, of all organic processes of the meninges possible in this region, that which we are now considering is the one present. It is the appearance of loss of motor power with muscular atrophy of root distribution which serves satisfactorily to answer the first of these questions; yet even then the second, concerning the nature of the morbid process, may be no nearer a satisfactory solution. Syphilitic meningo-myelitis, cervical caries, and tumours in the cervical region of the cord, may all result in paralysis with muscular atrophy, which has been preceded by pain and other phenomena indicative of irritation of sensory roots. Of these it may be possible to distinguish cervical caries alone by means of the angular curvature of the spine, which never occurs in the meningeal affection; by the presence, it may be, of tenderness greater in degree than is usual in pachymeningitis, evoked by pressure over a single vertebra, early in the course of the affection; and by the detection of tuberculous mischief in other organs. Yet all these signs may be absent, and the case may turn out to be one of caries after all.

As the symptoms produced by a pachymeningitis really depend on the meningo-myelitis, and as syphilis plays an important part in many cases of hypertrophic cervical pachymeningitis, it is obvious that even a syphilitic history does not help us to discriminate between this condition and syphilitic meningo-myelitis. A point in diagnosis, however, is that a

syphilitic affection of the meninges and cord is not wont to remain limited
to any one region; so that, while commonly affecting the cervical part
of the cord, it may show evidences nevertheless of invasion of other
levels, a state of things less likely to be met with in the pachymeningitis
of Charcot.

Where, as I have seen, new growth infiltrates the dura so as to produce a condition in all respects comparable with a hypertrophic pachymeningitis, symptoms of symmetrical implication of the nerve roots and
spinal cord make it quite impossible, in the absence of evidence of new
growth elsewhere in the body, to arrive at a correct diagnosis. Though
far from an infallible indication, symptoms of unilateral disease of nerve
roots and pressure on the spinal cord lend weight to the probability of
tumour, as opposed to pachymeningitis. The rate of progress may aid
us, for the course of a pachymeningitis is slower, as a rule, than that
of a tumour; but here, again, there are notable exceptions which rob
this indication of much of the value it would otherwise have.

Syringomyelia begins, as a rule, in the cervical region, and as it produces muscular atrophy and weakness of the upper limbs, with, it may
be, spastic phenomena in the lower, and as, moreover, pain may be a prominent feature in this disease, its exclusion in a differential diagnosis
may be attended with very great difficulty. In syringomyelia, while
tactile impressions are normally perceived, painful and thermic impressions are unfelt; this sign may, however, be absent in syringomyelia, and
it has been present in some cases of pachymeningitis. The presence
of painless whitlows and other trophic disturbances of the skin, and
the existence of lateral curvature, are points in favour of syringomyelia.
The course of the latter disease, again, is much more protracted, extending, as a rule, over a period of a great many years. As further
aids to the diagnosis of syringomyelia, careful inquiry should be made,
in the past history of the patient, for indifference to taking hold of
hot things; for burns that were not painful, for operations painless without an anæsthetic. Careful search should also be made for scars suggestive of former burns or operations.

Although the distribution of the muscular atrophy and weakness in
the arms could be explained equally well by a progressive muscular
atrophy, and while the added spastic phenomena in the lower limbs
suggest an amyotrophic lateral sclerosis, the complete absence of sensory
disturbances in these conditions, whether irritative or paralytic, serve to
exclude them. In any case the subsequent course of the case will settle
the question; for, whereas in progressive muscular atrophy and amyotrophic lateral sclerosis there may be a spread of the disease to the
medulla, giving rise to bulbar symptoms, this never occurs in hypertrophic cervical pachymeningitis.

In local neuritis the muscular and sensory defects correspond to
nerve and not to root distribution; moreover there is tenderness, and, it
may be, thickening of the nerve trunks, and an absence of pain and
stiffness in the neck. It may be difficult, however, in the absence of any

phenomena indicating pressure on the spinal cord, to exclude a neuritis of the cervical roots. In multiple neuritis a cause can usually be found in the shape of some toxic agent; notably alcohol, lead, or arsenic. Tenderness in the course of the nerves, and flaccid paralysis, in which the extensors suffer more than the flexors (the reverse of what obtains in hypertrophic pachymeningitis), with abolition of the tendon jerks both in the superior and inferior extremities, serve to distinguish these conditions; excepting in cases of lead neuritis, in which a certain degree of spasticity with exaltation of the tendon jerks may be present in the lower extremities. Concomitant evidence, in the shape of a history of lead intoxication, colic, the presence of the blue line along the gums, and the absence of any anæsthesia, serves to distinguish these cases.

Treatment. — Various measures may be tried for the relief of this disease; but, as a rule, some palliation is all we can expect. Counter-irritation to the spine is indicated; the milder forms of this, such as painting with iodine liniment, are of little use; the more energetic forms of counter-irritation are called for, such as repeated blisters, or Paquelin's or the actual cautery, which latter means is especially recommended by Joffroy.

In any case iodide of potassium should be given, and if there is any suspicion of syphilis, it may be advantageously combined with mercurial treatment. Where the evidence is in favour of syphilis a course of treatment by inunction, as recommended for syphilitic meningo-myelitis, should be carried out (see p. 899).

Warm baths and diaphoretic measures are of service; and for the wasting muscles massage and electrical treatment should be employed.

4. Syphilis of the spinal cord and its meninges.—In addition to secondary invasion of the spinal cord and its meninges by syphilitic affections of extra-spinal origin, such as gummatous periostitis with caries, the syphilitic poison is responsible for affections which are primarily intra-spinal in origin. To this class belong diffuse disease of the meninges, diffuse granulation tissue formation in the substance of the cord, circumscribed single or multiple gumma, affections of the vessels, and atrophy of the gray matter and of the nerve roots. Circumscribed tumour formations and multiple gumma in the spinal cord are much more rarely met with than the diffuse infiltrations of the meninges and cord. Such circumscribed gummata are in the meninges alone, or chiefly so; and compress the cord as any other tumour might do. The most common form of syphilitic affection is a meningo-myelitis; and the most prominent features are the affection of the meninges and the vessels to which the changes in the spinal cord are secondary; but it seems certain that a myelitic process may arise in the cord, secondary to vascular changes, without any concomitant affection of the spinal meninges. Moreover it is probable that such changes in the spinal cord may occur independently of syphilitic affection of the vessels. In 1892 Erb described a form of lateral sclerosis which he regards as a direct result of syphilitic infection. This subject will be considered under the head of Spastic Paralysis.

It is unusual for syphilitic affections of the nervous system to be limited to the spinal cord and its appendages; more frequently there is concomitant disease of the brain of a like character; though in some instances this gives rise to no definite signs, and is only recognised on the autopsy. In other cases, however, the cerebral symptoms may quite mask those of spinal origin. Parasyphilitic affections, such as tabes dorsalis and other indirect sequels of syphilis, do not, of course, come within the scope of this article.

Causation.—Though syphilis is the cause of the conditions of the spinal cord and its meninges which we are considering, other factors play an important part in the etiology of this form of affection. Cold, traumatic and other influences, which depress the nutrition of the nerve elements and render them less capable of resisting the action of toxic agents, favour the action of the syphilitic poison. On the other hand, a spinal cord, whose nutrition has been lowered by defect of blood-supply, consequent on syphilitic thickening of the coats of its vessels, is more prone to succumb to deleterious influences, such as cold and trauma. The modes of these influences, in the case of the spinal meninges, are much the same as in the cord.

Another important factor in the causation is the degree of thoroughness with which antisyphilitic treatment was carried out on the primary infection. In some cases there never was any such treatment; in others it was very imperfectly carried out. There does not appear, however, to be any proportion between the degree of severity of the previous manifestations of syphilis and the spinal cord affection; for in some cases the previous manifestations of the disease had been very severe, in others exceedingly slight. Probably, indeed, such previous attacks are often neglected on account of their mildness, and thus the virus is not neutralised.

These syphilitic affections are peculiarly prone to come on early. According to Oppenheim, most of them occur within the first six years from the time of the primary infection; and many observers are agreed that cases may be met with a year, or even six months, after infection. Whether there is a group of cases of which the morbid conditions belong to the secondary manifestations of syphilis, as opposed to those long recognised as tertiary manifestations, is an important question. The general blunting of sensibility which, according to Fournier, accompanies the exanthem stage of syphilis, does not concern us directly, as it probably depends on some influence on the peripheral nerves; it is rather the acute paraplegias coming on early in syphilis, and usually resulting in partial recovery, and certain cases of paresis of motion and sensation which may result in complete recovery, that we have here to consider. In opening a discussion on this subject at the Medical and Chirurgical Society, a few years ago, Mr. Jonathan Hutchinson brought forward evidence that such early manifestations of syphilis of the nervous system do occur; and that although most affections of the kind in the secondary period are the result of disease of the blood-vessels, there are other cases, including a form of paraplegia due to transverse myelitis, in which the lesion is the direct effect of the syphilitic poison on the nerve elements. He further expressed the belief that such early affections are invariably the result of neglect of treatment of the primary manifestations of syphilis. The general opinion seemed to be that such early affections of the nervous system do occur. That the clinical evidence of this opinion is strong, and that there is some pathological evidence in support of the contention also, there can be no question; but a great deal more post-mortem evidence is needed, more especially to determine whether such lesions are ever the result of a primary action of the syphilitic poison on the nerve elements, or whether they are always secondary to syphilitic disease of the blood-vessels. The known action of certain other toxins makes it possible that the syphilitic poison may act directly on the nerve elements; but pathological proof of this is still wanted. Two cases of acute paraplegia of this kind, which, by the kindness of Dr. Parkes Weber, I have had an opportunity of examining, have shown, besides signs of destruction of the nerve elements, round cell proliferation, thickening of the interstitial tissues, evidences of meningitis, with thickening of the vessels, well marked in one case and slight in the other. Moreover, in Lamy's case the nerve elements had escaped, and the chief changes were met with in connection with the perivascular spaces, especially those of the veins, some of which vessels were thrombosed and presented evidences of microscopic gummata. In a case mentioned by Dr. Mott, in the discussion already referred to, a diffuse small cell infiltration of the perivascular spaces was found; there was no sign of such a focal myelitis as the clinical phenomena suggested.

To the work of Gilles de la Tourette are we more especially indebted for a clear conception of the part that hereditary syphilis may play in the causation of lesions of the spinal cord. He divides such cases into three groups, according as the manifestations are produced during intra-uterine life, during infancy, or in the period of adolescence and later.

Morbid anatomy. — As a rule there are combined affections of the spinal meninges, cord, nerve roots, and vessels. The dura mater may show no signs of being affected, or it may be thickened to a variable extent.

Such thickening takes place especially on its inner surface, and the dura becomes intimately adherent to the pia-arachnoid over considerable areas, while it is free in other parts. The most pronounced changes are, however, to be seen in the thickening of the pia-arachnoid, which takes place throughout the greater extent of the spinal cord, though to a variable degree in different parts; in one part there may be scarcely any thickening, slight round cell infiltration alone being detected on microscopical examination, while in other parts the thickening is enormous. Between these two extremes we have all intermediate grades of intensity: the thickened membranes may be quite fibrous in consistence; on the other hand they may be quite soft, or have more of a thick gelatinous character. The thickened mass is richly infiltrated with round cells, and a marked feature in some cases is the abundance of blood-vessels.

In addition to these diffuse changes, single and multiple gummata occur in connection with the meninges, and, as in the case of other tumours, give rise to pressure on the spinal cord.

The vascular changes are naturally prominent features in the morbid anatomy of syphilitic affections of the nervous system. Various degrees of thickening of the walls of the arteries are met with up to complete obliteration of their lumen : this change takes place chiefly in the intima, constituting an endarteritis, or in the adventitia in the form of a periarteritis ; sometimes the one, sometimes the other coat of the vessel suffering the more, while the media is least affected. There has been considerable difference of opinion as to the primary seat of origin of the changes within the vessels (see p. 305).

The cell proliferation may be either diffuse or confined to certain parts of the circumference of the vessels ; but a true arteritis gummosa, in which circumscribed nodules are formed in the adventitia, is rare. The morbid process not only affects different vessels in different degrees, but also the same vessel is very differently affected in different parts of its course.

Apart from such primary affections the arteries may become involved in gummatous formations of the meninges, which lead secondarily to changes in them.

Thrombi may form in the vessels, and these in their turn may become vascularised.

Thickening of the walls of the veins by cell infiltration may occur, similar to that described in the arteries. Both Greiff and Siemerling have described such changes, and the former has shown that a phlebitis obliterans may occur.

Both the vessels of the meninges and those in the substance of the cord are affected ; according to some observers the latter is the result of extension of the morbid process along the vessels from the primary seat of their affection in the pia ; others, whose views commend themselves to me, regard the affection of the intra-medullary vessels as independent of that of the meninges, the only connection between the two being that they are both the result of the syphilitic poison.

A point of importance to which Siemerling has directed attention, is that the degree of alteration met with in the connective tissue does not at all necessarily correspond to the degree of affection of the vessels, for in one part the changes in the pia mater and spinal cord may predominate, while in another the change in the vessels is the marked feature.

Though the vessel changes form so important a part of these syphilitic affections of the spinal cord, it is not always possible to say with certainty, in any given case, that such changes are definitely syphilitic, as other conditions give rise to changes, both in arteries and veins, which are very similar to those met with in syphilis. The age of the patient is an important aid to diagnosis in such cases, for the younger the subject the more likely are such changes in the vessels to be syphilitic—the greatest degree of certainty being reached in the case of children with congenital syphilis.

The changes in the spinal cord consist in a round cell infiltration which results in increase of connective tissue rich in nuclei. Thickened wedge-shaped bands of pia mater penetrate for a variable depth into the substance of the cord—some being quite superficial, while others extend as deeply as the gray matter. Retrogressive changes may occur, as in true gummatous formations; while in some instances the change from the outset is a genuine gummatous proliferation in the substance of the spinal cord. Single and multiple gummata may originate in the spinal cord, but are much less common than the diffuse syphilitic changes. Apart from the breaking down of such gummatous formations, areas of softening occur which depend on the syphilitic arterial changes present; and hæmorrhages of various sizes are also met with in the substance of the cord.

The changes already described naturally lead to destruction of the nerve elements secondarily, notably of the nerve fibres, which are seen in all stages of degeneration up to complete destruction. According to the degree and extent of destruction of the white matter present, we meet with a correspondingly various degree of secondary ascending and descending degeneration. The gray matter may suffer, gummatous infiltration or hæmorrhages causing destruction of the ganglion cells,—an effect which also comes about occasionally as a result of softening consequent on the vascular changes. Further, it appears possible that the ganglion cells may suffer in a different way as the result of syphilis, for Mr. Jonathan Hutchinson has laid great stress on the importance of syphilis in the etiology of chronic ophthalmoplegia; and Sir William Gowers, who examined one of Mr. Hutchinson's cases, found atrophy of the cells of the ocular nuclei in every way identical with the atrophy met with in the ganglion cells of the ventral horns of the spinal cord in progressive muscular atrophy, an observation since abundantly confirmed. So too simple atrophy of the cells of the ocular nuclei in cerebro-spinal syphilis has been described by Oppenheim and Siemerling. Cases of atrophic paralysis have been published which had been regarded as syphilitic in origin, but the relationship to syphilis was not always clear; moreover, recovery prevented verification by autopsy. A case, published by Déjerine, some twenty-two years ago, showed atrophy and diminution of the number of ganglion cells of the ventral horns, the white matter being intact; but here again it is questionable what the previous attack of syphilis had to do with the changes in the gray matter.

Cases of central myelitis in syphilis have been recorded by Déjerine, Drummond, and Hayem; but it cannot be said that anything in the histological findings makes it certain that the lesions were syphilitic. The problem of Erb and Hayem is whether it is possible to get a myelitis the result of syphilis without the evidence of any specific characters.

In the presence of changes such as these in connection with the meninges, it will be readily understood that all degrees of implication of the anterior and posterior nerve roots may be met with. Where the changes in the pia-arachnoid are most pronounced, there, as a rule, the root affection is most severe. The nerve elements are destroyed by the pressure of the thickened membranes, and by cell infiltration and proliferation involving the peri- and endoneurium, extending along the vessels of the roots, and insinuating themselves between the nerve fibres. The roots are affected in an irregular manner, so that roots at various levels are affected, intermediate ones being intact, and often without any symmetry on the two sides; indeed, in one place a ventral, in another a dorsal root may be involved. It is surprising what a power of resistance is shown by the fibres of the nerve roots under such circumstances, so that, even where the root affection is most severe, a great many nerve fibres are quite intact, and are seen lying side by side with others that have been destroyed. Apart from the nerve fibres actually damaged by the local process in the roots, others of them degenerate secondarily as a result of interference with their trophic supply in the cord or dorsal root ganglia.

It seems probable that the multiple syphilitic root neuritis described by Kahler is a condition secondary to past spinal meningitis.

Symptoms.—After what has been said, it will be readily understood that the most varied clinical phenomena may be met with, including symptoms dependent on concomitant affection of structures within the cranial cavity. With the latter symptoms we are not now directly concerned, but since it is rare to meet with spinal syphilis without evidence of concomitant affection of the brain and its meninges, the symptoms of cerebral origin, when present, may give us great aid in diagnosis. They consist for the most part in headache, giddiness, vomiting, convulsions, optic atrophy or neuritis, inequality of pupils, loss of reflex action of the pupils, paralyses of ocular muscles, similar affection of other cranial nerves, especially the facial, hemiplegia which, when added to the paraplegia of spinal origin, makes up the clinical picture of a triplegia, aphasia, bulbar symptoms, dementia and the like. Polydipsia and polyuria have a similar significance in these cases.

The following description deals only with the manifestations which are of spinal origin :—

Sensory symptoms.—Pain may be the first, or at any rate one of the earliest symptoms, either in the form of girdle sensation or of shooting pains in the limbs. Occasionally there is pain in the back; and Charcot pointed out that often at the outset of a syphilitic meningo-myelitis this pain in the spinal column is troublesome at night, and is thus comparable to the night headache in cerebral syphilis. More often there is only a feeling of stiffness of the back without pain; and no tenderness is elicited on pressure along the spinal column. Paræsthesiæ, such as pins and needles or formications, occur in the extremities.

Hyperæsthesia may be present in the skin, and the muscles may be tender to pressure ; or may be painful on active or passive movement of the limbs. The more common objective defects of sensibility consist in a varying degree of abolition of tactile and painful sensibility ; the temperature sense being also affected occasionally. The temperature sense was affected alone in a case observed by Oppenheim, and remarkably in one recorded by Koppen. As. a rule the anæsthesia affects the legs and lower part of the trunk, though occasionally the arms are attacked also. The anæsthesia may be very patchy and irregular, and is often unsymmetrical ; sometimes it is limited to one side. Occasionally, though there is no distinct blunting of sensibility, there is distinct delay of conduction of sensory impulses.

The muscle sense may be affected, in which connection Romberg's sign may occasionally be met with, but usually only in slight degree.

Motor symptoms.—Most commonly there is a pronounced paresis of both legs ; but all variations may be met with from an exceedingly slight degree of weakness up to complete paraplegia. The lower limbs are much more commonly affected than the upper ; usually both lower limbs, though sometimes only one ; or while affecting both limbs the weakness may be much greater in one than in the other, or it may begin in one and subsequently involve the other also.

The onset of the paralysis may be either very slow or very rapid ; and even when gradual in onset there may at any time be a sudden exacerbation of it ; or it may progress by fits and starts. Feelings of weakness and stiffness in the legs may exist for a long time, and then paralysis of a much more pronounced character may suddenly set in. Every case of syphilitic affection of the spinal cord does not necessarily include motor weakness of the legs at the time of consultation, for this symptom may not arise until some later date.

In many cases the gait is only clumsy ; but it often presents characters due to a combination of weakness and spasticity ; and where only one leg is affected there is a tendency to drag it in walking.

As a rule more or less spasticity is combined with the paresis ; the muscles are more or less rigid ; and contracture sometimes exists. At times there is jerking of the limbs in association with greatly increased reflex irritability. In the later stages of the affection permanent contracture in the flexed position may result. But on the other hand there may be an absence of all spastic phenomena, the existing paralysis being quite flaccid. So, too, groups of muscles or individual muscles may present definite atrophy as a result of destruction of cells of the ventral horns, or inclusion of ventral roots in the lesion. Except where such atrophy exists the electrical reactions are normal ; but any atrophied muscles may, of course, show varying degrees of reaction of degeneration.

Reflexes.—There is nothing characteristic either in the superficial reflexes or the tendon jerks ; the former may be either active or abolished, and the same may be said of the latter. In most cases, however, the knee-jerks are exaggerated, and foot and rectus clonus may be present ; but a curious vacillation of the knee-jerks within wide limits is often observed.

Sphincters.—It is quite exceptional to meet with complete paralysis of the sphincters; even a slight defect is unusual. Retention is equally rare, so that cystitis and secondary kidney troubles are not to be feared. Constipation is generally troublesome. Loss of sexual power is occasionally met with.

Trophic disturbances.—These features are by no means prominent in the clinical picture. The occurrence of muscular atrophy has already been mentioned. Bedsores are not common, and are met with only in the most advanced stages of the disease.

Course.—These affections are usually slow, and, as aforesaid, it is characteristic of them that the symptoms advance by fits and starts, now an exacerbation, then a remission. An exacerbation may come on quite suddenly; or there may be a long period during which the patient steadily gets worse. Such periods of increase of the symptoms may be followed by intervals during which the disease appears to be stationary, or when actual improvement may occur. Most patients eventually improve; but anything like complete cure is only met with in very slight cases. Some cases run an acute course, with severe manifestations, including bedsore; but even in these, provided the disease be limited to the spinal cord, a fatal termination is exceptional.

Diagnosis.—With an entire absence of any evidence of concomitant affection of intracranial structures the diagnosis becomes extremely uncertain, as the manifestations are simply those of a meningo-myelitis with nothing distinctive of its syphilitic nature; if present the cerebral symptoms are all-important in diagnosis, even if, as sometimes happens, one or two signs only of their presence can be detected. These signs of intracranial syphilis are noted in another place (see special article in next volume). All that need be insisted on here is the importance of searching carefully for evidence of such manifestations, remembering that while in some cases many symptoms of concomitant intracranial mischief may be evident, in others only one or two may be present, and these perhaps in slight degree.

A history of previous syphilitic infection is naturally of great importance, but by no means decisive, for even with such a history the spinal cord affection need not necessarily be syphilitic; moreover, the absence of a history of the primary inoculation is far from precluding the possibility of its having occurred; nevertheless, where other facts make it probable that the affection is syphilitic in nature, a history of the primary infection is important.

The widespread distribution of the parts concerned, and the partial and irregular way in which they are affected, are very strongly in favour of a syphilitic origin. The patchy way in which sensation is affected, the unequal way in which motor power is lost on the two sides of the body, and so on, are all very characteristic. Of similar importance, from the point of view of diagnosis, is the prominence of meningitic and root symptoms in the clinical picture of the disease; more especially when these phenomena are considered in conjunction with other features which also suggest that the affection is syphilitic. Moreover, the ups and downs met with in the course of the disease are equally characteristic, as are the changes which occur in the several symptoms, the improvements and relapses, and the way symptoms spring up and progress in batches. The way in which paraplegia and anæsthesia may come on rapidly, or even suddenly, to be followed by spontaneous remission, is very significant. In this connection the variability of the knee-jerk is especially worthy of note ; its disappearance, subsequent return, and even increase, are all very suggestive. Of similar significance is the return of the pupil reflex after it has been lost.

This natural tendency to spontaneous remission makes it difficult to judge of the effects of specific remedies ; but if the improvement under their use be considerable the diagnosis is made a great deal more certain. It must be remembered, however, that non-syphilitic affections of the spinal cord also show improvement under anti-syphilitic treatment sometimes, while in some syphilitic cases not only is there no improvement under this mode of treatment, but the condition may even become worse.

It is easy to confound a simple myelitis with one of syphilitic origin, especially in the disseminated mode of the former affection. The absence of cerebral symptoms is important in so far as syphilitic cases of the kind are rare ; but since optic neuritis may occur in connection with a simple myelitis considerable difficulty may be experienced in coming to a decision. In the purely spinal form ántisyphilitic treatment alone may serve to clear up the doubt. The vacillation of certain of the symptoms, notably of the motor paralysis and the state of the knee-jerks, makes syphilis more probable, though not certain ; while the meningitic and root symptoms have a similar degree of significance.

It is obvious that disseminate sclerosis is especially difficult to differentiate in some cases, for in most of the varieties of this disease symptoms may indicate the existence of cerebral as well as spinal disorder ; and, further, great variation in the intensity of the symptoms is a very characteristic feature of this disease. The combination of spastic paraplegia with apoplectic attacks or with ocular changes is especially confusing. The following points are of chief importance as suggestive of disseminate sclerosis :—nystagmus, scanning utterance, tremor, and, as a rule, an absence of meningitic and root symptoms. On the other hand, although dementia, hemiplegia, and paralysis of ocular muscles may all occur in disseminate sclerosis, they are more common features of cerebral syphilis. In some cases, however, we have nothing but the effect of antisyphilitic treatment to guide us in our opinion.

Tumour of the spinal cord may not be easy to distinguish ; especially as in some cases of syphilis of the spinal cord Brown-Séquard's hemisection phenomena may be met with, though not usually in very pure form. The points to be relied on are the absence of cerebral symptoms, the presence of great rigidity, the more distinct anæsthesia, which is constant, and the negative result of antisyphilitic treatment.

The points which serve to distinguish a tuberculous from a syphilitic meningitis will be noted under the former affection in the next volume.

When sensory manifestations, together with ataxy and abolition of the knee-jerks, precede the motor phenomena, the case may be mistaken for one of tabes dorsalis. In some cases the picture may be even more like that of tabes, as there may be bladder trouble, paralysis of ocular muscles, and even bulbar symptoms. However, the subsequent paraplegia, in which, as a rule, motor power is definitely lost, serves to clear up any doubt that had formerly existed.

Prognosis.—In attempting to formulate a prognosis in syphilitic affections of the spinal cord, much depends on whether the condition be purely spinal; whether there are added signs of concomitant intracranial mischief; the amount of damage already done to the nerve elements; the length of time that the disease has existed untreated, and the response to antisyphilitic treatment.

The prognosis is best in the purely spinal form: when cerebral symptoms are added it becomes more unfavourable; and in such combined cases considerable improvement may be manifest as far as the spinal part of the affection goes, while the cerebral part of the disease pursues a totally different course. Where the clinical manifestations point to great mischief in the spinal cord itself, we know that irreparable damage is being done; and that, even if the morbid process be arrested under treatment, or if actual improvement occur, cicatricial changes and secondary degenerations must permanently disturb function in proportion to their extent. If the whole transverse section of the cord be affected, and paraplegia complete, the chances of improvement are very slight; yet even in severe cases of this kind a fair amount of improvement may come about. On the other hand, although the chances of amelioration are much greater in the slighter degrees of affection, this does not necessarily follow, as the effects even of slight damage may remain permanently.

The longer the disease remained untreated the worse the prognosis; again, if antisyphilitic treatment has been carried out for any length of time without amelioration of the symptoms the chances are poor, while they are correspondingly better in proportion to any degree of improvement. It is always well not to express any confident opinion until the effects of antisyphilitic treatment have been carefully tested for a time; we can thus formulate our prognosis with much more definiteness and accuracy.

In the very acute cases of syphilis of the spinal cord, according to Boettinger, death usually results in a few weeks or months.

Apart from these various considerations which should guide us in prognosis, it may be said in general terms that the majority of these patients improve; the degree of improvement, of course, varying in different cases: the prognosis is better indeed than in any other chronic affections of the spinal cord. The exact percentage of patients who do not die, or get practically quite well, is, of course, not easy to estimate, as the macroscopic and microscopic appearances are the only conclusive evidences of the nature of the morbid process.

Treatment.—Antisyphilitic treatment should be energetically carried out; and if we are fairly certain of our diagnosis it is well to give the treatment a prolonged trial, even if improvement do not appear, rather than discontinue it too soon. Mercury should always be employed; and as a rule it can be introduced into the system sufficiently rapidly and in large enough quantity by inunction, either of the blue ointment or the oleate; one to four drachms are to be rubbed in daily until the patient is well under the influence of the drug, and then in the amount necessary to keep him under its influence without producing toxic effects. Where there are special reasons for introducing the drug into the system more rapidly, as when the progress is very rapid, or especially where there is danger of implication of those parts of the central nervous system which govern the vital processes, subcutaneous or intra-venous injections may take the place of inunction.

Besides guarding the patient against the toxic effects of the mercury, care should be taken not to allow the drug to reduce him too much, as general nutrition is, of course, wont to suffer greatly under the treatment. Usually it is necessary to interrupt the treatment for several weeks, or even months, and then to persevere with it again; more than one such interruption and repetition of the treatment being often necessary, as in some cases the time is long before the good effects of the mercurial treatment become manifest. If such measures be adopted, and properly persevered in, great improvement results in the majority of the cases.

As a rule iodide of potassium is better reserved for the intervals when the mercurial treatment is interrupted, or as a therapeutic agent to be employed after the mercurial course; but in urgent cases it becomes necessary to combine the two forms of treatment from the beginning. The dose of the iodide necessarily varies a good deal according to the case; moreover, the drug is often badly borne. Usually ten grains three times a day is enough; but where no ill effects result from its use, and the case is obstinate, each dose may with advantage be increased to fifteen or twenty grains.

A warm bath should be given daily while the patient is under the mercurial treatment. There is no reason why the treatment should not be successfully accomplished at home; but when the patients' circumstances will allow of it they may be sent to Harrogate, Wiesbaden, or other thermal springs, to have the mercurial course carried out. Moreover, hydropathic measures are of advantage for the limbs, as in cases of chronic myelitis of non-specific origin. So, too, as a means of improving muscular nutrition and preventing contractures, massage with passive movements and electrical treatment should be carried out concomitantly with the other therapeutic measures, care being taken not to begin the electricity too early, but to reserve it rather for the later stages in the course of treatment, when gymnastics are also of advantage in re-educating the nerve centres and the muscles on which they act.

5. Leptomeningitis.—A. Acute leptomeningitis.—SYN. : *"Acute inter-*

nal meningitis," "Simple meningitis," "Purulent meningitis."—In this condition the inflammatory process involves the arachnoid and pia, as a rule; and in many cases the inner surface of the dura mater is affected also. According to some observers the process may, in rare instances, be limited to the arachnoid, without involving the pia.

The following account of the affection will not include epidemic cerebro-spinal meningitis, which has already been dealt with (see vol. i. p. 659), and the tuberculous variety of acute meningitis will be reserved for subsequent brief consideration (p. 911).

Causation.—Having excluded the epidemic cerebro-spinal and tuberculous varieties of acute meningitis, we are left with the following etiological factors, each of which appears capable of inducing a meningitis :—

(i.) Purulent cerebral meningitis, especially when affecting the base of the brain, is prone to extend to the spinal meninges.

A purulent process in connection with the spinal column, as in spinal caries, or an abscess of the soft parts in the neighbourhood of the spine may cause it; as may a deep bedsore over the sacrum perforating into the neural canal. So, too, suppurations in the pleura and mediastinum are said to have extended to the spinal meninges. On the other hand, the infective agent may be derived from some distant collection of pus or septic inflammation, as in pelvic suppuration (whether the result of puerperal sepsis or not); from cystitis, however induced, but especially when gonorrhœal; from a gonorrhœa without cystitis; or from a pyelitis. Similarly empyema, abscess of the lungs, and bronchiectasis may supply the infective agent, as may suppuration in any other organ. Carbuncle of the neck or back not uncommonly leads to a meningitis.

(ii.) A spinal meningitis may arise in the course of an infective disease, such as ulcerative endocarditis, septicæmia, erysipelas, and the like; in connection with the acute exanthems, pneumonia, acute rheumatism, or enteric fever.

(iii.) In sporadic cases of epidemic cerebro-spinal meningitis the mischief is sometimes restricted to the spinal cord. Such cases are of more moderate intensity than in the epidemic form. Although isolated instances occur, sometimes the number of such cases increases to such an extent as almost to constitute an epidemic.

(iv.) Injury, whether it be an injury to the spinal column or not, may lead to a meningitis. Without any fracture of the spine there may be tearing or contusion of the meninges; or injury to the spinal cord itself may form a suitable nidus for the multiplication of micro-organisms, which in their turn may give rise to a meningitis, in association, it may be, with a myelitis. The microbes may gain an entrance, under such circumstances, by way of an external wound; or, without any such, they may be derived from the intestinal or pulmonary tracts.

In this category must be mentioned operative procedures on the spine, and notably that for spina bifida which formerly was often attended with this result; or a spina bifida may be responsible for a meningitis by rupture of the sac.

(v.) Cold is said to cause meningitis; and instances have been recorded where this result has come about as an immediate consequence of great lowering of the surface temperature of the body, as from falling into water or sleeping in the open air. For my own part I prefer to regard the cold only in the light of a general depressing influence, creating a place of less resistance of which micro organisms take advantage, and thus give rise to the inflammatory process.

Morbid anatomy.—There is a good deal of variation in the extent of the spinal meninges affected in the long axis of the cord. In cases in which the inflammation has extended from the cranial cavity, only the upper few inches of the spinal meninges may show any change; or evidences of meningitis may be found as low down as some point corresponding to a change of direction in the spinal column, from a position more or less vertical above to one horizontal below, as the patient lay in bed. Herein we see how important is the part which gravity plays in the extension of the morbid process. If seen early in traumatic cases where there has been injury to the bones, or in cases of caries, or in abscess of the spinal cord, the meningitis may be limited in extent; but in all these cases the tendency is for rapid spread to occur from the seat of origin. That this should be so is scarcely to be wondered at when we remember how loose is the tissue of the arachnoid; but a second factor, which probably has a good deal to do with the spread of such inflammations, is the movement of the cerebro-spinal fluid, which must of necessity carry with it deleterious products from the seat of inflammation which are capable of causing irritation of other parts of the meninges; or it may be a specific virus is so carried, either a micro-organism or the toxins to which it gives origin. In cases of sporadic inflammation of an infective character the whole longitudinal extent of the meninges is usually affected, the morbid influence making itself felt simultaneously in all parts of the meninges; but even in these cases, as in all others where the membranes are involved in their whole extent, the evidences of inflammation are, as a rule, most marked on the dorsal aspect of the cord. No doubt gravity has much to do with this result, the recumbent posture facilitating the backward flow of the exudation whose ingredients are capable of inducing or increasing the inflammatory irritation.

As stated, the inner surface of the dura mater may be concomitantly affected; and, strange as it may seem, the pia, though usually affected in conjunction with the arachnoid, sometimes escapes; under these circumstances the spinal cord is also unaffected, but otherwise a varying degree of secondary affection of the spinal cord results. The nerve roots are, of course, liable also to secondary implication; but so great is their power of resistance that it is surprising how little change they may show, even when bathed in pus; indeed, under these circumstances they sometimes appear quite intact.

The morbid appearances depend a good deal on the length of time between the onset of symptoms and the death of the patient. In its earliest stages the only evidences of meningitis which the membranes

may present consist in pronounced hyperæmia, accompanied perhaps by
punctate extravasations of blood.   When dealing with congestion of the
spinal meninges, as stated in cases of acute meningitis, if death result
before the stage of exudation, all that may be found is this intense
hyperæmia of the membranes, which are of a rosy red hue, and the
vessels greatly engorged.   Similar appearances may be met with on the
inner surface of the dura mater and in the spinal cord.   Even at this
stage the cerebro-spinal fluid is cloudy.   It is rare to meet on necropsy
with these early indications of meningitis alone; far more commonly the
disease has passed beyond this stage: and though the appearances above
described are seen, there are added evidences of a more advanced inflammation.   Now the leptomeninges are of a milky appearance, or more
opaque, and distinctly thickened; and there is distinct exudation bathing
the outer surface of the arachnoid, lying in the meshes of this membrane,
and occupying the space between it and the pia.   All degrees of turbidity
of this exudate are seen, up to the most definite formation of pus, greenish
yellow in colour and creamy in consistence.   Even before such visible
evidences of pus, microscopic examination of the turbid exudate, or of the
meninges, reveals pus cells in abundance; a state of things that may be
found also in the pia and the inner layers of the dura.   Moreover, the
sheaths of the engorged vessels are infiltrated with similar cells.   As I
have said, the nerve roots frequently escape damage, even in purulent
meningitis; but, when affected, they may show macroscopic evidences of
this, in the shape of swelling and redness; and on microscopic examination
round cell infiltration is seen in conjunction with destruction of the
nerve elements.   Spread of the inflammatory mischief to the spinal cord
always takes place where the pia mater is affected; and the changes then
met with are those of a myelitis chiefly affecting the periphery of the
cord, and extending more deeply into its substance, in wedge-shaped
patches with their apices directed inward and their bases fusing at the
periphery.   Such extension into the deeper parts of the cord results from
spread of the inflammatory products along the perivascular spaces of the
pial vessels which dip into and supply the substance of the cord for a
considerable depth.   In some cases, however, instead of finding a
myelitis having so distinctly a marginal distribution, we may meet with
irregularly scattered minute foci of inflammation; as in the case, recorded by Dr. Buzzard and myself, to which reference has been made.
In such cases it is probable that the myelitis and the meningitis are produced independently by the same causative agent; or it may even be
that in some of these cases the myelitis may be primary in point of time,
and the meningitis induced secondarily by extension of the inflammatory
process to the surface of the cord at various parts.   When the cord is involved, softening and other macroscopic and microscopic changes common
to myelitis are met with, and need not be described here (see subsequent art. "Myelitis").   On the other hand, the spinal cord may be
intact, even in the presence of a purulent meningitis, provided the pia
be not involved; a state of things which, as I have said, is met with

sometimes. The cerebro-spinal fluid is increased in amount, is turbid, and contains flocculi of pus.

Bacteriological examinations in these cases yield results, as regards particular micro-organisms, which vary with the cause of the meningitis. The ordinary pus cocci are commonly met with; but other organisms have also been found, notably the diplococcus of pneumonia; while in the case to which I have already referred more than once, we found a diplococcus, pathogenetic to animals and having certain resemblances to the Diplococcus intra-cellularis of Weichselbaum, and to that of simple posterior basic meningitis described by Dr. Still, though in certain particulars differing from both of these organisms. The micro-organisms are found in the exudation, in the meninges, in the cord itself, and in the cerebro-spinal fluid; from all of which sources they may be cultivated on artificial media : or on microscopical examination they may be detected after suitable staining agents have brought them into view. In the case of the intra-cellularis the diplococci may be met with in the cells of the exudate; but otherwise the organisms lie free outside the cells, and in the tissues : they are especially plentiful in the immediate neighbourhood of vessels, the perivascular spaces sometimes containing large numbers of them; or they may even be met with in the interior of the vessels themselves, in the smaller branches of which they may produce embolic obstruction.

If, instead of death during the acute stage of the inflammatory disturbance, the patient survive, absorption of the inflammatory products takes place; but permanent changes remain by which the disease may be recognised on a subsequent necropsy. The meninges are cloudy and thickened, usually in an irregular manner; and a varying degree of matting together and adhesion is met with, not only of the arachnoid to the pia, but also of the former to the inner surface of the dura, and of the latter to the spinal cord. There is permanent excess of cerebro-spinal fluid in the arachnoid space; and a collection of this, shut in by adhesions, may give rise to the appearance known as hydrorrhachis. I have long wondered whether the shell-like calcareous plates not uncommonly met with in the meshes of the arachnoid, of which I have seen some beautiful examples, can possibly signify some past inflammatory condition of these membranes (see p. 917). Meningitis is usually so stormy in its manifestations that it is difficult to believe that these plates could be so frequently and accidentally met with at necropsies, without anything in the clinical history of the case to point to past meningitis.

When the spinal cord has been invaded, a varying degree of sclerosis, diffuse or circumscribed, will be met with corresponding to the parts previously damaged by the myelitic process; and, extending from these areas, ascending and descending secondary degenerations, the precise amount of which will depend on the degree to which the afferent and efferent tracts have been involved in the primary process.

Apart from epidemic cerebro-spinal meningitis, evidences of inflammation of the cerebral meninges are commonly associated with the spinal affection. Sometimes this is due, of course, to spread of the inflammatory process from the cerebral to the spinal meninges; but in others the reverse obtains, the spinal meninges being the primary seat of mischief. In some such cases there is no difficulty in tracing the continuity between the process in the neural canal and that in the intra-cranial cavity; in others the evidences of mischief in the membranes of the upper part of the cord are very indistinct, while the degree of meningitis, both below this and at the base of the brain, is much greater. The explanation of this probably is that the cerebro-spinal fluid is the means of conveying to the cerebral meninges the material capable in these cases of inducing inflammation of them. Where the cerebral meninges are involved secondarily to those of the spinal cord, the mischief is always most marked at the base of the brain, and especially at its posterior part. Some slight extension along the lower part of the convexity of the hemispheres may be met with; but well-marked meningitis at the upper part of the convexity is very rare under such circumstances.

Symptoms.—It will now be readily understood that, apart from the concomitant occurrence of symptoms due to invasion of structures within the cranial cavity, the clinical manifestations of the spinal condition may vary considerably, according as those which indicate affection of the meninges, irritation or destruction of the nerve roots, or invasion of the spinal cord predominate. As the manifestations of the last group are those of a myelitis to which meningitic symptoms are added, it would be superfluous to give a separate description of them here (see " Myelitis," vol. vii.); I propose therefore to confine my attention to the phenomena which indicate affection of the meninges, inseparable from which are those due to irritation, and, it may be, subsequent destruction of the nerve roots.

Premonitory symptoms, such as malaise and slight pain in the back, may precede the more characteristic symptoms of the condition, which consist in the acute and severe pain in the back in association with a rigor and elevation of temperature. The seat of the pain varies with the seat of the morbid process, but is frequently referred to the whole length of the spine; even then, however, it may be more intense at certain points than at others. This pain is often of the most violent character, and makes even the slightest movement of the patient quite unbearable; although constant it is prone to acute exacerbation. It is due, no doubt, to irritation of the nerves of the inflamed meninges. Pressure on the spinous processes of the vertebræ elicits tenderness over the seat of the inflammation, and a hot sponge applied to the skin of the back increases the pain.

Pain of a different character is also present, which is distinctly referable to irritation of the sensory spinal nerve roots. The pain is sharp, lancinating, or tearing in character; or again burning or constricting; this on the trunk gives rise to the well-known girdle sensation. It is paroxysmal, and radiates in the areas of distribution of the sensory roots of the trunk, or limbs, or both; according as the seat of the mischief in the meninges allows of irritation of one or both sets of nerve roots. The skin areas, corresponding to the distribution of these irritated sensory roots, may become markedly hyperæsthetic; and herpetic eruptions may appear in such areas. There is also tenderness of the muscles on pressure; this is especially marked in the legs, where it may be present when no discomfort results from similar pressure of the muscles of the arms. Interference with the vaso-motor nerves causes the hyperæmia which appears on stroking the skin with the finger-nail, or a pin, to be excessive in degree and to persist for an undue length of time; the phenomenon being known as the *tache spinale* or meningeal streak.

Equally characteristic of meningitis is the muscular spasm which usually accompanies the pain, and gives rise to varying degrees of rigidity, more especially of the neck and back, but it may be of the limbs also. The rigidity may be restricted to a small part of the back corresponding to the seat of inflammation, or the whole of the back muscles may be affected in a meningitis of more extensive distribution, giving rise to the most pronounced opisthotonos. Even if the whole back be not thus attacked there may be notable arching back of the neck, so that the occiput comes into close contact with the nape of the neck; and even when the rigidity afterwards becomes more general, it is often noticed first in the neck. The other trunk muscles commonly become involved, including those of the abdomen, spasm of which results in a boat-shaped retraction of the abdominal walls. The muscles of the limbs also become rigid, and paroxysms of painful recurring spasms occur in them, either spontaneously or on any attempts at movement. A rapid rhythmical tremor of the limbs may also occur; both this and the previous symptom being more commonly observed in the arms, while the legs may be persistently flexed at the knee, the patient being unable to overcome this contraction of the hamstring muscles. Some of the rigidity of the back may be in part the result of voluntary efforts to keep the spinal column fixed, owing to the intense suffering that the slightest movement occasions; but more important factors in this spasm, as well as in that of other parts of the trunk and the limbs, are irritation of the sensory nerve roots and the nerves of the meninges bringing about the spasm reflexly, while irritation of the motor roots brings it about directly.

In the early stages of the disease the reflexes are increased. There is spasmodic retention of urine, with irritable attempts on the part of the detrusor to expel the contents of the bladder. Constipation is usually troublesome. There is always some pyrexia, though this may be insignificant. The pulse is either rapid or abnormally slow. Respiration may be interfered with by spasm of the thoracic muscles so far as to cause dyspnœa, which may even become urgent.

When the cerebral meninges are involved there is headache, delirium, or somnolence passing on to coma; an event which may or may not be preceded by convulsions. "Cheyne-Stokes breathing" may occur in consequence of extension of the mischief to the medulla. The functions of some of the cerebral nerves may become disturbed, and notably squints, either irritative or paralytic, may appear.

The further progress of the case, in so far as the spinal symptoms are concerned, is marked by the subsidence of the signs of irritation, and their replacement by others indicative of destructive processes in the spinal cord and the nerve roots; though, owing to the great power of resistance which the nerve roots possess, evidences of the latter condition are rare. The anæsthesia and muscular atrophy of root distribution are therefore rare; and the anæsthesia with motor paralysis is to be attributed to extension of the mischief to the spinal cord; and the latter may become so great that scarcely any movement can be performed. As a rule the paralysis is at first of the spastic type, with exaggerated knee-jerks and ankle clonus; but in severe cases, and especially where the gray matter of the cervical and lumbar enlargements are invaded, flaccidity follows, and the tendon jerks are abolished. Under such circumstances it becomes a matter of difficulty to decide how much is to be accounted for by affection of the spinal cord, and how much may be due to destruction of nerve roots. Vaso-motor disturbances may be intense, so that even a slight prick or scratch may cause a large wheal to rise at the seat of irritation. Large bullæ may result from slight pressure on the skin, as by one leg lying for even a short time against its fellow; and bedsores are apt to appear. There may be considerable pyrexia; the heart becomes feeble; and death may result from asthenia, or from paralysis of the muscles of respiration.

Instead of this rapidly fatal course there may be an abatement in the severity of the symptoms; though the general tendency may still be that of slow progress in the wrong direction, suffering being thus prolonged, and death resulting after some weeks from bedsore, or from renal disease secondary to cystitis. In less severe cases, however, the irritation may gradually subside, and recovery may come about; though evidence of permanent damage to the spinal cord remains in the shape of anæsthesia and muscular paralysis, it may be with contracture or with muscular atrophy consequent on damage to the cord or nerve roots. Unfortunately, in some cases where the residual effects point to but slight permanent damage to the spinal cord, there may be subsequent increase of symptoms consequent on a chronic myelitis following the acute mischief. Then the best that can usually be hoped for is recovery with some persistence of spastic paraplegia, with or without some disturbance of the function of the bladder; yet in rare cases, where the disease has been slight, complete recovery may result.

The distribution of the symptoms which characterise an acute meningitis depends on the seat of the process and on its extent. In the majority of instances the affection of the meninges is widespread, and the symptoms are correspondingly wide in range; but in other cases the inflammatory mischief is circumscribed, and the symptoms are likewise limited, though not necessarily to the same extent as the morbid process on which they depend. When such circumscribed meningitis exists in the cervical region, prominent among the manifestations are those in connection with the upper limbs; respiration may be seriously interfered with, even to the degree of urgent dyspnœa. Dilatation or contraction of one or both pupils, with narrowing of the palpebral fissures, may be the result of interference with the pupillary fibres of the sympathetic. Deglutition often becomes very difficult, and the heart's action may be disturbed. When the thoracic region is chiefly affected, the pain and spasm are usually most marked in the trunk; though similar phenomena may also be met with in the lower limbs. And when the chief seat of the mischief is in the lumbar region, the symptoms are confined to the loins and lower extremities. Spread of the inflammation to the cerebral meninges is signalised by headache, vomiting, delirium, and even convulsions. Interference with the functions of various of the cranial nerves may result, notably those supplying the ocular muscles; but the earliest to suffer are, as might be expected, the spinal accessory and hypoglossal.

The course of the disease varies; but as a rule it is rapid, all the symptoms reaching a high degree of intensity, in severe cases, within twenty-four to forty-eight hours, and ending in death in a few days. Such a result is usually due to implication of the cerebral meninges leading to paralysis of the heart or asphyxia. In less severe cases the acute symptoms persist for a few weeks, and then end either in death or recovery; in others months elapse during which evidences of slow destructive processes going on in the spinal cord make themselves manifest.

Diagnosis.—Little difficulty is likely to be found in the diagnosis of a typical case of acute meningitis; pain in the back, rigidity of the neck and back, retraction of the head and opisthotonos, hyperæsthesia of the skin, and spasm of the muscles of the limbs coming on acutely and in association with pyrexia, leave no room for doubt as to the nature of the case. Evidence of irritation preceding paralytic symptoms is all-important in the diagnosis; and it is graver, of course, when symptoms indicative of cerebral meningitis coexist with those attributable to the spinal meninges. Further support is given to the diagnosis when a recognised cause for the meningitis can be established; when, for example, symptoms such as those detailed above come on in the course of one of the acute infective fevers, or when some purulent affection exists in some other organ, and is thus a possible source of infection, or where an injury preceded the onset of symptoms. The chief difficulty is when symptoms of irritation are absent, as is so often the case in the secondary purulent variety, in which, as we have seen, the nerve elements are usually but little disturbed.

As traumatism may be due either to a hæmorrhage into the spinal meninges or an inflammation of these structures, and as the former of these conditions may be followed by the latter in the same case, while, moreover, the manifestations of a hæmatorrhachis of necessity resemble those of a meningitis, the diagnosis may present some difficulties. As I have pointed out, reliance must be placed on the sudden occurrence of the symptoms, which, in the case of hæmatorrhachis, rapidly reach their height without the occurrence of pyrexia; while when due to meningitis, whether alone or following a hæmorrhage, such symptoms do not make their appearance until two or three days after the accident, and they are attended with pyrexia.

It is unlikely that a hæmorrhage into the spinal cord itself can be mistaken for a meningitis; for the two conditions have nothing in common, except pain in the back, which, in the case of hæmatomyelia, is limited to one spot. The sudden onset with pronounced paralytic phenomena should prevent any possibility of error.

Similarly, there is comparatively little difficulty in distinguishing a myelitis uncomplicated with meningitis from a meningitis uncomplicated with myelitis. In the former case pain in the back is either absent or but slight; there is an absence of spasm in the muscles of the limbs in the earliest stage; and paralysis of motion, and it may be of sensation also, is the prominent feature of the case from the outset. But, as meningitis and myelitis commonly occur together, sometimes one and sometimes the other being the primary affection, it will readily be understood how difficult it may be to arrive at a differential diagnosis in such cases. Whenever severe pain in the back exists, especially if accompanied by rigidity, we may feel sure that we are dealing with a meningitis, whether we have evidence of the coexistence of a myelitis or not; but where such symptoms precede those of a paralytic character the meningitis is the primary process.

The distinction of meningitis from tetanus must be based on the frequent absence of pyrexia in the latter condition, especially in its initial stage; on the increase of reflex irritability to a much greater degree, so that lightly stroking the patient's skin or even walking towards his bed is sufficient to evoke severe spasms, while in meningitis the spasms usually come on when the patient tries to move; and on the early occurrence of trismus. If the spinal meningitis be complicated by inflammation of the cerebral meninges trismus may occur, but under such circumstances it usually manifests itself much later than in tetanus; moreover, in tetanus this symptom is not accompanied by others of cerebral origin, such as delirium, convulsions, and coma. Any pain present in tetanus is due to the muscular spasm; there is an absence of radiating pains, of subjective sensations, and of hyperæsthesia of the skin.

Rheumatism of the muscles of the back may cause stiffness and pain on movement; and in children, if it is acute in onset and affects the cervical muscles, causing retraction of the head, the diagnosis may be difficult; but severe spontaneous and radiating pains are absent, and there is no spread of the spasm to the muscles of the limbs.

When hysteria simulates meningitis it is usually the cerebral rather than the spinal form which is manifested; in which case headache, vomiting, convulsions, and even what appears to be coma may be met with. Moreover, the pulse may become slow, and there may be spasm in the muscles of the back of the neck. Such cases may present a good deal of difficulty; but those experienced in the recognition of hysteria will, as a rule, be able to detect indications pointing to its existence;

notably that sleep is natural, the coma is factitious, and the various manifestations may be influenced psychically.

Having decided that meningitis is present, much difficulty may still be experienced in deciding the form of the affection. The recognition of the cause of the meningitis is all-important; thus when it occurs in the puerperal state, or under circumstances which favour the development of septicæmia, the purulent form is surely present. The onset is abrupt in these cases, and the manifestations, as a rule, stormy. In the tuberculous variety, on the other hand, there may be evidence of tuberculous disease in other organs, or a family history of such disease may be elicited; the onset is gradual, with indefinite symptoms at first, and, moreover, the coexistence of cerebral meningitis gives rise to symptoms which usually precede those of spinal origin. Quincke's lumbar puncture may be practised, for diagnostic purposes, when the matter is in doubt; the fluid from a tuberculous meningitis is usually clear, and tubercle bacilli may be found in stained cover-glass preparations; and even when these are negative the inoculation of guinea-pigs may yield positive results.

Prognosis.—The prognosis is always grave, except in those cases which, though occurring sporadically, resemble the epidemic cerebro-spinal form of the disease; in them recovery, either complete or partial, occurs in a large number of instances. The probable cause of the meningitis is a much better guide in prognosis than is the probable extent of the mischief; though, as far as the question of complete recovery is concerned, evidence of the degree to which the spinal cord is damaged secondarily is all-important. In the purulent form death almost always results sooner or later, whether secondary to some suppurative process about the spinal column, or metastatic in origin, the source of infection being situated at a distance. So too the prognosis is very bad in those cases which follow the acute infective fevers, or tuberculosis; and it is also serious in cases resulting from severe lesions of the spinal column, though in cases which are consequent upon the slighter traumatic influences the prognosis is much better; as it is also in those cases where cold appears to be the cause of the meningitis.

Although the causation is the most important factor in prognosis, valuable aid is obtained from other considerations; thus the higher the temperature, the more acutely the symptoms come on, and the more severe they become, the more serious the prognosis; and the early substitution of paralytic for irritative phenomena is of equally grave import. The prognosis further depends on the stage at which the case is seen; thus it becomes better if some days have elapsed since the onset; especially if there be any signs of abatement of the disease, such as diminution of pain and pyrexia, without the appearance of paralysis. Prognosis has to be guarded, however, even at this stage, in view of the many complications that may arise, and owing to the frequency of relapses; moreover, if paralytic phenomena are present, though life may be spared, the patient may be crippled by the persistence of this in association with spasticity or muscular atrophy. The age of the patient influences prognosis, as does his former state of health also; the chances of recovery are less in children and in old people than in those about the middle period of life; and debilitated subjects run a poorer chance than persons previously robust.

Treatment.—It is of primary importance that the patient should be kept at rest on a smooth water-bed; and, although it is harmful to have the back the most dependent part, yet this cannot well be avoided in most cases, as both the lateral and prone positions require a certain degree of muscular effort, sufficient, as a rule, to evoke attacks of spasm, which do more harm than the results of gravitation. Moreover, the prone position may seriously impede respiration in cases where the meninges of the upper parts of the cord are affected. Provided the spasms are not made worse to any extent, and that there is no reason to fear respiration, the prone or lateral positions are to be preferred to the dorsal. Mental as well as physical rest should be secured; the room should be cool and airy, darkened, and kept as quiet as possible. The greatest possible care is necessary to prevent the formation of bedsores, the most scrupulous cleanliness being called for in the nursing of such cases. The strength must be kept up by nourishing food, which, however, should not be stimulating; alcohol ought not to be given unless collapse threaten; and, while various mineral and other waters are allowed, where there is any weakness of the muscles of respiration the effervescing forms of water must be cautiously used, lest abdominal distension should seriously hamper the action of these muscles. Where deglutition is difficult, especially in children, it may be necessary to administer nourishment by the stomach tube. The bowels should, of course, be kept freely open.

Hydrotherapeutic measures are of advantage in some cases, if employed early in the course of the disease; and are especially indicated where the attack seemed to be due to exposure to cold. In such cases free diaphoresis should be induced at the outset, by means of the hot air or vapour bath; or wet packing may follow an ordinary warm bath. Packing may be employed with advantage later in the course of the disease when the warm bath is contra-indicated on account of the pain and spasm induced by movement. After all acute manifestations have subsided, and a more or less chronic stage of the affection is reached, bath treatment at Bath or Aix-les-Bains is of advantage.

Various local measures to the spine have been tried with a view to lessen the severity of the process within the neural canal. In the earliest stages dry and wet cupping are of advantage; the latter, and leeching, being, however, only permissible in robust patients. The practice of different physicians varies with regard to the use of heat or cold to the spine; but in cases of traumatic origin it will be found of most advantage on the whole to employ the latter in the shape of the ice-bag, especially when we suspect the existence of hæmorrhage; in other cases warmth is generally found to afford most comfort. Blistering and similar methods of counter-irritation should be avoided in the earlier stages of the disease; they may, however, prove useful later.

The only drug that appears to have any influence on the acute process is mercury, which may be given by inunction, or by the mouth ; but the former method is far superior to the latter. Half a drachm to a drachm of blue ointment should be rubbed in along the spine daily until the gums are slightly but distinctly touched. Iodide of potassium, useless at this stage, may be of advantage when the condition becomes more chronic, when quinine, iron, and even strychnine may be called for. Where cold applications are not capable alone of subduing the pain, morphia should be freely given by subcutaneous injection ; and, if the spasms be very severe, it may even be necessary to supplement the use of this drug by inhalations of chloroform, so intense is the suffering they induce. Belladonna or atropine has been found useful in mild cases. Of hypnotics chloral hydrate has a high reputation, and may be given alone or in combination with bromide. The various other hypnotics, such as chloralamide, sulphonal, trional, or paraldehyde, are of use in different cases.

Sequels such as contractions, muscular atrophies, and the like, call for massage, electrical, and other special treatments, according to the precise condition present.

B. **Cerebro-spinal meningitis** (see vol. i. p. 659).

C. **Tuberculous spinal meningitis.**—This form of meningitis is exceedingly rare except in combination with a similar condition of the cerebral meninges (vol. vii.) Seitz found this combination in twelve out of twenty cases of tuberculous cerebral meningitis in the adult. The spinal affection is commonly met with when the meninges at the base of the brain are affected ; indeed, according to Schultze, this is perhaps always the case. On the other hand, it seems possible that in some cases the affection of the spinal may precede that of the cerebral meninges.

Morbid anatomy.—As in other forms of leptomeningitis the dura mater may be quite normal and free, while in other instances there is some inflammatory infiltration of this membrane ; and it may be adherent in places to the arachnoid. The latter membrane is turbid-looking and thickened ; its vessels share in the inflammatory process, their walls being infiltrated and thickened ; and the subarachnoid space is filled with turbid fluid and fibrinous exudation. The pia mater is also very turbid-looking and thickened, and extremely hyperæmic. Miliary tubercles may be distinctly seen, but they are not nearly so commonly found as in the cerebral pia. On microscopical examination this membrane is seen to be infiltrated with large numbers of round cells, and, as in the case of the arachnoid, the walls of the vessels are infiltrated.

As the condition is so often secondary to a basal tuberculous meningitis, although the process may be met with throughout the whole length of the spinal cord, it may be limited to the cervical and upper thoracic regions. On the other hand, strange as it may seem, little or no evidence of implication of the meninges of the upper end of the cord may be found, while distinct evidences of tuberculous deposits may be seen in the lumbo-sacral region. Recently I examined a case in which with a basal meningitis, itself secondary to a tuberculous tumour removed from the cerebellum by Mr. Victor Horsley, the meninges of the upper cervical region showed least sign of implication; whereas the pia-arachnoid throughout the whole extent of the remainder of the spinal cord was distinctly affected.

The morbid changes are limited, as a rule, to the meninges of the dorsal aspect of the spinal cord; occasionally, however, the ventral aspect is involved also. In the case just referred to, the changes, though more pronounced dorsally, were present in slighter degree on the ventral aspect also.

As in ordinary acute leptomeningitis, so here the nerve roots and spinal cord may present evidences of secondary implication. The posterior roots are especially apt to suffer; round cell infiltration occurring in connection with the peri- and endoneurium. The periphery of the spinal cord naturally suffers most, a marginal or peri-myelitis, as it has been called, being the result. The infiltration of the spinal cord takes place by certain definite routes; as by the septa of the pia which dip into its substance, by the marginal vessels which have a similar course, and by the entering posterior roots. The consequent changes in the cord may be very irregular and diffuse; the neuroglia fibres are swollen, and varying degrees of destruction of the nerve elements are met with. Secondary degenerations naturally follow; but, in addition to this, there may be a degeneration in the posterior and lateral columns, in the ganglion cells of the ventral horns, and in the ventral roots, which, according to Leyden and Goldscheider, is an affection of the neurons, comparable to, and, indeed, the central homologue of the peripheral neuritis which occurs in tuberculosis.

Symptoms.—Clinically, the spinal symptoms may be quite overshadowed by those due to the concomitant affection of the cerebral meninges. Where such spinal symptoms exist they differ in no way from those which result from other forms of affection of the spinal leptomeninges, and need not be repeated here.

Neuralgic pains, sciatica, and the like, occurring in tuberculous subjects, should place us on our guard; such symptoms may indicate the existence of tuberculous spinal meningitis.

It is not common for the spinal form of tuberculous meningitis to progress rapidly; as a rule it runs a more or less subacute course. Indeed, in the majority of instances the limitation is determined by a concomitant cerebral affection, which in some cases appears in point of time to be secondary to the spinal meningitis.

Diagnosis.—Of primary importance in the diagnosis of this variety of meningitis is the detection of tuberculous lesions in other organs of the body, notably in the lungs and pleuræ. In the absence of such lesions there may be external evidences of scrofula; or the cachectic appearance of the patient may suggest the true nature of the condition. The detection of tubercles of the choroid on ophthalmoscopic examination would of course be conclusive; but, as a rule, this evidence is not forthcoming until the final stages of the disease.

This form of meningitis is especially apt to be confounded with the. syphilitic; but in the latter, besides the importance of the history of infection, we have the results of antisyphilitic treatment to aid us; moreover, the motor disorder is much greater than in the tuberculous variety.

In order to establish a diagnosis between this condition and purulent meningitis we have to rely on the rate of development of the symptoms and the degree of pyrexia present; for, although in some slight cases of purulent meningitis there may be little or no fever, the condition is usually more severe, and attended with marked pyrexia. In tuberculous meningitis, on the other hand, fever is absent, or only slight, and the early stage of the affection is protracted.

In Quincke's spinal puncture we have a procedure of the greatest possible value in the diagnosis of the nature of a spinal meningitis. The cerebro-spinal fluid withdrawn should be centrifuged, and cover-glass preparations made from the deposit and stained for tubercle bacilli. In the event of negative results inoculation experiments on guinea-pigs should be performed; for positive results are thus obtained when the examination of a large number of cover-glass preparations fail to detect the tubercle bacillus.

Prognosis.—The disease is nearly always fatal; even when it is apparently primarily spinal, the advance of cerebral symptoms may close the scene. It appears possible, however, for a circumscribed tuberculous spinal meningitis to end favourably, as in a case recorded by von Leube.

Treatment.—No measures hitherto adopted have been attended with any success; but in view of the satisfactory results obtained from laparotomy in connection with tuberculous peritonitis, it is possible that drainage and washing out of the subdural space, through one opening at the upper and another at the caudal end of the neural canal, may bring about better results in the future.

D. **Chronic leptomeningitis.**—There can be no question that chronic changes in the pia-arachnoid, consisting in diffuse or circumscribed thickenings and cloudiness, are commonly met with on autopsy; but it is equally certain that in the great majority of such cases nothing in the clinical manifestations had pointed to meningitis.

Such a condition of the leptomeninges is met with in hypertrophic cervical pachymeningitis, internal pachymeningitis hæmorrhagica, and syphilitic spinal meningitis; or in diseases such as tabes dorsalis, general paralysis of the insane, myelitis, and tumours.

Moreover, it is none the less clear that formerly a clinical diagnosis of chronic meningitis was often made without justification. Cases of so-called spinal irritation, neurasthenia, and hysteria, in all of which pain and tenderness of the back may be prominent features, were commonly so regarded. Injuries, such as railway accidents and the like, which are frequently responsible for such functional disturbances of the nervous system, supplied no small number of cases of supposed chronic meningitis. But organic disease of the spinal cord has been also so regarded, a myelitis with meningitis being looked on as one of the latter condition alone ; indeed, according to Sir William Gowers, the clinical picture now regarded as characteristic of spastic paraplegia used to be always considered as a chronic meningitis.

Making allowances for all these possible fallacies, two classes of cases still remain to be discussed : those in which the changes met with are the result of a former attack of acute meningitis, and those in which such thickenings are seen in the spinal leptomeninges of the subjects of chronic alcoholism and of senile degeneration. In the former class of cases some authors contend that such residual changes do not remain after acute meningitis, and that when recovery takes place from such an attack it is complete. With regard to the latter class of cases also it has been argued that though the condition of the meninges met with in chronic alcoholism and senile degeneration is regarded as inflammatory, there is no clinical evidence of this.

Morbid anatomy.—A diffuse change of the leptomeninges may be met with throughout the greater part of the long axis of the spinal cord ; but even when such is the case, the thickening is most pronounced on the dorsal aspect, and is most marked at the caudal extremity of the cord ; becoming less and less so as higher levels are reached. It may be so great that the surface of the cord is to be seen with difficulty through the meninges. Apart from this general tendency for the change to be most pronounced at the caudal end of the cord, the thickening is not uniform, but is irregular in distribution. The inner surface of the dura mater is, as a rule, also cloudy, and presents similar irregular thickenings and nodular formations. The microscopic appearances vary with the age of the process ; the proliferation of connective tissue may even show but little fibrous structure, while with more fibrous structure evident the cell elements may be still very scarce ; in the earlier stages the cells are naturally more plentiful. The septa, which extend from the pia mater into the substance of the cord, are similarly thickened ; and the margin of the cord may show a varying degree of sclerosis, with a little secondary ascending and descending degeneration as a result of the slight damage done to the nerve elements. Yet on the other hand, with chronic changes evident in the meninges, the interference with the spinal cord may not be sufficient to give rise to any recognisable secondary degenerations in it. The walls of the blood-vessels are thickened.

Symptoms.—I may repeat that, in the majority of instances in which this condition is met with, apart from any association with hypertrophic cervical pachymeningitis, internal pachymeningitis hæmorrhagica, syphilitic spinal meningitis, caries of the spine, tumours, myelitis, and chronic degenerative diseases of the spinal cord, no clinical manifestations have been present which could be attributed to chronic leptomeningitis. Where symptoms exist they are indistinguishable from those which result from chronic pachymeningitis, which have been fully dealt with already under that head. The affection runs a chronic course without febrile reaction. Pain and stiffness of the back are prominent features ; lancinating pains may occur in the trunk and limbs, and pain on movement of the spine may be present; as also may tender points on pressure along the spine— hyperæsthesia of the skin and muscles. Moreover, if sufficient damage have been done to the nerve roots, atrophic paralysis of limited extent may ensue, as may spastic changes in the legs when the spinal cord has been much interfered with.

III. TUMOURS OF THE SPINAL MENINGES.—No detailed description of tumours of the spinal meninges, and the effects to which they give rise, is called for here, in that they naturally come within the scope of a special article which deals with the whole subject of compression of the spinal cord (see p. 855).

Causation.—A few points require consideration as regards the etiology of tumours of the spinal meninges, as distinguished from new growths in general. Intra-dural lipomata are congenital, and extra-dural fatty growths are met with early in life, as are tuberculous tumours. From an analysis of twenty-six cases Herter finds that the tuberculous tumours occur most commonly between the ages of fifteen and thirty-five years, though they are occasionally met with in children. Myxoma occurs usually at the middle period of life; malignant growths, as a rule, are met with later.

Injury has been invoked as a cause, but the evidence is less convincing than in tumours of certain other parts. Cysts, the results of hæmorrhages, have been erroneously regarded as new growths of traumatic origin.

Where tumours seem to have followed exposure to cold or wet it is more likely that these factors aggravated morbid changes already commenced in the nerve elements by the pressure of a pre-existing growth; the damage previously done not having been sufficient to give rise to symptoms.

Of the various diatheses known to be associated with the development of new growths in general, tubercle and syphilis alone have any influence in the case of the spinal meninges.

Two forms of parasitic tumours are met with; the more common is the echinococcus, which occurs as a solitary cyst; the other variety, the cysticercus, occurs as multiple cysts.

Morbid anatomy.—Tumours which involve the meninges may originate outside the neural canal, and may make their way into it through the intervertebral foramina, so as to involve the dura mater and bring about secondary pressure effects on the spinal cord. I have examined a case, with Dr. Beevor, in which a large sarcoma of the neck passed into the neural canal in this way, and not only involved the external surface of the dura, but also spread along a nerve root so as to enter the subdural space as a small tumour compressing the spinal cord. In other instances the dura mater becomes affected secondarily to new growths arising from the bone of the spinal column.

New growths which begin in the meninges may either take their origin in the dura mater, the ligamentum denticulatum, the arachnoid, or the pia. They may be found chiefly in connection with the external surface of the dura mater occupying the peridural space; or they may be related to the inner surface of this membrane, in which case the subdural space becomes filled by new growth at the seat of the morbid change. Just as new growths originating outside the neural canal may make their way into it secondarily, so those originating in connection with the outer surface of the dura may make their way out by way of the intervertebral foramina, and give rise to tumours outside the neural canal: this occurs notably in connection with lipoma originating in the peridural cellular tissue. So too echinococci, situated between the bone and dura, may erode the former and appear externally as fluctuating tumours. But instead of the new growth involving chiefly the external or internal surface of the dura mater with tumour formation in one or other situation, there may be a general infiltration of the membrane by new growth, giving rise to a thickening of it resembling that of pachymeningitis. In a patient of Dr. Ormerod's, whom I examined, the new growth proved to be endothelioma; and it was associated with multiple growths of like character scattered over the surface of the parietal pleura, posterior mediastinum, and other parts.

Various forms of new growth have been found in the different situations already referred to; and an idea of their relative frequency may be gathered from some statistics compiled by Mr. Victor Horsley, who found that of 58 cases of tumour of the spinal meninges 20 were extra-dural and 38 intra-dural. Of the former class, 5 were sarcoma, 4 lipoma, 4 tubercle, 3 echinococcus, 1 myxoma, 1 fibro-chondro-lipoma, 1 fibro-sarcoma, and 1 carcinoma; while in the latter group were included 12 myxoma, 7 fibroma, 7 sarcoma, 4 psammoma, 4 tubercle, 2 syphilis, and 2 parasitic. In addition to these, certain other forms of tumour may be met with within the dura mater, such as multiple neuroma in connection with the roots of the cauda equina, and congenital lipoma; this may be associated with spina bifida, and sometimes contains striated muscle fibre (myolipoma); so too Taube has recorded a case in which a new growth of the pia mater proved to be a lymphangioma; and angio-sarcoma and true angioma also occur.

Tumours of the spinal meninges are usually solitary. A notable exception to this rule is met with in the case of neuroma; parasitic tumours again are not uncommonly multiple; and in some cases of sarcoma scattered nodules are present, such a multiple sarcomatosis being seen especially in connection with the pia mater.

These new growths of the meninges may apparently develop simultaneously in this situation and in some other part of the body; otherwise primary growths are more commonly met with than metastatic deposits. Such metastatic growths, when extra-dural, may spread out as a flat cake of deposit on the surface of the dura, and surround this membrane to a varying degree, or even completely.

Intra-dural tumours do not attain to any great size, and are usually oval or cylindrical in shape; the long axis corresponding to the long axis of the neural canal, as they have to adapt themselves to the characters of the space in which they are growing. They may, however, attain a much greater size in the region of the lumbo-sacral cord and cauda equina, where there is more room for their expansion. They are often situated laterally, a fact which accounts for the frequency with which they produce the Brown-Séquard symptom group by their pressure on the spinal cord. They are very rarely met with on the ventral aspect of the cord; but in some cases they may be situated dorso-laterally rather than laterally. As a rule the tumours do not destroy the meninges, so that it is rare to find an extra-dural tumour making its way into the neural canal by destroying the dura mater; and what is more remarkable is the rarity with which intra-medullary tumours are found piercing the pia mater, and attacking the spinal cord in this way.

The pressure effects produced by meningeal tumours are exerted on the spinal cord, the nerve roots, or the bone of the spinal column. The effects on the cord are usually preceded by those connected with the nerve roots; while the effects on the bone are the last to occur, and rarely become at all pronounced. The seat of the tumour has an important influence on the order of events, and on the rate at which they succeed each other. The cord becomes involved much earlier in the case of intra-dural tumours; while extra-dural growths, especially the metastatic variety which spreads itself out over the outer surface of the dura, may involve the nerve roots for a long time before exerting any deleterious influence on the spinal cord. It is sometimes remarkable how the root fibres resist the invasion of new growths, and in this respect remind us of their behaviour in inflammatory affections of the meninges.

IV. CALCIFICATION OF THE DURA AND ARACHNOID. — It is quite common to meet with this condition of the arachnoid, but it is very rare in the dura. In the arachnoid, irregularly circular or oval shell-like plates of varying sizes, with scalloped margins, are seen; they are of an opaque white colour, and thicker in the centre than at the periphery. They are usually met with in the lower thoracic and lumbo-sacral regions of the cord; they are rare in the cervical region, and when they do occur in the latter situation only a small platelet here and there is usually seen, and larger and more numerous plates will generally be found also in the lower thoracic and lumbo-sacral regions of the cord. They occur most commonly, and in greatest numbers, on the dorsal aspect of the spinal cord; though they may also be met with on the ventral aspect.

It is not clear how these platelets originate; for, though a previous meningitis might account for them, there is little to support this suggestion, either from the evidence of the morbid anatomy or of the clinical history. In the majority of cases of the kind that I have examined, even where the platelets have been numerous, and some of them large, there has been a total absence of any other condition attributable to meningitis. There has been no adhesion of the dura to the arachnoid, and the latter membrane, with its contained platelets, has been freely movable over the subjacent pia mater. In only one instance were there concomitant signs of chronic meningitis present; these consisted in adhesion of the dura to the arachnoid over limited areas, and of patches of thickening and matting together of the arachnoid and pia in places. In none of the cases was there anything in the clinical history to point to a previous inflammation. Meningitis of any intensity is usually so stormy in its manifestations that it is difficult to believe that this condition of the meninges, if dependent on a former meningitis, could be met with so frequently without any such clinical evidence. It is, of course, possible that a meningitis, slight in degree and more or less subacute or chronic, may run a latent course; or give rise only to symptoms of so slight a character that little attention is paid to them: but any degree of exudation in such cases would be uncommon, while these platelets in their characters rather suggest the remains of such an exudation.

V. PIGMENTATION OF THE SPINAL ARACHNOID. — This condition, first described by Valentin, has been very carefully studied by Virchow. It was formerly looked on as the remains of a previously existing hyperæmia, or inflammation of the membrane; but it has no pathological significance. In contradistinction to the condition last described, it is most commonly met with in the meninges of the cervical region, and on the ventral surface of the cord and medulla oblongata. Macroscopically the morbid change gives rise to a general slightly dark or black gray tint, which on closer inspection is seen to depend upon collections of black or brown specks. On microscopic examination the change is seen to be due to the presence of pigment cells similar to those of the choroid; they are spindle-shaped, or may be stellate; and possess a nucleus.

VI. HYDRORRHACHIS, or an excess of fluid in the arachnoid space, like the last condition, was formerly regarded as the result of venous congestion or inflammation of the meninges.

An excess of fluid is commonly met with in intra-cranial conditions associated with increase of the cerebro-spinal fluid; such as external or internal hydrocephalus, the various forms of meningitis, including the tuberculous variety, cerebral tumour, and cerebral abscess. So too in diseases attended with general dropsy, the arachnoid sac may contain an excess of fluid. In conditions of this kind more especially, although excess of fluid probably existed in the sac during life, it is not unlikely that a considerable accession is made during the final moments which precede total dissolution.

Formerly a definite group of symptoms was supposed to result from the pressure on the spinal cord occasioned by the excess of fluid in the arachnoid sac; but it is highly improbable that the fluid is ever present in sufficient amount to cause a degree of pressure capable of disturbing the functions of the spinal cord.

VII. VARICOSITY OF THE VEINS OF THE PIA MATER. — This condition calls for no special description except that care should be taken not to mistake for it the fulness of vessels so commonly seen at necropsies, after the cadaver has been in the dorsal position during the interval between death and the time of the examination.

J. S. RISIEN RUSSELL.

REFERENCES

Pachymeningitis: 1. ADAMKIEWICZ. *Pachymeningitis hypertrophica und der chronische Infarct des Rückenmarks.* Wien, 1890.—2. BRUBERGER. *Virchow's Archiv,* 1870-74, lx. p. 285.—3. BUTTERSACK. *Arch. f. Psych.* xvii.—4. CARTER. *Liverpool Med.-Chir. Journ.* 1896, xvi. p. 500.—5. CHARCOT. *Leçons sur les localisations dans les mal. du cerveau et de la moëlle épinière.* Paris, 1876-80.—6. FORESTIER. *Lyon méd.* 1897, lxxxiv. p. 109.—7. JOFFROY. *De la pachyméningite cervicale hypertrophique.* Paris, 1873.—8. KÖPPEN. *Arch. f. Psych.* 1895, xxvii. p. 918; 1896, xxviii. p. 293. —9. LEECH. *Brit. Med. Journ.* 1895, ii. 1299.—10. LUPI. *Il Morgagni,* 1898, xl. p. 210.—11. OPPENHEIM. *Charité-annalen,* 1884, xi. p. 409.—12. ROSENBLATH. *Deutsch. Archiv f. klin. Med.* 1893, li. p. 210.—13. SCHULZ. *Neurol. Centralbl.* 1891, x. p. 578.—14. WIETING. Inaug. Dissert. Marbourg, 1893. **Syphilis:** 15. ADAMKIEWICZ. *Wien. med. Presse,* 1895, xxxvi. p. 121; *Wien. med. Woch.* 1896, xlvi. pp. 2074, 2127, 2183.—16. ALZHEIMER. *Arch. f. Psych.* 1897, xxix. p. 63.—17. BARBOUR. *Med. News,* Phila. 1894, lxv. p. 37.—18. BARDURY. Thèse de Paris, 1896.—19. BEEVOR. *Tr. Clin. Soc. Lond.* 1893-4, xxvii. p. 28.—20. BIERNACKI. *Deutsch. Zeitschr. f. Nervenh.* 1897, vii. p. 173.—21. BRASCH. *Neurol. Centralbl.* 1891, x. pp. 489, 517, 552; *Deutsch. Zeitschr. f. Nervenh.* 1896, viii. p. 418.—22. BRISSAUD. *Progr. méd.* 1897, July 17 and Dec. 18, pp. 33 and 157.—23. CASSIRER. *Deutsch. Zeitschr. f. Nervenh.* 1897, ix. p. 99.—24. CLARKE, J. M. *Lancet,* 1894, i. p. 1297.—25. COLLINS. *The Post Graduate,* vol. xi. p. 287.—26. DÉJERINE. *Rev. de méd.* 1884, pp. 60, 76.—27. ERB. *Neurol. Centralbl.* 1892, xi. p. 161.—28. EWALD. *Berl. klin. Woch.* 1893, xxx. p. 284.—29. FOURNIER. *Ann. de dermat. et syph.* Paris, 1896, vii. p. 380.—30. FRANKE. *Deutsch. med. Woch.* 1895, No. 52.—31. GANITANO. *Arch. Ital. di clin. med.* 1894, xxxiii. p. 448.—32. GASNE. *Nouv. Iconograph. de la Salpêt.* 1896, Nos. 5 and 6; *Gaz. hebdom.* 1898, p. 1.—33. GERHARDT. *Berl. klin. Woch.* 1893, xxx. p. 1209.—34. GIANNULI. *Riv. sper. di freniatr.* 1897, p. 840.—35. GILBERT and LION. *Compt. rend. soc. de biol.* 1893, v. p. 430; Th. de Paris, 1893.—36. GILLES DE LA TOURETTE. *Bull. méd.* Paris, 1896, x. pp. 555, 567, 581; *Nouv. Icon. de la Salpêt.* Paris, 1896, ix. pp. 80, 109.—37. GOLDFLAM. *Wien. Klinik,* 1893, xix. p. 41.—38. GOWERS. *Syph. of Ner. Syst.* Lond. 1892.—39. HANOT and MEUNIER. *Nouv. Icon. de la Salpêt.* 1896, ix. No. 2.—40. HENRIQUES. *Contribution à l'étude de la syphilis médullaire.* Paris, 1894.—41. HOFFMANN. *Neurol. Centralbl.* 1894, xiii. p. 470.—42. HOPPE. *Berl. klin. Woch.* 1893, xxx. p. 233.—43. KALISCHER. *Archiv f. Kinderheilk.* 1897, p. 56. —44. KOWALEWSKY. *Arch. f. Psych.* 1894, xxvi. p. 552.—45. KUH. *Arch. f. Psych.* 1891, xxii. p. 699.—46. LAMY. *Nouv. Icon. de la Salpêt.* 1893, vi. pp. 86, 153, 205, 251; *Arch. de Neurol.* 1894, p. 464; *Ibid.* 1895, p. 63.—47. LANCEREAUX. *Leçons de clin. méd.* Paris, 1892, p. 217.—48. LEYDEN and GOLDSCHEIDER. Nothnagel's *specielle Path. u. Therap.* Wien, 1897, x. p. 324.—49. MARIE. *Semaine méd.* 1893, xiii. p. 34.—50. MENDIL. *Dermatolog. Zeitschr.* 1894; *Festschrift,* Georg Lewin, 5 Nov. 1895.—51. MÖLLER. *Arch. f. Dermat. u. Syph.* 1891, xxiii. p. 207.—52. MOUREK. *Monatsch. f. prakt. Dermat.* 1893, xvii. p. 217.—53. NAGEOTTE. *Arch. de Neurol.* 1895, p. 273.—54. NONNE. *Arch. f. Psych.* 1897, xxix. p. 695.—55. OLIVIER and HALIPRÉ. *Rev. Neurolog.* 1895, Nr. 16.—56. OPPENHEIM. *Berl. klin. Woch.* 1889,

xxvi. pp. 1033, 1064.—57. ORLOWSKI. *Ann. de dermat. et syph.* Paris, 1896, vii. p. 139.
—58. PICK. *Prag. med. Woch.* 1898, Nr. 18⁻20.—59. POLLAK. *Deutsch. med. Woch.*
1896, xxii. p. 28.—60. RAYMOND. *Arch. de Neurol.* 1894, xxvii. pp. 1, 112.—61.
ROMME. *Gaz. hebd. de Paris,* 1894, xxxi. p. 75.—62. ROSIN. *Ztschr. f. klin. Med.*
1896, xxx. p. 129.—63. RUMPF. *Die syph. Erkrank. d. Nervensyst.* Wiesbaden, 1887,
p. 340.—64. SACHS. *Brain,* 1893, xvi. p. 405.—65. SCALFATI. *La riforma medica,*
1895, i. p. 122.—66. SCHMAUS. *Deutsch. Arch. f. klin. Med.* 1889, xliv. p. 246.—67.
SCHULTE. Inaug. Dissert. Kiel, 1896.—68. SCHWARZ. *Ztschr. f. klin. Med.* 1898,
xxxiv. p. 469.—69. SIEMERLING. *Arch. f. Psych.* 1891, xxii. pp. 191, 257.—70.
SPILLER. *New York Med. Journ.* 1897, lxvi. p. 409.—71. SOTTAS. *Gaz. d. hôp.*
Paris, 1894, lxvii. p. 1401.—72. VOLPERT. *De la syphilis médullaire.* Nancy, 1894.
—73. WULLENWEBER. *Münch. med. Woch.* 1898, p. 1017.—74. WEYGANDT. *Arch. f.*
Psych. 1896, xxviii. p. 457.—75. WITTERN. *Munch. med. Woch.* 1898, p. 624.—76.
WILLIAMSON. *Brit. Med. Journal,* Dec. 31, 1898. **Tubercle:** 77. BEWLEY. *Brit.*
Med. Journ. 1892, ii. p. 129.—78. GOLDSCHEIDER. *Berl. klin. Woch.* xxviii. 1891.—79.
GOWERS. *Diseases of Nervous System,* 1891, i. p. 270.—80. HOCHE. *Arch. f. Psych.* 1888,
xix. p. 200.—81. HOLZ. *Festschrift des Stuttgarter ärztlichen Vereins,* 1897.—82.
JACOBÄUS. *Nord. med. Ark.* Stockholm, 1896, vi p. 1.—83. LIMBACH. *Deutsch. Ztschr.*
f. Nervnheilk. 1891, i. p. 319.—84. LONDE and BROUARDEL. *Arch. de méd. expér. et*
d'anat. prat. Paris, 1895, vii. p. 115.—85. MÜLLER. *Deutsch. Zeitschr. f. Nervenheilk.*
1897, x. p. 273 ; 1898, xii.—86. SCARPATELLI. *Jahrb. f. Psych. u. Neurol.* 1897, xv.
p. 310.—87. SCHAFFER. *Neurol. Centralbl.* 1898, xvii. p. 434.—88. SCHAMSCHIN. *Zeitschr.*
f. Heilk. 1895, xvi. p. 373.—89. SCHULTZE. *Deutsch. Arch. f. klin. Med.* 1880, xxv.
p. 297.—90. WEISS. Eulenburg's *Real - Encyclopaedia,* vol. xvii. p. 76.—91.
WILLIAMS. *Deutsch. Arch. f. klin. Med.* 1880, xxv. p. 292. **Tumours:** 92. BAILEY.
Journ. of Nerv. and Ment. Dis. N.Y. 1896, xxiii. p. 171.—93. BRUNS. *Neurol.*
Centralbl. 1894, xiii. p. 281.—94. *Idem. Arch. f. Psychiat.* 1896, xxviii. pp. 97,
280.—95. BRUNS and WINDSCHEID. *Twentieth Cent. Pract.* N.Y. 1897, xi. p. 563.
—96. BURGESS. *Quart. Med. Journ.* Sheffield, 1897-8, vi. p. 235.—97. CAPONOTTO.
Riforma med. Napoli, 1892, viii. p. 543.—98. CLADEK. *New York Med. Journ.* 1897,
lxvi. p. 205.—99. CLARKE, J. J. *Tr. Path. Soc. Lond.* 1891-2, xliii. p. 16.—100. CLARKE,
J. M. *Brain,* 1895, xviii. p. 256.—101. COLLET. *Arch. de méd. expér. et d'anat.*
path. Paris, 1894, vi. p. 966.—102. COLLINS and BLANCHARD. *Med. News,* N.Y.
1897, lxxi. p. 48.—103. ESKRIDGE. *Med. News,* N.Y. 1897, lxxi. p. 402.—104.
FLETCHER. *Brit. Med. Journ.* 1898, i. p. 1327.—105. GOWERS and HORSLEY. *Med.-*
Chir. Trans. Lond. 1886, lxxi. p. 377.—106. HERTER. *Boston M. and S. Journ.* 1893,
cxxviii. p. 220 ; *New York Med. Journ.* 1893, lvii. p. 225.—107. KUDZEWETZKY.
Ztschr. f. Heilk. 1892, xiii. p. 300.—108. KUMMELL. *Beilage zum Centralbl. f. Chir.*
1895, No. 27.—109. LENZ. *Beitr. z. path. Anat. u. z. allg. Path.* Jena, 1896, xix. p.
663.—110. MACALESTER. *Sarcom. des Rückenmarks.* Dissert. Zurich, 1891.—111.
MADER. *Wien. med. Bl.* 1898, xxi. p. 249.—112. MAGUIRE. *Brain,* 1888, x. p. 451.—
113. MILLS and LLOYD. Pepper's *Syst. of Med.* 1886, v. p. 1090.—114. MORTON. *Proc.*
Path. Soc. Phila. 1897-8, i. p. 2.—115. MULLER. *Deutsch. Arch. f. klin. Med.* 1895,
liv. p. 472.—116. OUSTANIOL. *Contribution à l'étude des tumeurs des méninges rachi-*
diennes. Paris, 1892.—117. PFEIFFER. *Deutsch. Zeitschrift f. Nervenheilk.* 1894, v.
p. 63.—118. POTTS. *Proc. Path. Soc. Phila.* 1897-8, i. p. 41.—119. QUENSEL. *Neurol.*
Centralbl. 1898, xvii. p. 482.—120. RANSOM and ANDERSON. *Brit. Med. Journ.* 1891,
ii. p. 1144.—121. RANSOM and THOMPSON. *Ibid.* 1894, i. p. 395.—122. RAYMOND and
NAGEOTTE. *Journ. de neurol. et d'hypnol. de Bruxelles,* 1896, Nos. 1 and 2.—123.
ROSS. *Med. Rec.* N.Y. 1893, xliv. p. 193.—124. ROUX and PAVIOT. *Arch. de*
Neurol. 1898, v. No. 38.—125. v. SCANZONI. *Zeitsch. f. Heilk.* 1897, xviii. p. 381.—126.
SCHLESINGER. *Beiträge zur Klinik der Rückenmarks und Wirbeltumoren,* Jena, 1898 ;
Neurol. Centralbl. 1898, xvii. p. 820.—127. SIEVEKING. *Jahrbücher d. Hamburger*
Statskrankenanstalten, 1896, iv.—128. STARR. *Am. Journ. of Med. Sc.* 1895, cix. p.
613.—129. SUDECK. *Jahrbücher d. Hamburger Statskrankenanstalten,* 1896, iv.—
130. WESTPHAL. *Arch. f. Psych.* 1894, xxvi. p. 770 ; *Neurol. Centralbl.* 1894, xiii. p.
498.—131. WOOD. *Intercolon. M. J. Australas.* Melb. 1896, i. p. 480.

J. S. R. R.

LIST OF AUTHORITIES

INDEX

ABDOMEN, aneurysms of arteries in, 435;
disease of organs of, and neuralgia, 748
Abdominal aneurysm, 407
Abdominal viscera in compression of spinal
cord, 861
• Abducens palsy, 772
Abductor paralysis of larynx, 378
Abscess in suppurative phlebitis, 292; in
tuberculous disease of the spine, 855;
treatment, 869
Abscess, cerebral, swelling of optic discs in,
843
Abscess, mediastinal, 72; course, 76;
diagnosis, 76; etiology, 73; symptoms,
74; treatment, 77
Accommodation, paralysis of, 781
Acromegaly and bitemporal hemianopsia,
761
Acupuncture in sciatica, 665
Adiposis dolorosa, 576
Ageusia in facial palsy, 797
Ague and Raynaud's disease, 602
Air-embolism, 254
Albuminuria and tricuspid incompetence,
25
Alcohol as cause of amblyopia, 845; as
cause of arterio-sclerosis, 320; as cause of
cardiac angina, 38
Alcoholic neuritis, 675
Alcoholism, chronic, spinal leptomeninges in,
914
Alimentary canal in compression of spinal
cord, 861
Amblyopia, "toxic," colour-sense in, 845
Amyotrophic lateral sclerosis with bulbar
palsy and ophthalmoplegia, 778
Amyotrophy, family, peroneal type of, 704
Anæmia and thrombosis, 200; as cause of
neuralgia, 740, 750; Varying susceptibility
of organs to, 240
Anæmia, cerebral, and arterio-sclerosis, 341
Anæsthesia in meningeal hæmorrhage, 877;
in spinal syphilis, 895; in alcoholic
neuritis, 677
Anæsthesia, retinal," 851
Analgesia in localisation of compression of

spinal cord, 864; in organic diseases of
spinal marrow and roots, plates, 866
Anastomoses in arterial embolism, 241
Anchylosis of shoulder joint, diagnosis from
paralysis of circumflex nerve, 657
Aneurysm of the aorta, 345; age in, 349;
application of X-rays to diagnosis of
internal, 408; as cause of compression of
spinal cord, 856; cardiac symptoms,
373, 405; diagnosis, 405; diagnosis from
intra-thoracic growth, 147; etiological
diagnosis, 365; etiology, 348; hæmorrhage, 380; laryngeal symptoms, 374,
405; physical diagnosis, 387; prognosis,
409; respiratory symptoms, 374, 406;
sex in, 350, 353; symptomatic diagnosis,
369; symptoms, physical signs, diagnosis,
363; treatment, medical, 423; treatment,
surgical, 411; Varicose, 399
Aneurysm, rupture of, as cause of meningeal
hæmorrhages, 874, 875
Aneurysma mycotico-embolicum," 251
Aneurysmal impulse, 390; sounds and
murmurs, 391
Aneurysmal sac, 381; filipuncture of, 417;
rupture of, 383, 410
Aneurysms and atheroma, 331, 350
Aneurysms, embolic, 251; Verminous, 252;
miliary, 333; relation of, to arterio-
sclerosis, 334
Aneurysms of arteries in the abdomen, 435;
of the branches of the cœliac axis, 435;
of the coronaria Ventriculi artery, 437;
of the hepatic artery, 435; of the
inferior mesenteric artery, 438; of the
renal arteries, 438; of the splenic artery,
437; of the superior mesenteric artery,
437
Angina Ludovici as cause of external spinal
pachymeningitis, 882
Angina pectoris, 26; and coronary sclerosis,
341; forms, 27; history, 26
Angina pectoris gravior, 38; cases, 48;
diagnosis, 52; primary, 41; prognosis,
54; secondary, 38; symptomatology 47;
treatment, 54

END OF VOL **VI**

Works on Medicine and Surgery

...PUBLISHED BY...

THE MACMILLAN COMPANY

66 FIFTH AVENUE, NEW YORK

ALLCHIN

A Manual of Medicine. Edited by W. H. ALLCHIN, M.D. (Lond.), F.R.C.P., F.R.S.E., Senior Physician and Lecturer on Clinical Medicine, Westminster Hospital, Examiner in Medicine in the University of London, and to the Medical Department of the Royal Navy. In five volumes.

Vol. I. General Diseases. Diseases excited by atmospheric influences, the Infections. 12mo. Cloth. Colored Plates. pp. x + 442. Price $2.00 *net.*

Vol. II. General Diseases (continued). Diseases caused by Parasites, Diseases determined by Poisons, introduced into the Body, Primary Perversions of General Nutrition, Diseases of the Blood. 12mo. Cloth. Colored Plates and 21 other illustrations. pp. viii + 380.
Price $2.00 *net.*

Vol. III. Diseases of the Nervous System. Organic Disease of the Brain and its Membranes, Diseases of the Spinal Cord, Functional Diseases of the Nervous System. 12mo. Cloth. Colored Plates and 27 other illustrations. pp. x + 417. Price $2.00 *net.*

Vol. IV. Diseases of the Respiratory and of the Circulatory Systems. 12mo. Cloth. Colored Plates and numerous other illustrations. pp. xiv + 493. Price $2.00 *net.*

Vol. V. Diseases of the Digestive System and of the Liver, Diseases of the Peritoneum and of the Vessels of the Abdomen, Diseases of the Kidneys, Diseases of the Ductless Glands. 12mo. Cloth. Colored Plates and numerous other illustrations. pp. xii + 687.
Price $2.00 *net.*

BRUNTON

On Disorders of Digestion: Their Consequences and Treatment. By Sir T. LAUDER BRUNTON. 8vo. Cloth. Illustrated. pp. xvi + 389. Price $2.50.

By the Same Author

An Introduction to Modern Therapeutics. Being the Croonian Lectures on the relationship between Chemical Structure and Physiological Actions in relation to the Prevention, Control, and Cure of Disease. Delivered before the Royal College of Physicians in London. By Sir T. LAUDER BRUNTON. 8vo. Cloth. Illustrated. pp. vii + 195.
Price £1.50.

Lectures on the Action of Medicines. Being the Course of Lectures on Pharmacology and Therapeutics delivered at St. Bartholomew's Hospital during the Summer Session of 1896. By Sir T. LAUDER BRUNTON, M.D., D.Sc. (Edin.), LL.D. (Hon.) (Aberd.), F.R.S., etc. 8vo. Cloth. 144 Illustrations. pp. xv + 673. Price $4.00 *net.*
Sheep binding. Price $5.00 *net.*

Lectures on Disorders of Assimilation, Digestion, etc. By Sir T. LAUDER BRUNTON. 8vo. Cloth. pp. xx + 495. Price $4.00 *net.*

DAVIS

The Refraction of the Eye. Including a Complete Treatise on Ophthalmometry. A Clinical Text-Book for Students and Practitioners. By A. EDWARD DAVIS, A.M., M.D., Adjunct Professor of Diseases of the Eye in the New York Post-Graduate Medical School and Hospital, etc. 8vo. Cloth. 119 Illustrations. pp. xii + 431. Price $3.00 *net.*

DEFENDORF

Clinical Psychiatry. A Text-Book for Students and Physicians. Abstracted and adapted from the Sixth German Edition of Kraepelin's "Lehrbuch der Psychiatre." By A. Ross DEFENDORF, M.D., Lecturer in Psychiatry in Yale University. Illustrated. 8vo. Cloth. pp. xii + 420.   Price $3.50 *net.*

ESMARCH and KOWALZIG

Surgical Technic: A Text-Book on Operative Surgery. By FR. VON ESMARCH, M.D., Professor of Surgery at the University of Kiel, and Surgeon-General of the German Army, and E. KOWALZIG, M.D., late First Assistant at the Surgical Clinic of the University of Kiel. Translated by Professor LUDWIG H. GRAU, Ph.D., formerly of Leland Stanford Junior University, and WILLIAM N. SULLIVAN, M.D., formerly Surgeon of U.S.S. "Corwin," Assistant of the Surgical Clinic at Cooper Medical College, San Francisco. Edited by NICHOLAS SENN, M.D., Professor of Surgery at Rush Medical College, Chicago. With 1497 Illustrations and 15 Colored Plates. 8vo. Cloth. pp. xl+866. Price $7.00 *net.*
                                     Half morocco. Price $8.00 *net.*

FOSTER

A Text-Book of Physiology. By M. FOSTER, M.A., M.D., LL.D., F.R.S., Professor of Physiology in the University of Cambridge, etc. Revised and abridged from the Author's Text-Book of Physiology in Five Volumes. With an Appendix on the Chemical Basis of the Animal Body, by A. SHERIDAN LEA, M.A., D.Sc., F.R.S., University Lecturer in Physiology in the University of Cambridge. 8vo. Cloth. 234 Illustrations. pp. xlix + 1351.   Price $5.00 *net.*
                                     Sheep binding. Price $6.00 *net.*

By the Same Author

A Text-Book of Physiology. In Five Volumes.
Part I. Blood; The Tissues of Movement; Vascular Mechanism.   Price $2.60 *net.*
Part II. The Tissues of Chemical Action; Nutrition.   Price $2.60 *net.*
Part III. The Central Nervous System.   Price $2.50 *net.*
Part IV. The Central Nervous System (concluded); The Tissues and Mechanism of Reproduction.   Price $2.00 *net.*
Part V. The Chemical Basis of the Animal Body. By LEA.   Price $1.75 *net.*
Lectures on the History of Physiology during the Sixteenth, Seventeenth, and Eighteenth Centuries. By Sir M. FOSTER, K.C.B., M.P., M.D., D.C.L., Sec. R.S., Professor of Physiology in the University of Cambridge, and Fellow of Trinity College, Cambridge. 8vo. Cloth. pp. 310.   Price $2.25 *net.*

FULLER

Diseases of the Genito-Urinary System. A Thorough Treatise on Urinary and Sexual Surgery. By EUGENE FULLER, M.D., Professor of Genito-Urinary and Venereal Diseases in the New York Post-Graduate Medical School; Visiting Genito-Urinary Surgeon to the New York Post-Graduate Hospital. 8vo. Cloth. 137 Illustrations. pp. ix + 774.
                                     Price $5.00 *net.*
                     Sheep. ·   Price $6.00 *net.*
                     Half morocco. Price $6.50 *net.*

GIBBONS

The Eye. Its Refraction and Diseases. The Refraction and Functional Testing of the Eye, complete in itself, in Twenty-eight Chapters, with Numerous Explanatory Cuts and Diagrams. By EDWARD E. GIBBONS, M.D., Assistant Surgeon of the Presbyterian Eye, Ear, and Throat Hospital, Demonstrator and Chief of Clinic of Eye and Ear Diseases in the University of Maryland, Baltimore. 8vo. Cloth. pp. ix + 472.   Price $5.00 *net.*

KIMBER

Text-Book of Anatomy and Physiology for Nurses. Compiled by DIANA CLIFFORD KIMBER, Graduate of Bellevue Training School; Assistant Superintendent New York City Training School, Blackwell's Island, N.Y., formerly Assistant Superintendent Illinois Training School, Chicago, Ill. 8vo. Cloth. 137 Illustrations. pp. xvi + 268.
                                     Price $2.50 *net.*

KLEMPERER

The Elements of Clinical Diagnosis. By Professor Dr. G. KLEMPERER, Professor of Medicine at the University of Berlin. Second American from the Seventh (last) German Edition. Authorized Translation by NATHAN E. BRILL, A.M., M.D., Attending Physician, Mount Sinai Hospital, New York City, and SAMUEL M. BRICKNER, A.M., M.D., Assistant Gynæcologist, Mount Sinai Hospital, Out-Patient Department. 12mo. Cloth. 61 Illustrations. pp. xvii + 292. Price $ 1.00 *net.*

KOCHER

Text-Book of Operative Surgery. By Dr. THEODOR KOCHER, Professor of Surgery and Director of the Surgical Clinic in the University of Bern. Authorized Translation from the Fourth German Edition. By HAROLD J. STILES, M.B., F.R.C.S. (Edin.), Surgeon to the Royal Edinburgh Hospital for Sick Children, Late Assistant Surgeon, Edinburgh Royal Infirmary, Examiner in Anatomy, Royal College of Surgeons, Edinburgh. With 255 Illustrations. pp. xx + 440. 8vo. Cloth. Price $ 5.00 *net.*
Half morocco. Price $ 6.50 *net.*

LILIENTHAL

Imperative Surgery. For the General Practitioner, the Specialist, and the Recent Graduate. By HOWARD LILIENTHAL, M.D., Attending Surgeon to Mount Sinai Hospital, New York City. 8vo. Cloth. 153 Illustrations. pp. xvi + 412. Price $ 4.00 *net.*
Half morocco. Price $ 5.00 *net.*

MUIR and RITCHIE

Manual of Bacteriology. By ROBERT MUIR, M.A., M.D., F.R.C.P. (Edin.), Professor of Pathology, University of Glasgow, and JAMES RITCHIE, M.A., M.D., B.Sc., Reader in Pathology, University of Oxford. American Edition (with Additions), Revised and Edited from the Third English Edition. By NORMAN MACLEOD HARRIS, M.B. (Tor.), Associate in Bacteriology, the Johns Hopkins University, Baltimore. With 170 Illustrations. pp. xx + 565. 8vo. Cloth. Price $ 3.75 *net.*

OPPENHEIM

The Development of the Child. By NATHAN OPPENHEIM, Attending Physician to the Children's Department of Mount Sinai Hospital Dispensary. 12mo. Cloth. pp. viii + 296. Price $ 1.25 *net.*

By the Same Author

The Care of the Child in Health. 12mo. Cloth. pp. vii + 308. Price $ 1.25.
The Medical Diseases of Childhood. By NATHAN OPPENHEIM, A.B. (Harv.), M.D. (Coll. P. & S., N.Y.). 8vo. Cloth. 101 Illustrations and 19 Charts. pp. xx + 653.
Price $ 5.00 *net.*
Sheep. Price $ 6.00 *net.*
Half morocco. Price $ 6.50 *net.*

SCHÄFER

Text-Book of Physiology. Edited by E. A. SCHÄFER, LL.D., F.R.S., Professor of Physiology, University of Edinburgh. Cloth. 8vo.
Vol. I. 27 Plates and 92 Text Illustrations. pp. xviii + 1036. Price $ 8.00 *net.*
Vol. II. 499 Illustrations. pp. xxiv + 1365. Price $ 10.00 *net.*

SEDGWICK

Principles of Sanitary Science and the Public Health. With Special Reference to the Causation and Prevention of Infectious Diseases. By WILLIAM T. SEDGWICK, Ph.D., Professor of Biology and Lecturer on Sanitary Science and the Public Health in the Massachusetts Institute of Technology, Boston, sometime Biologist to the State Board of Health of Massachusetts. 8vo. Cloth. pp. xix + 368. Price $ 3.00 *net.*

SMITH

Introduction to the Outlines of the Principles of Differential Diagnosis, with Clinical Memoranda. By FRED J. SMITH, M.A., M.D. (Oxon.), F.R.C.P. (Lond.), Physician and Senior Pathologist to the London Hospital. 12mo. Cloth. pp. ix + 353.

Price $ 2.00 *net.*

SUTER

Handbook of Optics. For Students of Ophthalmology. By WILLIAM NORWOOD SUTER, B.A., M.D., Professor of Ophthalmology, National University, and Assistant Surgeon, Episcopal Eye, Ear, and Throat Hospital, Washington, D.C. 12mo. Cloth. 54 Illustrations. pp. viii + 209.

Price $ 1.00 *net.*

VERWORN

General Physiology: An Outline of the Science of Life. By MAX VERWORN, M.D., Ph.D., A.O., Professor of Physiology in the Medical Faculty of the University of Jena. Translated from the Second German Edition and edited by FREDERIC S. LEE, Ph.D., Adjunct Professor of Physiology in Columbia University. With 285 Illustrations. 8vo. Cloth. pp. xvi + 615.

Price $ 4.00 *net.*

WARNER

Three Lectures on the Anatomy of Movement. A Treatise on the Action of Nerve-Centres and Modes of Growth. Delivered at the Royal College of Surgeons of England. By FRANCIS WARNER, M.D. 12mo. Cloth. 18 Illustrations. pp. xiv + 135.

Price 75 cents *net.*

By the Same Author

The Nervous System of the Child: Its Growth and Health in Education. By FRANCIS WARNER, M.D. (Lond.), F.R.C.P., F.R.C.S. (Eng.), Physician to and Lecturer at the London Hospital, etc. 12mo. Cloth. pp. xvii + 233.   Price $ 1.00 *net.*
The Study of Children and Their School Training. By FRANCIS WARNER, M.D. 12mo. Cloth. pp. xix + 264.   Price $ 1.00 *net.*

WILLIAMS

The Roentgen Rays in Medicine and Surgery as an Aid in Diagnosis, and as a Therapeutic Agent. By FRANCIS H. WILLIAMS, M.D. 391 Illustrations. 8vo. Cloth. pp. xxx + 658.

Price $ 6.00 *net.*

Half morocco. Price $ 7.00 *net.*

WILSON

The Cell in Development and Inheritance. By EDMUND B. WILSON, Ph.D., Professor of Zoölogy, Columbia University. Second Edition, Revised and Enlarged. 8vo. Cloth. 194 Illustrations. pp. xxi + 483.

Price $ 3.50 *net.*

ZIEGLER

A Text-Book of Special Pathological Anatomy. By ERNST ZIEGLER, Professor of Pathology in the University of Freiburg. Translated and edited from the Eighth German Edition by DONALD MACALISTER, M.A., M.D., Linacre Lecturer of Physic and Tutor of St. John's College, Cambridge, and HENRY W. CATTELL, M.A., M.D., Demonstrator of Morbid Anatomy in the University of Pennsylvania. 8vo. 562 Illustrations.

Sections I–VIII. pp. xix + 575 + xxxii. Cloth.   Price $ 4.00 *net.*

Sheep. Price $ 5.00 *net.*

Sections IX–XV. pp. xv + 576–1221 + xxxi. Cloth.   Price $ 4.00 *net.*

Sheep. Price $ 5.00 *net.*

THE MACMILLAN COMPANY

66 FIFTH AVENUE, NEW YORK